ATLAS OF
PEDIATRIC
PHYSICAL
DIAGNOSIS

ATLAS OF PEDIATRIC PHYSICAL DIAGNOSIS

Fifth Edition

Basil J. Zitelli, MD
Edmund R. McCluskey Professor of Pediatrics
University of Pittsburgh School of Medicine
Director, The Paul C. Gaffney Diagnostic Referral Service
Children's Hospital of Pittsburgh
Pittsburgh, Pennsylvania

Holly W. Davis, MD
Associate Professor of Pediatrics, Emeritus
University of Pittsburgh School of Medicine
Children's Hospital of Pittsburgh
Pittsburgh, Pennsylvania

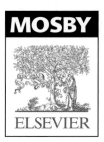

MOSBY

ELSEVIER

1600 John F. Kennedy Blvd
Suite 1800
Philadelphia, PA 19103-2899

ATLAS OF PEDIATRIC PHYSICAL DIAGNOSIS ISBN: 978-0-323-04878-1

Notice

Knowledge and best practice in this field are constantly changing. As new research and experience broaden our knowledge, changes in practice, treatment, and drug therapy may become necessary or appropriate. Readers are advised to check the most current information provided (i) on procedures featured or (ii) by the manufacturer of each product to be administered to verify the recommended dose or formula, the method and duration of administration, and contraindications. It is the responsibility of the practitioner, relying on their own experience and knowledge of the patient, to make diagnoses, to determine dosages and the best treatment for each individual patient, and to take all appropriate safety precautions. To the fullest extent of the law, neither the Publisher nor the Editors assume any liability for any injury and/or damage to persons or property arising out of or related to any use of the material contained in this book.

The Publisher

Library of Congress Cataloging-in-Publication Data

Atlas of pediatric physical diagnosis / [edited by] Basil J. Zitelli, Holly W. Davis.—5th ed.
    p. ; cm.
  Includes bibliographical references and index.
  ISBN 978-0-323-04878-1
  1. Children—Diseases—Diagnosis. 2. Physical diagnosis. 3. Children—Medical examinations. I. Zitelli, Basil J. (Basil John). II. Davis, Holly W. III. Title: Pediatric physical diagnosis.
  [DNLM: 1. Diagnosis—Atlases. 2. Child. 3. Infant. 4. Physical Examination—Atlases. WS 17 A881 2007]
  RJ50.A86 2007
  618.92′00754—dc22   2006025411

Publishing Director: Judith Fletcher
Developmental Editor: Joanie Milnes
Publishing Services Manager: Frank Polizzano
Senior Project Manager: Robin E. Hayward
Multimedia Producer: David Wisner
Cover Design Direction: Steven Stave
Interior Designer: Steven Stave

Printed in China.

Last digit is the print number: 9 8 7 6 5 4 3 2 1

Working together to grow
libraries in developing countries

www.elsevier.com | www.bookaid.org | www.sabre.org

ELSEVIER   BOOK AID International   Sabre Foundation

Contributors

EDWARD M. BARKSDALE, JR., MD
Professor of Surgery, Case Western Reserve School of Medicine; Robert J. Izant, Jr., MD Professor and Chief, Division of Pediatric Surgery, Rainbow Babies and Children's Hospital, University Hospitals of Cleveland, Cleveland, Ohio
Surgery

CAROLYN A. BAY, MD
Associate Professor of Pediatrics; Chief, Division of Clinical/Biochemical Genetics and Dysmorphology, University of Kentucky, Lexington, Kentucky
Genetic Disorders and Dysmorphic Conditions

LEE B. BEERMAN, MD
Professor of Pediatrics, University of Pittsburgh School of Medicine; Director of Electrophysiology, Children's Hospital of Pittsburgh, Pittsburgh, Pennsylvania
Cardiology

MARK F. BELLINGER, MD
Clinical Professor, University of Pittsburgh School of Medicine; Pediatric Urologist, Children's Hospital of Pittsburgh, Pittsburgh, Pennsylvania
Urologic Disorders

MICHAEL L. BENTZ, MD
Professor of Surgery, Pediatrics, and Neurosurgery; Chair, Division of Plastic Surgery; Vice Chair, Clinical Affairs, University of Wisconsin School of Medicine and Public Health, Madison, Wisconsin
Craniofacial Anomalies

ALBERT W. BIGLAN, MD
Adjunct Professor of Ophthalmology, University of Pittsburgh School of Medicine, Pittsburgh, Pennsylvania
Ophthalmology

CHERYL BLANK, DO
Assistant Professor of Pediatrics, University of Pittsburgh School of Medicine; Department of Gastroenterology, Children's Hospital of Pittsburgh, Pittsburgh, Pennsylvania
Nutrition and Gastroenterology

DEBRA L. BOGEN, MD
Assistant Professor of Pediatrics, University of Pittsburgh School of Medicine; Director, General Academic Pediatric Fellowship, Children's Hospital of Pittsburgh, Pittsburgh, Pennsylvania
Neonatology

BEVERLY S. BROZANSKI, MD
Professor of Pediatrics, University of Pittsburgh School of Medicine; Clinical Director, Neonatal Intensive Care Unit, Children's Hospital of Pittsburgh, Pittsburgh, Pennsylvania
Neonatology

MARY M. CARRASCO, MD
Clinical Associate Professor of Pediatrics, University of Pittsburgh School of Medicine; Director of International and Community Health, Mercy Children's Medical Center, Pittsburgh, Pennsylvania
Child Abuse and Neglect

KENNETH P. CHENG, MD
Clinical Instructor of Ophthalmology, University of Pittsburgh School of Medicine; Attending Physician, Children's Hospital of Pittsburgh, Magee-Women's Hospital, and University of Pittsburgh Medical Center, Pittsburgh, Pennsylvania
Ophthalmology

BERNARD A. COHEN, MD
Professor of Dermatology, Johns Hopkins School of Medicine; Interim Chair, Dermatology, Johns Hopkins Hospital, Baltimore, Maryland
Dermatology

HOLLY W. DAVIS, MD
Associate Professor of Pediatrics, Emeritus, University of Pittsburgh School of Medicine; Children's Hospital of Pittsburgh, Pittsburgh, Pennsylvania
Child Abuse and Neglect; Dermatology; Genetic Disorders and Dysmorphic Conditions; Infectious Disease; Oral Disorders; Orthopedics; Otolaryngology; Pediatric and Adolescent Gynecology

VINCENT F. DEENEY, MD
Assistant Professor of Orthopedics, University of Pittsburgh School of Medicine; Program Director, Orthopedic Residency, Children's Hospital of Pittsburgh, Pittsburgh, Pennsylvania
Orthopedics

DEMETRIUS ELLIS, MD
Professor of Pediatrics and Nephrology, University of Pittsburgh School of Medicine; Director, Pediatric Nephrology, Children's Hospital of Pittsburgh, Pittsburgh, Pennsylvania
Nephrology

HEIDI M. FELDMAN, MD, PhD
Professor of Pediatrics, Stanford University School of Medicine; Medical Director, Development and Behavior Unit, Lucile Packard Children's Hospital, Palo Alto, California
Developmental-Behavioral Pediatrics

JONATHAN D. FINDER, MD
Associate Professor of Pediatrics, University of Pittsburgh School of Medicine; Pediatric Pulmonologist, Children's Hospital of Pittsburgh, Pittsburgh, Pennsylvania
Pulmonary Disorders

J. CARLTON GARTNER, JR., MD
Professor of Pediatrics, Jefferson Medical College of Thomas Jefferson University, Philadelphia, Pennsylvania; Pediatrician in Chief, Alfred I. duPont Hospital for Children, Wilmington, Delaware
Nutrition and Gastroenterology

ROBIN P. GEHRIS, MD
Clinical Assistant Professor of Dermatology and Pediatrics, University of Pittsburgh School of Medicine; Children's Dermatology Services, Children's Hospital of Pittsburgh, Pittsburgh, Pennsylvania
Dermatology

JACQUELINE KREUTZER, MD
Assistant Professor of Pediatrics, University of Pittsburgh School of Medicine; Director, Cardiac Catheterization, Children's Hospital of Pittsburgh, Pittsburgh, Pennsylvania
Cardiology

JOSEPH E. LOSEE, MD
Program Director, Plastic Surgery Residency, University of Pittsburgh School of Medicine; Chief, Division of Pediatric Plastic Surgery, and Director, Pittsburgh Cleft-Craniofacial Center, Children's Hospital of Pittsburgh, Pittsburgh, Pennsylvania
Craniofacial Anomalies

KECHA A. LYNSHUE, MD
Fellow, Pediatric Endocrinology, University of Pittsburgh School of Medicine; Children's Hospital of Pittsburgh, Pittsburgh, Pennsylvania
Endocrinology

ANDREW MACGINNITIE, MD, PhD
Assistant Professor of Pediatrics, University of Pittsburgh School of Medicine; Children's Hospital of Pittsburgh, Pittsburgh, Pennsylvania
Allergy and Immunology

J. JEFFREY MALATACK, MD
Professor of Pediatrics, Jefferson Medical College of Thomas Jefferson University, Philadelphia, Pennsylvania; Director, Diagnostic Referral Service, Alfred I. duPont Hospital for Children, Wilmington, Delaware
Hematology and Oncology

BRIAN S. MARTIN, DMD
Clinical Assistant Professor, University of Pittsburgh School of Dental Medicine; Chief, Division of Pediatric Dentistry, Children's Hospital of Pittsburgh, Pittsburgh, Pennsylvania
Oral Disorders

A. CORDE MASON, MD
Associate Professor of Plastic Surgery and Pediatrics, The University of Texas Health Science Center at San Antonio; Director, Center for Reconstructive Pediatrics, CHRISTUS Santa Rosa Children's Hospital, San Antonio, Texas
Craniofacial Anomalies

TIMOTHY P. MCBRIDE, MD
Fairfax, Virginia
Otolaryngology

SARA C. MCINTIRE, MD
Professor of Pediatrics, University of Pittsburgh School of Medicine; The Paul C. Gaffney Diagnostic Referral Service, Children's Hospital of Pittsburgh, Pittsburgh, Pennsylvania
Rheumatology

DAVID H. MCKIBBEN, DMD, MDS
Adjunct Associate Professor, University of Pittsburgh School of Dental Medicine; Director, Pediatric Dental Residency Program, Children's Hospital of Pittsburgh, Pittsburgh, Pennsylvania
Oral Disorders

MARIAN G. MICHAELS, MD, MPH
Associate Professor of Pediatrics and Surgery, University of Pittsburgh School of Medicine; Division of Allergy, Immunology, and Infectious Diseases, Children's Hospital of Pittsburgh, Pittsburgh, Pennsylvania
Infectious Disease

MOREY S. MORELAND, MD
Professor of Orthopedic Surgery, University of Pittsburgh School of Medicine; William F. and Jean W. Donaldson Professor, Children's Hospital of Pittsburgh, Pittsburgh, Pennsylvania
Orthopedics

PAMELA J. MURRAY, MD, MPH
Associate Professor of Pediatrics and Obstetrics/Gynecology, Assistant Professor of Obstetrics, Gynecology, and Reproductive Health Services, University of Pittsburgh School of Medicine; Division Chief and Fellowship Director, Department of Pediatrics, UPSOM, and Adolescent Medicine, Children's Hospital of Pittsburgh, Pittsburgh, Pennsylvania
Pediatric and Adolescent Gynecology

DAVID NASH, MD
Assistant Professor of Pediatrics, University of Pittsburgh School of Medicine; Children's Hospital of Pittsburgh, Pittsburgh, Pennsylvania
Allergy and Immunology

MAMOUN M. NAZIF, DDS, MDS
Clinical Professor of Pediatric Dentistry, Emeritus, University of Pittsburgh School of Dental Medicine; Emeritus Staff, Children's Hospital of Pittsburgh, Pittsburgh, Pennsylvania
Oral Disorders

SANG C. PARK, MD
Professor of Pediatrics, University of Pittsburgh School of Medicine; Attending Physician, Children's Hospital of Pittsburgh, Pittsburgh, Pennsylvania
Cardiology

A. KIM RITCHEY, MD
Professor of Pediatrics, University of Pittsburgh School of Medicine; Chief, Pediatric Hematology/Oncology, Children's Hospital of Pittsburgh, Pittsburgh, Pennsylvania
Hematology and Oncology

PAUL ROSEN, MD, MPH
Assistant Professor of Pediatrics, University of Pittsburgh School of Medicine; Clinical Director, Division of Rheumatology, Children's Hospital of Pittsburgh, Pittsburgh, Pennsylvania
Rheumatology

MARK W. STEELE, MD*
Associate Professor of Pediatrics, Emeritus, University of Pittsburgh School of Medicine; Former Director, Medical Genetics, Children's Hospital of Pittsburgh, Pittsburgh, Pennsylvania
*Retired
Genetic Disorders and Dysmorphic Conditions

JEAN M. TERSAK, MD
Assistant Professor of Pediatrics, University of Pittsburgh School of Medicine; Division of Hematology/Oncology and BMT, Children's Hospital of Pittsburgh, Pittsburgh, Pennsylvania
Hematology and Oncology

RAJIV VARMA, MD
Clinical Associate Professor of Pediatrics and Neurology, University of Pittsburgh School of Medicine; Children's Hospital of Pittsburgh, Pittsburgh, Pennsylvania
Neurology

W. TIMOTHY WARD, MD
Executive Vice Chair and Professor of Orthopedic Surgery, University of Pittsburgh School of Medicine; Chief, Department of Orthopedic Surgery, Children's Hospital of Pittsburgh, Pittsburgh, Pennsylvania
Orthopedics

HENRY B. WESSEL, MD
Clinical Associate Professor of Pediatrics and Child Neurology, University of Pittsburgh School of Medicine; Director, MDA Clinic, Children's Hospital of Pittsburgh, Pittsburgh, Pennsylvania
Neurology

SHELLEY D. WILLIAMS, MD
Associate Professor of Pediatrics and Child Neurology, University of Pittsburgh School of Medicine; Children's Hospital of Pittsburgh, Pittsburgh, Pennsylvania
Neurology

SELMA F. WITCHEL, MD
Associate Professor of Pediatrics, University of Pittsburgh School of Medicine; Children's Hospital of Pittsburgh, Pittsburgh, Pennsylvania
Endocrinology

ROBERT F. YELLON, MD
Associate Professor of Otolaryngology, University of Pittsburgh School of Medicine; Department of Pediatric Otolaryngology, Children's Hospital of Pittsburgh, Pittsburgh, Pennsylvania
Otolaryngology

Foreword

For most people, visual images are the key to permanent memory. Although physicians develop numerous systems for memorizing medical facts, visual recognition continues to be the most powerful memory hook. Only direct patient care is a better teacher. Isn't that why we "round up the residents" when we have a patient with an interesting physical finding?

This book is a visual encyclopedia of pediatrics. We expect dermatology, infectious disease, and child abuse to be highlighted in an atlas, but in this comprehensive work, every pediatric subspecialty is covered in depth. Even child development is captured in photographs and drawings.

Herein are included more visual diagnoses than any pediatrician will see in a lifetime of practice. Radiographs, CT scans, and MRI views of basic conditions are also included. This atlas is a gold mine for medical students and residents who need to explore and categorize their physical findings. No teaching clinic should be without a copy. Doctors Zitelli and Davis are to be commended for giving us the ultimate *Atlas of Pediatric Physical Diagnosis*. Sharpen your diagnostic acumen, good reader.

Barton D. Schmitt, MD
Professor of Pediatrics
University of Colorado School of Medicine
Denver, Colorado

Preface

For many disorders, visual recognition is the major factor in making a correct diagnosis. The experienced clinician who has seen a wide spectrum of different disorders carries a wealth of information for diagnosis and teaching.

This book was envisioned by teachers and was developed to aid students, residents, nurses, and practitioners who care for children in the recognition and diagnosis of pediatric disorders. Our goal is to broaden the visual experience of the student and the clinician through rapid visual examination or review of simple laboratory tests and imaging studies.

The enthusiastic response to the previous editions of the *Atlas* led us to believe that a fifth edition was not only possible but also necessary. Many readers offered helpful suggestions for photos and topics to be included. Every chapter has been reviewed, revised, and updated. Some chapters have been entirely rewritten. New information and diagnostic techniques have been incorporated.

Emphasis has been placed on physical examination techniques in each chapter. Additional contributors have provided greater depth and dimension. The *Atlas* is by no means encyclopedic but rather presents an overview of clinical disorders that lend themselves to visual diagnosis. The accompanying text deliberately emphasizes pertinent historical factors, examination techniques, visual findings, and diagnostic methods rather than therapy. We firmly believe that a careful history and physical examination provide the foundation for any clinical assessment. We have attempted to select disorders that are common or important, and, when relevant, to describe the spectrum of clinical findings. It is our hope that this *Atlas* continues to serve as a useful and practical reference for anyone who cares for children.

Basil J. Zitelli, MD
Holly W. Davis, MD

Acknowledgments

The *Atlas* results from the untiring efforts of many dedicated people who contributed not only to the current edition but also to all previous editions. Although each chapter has been reviewed and some have been totally rewritten, each chapter is in some way built on the foundation of previous editions. All contributors from the first edition onward have left their mark, and their contributions continue to be felt. We recognize their efforts and work: Michael J. Balsan and Ian R. Holzman (Neonatology); Philip Fireman, Deborah Gentile, and David Skoner (Allergy and Immunology); F. Jay Fricker and Cora C. Lenox (Cardiology); Andrew H. Urbach (Rheumatology); Julie Blatt and Lila Penchansky (Hematology and Oncology); David Finegold (Endocrinology); Raymond B. Karasic (Pediatric Infectious Disease); Blakeslee E. Noyes and David M. Orenstein (Pulmonary Disorders); David A. Lloyd and Don K. Nakayama (Surgery); Melissa Hamp (Pediatric and Adolescent Gynecology); David A. Hiles (Ophthalmology); Mary Ann Ready and Apostole Vanderas (Oral Disorders); Edward N. Hanley, Jr., and Greg Bisignani (Orthopedics); and James S. Reilly (Otolaryngology).

Many people at Children's Hospital of Pittsburgh have contributed in countless ways to the *Atlas*. First and foremost, we appreciate the generosity of our patients and their families who graciously allowed us to photograph them for the education of those who care for children. Secretaries, radiology technicians, file clerks, librarians, medical media staff, and many unnamed colleagues who provided constructive criticism all have given freely of themselves to help us with the *Atlas*. We could not have succeeded without them. Among these, special recognition goes to Diane Weidner, Susan Gelnett, Jonathan Bickel, and Sophie Davis for their tireless work, expertise, and unflagging support.

Our colleagues at Elsevier have been patient, understanding, and accommodating in guiding us through the publication process. Special thanks go to Judy Fletcher, Joanie Milnes, Robin Hayward, and other staff who worked countless hours in design, layout, and production of the final product.

Finally, we thank the many thousands of readers who have found the previous editions of the *Atlas* useful for their praise, support, and suggestions. We hope that their thoughts and our efforts have resulted in an improved work that benefits them and their patients.

Basil J. Zitelli, MD
Holly W. Davis, MD

Contents

Chapter 1

Genetic Disorders and Dysmorphic Conditions 1
CAROLYN A. BAY, MARK W. STEELE, AND HOLLY W. DAVIS

Chapter 2

Neonatology 33
BEVERLY S. BROZANSKI AND DEBRA L. BOGEN

Chapter 3

Developmental-Behavioral Pediatrics 65
HEIDI M. FELDMAN

Chapter 4

Allergy and Immunology 93
ANDREW MACGINNITIE AND DAVID NASH

Chapter 5

Cardiology 127
LEE B. BEERMAN, JACQUELINE KREUTZER, AND SANG C. PARK

Chapter 6

Child Abuse and Neglect 161
HOLLY W. DAVIS AND MARY M. CARRASCO

Chapter 7

Rheumatology 241
PAUL ROSEN AND SARA C. MCINTIRE

Chapter 8

Dermatology 275
BERNARD A. COHEN, HOLLY W. DAVIS, AND ROBIN P. GEHRIS

Chapter 9

Endocrinology 347
KECHA A. LYNSHUE AND SELMA F. WITCHEL

Chapter 10

Nutrition and Gastroenterology 375
CHERYL BLANK AND J. CARLTON GARTNER, JR.

Chapter 11

Hematology and Oncology 403
JEAN M. TERSAK, J. JEFFREY MALATACK, AND A. KIM RITCHEY

Chapter 12

Infectious Disease 443
HOLLY W. DAVIS AND MARIAN G. MICHAELS

Chapter 13

Nephrology 509
DEMETRIUS ELLIS

Chapter 14

Urologic Disorders 535
MARK F. BELLINGER

Chapter 15

Neurology 563
RAJIV VARMA, SHELLEY D. WILLIAMS, AND HENRY B. WESSEL

Chapter 16

Pulmonary Disorders 597
JONATHAN D. FINDER

Chapter 17

Surgery 623
EDWARD M. BARKSDALE, JR.

Chapter 18

Pediatric and Adolescent Gynecology 675
PAMELA J. MURRAY AND HOLLY W. DAVIS

Chapter 19

Ophthalmology 713
KENNETH P. CHENG AND ALBERT W. BIGLAN

Chapter 20

Oral Disorders 755
MAMOUN M. NAZIF, BRIAN S. MARTIN, DAVID H. MCKIBBEN, AND HOLLY W. DAVIS

Chapter 21

Orthopedics 781
VINCENT F. DEENEY, MOREY S. MORELAND, W. TIMOTHY WARD, AND HOLLY W. DAVIS

Chapter 22

Craniofacial Anomalies 867
A. CORDE MASON, JOSEPH E. LOSEE, AND MICHAEL L. BENTZ

Chapter 23

Otolaryngology 889
ROBERT F. YELLON, TIMOTHY P. MCBRIDE, AND HOLLY W. DAVIS

Index 939

CHAPTER 1

Genetic Disorders and Dysmorphic Conditions

Carolyn A. Bay, Mark W. Steele, and Holly W. Davis

The field of pediatric genetics and dysmorphology is complex, interesting, and rapidly evolving. Our knowledge base is gleaned from the careful observations of master clinicians and scientists who recognized clinical characteristics and patterns of malformation in individuals with genetic, teratogenic, developmental, and metabolic problems. They have provided us with a framework for the investigation of patients from clinical and laboratory perspectives. Recent advances in laboratory technology have greatly assisted evaluation, enabled far greater understanding of the molecular and physiologic basis of these disorders, and have greatly increased the rate of diagnosis of children with genetic and metabolic disorders. However, even with the availability of an ever widening array of confirmatory tests, clinical evaluation of patients remains an essential component of the complete assessment of children and adults with genetic diseases and dysmorphic conditions. This stems from the fact that careful evaluation can substantially reduce the number of differential diagnostic possibilities and, thereby, the number of diagnostic tests and the total expense.

Visual identification of dysmorphic features, combined with recognition of patterns of malformation and behavioral phenotypes, remains an integral part of the diagnostic algorithm. As in pediatrics in general, genetic disorders should be investigated using a careful history, with a family pedigree and a thorough physical examination including evaluation for the presence of major and minor anomalies, and thoughtful laboratory testing. This chapter is designed to present clinicians who care for children with background on the general principles of genetics and dysmorphology, as well as updated information about important advances in our field. Although not exhaustive, it provides a framework for the broad categories of genetic diseases and discusses an approach to the evaluation of the dysmorphic child. Definitions and examples of the types of disorders resulting in genetic and/or congenital anomalies in children are described including malformations, deformations, disruptions, associations, and sequences. We include examples of disorders inherited through classic mendelian inheritance patterns, including single gene mutations, such as Marfan syndrome and Smith-Lemli-Opitz syndrome, as well as examples of nonmendelian disorders such as teratogenic exposures in utero and disruptions or deformations of previously normal fetal structures. New etiologic mechanisms of diseases such as imprinting abnormalities and expansions of trinucleotide repeats in nuclear deoxyribonucleic acid (DNA) are presented. Finally, a newly evolving area of genetics, the investigation of disorders of mitochondrial DNA and/or mitochondrial function, is discussed.

Common Chromosomal Disorders

General Principles

The Nature of Chromosomes

Productive insights gleaned from the results of the recently completed Human Genome Project are likely to dramatically change our understanding in the near future of how the human genome functions. However, it is important to introduce to the reader our current understanding of the subject matter. Human hereditary factors are located in genes (the genome). Approximately 10% are genes that code for proteins that are assembled to form tissue structures or to form enzymes that catalyze chemical reactions within cells. The other 90% have functions that are currently not clear (see also "The Nature of Genes and Single Gene Disorders" later). The genes are composed of DNA and are stored in intranuclear cell organelles called *chromosomes*. Each chromosome contains one linear DNA molecule folded over onto itself several times, as well as ribonucleic acid (RNA) and proteins. Because all genes exist in pairs, all *chromosomes* must likewise exist in pairs. The members of each pair of genes are called *alleles,* and the members of each pair of chromosomes are known as *homologues*. The conventional depiction of the constitution of homologues in the nucleus is called the cell's *karyotype* (Fig. 1-1). If at any gene locus the alleles are identical, that gene locus is *homozygous*. If the alleles are not identical, the gene locus is *heterozygous*.

Except for gametes, normal human cells contain 23 pairs of chromosomes, 46 in all. One of these pairs is concerned in part with inducing the primary sex of the embryonic gonads. These sex chromosomes are called the *X and Y chromosomes,* and they are not genetically homologous except in a few areas. Women have two X chromosomes, whereas men have an X and a Y chromosome. The remaining 22 pairs are called *autosomes* and determine non–sex-related (somatic) characteristics.

During most of a cell's life cycle, chromosomes are diffusely spread throughout the nucleus and cannot be identified by morphologic means. Only when the cell divides does chromosome morphology become apparent (Fig. 1-2). The in vitro life cycle and the cellular division, or

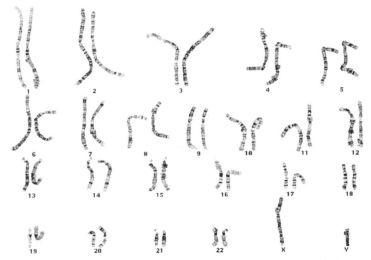

Figure 1-1. Photomicrographs show that this is a G-banded male karyotype (a female would have two X chromosomes and no Y chromosome). The horizontal banding produced by the Giemsa staining technique allows for precise identification of homologous chromosomes. (Courtesy Urvashi Surti, PhD, Pittsburgh Cytogenetics Laboratory.)

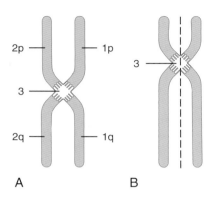

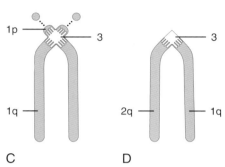

Figure 1-2. Morphology of a chromosome during metaphase. **A,** Metacentric chromosome with centromere (3) in middle. **B,** Submetacentric chromosome with centromere off-center. **C,** Acrocentric chromosome with centromere near one end. **D,** Telocentric chromosome (not found in humans) with centromere at one end. The DNA of the chromosome has replicated to form two chromatids: *1p* and *1q* represent one complete chromatid, *2p* and *2q* the other complete chromatid (*p* refers to the short arm and *q* refers to the long arm). The chromosome will then divide longitudinally, as shown in **B.**

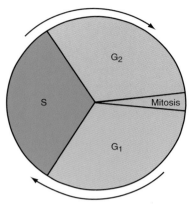

Figure 1-3. The in vitro life cycle of a somatic cell. The interphase lasts 21 hours and can be divided into the following three stages: G_1 (7 hours)—cell performs its tasks; S (7 hours)—DNA replicates; G_2 (7 hours)—cell prepares to divide. Then mitosis occurs.

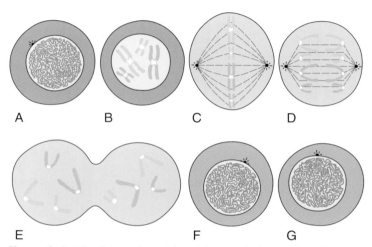

Figure 1-4. Mitosis lasts about 1 hour, during which time the cell divides. **A,** Interphase cell at end of G_2. **B,** Prophase-replicated DNA condenses and is visible. **C,** Metaphase-46 duplicated chromosomes align randomly on spindle and can be photographed for karyotyping. **D,** Anaphase-chromosomes divide longitudinally, and half of each one moves to the opposite pole of the cell. **E,** Telophase-cell wall divides. **F** and **G,** Interphase at G_1-two daughter cells each with 46 chromosomes.

mitosis, of a somatic cell are illustrated in Figures 1-3 and 1-4, respectively. The life cycle and divisions, or meiosis, of a germ cell are much more complex and are not suitable for ordinary clinical evaluation.

Any somatic cell that can divide in tissue culture can be used for chromosomal (cytogenetic) analyses. The most convenient tissue source is peripheral blood from which lymphocytes can be stimulated to divide during 2 or 3 days of incubation in tissue culture media. Fibroblasts obtained from skin remain a frequently used alternative when peripheral blood lymphocytes are not clinically suitable, but fibroblasts require an incubation period of 4 to 6 weeks. After death, lung tissue is the best tissue to culture for chromosomal analyses, although the process also requires a 4- to 6-week incubation period. Alternatively, skin fibroblasts are frequently obtained postmortem for various enzymatic and cytogenetic analyses, which may be used to confirm a clinical diagnosis. When a treatment decision requires urgency, preliminary chromosomal evaluation can be made within 4 to 24 hours using uncultured bone marrow aspirate or within 48 to 72 hours using rapid culturing and diagnostic techniques. This is an ever-evolving area, and pediatric clinicians are advised to discuss clinical and laboratory investigations with clinical geneticists and/or laboratory directors before the initiation of tissue sampling to ensure the most productive use of samples and rapid testing methods.

Aneuploidy

An abnormality in chromosome number different from an even multiple of 23 (the haploid number) is called *aneuploidy* (Fig. 1-5). Usually, in aneuploidy there are 45

or 47 chromosomes instead of the usual 46. Rarely, multiples of the X or Y chromosome result in individuals with 48 or 49 chromosomes. If aneuploidy occurs in a gamete as a result of an error of chromosomal division (nondisjunction or anaphase lag) during meiosis, all cells are affected in the fertilized embryo. With subsequent pregnancies, the risk for another chromosomal abnormality in the offspring is increased approximately 1% to 2% overall, in addition to the general background risk of abnormalities. The couple would be at risk for aneuploidy states of many types, not just the particular aneuploidy in their affected child. We are not yet aware of the underlying mechanism for the increased risk; however, families may benefit from an understanding of the possibilities for prenatal diagnosis in their individual case and may want to be referred for genetic counseling before the conception of another child.

Mosaic Aneuploidy States. Mosaicism, the presence of two or more genetically different cell lines within an individual, can result from an error in division during either meiosis or mitosis. In one possible scenario aneuploidy originates during meiotic division (i.e., before conception). In such cases the fetus starts out with an aneuploid chromosomal number and, subsequently, a

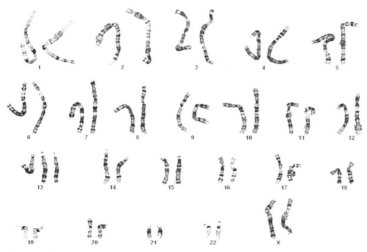

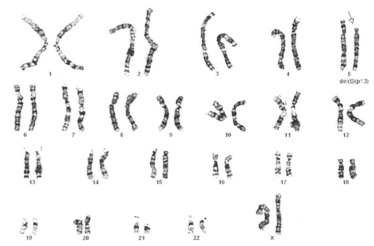

Figure 1-5. Karyotype of a patient with trisomy 13 demonstrates aneuploidy. Note the extra chromosome 13, causing the cell to have 47 instead of 46 chromosomes. (Courtesy Urvashi Surti, PhD, Pittsburgh Cytogenetics Laboratory.)

Figure 1-7. Deletion *(arrow)* of the p arm of chromosome 5 (cri du chat syndrome). (Courtesy Urvashi Surti, PhD, Pittsburgh Cytogenetics Laboratory.)

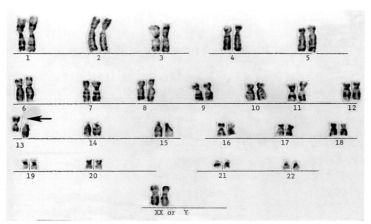

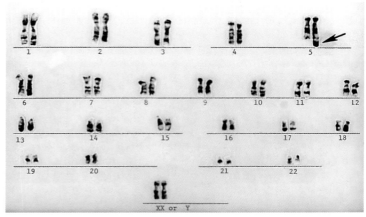

Figure 1-6. Pericentric inversion *(arrow)* of chromosome 13.

Figure 1-8. Unbalanced translocation. The additional DNA was translocated onto the q arm of chromosome 5. The abnormality was inherited from a normal carrier father (see Fig. 1-9) with a balanced reciprocal translocation between the q arms of chromosome 3 and chromosome 5. The patient died of multiple birth defects and in essence had a partial trisomy of the distal portion of the q arm of chromosome 3.

division error occurs, resulting in formation of another cell line that is chromosomally normal. In other cases of mosaicism the one-celled embryo (zygote) is chromosomally normal and a division error occurs after fertilization during mitosis of an embryonic somatic cell, resulting in aneuploidy. Most individuals with mosaicism have only two or three different lines of embryonic cells. It requires considerable laboratory investigation to distinguish the meiotic or mitotic types. Generally speaking, parents are given a 1% to 2% recurrence risk due to the possibility of mosaicism present in a parental gonad, which is not identifiable in usual tissue sample analyses.

Abnormalities of Chromosome Structure

Chromosomes can be normal in number (diploid) but still be abnormal in structure. Inversions (Fig. 1-6), deletions (Fig. 1-7), and translocations (Fig. 1-8) of genetic material are examples of structural chromosomal abnormalities. These can arise as new (sporadic) mutations in the egg or sperm from which the embryo was formed, in which case the parents' recurrence risk for another child with a chromosomal abnormality is again 1% to 2%. However, the abnormality may also be inherited from a phenotypically normal parent who is a "carrier" of a structural chromosomal abnormality (Fig. 1-9).

About 1 in 520 normal individuals carries a balanced but structurally abnormal set of chromosomes (Smith),

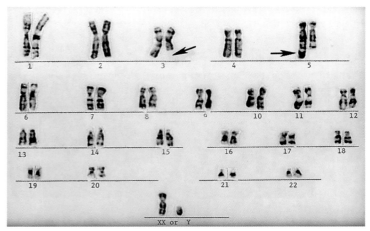

Figure 1-9. A "balanced" reciprocal translocation from chromosomes 3 to 5 in a normal man (the father of the chromosomally defective newborn whose karyotype is shown in Fig. 1-8).

called a *chromosome translocation.* The term *balanced,* for the purposes of this chapter, means that on cytogenetic analysis the structural abnormality does not appear to have resulted in any net loss or gain of genetic material. If the balanced chromosomal abnormality has been transmitted by other members of the family who are apparently phenotypically normal, it is considered a familial balanced translocation. Data suggest that a small percentage of individuals with apparently "balanced" translocations are actually mildly affected clinically by variable degrees of cognitive and physical deficits (Warburton). Thus high-resolution chromosome analyses are warranted in these instances including, as needed, in situ hybridization techniques using DNA probes to completely characterize the location of the chromosome breakpoints and to determine on a molecular level whether any genetic material is missing, or comparative genomic hybridization array (CGH).

A frequent way in which families with apparently balanced chromosome translocations present for evaluation occurs when a child is born with structural malformations and on karyotyping is found to have an unbalanced chromosome translocation. This may have occurred de novo in the child's chromosomes only or may be due to a previously undiagnosed familial balanced chromosomal translocation in a parent. Parental karyotypes are used to distinguish the etiology and are crucial in providing accurate genetic counseling regarding future pregnancies for that couple.

Incidence of Chromosomal Abnormalities

Recent data from Hook suggest that upwards of 50% of human conceptions terminate in a spontaneous abortion. Most of these miscarriages occur so early during gestation that the pregnancy is never recognized. The earlier the abortion occurs, the more likely it is that the miscarried embryo had a chromosomal abnormality. Of recognized first-trimester abortuses, 50% are chromosomally abnormal, compared with 5% of later embryos. Among the chromosomally abnormal abortuses, the most frequent abnormalities are triploidy (69 chromosomes), trisomy 16, and 45,X (Turner syndrome) (Table 1-1). Generally speaking, triploidy and trisomy 16 are not compatible with life and are only occasionally seen among liveborn infants.

Table 1-1	Occurrence of Chromosomal Abnormalities

AMONG SPONTANEOUS ABORTUSES	INCIDENCE (%)
Overall Incidence	32.0
First trimester	52.0
After first trimester	5.8
Type of Abnormality Seen in Spontaneous Abortions	
Trisomy 16	
Other trisomies	
Triploidy	
45X	
Miscellaneous	

AMONG LIVEBORNS	NO. OF CASES PER 1000
Overall Incidence	6.20
Abnormality of Autosomes (Males and Females)	4.19
Trisomies	
Balanced rearrangements	
Unbalanced rearrangements	
Abnormality of Sex Chromosomes (Males and Females)	2.03
In males XXY, XYY, mosaics	
In females 45,X (0.08) XXX, mosaics (1.43)	

About one quarter of all conceptuses are chromosomally abnormal. About 50 in 1000 stillborns have a chromosomal abnormality.

Despite the fact that Turner syndrome is relatively common among liveborn infants, the majority of conceptuses with 45,X also abort spontaneously. The incidence of chromosomal abnormalities among liveborn infants in general is about 6 in 1000. Among a group including both stillborn infants and infants who die in the immediate perinatal period, the number is increased to approximately 50 in 1000.

When to Suspect a Chromosomal Abnormality

Chromosomal abnormalities of either number or structure are likely to have a detrimental effect on the phenotype of an affected individual. Aneuploidy of an autosome, or nonsex chromosome, generally significantly impairs physical and cognitive development. However, aneuploidy of a sex chromosome may have little or no apparent effect on the phenotype. One should look for clustering of abnormalities in family members to suggest a problem, although their absence does not rule out a chromosomal abnormality.

Carriers of an inherited or a de novo reciprocal translocation are usually genetically balanced and are subsequently normal. However, their conceptuses are likely to be genetically unbalanced and may abort spontaneously or be born with major congenital anomalies. A history of unexplained infertility, multiple spontaneous abortions (three or more), and particularly of previous birth to the couple or to a close relative of a child with dysmorphic findings and/or major anomalies may be an indication that one of the parents carries a balanced chromosomal translocation or rearrangement. A chromosome study on the couple is thus indicated, and if translocation is found, they should seek antenatal genetic counseling. This may also be advisable for extended family members.

A normal person who carries a balanced reciprocal translocation can commonly produce six chromosomal types of gamete. On fertilization, these gamete types can result in several possible fertilized embryos: a normal conceptus, a carrier conceptus like the normal carrier parent, two types of immediately lethal conceptus resulting from gross chromosomal imbalances (i.e., too much or too little DNA), or two types of abnormal conceptus caused by lesser chromosomal imbalances. Whether the latter two types abort spontaneously or come to term as liveborns cannot be predicted in advance solely on theoretical grounds. Therefore genetic counseling in such situations depends somewhat on analysis of what has occurred within the individual family and in other families with similar rearrangements. Rarely, other types of chromosomal imbalances are found in conceptuses of such carrier parents.

Experience suggests the following: If a carrier has already produced a chromosomally unbalanced liveborn child, then it is apparent that it is possible for this to occur again in future pregnancies and the risk that the translocation carrier might have another chromosomally unbalanced liveborn infant can be as high as 20%. However, if the translocation carrier parent has either produced only healthy liveborn infants or spontaneous miscarriages, then it is less likely that the chromosomally unbalanced gametes are viable. Consequently, that person's risk for producing a chromosomally unbalanced liveborn is only about 4%. Finally, if a couple of whom one spouse is a carrier has not yet experienced any pregnancies, their risk for a chromosomally abnormal liveborn is estimated to be about 10%.

New Technologies

Fluorescence in Situ Hybridization

Fluorescence in situ hybridization (FISH) is a dramatic new laboratory technology that has revolutionized the diagnostic capabilities of clinical cytogenetic laboratories. In this technique a DNA probe is tagged with a label that fluoresces when viewed under a special microscope. The probe is applied to slides of metaphase chromosomes, to which it binds, but the probe also binds to interphase nuclei on the slide (Fig. 1-10A to J). The probe can be a cosmid probe for a small segment of single-copy DNA, such as part of a specific gene, or an anonymous bit of chromosomal DNA. The probe can be an alpha or beta

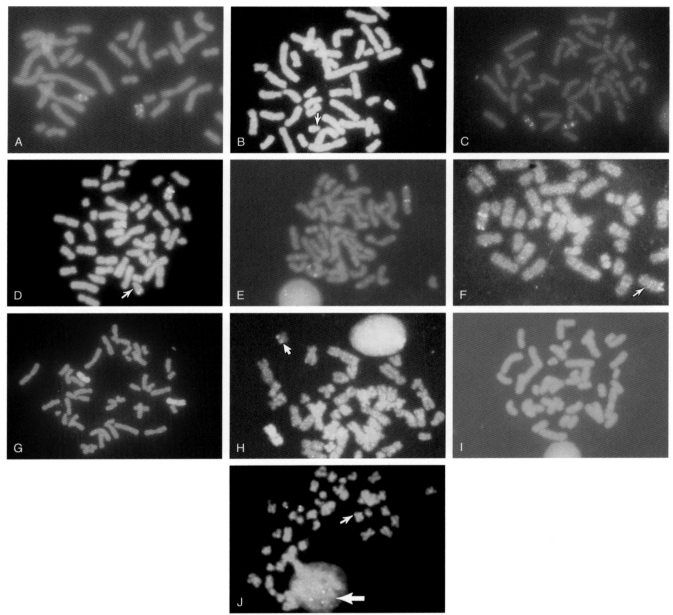

Figure 1-10. Fluorescence in situ hybridization (FISH) technology. **A,** Two normal chromosomes 22. The more distal yellow fluorescence on each chromosome is a cosmid probe for chromosome 22. The more central fluorescence on each chromosome is a cosmid probe for the DiGeorge sequence critical region. The general chromosome-DNA background stains orangish red. **B,** Patient with DiGeorge sequence. The normal chromosome 22 is at 4 o'clock. The arrow points to the chromosome 22 with deleted DiGeorge critical region. **C,** Two normal chromosomes 15. The lower fluorescence on each chromosome is a cosmid probe for chromosome 15. The upper fluorescence on each chromosome is a cosmid probe for the Prader-Willi syndrome critical region. **D,** Patient with Prader-Willi syndrome. The normal chromosome 15 is at 1 o'clock. The arrow points to the chromosome 15 with deleted Prader-Willi syndrome critical region. **E,** Two normal chromosomes 7. The more distal fluorescence on each chromosome is a cosmid probe for chromosome 7. The more central fluorescence on each chromosome is a cosmid probe for the Williams syndrome critical region. **F,** Patient with Williams syndrome. The normal chromosome 7 is at 9 o'clock. The arrow points to the chromosome 7 with deleted Williams syndrome critical region. **G,** Two normal X chromosomes each fluorescing end to end with an X chromosome FISH paint in a normal female. **H,** Male patient with a pericentric inversion of the Y chromosome determined by FISH and molecular analyses. An X chromosome FISH paint fluoresces the normal X chromosome at 7 o'clock. The arrow points to a fluorescence on the p arm end of the Y chromosome, which fluoresces because the p arm ends of the X and Y chromosomes normally are genetically homologous. **I,** Two normal chromosomes 21. The fluorescence on each chromosome is a cosmid probe for the Down syndrome critical region. **J,** Patient with Down syndrome caused by a cryptic translocation involving the Down syndrome critical region. The two normal 21 chromosomes are at 10 o'clock. The small arrow points to a chromosome 12 with fluorescence from the Down syndrome critical region on its end. The large arrow points to a nearby interphase nucleus with three fluorescent areas because of the trisomy for the Down syndrome critical region. The patient's conventional chromosome test (karyotype) on both blood and cultured skin fibroblasts was normal. (Courtesy Sharon L. Wenger, PhD, West Virginia University, and Mr. James H. Cummins, Children's Hospital of Pittsburgh.)

Table 1-2	Some Syndromes Identifiable by FISH Probe	
SYNDROME	**MAJOR FINDINGS**	**COMMENTS**
Cri du chat Deletion 5p15.2	Microcephaly, round face, downward-slanting palpebral fissures, epicanthal folds, hypertelorism, catlike cry in infancy	
Isolated lissencephaly	Lissencephaly	Approximately 30% have deletion 17p13.3
Miller-Dieker phenotype with lissencephaly	Microcephaly, incomplete development of brain with smooth surface (lissencephaly), variable high forehead, vertical furrowing of central forehead, low-set ears, small nose with anteverted nostrils, congenital heart disease, poor feeding	Deletion 17p13.3 in vast majority
Deletion 22q11.2	Phenotypes Velocardiofacial syndrome DiGeorge sequence Some cases of Opitz syndrome Conotruncal type of congenital heart disease (in an infant with dysmorphic features)	Appears to be a common deletion and should be considered in the differential diagnosis of children with multiple anomalies even if the features are not classic to any one phenotype
Wolf-Hirschhorn Deletion 4p16.3	Moderate to severe cognitive impairment, hypertelorism, preauricular pit or tag, broad nasal bridge, micrognathia, cleft palate, short philtrum, growth deficiency	
Smith-Magenis Deletion 17p11.2	Brachycephaly, flat facies, broad nasal bridge, short stature	Self-hugging behaviors, sleep disturbances

satellite probe for repetitive DNA sequences, such as those found in the centromeric area of a chromosome, or it can be a probe specific for repetitive DNA at the telomeric end of a chromosome. Finally, a cocktail of many repetitive DNA probes blanketing a specific chromosome from end to end can be obtained. This is called a *FISH paint*. Using special microscope filters, a clinician can simultaneously FISH paint a slide with probes fluorescing in two or three different colors.

FISH paints specific for all chromosomes are available. Technology is advancing quite rapidly to allow the identification of specific segments of chromosomes. This in turn allows characterization of specific regions of additional or deleted chromosomal material, which is extremely useful to clinicians in determining the clinical prognosis on the basis of similar cases in the literature. FISH probes are currently routinely available for chromosome microdeletion syndromes, including:

- Angelman syndrome del 15q11-13
- Prader-Willi syndrome del 15q11-13
- Cri du chat syndrome del 5p15.2
- DiGeorge sequence/velocardiofacial syndrome del 22q11.2
- Miller-Dieker/lissencephaly syndromes del 17p13.3
- Williams syndrome del 7q11.23
- Smith-Magenis syndrome del 17p11.2
- Wolf-Hirschhorn syndrome del 4p16.3
- Severe X-linked Ichthyosis del Xp22.3

In cases of disorders with several etiologic mechanisms such as Angelman syndrome, the absence of a deletion does *not* mean the child does not have the condition. An alternative mechanism that can result in a similar, possibly milder, clinical phenotype may be the source.

DiGeorge sequence is discussed in Chapter 4, Williams syndrome is discussed in Chapter 5, and Angelman and Prader-Willi syndromes are covered later in this chapter. The remaining syndromes are outlined briefly in Table 1-2.

Approach to the Evaluation of a Dysmorphic Child

Approximately 2% to 3% of liveborn infants have an observable structural abnormality. This number rises to about 4% to 5% by the time the child is old enough to

Table 1-3	Examples of Congenital Anomalies	
CATEGORY	**MAJOR**	**MINOR**
Craniofacial	Choanal atresia	Plagiocephaly Flat occiput
Eyes	Coloboma of iris	Epicanthal folds
Ears	Microtia	Preauricular pit
Hand	Polydactyly Absent thumbs	Single transverse palmar crease Clinodactyly

attend school. Structural differences can be determined to be either major or minor in character (Table 1-3; Figs. 1-11 and 1-12). Major structural anomalies have functional significance. Examples are polydactyly, colobomas of the iris (see Fig. 19-69), meningomyelocele, and cleft lip. Minor anomalies are usually of cosmetic importance only. Examples are epicanthal folds of the eyes, single transverse palmar creases, and supernumerary nipples. The incidence of isolated major anomalies in the general newborn population is approximately 1%, and the incidence of minor anomalies is approximately 14%. Both are more common in premature newborns.

The probability of an infant having a major anomaly increases with the number of minor anomalies found. Thus all children with multiple minor anomalies warrant a careful clinical assessment in order to find potentially significant occult major anomalies. Once an anomaly is identified, assessing its significance begins with a determination of whether the anomaly in question is a single localized error in morphogenesis or one component of a multiple malformation syndrome. An understanding of the pathophysiological mechanisms that produce structural abnormalities or differences provides an opportunity to define the types of structural abnormalities seen. This also assists the process of identifying the etiology and arriving at a specific diagnosis, which then can be useful in determining the prognosis and estimating the risk of recurrence of a similar problem in future pregnancies.

Definitions of the classifications of structural anomalies aid in communication between clinicians and in the process of evaluation and are summarized from Jones (see Bibliography):

Malformation This is an abnormality of embryonic morphogenesis of tissue. It usually results from genetic,

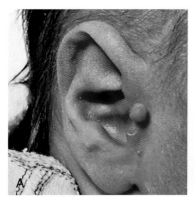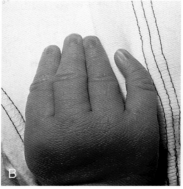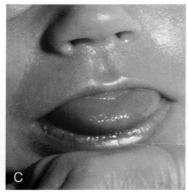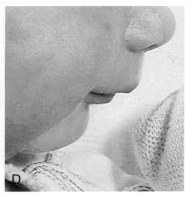

Figure 1-11. Clinical photographs show several minor anomalies seen at birth. **A,** Preauricular skin tag. **B,** Clinodactyly of the fifth finger. **C,** Macroglossia. **D,** Microretrognathia. (Courtesy Christine L. Williams, MD.)

chromosomal, or teratogenic influences, but it can be of multifactorial etiology. Malformations are divided into two main categories: those that constitute a *single primary defect in development* and those that represent a single component of a *multiple malformation syndrome.* A *multiple malformation syndrome* can be defined as one having several observed structural defects in development involving multiple organ systems that share the same known or presumed etiology. Malformations often require surgical intervention.

Deformation This represents an alteration (often molding) of an intrinsically normal tissue due to exposure to unusual extrinsic forces. A classic example is clubfoot, which may be the result of uterine constraint from crowding associated with a multiple gestation. A more severe example is the compressed facial features ("Potter facies") of a child exposed to severe uterine constraint associated with oligohydramnios, due to renal agenesis (see Fig. 13-37). The vast majority of deformations respond to medical therapy alone and have a relatively good prognosis in contrast to malformations, which frequently require surgical intervention.

Disruption This represents a breakdown of normally formed tissue, which may be the result of vascular accidents or exposure to adverse mechanical forces that are usually more severe than those that produce deformation. A classic example is the combination of clefting, constriction bands, and limb reduction defects associated with the presence of amniotic bands (see Fig. 2-46). The earlier these vascular accidents or abnormal forces occur during embryogenesis, the more severe the resulting defects.

Dysplasia This is characterized by abnormal organization of cells within tissue, which usually has a genetic basis. An example is achondroplasia, the most frequent form of skeletal dysplasia.

Each of these categories can have a *sequence* associated with it.

Sequence This term refers to a recognizable pattern of multiple anomalies that occurs when a single problem in morphogenesis cascades, resulting in secondary and tertiary errors in morphogenesis and a corresponding series of structural alterations. A classic example is the Robin malformation or Pierre Robin sequence, in which the single primary malformation is microretrognathia (see Fig. 23-63). The resulting glossoptosis, or posterior placement of the tongue in the oropharynx, interferes with normal palatal closure if the lingual displacement occurs before 9 weeks' gestation. The resulting cleft palate is U-shaped, rather than having the V shape that

is usually seen in classic cleft palate, a finding that aids in recognition.

Association An association is a pattern of malformations that occurs together too frequently to be due to random chance alone, but for which no specific etiology is yet recognized.

The approach to the evaluation of a child with a dysmorphologic abnormality is similar to a careful diagnostic evaluation of most pediatric problems, starting with a complete history and careful physical examination. In obtaining these it is helpful to remember that there are six broad etiologic categories to be considered in the differential diagnosis: a known syndrome, an unknown syndrome, a chromosomal abnormality, a teratogen, congenital infection, and maternal disease and/or placental abnormalities.

The history should include the following:
- Course of the pregnancy, complications including possible infections or environmental exposures, medications/substance abuse
- Prior pregnancies, spontaneous abortions, stillborns or infant/child deaths for this couple
- Labor/delivery/perinatal problems
- Past medical history
- Growth and development
- Meticulous family history with family tree going back three generations and including the following:
  Familial traits and growth characteristics
  Familial physical or developmental disorders
  Spontaneous abortions, stillborns, infant/child deaths in extended family

The physical examination entails the following:
- Thorough general examination
- A search for major and/or minor anomalies
- Neurodevelopmental assessment

In addition, focused examination of immediate family members for physical characteristics and growth parameters and review of family photo albums may be helpful.

Determining how the child fits into the norms for growth and development for the general population, for the family's ethnic group(s), and for the extended family is important. One continuing challenge is to determine whether the norms for the family are truly in the normal range for the general population and ethnic background or, in fact, constitute variability of a genetic trait present in its severe expression in the child or family member seen for evaluation.

The *identification of a recognizable pattern of both major and minor anomalies* provides the clinical dysmorphologist with a diagnosis, or a short list of differential diagnostic possibilities. Thus the detection of major and minor

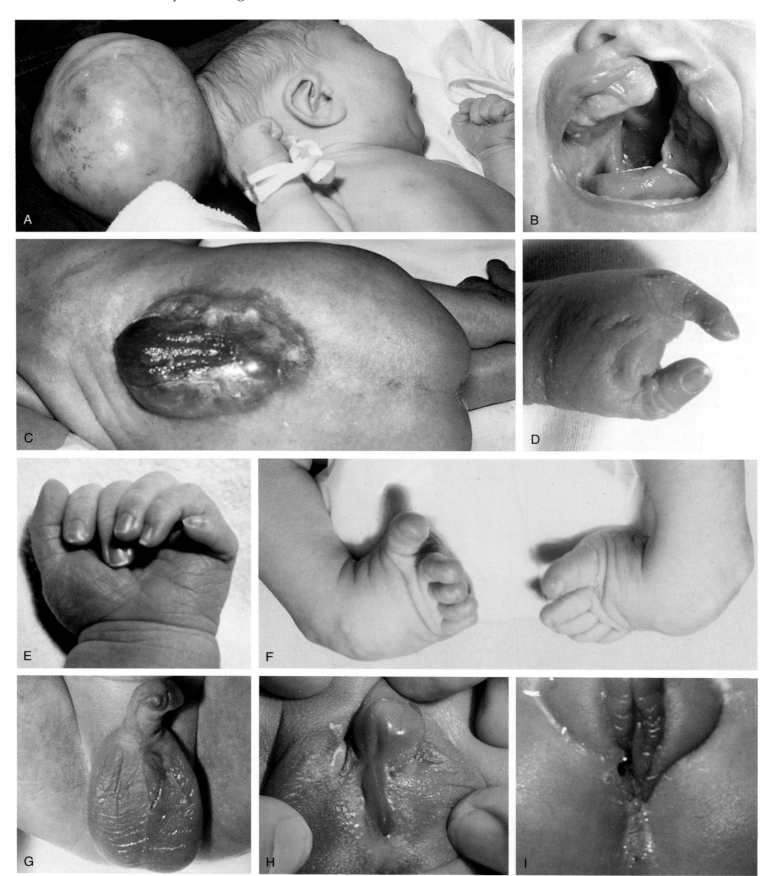

Figure 1-12. Clinical photographs show several major anomalies seen at birth. **A,** Encephalocele. **B,** Cleft lip and palate. **C,** Meningomyelocele. **D,** Ectrodactyly (previously termed lobster-claw deformity). **E,** Polydactyly (postaxial). **F,** Bilateral clubfoot. **G,** Hypospadias. **H,** Fused labia with enlarged clitoris. **I,** Imperforate anus. (Courtesy Christine L. Williams, MD.)

anomalies is critical in the diagnostic process. Identification of specific and unusual malformations that are uncommon and occur in only a few syndromes can be especially helpful. For example, finding that a child has long palpebral fissure length and pronounced fingertip fat pad size in combination with the pattern of anomalies typical of the Kabuki syndrome make it extremely likely that the diagnosis is the Kabuki syndrome. Training in dysmorphology emphasizes the recognition of key components in patterns of malformation, as well as the specific findings useful in distinguishing syndromes with similarities from one another. Texts that outline currently recognized patterns of malformations can be helpful in assisting the clinician in the identification of specific features that can rule a diagnosis in or out. Commercial computer-based programs exist for syndrome identification; however, these are often more effectively used by experts in the field due to complexity of terminology and the need for exacting descriptions of the anomalies present in a given child.

A chromosome study should be performed on each child with a syndrome of congenital anomalies. Such a study may establish or confirm the diagnosis of a chromosomal disorder and its hereditary potential and may possibly help map the chromosomal location of genes for those syndromes known to be simple mendelian disorders.

Abnormalities of Autosomes

Down Syndrome

The worldwide incidence of Down syndrome among liveborns is approximately 1 in 660, with 45% of affected individuals born to women older than 35 years of age. The incidence of Down syndrome among conceptuses is far greater than among liveborns because the majority of Down syndrome fetuses spontaneously abort.

No single physical stigma of Down syndrome exists; rather, the clinical diagnosis rests on finding a recognizable constellation of clinical characteristics including a combination of major and minor anomalies (Fig. 1-13).

The most frequent features are upslanting palpebral fissures and small external ears (by length). Several major anomalies are commonly associated with Down syndrome. Congenital heart disease is found in 45% of cases, particularly atrioventricular communis and ventricular septal defects. Hence all newborns with Down syndrome should undergo cardiac evaluation with echocardiogram. About 5% have a gastrointestinal anomaly, most commonly duodenal atresia or Hirschsprung disease. An increased incidence of thyroid disorders also exists, particularly of the autoimmune type. Thus regular testing of thyroid function is recommended. Acute and neonatal leukemias occur 15 to 20 times more frequently in people

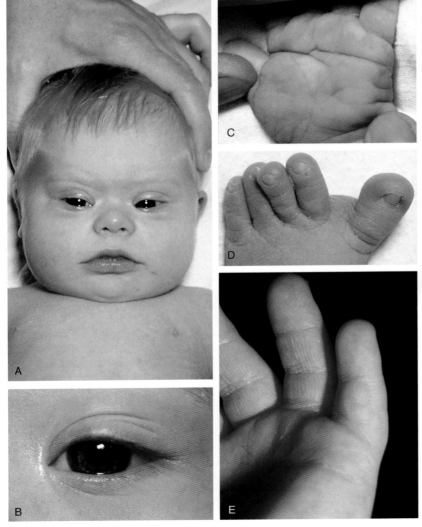

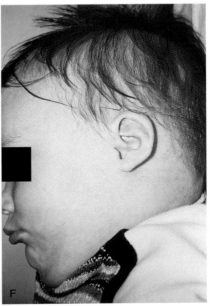

Figure 1-13. Down syndrome. Clinical photographs show several minor anomalies associated with this disorder. **A,** Characteristic facial features with upward-slanting palpebral fissures, epicanthal folds, and flat nasal bridge. **B,** Brushfield spots. **C,** Bridged palmar crease, seen in some affected infants. Two transverse palmar creases are connected by a diagonal line. **D,** Wide space between first and second toes. **E,** Short fifth finger. **F,** Small ears and flat occiput.

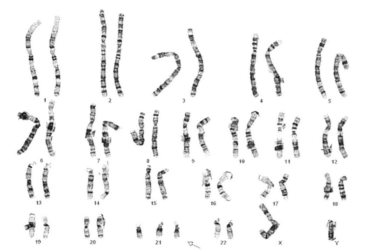

Figure 1-14. Karyotype of a patient with Down syndrome indicates trisomy 21. (Courtesy Urvashi Surti, PhD, Pittsburgh Cytogenetics Laboratory.)

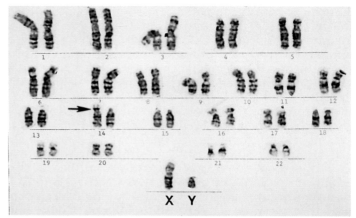

Figure 1-15. Karyotype of a patient with Down syndrome shows 14/21 centric fusion translocation.

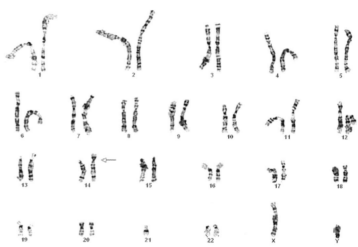

Figure 1-16. Karyotype of a normal female 14/21 centric fusion translocation carrier. (Courtesy Urvashi Surti, PhD, Pittsburgh Cytogenetics Laboratory.)

with Down syndrome than in the general population. In newborns, much of this is represented by transient leukemoid reactions with complete remission being the most frequent outcome. Quantitative abnormalities are found in many enzyme systems. People with Down syndrome are shorter than family members and the general population and have premature graying of hair. As adults, most males are infertile, but females may reproduce and can have children who will also have Down syndrome approximately one third of the time.

Minor anomalies include brachycephaly; inner epicanthal folds; Brushfield spots; flat nasal bridge; a small mouth with protruding tongue that fissures with age; a short neck with redundant skinfolds; single transverse palmar (simian) creases; clinodactyly of the fifth fingers, with single digital crease caused by hypoplasia of the middle phalanx; and wide spacing between the first and second toes. The number of such anomalies varies in any particular case.

With rare exceptions, individuals with Down syndrome are cognitively impaired. The degree of impairment varies, with intelligence quotients (IQs) ranging from 20 to 80. Most individuals function in the mild to moderate range of developmental delay. The advent of individualized programs of early intervention therapy, education, and sporting activities has resulted in much improved outcomes and individuals who are much more likely to function at the maximum of their developmental capabilities. Autopsy analyses of brains from individuals with Down syndrome have revealed the neuropathologic changes of Alzheimer disease in 100% of those older than 40 years. Nevertheless, only about 25% of older individuals with Down syndrome exhibit clinical manifestations of Alzheimer disease. The reason for the clinical-pathologic discordance is not known. However, there does tend to be a progressive loss of cognitive functioning after the fourth decade of life. Longevity, though less than that of the general population, has steadily increased over the years. Individuals with Down syndrome who do not have congenital heart disease may expect to live well into their 60s. The principal causes of death in children with Down syndrome are infection, congenital heart disease, and malignancy.

The etiology of Down syndrome is trisomy 21, the presence of an extra chromosome 21 either as a simple trisomy (Fig. 1-14) or as part of a chromosome 21 fused with another chromosome (Fig. 1-15). These fused chromo-

Table 1-4	Maternal Age–Specific Risk for Trisomy 21 at Live Birth
MATERNAL AGE	**PREVALENCE AT LIVE BIRTH**
25	1/1350
30	1/890
35	1/355
40	1/97
45	1/23

somes are often robertsonian translocation chromosomes or isochromosomes. Cases of mosaicism, in which trisomy 21 cell lines coexist with cell lines with the standard 46 chromosomes, exist as well and may range in phenotype from normal to that typical of complete trisomy 21. An association between trisomy 21 and advanced maternal age is clear (Table 1-4).

About 5% of Down syndrome cases represent a centric fusion translocation between the long arm of a chromosome 21 and those of a 14, 15, 13 (see Fig. 1-15) or a 21/22 acrocentric chromosome. Of these, about one third are inherited from a clinically normal, balanced carrier parent (Fig. 1-16); in the remaining two thirds the translocation is new in the affected child. Chromosome studies should therefore be performed on the parents and appropriate family members of an individual with translocation Down

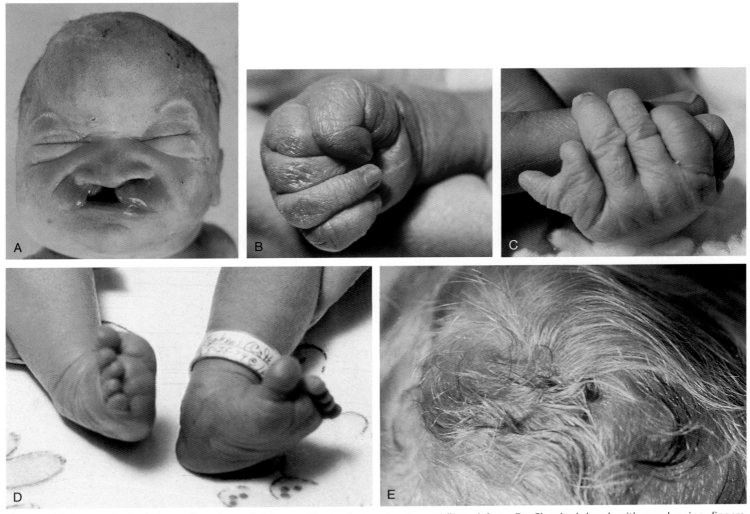

Figure 1-17. Several physical manifestations of trisomy 13. **A,** Facies showing midline defect. **B,** Clenched hand with overlapping fingers. **C,** Postaxial polydactyly. **D,** Equinovarus deformity. **E,** Typical punched-out scalp lesions of aplasia cutis congenita. (**A,** Courtesy T. Kelly, MD, University of Virginia Medical Center, Charlottesville; **B** to **E,** courtesy Kenneth Garver, MD, Pittsburgh.)

syndrome. If a parent carries a 21/21 translocation, all liveborns will have Down syndrome; for the remaining 21/centric fusion translocations, the empirical recurrence risk for a Down syndrome liveborn is less than 2% if the father is the carrier and roughly 15% if the mother is the carrier. The parents of children with trisomy 21 may benefit from genetic counseling to determine their individual risk of having another child with Down syndrome or with other chromosomal abnormalities in future pregnancies.

Trisomy 13

Trisomy 13 is a relatively rare (1 in 5000) genetic condition caused by the presence of additional chromosome material from all or a large part of chromosome 13. The vast majority of embryos with classic trisomy for a complete 13th chromosome abort spontaneously, but approximately 5% survive to be liveborn. They have a severe, recognizable pattern of malformation that allows clinicians to suspect this etiology immediately (Fig. 1-17). The hallmark features are defects of forebrain development related to those seen in holoprosencephaly, aplasia cutis congenita, polydactyly (most frequently of the postaxial type), and narrow hyperconvex nails. A broader listing of features is outlined in Table 1-5, which can be useful in

Table 1-5	Physical Abnormalities in Trisomy 13 and 18 Syndromes	

ABNORMALITY	TRISOMY 13	TRISOMY 18
Severe developmental retardation	††††	††††
Approximately 90% die within first year	††††	††††
Cryptorchidism in males	††††	††††
Low-set, malformed ears	††††	††††
Multiple major congenital anomalies	††††	††††
Prominent occiput	†	††††
Cleft lip and/or palate	†††	†
Micrognathia	††	†††
Microphthalmos	†††	††
Coloboma of iris	†††	†
Short sternum	†	†††
Rocker-bottom feet	††	†††
Congenital heart disease	††	††††
Scalp defects	†††	†
Flexion deformities of fingers	††	††††
Polydactyly	†††	†
Hypoplasia of nails	††	†††
Hypertonia in infancy	†	†††
Apneic spells in infancy	†††	†
Midline brain defects	†††	†
Horseshoe kidneys	†	†††

Relative frequency: ††††, usual; †, rare.

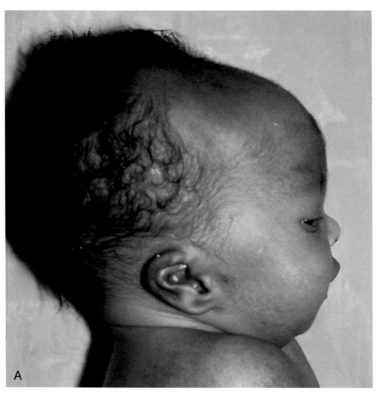

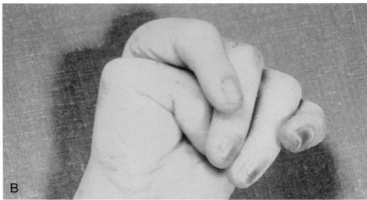

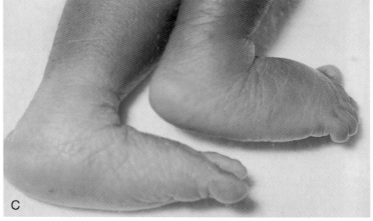

Figure 1-18. Several physical manifestations of trisomy 18. **A,** Typical profile reveals prominent occiput and low-set, posteriorly rotated malformed auricles. **B,** Clenched hand showing typical pattern of overlapping fingers. **C,** Rocker-bottom feet. (Courtesy Kenneth Garver, MD, Pittsburgh.)

comparing the features frequently seen in infants with trisomy 13 to those seen in trisomy 18. As with many syndromes, trisomy 13 and trisomy 18 share structural abnormalities; however, they usually are distinguishable on the basis of the pattern of anomalies present. Liveborn infants with trisomy 13 represent those who have the least severe structural abnormalities of major organs. Of these, about 5% survive the first 6 months of life. Thus discussions with parents about surgical interventions must take into account the small possibility of long-term survival and require sensitivity to the needs of child and family.

Milder chromosome abnormalities involving extra material determined to originate from chromosome 13 must be identified and distinguished from classic trisomy 13 because the clinical phenotype and prognosis may be different and, in some cases, less severe. Children with mosaicism, that is, with a normal cell line and a trisomy 13 cell line, as well as those with trisomy of part of chromosome 13, can be identified by chromosome analysis. Careful laboratory investigation must be carried out to identify the exact chromosomal abnormality. The advent of FISH technology has dramatically increased the ability of laboratory specialists to characterize chromosome rearrangements, with the goal being to identify the exact breakpoints of the chromosomes involved in the rearrangements. Molecular studies then may be possible to determine any potential impact of the rearrangement on individual genes and their products. This information is extremely helpful to clinicians in determining prognosis and in providing more realistic information when discussing treatment options. Rarely, children who have the recognizable pattern of clinical features of trisomy 13 have normal chromosomes. If a geneticist/dysmorphologist is not already involved, a consultation is warranted to aid in

diagnosis and prognosis counseling and to determine any recurrence risks for the parents in future pregnancies.

Trisomy 18

This chromosomal disorder occurs in approximately 3 in 10,000 newborns, and females are more likely to be liveborn. Affected infants are small for gestational age and have a frail appearance, and the face tends to appear petite relative to the rest of the craniofacial contour (Fig. 1-18A). They also have a recognizable pattern of malformation, but in these infants hallmark features—clenched hands with overlapping fingers (see Fig. 1-18B), short sternum, and "low arch" fingerprint patterns—are minor anomalies. Major anomalies, especially congenital heart disease, are generally present as well and are the source of significant morbidity and mortality. Other common findings include a prominent occiput, low-set and structurally abnormal ears, micrognathia, and rocker-bottom feet (Fig. 1-18C). Table 1-5 presents a broader listing of clinical features that can be useful in distinguishing trisomy 18 from trisomy 13, which shares many of the same structural abnormalities.

Trisomy 18 was previously thought to be almost invariably fatal in the neonatal period; however, recent data suggest that a small percentage of children can live longer, and that between 5% and 10% will be alive at their first birthday. Survivors are more frequently female and have less severe structural abnormalities of major organs than most affected infants. Even with optimal neonatal, pediatric, and surgical management and excellent home-based care, children with classic trisomy 18 often "fail to thrive" and have significant developmental and cognitive impairments. Discussions with parents about interventions must take into account the slim possibility of long-term survival and require sensitivity to the needs of child and family. Great care must be taken in providing a balanced picture to the family when discussing treatment options.

Chromosome analysis allows clinicians to evaluate the etiology of the trisomy and can help determine prognosis. Results can demonstrate classic trisomy 18 due to a complete extra chromosome 18, mosaicism for trisomy 18, or a complex chromosome abnormality involving one or more chromosomes. Children with chromosomal rearrangements that result in partial rather than complete trisomy 18 may have a milder clinical outcome. Trisomy limited to the short arm of chromosome 18 is associated with a significantly milder prognosis, whereas trisomy of the entire long arm of chromosome 18 may be indistinguishable from an individual with classic trisomy 18. Smaller areas of trisomy for the long arm of chromosome 18 may show some, but not all, of the features of classic trisomy 18. Thus chromosomal study of each child is essential.

If a complex chromosome rearrangement is identified in a child, further parental chromosome studies are indicated. Chromosome analysis of the parents will determine if the rearrangement is new in the child or is evidence of a familial balanced translocation. Full characterization of the extent of a chromosome rearrangement also allows clinicians the opportunity to find similar cases if they exist and to provide more accurate information regarding prognosis, treatment options, and recurrence risk to the family. If a familial balanced translocation is present in one of the parents and appears to be the explanation for the triplicated chromosome 18 material in the child, other family members may benefit from genetic counseling to determine what options are available to them when they consider having additional children.

It has been our experience that parent support organizations can be extremely helpful to family members in the long process of adjustment to having a child with a chromosome problem. If the child expires, they can be helpful as a resource to the parents because of the similarity of their collective experience and can help them through the grieving and healing process. They can also be a source of ongoing support and information to parents of a child with trisomy 13 or trisomy 18 who may live but who will face major medical and developmental challenges due to the chromosomal abnormality.

Abnormalities of Sex Chromosomes

Turner Syndrome

Turner syndrome is one of the three most common chromosomal abnormalities found in early spontaneous abortions. The phenotype is female. About 1 in 2000 liveborn females has Turner syndrome. Primary amenorrhea, sterility, sparse pubic and axillary hair, underdeveloped breasts, and short stature ($4^1/_2$ to 5 ft) are the usual manifestations. Other external physical features may include webbing of the neck; cubitus valgus; a low-set posterior hairline; a shield chest with widely spaced nipples; and malformed, often protruding, ears (Fig. 1-19A-E). Internally, renal anomalies may be present along with congenital heart disease, particularly bicuspid aortic valve (in 30% of cases) and coarctation of the aorta (in

10% of cases). Affected women have an infantile uterus, and their ovaries consist only of strands of fibrous connective tissue. Newborns often have lymphedema of the feet and/or hands (Fig. 1-19D and E), which can reappear briefly during adolescence. Mental development is usually normal. Schooling and behavioral problems seem to be the same as in age-matched control subjects, though difficulty with spatial orientation such as map reading may be a problem. The classic physical findings of Turner syndrome may be absent, or the abnormalities may be so minimal in the newborn that the diagnosis is missed. The first indication may be unexplained short stature in later childhood or failure to develop secondary sex characteristics by late adolescence. Thus a chromosome study is indicated as part of the diagnostic workup of adolescent girls with these complaints.

The karyotype in the majority of individuals with Turner syndrome is 45,X. Most often, the missing sex chromosome is paternally derived, so the risk of Turner syndrome does not increase with parental age. Another 15% of individuals with Turner syndrome are mosaics (XO/XX, XO/XX/XXX, or XO/XY). The physical stigmata may be less marked in mosaics, some of whom may be fertile. If an XY cell line is present, the intra-abdominal gonads should be removed because they are prone to malignant change. The remaining cases of Turner syndrome have 46 chromosomes including one normal plus one structurally abnormal X. The latter may have a short (p) arm deletion or may be an isochrome duplication of the long (q) arm of the X chromosome; usually it is paternally derived. Cases of Turner syndrome with one normal and one abnormal X chromosome are more likely to have other, more serious major anomalies including cognitive deficits. A structurally abnormal X chromosome may lead to abnormal X inactivation (see Fig. 1-22), resulting in a deleterious dosage effect for X-linked genes. Karyotypes such as 46,XYp-or 46,Xi(Yq) result in a female with Turner syndrome.

Whereas loss of the short arm of an X chromosome results in full-blown Turner syndrome, deletion of the long arm usually produces only streak (fibrous) gonads with consequent sterility, amenorrhea, and infantile secondary sex characteristics without the other somatic stigmata of Turner syndrome. If the diagnosis is clinically suspected, a chromosome study should be ordered. Should the affected child be 45,X or a mosaic, the parental risk for recurrence of a chromosomally abnormal liveborn is 1% to 2% but may be higher if a parent carries a structurally abnormal X chromosome.

Antenatal diagnosis of chromosomally abnormal fetuses should be discussed with the parents, and the relatively good prognosis for Turner syndrome liveborns should not be overlooked. Girls with Turner syndrome should receive appropriate hormone therapy during adolescence to enable development of secondary sex characteristics and stimulate menses. Rarely, 45,X women with Turner syndrome have been fertile for a limited number of years.

Klinefelter Syndrome

One in 500 newborn boys has Klinefelter syndrome. The physical stigmata are subtle and usually not obvious until puberty, at which time the normal onset of spermatogenesis is blocked by the presence of two X chromosomes. Consequently the germ cells die, the seminiferous tubules become hyalinized and scarred, and the testes

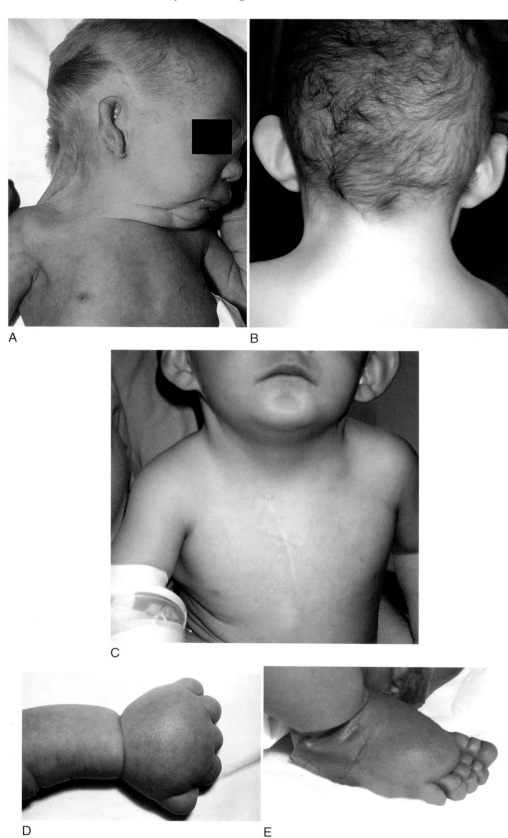

A

B

C

D

E

Figure 1-19. Clinical photographs show several physical manifestations associated with Turner syndrome. **A,** In this newborn a webbed neck with low hairline, shield chest with widespread nipples, abnormal ears, and micrognathia are seen. **B,** The low-set posterior hairline can be better appreciated in this older child who also has protruding ears. **C,** In this frontal view mild webbing of the neck and small widely spaced nipples are evident, along with a midline scar from prior cardiac surgery. The ears are low set and prominent, protruding forward. **D** and **E,** The newborn shown in **A** also had prominent lymphedema of hands and feet.

become small. Testosterone levels are below normal adult male levels, though the level varies from case to case (the average being about half as much as normal). Hence there is a wide range in degree of virilization. At one extreme is the man with a small penis and gynecomastia (Fig. 1-20); at the opposite extreme is the virile mesomorph with a normal penis. Scoliosis may develop during adolescence. The average full-scale IQ of men with Klinefelter

syndrome is 98, which is about the same as the general population. Behavioral problems may be more common than in the population at large, however.

The karyotype in Klinefelter syndrome is XXY in 80% of cases and mosaic (XY/XXY) in the other 20%. Rarely the latter type may be fertile. About 60% of cases reflect a chromosome error in oogenesis, and in 40% an error in spermatogenesis. The risk of having an affected child

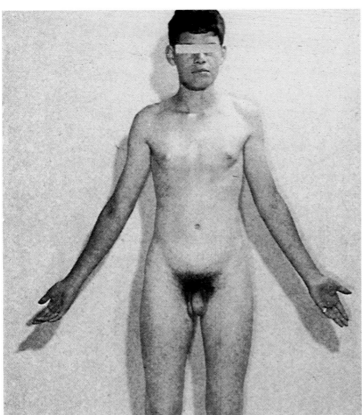

A

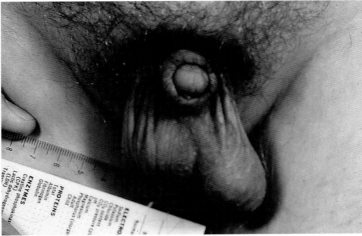

B

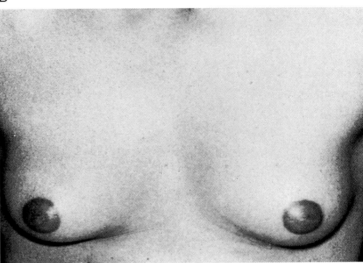

C

Figure 1-20. Clinical photographs show several physical manifestations of Klinefelter syndrome. **A,** Relatively narrow shoulders, increased carrying angle of arms, female distribution of pubic hair and normal penis but with small scrotum due to small testicular size. **B,** Small testes and penis. **C,** Gynecomastia. (**B,** Courtesy Peter Lee, MD, Hershey Medical Center; **C,** from Gardner LI [ed]: Endocrine and Genetic Diseases of Childhood, 2nd ed. Philadelphia, WB Saunders, 1975.)

increases with maternal age. Males with more than two X chromosomes (XXXY, XXXXY) are usually cognitively impaired and are more likely to have skeletal and other major congenital anomalies such as cleft palate, congenital heart disease (particularly a patent ductus arteriosus), and microcephaly. The parents' recurrence risk for another chromosomally abnormal liveborn is 1% to 2%; antenatal diagnosis with subsequent pregnancies is possible.

XXX and XYY

Triple X females have a karyotype result of 47,XXX. Incidence is approximately 1 in 1000 liveborn females. Affected individuals have no characteristic abnormal physical features. Although usually within the normal range of intelligence, their IQ scores may be lower than those of their normal siblings, delays in development of motor skills and coordination are common, and approximately 60% require some special education classes. Behavior problems occur in approximately 30% and are usually mild. XXX women are fertile, and their children are usually chromosomally normal.

XYY males have a karyotype result of 47,XYY. Incidence is 1 in 840 among liveborn males. They tend to be tall in comparison with their own family members, but generally their phenotypic appearance is normal. As in 47,XXX females, IQ is usually within the normal range but may

be lower than that of siblings. Affected boys often come to medical attention because of problems with fine motor coordination, speech disorders, and learning disabilities. Early reports raised concerns about significant behavioral problems; however, long-term prospective studies now suggest that these boys do not have any greater incidence of problem behaviors than the general population.

The risk of recurrence for a couple with a child with XXX or XYY depends on many factors including the parents' own karyotype results and on advancing maternal age. Therefore it is recommended that they be referred for individualized genetic counseling when considering future pregnancies.

Molecular Cytogenetic Syndromes

Advances in molecular genetics have provided new insights into the genetic pathogenesis of several syndromes often associated with specific cytogenetic abnormalities.

Fragile X Syndrome

It has long been recognized that there is a significant excess of males in moderately to severely mentally retarded

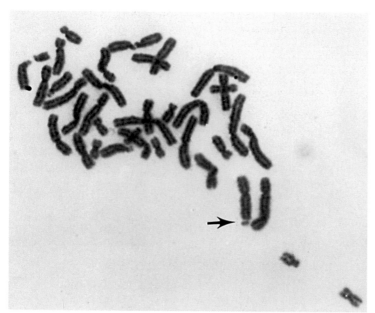

Figure 1-21. Fragile X chromosome marker in lymphocyte culture. Partial metaphase plate shows the chromosome break at Xq27 *(arrow)* characteristic of fragile X syndrome (solid Giemsa stain).

X-CHROMOSOME INACTIVATION

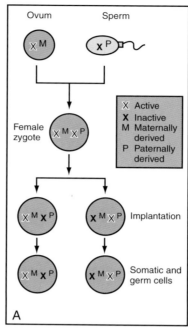

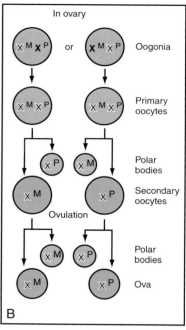

Figure 1-22. Functional behavior of the X chromosome in XX females. **A,** Somatic and premeiotic germ cells. Implantation occurs 5 days after conception, at which time in each female cell either X^M or X^P is randomly genetically inactivated and remains so in each of the cell's descendants. Because the process is random, by determining the proportion of cells with an inactive X^M or inactive X^P in each of a large population of women, a gaussian population distribution of women is generated. That is, most women in the population will have an approximate 50/50 mix of cells, in which each cell expresses either X^M or X^P. However, some women will by chance have more cells with an inactive X^M and vice versa. **B,** Meiotic germ cells. When a female germ cell enters first prophase of meiosis, X inactivation is abolished; both X chromosomes become genetically active through fertilization and continue so until embryonic uterine implantation. Then, as in **A,** random X inactivation in XX females occurs all over again.

populations. Much of this inordinate male representation is the result of altered X-linked recessive genes. These may represent new mutations or inheritance of the abnormal gene from normal heterozygous (carrier) mothers. About 1 in 150 individuals, usually male, has some form of X-linked mental retardation. Of these it is estimated that between 30% and 50% have fragile X syndrome.

In 1969 Herbert Lubs noted the in vitro cytogenetic marker now called *fragile X* in short-term lymphocyte cultures. However, its clinical significance was not realized until a 1977 report by G. R. Sutherland in Australia. Under tissue culture conditions that starve the cell of its ability to synthesize thymidylic acid, a chromosome break at Xq27, the distal part of the long arm of the X chromosome (Fig. 1-21), is visible in cells of individuals clinically affected with fragile X syndrome. By pedigree analysis, about 1 in 4000 males has the Fragile X gene.

Fragile X syndrome is the first recognized example of a *trinucleotide* repeat disorder. The gene involved, located at Xq27.3, is called *FMR1* and is active in brain cells and sperm. At the start of the gene is the DNA trinucleotide CGG, which in the general population is normally linearly repeated about 5 to 50 times (the average being 30). Presence of from 55 to 200 linear CGG repeats is considered a Fragile X *premutation.* Individuals with a premutation appear clinically normal. The finding of more than 200 linear CGG repeats is considered a *full mutation* and in males results in fragile X syndrome. In females with more than 200 linear CGG repeats, there are clinical effects in 50% and apparently little or no effect in 50%. The explanation for this disparity in females most likely is the phenomenon known as *X chromosome inactivation* (Fig. 1-22). Premutation and, in females, random X inactivation explain the lack of penetrance of the Fragile X gene.

No cases of new mutations for these *FMR1* gene CGG trinucleotide expansions or repeats have been found. That is, all such expansions are inherited from a parent. A man with a premutation passes it on to all of his daughters as a premutation. Men with a full mutation generally do not reproduce. Men with premutations don't pass them to

Table 1-6	Relative Risk of Maternal Transmission of a Fragile X Premutation to Her Offspring as a Full Mutation
NUMBER OF CGG REPEATS IN MOTHER'S PREMUTATION	**RISK OF EXPANSION TO FULL MUTATION IN OFFSPRING (%)**
55-59	3.7
60-69	5.3
70-79	31.1
80-89	57.8
90-99	80.1
100-109	100
110-119	98.1
120-129	97.2

From Saul RA, Tarleton JC: *FMR1*-related disorders, 2006. Gene Reviews (www.genetests.org).

their sons because they give their Y chromosome to their sons.

Women heterozygous for either a premutation or full mutation have a 50% chance of passing it on to each child as follows: If she has a full mutation, she passes it on as a full mutation in most instances; if she has a premutation, she passes it on to her child either as a premutation or expanded into a full mutation, depending on the size of her own premutation. As the number of repeats in the premutation increases, the greater the likelihood that her premutation will expand to a full mutation in her offspring. The relative risk is shown in Table 1-6.

Males affected with fragile X syndrome have cognitive impairment, ranging from severe to borderline in degree.

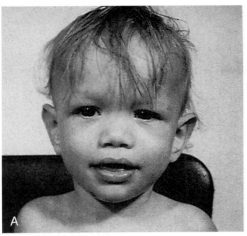 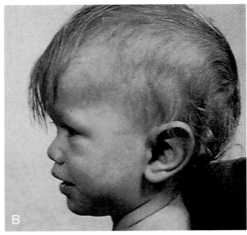 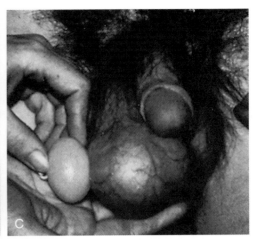

Figure 1-23. Physical findings in fragile X syndrome. **A** and **B,** Note the long, wide, and protruding ears, elongated face, and flattened nasal bridge. **C,** Macro-orchidism in adult man with fragile X syndrome. (**A** and **B,** From Simko A, Hornstein L, Soukup S, Bagamery N: Fragile X syndrome: Recognition in young children. Pediatrics 83:547-552, 1989; **C,** from Hagerman RJ: Fragile X syndrome. In Lockhart JD [ed]: Current Problems in Pediatrics, vol 17, no 2. Chicago, Year Book Medical Publishers, 1987.)

The majority have an IQ between 20 and 49, and the remainder fall in the 50 to borderline IQ range. Furthermore, IQ may decline with age. The majority have speech delay, short attention span, hyperactivity, persistence of mouthing objects, and poor motor coordination. Many exhibit a variety of disordered behaviors including disciplinary problems, temper tantrums, poor eye contact, perseverative speech, hand flapping, avoidance of socialization, and rocking. Physical stigmata may include long, wide, or protruding ears; long face; a prominent jaw; flattened nasal bridge (Fig. 1-23A and B); "velvety" skin; hyperextensible joints; and mitral valve prolapse. Relative macrocephaly is more likely than microcephaly. Macro-orchidism is found in most mature males (Fig. 1-23C).

Approximately 50% of females affected with fullmutation Fragile X are clinically normal. The 50% who are affected usually have lesser degrees of cognitive impairment than males; about 35% fall in the 20 to 49 IQ range and the remainder fall in the 50 to borderline range. However, learning disabilities, mood disorders, schizoid personality, and significant disturbances in affect, socialization, and communication are common. The physical features often seen in males with fragile X syndrome are less common in females.

Laboratory testing for Fragile X mutations is done using molecular genetic techniques. The standard molecular genetic test is Southern blot analysis of DNA extracted from cells, usually in blood (Fig. 1-24). Another molecular genetic technique, polymerase chain reaction (PCR) analysis of DNA, can be done with less blood. These techniques can also be applied to fetal cells for the purpose of antenatal diagnosis. However, if the fetus is a female with a full mutation, it is impossible to predict with certainty whether the child will be clinically affected with fragile X syndrome after birth because of the influence of X inactivation.

Rarely, an individual may seem to have a mild form of fragile X syndrome but tests are negative using these molecular genetic laboratory techniques. Another Fragile X gene site (FRAXE) distal to the Fragile X gene on Xq is associated with mild mental retardation and a positive Fragile X cytogenetic laboratory test.

The number of known trinucleotide expansion disorders is increasing. Three other examples are Huntington

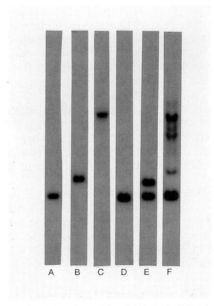

Figure 1-24. Fragile X Southern blot DNA test. DNA is extracted from cells (usually blood), digested with a restriction enzyme, and then placed in slots at the top of an agarose gel. The smaller the DNA segment, the farther down the gel it moves when an electric current is applied to the gel. Next, the electrophoresed DNA is transferred from the gel to a nylon membrane and hybridized with a radioactive-labeled DNA probe for part of the *FMR1* gene, which includes the CGG repeat region. Then, x-ray film is applied to the nylon membrane for several days and an autoradiograph results. By comparing the DNA migration to that of a standard, its number of CGG repeats can be calculated. **A,** Normal male; **B,** premutation male; **C,** full mutation male; **D,** normal female; **E,** premutation female showing one normal allele *(bottom)* and one premutation allele *(top);* **F,** full mutation female showing one normal allele *(bottom)* and a full mutation allele *(above),* which has broken down postconception into several alleles of different size. Any one cell, however, would contain only two alleles: the one normal allele and one of the several-sized abnormal alleles. Note that the lower one of the latter shown here is in the premutation size range. (Courtesy James H. Cummins, Children's Hospital of Pittsburgh.)

disease, caused by a linear CAG trinucleotide expansion in its gene at the end of chromosome 4p; myotonic dystrophy, resulting from a linear CTG expansion in its gene on chromosome 19q; and spinobulbar muscular atrophy caused by a linear CAG expansion in its gene on the proximal part of chromosome Xq.

Disorders of Imprinting—Prader-Willi and Angelman Syndromes

Etiologic Mechanisms

Prader-Willi and Angelman syndromes are disorders that derive from abnormalities of imprinted genes. The concept of imprinting refers to the fact that the function of certain genes is dependent on their parental origin: maternal versus paternal. This appears particularly true of the 15q11-q13 region of chromosome 15, a region that contains several imprinted genes that, when abnormal, result in recognizable constellations of physical and behavioral problems.

Mechanisms that can produce the Prader-Willi phenotype include the following:
1. A chromosome deletion of 15q11-q13 including the Prader-Willi critical region of the paternally derived chromosome 15 (majority of cases).
2. A structural chromosome abnormality involving the Prader-Willi critical region of 15q11-q13 (translocation, etc.).
3. Maternal uniparental disomy (UPD) in which the child has two maternally derived chromosome 15s and no paternally contributed 15 (25% of cases).
   Note: The association of UPD with older maternal age suggests that in these cases the fetus may originally have had trisomy 15 but that owing to a phenomenon known as *trisomic rescue,* one of the three chromosome 15s was lost, returning the fetus to the normal chromosome number. If the "lost" chromosome is paternally derived, then UPD-derived Prader-Willi results.
4. Mutations of imprinting control center genes (1% of cases).

The critical region of chromosome 15 for Angelman syndrome is located adjacent to the Prader-Willi critical region. However, when deletion of the Angelman critical region is causative, it is the maternally derived chromosome that is deleted. The six currently identified etiologic mechanisms of Angelman syndrome include the following:
1. A large chromosome deletion of the 15q11-q13 including the Angelman critical region of the maternally derived chromosome 15 (68% of cases).
2. A structural chromosome abnormality involving the Angelman critical region of 15q11-q13 (translocation, etc.).
3. Paternal UPD of chromosome 15 (7% of cases).
4. Mutations of imprinting control center genes (3% of cases).
5. Mutations of the ubiquitin-protein ligase gene (*UBE3A*) (11% of cases).
6. Classic phenotype, with no identifiable etiologic mechanisms but a positive family history of other affected individuals (11% of cases).
   Note: 4, 5, and 6 account for approximately 25% of cases of Angelman syndrome cases.

Because of etiologic variability and complexity of the diagnostic process, families of children suspected of having either of these disorders should be referred for genetic evaluation and diagnostic testing to ensure the most accurate determination of etiologic mechanism, and therefore, of recurrence risk.

Current diagnostic testing for these disorders includes the following:
1. Karyotype with high-resolution cytogenetic technology (Fig. 1-25).

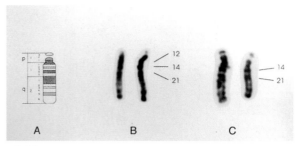

Figure 1-25. High-resolution banding in Prader-Willi syndrome. The diagram of a high-resolution analysis of chromosome 15 is shown on the left (**A**). In **B**, both chromosomes are normal, whereas in **C** the band q12 is deleted from the paternally derived chromosome 15 *(on the right)* in a patient with Prader-Willi syndrome. In higher-resolution chromosome preparations, banding patterns become more and more subdivided. This allows detection of increasingly smaller structural abnormalities. However, as the number of bands increases, cytogenetic analysis becomes progressively more difficult. To avoid error, the clinician should provide sufficient medical information to help laboratory personnel decide specifically where to look for small structural abnormalities in the patient's karyotype.

2. Methylation studies, which determine whether genes within the 15q11-q13 critical region are functional.
3. Appropriate DNA FISH probes (e.g., SNRPN for Prader-Willi syndrome [see Fig. 1-10C and D] and D15S10 for Angelman syndrome).
4. In some cases of Angelman syndrome, direct analysis of the *UBE3A* gene.

Clinical Findings in Prader-Willi Syndrome

Newborns affected with Prader-Willi syndrome usually are markedly hypotonic and often have a history of decreased fetal movement in utero and breech fetal position. Although birth is usually at term, birthweights tend to be below 3000 g. In neonates, in addition to hypotonia, poor sucking and swallowing are common and predispose to choking episodes that can cause respiratory problems. Although the baby's cry may be weak and Moro and deep tendon reflexes are often decreased, the neurologic evaluation is otherwise unremarkable. Subsequently motor development is delayed, speech even more so, and most patients have cognitive impairment in the mild to moderate range. Hypotonia abates over the first 2 to 3 years, and patients develop an insatiable appetite that rapidly results in morbid obesity. The distribution of excess fat is particularly prominent over the lower trunk, buttocks, and proximal limbs (Fig. 1-26A). Although the facies are not particularly dysmorphic, they are similar in most Prader-Willi patients. The bifrontal diameter is narrow, the eyes are often described as "almond shaped," and strabismus is not unusual. Hypopigmentation is common, the patient usually having blond to light brown hair, blue eyes, and sun-sensitive fair skin. Picking of skin sores can become a problem. Hands and feet are noticeably small from birth (Fig. 1-26B), and the stature of the older child and adult is short. The penis and testes are hypoplastic in males with Prader-Willi syndrome (Fig. 1-26C), although the penile size can be enlarged by testosterone therapy. If the testes are cryptorchid, surgical correction should be attempted. Menarche in females is delayed or absent, and menses, when present, are sparse and irregular. Gonadotropic hormone levels are reduced in both sexes. Infertility is the ruke, but there are two known exceptions.

Of particular concern in older children with Prader-Willi syndrome are problems of emotional lability and

Figure 1-26. Prader-Willi syndrome. **A,** This patient demonstrates the marked obesity characteristic of Prader-Willi syndrome. Excess fat is distributed over the trunk, buttocks, and proximal extremities. **B** and **C,** Small hands (and feet) and a hypoplastic penis and scrotum are other typical features. (**A,** Courtesy Jeanne M. Hanchett, MD, Pittsburgh, Pa.).

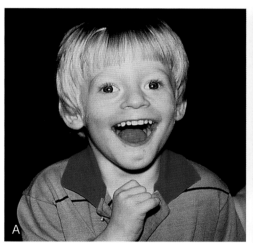
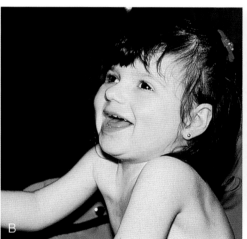
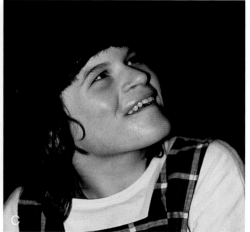

Figure 1-27. Angelman syndrome. **A-C,** Three patients with typical facies. Note the maxillary hypoplasia, large mouth (often with a protruding tongue), and prognathism. (Courtesy C. A. Williams, MD, and J. Hendrickson, MD.)

extreme temper tantrums. These conditions and the over-eating often can be partly ameliorated by intensive in-patient behavioral modification programs followed by longitudinal parental support and follow-up in the home. Interestingly, despite a normal basal metabolic rate, weight reduction requires significantly more severe caloric restriction in these patients than in normal persons. Diabetes mellitus can develop in the older child, and its incidence is correlated with the severity of obesity. Although it tends to be insulin resistant, the condition responds well to treatment with oral hypoglycemic agents. Life expectancy can be shortened by cardiorespiratory complications related to the extreme obesity (pickwickian syndrome).

Clinical Findings in Angelman Syndrome

Angelman syndrome, first recognized in 1956, has an incidence of 1 in 15,000 to 1 in 20,000 live births. Except for the tendency to have hypopigmentation, the clinical phenotypes of Prader-Willi and Angelman syndromes are quite different. The latter have severe cognitive deficits; speech is impaired or absent; and inappropriate paroxysms of laughter are common. Physical features include microbrachycephaly, maxillary hypoplasia, large mouth, prognathism, and short stature (in adults) (Fig. 1-27A to C). The gait is ataxic, with toe-walking and jerky arm movements. Akinetic or major motor seizures are common. Although survival to adulthood is possible, to date only one patient with Angelman syndrome has been known to reproduce.

The Nature of Genes and Single Gene Disorders

A gene consists of a sequence of DNA that contains the code for production of a "functional product" along with sequences that ensure "proper expression" of the gene. Its product may be an RNA molecule or a polypeptide chain or protein that ultimately becomes a structural component of a cell or tissue, or of an enzyme. The latter may catalyze a step in formation or modification of another product, a step in cell metabolism, or one of a number of steps involved in the breakdown or degradation of molecules that are no longer necessary. "Proper expression" includes production of the product at the right time, in the needed amount, in the correct cell type and ensures its transport to its proper site of biological action.

Approximately 30,000 genes are arranged in linear fashion on the chromosomes, all having their own specific locus. Genes range in length from about 1000 to hundreds of thousands of bases in length (any of which can be subject to mutation). Coding sequences for the gene's product, termed *exons*, vary in length and are not continuous but occur in sections with noncoding sequences, termed *introns*, interspersed between them. Exons are further subdivided into triplets of bases, termed *codons*, each of which codes for a specific amino acid within the polypeptide product. Because there are 64 possible triplet combinations of the 4 nucleotide bases (adenine, guanidine, thymine and cytosine) and 20 amino acids (AA), most AAs have more than one codon that can specify them, the exceptions being methionine and tryptophan, which have only one specific codon each. In addition, three triplets code for stop codons in mRNA that signal for termination of mRNA translation.

The process of going from DNA code to polypeptide product has many steps and begins with *transcription*, during which the DNA of the gene serves as a template for formation of a messenger RNA (mRNA) molecule. RNA synthetase, proteins called transcription factors, and regulatory elements all participate in this process, which is initiated and concluded by DNA sequences that signal where to start and stop transcription. Following this, both ends of the mRNA molecule undergo modification. Thereafter, the introns are excised and the exons spliced together. Then the mRNA is transported to the rough endoplasmic reticulum within the cytoplasm, where it attaches to ribosomes, and the process of *translation* from mRNA template to polypeptide chain begins. During translation transfer RNA (tRNA) molecules, each of which is specifically designed to attach to a particular amino acid, find their target moieties and bring them into position at the correct time over a codon on the mRNA that specifies for their particular amino acid.

Following assembly, the polypeptide chain is released from its template and then may be subject to *"post-translational modification."* Steps may include folding, bonding into a three-dimensional conformation, being combined with another or other polypeptide chains as part of a protein complex, being split into smaller segments, and addition of phosphate or carbohydrate moieties. Thereafter, it is transported to its site of action via directional terminal sequences, which are then cleaved from the finished product. Mutation of a gene coding for the polypeptide product or for any molecule used at any step along the entire process can adversely influence the end product.

A single gene mutation produces a permanent change in a gene's DNA sequence and may involve anywhere from one to several thousands of nucleotides. Most appear to affect only one to a few to several base pairs via substitution of one base for another or by deletion or insertion of one or more bases.

Some mutations have no effect on phenotype or cell function. One example is a base substitution within a codon for an amino acid that changes it to another codon specifying for the same amino acid. Still other mutations have no adverse effect but rather code for normal variations in human characteristics (e.g., eye or hair color). Other mutations do have adverse effects and are causative in disease. Examples of these include: *missense* mutations in which a base substitution changes a codon specific for one amino acid into one specifying another; *frameshift* mutations in which a deletion or insertion is not an exact multiple of three bases, and thereby shifts the reading frame for transcription (and later translation) from that point on; and *nonsense* mutations in which a base substitution changes a codon for an amino acid into one specifying one of the three possible stop codons in mRNA, thereby stopping translation prematurely.

A single gene disorder is the result of a mutation altering the DNA sequence within a single gene on one (dominant) or both (recessive) of a pair of chromosomes. Correspondingly, this change may result in alteration of the amount of the gene's product, failure to produce the product at all, and/or compromise of its functional integrity. The greater the degree of functional loss is, the more severe the clinical manifestations of the disorder and often the earlier their onset.

The family of disorders known as *osteogenesis imperfecta* (OI, see also Chapter 21) provides a good example of the effects of mutations that alter the precursors of a structural protein, type I collagen. Collagen is a triple helix made up of two pro α-1 chains and one pro α-2 chain. The latter are composed of hundreds of amino acid triplet repeats with glycine (the smallest amino acid) being the first member of each triplet and forming the apex of each bend in the helical structure. A base substitution in a codon specifying glycine at any one of the hundreds of such points along either the COL1A1 (on band 17q21) or COL1A2 (on band 7q22.1) genes may result in production of an unstable mRNA molecule that is degraded in the nucleus or in the production of structurally abnormal pro α-1 or α-2 chains. The assembly of these may be slowed; they may be subject to excessive post-translational modification, may be unstable and subject to degradation, or may have difficulty conforming and associating with other pro chains to form the triple helix. The earlier the altered mRNA codon appears in the translation process, the more abnormal is the resulting pro chain structure, and the greater is the degree of compromise of collagen strength and function within connective tissues. Also, because there are two pro α-1 chains for each pro α-2 chain, mutations in the COL1A1 gene are more likely to be deleterious. These types of mutations, which result in synthesis of structurally abnormal product, are the basis for clinical abnormalities found in types II to IV OI.

In type I OI, the causative mutations in the COL1A1 gene (often nonsense or splicing mutations) usually result in production of mRNA that is so abnormal it is degraded before it can leave the nucleus and be translated or in synthesis of a prochain that is unstable and degraded.

Hence the mutant gene is unexpressed, a *null mutation*. The end result of this is that the patient can only make 50% of the expected amount of type I collagen, although all of that product is structurally normal. Being the mildest form OI, it demonstrates the fact that in many cases of mutations involving genes that code for structural polypeptides or proteins, it can be better to have no gene product than to have an abnormal one.

The phenomenon of excessive post-translational modification of a structurally abnormal gene product is also seen in some types of Ehlers-Danlos syndrome (see later).

When the gene product is an enzyme or a component of an enzyme, this results in interruption of its step in a chain of reactions that may be involved in formation or modification of a product, a step in cell metabolism, or in the degradation of molecules no longer needed by the cell. The missed step results in buildup of substrate from the step preceding the one in which the affected enzyme acts. In some instances this accumulated substrate can be toxic, as in phenylketonuria. In others, ever-expanding storage of substrate can adversely affect cell function, as in the lysosomal storage diseases.

Connective Tissue Disorders of Genetic Origin

Marfan Syndrome

Marfan syndrome is a genetic disorder of connective tissue that is inherited as an autosomal dominant trait, although approximately 25% of cases represent new mutations. The site of the genetic abnormality or mutation is the Fibrillin gene *(FBN1)* located at band 15q21.1 on chromosome 15. As a result, the molecular structure of the protein fibrillin, an intrinsic component of connective tissue, is abnormal. Clinical consequences are most notable in the musculoskeletal, cardiovascular, and ocular systems. Classic phenotypic findings include arachnodactyly (Fig. 1-28A and B), joint hyperextensibility due to ligamentous laxity (see Fig. 5-8B); tall stature with long, thin extremities; a decreased upper-to-lower segment ratio; an arm span that exceeds height; and moderate to severe pectus excavatum or carinatum (Fig. 1-28C). Pes planus and thoracolumbar kyphoscoliosis are other common skeletal features (Fig. 1-28D). A defect in the suspensory ligaments of the eye is responsible for subluxation of the lens (seen in 50% to 60% by age 10), which is usually displaced in an upward direction. Myopia and astigmatism are common, and affected individuals are also at risk for developing glaucoma, cataracts, and retinal detachment in adulthood. Mitral valve prolapse (MVP) may progress to mitral insufficiency (at times associated with arrhythmias). Of great concern is progressive aneurysmal dilatation of the ascending, less commonly, the thoracic or abdominal aorta. The latter is the major source of morbidity and mortality because it can result in acute dissection and death. Presence of a high arched palate is common. The incidence of hernias, both inguinal and femoral, is increased, and patients often have striae of the skin in unusual places such as the shoulder. Although most Marfan individuals are of normal intelligence, an occasional patient may have learning disabilities.

Currently the disorder is diagnosed primarily on clinical grounds because molecular testing of all individuals clinically suspected of having Marfan syndrome, although available, is not usually necessary to feel confident of the diagnosis. Because it takes time for a number of the major abnormalities to develop or become clinically evident, a firm diagnosis is generally impossible in early childhood, especially in the absence of a positive family history. Recurrence risk for affected individuals to their offspring is 50%.

When the diagnosis of Marfan syndrome is strongly suspected or confirmed, patients should be monitored closely during growth spurts for signs of onset and progression of kyphoscoliosis, undergo regular ophthalmologic evaluations, and have regular echocardiograms and electrocardiograms. When aortic dilatation is detected, administration of β-blockers can slow progression by decreasing blood pressure and the force of myocardial contractions. Subacute bacterial endocarditis (SBE) prophylaxis is indicated for patients with evidence of cardiovascular involvement. Patients also should be cautioned to avoid weight lifting and contact sports.

The differential diagnosis of Marfan syndrome includes Beals congenital contractural arachnodactyly (Fig. 1-29); homocystinuria; the MASS phenotype, MASS being an acronym for *M*VP, borderline nonprogressive *a*ortic dilatation, *s*triae and marfanoid *s*keletal features, without ocular findings; familial ectopia lentis; Klinefelter syndrome; and syndromes characterized by joint hypermobility.

Ehlers-Danlos Syndrome

Ehlers-Danlos syndrome (EDS) is composed of a group of inherited connective tissue disorders, the major features of which consist of hyperextensibility and fragility of the skin and ligamentous laxity with secondary joint hypermobility. Each type stems from a defect in synthesis of types I, III, or V collagen resulting in decreased tensile strength of connective tissues. Previously divided into types I to XI, it has been reclassified into six major subgroups on the basis of their predominant clinical features; mode of inheritance; and, when known, underlying defect. Table 1-7 presents these along with their estimated incidence. Given limitations of space, we focus on the clinical features of the four most common types.

Ehlers-Danlos Syndrome—Classical Type

Known as the classical form of EDS, cutaneous manifestations are especially prominent in this type, although they may have a wide spectrum of severity. Skin hyperextensibility is prominent (Fig. 1-30A); the texture smooth and "velvety"; and the skin abnormally fragile, bruising and tearing easily. Wound healing is impaired and slower than average, often resulting in formation of unusually wide atrophic scars that have a thin papery quality, sometimes likened to cigarette paper (Fig. 1-30B).

When these children incur lacerations necessitating wound closure, use of glue or tape is preferable to sutures because the latter tend to tear away from the fragile skin. Staples are better tolerated for closure of operative incisions, and postoperatively development of incisional hernias is not uncommon.

Two features unique to this type are the tendency to form pseudotumors under scars located over bony prominences and to develop subcutaneous fatty tumors over the forearms and shins.

Although usually not as severe as in the hypermobility type, ligamentous laxity and joint hypermobility also are

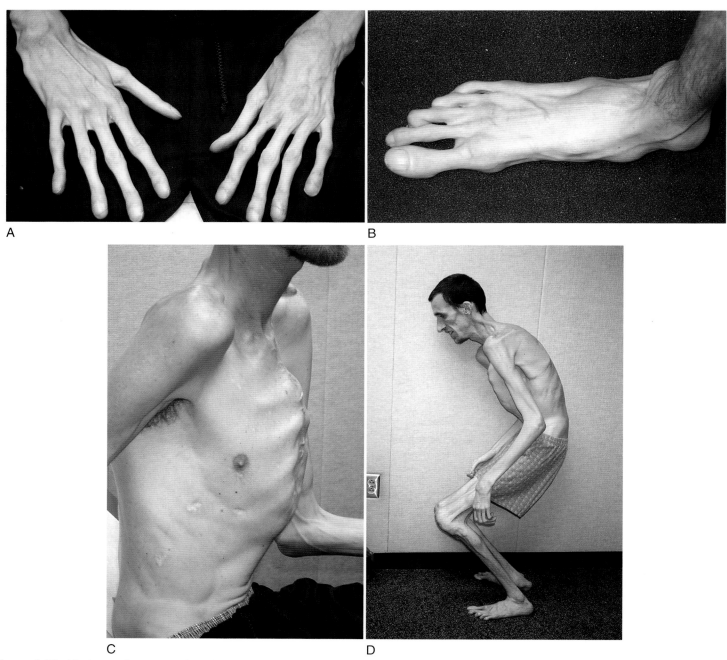

Figure 1-28. Marfan syndrome. **A** and **B,** This young man has prominent arachnodactyly of both fingers and toes. Note the clubbing due to associated cardiopulmonary problems and the flattening of the arch of his foot. **C,** He also has severe pectus carinatum and **D,** significant kyphosis and joint contractures. Also note his long arms.

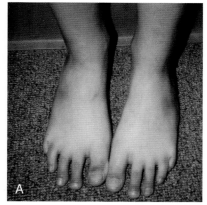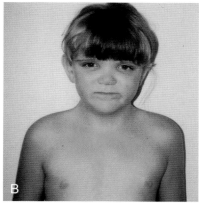

Figure 1-29. Beals syndrome variant. This child was found to have an abnormality of fibrillin 2 secretion in fibroblasts. **A,** She was tall and had arachnodactyly with contractures. **B,** Her broad forehead and hypertelorism are physical features that help distinguish her case from classic Beals syndrome and Marfan syndrome.

Table 1-7   Classification of Types of Ehlers-Danlos Syndrome

TYPE	FORMER TYPE	MODE OF INHERITANCE	APPROXIMATE INCIDENCE	UNDERLYING ABNORMALITY
Classical	I & II	AD	1/20-40,000	Abnormal electrophoretic mobility of pro α-1 & 2 chains of type V collagen
Hypermobility	III	AD	1/10-15,000	No specific biochemical defect identified
Vascular	IV	AD	1/100-200,000	Mutation in COL3A1 gene resulting in structurally abnormal pro α-1 chain of type III collagen, posttranslational overmodification, thermal instability, or increased sensitivity to proteases
Kyphoscoliotic	VI	AD	Rare	Deficiency of the collagen-modifying enzyme lysylhydroxylase
Arthrochalasia	VII A & B	AD	Very rare	Mutations resulting in deficient processing of amino-terminal ends of pro α-1 or 2 chains of type I collagen
Dermatosparaxis	VI C	AR	Very rare	Deficiency of pro collagen 1 amino-terminal peptidase

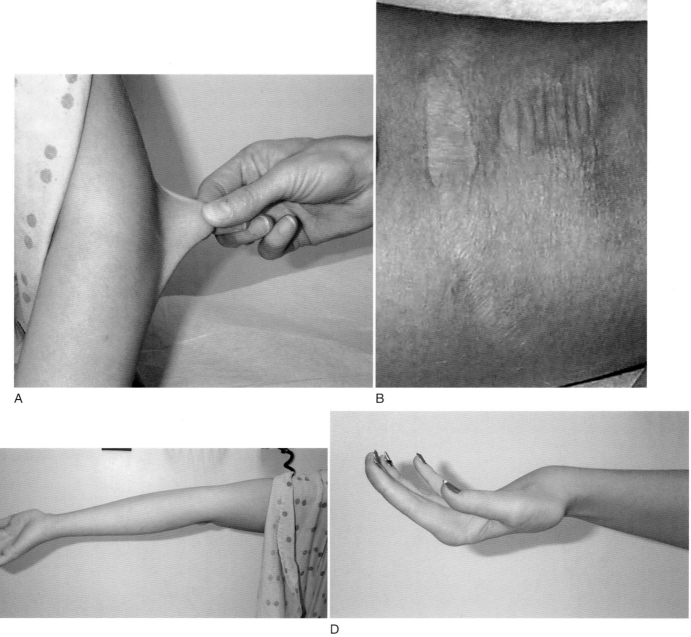

A   B

C   D

Figure 1-30. Ehlers-Danlos syndrome—classical type. **A,** Note the marked hyperextensibility of the skin over this child's arm. **B,** These widened atrophic scars have the thin papery texture that is characteristic. **C** and **D,** Hyperextensibility of the joints of the elbow and fingers is seen as well.

features (Fig. 1-30C and D) and predispose to sprains, subluxations, and dislocations, and to early onset of chronic musculoskeletal pain.

Hypotonia and gross motor delays are seen in some infants and young children with this type of EDS.

Ehlers-Danlos Syndrome—Hypermobility Type

In this, the most common type, ligamentous laxity and attendant joint hypermobility are the major source of symptomatology. All joints, large and small, are affected, and patients are prone to frequent and recurrent subluxations and dislocations, especially of the patella, shoulder, and temporomandibular joints. Chronic limb and joint pain due to the excessive pull placed on periarticular structures and to the sequelae of dislocations develops early on and can become increasingly debilitating over time.

Cutaneous manifestations vary widely in severity and include a smooth "velvety" texture, hyperextensibility, and easy bruisability.

Ehlers-Danlos Syndrome—Vascular Type

This is the most serious form of EDS because fragility of vascular and visceral tissues accompany cutaneous and joint abnormalities. Many affected children are born with clubfeet, and they tend to have rather characteristic facial features that include prominent eyes and sunken cheeks (due to decreased subcutaneous facial fat), a thin nose, small chin, and lobeless external ears. Scalp hair is sparse in some.

In this type the skin is thin and appears translucent, giving prominence to the underlying venous pattern, especially over the chest and abdomen. Easy bruisability and skin fragility are significant features, and postoperative wound dehiscence is not unusual. Premature aging of the skin over the distal extremities and early development of varicose veins are also seen. Joint hypermobility is present but is limited to the small joints of the fingers and toes.

As noted earlier, the features that make this type of EDS so serious clinically are fragility of the walls of medium size arteries, the intestines, and the uterus. This predisposes to wall rupture with potentially catastrophic results. Arterial and intestinal rupture are heralded by sudden onset of severe abdominal and/or flank pain, which is promptly followed by signs of shock. Risk of uterine rupture is greatest intrapartum and is associated with significant hemorrhage. Other reported problems include pneumothoraces and development of arteriovenous fistulas.

Because the major complications of this form of EDS tend to not occur until the third or fourth decade, exact diagnosis in early childhood can be difficult in patients without a positive family history whose other clinical findings are subtle.

Ehlers-Danlos Syndrome—Kyphoscoliosis Type

Newborns with this form of EDS tend to have severe hypotonia with delayed gross motor development and congenital scoliosis, which is progressive. Some patients develop a Marfanoid body habitus with growth. Generalized ligamentous laxity and joint hypermobility may be so severe that the ability to ambulate is lost in the teens or twenties. Osteopenia is seen radiographically, perhaps partly from disuse.

Other features include easy bruisability, skin fragility, and formation of atrophic scars. In contrast to other forms of EDS, children with this type have scleral fragility, which

places them at risk for globe rupture following even minor trauma. High myopia and microcornea are seen in some.

Diagnosis

The diagnosis of EDS should be suspected in children who present with unusually distensible skin, especially when atrophic scars are seen, and in those with unusual degrees of joint hypermobility who suffer recurrent joint dislocations. Presence of skin hyperextensibility is best tested over the volar forearm by grasping the skin and pulling until resistance is felt. Evidence of significant joint hypermobility includes the following:

- Ability to touch palms to the floor on forward bending
- Hyperextensibility of knees and elbows greater than 10 degrees
- Ability to appose thumb to the volar forearm
- Passive dorsiflexion of the fifth fingers past 90 degrees

Finding these and other clinical features described earlier in a child with a positive family history is especially helpful. With the exception of the kyphoscoliotic type, for which a urine test is available, confirmatory diagnostic tests usually require skin biopsy.

Depending on type, differential diagnostic considerations may include Marfan syndrome and cutis laxa. Easy bruisability can be mistaken for child abuse.

Osteogenesis Imperfecta

OI is a family of genetic connective tissue disorders characterized predominantly by brittle bones. The four major types and the vast majority of patients have been found to have mutations that either reduce the amount or alter the structure of type I collagen. A description of some of the many causative mutations and their structural consequences is presented in the section above on The Nature of Genes and Single Gene Disorders. Clinical features are presented in Chapter 21.

Recognizable Patterns of Malformation Due to an Inborn Error of Metabolism

An inborn error of metabolism is a genetically determined disorder in which an altered or abnormal gene codes for the production of an abnormal polypeptide product, which is usually an enzyme or a cofactor necessary to the normal operation of a metabolic process. For example, when an enzyme needed for a step in a chain of chemical reactions is nonfunctional, the product of that and those of subsequent steps including the end product are not made or are nonfunctional. The absence of this end product tends to have a significant adverse effect on function and/or structure. Furthermore, precursors to the blocked step tend to build up. In some cases, their accumulation may be a source of toxicity, and in others they are stored in ever-increasing amounts in cells of certain tissues, adversely affecting their function (as in the lysosomal storage diseases).

Smith-Lemli-Opitz Syndrome

Smith-Lemli-Opitz syndrome (SLOS), an autosomal recessive, mendelian genetic disorder, is an example of

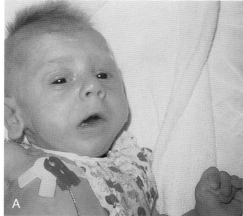
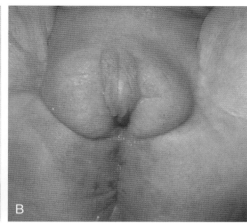

Figure 1-31. Smith-Lemli-Opitz syndrome. **A,** Note the anteverted nostrils, low-set ears, small chin, and clenched hand. **B,** Hypospadias, cryptorchidism, or ambiguous genitalia as shown here may also be seen. (Courtesy W. Tunnessen, MD.)

an inborn error of metabolism that results in a multiple malformation syndrome. Approximately 1 in 20,000 live births is affected. The discovery of an abnormality in cholesterol biosynthesis in patients with SLOS has enabled development of a confirmatory laboratory test. This block in the final step of cholesterol biosynthesis results in cholesterol deficiency and an excess of possibly toxic cholesterol precursors, particularly 7-dehydrocholesterol (DHC). The deficiency of cholesterol and the toxicity of DHC are hypothesized to cause the clinical features of SLOS, particularly abnormal central nervous system development. Affected infants tend to be small for gestational age and often are born via breech presentation after a pregnancy noted for decreased fetal movements. Patients have microcephaly with a prominent occiput and narrow bifrontal diameter. Facial stigmata include eyelid ptosis, epicanthal folds, strabismus, low-set or posteriorly rotated ears, broad nasal tip with upturned nares, and micrognathia (Fig. 1-31A). Single transverse (simian) creases of the palms and syndactyly of the second and third toes are characteristic; in males, hypospadias with cryptorchidism and even ambiguous genitalia are other typical findings (Fig. 1-31B). Clenched hands, digital abnormalities, cataracts, cleft palate, and bifid uvula are seen in some cases. Structural abnormalities of the central nervous system (at times associated with seizures), heart, gastrointestinal tract, and/or kidneys are common. Initial hypotonia progresses to hypertonia with irritable behavior, shrill screaming, and feeding problems, and affected infants fail to thrive. The majority are moderately to severely mentally retarded. However, with the advent of biochemical testing, cases with milder phenotypic expression are now being identified. Reports on the use of oral cholesterol therapy suggest some improvement, especially with regard to quality of life.

Because SLOS is an autosomal recessive disorder, the recurrence risk for a couple with an affected child is 25% for each subsequent conception. Antenatal diagnosis is possible by molecular testing of DNA, if mutations are known, or by biochemical analysis of amniotic fluid and cultured amniocytes obtained through amniocentesis. Parents of affected children may benefit from genetic counseling.

Lysosomal Storage Diseases

The lysosomal storage diseases (LSDs) are a heterogeneous group of heritable disorders that are the result of mutations in genes that code for production of lysosomal enzymes or for their interacting nonenzymatic proteins.

Lysosomes are membrane-bound cytoplasmic organelles that serve as the digestive or recycling plants of cells, their major purposes being to break down cellular waste products and debris and to degrade macromolecules that are no longer needed into smaller components. They perform this function with an array of hydrolytic enzymes that degrade their target molecules in a stepwise fashion. Once the process of degradation is completed, the residual material is transported to the cytoplasm for recycling (as new molecular building blocks) or to the cell membrane for removal.

A mutation that results in malfunction of a lysosomal enzyme leads to accumulation of substrate formed in the step prior to the one in which the affected enzyme would normally act. Over time the volume of the undegraded substrate increases, progressively distending the lysosome, and ultimately, this impairs cell function. Concurrently, clinical signs and symptoms become evident and increase in severity. In the brain this phenomenon tends to cause progressive neurodegeneration, and in other organs or tissues progressive enlargement or thickening.

Causative mutations may inactivate an enzyme, reduce its amount or level of activity, impede its transport to its proper site of action, or otherwise impair its function. Inactivation or severe inhibition of enzyme activity results in more rapid accumulation of substrate and in earlier onset and more rapid progression of clinical signs and symptoms. Lesser degrees of functional alteration or impairment result in phenotypes of lesser clinical severity and/or later onset. The clinical picture also depends on the type of substrate that is accumulated and the sites or cell types in which the original macromolecule is most likely to play a role, structurally or functionally.

More than 40 different LSDs have been identified, and their classification is based on the enzyme or nonenzymatic protein involved, the substrate that progressively collects, or (less often) other abnormalities of lysosomal function (Table 1-8). Many of these disorders have characteristic physical features, enabling clinical diagnosis, whereas others are less classic. Depending on the disorder, diagnostic or confirmatory tests are available and include newborn screening batteries; urine, blood, and white blood cell analyses; and, in some cases, examination of fibroblasts cultured from skin biopsy specimens. Prenatal diagnosis is frequently possible using enzymatic and molecular testing of amniocytes or chorionic villous

Table 1-8	Classification of Lysosomal Storage Disorders

DISORDER CLASS	UNDERLYING DEFECT
Mucopolysaccharidoses	Defective metabolism of glycosaminoglycans
Sphingolipidoses and sulfatidoses	Defective degradation of sphingolipids and their components
Glycogen storage diseases	Defective degradation of glycogen
Oligosaccharidoses	Defective degradation of the glycan portion of glycoproteins
Mucolipidoses	Defective degradation of acid mucopolysaccharides, sphingolipids and/or glycolipids
Defects in degradation or transport of cholesterol, cholesterol esters, and other complex lipids	
Lysosomal transport and trafficking defects	

Table 1-9	The Mucopolysaccharidoses

TYPE	DISORDER	ENZYME DEFICIENCY
MPS I	Hurler syndrome	α-L-iduronidase
	Hurler-Scheie syndrome	
	Scheie syndrome	
MPS II	Hunter syndrome	Iduronate sulfatase
MPS III	Sanfilippo disease	
	Type A	Heparan N-sulfatase
	Type B	α-N-acetylglucosaminidase
	Type C	Heparan-N-acetyltransferase
MPS IV	Morquio disease	
	Type A	N-Acetylgalactosamine-6 sulfate sulfatase
	Type B	β-Galactosidase
MPS VI	Maroteaux-Lamy disease	Arylsulfatase B
MPS VII	Sly disease	β-Glucuronidase

samples. Genetic evaluation and counseling are advisable to provide parents with education regarding relative risk to future children, home management of their affected child, and support services.

The Mucopolysaccharidoses

Among the most well known of the lysosomal storage disorders are the mucopolysaccharidoses (MPSs). They are characterized by absence or functional impairment of 1 of the 11 lysosomal enzymes needed for the breakdown of glycosaminoglycans (mucopolysaccharides). These macromolecules consist of long chains of repeating disaccharide units that are synthesized by connective tissue cells as structural constituents of connective tissues, bone, cartilage, and synovial fluid; skin; the cornea; and the reticuloendothelial system. Degradation involves stepwise removal of monosaccharides by the lysosomal enzymes acting in sequence. Deficiency or malfunction of one of the enzymes results in accumulation of one or more glycosaminoglycans. As lysosomes become increasingly distended, clinical effects make their appearance and progress. These may include alterations in facial features, body habitus, joint structure and function, and cognitive abilities and vary depending on the enzyme involved and the degree of functional impairment.

Seven major types and a number of subtypes have been identified, each associated with a specific enzymatic defect (Table 1-9). All of these disorders have a chronic and progressive course and involve multiple systems, and all are autosomal recessive with the exception of Hunter syndrome, which is X-linked. Because of space limitations, we focus on MPS type I, which is considered a prototypical lysosomal disorder.

Mucopolysaccharidosis I. MPS type I is due to a mutation in the gene that codes for α-L-iduronidase (located on chromosome 4p16.3), which results in impaired degradation of dermatan and heparan sulfate. It is divided into three subtypes—MPSIH or Hurler syndrome, Hurler-Scheie syndrome, and Scheie syndrome—on the basis of clinical severity.

Hurler syndrome is the most severe and was the first described. Affected newborns appear normal. Many are above average in size and are born with umbilical and inguinal hernias. Initially growth and development are on target, but between 6 and 24 months (usually by 12 months), growth rate decreases and signs of developmental delay begin to appear. Growth ceases around 3 or 4 years, resulting in short stature with an especially foreshortened trunk. Development peaks at the 2- to 4-year level, after which there is a gradual and progressive regression in cognitive abilities and developmental milestones. Concurrently, these children experience coarsening of facial features, ultimately characterized by prominence of the forehead, flattening of the midface, a broad nose with a flattened nasal bridge, and enlargement and protrusion of the tongue (Fig. 1-32A). Facial changes are often accompanied by tonsillar and adenoidal hypertrophy and combine to predispose the child to recurrent upper respiratory, ear and sinus infections, noisy respirations, chronic upper airway obstruction, and sleep apnea. Progressive hepatosplenomegaly results in a protuberant abdomen and further increases the likelihood of hernias. Skeletal manifestations include dysostosis multiplex and progressive joint stiffness, eventually limiting mobility and resulting in contractures. The hands become broad, and fingers are short and ultimately become clawed (Fig. 1-32B). Radiographically, widening of the ribs into an oar shape is evident. Other manifestations include thickening of the skin with hirsutism; corneal clouding, sometimes accompanied by retinal degeneration or glaucoma; communicating hydrocephalus; peripheral nerve and nerve root compression; chronic hearing loss; and cardiomyopathy with asymmetric hypertrophy of the ventricular septum, associated with thickening of the aortic and mitral valves, which may progress to valvular insufficiency.

Life expectancy is shortened to between 5 and 10 years with death usually due to infection, airway obstruction, or cardiac complications.

Hurler-Scheie syndrome is intermediate in severity and has its onset between 3 and 8 years. Changes in physical features are milder than in Hurler syndrome; cognitive deficits are in the moderate range; and patients have a life expectancy to the teens or twenties. Scheie syndrome is the mildest variant with onset after age 5, normal or mildly decreased cognitive abilities, and survival well into adulthood. Treatment for Hurler syndrome is now possible using enzyme replacement therapy, and requires early diagnosis for maximum benefit.

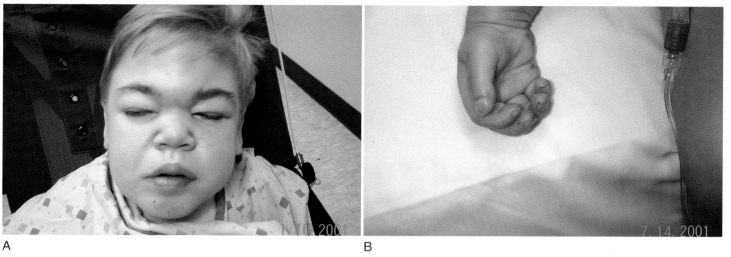

Figure 1-32. Hurler syndrome. **A,** The coarsening of facial features characteristic of this disorder includes prominence of the forehead, a flattened nasal bridge, a short broad nose, and widening of the lips. Features appear puffy due to thickening of the skin. **B,** Progressive joint stiffness and contractures lead to clawing of the hand.

Figure 1-33. CHARGE association. **A,** Note the short palpebral fissures and ptosis; low-set, dysplastic ears; and small chin. Choanal atresia necessitated tracheotomy. **B,** Another example of an infant with CHARGE association has clinical features that include a prominent forehead, hypertelorism, narrow palpebral fissures, hypoplasia of the right naris, low-set ears, and a cupid's-bow mouth. (**A,** Courtesy W. Tunnessen, MD. **B,** Courtesy Timothy McBride, MD, Fairfax, Va.)

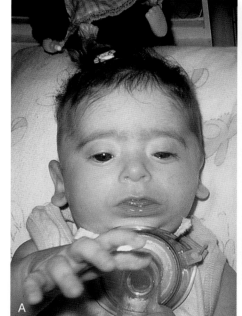

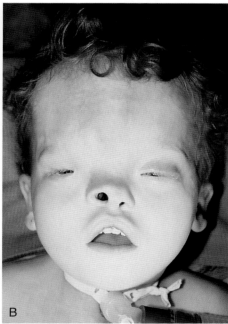

Associations

As noted earlier, an *association* is a pattern of malformations that occurs together too often to be the result of chance alone, but for which no specific cause has yet been identified.

CHARGE Association

CHARGE is an acronym for a nonrandom association of features including **c**oloboma of the retina, less commonly the iris; **h**eart abnormalities; **a**tresia of the choanae; **r**etarded growth and mental development; **g**enital hypoplasia in males; and **e**ar anomalies that can include deafness. The minimal diagnostic criteria should include abnormalities in four of the six categories, at least one of which must be coloboma or choanal atresia. Cleft lip and/or palate and renal abnormalities are sometimes found. The association includes congenital heart disease, particularly abnormalities of the aortic arch, right subclavian artery, or ventricular septal defect; agenesis or hypoplasia of the thymus with decreased T-cell production and impaired cell-mediated immunity; partial or less often complete absence of the parathyroid glands, manifest by hypocalcemia and neonatal tetany; and often a facies characterized by wide-spaced, slightly down-slanting palpebral fissures, anteverted nares, a short philtrum, and small, dysmorphic ears (Fig. 1-33). Infants with CHARGE association often die early as a result of their congenital anomalies, but many survive to adulthood. Although developmental delay exists, the IQ range is broad (<30 to 80).

CHARGE has recently been found to be related to mutations in the *CHD7* gene located on chromosome 8q12. In the neonate, CHARGE association must be differentiated from other chromosomal disorders, such as deletion

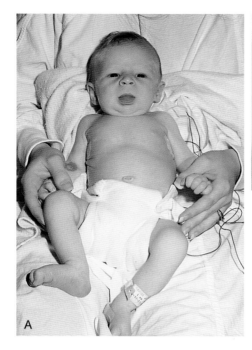

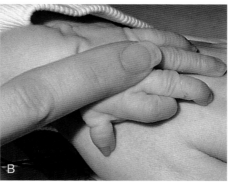

Figure 1-34. This child with VATER association **(A)** has facial features that are not dysmorphic, but he has preaxial polydactyly of the thumb **(B)**, which was associated with radial dysplasia.

22q11.2 or trisomy 13 or 18, and from the more benign nonchromosomal VATER association. When the DiGeorge sequence is present in patients with CHARGE association, a small interstitial deletion of chromosome 22 at q11 is occasionally found with high-resolution cytogenetic techniques and FISH DNA probe (see Fig. 1-10A and B).

The etiology of CHARGE association is most likely heterogeneous. Although most cases are sporadic, instances of affected siblings and an affected parent and offspring have been reported. The risk of recurrence must be determined after genetic evaluation and ranges from 4% to 6% to as high as 50%.

VATER Association

VATER is another acronym for a nonrandom association of *v*ertebral and *a*nal anomalies, *t*racheoesophageal fistula with *e*sophageal atresia, and *r*adial and/or renal abnormalities. Most affected newborns have anomalies in all five categories. The acronym can be expanded to VACTERL to include *c*ongenital heart disease (particularly ventricular septal defect) and, less often, other *l*imb defects. Vertebral anomalies include hemivertebrae and sacral abnormalities. Limb deformities consist of ray abnormalities such as radial aplasia or hypoplasia, abnormal thumbs, preaxial polydactyly, and syndactyly (Fig. 1-34). Renal abnormalities include unilateral agenesis and less commonly ectopic or horseshoe kidney. The etiology of VATER association is unknown. Virtually all cases are sporadic. Detection of an abnormal karyotype rules out this disorder. The prognosis for growth and development in newborns who survive infancy is good. Most have normal intelligence and eventually achieve normal stature. Consequently, to make optimal management decisions, it is important to distinguish VATER syndrome from more dire chromosomal abnormalities (such as trisomy 18) or nonchromosomal disorders (such as CHARGE association).

For the purpose of genetic counseling, VATER association must also be differentiated from Townes-Brocks syndrome, an autosomal dominant, simple mendelian genetic disorder that shares some features. However, in Townes-

Brocks syndrome there is often a positive family history of autosomal dominant inheritance of ear, thumb, and anal abnormalities, whereas vertebral anomalies and tracheoesophageal fistula are unusual. The prognosis for growth and development in Townes-Brocks syndrome patients is good. However, the risk for recurrence of Townes-Brocks syndrome with a positive family history may be up to 50%, whereas for VATER association the risk may be less than 2%. Antenatal diagnosis for both conditions depends on detecting structural anomalies in the fetus by high-resolution ultrasound.

Other disorders in the list of differential diagnostic possibilities include Fanconi anemia and Holt-Oram syndrome (see Fig. 5-7). Once chromosome studies are completed and found to be normal, when other disorders are deemed less likely, and a child has the pattern of malformation characteristic of the VATER association, the diagnosis (which remains one of exclusion) can be made.

Recognizable Multiple Malformation Syndromes

De Lange, Cornelia de Lange, or Brachmann–de Lange Syndrome

De Lange syndrome is characterized by intrauterine growth retardation, persistent postnatal failure to thrive, moderate to severe cognitive impairment, and microcephaly with a flat occiput and low hairline. Facial features are quite distinctive and include long eyelashes; a fine, almost "brushed-on" appearance of the arch to the eyebrows; occasional synophrys due to hirsutism; small nose with anteverted nostrils; long philtrum; downturned upper lip with cupid's-bow shape; and micrognathia (Fig. 1-35A and B). Extremities are notable for small hands and feet, and varying abnormalities can include proximally placed thumbs (Fig. 1-35C), flexion contractures of the elbows, hypoplastic limbs, and even overt phocomelia. Hirsutism is generalized and distinctive, and cutis marmorata is a frequent feature. In males, hypospadias with

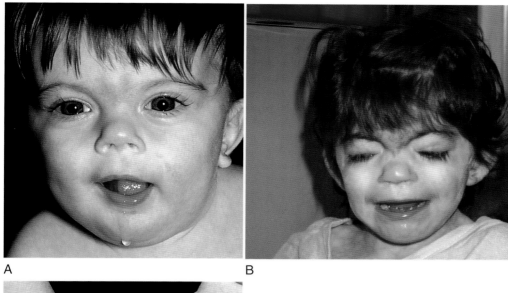

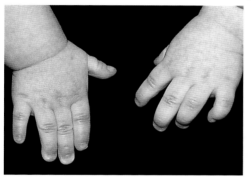

Figure 1-35. Cornelia de Lange syndrome. **A** and **B,** Facial features seen in an infant and an older child include finely arched heavy eyebrows, long eyelashes, small upturned nose, long smooth philtrum, and Cupid's-bow mouth. **C,** Small hands, hypoplastic proximally placed thumb, and short fifth finger with mild clinodactyly are examples of commonly associated extremity anomalies. (**A** and **C,** Courtesy A. H. Urbach, MD, Children's Hospital of Pittsburgh, Pa.)

cryptorchidism is common, and females may have a bicornuate uterus. Most affected adults are quite short in stature.

Generally, most cases are believed to be the result of new autosomal dominant mutations, and recently mutations in the *NIPBL* gene on chromosome 5p13 have been identified as responsible for approximately 50% of cases of classical De Lange syndrome. In evaluating cases, careful physical examination of family members must be performed to determine recurrence risks for individual families. Clearly, this disorder can be so mild in expression that many cases may go unrecognized. Families have been identified with severely affected children whose parents have been determined to be subtly affected. In those families autosomal dominant inheritance would apply, with a 50% recurrence risk for any affected individual to have a child with the same disorder. If parents are not thought to be affected, the recurrence risk has been shown to range from 1% to 5%. A few individuals have somewhat similar features, most notably synophrys, and have been found to have an abnormality of the short arm of chromosome 3; thus careful high-resolution chromosome studies are indicated, with particular attention to chromosome 3.

Noonan Syndrome

Noonan syndrome is an autosomal dominant, simple mendelian genetic disorder that shares a number of clinical features with 45,X (Turner syndrome). Recently the disorder has been found to be associated with mutations in the *PTPN11* gene on chromosome 12q24.1 (in 50% of classic cases) and in the *KRAS* gene on 12p12.1 in 5 to 10% of the cases that are negative for the *PTPN11* mutation. Thus a chromosome study should be performed on any individual in whom this diagnosis is suspected. It is relatively common and thought to be present in 1 in 1000 to 1 in 2500 individuals. Like many other autosomal dominant disorders, it is seen in both males and females and there is significant variability in clinical expression. Hence careful examination of close relatives of an index case may identify other affected individuals within the extended family, which is helpful when attempting to determine recurrence risks, as that risk would be 50% for offspring of an affected individual. In cases in which the child is considered to be the first in the family with Noonan syndrome, the empiric recurrence risk to apparently unaffected parents is 5%.

The pattern of malformations in Noonan syndrome is characterized by webbing of the neck, sternal abnormalities, pulmonic stenosis, and cryptorchidism in males. Facial characteristics include widely spaced eyes with down-slanting palpebral fissures, ptosis, and retrognathia (see Fig. 5-9). Ears are often low set and can be posteriorly rotated. Hair can be coarse and curly, and the posterior hairline is often low. Sternal abnormalities include both pectus excavatum and carinatum, and often there are differences in the number of sternal ossification centers. Many have congenital heart disease with pulmonary valvular stenosis being the most common, followed by septal hypertrophy or defects. Hypertrophic cardiomyopathy is found in approximately 20% and can be sufficiently severe as to necessitate cardiac transplantation. Coagulation abnormalities are found in approximately one third of cases.

Puberty can be delayed in individuals with Noonan syndrome. Cryptorchidism, when present in males, can result in sterility. Females are fertile. Stature is often less than the third percentile, but head circumference and intelligence are usually normal.

Several recognizable patterns of malformation share features in common with Noonan syndrome. Cardio-facio-cutaneous syndrome has additional features suggesting abnormal development of tissues derived from ectoderm, and affected individuals usually have significant central nervous system abnormalities. The phenotypic features of Noonan syndrome and neurofibromatosis type I may overlap (Watson syndrome). In the Costello syndrome, macrocephaly; coarse facial features; papillomas in the oral, nasal, and anal areas; cutis laxa; and cognitive impairments are seen in addition to findings shared with Noonan syndrome. The differential diagnosis also includes several well-known teratogenic exposures including fetal hydantoin syndrome and fetal alcohol syndrome (see Fig. 1-36). Hence careful dysmorphologic assessment of all individuals suspected of having Noonan syndrome is indicated before making a final diagnosis.

Patterns of Malformation Associated with In Utero Teratogen Exposure

Fetal Alcohol Syndrome

The effect of exposure to significant levels of serum alcohol during gestation results in a pattern of microcephaly, prenatal and postnatal growth deficiency, short palpebral fissures, long smooth philtrum; and a thin upper lip (Fig. 1-36). Other features include a short nose and hypoplasia of the nails and distal phalanges (particularly the fifth toes). Occasionally, affected infants have eyelid ptosis, epicanthal folds, strabismus, small raised hemangiomas, cervical vertebral abnormalities, and congenital heart disease.

Newborns with fetal alcohol syndrome are small for gestational age and have poor catch-up growth postnatally. They may have increased or decreased muscle tone

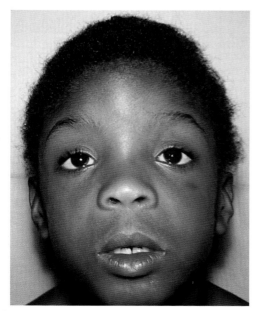

Figure 1-36. Fetal alcohol syndrome. Note the short palpebral fissure length, mild ptosis, and long simple philtrum.

and can be irritable and tremulous. Most older children tend to be thin and hyperactive, and more than 80% have some delay in development, especially fine motor function.

The diagnosis of fetal alcohol syndrome should be reserved for those infants who have a history of in utero exposure to large amounts of alcohol and who have the characteristic physical features of the disorder. The past practice of labeling children with developmental disorders who do not have the clinical stigmata as having fetal alcohol effects should be abandoned.

Although there may be no absolutely safe level of maternal alcohol consumption throughout pregnancy (particularly in the first trimester), the risk of teratogenesis increases dramatically with increasing degrees of maternal ethanol consumption. Major evidence of fetal alcohol syndrome is observed in 30% to 50% of offspring of mothers who are chronic severe alcoholics, whereas more subtle effects result from ingestion of lesser quantities of alcohol. The risk to the fetus of occasional maternal alcoholic binges is not clear, but such drinking is best avoided. Why some babies are affected and others are not, despite equivalent degrees of maternal alcoholism, is also unclear.

Other examples of teratogen-induced disorders include fetal hydantoin syndrome and fetal retinoic acid (Accutane) embryopathy.

Disorders Associated with Deficient Energy Production and Mitochondrial (Maternal Cytoplasmic) Inheritance

A group of diseases receiving increased recognition and better clinical delineation is that of the disorders of energy metabolism which involve insufficient availability of energy to tissues. This is a large and complex group of individual disorders that share a recognizable phenotype of systemic illness, often associated with lactic acidosis. They are most easily recognized either when classic clinical features are present, such as strokes (seen in children with the MELAS A3243G point mutation), or when a family history with construction of a three-generation family tree provides clues suggestive of a maternally inherited mitochondrial DNA (mtDNA) point mutation.

Mitochondria are membrane-bound cytoplasmic organelles that, in essence, serve as the power plants of cells. Because all of one's mitochondria are derived from those present in the oocyte (those of the sperm having been destroyed on fertilization), all mtDNA is inherited from one's mother. mtDNA is found in mitochondria within a small circular chromosome that contains about three dozen genes. These code for production of two types of ribosomal RNA (rRNA), 22 transport RNA (tRNA) molecules, and approximately 15% of the polypeptide chains that comprise subunits of the enzymes used in oxidative phosphorylation. The genes that code for about 85% of the polypeptide chains or proteins that operate within the electron transport chain of mitochondria are, however, nuclear, not mitochondrial genes. Hence some of these disorders stem from mutations of nuclear DNA, whereas others are the result of mtDNA mutations. The actions of the enzymes involved within the process of oxidative phosphorylation being the major source of energy for the cell, mutations that alter their structure, reduce their production, or impair their function have deleterious effects on energy production. Correspondingly, the effects of these alterations have their greatest expression in cells or

Table 1-10	Clinical Clues Suggestive of Mitochondrial Diseases

Neurologic	**Ophthalmologic**	**Gastrointestinal**
Neuropathy	Retinitis pigmentosa	Pancreatitis
Seizures	Progressive external ophthalmoplegia	Pseudo-obstruction
Dementia	Optic atrophy	Dysmotility
"Cerebral palsy"	Reversible visual field deficits	Hepatitis/hepatic failure (while taking valproic acid, with certain
Neurodegenerative picture	Ptosis	viral illnesses)
Strokelike episodes	**Renal**	Food intolerances
Myoclonic epilepsy	Glomerulopathy	Atypical irritable bowel
Mental retardation	**Cardiac**	**Audiologic**
Ataxia, dystonia	Cardiomyopathy	Sensorineural hearing loss
EEG: hypsarrhythmia	Cardiac conduction defects	**Endocrine**
Migraines		Short stature
Fatigability		Diabetes mellitus
Pathologic		**Pedigree consistent with:**
Mitochondrial proliferation		Sporadic inheritance
Ragged red fibers		Maternal-line systemic disease
MtDNA depletion		Autosomal recessive inheritance
Hematologic		Autosomal dominant inheritance
Sideroblastic anemia		X-linked recessive inheritance
Neutropenia		**Rare but Useful Clinical Symptoms**
Metabolic		**Suggestive of a Mitochondrially**
Increased lactate/pyruvate		**Based Disorder**
Normal lactate (in some cases)		Multiple lipomas
Hyperalaninemia		Myoglobinuria
Episodic illness		Adrenal insufficiency
Severe response to routine illness		

EEG, electroencephalogram.

tissues with high energy demands. This accounts for the relatively high incidence of neural, muscular, and ocular symptomatology seen among these disorders.

At this time, most of the nuclear genes responsible for disorders of energy metabolism are just beginning to be identified. An example of a causative nuclear gene mutation is one that involves a gene located on the X chromosome (inherited as an X-linked recessive trait), which affects the E1 subunit of the pyruvate dehydrogenase enzyme complex (PDC). This results in PDC deficiency, the most common inborn error of metabolism characterized by lactic acidosis.

In contrast to disorders caused by abnormalities in nuclear genes, a considerable number of diseases due to mtDNA point mutations have been identified more recently, due in part to the fact that family trees demonstrating maternal-line inheritance patterns have made it relatively simple to identify these mutations. In such cases the maternal family tree tends to be dotted with a number of individuals, each of whom has one or more of a wide variety of relatively unusual symptoms or problems. Among these are neurodegenerative diseases, myopathies, weakness, seizures, migraine headaches, diabetes, multiple lipomas, gastrointestinal dysmotility or pseudo-obstruction, and arrhythmias. In each affected family a variety of these problems or symptoms are represented. Features seen frequently in individual patients and families are outlined in Table 1-10.

The age of onset of disorders of energy metabolism that are characterized by lactic acidosis can be quite variable and may be used in part to distinguish among different types. Most commonly, those presenting with symptoms in infancy involve defective glycolysis and/or gluconeogenesis, whereas patients with mtDNA point mutations are more likely to become symptomatic at older ages.

Given the fact that other more easily recognized inborn errors of metabolism can share common presenting features (including lactic acidosis), disorders of amino acid, organic acid, and biotin metabolism, as well as of fatty acid oxidation, should be ruled out. In investigation of mitochondrial disorders, determination of sufficiency of mtDNA content and functional activity of the electron transport chain is often necessary. This requires the use of laboratories that are expert in the analysis of mtDNA mutations to confirm clinical suspicion. Tests often require considerable time, for both sample preparation and actual testing. In seriously affected individuals, samples for analysis may be obtained by muscle biopsy or from autopsy specimens.

The most common mitochondrial point mutations currently known are listed as follows:

1. A3243G associated with MELAS, an acronym for a disorder characterized by *m*itochondrial *e*ncephalopathy, *l*actic *a*cidosis, and *s*troke (Fig. 1-37)
2. A8344G associated with MERRF, an acronym for *m*itochondrial *e*ncephalopathy with *r*agged *r*ed *f*ibers (Fig. 1-38)
3. T8993C associated with NARP, an acronym for *n*europathy, *a*taxia, and *r*etinitis *p*igmentosa

When an individual is determined to be positive for a maternal-line mtDNA point mutation, test results usually describe the percentage of heteroplasmy, or mutation, that the individual has in the tissue sample tested because most individuals have a mix of normal and mutated mtDNA. In general, for most of these diseases, the higher the rate of heteroplasmy, the earlier the age of onset of symptoms in the affected individuals, and the more severe the symptoms.

Due to the multiple modes of inheritance possible in this group of disorders, accurate diagnosis is essential before the provision of genetic counseling.

Newborn Screening for Genetic Disorders

A new era is developing in the provision of neonatal screening. The advent of methodologies, particularly Tandem Mass Spectroscopy, provides an inexpensive mechanism to screen for a much larger number of disorders than was previously routine. At present, individual

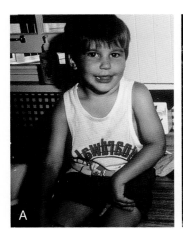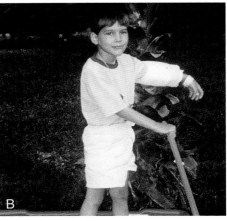

Figure 1-37. MELAS syndrome. This boy presented with mild cognitive delay, short stature, neutropenia, and Wolff-Parkinson-White syndrome. **A,** At age 4 he appears healthy. **B,** By age 6 he had muscle weakness and visual and hearing impairment as a result of a series of strokes.

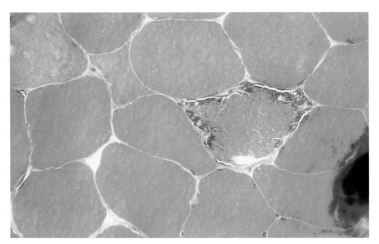

Figure 1-38. Ragged red fibers as seen in this muscle biopsy can be found in patients with a variety of mitochondrial DNA point mutations such as MERRF syndrome.

states determine the appropriate diseases for screening. However, a national effort is under way to standardize testing and determine appropriate new screening tests to be included in a single newborn screening panel. A major increase in the number of screenable disorders is anticipated in the next few years and will ultimately lead to development of new treatment modalities for use in patients with genetic disorders, which can be implemented before the onset of many of their signs and symptoms.

Bibliography

Buyse ML (ed): Birth Defects Encyclopedia. Cambridge, Mass, Blackwell Scientific, 1990.

Cooley WC, Graham JM: Down syndrome—an update and review for the primary pediatrician. Clin Pediatr 30:233-253, 1991.

Epstein CJ: Down syndrome (trisomy 21). In Scriber CR, Beaudet AL, Sly WS, Valle D (eds): The Metabolic and Molecular Basis of Inherited Disease, 8th ed. New York, McGraw-Hill, 2001, pp 1223-1256.

Francke U: Prader-Willi syndrome: Chromosomal and gene aberrations. Growth, Genetics and Hormones 10:4-7, 1994.

Gorlin RJ, Cohen MM Jr, Hennekam RCM: Syndromes of the Head and Neck, 4th ed. New York, Oxford University Press, 2001.

Graham JM Jr: Smith's Recognizable Patterns of Human Deformation, 2nd ed. Philadelphia, WB Saunders, 1988.

Hook EB: Chromosome abnormalities: Prevalence, risks, and recurrence. In Brock BJH, Rodeck CH, Ferguson-Smith MA: Prenatal Diagnosis and Screening. New York, Churchill Livingstone, 1992, pp 351-392.

Johns DR: Mitochondrial DNA and disease. N Engl J Med 333:638-644, 1995.

Jones KL: Smith's Recognizable Patterns of Human Malformation, 6th ed. Philadelphia, Elsevier Saunders, 2006.

Nussbaum RL, McInnes RR, Willard HF: Thompson and Thompson Genetics in Medicine, 6th ed. Philadelphia, WB Saunders, 2004.

Online Mendelian Inheritance in Man, OMIM. McKusick-Nathans Institute for Genetic Medicine, Johns Hopkins University (Baltimore, Md) and National Center for Biotechnology Information, National Library of Medicine (Bethesda, Md), 2000. Available at http://www.ncbi.nlm.nih.gov/omim/

Patton MA: Noonan syndrome: A review. Growth, Genetics and Hormones 10:1-3, 1994.

Robinson BH: Lactic acidemia: Disorders of pyruvate carboxylase and pyruvate dehydrogenase. In Scriber CR, Beaudet AL, Sly WS, Valle D (eds): The Metabolic and Molecular Basis of Inherited Disease, 8th ed. New York, McGraw-Hill, 2001, pp 2275-2295.

Ryan AK, Goodship JA, Wilson DI, et al: Spectrum of clinical features associated with interstitial chromosome 22q11 deletions: A European collaborative study. J Med Genet 34:798-804, 1997.

Shepard TH, Lemire RJ: Catalog of Teratogenic Agents, 11th ed. Baltimore, Johns Hopkins University Press, 2004.

Stalker HJ, Williams CA: Genetic counseling in Angelman syndrome: The challenges of multiple causes. Am J Med Genet 77:54-59, 1998.

Stevenson RE, Hall JG, Goodman RM (eds): Human Malformations and Related Anomalies, 2nd ed. New York, Oxford University Press, 2006.

Sutherland GR, Gecz J, Mulley JC: Fragile X syndrome and other causes of X-linked mental handicap. In Rimoin DL, O'Connor JM, Pyeritz RE, Korf BR (eds): Emery and Rimoin's Principles and Practice of Medical Genetics, 5th ed. Philadelphia, Churchill Livingstone, 2006, pp 2801-2826.

Trask BJ: Fluorescence in situ hybridization. Trends Genet 7:149-154, 1991.

Wenger SL, Steele MW, Boone LY, et al: "Balanced" karyotypes in six abnormal offspring of balanced reciprocal translocation normal carrier parents. Am J Med Genet 55:47-52, 1995.

Willard HF, Ferguson-Smith MA, Goodfellow PN, et al: Chromosomes and autosomes. In Scriver CR, Beaudet AL, Sly WS, Valle D (eds): The Metabolic and Molecular Bases of Inherited Disease. New York, McGraw-Hill, 1995.

www.genetests.org (gene reviews)

www.mayoclinic.com

www.mghlysosomal.org

www.ninds.nih.gov

CHAPTER 2

Neonatology

Beverly S. Brozanski and Debra L. Bogen

General Techniques of Physical Examination

Assessment of the Newborn

The purposes of the routine newborn assessment are to determine the infant's gestational age, document normal growth and development for a given gestational age, uncover signs of birth-related trauma or congenital anomalies, and evaluate the overall health and condition of the infant. The assessment begins with the establishment of a historical database. Information may be obtained from antenatal, labor, delivery, and postpartum records and a brief interview with the parents (Fig. 2-1). The aim of this data gathering is to assess the fetal and neonatal responses to pregnancy, labor, and delivery; estimate the risk for hereditary or congenital diseases; and identify the potential for future difficulties by reviewing the family's social history and observing maternal-infant interactions. This background is recorded in the infant's medical record and serves as a guide to the subsequent physical examination (Table 2-1).

Whenever possible, it is preferable that the newborn be examined in the presence of one or both parents to reassure them regarding normal variations and to discuss any abnormal findings. The baby should remain at least partially clothed through as much of the examination as possible, although a complete and thorough examination is imperative. The examiner's hands should be warm to minimize the chance that the infant will become uncomfortable because of heat loss.

Observation must be done before the quiet infant is disturbed by the examination. By visual inspection the clinician can assess skin and facies; general tonus and symmetry of movement; respiratory rate, retractions, and color; and abdominal contour. Auscultation of the heart and lungs should be done before more stressful portions of the examination, which are likely to make the infant fussy. Allowing the infant to suck on a gloved finger can help quiet the infant and permit assessment of sucking strength and palate integrity. Lifting the infant under the arms (Fig. 2-2) and gently rocking him or her (such that the head swings toward and away from the examiner) is usually calming. This maneuver also induces a reflexive opening of the eyes, which assists the ophthalmologic examination. Sucking also induces eye opening. Such maneuvers may be necessary to convince the examiner that the patient does not have a congenital cataract or an intraorbital mass (see Chapter 19) requiring prompt intervention.

When the abdomen is examined, it often helps to gently flex the hip on the side being examined because this relaxes the abdominal muscles. Most structures in the abdomen are smaller (pyloric olive), softer (liver), more superficial (spleen tip), or deeper (kidneys) than expected. The use of any part of the hand other than the fingertips should be discouraged because maximal sensitivity is essential.

Careful evaluation of the hip joints is a crucial part of each newborn examination because identification and early treatment of congenital dislocation can prevent later disability. Although asymmetry of the buttocks and skin creases or asymmetry of femoral length can be clues to dislocation, the performance of at least one of a number of active motion tests is essential. The Ortolani maneuver involves placing the third or fourth finger over the greater trochanter and the thumb on the medial aspect of the thighs (Fig. 2-3). The thighs are first adducted to try to dislocate a dislocatable hip and then abducted with the fingers pushing toward the midline and the thumbs away from midline to relocate a dislocated hip. A definite "clunk" can be felt and often heard if the femoral head has been dislocated and clunks back into the acetabulum. Often, higher-pitched clicks and snaps that represent nothing more than tendons passing over bone or cartilage can be heard and felt.

Assessment of Gestational Age

One of the unique considerations in the examination of the newborn is the assessment of gestational age. Accurate determination should be the first part of any newborn examination because this provides the context for the remainder of the evaluation. No differential diagnosis of newborn disease can be made without knowing whether the patient is premature or full term and whether he or she is small, large, or appropriate for gestational age. Although an accurate menstrual and pregnancy history usually provides firm evidence of gestational age, there are many cases in which data such as the date of the last menses and the date of the onset of fetal movement are unavailable or unreliable.

Many investigators have developed examination criteria, both morphologic and neurologic, for the assessment of gestational age. Although these criteria are generally useful because of the ordered patterns of fetal development, the clinician cannot rely on any single feature or even small group of features to develop at the same rate in all infants. In fact, assessment of paired structures, such as ears, may reveal slightly different degrees of maturation from one side to the other. Thus all of the available methods involve numerous physical and neurologic items and have, at best, a 2-week range of error.

Although morphologic criteria tend to be uninfluenced by events occurring around the time of delivery, neurologic findings may be unreliable in the presence of a number of conditions including depression secondary to medication, asphyxia, seizures, metabolic diseases, infections, and severe respiratory distress. Even morphologic criteria may be inaccurate if the infant is born with severe edema or growth retardation or side effects from maternal drug use. Such factors must be considered in estimating gestational age.

The Ballard assessment for gestational age determination of newborns uses six morphologic and six neurologic criteria to estimate gestational age on the basis of an examination performed at 12 to 24 hours of life (Fig. 2-4). Individual findings are scored on a scale of 0 to 5, and the total score is compared with the chart shown in Figure 2-4.

Physical Maturity

One of the most striking differences among newborns of various gestational ages is the quality of the skin. The

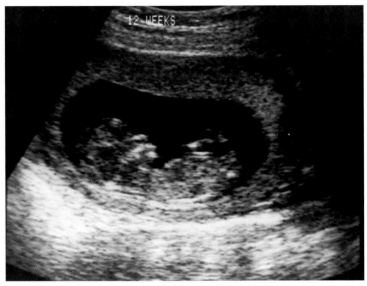

Figure 2-1. Antenatal assessments. This infant has a normal sonographic appearance at 12 weeks' gestation. Knowledge of the results of in utero evaluations may assist in the provision of appropriate antenatal and postnatal care. (Courtesy Lyndon Hill, MD, Pittsburgh.)

Table 2-1	Newborn Historical Database

Antenatal Record
Maternal age
Maternal medical history
Obstetric history
  Number of previous pregnancies
  Number of term/preterm deliveries
  Outcomes of previous pregnancies
Estimations of gestational age
Antenatal ultrasound or fetal surveillance results (if available)
Complications of pregnancy
Adequacy of antenatal care

Labor and Delivery Record
Date and time of delivery
Duration of labor
Time of the rupture of membranes
Complications or abnormalities of labor
Method of delivery or type of anesthesia
Placental weight and morphologic condition
Birthweight
Need for resuscitation and Apgar scores
Maternal blood type

Postpartum Record
Maternal postpartum complications
Newborn vital sign records
Nursing documentation of the activity and condition of the infant
  On admission to the nursery
  Since admission to the nursery
Abnormal physical findings noted by the nursing staff
Feeding, voiding, and stool history
Observations of maternal-infant interactions

Parental Interview
Parental perceptions of
  Pregnancy
  Labor
  Delivery
History of parental and family illnesses
Health status and growth and development of siblings and other
  family members
Degree of education, preparation, and planning for newborn care
Available social support systems
Medical follow-up plans

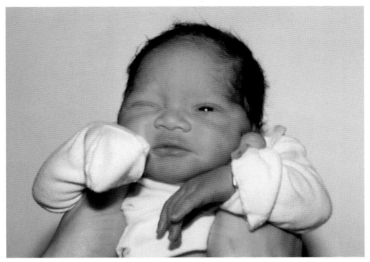

Figure 2-2. Examination techniques. Holding an infant under the arms and gently rocking calms the infant and reflexively induces eye opening.

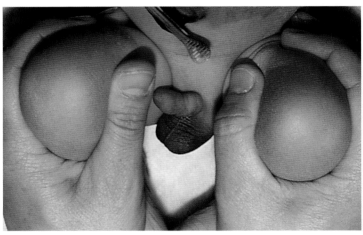

Figure 2-3. Ortolani maneuver. The proper hand positioning for this maneuver is demonstrated. Abducting the femur produces a palpable clunk in the infant with congenital hip dislocation.

chemical nature of skin changes during intrauterine development with a gradual decrease in water content and a thickening of the keratin layer. Very premature infants (24 to 28 weeks) have nearly translucent, paper-thin skin (Fig. 2-5) that is easily abraded. A diffuse red hue and a promi-nent venous pattern are characteristic. At term, the skin no longer appears thin, and the general color is a pale pink. Some superficial peeling and cracking around the ankles and wrists may be visible. Post-term infants (42 to 44 weeks) often have more diffuse peeling and crack-ing of the skin because the outermost layers are sloughed (Fig. 2-6).

The general quality of scalp hair changes during devel-opment from rather fine, thin hair (24 to 28 weeks) to coarser, thicker hair (term). Racial differences in hair quality can make this change difficult to assess. A second type of hair, known as lanugo, appears and disappears during development. Lanugo is fine body hair that re-sembles peach fuzz. It is absent before weeks 20 to 22, becomes diffuse until weeks 30 to 32, and then begins to thin. Assessment of the presence and extent of lanugo is best accomplished by observing the back tangentially (Fig. 2-7).

Transverse creases begin to appear on the anterior portion of the soles of the feet at approximately 32 weeks (Fig. 2-8). By 36 weeks the anterior two thirds of the sole is covered with creases. For adequate assessment of this feature, it is necessary to stretch the skin over the sole gently to distinguish wrinkling from true creases. Infants with congenital neurologic dysfunction involving the

Physical maturity

	0	1	2	3	4	5
Skin	Gelatinous, red, transparent	Smooth, pink, visible veins	Superficial peeling and/or rash, few veins	Cracking, pale area, rare veins	Parchment, deep cracking no vessels	Leathery, cracked, wrinkled
Lanugo	None	Abundant	Thinning	Bald areas	Mostly bald	
Plantar creases	No crease	Faint red marks	Anterior transverse crease only	Creases anterior two thirds	Creases cover entire sole	
Breast	Barely perceptible	Flat areola, no bud	Stippled areola, 1–2 mm bud	Raised areola, 3–4 mm bud	Full areola, 5–10 mm bud	
Ear	Pinna flat, stays folded	Slightly curved pinna, soft, slow recoil	Well-curved pinna, soft but ready recoil	Formed and firm with instant recoil	Thick cartilage, ear stiff	
Genitals: male	Scrotum empty, no rugae		Testes descending, few rugae	Testes down, good rugae	Testes pendulous, deep rugae	
Genitals: female	Prominent clitoris and labia minora		Majora and minora equally prominent	Majora large, minora small	Clitoris and minora completely covered	

Maturity rating

Score	Weeks
5	26
10	28
15	30
20	32
25	34
30	36
35	38
40	40
45	42
50	44

Neuromuscular maturity

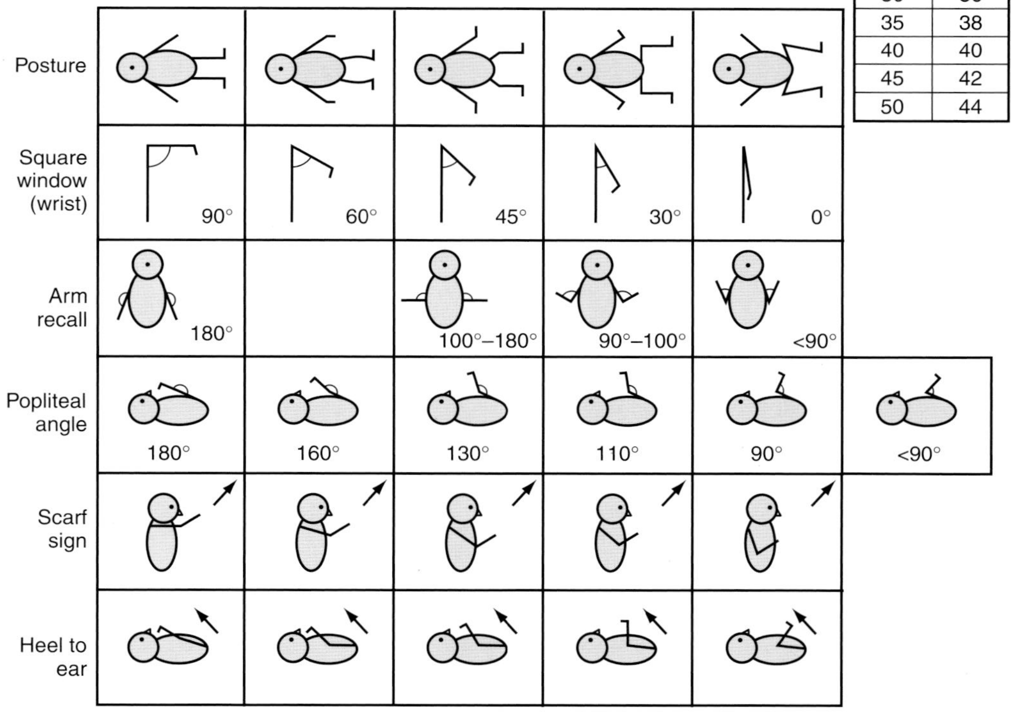

	0	1	2	3	4	5
Posture						
Square window (wrist)	90°	60°	45°	30°	0°	
Arm recall	180°		100°–180°	90°–100°	<90°	
Popliteal angle	180°	160°	130°	110°	90°	<90°
Scarf sign						
Heel to ear						

Figure 2-4. Gestational age assessment. The six morphologic and six neurologic criteria, in aggregate, yield an estimation of gestational age. (From Ballard J, Novak KK, Driver M, et al: A simplified score of assessment of fetal maturation of newly born infants. J Pediatr 95:769-774, 1979.)

lower extremities and infants with pedal edema may lack normal creases.

Breast tissue, which is responsive to maternal hormonal influences, shows progressive increase in size as gestational age advances. Infants born at younger than 28 weeks' gestation have barely perceptible breast tissue (see Fig. 2-5). With advancing age, breast tissue increases in size (see Figure 2-6) and, occasionally, a term infant has active glandular secretions, which resolve spontaneously. Breast tissue can remain palpable for 2 to 3 months.

Cartilaginous development proceeds in an orderly manner during gestation and can be assessed by examination of the external ear. Although the normal incurving of the upper pinnae begins at 33 to 34 weeks and is complete at term, it is more reliable to assess the extent of cartilage in the pinnae by feeling its edge and folding the

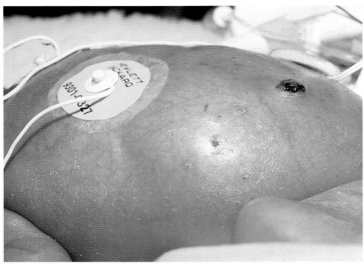

Figure 2-5. Premature skin. This premature infant demonstrates translucent, paper-thin skin with a prominent venous pattern.

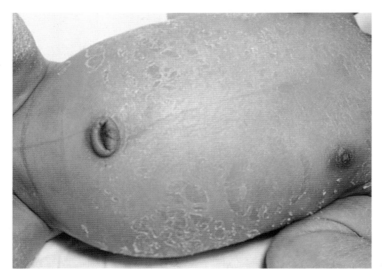

Figure 2-6. Post-term skin. Peeling and cracking of the skin are characteristics of the infant delivered after 42 weeks' gestation.

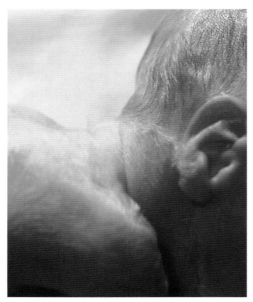

Figure 2-7. Lanugo. This fine body hair resembling peach fuzz is present on infants of 24 to 32 weeks' gestation.

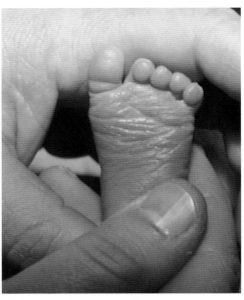

Figure 2-8. Sole creases. Transverse sole creases cover approximately half the sole in this infant, indicating a gestational age of approximately 34 weeks.

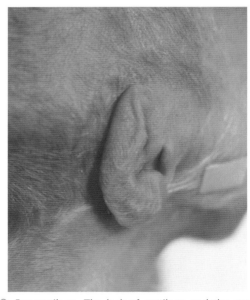

Figure 2-9. Ear cartilage. The lack of cartilage and the easy foldability (lack of recoil) are evident in the ear of this premature infant at 26 weeks.

ear (Fig. 2-9). Until approximately 32 weeks, there is only minimal recoil of a folded ear, but by term there is instant recoil.

The appearance of the genitalia can be used to assess gestational age. In a boy the testes descend into the scrotum during the last month of gestation, but they are often palpable in the inguinal canal by 28 to 30 weeks. The appearance of rugae on the scrotum parallels testicular migration, appearing first on the anterior scrotum at 36 weeks and covering the entire scrotal sac by 40 weeks. Absence of testicular descent alters the appearance of the scrotum at term. Clearly, congenital cryptorchidism complicates this evaluation. In a girl the labia majora tend to be overshadowed by the clitoris and labia minora until 34 to 36 weeks (Fig. 2-10). In cases of fetal malnutrition, lack of subcutaneous fat, which should normally be present in the latter part of gestation, can interfere with assessment of the female genitalia.

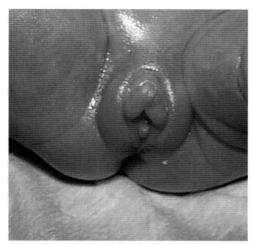

Figure 2-10. Premature female genitalia. Prominence of the labia minora in a premature female infant at 28 weeks.

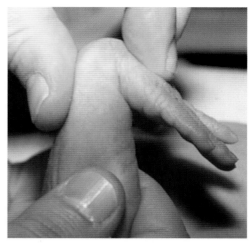

Figure 2-12. Square-window test. The position for assessing the square window is shown. The 45-degree angle seen between the palm and forearm is consistent with a gestational age of 30 to 32 weeks.

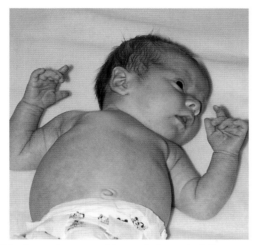

Figure 2-11. General posture. The typical, marked flexor posture of the term infant.

Neuromuscular Maturity

Numerous neurologic tests and observations can be used to assess gestational age. Most examiners use the tests that seem to best cover the various facets of neurologic function including range of motion, tone, reflexes, and posture. None is particularly reliable in the presence of illness, and the entire neurologic examination is best done between 12 and 24 hours after birth to allow recovery from the stress of delivery.

The resting supine posture of infants changes with advancing gestational age. The mature infant exhibits a marked flexor posture of the extremities compared with the extensor posture of the premature infant (Fig. 2-11).

Tests for flexion angles assess a combination of muscle tone, ligament and tendon laxity, as well as flexion-extension development. The inexperienced examiner usually assumes that the very premature infant is the most flexible, but observation of flexion angles demonstrates that this is false. The square-window test of the wrist (Fig. 2-12) is performed by gently flexing the hand on the wrist and assessing the resultant angle. The wrists of babies younger than approximately 32 weeks can be flexed only to 45 to 90 degrees, whereas the wrists of term infants undergo full flexion. Sometime between birth and adulthood this flexion ability is lost. Examination of the flexion of the knees reveals a different pattern of development, with decreasing flexibility as gestational age increases (Fig.

2-13). Gentleness is *essential* in these evaluations because any result can be achieved if the examiner applies undue force.

Examination of arm recoil can assess active tone and reflex responsiveness. In this maneuver the supine infant's forearms are fully flexed for 5 seconds, extended by pulling on the hands, and then released. As gestational age increases, the flexion response is more pronounced.

The resting tone of the upper extremities can be assessed by eliciting the scarf sign. Gentle traction of the upper extremities across the chest in a rostral direction ("placing a scarf on the infant") while examining the position of the elbow reveals a decreasing displacement of the elbow as gestational age increases (Fig. 2-14).

In a similar manner the resting tone of the lower extremities can be assessed by the heel-to-ear maneuver. With the baby on the back and the pelvis flat, a foot is moved as near to the ipsilateral ear as possible without exerting undue force. Very premature infants can easily touch their heels to their ears (Fig. 2-15). This becomes somewhat more difficult after 30 weeks and impossible by week 34 of gestation.

Abnormalities of Growth

Intrauterine growth restriction (IUGR) is a deviation in the expected fetal growth pattern, complicates up to 8% of all pregnancies, and is associated with an increase in perinatal morbidity and mortality. Infants with IUGR may appear long and thin and often have an obvious loss of subcutaneous tissue, which is best seen as redundant skin-folds over the buttocks, thighs, and knees. The etiology of IUGR is multifactorial and includes fetal, placental, or maternal factors that inhibit normal fetal growth. The conditions IUGR and small for gestational age (SGA) are related but not synonymous. The diagnosis of SGA is based on population norms and includes infants who weigh less than a predetermined cutoff value (Fig. 2-16). There is no universal agreement in the definition of SGA or large for gestational age infant (LGA). Similarly, appropriate for gestational age (AGA) infants have growth parameters within two standard deviations of the mean or between the 10th and 90th percentiles or between the 3rd and 97th percentiles.

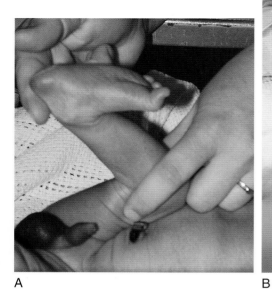

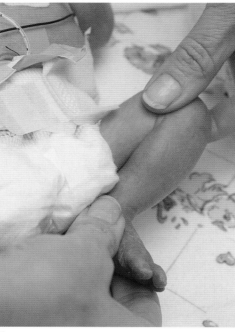

A   B

Figure 2-13. Knee flexion. The position for assessing knee flexion is shown. Note the decreased knee flexibility of this term infant **(A)** compared with preterm infant of 29 weeks' gestation **(B).**

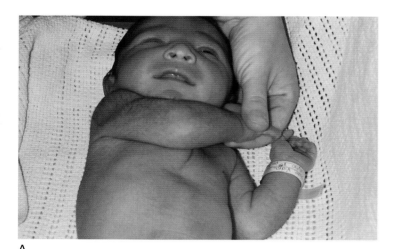

A

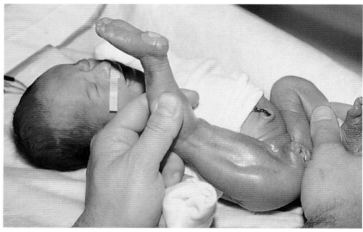

Figure 2-15. Heel-to-ear maneuver. The position for assessing the heel-to-ear maneuver is demonstrated. The degree of extension seen is consistent with a 28- to 30-week infant.

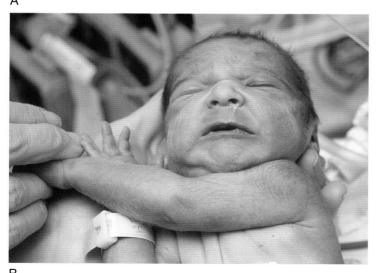

B

Figure 2-14. Scarf sign. The elbow cannot be drawn, with gentle traction on the upper extremity, across this term infant's chest **(A).** This is in contrast to the marked flexibility of a preterm infant of 29 weeks' gestation **(B).**

The relationship among weight, length, and head circumference can be useful in understanding the etiology of the small size (see Fig. 2-16). By comparing length or head circumference percentiles with the weight percentile at any given gestational age, the clinician can detect growth retardation even if the actual weight still falls within two standard deviations of normal. Conditions that affect growth during the third trimester of pregnancy, such as preeclampsia, tend to interfere with the normal acquisition of fatty tissue while sparing brain growth (and thus head circumference) and linear growth. These newborns have an asymmetrical form of growth retardation. Often postmature infants (>42 weeks) have some decrease in weight compared with length or head circumference. Problems beginning earlier than the third trimester tend to produce generalized growth retardation (Fig. 2-17) because head circumference, weight, and length are affected to equivalent degrees. Historically, infants with symmetrical IUGR have higher rates of chromosomal disorders, dysmorphic syndromes, and congenital infection and are associated with higher rates of prematurity

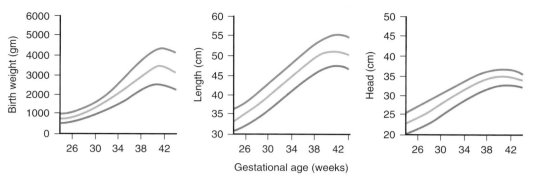

Figure 2-16. The mean (±2 standard deviations) weight, length, and head circumference for infants born at various gestational ages. Infants above or below the curves are considered too large or too small for gestational age, respectively. (From Usher R, McLean F: Intrauterine growth of liveborn Caucasian infant at sea level. J Pediatr 74:901-910, 1969.)

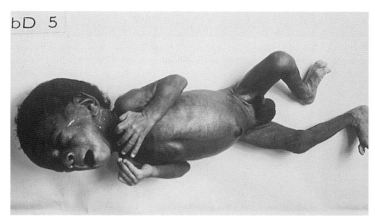

Figure 2-17. Intrauterine growth retardation. This term baby weighed only 1.7 kg. The head appears disproportionately large for the thin, wasted body. This resulted from placental insufficiency late in pregnancy. Hypoglycemia may be a complication. (Courtesy TALC, Institute of Child Health, Bethesda, Md.)

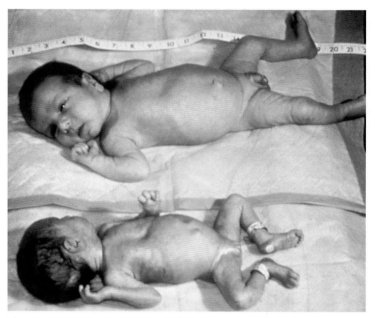

Figure 2-18. Discordant twins. This is a pair of markedly discordant dizygotic twins. Disturbed placentation accounted for the marked reduction in size of the smaller twin.

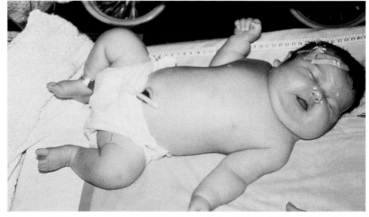

Figure 2-19. Large-for-gestational-age infant. This infant of a diabetic mother weighed 5 kg at birth and exhibits the typical rounded facies.

and neonatal mortality. In very premature infants, global decreases in growth often complicate assessment of gestational age because the tools are rather limited in babies born at 24 to 28 weeks' gestation. A thorough investigation should be undertaken in any unexplained instance of growth retardation.

Multiple-gestation pregnancies often produce newborns who are premature and symmetrically small. Fetal growth decreases as the number of fetuses increases. Although multiple factors interfere with growth in these pregnancies, uterine constraint appears to occur when the combined fetal size approximates 3 kg. Size discordance (>10% difference in weight) between identical twins occurs because their placentas can share vascular connections, resulting in overperfusion of one twin and underperfusion with subsequent growth restriction of the other. Discordance may also occur in dizygotic twins (Fig. 2-18) if one has placental insufficiency. Rarely, only one twin will be afflicted with a chromosomal abnormality or congenital infection.

Newborns who are large for gestational age (LGA) are often the products of pregnancies in diabetic or "prediabetic" mothers. The effect is usually noted during the third trimester, with infants at term who weigh more than 4 kg (8 lb 13 oz). Weight is the most affected parameter, but length and head circumference are often increased as well. Infants of diabetic mothers are often identifiable by macrosomia, round facies (Fig. 2-19), and sometimes plethora and hirsutism (especially of the pinnae). Maternal hyperglycemia causes glycogen deposition in the newborn resulting in visceromegaly, most notable in the liver and heart. Although babies weighing more than 8 lb are more likely to be from diabetic pregnancies, a signifi-

cant number of large full-term newborns are the product of normal pregnancies. Nevertheless, all LGA infants should be routinely screened for hypoglycemia and their mothers investigated for the possibility of undiagnosed diabetes mellitus.

Two fairly unusual syndromes can also cause excessive size: (1) cerebral gigantism, or Solo syndrome, with macrosomia, macrocephaly, large hands and feet, poor coordination, and variable mental deficiency; and (2)

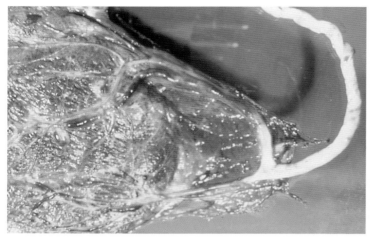

Figure 2-20. Velamentous cord insertion. The umbilical cord is inserted into the amniotic membranes rather than into the placental disk. This leaves the umbilical vessels relatively unprotected and predisposes them to rupture.

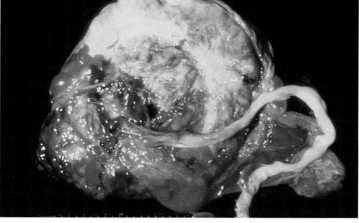

Figure 2-21. Circumvallate placenta. Extension of villous tissue exists beyond the chorionic surface, with a well-defined hyalinized fold at the edge of the chorionic plate.

Beckwith-Wiedemann syndrome with macrosomia, macroglossia, omphalocele, linear ear fissures, and neonatal hypoglycemia (see Chapter 9).

Placenta

Careful examination of the placenta can aid in the diagnosis and treatment of many conditions and diseases. Unfortunately the placenta has been relegated to the afterbirth and is often immediately discarded without knowing the condition of the offspring. After the membranes and cord are trimmed, the normal ratio of fetal-to-placental weight is approximately 4.7:1. The configuration, color, condition of the membranes, insertion of the cord, and condition of the fetal and maternal surfaces are all relevant.

The insertion of the umbilical cord into the placenta, which can be central, eccentric, marginal, or velamentous, can be important in understanding unexplained asphyxia or blood loss. In a velamentous insertion (Fig. 2-20), the cord is inserted into the membranes rather than into the placental disk, leaving the umbilical vessels unprotected for a variable distance. These vessels are more prone to rupture, with resultant fetal hemorrhage (vasa praevia).

At times, placentation itself is abnormal. In a circumvallate placenta (Fig. 2-21), the villous tissue projects beyond the chorionic surface, with a hyalinized fold at the edge of the chorionic plate. This type of placentation may cause antepartum bleeding, premature labor, and increased perinatal mortality.

Premature placental separation (abruptio placentae) can lead to an accumulation of blood behind the placenta (Fig. 2-22). Although the bleeding is usually of maternal origin, rare fetal blood loss may also occur. Large abruptions may lead to poor growth, fetal asphyxia, or even death. Distinguishing a true abruption, in which an adherent clot compresses the maternal surface, from the nonadherent collection of blood that forms on normal placental separation is important.

Placental infarctions (Fig. 2-23) tend to occur along the margin of the placenta, can vary in color from red to yellowish white, and are most common in pregnancies complicated by hypertension. Small placental infarcts (<30% of placental volume) are usually of little significance. However, large central infarcts can reduce the placental

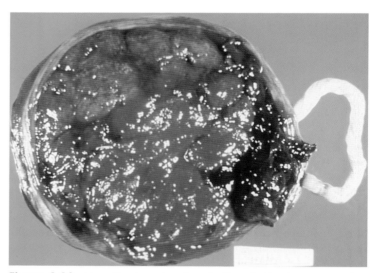

Figure 2-22. Abruptio placentae. Examination of this placenta reveals a small abruption site, with an adherent blood clot along the margin.

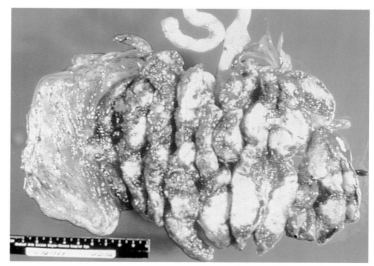

Figure 2-23. Infarcted placenta. A massive placental infarction making up the majority of the villous surface is shown. Such an extensive infarction compromises fetal nutrition and oxygenation.

surface available for fetal oxygenation and nutrition and can result in aberrations in fetal growth.

Chorioamnionitis (Fig. 2-24), or inflammation of the fetal membranes, is an immediate clue to potential neonatal infection. On gross examination the membranes lack their normal sheen and translucency, appearing gray or yellow. Inflammation, confirmable by microscopic examination, can also be found in the fetal vessels of the chorionic plate and umbilical cord.

In pregnancies in which the quantity of amniotic fluid is decreased (oligohydramnios), examination of the amnion may also reveal shiny, gray, flat nodules known as *amnion nodosum* (Fig. 2-25). The presence of these nodules can be an immediate indication of the diagnosis of renal dysfunction or renal agenesis in the newborn (or the newborn may have normal renal function). Because such infants may also have hypoplastic lungs and dysmorphic features (such as occurs in Potter syndrome), early diagnosis can be helpful to the physician and family.

In multiple-gestation deliveries, a careful placental evaluation is crucial to determine chorion number and to distinguish between monozygotic and dizygotic twins. The major distinction to be made is whether there is a single chorion, or outer layer of the fetal membranes. When twins with a single chorion are present in a single amniotic cavity (Fig. 2-26), monozygosity is ensured. For all practical purposes, a single chorion that bridges two amniotic sacs is also evidence of monozygotic twins. In this instance it is essential to examine the membranes at the site of connection of the two amniotic sacs. When two chorions and two amnions (or a total of four membranes at their interface) are present (Fig. 2-27), twins may be monozygotic or dizygotic. Approximately 36% of monozygotic twins are dichorionic. Monochorionic twin (MC) placentas, developed for a singleton pregnancy, may not adapt to the demands of twin circulations. The majority of MC twin placentas have connecting vessels, which account for higher rates of complications.

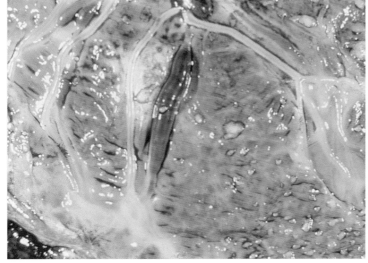

Figure 2-24. Chorioamnionitis. This is a placental specimen from a pregnancy with documented amniotic fluid infection. The surface of the membranes is opaque and shows yellowish discoloration.

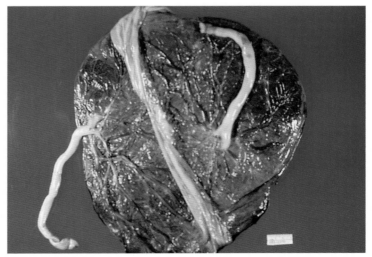

Figure 2-26. Monochorionic, monoamniotic placenta. Examination of this placenta from monozygotic twins reveals no dividing membranes, thus assuring monozygosity.

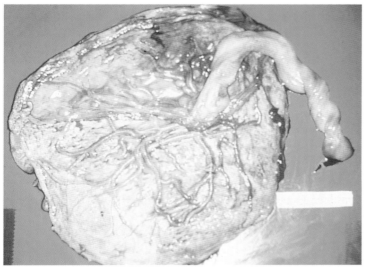

Figure 2-25. Amnion nodosum. The fetal surface of this placenta from a pregnancy with oligohydramnios demonstrates multiple nodules consistent with amnion nodosum. This finding suggests a strong possibility of renal agenesis or dysgenesis.

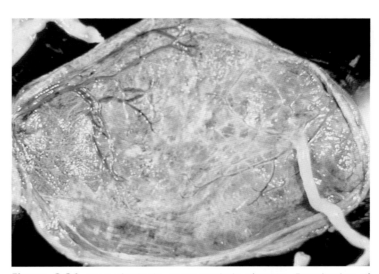

Figure 2-27. Dichorionic, diamniotic placenta. The presence of two amniotic sacs and separate chorions in this twin placenta precludes determination of zygosity.

Birth Trauma

In the majority of cases a newborn is relatively unscathed by the birth process. However, sometimes transient and permanent stigmata of birth trauma are evident. Prompt identification of such injuries is important for good management and can also prevent inappropriate speculation, diagnostic testing, and treatment.

Caput Succedaneum

Normal transit of the fetal head through the birth canal induces molding of the skull and scalp edema, especially if labor is prolonged. The edema, which can be massive, is known as a *caput succedaneum* (Fig. 2-28). Much of this edema is present at birth and tends to overlie the occipital bones and portions of the parietal bones bilaterally. In some cases, bruising of the scalp may also be present (especially if a vacuum extractor was used). The presence of a caput requires no therapy, and spontaneous resolution within a few days is the rule. Distinguishing caput from a subgaleal (subaponeurotic) hematoma, a rare but serious complication of delivery, is important. A subgaleal hematoma is a collection of blood within scalp tissues extending beneath the epicranial aponeurosis. Palpation of a large caput succedaneum reveals firm nonpitting swelling. In contrast, the cranial swelling of subgaleal bleeding is boggy due to the palpation of clotted blood just beneath the epicranial aponeurosis (Fig. 2-29). The collection of

blood in this potential space can be quite large, and these infants must be followed for signs of hypovolemia. Serial exams which can include measurement of head circumference and hematocrit are important to identify ongoing blood loss.

Cephalhematoma

Often, confusion arises between the diagnosis of a caput and that of a cephalhematoma. The latter is a localized collection of blood beneath the periosteum of one of the calvarial bones; it may be bilateral, but is most often unilateral (Fig. 2-30). It is distinguished from a caput by the fact that its borders are limited by suture lines, usually those surrounding the parietal bones (see Fig. 2-29). However, diagnosis can be difficult in the immediate newborn period, when there may be overlying scalp edema. On palpation, the border may feel elevated and the center depressed. Most patients have an uncomplicated course of slow resolution over one or more months, although calcification may occur. Occasionally these infants may develop jaundice from the breakdown and resorption of the large hematoma. Underlying hairline skull fractures occur with some regularity but are rarely of clinical significance. The exception is the uncommon development of a leptomeningeal cyst. Radiologic investigation for an underlying depressed fracture is indicated in infants whose histories suggest significant trauma and those having depressed levels of consciousness *or* neurologic abnormalities on examination. Infection is another potentially serious but rare complication, which is more likely when the integrity of the overlying skin is broken.

Clavicle Fracture

Fracture of a clavicle can occur during delivery when the infant is large, in breech position, or if there is fetal distress requiring rapid extraction. If undisplaced, the fracture may not be painful, and the infant may be asymptomatic. The diagnosis may be suspected by palpation of crepitus or an asymmetrical Moro reflex. If there is pain or discomfort with routine handling, the fracture can be treated by immobilization of the ipsilateral limb and

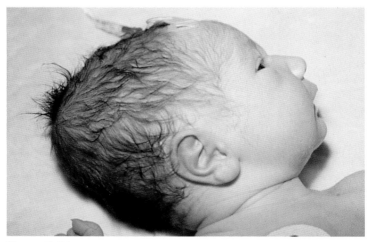

Figure 2-28. Caput succedaneum. This infant has significant scalp edema as a result of compression during transit through the birth canal. The edema crosses suture lines.

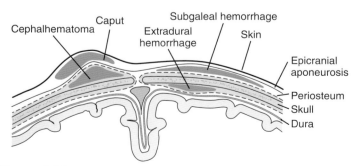

Figure 2-29. Sites of extracranial (and extradural) hemorrhages in the newborn. Schematic diagram of the important tissue planes from skin to dura. (Modified from Pape KE, Wigglesworth JS: Haemorrhage, Ischaemia and the Perinatal Brain. Philadelphia, JB Lippincott, 1979.)

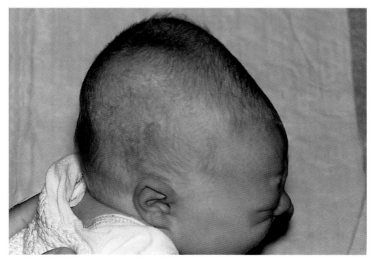

Figure 2-30. Cephalhematoma. In this infant with bilateral cephalhematomas, the midline sagittal suture remained palpable, confirming the subperiosteal location of the hematomas.

shoulder with the elbow flexed 90 degrees. Immobilization can be discontinued when a callus is palpable at 8 to 10 days. Many nondisplaced clavicle fractures are not diagnosed until the first newborn outpatient follow-up visit when you can palpate a large, firm callus along the clavicle. If the child has an otherwise normal physical and neurological examination at this time, a radiograph is not indicated. Radiographs would be indicated to help differentiate if decreased arm movement is secondary to pain (clavicle fracture) or nerve injury (Erb palsy).

Meconium Staining

Meconium is noted in the amniotic fluid in as many as 10% of deliveries. The meconium may have been recently expelled or may have been present in the amniotic fluid for hours or days. Because the timing of the passage of meconium may have significance for the diagnosis of fetal distress, it is useful to examine infants for the presence of meconium staining. It takes at least 4 to 6 hours of contact before staining of the umbilicus, skin, and nails occurs (Fig. 2-31). Often, the meconium-stained infant is postmature and has diffuse peeling of the skin and a shriveled, stained umbilical cord.

Bruises and Petechiae

Superficial bruising can occur when delivery is difficult. This is relatively common with breech presentations (Fig. 2-32) and can include swelling and discoloration of the labia or scrotum (to be distinguished from an incarcerated inguinal hernia). When bruises are extensive, significant secondary jaundice may develop as the extravasated blood is broken down and resorbed. In an infant in whom a nuchal cord is found at delivery, the presence of diffuse petechiae around the head and neck is common and does not warrant further investigation. In addition, petechiae found on the presenting body part are normal. The appearance of new bruises or petechiae after delivery should alert the physician and nurse to the possibility of a bleeding disorder or infection.

Fat Necrosis

Many infants delivered with the aid of forceps show forceps marks after delivery. These marks tend to fade over 24 to 48 hours. Occasionally, a well-circumscribed, firm nodule with purplish discoloration may appear at the site of a forceps mark. This may represent fat necrosis (Fig. 2-33) and resolves spontaneously over weeks to months. The phenomenon may also occur at other sites of trauma.

Nasal Deformities

Abnormalities of the nose are common after delivery, the majority consisting of transient flattening or twisting induced during transit through the birth canal. Less than 1% of nasal deformities are due to actual dislocations of the triangular cartilage of the nasal septum. These can be differentiated from positional deformities by manually moving the septum to the midline and observing the resultant shape of the nares. In a true dislocation, marked asymmetry of the nares persists (Fig. 2-34). Returning the

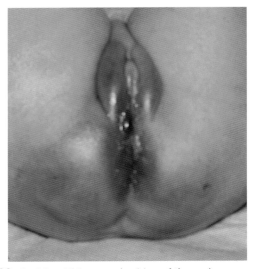

Figure 2-32. Bruising. This severe bruising of the perineum was the result of a difficult breech labor and delivery.

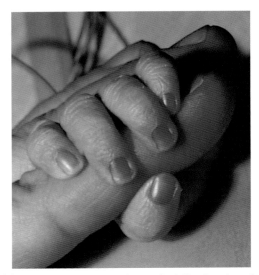

Figure 2-31. Meconium staining. The marked discoloration of this infant's fingernails resulted from long-standing meconium staining of the amniotic fluid before delivery.

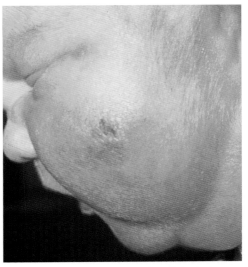

Figure 2-33. Fat necrosis. This discolored nodular lesion on the cheek is characteristic of subcutaneous necrosis of fat secondary to forceps trauma.

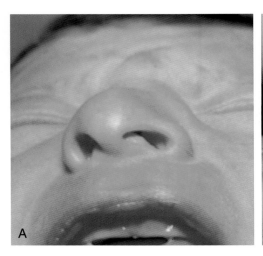

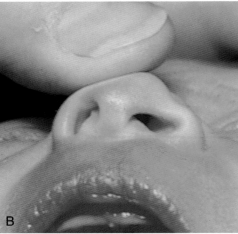

Figure 2-34. Nasal deformity. This infant incurred dislocation of the triangular cartilage of the nasal septum during delivery. Inspection of the nose reveals deviation of the septum to the right and asymmetry of the nares **(A)**. When the septum is manually moved toward the midline, the asymmetry persists, confirming the dislocation **(B)**.

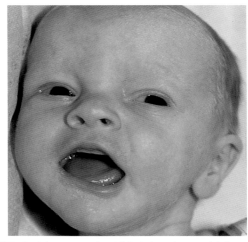

Figure 2-35. Facial nerve palsy. This infant incurred injury to the right facial nerve, resulting in loss of the nasolabial fold on the affected side and asymmetrical movement of the mouth. The side of the mouth that appears to droop is the normal side.

septum to its proper position can be accomplished in the nursery with the guidance of an otolaryngologist. Failure to recognize and treat dislocation may lead to permanent deformity.

Peripheral Nerve Damage

Injury to the peripheral nervous system, especially the facial and brachial nerves, is one of the more common serious occurrences related to birth. Unilateral facial nerve palsy is the most common peripheral nerve injury, with an incidence as high as 1.4 per 1000 live births. Injury can result from direct trauma from forceps or from compression of the nerve against the sacral promontory while the head is in the birth canal. With pronounced nerve injury, there is decreased facial movement and forehead wrinkling on the side of the palsy, eyelid elevation, and flattening of the nasolabial folds and corner of the mouth (Fig. 2-35). Crying accentuates the findings, with the most obvious sign being asymmetrical movement of the mouth. The side that appears to droop when crying is the normal side. The differential diagnosis includes Möbius syndrome (usually bilateral) and absence of the depressor anguli oris muscle, which may be associated with cardiac anomalies. The latter condition is distinguishable from facial nerve

palsy by the absence of involvement of the forehead, eyelid, or nasolabial area. The prognosis for facial nerve palsies is excellent, and recovery usually occurs within the first month. In the meantime, prevention of corneal drying is essential. Surgery is reserved for cases in which clear-cut severing of the facial nerve has occurred. Referral should be made if there is no improvement after 2 to 3 months.

The incidence of brachial plexus trauma with current obstetric management is approximately 0.7 per 1000 live births. The mechanism of injury in most instances is traction on the plexus during delivery. Although lesions have classically been divided into those affecting upper spinal segments (Erb palsy) and those affecting lower segments (Klumpke palsy), the distinction may not be clear-cut in some cases. Injury to the C5 and C6 fibers is most often identified by the child's arm hanging limply adducted and internally rotated at the shoulder and extended and pronated at the elbow (Fig. 2-36A). Injury affecting the lower segments of C7 and T1 rarely occurs in isolation, causing weakness of the wrist and hand, and ultimately leads to a claw-hand deformity (Fig. 2-36B, C). There may be sensory loss along the ulnar side of the hand and forearm in the distribution of the T1 dermatome. If the T1 root is affected with interruption of the sympathetic innervation at that level, Horner syndrome may be apparent. Appropriate deep-tendon reflexes are absent. It may be difficult to confirm sensory deficit, and autonomic fibers are often intact. Diagnosis is made clinically, but electromyography may be indicated to assess the severity of the injury and determine the prognosis in patients not showing improvement after 6 to 8 weeks. Treatment should be deferred for at least 7 to 10 days; then specific physical therapy and splinting should be undertaken. Most infants with brachial plexus palsies demonstrate complete recovery in the first few months of life. Earlier recovery suggests better long-term prognosis.

Congenital Anomalies

Innumerable congenital anomalies, many of a minor nature, can be noted at birth. Although any single minor malformation may be of little medical consequence, the identification of three or more in a single infant may be a clue to more serious errors of morphogenesis. A careful family history including examination of the parents and siblings can often place these malformations in proper perspective.

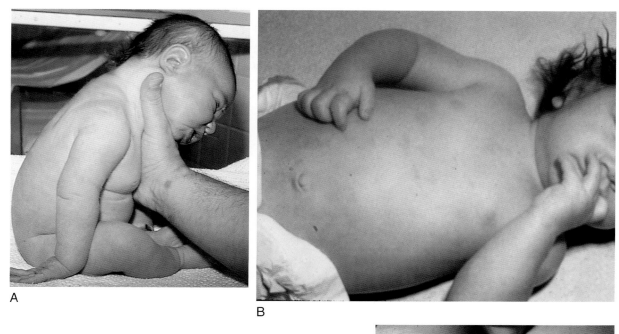

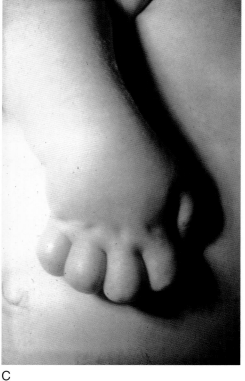

Figure 2-36. Brachial plexus injury. **A,** Traction injury to C5, C6, and C7 spinal cord segments produces this (Erb) palsy. This infant demonstrates the characteristic posture of the limply adducted and internally rotated arm. **B** and **C,** Infant with a Klumpke palsy involving lower segments of C7 and T1. Note the different posture of the arm compared with the Erb palsy and the claw-hand deformity. (**B** and **C** Courtesy of Dr. Michael Painter, Children's Hospital of Pittsburgh.)

Hands and Feet

The majority of minor external anomalies involve the hands, feet, and head. One of the more common abnormalities of digitation, especially in African American infants, is the presence of a supernumerary digit (Fig. 2-37), which is most often located lateral to the fifth digit on the hand or foot. This condition is distinguishable from true polydactyly because of the small pedicle that attaches the extra digit to the fifth digit. The supernumerary digit may have a fingernail but often lacks bones. Although usually of no consequence, a supernumerary digit has, on occasion, been associated with major central nervous system (CNS) malformations. Removal may be accomplished by applying a ligature around the pedicle

(assuming that it is thin and lacks palpable bony tissue) as close as possible to the surface of the fifth digit and allowing for the extra digit to fall off naturally. This usually takes approximately 1 week. Care should be taken to observe for infection.

True polydactyly (duplication of digits) may also be seen (Fig. 2-38). It is most common on the feet but can also occur on the hands. A family history of this anomaly may exist, or it may occur in association with other, more serious patterns of malformation. Although removal is not required, it may be indicated cosmetically.

Syndactyly, fusion of the soft tissues between digits, is relatively common (Fig. 2-39). Once again, a family history can be helpful to determine association with other anomalies. Surgical correction of the syndactylism is usually

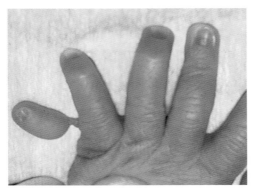

Figure 2-37. Supernumerary digit. This is the common position for a sixth digit. The thin pedicle distinguishes this anomaly from true polydactyly.

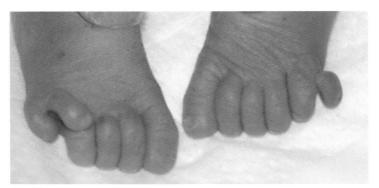

Figure 2-38. Polydactyly. True bilateral polydactyly of the fifth toe is seen in this infant.

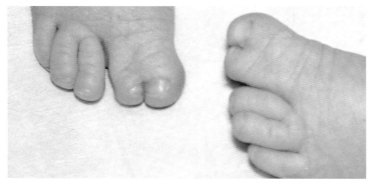

Figure 2-39. Syndactyly. This child demonstrates bilateral fusion of the soft tissue between the first and second toes.

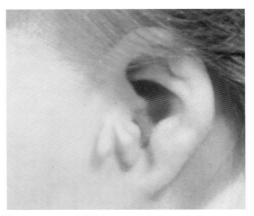

Figure 2-40. Ear tags. Multiple preauricular skin tags were seen as an isolated finding in this patient.

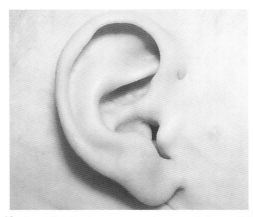

Figure 2-41. Aural fistula. A pronounced congenital ear pit is seen anterior to the tragus. Its only significance is that it may become infected.

postponed until 3 years of age unless there is a synchondrosis (cartilaginous union) or synostosis (bony union) that may interfere with growth.

Palmar creases occur as a consequence of flexion of the thickened skin of the hand. Alterations in folding of the palmar plane may be affected by the slope of the 3rd, 4th, and 5th metacarpal-phalangeal joints or relative shortness of the palm. A single, unilateral, midposition plane of flexion, *single palmar crease,* is found in 4% of the population (bilateral in 1% of the population).

External Ear

Careful morphologic examination of the external ear may reveal a number of minor anomalies. One of the more common is the presence of preauricular skin tags located anterior to the tragus (Fig. 2-40). These tags may be uni-

lateral or bilateral and represent remnants of the first branchial arch. Although often of little consequence, they may be seen in serious malformations of branchial arch development involving multiple structures of the head and neck. Surgical removal may be indicated for cosmetic purposes.

A second, often overlooked malformation is the presence of ear pits or congenital aural fistulas located anterior to the tragus (Fig. 2-41). These may be familial, occur twice as often in girls, and are more common in African Americans. They are of little consequence beyond the fact that they may become infected.

Midline Defects

Although major malformations of the spinal column, such as myelomeningocele, are readily identifiable (see Chapter 15), diagnostic differentiation between two other midline defects—pilonidal sinuses and congenital dermal sinuses of the lumbar and sacral spine—can be difficult. A pilonidal sinus tends to be located over the sacrum (Fig. 2-42). The surface opening is usually larger than that of a dermal sinus, but the tract rarely extends into the spinal canal; therefore although infection can occur, CNS extension is unlikely. A congenital dermal sinus is usually located over the lower lumbar region, with a sinus tract that can extend farther down the spinal column. The external orifice may be a small dimple or an easily visible opening surrounded by hair. Recognition is important because there may be an underlying spinal dysraphism,

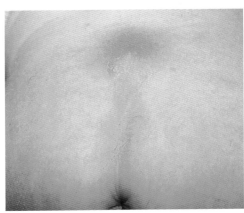

Figure 2-42. Pilonidal sinus. This midline sinus overlying the sacrum did not extend to the spinal cord.

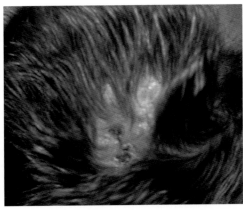

Figure 2-44. Localized ectodermal dysplasia. An extensive punched-out area lacking all normal dermal elements is seen in the midline of the scalp of this child with trisomy 13.

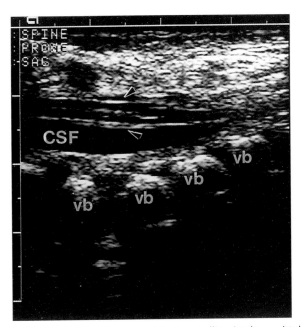

Figure 2-43. Transducer is centered in the midline in the sagittal plane over the lower lumbar spine. The lumbar spinal cord (arrowheads) extends into the sacral portion of the spinal canal and is dorsally displaced. The conus terminate at the approximate level of S2. CSF, cerebrospinal fluid; vb, vertebral body. (Courtesy A'Delbert Bowen, MD, Children's Hospital of Pittsburgh.)

and infection of the tract can extend to the CNS. These abnormalities can herald an occult tethered spinal cord, which may occur with minimal or no neurologic signs. Failure to recognize the possible association of these cutaneous abnormalities with an occult tethered cord could result in later neurologic abnormalities including foot and lower extremity deformities, decreased sensation, weakness, abnormal gait, and bladder dysfunction. Diagnosis can be made by ultrasound, optimally in the newborn period because the acoustic window gets smaller as the child grows (Fig. 2-43).

Another form of midline defect may occur over the posterior parietal scalp and consists of a localized area of ectodermal dysplasia (Fig. 2-44). This lesion appears "punched out" and lacks all normal dermal elements. It may be associated with chromosomal anomalies, especially trisomy 13, but may be present in otherwise normal infants. Similar lesions, often located on the extremities, should be distinguished from those on the scalp because they often represent a dermatologic defect known as *cutis aplasia*.

Congenital Hip Dislocation

Congenital hip dislocation occurs six times more frequently in females than in males, with an overall incidence of 1.5 in 1000 live births. Associated factors include breech presentation, oligohydramnios, and first-born infants. The pathologic anatomy involves superior capsular laxity and a shallow acetabulum due to limited concentric contact with the femoral head. The key diagnostic sign on physical examination of the newborn is hip instability with the capacity for hip dislocation and subsequent relocation. Only one hip should be examined at a time. Examining both hips simultaneously may impair proprioception such that soft tissue "clicks," due to movement of fascia over the greater trochanter, may be mistaken for the dull "clunk" of dislocation. In experienced hands the diagnosis can easily be confirmed by ultrasonography, which is a sensitive procedure for detecting hip dysplasia (Fig. 2-45) in the immediate newborn period. Screening ultrasound, however, should not be performed before 2 weeks of life because physiologic laxity of the ligaments may result in a high false-positive rate. Ideally, orthopedic consultation for treatment should be obtained within the first 6 months of life.

Amniotic Bands

A number of serious structural deformations can result from early in utero amniotic rupture and subsequent bandline compression or amputation. The band-induced abnormalities generally affect the limbs, digits, and craniofacial structures (Fig. 2-46). This phenomenon is usually sporadic.

Umbilical Hernia

An umbilical hernia is a common finding, especially in African American infants (Fig. 2-47). The incidence of this defect of the central fascia beneath the umbilicus is also higher in premature infants and those with congenital thyroid deficiency. Distinguishing between this relatively benign fascial defect and the more serious defects of the somites that form the peritoneal, muscular, and ectodermal layers of the abdominal wall underlying the umbilicus, resulting in an omphalocele, is important. In the

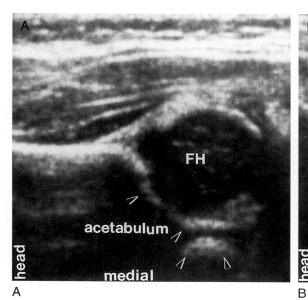

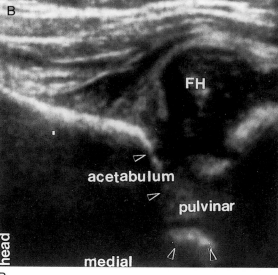

Figure 2-45. Coronal flexion images with the transducer over the posterolateral aspect of the hip joint, centered on the femoral head (FH). **A,** Normal cartilaginous femoral head is shown well-seated in the acetabulum *(arrowheads)*. **B,** Congenital dislocation with the femoral head markedly subluxed laterally and the invagination of fatty tissue (pulvinar) that occupies the space between the femoral head and the acetabulum *(arrowheads)*. (Courtesy A'Delbert Bowen, MD, Children's Hospital of Pittsburgh.)

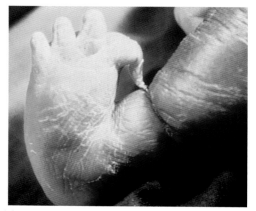

Figure 2-46. Amniotic bands. A lower extremity amniotic band caused amputation of the toes and constriction around the lower leg.

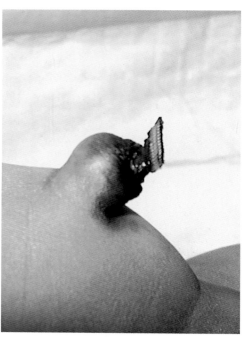

Figure 2-47. Umbilical hernia. This prominent umbilical hernia was noted at birth in an otherwise normal African American infant.

latter condition, a portion of the intestine is located outside the abdominal wall (see Chapter 17). When large, the distinction is obvious, but in its mildest form, an omphalocele resembles a fixed hernia of the umbilicus. True umbilical hernias usually require no therapy, and spontaneous resolution occurs within the first few years of life. Those that remain after the age of 3 years can be surgically repaired. Attempts to reduce the hernia with tape or coins are ineffective and may result in side effects such as adhesive reaction/allergy. Incarceration is rare.

Scrotal Swelling

Swelling of the scrotum in the neonate is relatively common, especially in breech deliveries. Although the differential diagnosis includes hematomas, infections, testicular torsion, and tumors, the majority of cases are attributable to hydroceles or fluid accumulation in the tunica vaginalis. Palpation reveals an extremely smooth, firm, egg-shaped mass that brightly transilluminates (Fig. 2-48). When the hydrocele is noncommunicating, the clinician can often palpate above the mass with the thumb and finger and feel a normal spermatic cord. The testicle

may be difficult to palpate but is usually visible on transillumination. With inguinal hernias, the prolapsed intestine may transilluminate as well, but it usually presents visible septa under high-intensity light. Furthermore, on palpation there is significant thickening of the spermatic cord. Although a hydrocele may persist for months, the majority resolve spontaneously. There is a high association with inguinal hernias, especially in hydroceles that persist. In such cases the spermatic cord is often noticeably thickened. Given the association with hernias, the possibility of bowel incarceration should be kept in mind. Surgical repair is indicated when a hydrocele persists for more than 6 months or when it is associated with findings suggestive of an inguinal hernia such as a communicating hydrocele. These hydroceles will randomly appear to get smaller and larger over time. (See Chapter 17 for a more detailed discussion of inguinal hernias.)

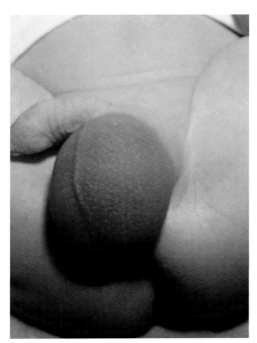

Figure 2-48. Scrotal swelling. This infant demonstrates a unilateral hydrocele that was noted at birth. Transillumination was consistent with the diagnosis.

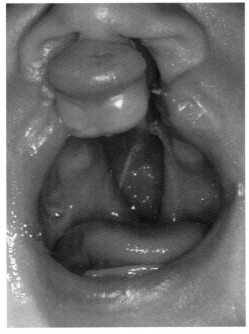

Figure 2-49. Cleft lip. A prominent bilateral cleft lip with a complete cleft palate is seen in an infant with trisomy 13. The cleft extends from the soft to the hard palate, exposing the nasal cavity.

Oral Clefts

Cleft lip and palate are among the most common facial anomalies (Fig. 2-49). These defects represent failure of lip fusion (at 35 days' gestation) and, in some cases, subsequent failure of closure of the palatal shelves (at 8 to 9 weeks' gestation). Although many cases occur spontaneously, others appear to be inherited, and in a minority of instances the defect is one manifestation of a chromosomal disorder. Adequate assessment necessitates careful examination of all structures of the head and neck and their relationship to each other. For example, cleft palate

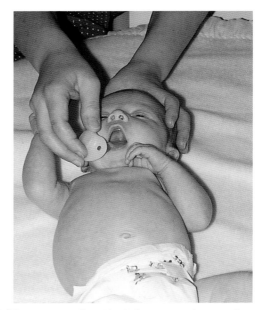

Figure 2-50. Rooting reflex. The infant opens the mouth and turns the head toward the pacifier stimulating the cheek.

may be coupled with mandibular hypoplasia (Pierre Robin sequence), resulting in significant respiratory obstruction. Because of associated eustachian tube dysfunction, otitis media is an almost invariable complication of cleft palate. Specialized feeding techniques are often necessary for these infants. Even in the absence of an overt cleft, palpation and visualization of the palate and uvula should be routine because clefts of the soft palate (associated with a bifid uvula and a midline notch at the posterior border of the hard palate) can lead to later speech problems (see Chapters 22 and 23).

Primitive Reflexes

Normal newborns exhibit a large number of easily elicited primitive reflexes that are often altered or absent in the infant with neurologic impairment. These reflexes may be transiently depressed in the infant who has experienced difficulty in achieving the transition between intrauterine and extrauterine existence. The persistent absence or asymmetry of one or more of these reflexes may be a clue to the potential presence of neuromuscular abnormalities requiring further investigation (see Chapter 3).

The rooting reflex may be elicited by lightly stimulating the infant's cheek and observing the reflexive attempts to bring the stimulating object to the mouth (Fig. 2-50). The sucking reflex is activated by placing an object in the infant's mouth and observing the sucking movements (Fig. 2-51). In the grasp reflex (Figs. 2-52 and 2-53), transverse stimulation of the midpalm (without touching the back of the hand) or midsole leads to flexion of the digits or toes around the examiner's fingers.

The Moro reflex (Fig. 2-54) evaluates vestibular maturation and the relationship between flexor and extensor tone. Elicitation of the reflex involves a short (10 cm), sudden drop of the head when the infant is supine. The full response involves extension of the arms, "fanning" of the fingers, and then upper extremity flexion followed by a cry. An incomplete but identifiable reflex becomes apparent at approximately 32 weeks' gestation, and by 38 weeks it is essentially complete. Very immature infants

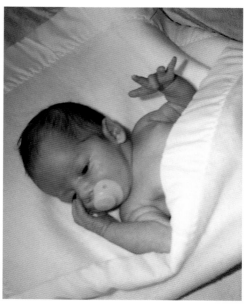

Figure 2-51. Sucking reflex. Vigorous sucking movements are initiated when an object is placed in the infant's mouth.

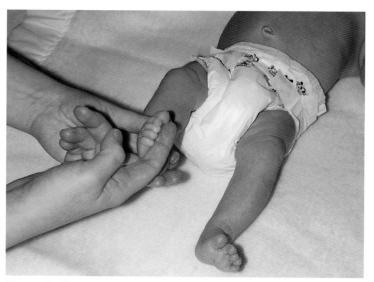

Figure 2-53. Grasp reflex (sole). Transverse stimulation of the midsole triggers a grasp by the infant.

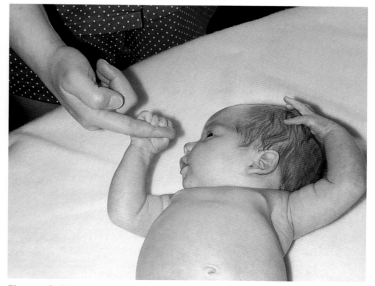

Figure 2-52. Grasp reflex (palm). Transverse stimulation of the midpalm leads to a grasp by the infant.

demonstrate extension of the arms and fingers but do not show true flexion or make a sustained cry. Marked asymmetry of response may be associated with focal neurologic impairment.

These reflexes and a host of other less commonly used reflexes are termed *primitive* because they are present at or shortly after birth and normally disappear after the first few months of life. Just as their absence may indicate neurologic impairment at birth, their abnormal persistence may also be a cause for concern and further evaluation.

Respiratory Distress

The differential diagnosis and the subsequent management of the infant with respiratory distress are the most frequent challenges encountered by the practitioner of newborn medicine. Problems posed by prematurity, the

failure of the necessary transition to extrauterine existence, infectious complications, metabolic derangements, and various congenital and acquired abnormalities of the cardiopulmonary system may all lead to a similar presentation in the newborn period.

Infants with respiratory distress may present with tachypnea or cyanosis (Fig. 2-55), or both, and varying degrees of a triad of signs, which include *grunting, flaring,* and *retractions (GFR)*. *Grunting* is a characteristic involuntary guttural expiratory sound made by infants as they exhale against a closed glottis in an attempt to maintain expiratory lung volume. *Flaring* refers to the reflexive opening of the nares during inspiration (Fig. 2-56). *Retractions* are the result of increased respiratory effort with high negative intrathoracic pressures leading to an inward collapse of the relatively compliant chest wall of the newborn during inspiration (Fig. 2-57).

Classic respiratory distress syndrome (RDS) is caused by a combination of lung immaturity secondary to preterm delivery and surfactant deficiency. The radiographic findings (Fig. 2-58) in such infants consist of a ground-glass appearance (small airway and alveolar atelectasis) and "air bronchograms" (an outline of the large airways superimposed on the relatively airless lung parenchyma). Infants with RDS usually need supplemental oxygen therapy and often require mechanical ventilatory assistance.

Most infants with RDS recover without sequelae. However, a small proportion develop a chronic lung condition known as *bronchopulmonary dysplasia*. Histologically, this condition is characterized by varying degrees of inflammation and fibrosis (Fig. 2-59). The chest x-ray studies of such infants exhibit areas of hyperinflation alternating with atelectasis (Fig. 2-60).

The most common cause of respiratory distress in term infants is transient tachypnea of the newborn (TTN). Thought to be related to the delayed removal of fetal lung fluid, this condition is more common in infants born by cesarean section. Radiographic findings may include streaky perihilar shadows caused by dilated lymphatics or visible fluid densities within the intralobar fissures (Fig. 2-61), or both. As its name implies, TTN resolves over time, usually with minimal supportive care.

Unfortunately for the clinician, the early clinical and radiographic findings in infants with potentially life-threatening congenital pneumonias may mimic those

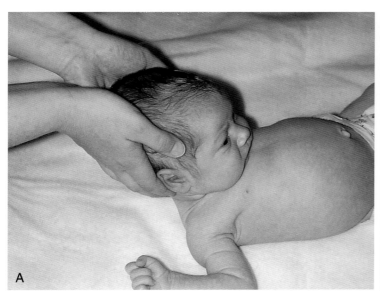

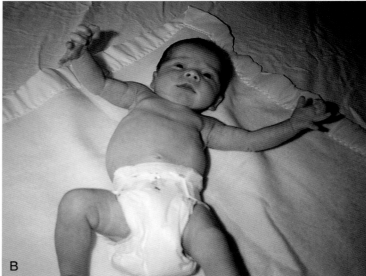

Figure 2-54. Moro reflex. **A,** To elicit the reflex, the head is supported and allowed to drop to the level of the bed. The initial extension response to vestibular stimulation is shown in **B.** The complete response includes secondary flexion and cry.

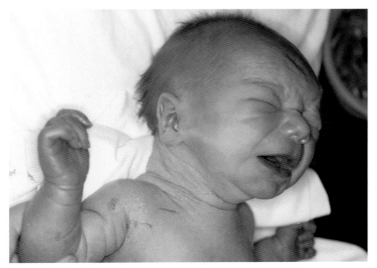

Figure 2-55. Cyanosis. This critically ill infant exhibits cyanosis and poor skin perfusion.

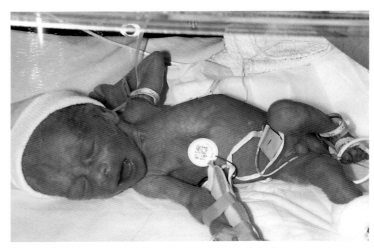

Figure 2-57. Retractions. The inward collapse of the lower anterior chest wall can be seen in this premature infant with respiratory distress syndrome.

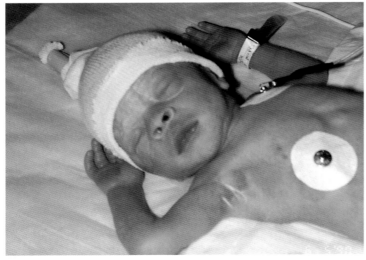

Figure 2-56. Flaring. Reflexive widening of the nares may be seen in infants with respiratory distress.

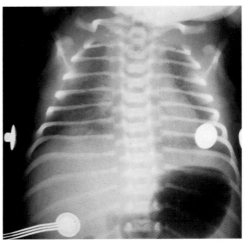

Figure 2-58. Respiratory distress syndrome. Note the ground-glass appearance and the presence of air bronchograms.

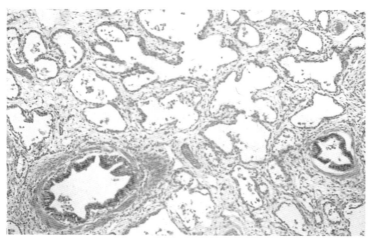

Figure 2-59. Bronchopulmonary dysplasia. Histologic features include inflammation and fibrosis.

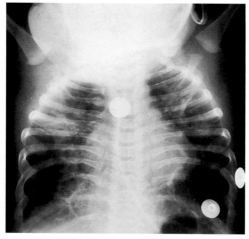

Figure 2-60. Bronchopulmonary dysplasia. Note the alternating areas of hyperinflation and atelectasis.

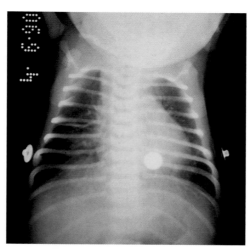

Figure 2-61. Transient tachypnea of the newborn. Radiograph reveals a number of streaky perihilar densities and a visible fluid density in the right major fissure.

seen in RDS or TTN (Fig. 2-62). This diagnostic uncertainty leads to early treatment with antibiotics until bacterial cultures, serial chest radiographs, and clinical improvements reassure the practitioner that the discontinuation of such antibiotics is warranted.

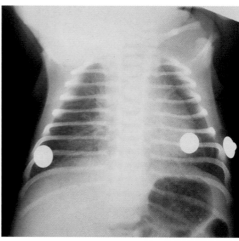

Figure 2-62. Congenital pneumonia. Cultures from the lungs of this infant were positive for group B streptococci. Note the similarity to Figure 2-61, with streaky perihilar densities and visible fluid density in the right major fissure.

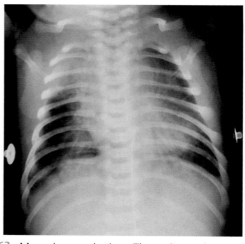

Figure 2-63. Meconium aspiration. The radiograph reveals irregularly distributed areas of hyperaeration and consolidation.

Meconium aspiration elicits an inflammatory response within the lungs and may also present as respiratory distress. The radiographic findings consist of irregularly distributed areas of hyperaeration and consolidation throughout the lung parenchyma (Fig. 2-63).

Congenital heart disease (see Chapter 5) and various anomalies of the thoracic cavity or lungs (see Chapter 16) also commonly manifest in the newborn with signs of respiratory distress and should be included in the differential diagnosis.

Newborn Stools

An infant's first few bowel movements consist of accumulated intestinal cells, bile, and proteinaceous material formed during intestinal development. The material, termed *meconium* (Fig. 2-64), is a sticky greenish black product mirroring the shape of the fetal intestine. When passed into the amniotic fluid before delivery, it can, if aspirated into the lung, cause an inflammatory pneumonitis. Early passage of meconium is generally precipitated by fetal distress or asphyxia. Failure to pass meconium in the first 2 days of life may indicate intestinal obstruction resulting from stenosis, atresia, or Hirschsprung disease.

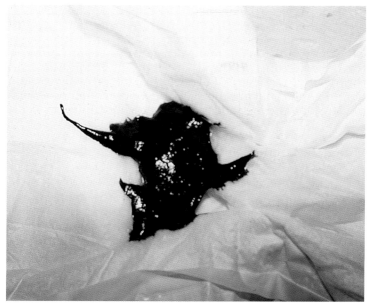

Figure 2-64. Meconium. A typical, sticky, greenish black meconium stool consists of accumulated intestinal cells, bile, and proteinaceous material formed during intestinal development.

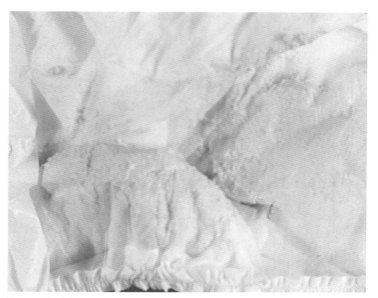

Figure 2-66. Breast-milk stool. The stools of breast-fed infants are usually yellow, soft, and mild-smelling and typically have the consistency of pea soup. Breast milk stools can also be watery.

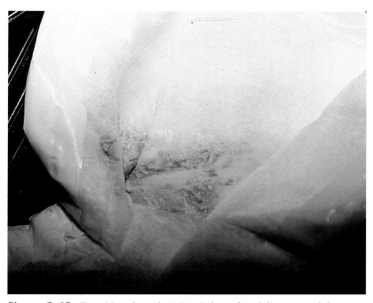

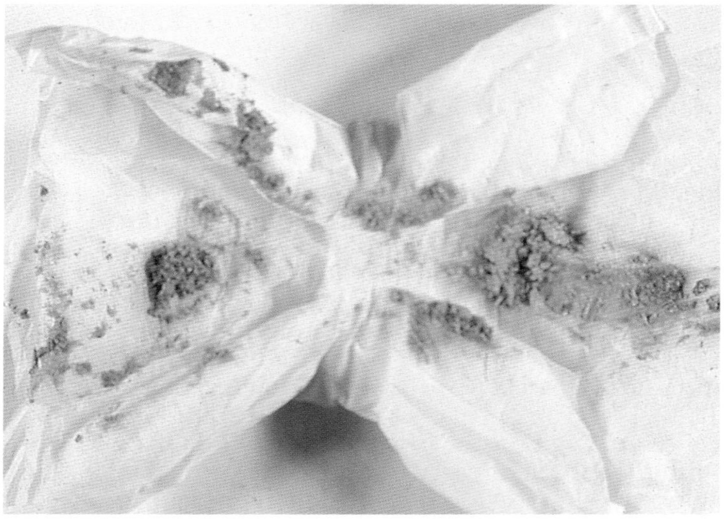

Figure 2-65. Transitional stool. At 2 to 3 days after delivery, stools become greenish brown and may contain some milk curds.

Figure 2-67. Formula stool. Infants fed commercial formulas typically have darker, firmer stools than breast-fed infants.

The possibility of cystic fibrosis with a meconium ileus should also be considered. In premature infants, failure to pass meconium may reflect meconium plug syndrome (small left colon syndrome), which appears to be a disorder of maturation of intestinal motility. In most cases a Gastrografin enema leads to prompt passage of meconium without recurrence.

By the third day of life, stools change in character and become known as *transitional* stools (Fig. 2-65). They are greenish brown to yellowish brown, are less sticky than meconium, and may contain some milk curds. In some infants who are fed generous quantities of milk during the first few days, the stool may have an increased liquid component that contains undigested sugar. This diarrheal stool resolves with moderation in the quantity of feeding because it is caused by the osmotic effect of undigested lactose.

After the third to fourth day, the quality and frequency of stool are often functions of the type of milk ingested. Breast-fed infants have stools that are yellow to golden, mild smelling, and vary from pasty to watery in consistency (Fig. 2-66). Infants fed commercial formulas have pale yellow to light brown stools that are firm and somewhat more offensive in odor (Fig. 2-67). A wide range of normal stool frequency exists in formula-fed neonates. Many infants have a stool after each feeding for the first several weeks, which is due to an active gastrocolic reflex; other infants may have one stool every few days. Breast-fed infants should have at least six stools per day by the third day of life, and this should persist for the first few weeks of life. Infrequent passage of stool in the breast-fed infant is a sign of inadequate feeding in the first weeks of life.

A careful history, with emphasis on an infant's stool pattern, feeding history, and any parental attempts (laxatives, rectal manipulation) to induce bowel movements, can be extremely important. Normal weight gain in the presence of true diarrhea is unusual. Difficulty passing stools (straining, crying, decreased frequency) may reflect local irritation from anal fissure formation rather than true constipation. Constipation is defined by hard pellet stools rather than frequency. The use of a topical lubricant and stool softeners can be recommended to resolve constipation. Failure of such measures suggests the possibility of a significant pathologic condition (see Chapter 17 for further discussion).

Breastfeeding

Breast milk is the optimal food for almost all infants in the first year of life. In 2003, 71% of women initiated breastfeeding, but only 36% were still feeding their infant any breast milk at 6 months compared with the national public health objectives of 75% and 50%, respectively. Health care providers play an important role in a woman's decision to breast-feed and can also have a significant impact on a woman's success with breastfeeding. Therefore it is important that health care providers learn about breastfeeding in order to provide appropriate support and information. Providers should know the benefits of breastfeeding, the normal patterns of feeding, elimination, and growth, and be able to assist a woman with latch, positioning, and commonly encountered breastfeeding problems.

Breast milk is biologically complex, species specific, and serves both as a source of nutrition and immunological support for the developing infant. It contains hundreds of bioactive substances including entire white blood cells (e.g., macrophages, T cells, B cells, and neutrophils); proteins such as immunoglobulins (IgA, D, G, M) and immune-modulating factors (e.g., lactoferrin, lysozyme, lactoperoxidase); hormones (e.g., thyrotropin-releasing hormone, thyroxine, cortisol, insulin-like growth factor 1); growth factors (e.g., epidermal growth factor, human-milk growth factors I, II, III); enzymes; and cholesterol. These bioactive agents, which are not found in commercially prepared formulas, augment the infant's immature immune system. Breast milk changes during feedings and across time in order to meet the changing nutritional and immunological needs of infants.

Breast milk provides both immediate and long-term benefits to infants. Breast-fed infants have a decreased risk of gastroenteritis, respiratory tract infections, urinary tract infections, and serious bacterial infections. Data suggest that breastfeeding also reduces the risk of childhood diseases after weaning including type I diabetes mellitus, Crohn's disease, juvenile rheumatoid arthritis, lymphoma, allergies, and others. Mothers also benefit from breastfeeding. Women who breast-feed have less postpartum bleeding, more rapid involution of the gravid uterus, earlier return to their prepregnancy figure, and possibly decreased risk of ovarian cancer, breast cancer, and osteoporosis.

Research has shown that women usually choose an infant feeding method before or in the first trimester of pregnancy but that their obstetrician and a prenatal visit with a pediatrician can affect this decision. Therefore it is essential that the benefits of breastfeeding be discussed in the early reproductive years and reinforced early in pregnancy in order to increase the rates of breastfeeding. The benefits of breastfeeding can be discussed in multiple settings, such as school-based education, family planning and obstetric clinics, prenatal visits, and public health campaigns. Health care providers can help a mother-baby dyad succeed at breastfeeding by providing both clinical expertise and emotional support.

The role of the pediatric health care provider in supporting breastfeeding begins at either the prenatal visit or in the newborn nursery. The health care provider should obtain a maternal and birth history, observe a breastfeeding session, and provide appropriate education.

Prenatal Maternal History

During a prenatal visit or at the time of delivery, a pediatric health care provider should ask a woman a few key questions to make sure that breastfeeding is feasible and appropriate. Women should be asked if they have experienced the normal breast changes of pregnancy, that is, breast enlargement, darkening of the areola, and increased prominence of the Montgomery glands around the areola. These breast changes in the first and second trimesters of pregnancy are reassuring that the breasts are preparing for lactation. When these breast changes do not occur, it is important to closely monitor breastfeeding and watch for signs of inadequate milk production. Although rare, some women may have insufficient glandular tissue (Fig. 2-68A and B) that is associated with insufficient milk supply, resulting in an inability to exclusively breast-feed. However, most of these women can breast-feed and supplement with formula.

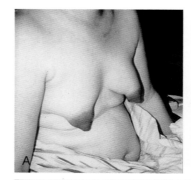
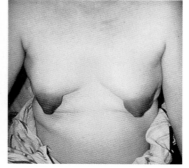
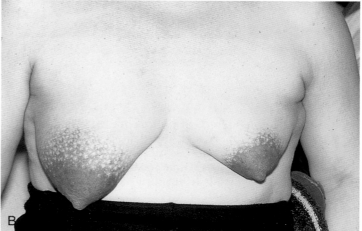

Figure 2-68. Insufficient breast glandular tissue. Tubular breast shape, little to no breast enlargement, and little areolar darkening with pregnancy may indicate insufficient glandular tissue. There is often a family history of inadequate milk supply. Women with this condition may benefit from a referral to a lactation consultant. **A,** A 26-hour postpartum woman with tubular-shaped breasts without any fullness. **B,** A woman with insufficient glandular tissue and significantly different breast size who has insufficient milk supply. (Courtesy Susan Costanza, RN, IBCLC, Rochester General Hospital, Rochester, NY.)

Breast size is not associated with breastfeeding success. Breast reduction surgery can negatively affect a woman's ability to exclusively breast-feed her infant because of disruption of nerves and milk ducts. However, newer surgical techniques result in fewer problems and therefore women who have had breast reduction surgery should be encouraged to try breastfeeding. Augmentation does not usually affect breastfeeding success, although excessively large implants could interfere. Women who have had breast surgery should be followed closely in the first few weeks after delivery for evidence of low milk supply and inadequate infant weight gain.

Most, but not all, medications are safe to take during lactation. The American Academy of Pediatrics publishes a policy statement, *The Transfer of Drugs and Other Chemicals into Human Milk,* which summarizes current information on the safety of medication use during pregnancy. Another resource is *Medications and Mother's Milk,* by Thomas Hale, which is updated and published every 2 to 3 years and provides up-to-date information about medication use during lactation. Women with some infections (e.g., HIV, untreated tuberculosis) and women who use illicit drugs should not breast-feed. Mothers who smoke tobacco should be encouraged to smoke outside and to decrease cigarette use or preferably to stop smoking. Because nicotine readily passes into breast milk, at a minimum, women who smoke should be told to do so after feedings to minimize the transfer of nicotine into breast milk.

Special breast care is not necessary to prepare for lactation. Women should be instructed to avoid the use of soap and lotions on the breast toward the end of pregnancy because they interfere with the natural lubricants and scents produced by the breast. Nipple manipulation and scrubbing should be discouraged because of the potential for inducing preterm labor.

Breastfeeding Evaluation

Pediatric health care providers should be comfortable observing and assisting women with breastfeeding, especially during the neonatal period, the first health maintenance examination, and when problems arise such as poor weight gain or painful nursing. A thorough evaluation includes a history, examination of the mother's breasts, observation of the latch, and positioning and assessment of milk transfer. Some health care providers may find it more comfortable to perform the physical examination of the maternal breast with a chaperone, as is done with examinations of the genitalia.

History. The history should be appropriate for the visit. At the neonatal and first postpartum visits it should include pregnancy and birth history, frequency, duration and pattern of nursing, frequency of voids, frequency and character of stools, weight change, jaundice, pain with nursing, and maternal concerns. See American Academy of Pediatrics Task Force on Breastfeeding, Breastfeeding Health Supervision for a visit-by-visit assessment.

Breast Examination. If a woman is having difficulty latching the baby in the neonatal period or she complains of pain at any time, her breasts should be examined. For latching problems, it is important to determine if a woman has flat or inverted nipples. Nipple inspection alone does not answer this question, and the pinch test must be performed (Fig. 2-69). The nipple is normally everted if the nipple protrudes when the areola is compressed, inverted when it retracts toward the breast when the areola is

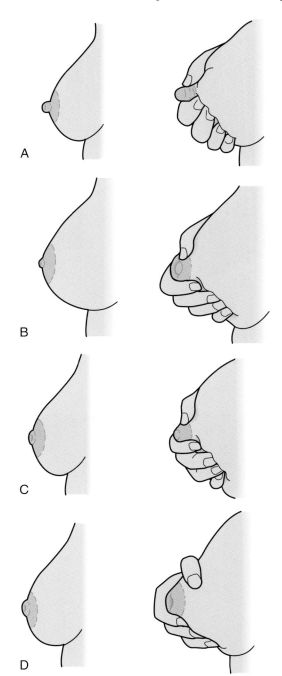

Figure 2-69. Nipple evaluation with the pinch test. **A,** Protracting normal nipple. **B,** Moderate to severe retraction. **C,** Inverted-appearing nipple, which, when compressed using the pinch test, either inverts farther inward or protracts forward. **D,** True inversion: nipple inverts further using pinch test. (Reprinted with permission from Riordan J, Auerbach K [eds]: Breastfeeding and Human Lactation, 2nd ed. Sudbury, Mass, Jones and Bartlett Publishers, 1999, p 99; www.jbpub.com)

squeezed, and flat when it neither protrudes nor retracts. Although flat or inverted nipples may make it more difficult for the infant to latch in the first few days, women with flat or inverted nipples should not be discouraged about breastfeeding because in many cases of flat and inverted nipples, babies latch without difficulty. However, if an infant has difficulty latching, the mother-infant dyad should be seen within the first day of birth by someone experienced in lactation support. The adhesions that cause the nipple to flatten or invert can usually be broken. Having the mother use a manual or electric breast pump for a few minutes before the baby latches to draw out the nipple can do this. Another option is to use a nipple shield (Fig. 2-70) for a short time to allow the baby

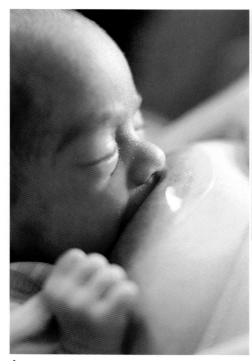

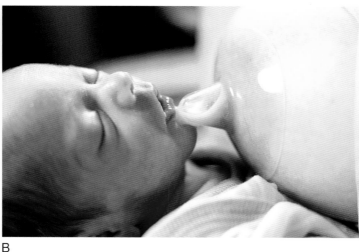

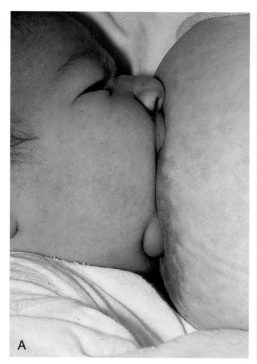

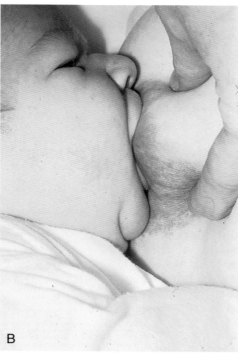

Figure 2-70. **A,** A preterm infant is breastfeeding with nipple shield in place. Nipple shields can be used for preterm or term infants who have difficulty with latch due to a variety of reasons, such as maternal flat or inverted nipples and engorgement. They are not intended for long-term use and should be used under the supervision of a person well trained in lactation support. **B,** A preterm infant is full and satisfied after breastfeeding with a nipple shield in place. The nipple shield has multiple fenestrations, so the milk comes out as it does from the mother's nipple.

Figure 2-71. **A** and **B,** Good latch. A good latch is characterized by a wide-open mouth, everted lips, and high position on the mother's areola. The angle between the baby's two lips should be close to 180 degrees. (Courtesy Susan Costanza, RN, IBCLC, Rochester General Hospital, Rochester, NY.)

to latch more easily. If a nipple shield is offered, it should be done under the supervision of someone experienced in lactation support because it is not intended for long-term use. Flat and inverted nipples usually improve with nursing and are rarely a problem with subsequent pregnancies. The use of breast shells during pregnancy has not been shown to improve flat and inverted nipples. Prepregnancy use of shells may undermine a woman's confidence in her ability to nurse her infant and thus may impede successful breastfeeding.

Latch. A key factor in the success of breastfeeding is an appropriate latch (Fig. 2-71A and B) because it affects both milk supply and comfort. When a baby is properly latched

on the breast, the baby's mouth is wide open with the angle between the baby's upper and lower lips close to at least 90 degrees but up to 180 degrees. The upper and lower lips should be everted with the baby's lips as far back on the areola as possible and the nipple in the back of the baby's mouth. Because of the wide variability in the size of babies' mouths and mothers' nipples and areolas, the amount of the areola visible during an effective latch is highly variable. When the latch is inadequate (Fig. 2-72), the mother may experience discomfort and the baby may not be able to empty the breast effectively and efficiently. Some women experience normal discomfort just as the baby latches that resolves in less than a minute. However,

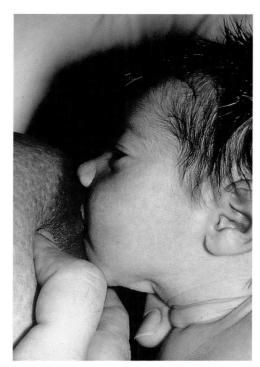

Figure 2-72. Inadequate latch is characterized by a partially closed mouth with the angle between the baby's lips less than 90 degrees, often with the lips near the base of the mother's nipple. (Courtesy Susan Costanza, RN, IBCLC, Rochester General Hospital, Rochester, NY.)

if a woman experiences persistent pain with breastfeeding she should unlatch the baby from the breast by inserting a finger into the corner of the baby's mouth and between the gums and gently press down toward the baby's chin. The baby should then be repositioned and a proper latch attempted again. If the pain continues, the mother-baby dyad should be observed during a feeding by a person experienced in breastfeeding assessment. An inadequate latch can result in nipple trauma (Fig. 2-73A and B) and, over time, can compromise milk supply.

Holding Positions

Optimally, all babies should be placed at the breast within the first 30 minutes of life when they are wide awake from the adrenaline surge that occurs at the time of delivery. Placing the baby near the breast early helps to establish attachment and allows the baby the opportunity to latch when ready. The four main breastfeeding positions for the newborn are the football (Fig. 2-74A and B), cross-cradle (Fig. 2-75), classic cradle (Fig. 2-76), and side-lying (Fig. 2-77) positions. Each nursing mother should find the positions that are comfortable for her. Pillows and foot rests can be used to increase comfort. Pillows can be used to raise the baby to the level of the mother's breast for optimal support. In all the positions, it is helpful to support the baby so that he or she feels secure, without a sense of falling. The angle between the baby's neck and chin should be about 90 degrees. The midline of the chin should be aligned with the center of the chest, thus placing the baby's head, neck, and anterior chest in alignment for ease in swallowing. To initiate the latch, the mother can touch her nipple to the baby's upper lip. This stimulates the baby to open the mouth and lower and extend the tongue. When the baby opens widely, the mother should place the baby's open mouth past the nipple and as far

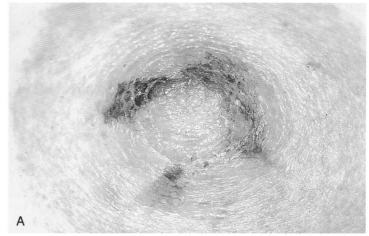

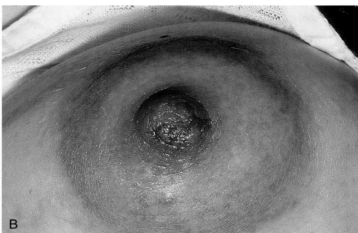

Figure 2-73. **A** and **B,** Cracked, abraded, bruised nipples and areola. These result from improper latch and positioning. An experienced clinician should assess the mother's technique for holding and latching the baby. (Courtesy Susan Costanza, RN, IBCLC, Rochester General Hospital, Rochester, NY.)

back onto the areola as possible with the nipple aimed toward the hard palate. The baby's chin and lower lip should make first contact with the breast. Many women have to hold their breast as the baby initially latches. Either the C hold, with the thumb on top of the breast and the other four fingers below, or the scissor hold, with the thumb and index finger on top of the breast and the other three fingers below, can be used. With either hold, the fingers should be off the areola so that they do not interfere with the latch. After the baby is well latched, some women may be able to release the hold on the breast. For women with large breasts, a rolled washcloth can be placed under the breast for support so that the breast doesn't have to be held for the entire feeding.

Football Hold (see Fig. 2-74A and B). The football hold is especially good for women with large breasts and women who have had a cesarean section and cannot tolerate abdominal pressure. Because it allows good visualization of the latch and good head control, it is also an excellent position for premature infants and for new mothers. The mother holds the baby in the same arm as the breast she intends to feed from. The heel of the mother's hand should rest approximately between the baby's scapulae, and her thumb and index finger should be placed on the baby's mastoid processes. The baby's back should rest on the mother's forearm, and the baby's bottom should be firmly tucked under her upper arm. The baby's head should be tipped back just slightly. The mother takes her opposite hand and grasps the breast behind the areola. A pillow

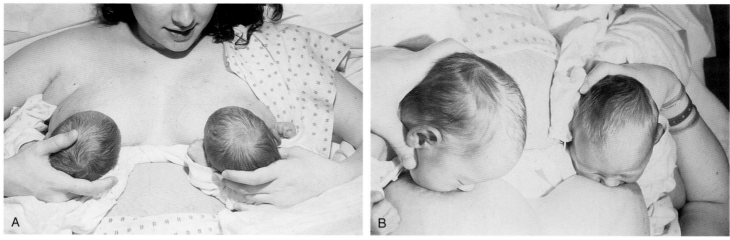

Figure 2-74. A and **B,** Football position. This position is especially good for women with large breasts, women who have had a cesarean section, and new mothers because it allows good visualization of the latch and good head control. It is also the position of choice for twins. (Courtesy Susan Costanza, RN, IBCLC, Rochester General Hospital, Rochester, NY.)

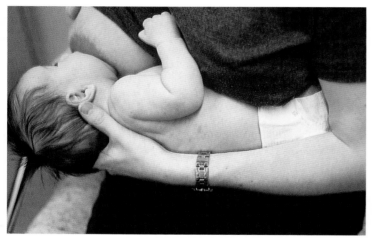

Figure 2-75. Cross-cradle position. This is an excellent position to use in the young infant because it allows good visualization of the latch and provides firm head control of the neonate. The mother's hand is under the baby's neck. The baby's chin but not the nose is in the mother's breast. More of the areola is covered by the lower lip than by the upper lip, which is characteristic of a normal, asymmetrical latch. (Courtesy J. Newman, MD, FRCPC, Hospital for Sick Children, Toronto.)

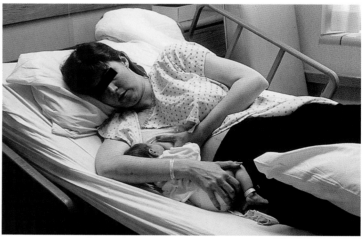

Figure 2-77. Side-lying position. This is suitable for mothers who have had a cesarean section, are tired, have a sore perineum, have a sleepy baby, and for nighttime feeding. The mother and baby are belly to belly, and the baby is held on the side by the mother's hand. A receiving blanket can be rolled up and placed behind the infant's back to hold the baby in the position if the mother prefers. (Courtesy Susan Costanza, RN, IBCLC, Rochester General Hospital, Rochester, NY.)

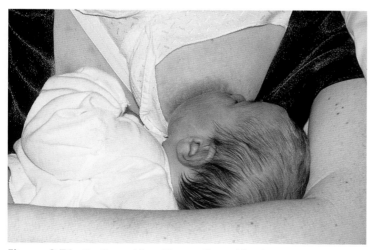

Figure 2-76. Cradle position. The cradle position is easier to use when the baby has developed a modicum of head control but can also be used in the newborn if the mother finds it comfortable. The infant's nose, chin, and chest are aligned, and the mother and baby are belly-to-belly. (Courtesy Susan Costanza, RN, IBCLC, Rochester General Hospital, Rochester, NY.)

can be placed under the mother's arm for her support. Depending on the size of the mother's breasts and the length of her arms, the baby may be facing the ceiling or be turned on the side with the baby's abdomen in contact with the mother's ribs. Either position is acceptable as long as the mother is comfortable and the baby's nose, chin, and midchest are all in alignment with the neck slightly extended.

Cross-Cradle (see Fig. 2-75). The cross-cradle is an excellent position because it allows good visualization of the latch and provides firm head control for the neonate. When the baby is several weeks old and has developed a good latch and improved head control, many women transition to the classic cradle hold. In the cross-cradle position, the baby is held by the mother in the arm opposite to the breast she intends to feed from. The baby is turned belly to belly with the mother so that the umbilicus and knees are touching the mother's abdomen. The baby's nose, chin, and midchest are aligned, and the neck is slightly extended. The heel of the mother's hand should rest approximately between the baby's scapulae, and her thumb and index finger should be placed on the baby's mastoid processes. The mother's forearm should rest along the baby's spine, and the baby's bottom should be firmly tucked under the mother's elbow and upper arm, with the baby's head tipped back slightly. When the baby is well latched, the mother can release her hold of the breast and use her arm for additional support of the baby.

Classic Cradle (see Fig. 2-76). The classic cradle position is easier to use when the baby has developed a modicum of head control, but it can also be used in the newborn if the woman finds it comfortable. The classic cradle has the baby's head in the bend of the mother's arm on the same side as the breast she is offering. The baby's umbilicus and knees should be facing the mother's abdomen. The mother can use her other hand to hold her breast behind the areola to guide it to the baby's mouth.

Side-Lying Position (see Fig. 2-77). This position is good for mothers who have had a cesarean section, have a sore perineum, are tired, or at nighttime after breastfeeding is well established. It may be helpful to place a pillow behind the mother's low back for support and between her legs if desired for comfort. A rolled receiving blanket can be placed behind the infant to keep the baby in a side-lying position. The mother may initially need assistance getting her baby latched in this position if she has limited agility after delivery and because she may not be able to completely visualize the latch. The baby should be turned so that the infant's abdomen is touching the mother's abdomen.

Breast Problems

Engorgement. Engorgement is painful breast fullness caused by vascular congestion, edema, or milk accumulation in the breast tissue. It may be mild to severe and most commonly occurs 2 to 7 days after delivery. Engorgement can be prevented in many cases by encouraging frequent feedings (10 to 14 per day) and proper latch. Despite these preventive efforts, engorgement still occurs and physicians must recognize the signs and symptoms promptly. The signs are firm, sometimes lumpy, tender breasts with increased vascular markings in the face of a maternal sense of fullness to the point of discomfort. If not relieved, engorgement can make it difficult for the baby to latch, result in decreased milk production, and contribute to the development of mastitis. Treatment is frequent emptying of the breasts and symptomatic care. Infants should be nursed frequently, or milk should be expressed manually or with a pump. Warm compresses to soften the breast tissue and manual expression of milk before putting the baby to the breast may make it easier for the baby to latch properly. Cool compresses after feedings may help to decrease vascular congestion.

Sore, Bruised, or Cracked Nipples (see Fig. 2-73A and B). These can occur when a baby is not latched properly. The pain caused by these conditions is the reason that many mothers become discouraged and stop breastfeeding. Improper latch, usually too close to the nipple, is the leading cause of sore nipples. Mothers should not be told to grin and bear the pain. They should be promptly referred to an experienced clinician to assess the latch and positioning. Milk pores at the end of the nipple can become plugged (Fig. 2-78), causing acute pain with breastfeeding. This should be treated by unroofing the pore with a needle held horizontal to the tip of the nipple. Pain relief is instant when milk is released from the duct.

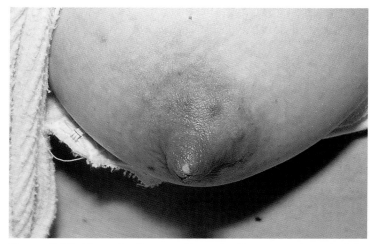

Figure 2-78. Plugged milk pores. Plugged milk pores at the end of the nipple cause acute pain with breastfeeding. This should be treated by unroofing the pore with a needle held horizontal to the tip of the nipple. Pain relief is instant when milk is released from the duct. (Courtesy Susan Costanza, RN, IBCLC, Rochester General Hospital, Rochester, NY.)

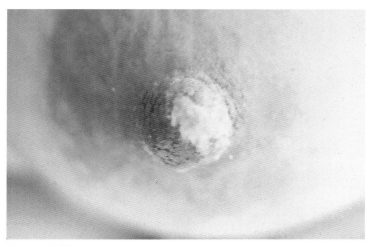

Figure 2-79. *Candida* infection. Fungal infection of the breast to this degree is uncommon, but more subtle presentations are common. Women with candidal infection of the breast complain of burning or stabbing pain during or after breastfeeding. Most often the mother's breast appears normal or slightly red, but the breastfeeding baby has oral or diaper candidiasis. In this case both mother and baby should be treated. (Courtesy J. Newman, MD, FRCPC, Hospital for Sick Children, Toronto.)

Yeast Infections (Fig. 2-79). Yeast infections of the mother's breast and baby's oropharynx or diaper area are common after the first week or two of life. The signs of thrush in the baby include white plaques on the gingiva and tongue that do not wipe off and are present before and after feeding. Babies may pull on and off the breast when they have thrush, likely due to mouth soreness. Mothers may experience a variety of symptoms from yeast infection of the breast including sharp, stabbing, or burning pain during and after feeding, as well as red, cracked, and sore nipples. If a breast-fed baby has thrush, both mother and baby should be treated even if the mother is asymptomatic at the time of the visit. A number of treatment options exist. The mother can be treated with nystatin ointment or another antifungal agent applied to the nipple and areola after each feeding, and the baby can be treated with 1 mL of oral nystatin solution (100,000 IU/mL) four times a day. Treatment should continue for several days after both are without obvious lesions. The second option is to treat both mother and baby with 0.5%

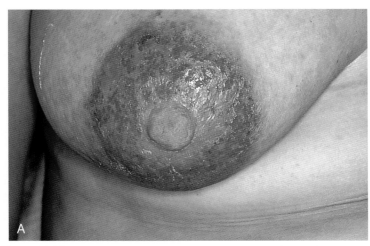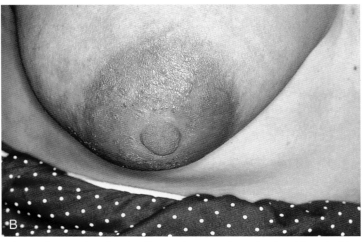

Figure 2-80. Impetigo of the breast before treatment **(A)** and after treatment **(B)** with an oral antibiotic. The mother experienced pain with and without nursing. (Courtesy Nancy G. Powers, MD, Medical Director of Lactation Services, Wesley Medical Center, Wichita, Kan.)

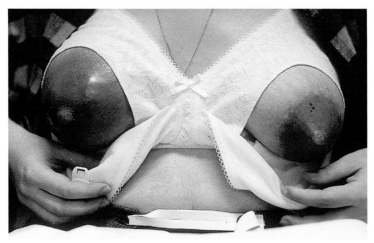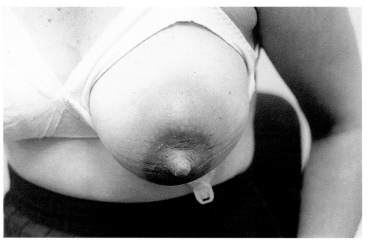

Figure 2-81. Mastitis, an infection of the breast, often presents as acute onset of fever, chills, and extreme breast tenderness over an area of induration and firmness. This is not a reason to cease breastfeeding. In fact, the treatment includes frequent emptying of the breast and oral antibiotics to cover both staphylococcal and streptococcal species. (Courtesy J. Newman, MD, FRCPC, Hospital for Sick Children, Toronto.)

Figure 2-82. Breast abscess is a localized breast infection that requires incision and drainage and treatment with an antibiotic to cover staphylococcal and streptococcal infection. It can occur as a complication of inadequately treated mastitis. (Courtesy J. Newman, MD, FRCPC, Hospital for Sick Children, Toronto.)

to 1% topical gentian violet once daily for no more than 3 days. Prolonged use can result in mouth ulcers. Combined therapy can be used. For example, you can apply the gentian violet one time in the office and continue at home treatment with antifungal agents. Finally, both mother and infant can be treated with oral fluconazole for 10 to 14 days if they are not responding to the other treatments or in the case of recurrent infections. As with all cases of thrush, all artificial nipples should be properly cleaned.

Impetigo (Fig. 2-80A and B). Impetigo can also occur on the breast. It should be treated with an oral antibiotic (e.g., cephalexin) if widespread or with a topical antibiotic (e.g., mupirocin) if fairly localized.

Mastitis (Fig. 2-81). Mastitis is a bacterial infection of the breast. It can result from blocked ducts or from ascending infection due to cracked nipples. Mastitis often presents as acute onset of fever, chills, and extreme breast tenderness over an area of induration and firmness usually on one breast. This is not a reason to cease breastfeeding. In fact, the treatment includes frequent emptying of the breast, oral antibiotics to cover penicillin resistant staphylococcal and streptococcal species (e.g., first-generation cephalosporin or dicloxacillin), analgesics, rest, and ade-

quate fluid intake. However, mastitis can progress to breast abscess (Fig. 2-82), which requires incision and drainage and antibiotics. This can often be done as an outpatient with close follow-up.

Assessing Milk Transfer

Many women are concerned that their baby is not getting enough to eat, especially in the first few days when they have colostrum. Many women believe that all the milk for a given meal is ready and waiting in the breast for the baby and worry that if their breast is soft the baby will not get more milk. That is not true. Only a small volume of milk is in the breast at the start of a feeding; most of the milk for each feeding is synthesized and secreted during infant suckling. Mothers can be reassured that there are ways to assess adequate intake without actually measuring anything in a bottle, including elimination patterns, weight changes, breast changes, and frequency and duration of feedings. Babies should have increasing numbers of voids and stools with each day. By day 3 of life, babies should have at least four to five voids and transitional stools a few times per day. By day 4 to 5,

Table 2-2	Assessing Milk Transfer			
	DAY 0	**DAY 1-2**	**DAY 3-4**	**DAY 5-6**
Voids	≥1	≥2	≥4	≥5
Stools				
Number	≥1	≥2	≥3	≥5
Color	Meconium	Meconium	Transitional	Yellow/seedy
Weight compared with birth weight	—	≤5% loss	≤10% loss	No further weight loss
Frequency of feeds	2-8	4-10	8-12	8-12
Duration of feeds (minutes)	5-40	15-45	20-45	20-45

babies should have more than five voids per day and transitional to yellow stools at least four to five times per day. By day 6 of life, babies should have at least six to eight voids per day and at least four loose to watery yellow stools per day. Babies should not lose more than 10% from birthweight in the first 3 days of life. Excessive weight loss is a sign of some breastfeeding problem.

When a mother senses that her breasts are fuller, heavier, and warmer, this is a sign that the volume of milk she is producing is increasing. This should occur as early as day 2 but may be as late as day 5 to 7. After this happens, babies should no longer lose weight and should begin to gain at least 15 to 30 g per day. A mother should notice that her breast feels full and heavy before the baby nurses and softer after the baby is finished. For the first 24 to 48 hours after birth, a baby's nursing frequency is highly variable. However, after that, most babies nurse 10 to 12 times per day (Table 2-2). The baby should be satisfied after the feeding and be content and often asleep. If the baby is not meeting these assessment goals, the mother should also be told to seek professional assistance with breastfeeding. According to the American Academy of Pediatrics, all breastfeeding infants should be assessed within 48 to 72 hours of hospital discharge.

Premature Infants

Among the many benefits to providing breast milk to premature infants are decreased risk of perinatal infections and necrotizing enterocolitis, shorter hospital stays, and improved developmental outcomes. With adequate support and close follow-up, babies as small as 1500 g can feed well at the breast. However, most premature babies must be assessed and stabilized before they are put to the breast, which can be days or weeks. In any case, there are some important ways that mothers can be supported to breast-feed their premature infants. The most important is to create an environment in the neonatal intensive care unit (NICU) or newborn nursery in which breastfeeding is encouraged and supported. This includes allowing flexible visiting hours to encourage breastfeeding, as well as knowledgeable and supportive staff.

A mother should be asked about the desire to breast-feed on the day of delivery. To stimulate breast-milk supply, she should be given access to a high-grade electric breast pump and instructed on how to use it as soon as possible. Most insurance companies will cover a breast pump rental for infants in the NICU. In the first few days of pumping, only small amounts of yellow to white colostrum are expressed, as little as a teaspoon per pumping. This is normal. Occasionally the early milk looks rusty or bloody, dubbed the "rusty pipe syndrome" (Fig. 2-83), which is also normal and can be used without concern. However, if the rusty milk continues for more than a week, the

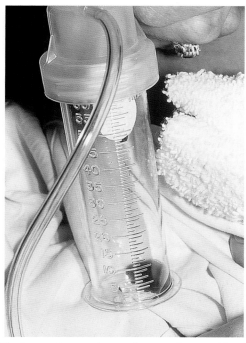

Figure 2-83. Rusty pipe syndrome. Rusty or brown, bloody-appearing early milk. This uncommon finding usually occurs in primiparous women early in lactogenesis. They experience painless breastfeeding, and the nipples are not cracked and bleeding. The etiology is uncertain, but the condition may be caused by internal bleeding due to edema and engorgement. This milk is safe and can be used without concern. (Courtesy Susan Costanza, RN, IBCLC, Rochester General Hospital, NY.)

mother should be referred for further evaluation. Mothers should be instructed to double-pump (both breasts at the same time) (Fig. 2-84) at least six times per day, with at least one period of 5 to 6 hours of uninterrupted sleep. The volume of milk expressed should increase 3 to 5 days after delivery. Stress can definitely delay and decrease milk production, a common problem for mothers with a baby in the NICU. Women should be encouraged to keep pumping. Pumped milk should be frozen in small volumes and thawed as needed. The milk should have the date on the label so that the first bottles into the freezer are the first to be used to avoid spoilage and because the milk composition changes over time. Before babies are put to the breast, they can be placed in kangaroo care (placed on the mother's chest in skin-to-skin contact) to encourage bonding and to begin movement toward breastfeeding.

A baby who is ready to bottle-feed is also ready to breast-feed. Premature babies fed at the breast have on average lower heart rate, lower respiratory rate, and higher pulse oximetry measurement compared with bottle-fed infants. The first few times a mother offers her baby the breast, she should be observed and supported. The baby may just lick the breast and snuggle or may latch well. Again, either

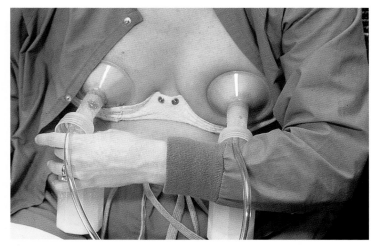

Figure 2-84. Double pumping of the breasts. This is the most efficient and effective way for women to maintain a milk supply when they are unable to breast-feed directly. The pump should initially be set at the minimum setting and gradually increased to a level of comfort for the mother. (Courtesy Susan Costanza, RN, IBCLC, Rochester General Hospital, Rochester, NY.)

is normal. If there is concern that the baby is not getting enough milk at the breast or that the infant requires some fortified breast milk or formula, there are several options. First, the baby can be weighed three times on a gram scale before the feeding, wearing a clean diaper and the clothes to be worn during the feeding. The baby is then fed and reweighed two more times without a change in the diaper or clothes after feeding. The difference between the average postfeed weight and the prefeed weight is the grams of breast milk consumed—the same as the volume consumed. If the baby has not taken "enough," the baby can then be fed by an alternate feeding method to supplement, such as cup (Fig. 2-85) or finger feeding (Fig. 2-86). Second, a supplemental nursing system (SNS) (Fig. 2-87A and B) filled with expressed breast milk, fortified breast milk, or appropriate formula can be attached to the breast so that the baby receives both breast milk and the supplement. The tip of the tubing must be placed about a quarter

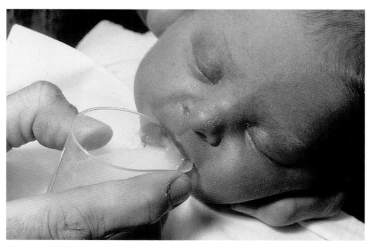

Figure 2-85. Cup feeding is an alternate feeding method for infants. A small medicine cup or one designed specifically for this purpose can be used. The cup is placed at the margin of the infant's lower lip and tipped gently toward the mouth. The infant should extrude the tongue and assist feeding by lapping the milk as small amounts are poured between the lower lip and gum. Cup feeding is widely used in underdeveloped countries when mothers are unable to feed their infants from the breast. (Courtesy Susan Costanza, RN, IBCLC, Rochester General Hospital, Rochester, NY.)

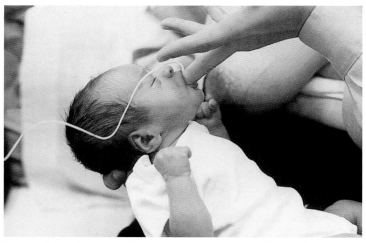

Figure 2-86. Finger feeding is an alternative method for feeding infants. The largest finger that is convenient for the feeder should be used. The finger used should be held flat and placed far back in the infant's mouth so that the infant's tongue is forward and curved around the sides of the finger. A 5-French, 36-inch feeding tube is convenient because the thin caliber provides a slow flow rate and the length allows some flexibility with positioning. Among the available alternative feeding methods, finger feeding has the added benefit of training the infant with a weak or immature suck to suck in a similar fashion as during breastfeeding. The one drawback to finger feeding is that it is relatively slow. (Courtesy J. Newman, MD, FRCPC, Hospital for Sick Children, Toronto.)

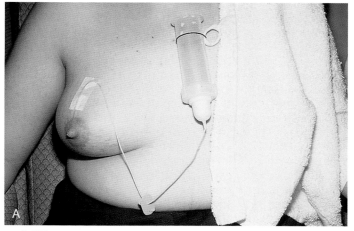
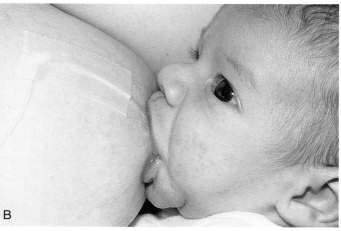

Figure 2-87. **A** and **B,** Supplemental nursing system (SNS). SNS allows a baby to receive additional nutrients while still breastfeeding and thus provides stimulation to the breast. It does not interfere with breastfeeding technique and latch. The tip of the SNS tubing should protrude past the end of the nipple about a quarter of an inch. (Courtesy Susan Costanza, RN, IBCLC, Rochester General Hospital, Rochester, NY.)

inch past the end of the mother's nipple so that it remains in the back of the oropharynx as the nipple is lengthened in the infant's mouth. The reasons to go directly to the breast from gavage feeding are multiple. Bottle-feeding and breastfeeding require the use of different oral muscles and sucking mechanics. Premature babies may get used to bottle-feeding and may not breast-feed well as a result. Therefore it is ideal to feed infants by alternate feeding methods when a mother is not available to breast-feed.

Finger feeding is inexpensive and mimics breastfeeding well but is also time consuming. Finger feeding may be accomplished with a 5-French, 36-inch feeding tube. One end of the feeding tube is placed into a bottle of breast milk or supplement, and the other end is placed in a clean (gloved if not the parent) hand with the tip about a quarter of an inch past the end of the index finger. As the baby draws the finger into the back of the mouth and begins to suck, the milk is drawn up into the feeding tube. Finger feeding also helps prepare the baby to suck properly at the breast with a rounded tongue, and milk is provided deep into the baby's mouth.

Cup feeding is another alternative feeding method. The milk can be dispensed from a small medicine cup. The cup is placed near the baby's lower lip so that the milk can be lapped up. It can also be slowly poured between the lower lip and gums. A variety of cups are made specifically to cup-feed infants, such as the Foley cup and Haberman feeder. This method of feeding is more time efficient than finger feeding and usually is used when the mother is not available to feed the baby herself.

Most infants can transition to full feeds at the breast exclusively by 36 to 40 weeks. However, the transition to full breastfeeding should begin as soon as possible. Now that infants are discharged well before term, pediatricians, family practitioners, and lactation consultants in the outpatient setting often provide this education and support. Advice should be individualized to each mother-baby dyad. A general approach is to have the mother dual-pump with a high-grade electric pump every time she offers the baby milk other than at the breast, including if she is using an SNS to provide the supplement. Initially the mother may need to pump after every feeding, especially if the baby has not yet reached term, has a weak suck, or is a sleepy baby. This will help to match her milk supply and her baby's increasing needs. Every few days, she can increase the number of feedings at the breast without supplement. The baby's stool and urine output should be monitored to ensure adequate intake, and the baby's weight should be monitored to ensure adequate growth during the transition.

Significant and long-lasting health benefits are associated with breastfeeding both for the individual mother-baby dyad and society. Breastfeeding is the ideal way to feed babies; however, it is not always easy. Mothers must receive adequate support in order to breast-feed successfully. This support and education are most certainly within the role of the pediatric health care provider. Excellent references including textbooks, journals, Web sites, books, printed materials, and videos are devoted to breastfeeding for those interested in more in-depth information.

Bibliography

Academy of Breastfeeding Medicine. Available at http://www.bfmed.org

American Academy of Pediatrics, Committee on Infectious Diseases: 2000 Red Book: Report of the Committee on Infectious Diseases, 25th ed. Elk Grove Village, Ill, American Academy of Pediatrics, 2000.

American Academy of Pediatrics, Committee on Nutrition: Pediatric Nutrition Handbook, 4th ed. Kleinman R (ed). Elk Grove Village, Ill, American Academy of Pediatrics, 2000.

American Academy of Pediatrics, Task Force on Breastfeeding 1999-2000: Breastfeeding Health Supervision. Elk Grove Village, Ill, American Academy of Pediatrics, 1999.

American Academy of Pediatrics, Work Group on Breastfeeding: Breastfeeding and the use of human milk. Pediatrics 100:1035-1039, 1997.

Avery GB (ed): Neonatology: Pathophysiology and Management of the Newborn, 3rd ed. Philadelphia, JB Lippincott, 1987.

Ballard JL, Novak KK, Driver M, et al: A simplified score for assessment of fetal maturation of newly born infants. J Pediatr 95:769-774, 1979.

Case Western Reserve University, University Hospitals of Cleveland. Available at http://www.breastfeedingbasics.org

Dick EA, de Bruyn: Ultrasound of the spinal cord in children: Its role. Eur Radiol 13:552-562, 2003.

Dubowitz LV, Dubowitz C, Goldburg C: Clinical assessment of gestational age in the newborn infant. J Pediatr 77:1-10, 1970.

Fox H: Pathology of the placenta. In Major Problems in Pathology, vol 7. Philadelphia, WB Saunders, 1978.

Jones KL: Smith's Recognizable Patterns of Human Malformation, 4th ed. Philadelphia, WB Saunders, 1988.

La Leche League, International. Available at http://www.lalecheleague.org

Lawrence RA, Lawrence RM: Breastfeeding: A Guide for the Medical Profession, 8th ed. St Louis, Mosby, 1999.

Painter MJ, Bergman I: Obstetrical trauma to the neonatal central and peripheral nervous system. Semin Perinatol 6(1):89-104, 1982.

Riordan J, Auerbach K: Breastfeeding and Human Lactation, 2nd ed. Sudbury, Mass, Jones & Bartlett, 1999.

Scanlon JW, Nelson T, Grylack U, Smith VF: A System of Newborn Physical Examination. Baltimore, University Park Press, 1979.

CHAPTER 3

Developmental-Behavioral Pediatrics

HEIDI M. FELDMAN

Pediatricians are frequently called on to distinguish among normal development, individual differences, and developmental or behavioral delays and disorders. Once developmental or behavioral delays have been identified, the pediatrician conducts a diagnostic workup, initiates management, refers to appropriate services, counsels families, and coordinates care. The goal of this chapter is to review the developmental-behavioral issues faced in routine pediatric practice. In the first half, the fundamental principles of development are applied to each major domain of functioning. Within each domain, discussion centers on the major developmental milestones, methods of assessment, signs of developmental variation, and approaches to children who show developmental or deviant patterns. In the second half, several developmental disorders are described including definitions, diagnostic criteria, the role of physical examination in evaluation, physical findings, and prognosis.

Principles of Normal Development

For ease of description and investigation, development is commonly discussed in terms of domains of function. Gross motor skills refer to the use of the large muscles of the body; fine motor skills refer to the use of small muscles of the hands; cognition means the use of higher mental processes including thinking, memory, and learning; language refers to the comprehension and production of meaningful symbolic communication; and social and emotional functioning refers to emotional reactions to events and interactions with others. In fact, these domains are interdependent. Cognitive abilities in infancy cannot readily be distinguished from sensorimotor functioning. Similarly, mature social functioning depends on competent language abilities. Within each domain, developmental change is generally orderly and predictable. Early reflex patterns and congenital sensory and motor capabilities are the building blocks of higher-order skills.

Developmental Assessment

A central component of health maintenance is the prompt identification of developmental problems and the promotion of development. *Developmental surveillance* is the term that has been used to encompass the longitudinal, continuous processes by which physicians and other professionals use all available clinical tools—review of parental concerns, routine developmental history, physical examination, observations, screening tests, review of teacher and daycare provider concerns, and other assessment techniques—to determine a child's developmental status. Frequent routine assessments promote a longitudinal view of the child and allow parental concerns to be addressed in a timely manner. A formal developmental assessment can be arranged if there are severe or persistent concerns.

Standardized screening methods, such as the Ages and Stages Questionnaires (ASQ), second edition, and the Parents' Evaluation of Developmental Status (PEDS), rely on parental reports. The Denver Developmental Screening Test and the Battelle Developmental Inventory (BDI-2) Screening Test elicit behavior from the child. Physicians should consider using screening instruments as part of surveillance at a few selected health maintenance visits, such as the 9-, 18-, 24-, and 36-month visits. These tests substantially improve the clinicians' abilities to accurately detect developmental delays and disorders in unselected populations. However, they are inappropriate instruments for populations at risk, who require comprehensive assessment. The sensitivity and specificity of these instruments range from 70% to 90%. Children who are developing normally may fail a screening test because of shyness, unfamiliarity with the examiner or the materials, or other factors unrelated to developmental competence. Screening tests can be used to confirm parental concerns but are not appropriate for diagnosing the nature of the problem. If parental concerns persist despite negative findings, a full evaluation is advisable because of the limited sensitivity of the tests. To ensure that the performance is representative of the child's ability, screening tests should be performed when the child is physically well, familiar with the setting and examiner, and under minimal stress.

Gross Motor Development

Early Reflex Patterns

At birth, a neonate's movements consist of alternating flexions and extensions that usually are symmetrical and vary in strength with the infant's state of wakefulness. In addition, involuntary reflexes can be elicited; they indicate that the patterns of movement requiring the integrated activity of multiple muscle groups are present even at birth.

Perhaps the best known of these reflex patterns is the Moro response. This reflex can occur spontaneously after a loud noise, but typically it is elicited during the course of physical examination by an abrupt extension of the infant's neck. The first phase of the response consists of symmetrical abduction and extension of the arms with extension of the trunk (Fig. 3-1). The second phase is marked by adduction of the upper extremities, as in an embrace, and frequently is accompanied by crying (Fig. 3-2). The Moro reflex gradually disappears by 4 months of age, associated with the development of cortical functioning. In children up to 4 months of age, the Moro response can be used to evaluate the integrity of the central nervous system and to detect peripheral problems, such as congenital musculoskeletal abnormalities or neural plexus injuries.

Another early reflex pattern is called the *asymmetrical tonic neck reflex (ATNR)* (Fig. 3-3). A newborn's limb motions are strongly influenced by head position. If the head is directed to one side, either by passive turning or by inducing the baby to follow an object to that side, tone in the extensor muscles increases on that side and in the flexor muscles on the opposite side. This response is not often seen immediately after birth, when the newborn has high flexor tone throughout the body, but it usually

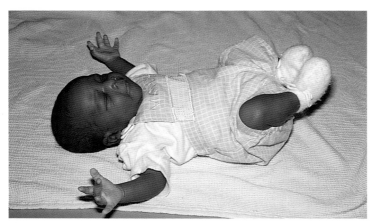

Figure 3-1. First phase of the Moro response. Symmetrical abduction and extension of the extremities follow a loud noise or an abrupt change in the infant's head position.

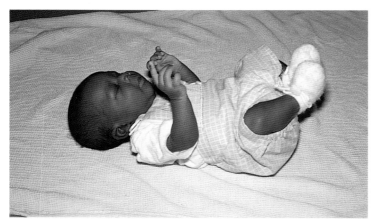

Figure 3-2. Second phase of the Moro response. Symmetrical adduction and flexion of the extremities, accompanied by crying.

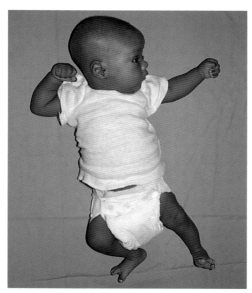

Figure 3-3. Asymmetrical tonic neck reflex (ATNR). Flexion of the arm and leg on the occipital side and extension on the chin side create the "fencer position."

appears by 2 to 4 weeks of age. The ATNR allows the baby to sight along the arm to the hand and is considered one of the first steps in the coordination of vision and reaching. This reflex disappears by 6 months of age, associated with the development of cortical functioning. Other primitive reflexes are listed in Table 3-1.

Table 3-1	Primitive Reflexes and Protective Equilibrium Responses	
REFLEX	**APPEARANCE***	**DISAPPEARANCE***
Moro	Birth	4 months
Hand grasp	Birth	3 months
Crossed adductor	Birth	7 months
Toe grasp	Birth	8-15 months
ATNR	2 weeks	6 months
Head righting	4-6 months	Persists voluntarily
Protective equilibrium	4-6 months	Persists voluntarily
Parachute	8-9 months	Persists voluntarily

*Different sources may vary on the precise timing of the appearance and disappearance of these primitive and equilibrium responses.
ATNR, asymmetrical tonic neck reflex.

With the emergence of voluntary control from higher cortical centers, muscular flexion and extension become balanced. Primitive reflexes are replaced by reactions that allow children to maintain a stable posture, even if they are rapidly moved or jolted. A timetable listing the expected emergence and disappearance of some of the protective equilibrium responses also is presented in Table 3-1.

Antigravity Muscular Control

Head Control

The infant's earliest control task is to maintain a stable posture against the influence of gravity. This control develops in an organized fashion, from head to toe, or in a cephalocaudal progression, paralleling neuronal myelination. For example, neck flexors allow head control against gravity when a child is pulled from the supine to the sitting position. Neonates show minimal control of the neck flexors, holding their heads upright only briefly when supported in a sitting position. When an infant is pulled to a sitting position, the head lags behind the arms and shoulders. At 5 to 6 months of age the infant anticipates the direction of movement of the pull-to-sit maneuver and flexes the neck before the shoulders begin to lift (Fig. 3-4).

Trunk Control and Sitting

In the prone position a newborn remains in a tightly flexed position and can simply turn the face from side to side along the bedsheets. Progressive control of the shoulders and upper trunk in the first few months of life, plus a decrease in flexor tone, enables the young infant to hold the chest off the bed with the weight supported on the forearms (Fig. 3-5). Evolution of trunk control down the thoracic spine can also be observed with the infant in a sitting position (Fig. 3-6). As control reaches the lumbar area, the lumbar lordotic curve can be seen when the child is standing (Fig. 3-7).

Head Righting and Parachute Response

Balance and equilibrium reactions also emerge in a cephalocaudal sequence. *Head righting* refers to the infant's ability to keep the head vertical despite a tilt of the body. A 4-month-old infant typically demonstrates this ability in vertical suspension when gently swayed from side to side. As control moves downward, protective equilibrium responses can be elicited in a sitting infant by abruptly but gently pushing the infant's center of gravity past the midline in one of the horizontal planes. This reflex

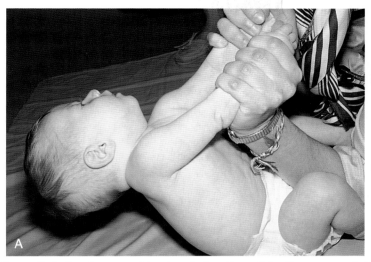

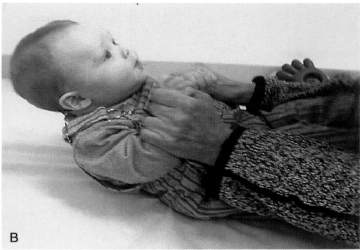

Figure 3-4. Development of head control on the pull-to-sit maneuver. **A,** At 1 month of age the head lags after the shoulders. **B,** At 5 to 6 months the child anticipates the movement and raises the head before the shoulders.

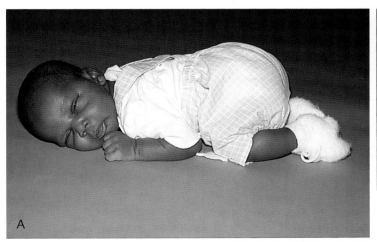

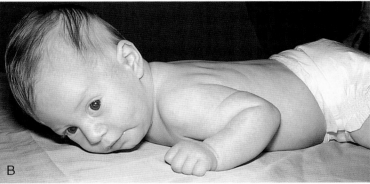

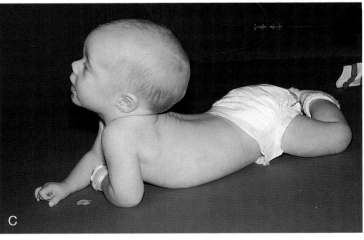

Figure 3-5. Development of posture in the prone position. **A,** The newborn lies tightly flexed with the pelvis high and the knees under the abdomen. **B,** At 2 months of age, the infant extends the hips and pulls the shoulders slightly. **C,** At 3 to 4 months, the infant keeps the pelvis flat and lifts the head and shoulders.

response, which involves increased trunk flexor tone toward the force and an outreached hand and limb away from the force, usually emerges by 6 months of age (Fig. 3-8). At 10 months the child develops the parachute response, an outstretching of both arms and legs when the body is abruptly moved head first in a downward direction (Fig. 3-9). The acquisition of this equilibrium response demonstrates the integrity of the sensations and motor responses of the central nervous system, which allows independent sitting and standing in children developing normally and those with motor impairment.

Development of Locomotion

Gross motor milestones can also be described in terms of locomotion (Table 3-2). Prone-to-supine rolling may be accomplished by 3 to 4 months of age, after the child gains sufficient control of shoulder and upper trunk musculature to prop up on the arms. Supine-to-prone rolling requires control of the lumbar spine and hip region, as well as the upper trunk; this is usually present by 5 to 6 months of age. Because most children are now placed in

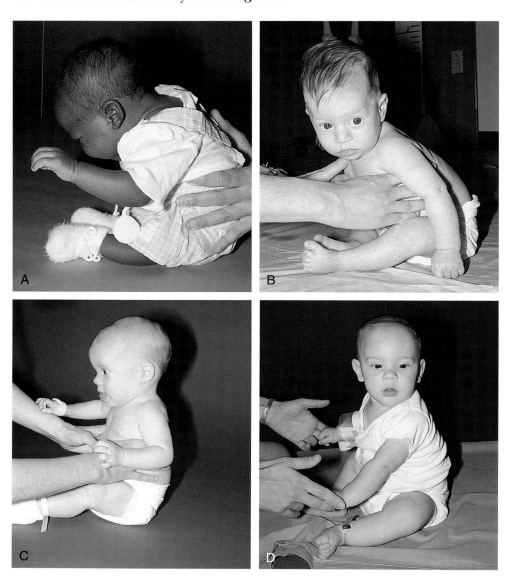

Figure 3-6. Development of sitting posture. **A,** At 1 to 2 months of age the head is held up intermittently, but trunk control is lacking. **B,** At 2 to 3 months of age the infant raises the head and shoulders well but lacks control of the thoracolumbar area. **C,** At 3 to 4 months, support in the lumbar area is required to sit. **D,** At 5 to 6 months the infant holds the head erect and the spine straight.

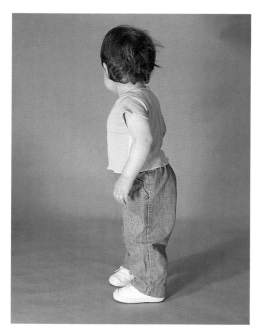

Figure 3-7. Standing. By 1 year of age, the lordotic curve, exaggerated here by a diaper, is evident.

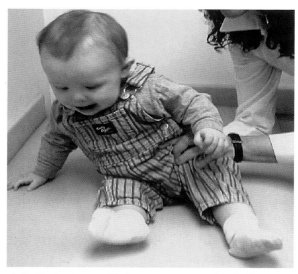

Figure 3-8. Protective equilibrium response. As the child is pushed laterally by the examiner, he flexes his trunk toward the force to regain his center of gravity while one arm extends to protect against falling (lateral propping).

the recommended supine position to sleep, supine-to-prone rolling may precede prone-to-supine rolling, demonstrating the impact of experience on gross motor skills. Early commando crawling, accomplished at 5 to 6 months of age (Fig. 3-10A), involves coordinated pulling with upper arms and passive dragging of the legs, akin to a soldier trying to keep the body out of the line of fire. By 6 to 9 months of age, as voluntary control moves to the hips and legs, the child is capable of getting up on the hands and knees, assuming a quadruped position, and creeping (Fig. 3-10B). The next developmental milestone is supported standing. By 9 to 10 months of age, many children like to demonstrate this new skill by holding on to a parent or by walking independently while holding on to furniture. This is called *cruising* (Fig. 3-10C). Increased control to the feet and disappearance of the plantar grasp

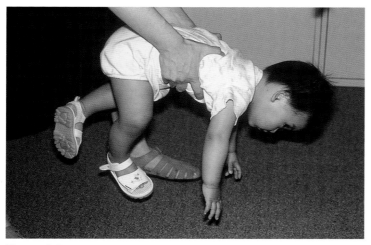

Figure 3-9. Parachute response. As the examiner allows the child to free fall in ventral suspension, the child's extremities extend symmetrically to distribute his weight over a broader and more stable base on landing.

Table 3-2	Early Gross Motor Milestones in the Normal Child
TASK	**AGE RANGE***
Sits alone momentarily	4-8 months
Rolls back to stomach	4-10 months
Sits steadily	5-9 months
Gets to sitting	6-11 months
Pulls to standing	6-12 months
Stands alone	9-16 months
Walks three steps alone	9-17 months

*Wide ranges in the attainment of these gross motor milestones in healthy children are the rule rather than the exception.

From Bayley N: Bayley Scales of Infant Development, 2nd ed. San Antonio, Tex, Psychological Corp, Harcourt Brace, 1993.

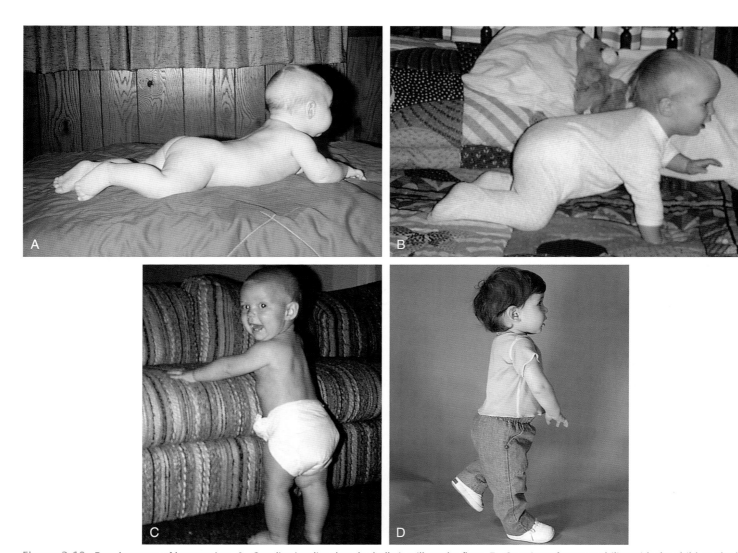

Figure 3-10. Development of locomotion. **A,** *Crawling* implies that the belly is still on the floor. **B,** *Creeping* refers to mobility with the child on the hands and knees (quadruped). **C,** *Cruising* refers to standing with two-handed support on stationary objects before moving with steps. **D,** Early free walking.

reflex allow the child to walk independently. Walking three steps alone occurs at a median age of about 12 months, with a range of 9 to 17 months of age (Fig. 3-10D).

Development of Complex Gross Motor Patterns

Further progress in gross motor skills continues throughout childhood. The developmental sequence beyond walking incorporates improved balance and coordination and progressive narrowing of the base of support. The sequence of milestones is as follows: running, jumping on two feet, balancing on one foot, hopping, and skipping. The child simultaneously learns to use muscle groups in timed sequences. By $13^{1}/_{2}$ months the child walks well, and by 36 months he or she can balance on one foot for 1 second. Most children can hop by age 4. They can throw a ball overhead by $22^{1}/_{2}$ months, but catching develops later, at almost 5 years.

Gross Motor Assessment during Health Maintenance Visits

The evaluation of gross motor skills can often begin when the pediatrician enters the office for a well-child visit. The typical 2-month-old infant is cradled in the parent's arms; the 6-month-old child is sitting with minimal support on the parent's lap or on the examination table next to the parent; the 12-month-old is cruising or toddling through the room. Although there is a wide age range in the onset and duration of each stage, the 6-month-old infant who lacks head control on the pull-to-sit maneuver, who cannot clear the table surface with the chest by supporting weight on the arms when prone, who shows no head righting, or who has persistent primitive reflexes such as a complete Moro response or ATNR is at sufficient variance from peers to warrant evaluation for a possible neuromuscular disorder. In addition, when gross motor delays are found in association with verbal and social delays, asymmetrical use of one limb or one side of the body, or loss of previously attained milestones, diagnostic evaluation is indicated.

Evaluation of the older infant or toddler who has mastered walking can occur in the course of the physical and neurologic evaluation. Many children enjoy showing off their abilities to jump, balance on one foot, hop, and skip. Some pediatricians use gross motor testing to establish rapport at the outset of a physical examination. However, because an aroused preschooler may not cooperate with a sedentary evaluation of heart or ears, many pediatricians hold off on motor evaluation until the conclusion of the examination. Developmental screening tests include assessment of motor skills.

At the discovery of delayed or atypical development, the pediatrician's first task is to develop a differential diagnosis and a plan to establish the specific diagnosis. Potential causes of delayed gross motor development are listed in Table 3-3. Another equally important task is to recommend a treatment program. Early intervention programs or physical therapy should be actively considered for children with motor difficulties during infancy through preschool. Adaptive physical education programs are available for older children with mild problems that do not seriously impair function.

Fine Motor Development

Involuntary Grasp

At birth the neonate's fingers and thumb are typically tightly fisted. A newborn grasps reliably and reflexively at any object placed in the palm (Fig. 3-11) and cannot release the grasp. Because of this reflex, the newborn's range of upper extremity motion is functionally limited. Normal development leads to acquisition of a voluntary grasp.

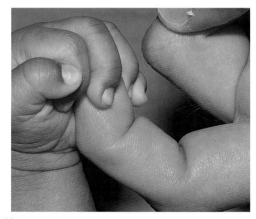

Figure 3-11. Reflex hand grasp. A newborn reflexively grasps at a finger placed in the palm.

Table 3-3	Potential Causes of Delayed Gross Motor Development	
GLOBAL DEVELOPMENTAL DELAY	**MOTOR DYSFUNCTION**	**MOTOR INTACT BUT OTHERWISE RESTRICTED**
Genetic syndromes and chromosomal abnormalities	Central nervous system damage—kernicterus, birth injury, neonatal stroke, trauma, prolonged seizures, metabolic insult, infection	Congenital malformations—bony or soft tissue defects
Brain morphologic abnormalities		Diminished energy supply—chronic illness, severe malnutrition
Endocrine deficiencies—hypothyroidism, prolonged hypoglycemia	Spinal cord dysfunction—Werdnig-Hoffmann disease, myelomeningocele, polio	Environmental deprivation—casted, non–weight bearing
Neurodegenerative diseases	Peripheral nerve dysfunction—brachial plexus injury, heritable neuropathies	Familial and genetic endowment—slower myelination
Congenital infections		Sensory deficits—blindness
Idiopathic mental retardation	Motor end-plate dysfunction—myasthenia gravis	Temperamental effects—low activity level, slow to try new tasks
	Muscular disorders—muscular dystrophies	Trauma—child abuse
	Other—benign congenital hypotonia	

Voluntary Grasp

The reflexive palmar grasp gradually disappears at about 1 month of age. From that point, the infant gains control of fine motor skills in an orderly progression, from the midline to the periphery or from proximal to distal. In the second or third month of life, the infant initially brings both hands together for midline hand play (Fig. 3-12). Shortly after that, the baby begins to swipe at objects held in or near the midline (Fig. 3-13). At this early stage, swiping is in fact a gross motor activity that involves the entire upper extremity as a unit. However, it is through swiping that the infant increases the exploratory range and fine tunes the small muscles of the wrist, hand, and fingers.

Improvements in fine motor control increase sensory input from the hands and permit greater hand manipulation through space. By 2 to 3 months of age, the hands are no longer tightly fisted, and the infant may begin sucking on a thumb or individual digit rather than the entire fist for self-comfort. A 3-month-old is usually able to hold an object in either hand if it is placed there, although the ability to grasp voluntarily or to release that object is limited. At approximately 4 to 5 months of age, infants begin to use their hands as entire units to draw objects toward them. Neither the hand nor the thumb functions independently at this point and, consequently, the child uses the hand like a rake.

Next, the child develops the ability to bend the fingers against the palm (palmar grasp), squeeze objects, and obtain them independently for closer inspection. Differentiation of the parts of the hand develops in association with differentiation of the two hands. Between 5 and 7 months of age, the infant can use hands independently to transfer objects across the midline. Further differentiation of the plane of movement of the thumb allows it to adduct as the fingers squeeze against the palm in a radial-palmar or whole-hand grasp. With time, the thumb moves from adduction to opposition. The site of pressure of the thumb against the fingers moves away from the palm toward the fingertips in what is called an *inferior-pincer* or *radial-digital grasp,* seen around 9 months of age (Fig. 3-14). By 10 months of age, differentiated use of the fingers allows the child to explore the details of an object.

Between 9 and 12 months of age, the fine pincer grasp develops, allowing opposition of the tip of the thumb and the index finger (see Fig. 3-14). This milestone enables the precise prehension of tiny objects (Fig. 3-15). The infant uses this skill in tasks such as self-feeding and exploration of small objects. By 1 year, the infant can position the hand in space to achieve vertical or horizontal orientation before grasping or releasing an object.

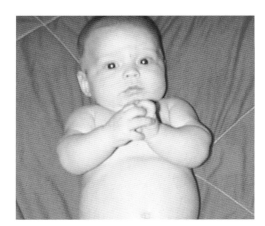

Figure 3-12. Midline hand play. A 2-month-old infant brings the hands together at the midline.

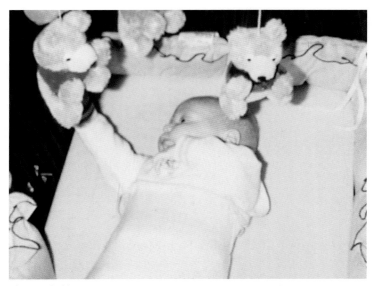

Figure 3-13. Reaching and swiping. A 3-month-old infant uses his entire upper extremity as a unit in interacting with the toy.

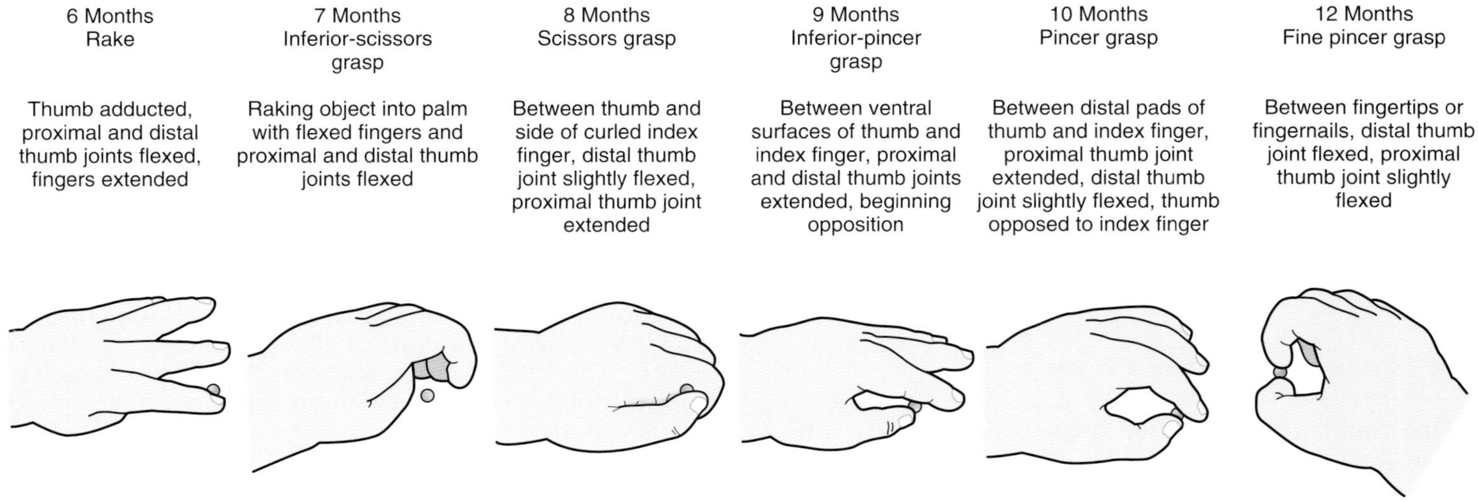

6 Months Rake	7 Months Inferior-scissors grasp	8 Months Scissors grasp	9 Months Inferior-pincer grasp	10 Months Pincer grasp	12 Months Fine pincer grasp
Thumb adducted, proximal and distal thumb joints flexed, fingers extended	Raking object into palm with flexed fingers and proximal and distal thumb joints flexed	Between thumb and side of curled index finger, distal thumb joint slightly flexed, proximal thumb joint extended	Between ventral surfaces of thumb and index finger, proximal and distal thumb joints extended, beginning opposition	Between distal pads of thumb and index finger, proximal thumb joint extended, distal thumb joint slightly flexed, thumb opposed to index finger	Between fingertips or fingernails, distal thumb joint flexed, proximal thumb joint slightly flexed

Figure 3-14. Development of prehension. (Modified from Erhardt RP: Developmental Hand Dysfunction: Theory, Assessment, Treatment, 2nd ed. San Antonio, Tex, The Psychological Corporation, 1994. Copyright © 1982, 1989, 1994 by Rhoda P. Erhardt. All rights reserved.)

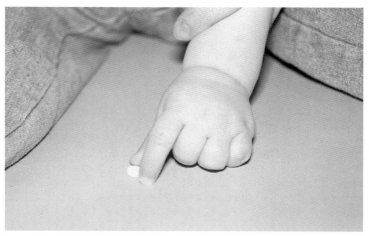

Figure 3-15. Fine pincer grasp. A 12-month-old child lifts a pill.

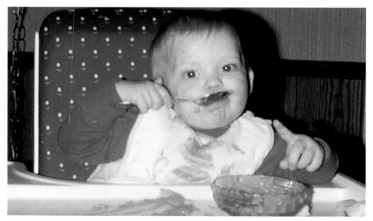

Figure 3-16. Independent feeding. A 15-month-old child employs fine motor skills to use a spoon independently.

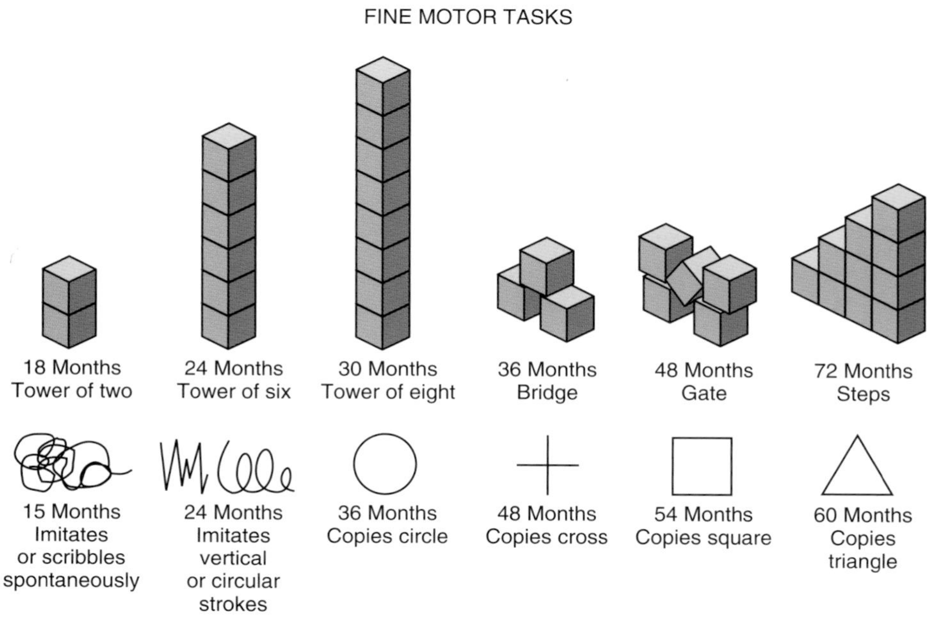

FINE MOTOR TASKS

18 Months Tower of two	24 Months Tower of six	30 Months Tower of eight	36 Months Bridge	48 Months Gate	72 Months Steps

Figure 3-17. Development of fine motor skills.

15 Months Imitates or scribbles spontaneously	24 Months Imitates vertical or circular strokes	36 Months Copies circle	48 Months Copies cross	54 Months Copies square	60 Months Copies triangle

Development of Complex Fine Motor Skills

Early in the second year of life the young child uses the grasp to master tools and to manipulate objects in new ways. Dropping and throwing, stacking, and putting objects in and out of receptacles become favorite pastimes. Mastery of the cup and spoon supplement or replace finger feeding as a more efficient and less messy means of eating (Fig. 3-16).

Advancements in fine motor planning and control can be demonstrated through the child's ability to stack small cubes. After children master stacking, they show consistent patterns of improvement in reproducing structures that they have watched the examiner assemble (Fig. 3-17). The child's ability to copy a variety of drawings also improves during this period.

Fine Motor Evaluation and Testing

Fine motor testing can be incorporated readily into a physical examination and may uncover problems with vision, neuromuscular control, or perception, in addition to difficulties with attention or cooperation. The 4-month-old child usually can be encouraged to grasp a tongue depressor. By 6 to 9 months of age, two tongue depressors should be offered, one for each hand, because the child can operate the hands independently. At 9 to 12 months the child spontaneously points with an isolated index finger or picks up small objects with a fine-pincer grasp. Children younger than 18 months of age generally use both hands equally well. Therefore the child who develops consistent handedness with neglect of the other limb before that time should have a neurodevelopmental assessment. The child who has not developed use of the thumb and pincer grasp by 1 year of age deserves further evaluation, as does the child who is unable to copy vertical or horizontal lines by age 3 or circles by age 4.

Fine motor activities can be engaging and nonthreatening to the preschool and school-age child; these activities allow the physician to make valuable observations and to establish a rapport. The physician can routinely request that the child use the waiting time or the period of history-taking to draw a self-portrait. These drawings provide a wealth of information not only on the child's capacities for fine motor control, but also on cognitive development and social and emotional functioning. A quick method for analyzing the age level of a drawing is to count the number of features in the drawing. The child receives one point for each of the following features: two eyes, two ears, a nose, a mouth, hair, two arms, two legs, two hands, two feet, a neck, and a trunk. Each point converts to the value of $1/4$ year added to a base age of 3 (Fig. 3-18). Screening tests and standardized measures, such as the *Beery-Buktenica Developmental Test of Visual Motor Integration,* fifth edition, can also be used to assess fine motor skills.

Children with brain damage are at particular risk for problems with perceptual–fine motor integration, even in the absence of visual problems and with minimal involvement of the upper extremities (Fig. 3-19).

Fine motor skills figure prominently in self-care activities. The child who lacks the dexterity to complete simple daily activities such as zipping, buttoning, or cutting with a knife may lack the self-esteem that accompanies independent self-care. Furthermore, children who continually depend on parents or teachers may be viewed by peers; teachers; or, perhaps most damagingly, by themselves as less mature. In the school-age child, inefficient fine motor skills can have a significant impact on the ability to write

legibly or to compete with peers in timed tasks, even if the child has sound academic and conceptual skills. Occupational therapy and special education may enhance fine motor skills and emotional development in these children.

Cognitive Development

Early Sensory Processing

Innate sensory capabilities serve as the building blocks of cognitive development. Even at birth the healthy neonate responds to visual and auditory stimuli. These responses, like the primitive reflexes, take the form of integrated patterns of activity.

The visual acuity of the full-term infant is estimated to fall between 20/200 and 20/400 and improves rapidly over the first year of life. Even at birth, it is possible to get the full-term newborn to fix on faces 9 to 12 inches from the face and to track objects horizontally at least 30 degrees (Fig. 3-20). Some neonates, if assessed when calm and fully alert, can track objects 180 degrees across the visual field. Newborns also respond to sound, typically quieting to a human voice, rattles, or music. In the first days of life, many infants turn to the source of sound and search for it with their eyes. These maneuvers, found on the Brazelton Neonatal Behavioral Assessment Scale, are useful in demonstrating neurobehavioral characteristics of newborns.

Examination must take place at optimal times, when the infant is alert; if the infant is drowsy or agitated, the ability to track visually or to search for sounds is severely compromised. If, when assessed under optimal circumstances and when fully alert, infants do not demonstrate horizontal tracking of objects, do not look at the toys or people with whom they are involved, or hold their heads in unusual positions, the physician should recommend prompt evaluation for abnormal visual perception or central nervous system development.

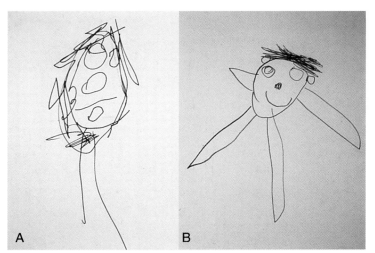

Figure 3-18. Development of skill at drawing a person. **A,** This drawing by a 4-year-old child includes five features: eyes, nose, mouth, hair, and legs. To calculate an age equivalent, the child earns $1/4$ year for each of the five features, added to a base age of 3 years. This drawing has an age equivalent of $4^{1}/_{4}$ years. **B,** A drawing by the same child at age 5. Note the inclusion of ears and arms, as well as improvements in proportion. This drawing has an age equivalent of $4^{3}/_{4}$ years.

Development of Sensorimotor Intelligence

During the first 2 years of life, the sensorimotor period of development, the young child's cognitive abilities can

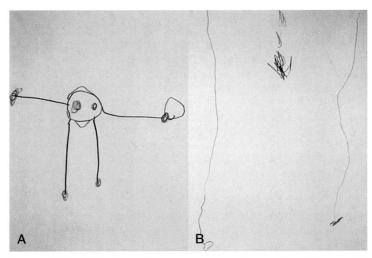

Figure 3-19. Difficulties with visual–fine motor integration skills in a child with cerebral palsy. **A,** Drawing by a bright 4-year-old who was born prematurely but showed no developmental delays. Note the inclusion of seven features: eyes, hair, mouth, arms, hands, legs, and feet. The age equivalent for this drawing is $4^{3}/_{4}$ years. **B,** Drawing by a 4-year-old child with spastic diplegia. Difficulties in organization appear related to visuomotor integration skills rather than to problems with fine motor skills.

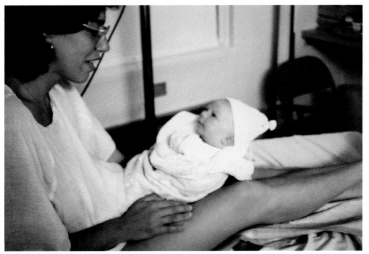

Figure 3-20. Early social skills. A newborn within an hour of birth fixates on the face of the mother.

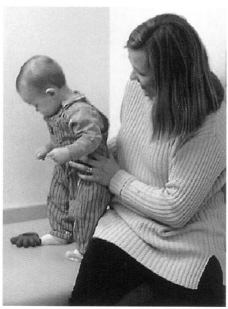

Figure 3-21. Early object permanence. A 6-month-old infant was able to track his toy through a vertical fall and to search for it on the floor even after his gaze had been interrupted.

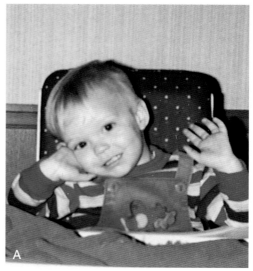

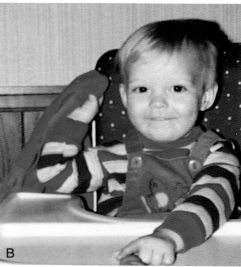

Figure 3-22. Object permanence. **A** and **B**, An 11-month-old child can locate a small, hidden object even if no part of it remains visible. In doing so, he is demonstrating his understanding that objects are permanent.

be surmised only through use of the senses and through the physical manipulation of objects. The nature of an infant's thinking is assessed through concrete interaction with the environment. During this period, the child develops an understanding of the concept of object permanence, the ability to recognize that an object exists even when it cannot be seen, heard, or felt. Simultaneously, the child develops an understanding of cause-and-effect relationships. Progress in the child's development of these concepts is an important prerequisite to the development of pure mental activity, reflected in the ability to use symbols and language.

Early progress in the development of object permanence is indicated by the infant's continued though brief gaze at the site where a familiar toy or face has disappeared. At this point, children also repeat actions that they have discovered will produce interesting results. Between 4 and 8 months of age, infants become interested in changes in the position and appearance of toys. They can track an object visually through a vertical fall (Fig. 3-21) and search for a partially hidden toy. They also begin to vary the means of creating interesting effects. In these early months the baby's play consists of exploring toys to gain information about their physical characteristics. Activities such as mouthing, shaking, and banging can provide sensory input about an object beyond its visual features. However, when mouthing of toys persists as the predominant mode of exploration after 12 to 18 months of age, assessment of cognitive function is warranted.

At approximately 9 to 12 months of age, infants can locate objects that have been completely hidden (Fig. 3-22). Not surprisingly, peekaboo becomes a favorite pastime at this point. Later, the infant can crawl away from the mother and recall where to return to find her.

As children near 1 year of age, interest in toys extends beyond physical properties (e.g., color, texture). These children may begin to demonstrate their awareness that different objects have different purposes. For example, a child might touch a comb to the hair in a meaningful nonpretend action, typical of the 9- to 12-month age range. Beyond 1 year of age, children begin to vary their behavior to create novel effects. They no longer need to

be shown how to work dials or knobs on a busy box, nor do they need to hit something by accident to discover the interesting effect that will result.

By 18 months of age, children can deduce the location of an object even if they have not seen it hidden from view. They can maintain mental images of desired objects and develop plans for obtaining them. The child's understanding of causality also advances; cause-and-effect relationships no longer need to be direct to be appreciated (Fig. 3-23). These developments herald the beginning of a new stage in cognitive development, that of symbolic thinking. They also indicate that distraction may not succeed to draw a child away from a desired object and a direct request is required.

Development of Symbolic Capabilities

In the second year of life the child demonstrates mental activity independent of sensory processing or motor manipulation. For example, the child observes a television superhero performing a rescue mission and hours later reenacts the scene with careful precision. Clearly, the child has a mental image of the event and uses it to generate the delayed imitation.

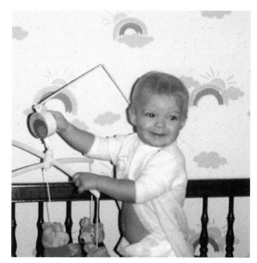

Figure 3-23. Mature means-end reasoning. A 15-month-old child turns the key of the music box atop the mobile to make it play. The child's understanding has advanced beyond that of direct causality, such as pulling a toy to bring it closer.

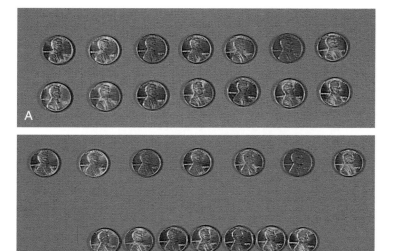

Figure 3-24. Experimental design to demonstrate preoperational logic. The 3- or 4-year-old child agrees that the two rows in **A** have the same number of pennies. After seeing the pennies moved into the configuration in **B**, the child claims that the top row has more because it is longer.

As children develop the capacity for pure mental activity, they use objects to represent other objects or ideas. Genuine pretending begins; the child engages in playful representation of commonplace activities, using objects for their actual purpose but accompanied by exaggerated sounds or gestures. Pretend actions are combined into a series of events. For example, the child may hold a phone to the ear and then to a doll's ear or may feed a teddy bear and then put the bear to bed.

The next stage in development allows the child to plan pretend activities in anticipation of the play theme to come, combining many steps into the play. Preparing for play indicates an advance in pretending beyond that of improvising with the objects at hand. For example, the child might be seen preparing the play area or searching for needed objects and announcing what the objects are meant to represent.

Development of Logical Thinking

The preschool child has well-developed capabilities for mental representation and symbolic thinking. However, the dominance of sensory input, limited life experience, and a lack of formal education lead to a unique and charming logic during this period. Preschoolers often assume that all objects are alive like themselves. A car and a tricycle, for example, may be seen as alive, perhaps because they are capable of movement. Similarly, children claim that the moon follows them on an evening walk.

The logic of the preschooler is in large part influenced by the appearance of objects. Because an airplane appears to become smaller as it takes off, the preschooler may assume that all the people on the plane become smaller as well. Piaget demonstrated that preschoolers seem to think that number and quantity vary with appearance (Fig. 3-24). Under certain circumstances a 4-year-old child may show understanding that a quantity remains invariant unless something is added or subtracted. That same child, however, may insist that two rows of pennies are different in number simply because of a compelling visual difference between them.

The immature logic of the preschooler is gradually replaced by conventional logic and wisdom. School-age children follow logic akin to adult reasoning, at least when the stimuli are concrete. Faced with the same question about the pennies, they readily acknowledge that the two rows have the same number regardless of their visual appearance (see Fig. 3-24). They also know that the airplane just looks smaller because it has moved farther from the viewer, and they giggle at the suggestion that the people on the plane have shrunk. Their logical limitations become obvious when they must reason about the hypothetical or the abstract.

Adolescents, particularly those with the benefits of formal education, tend to extend logical principles to increasingly diverse problems. They can generate multiple logical possibilities systematically when faced with scientific experiments, and they can also consider hypothetical problems. These principles of reasoning are applied not only to schoolwork but also to social situations. For example, the adolescent may think about who will go with whom to the school prom: "She thinks that I think that she wants to go with him, but I know that she wants to go with me."

Assessing Cognitive Development

Because the observations necessary to assess cognitive abilities in the preverbal period are less well known by the general public than the major motor milestones, parents often rely on physicians for guidance. Simple observation of the child's use of toys or objects can help to determine cognitive progress. The pediatrician can induce the infant to look for a hidden toy or to play a game of peekaboo; the infant's anticipation of reappearance indicates the development of the concept of object permanence. Similarly, the toddler's ability to play with a toy telephone indicates the emergence of symbolic thought. Beyond the toddler stage the physician typically relies on conversation and language ability to assess levels of cognitive skill. Screening tests are particularly useful for determining if cognitive and language skills are within the normal range. Children with language delays may need a formal nonverbal assessment of cognitive abilities by a psychologist.

For the parents, a delay in a child's attainment of a well-known milestone may create tremendous fear about ultimate learning potential. In many cases, such parental concerns are put to rest when the physician determines that the child's learning to date is age-appropriate. If a child does show delays in cognitive development, the physician should generate a differential diagnosis (Table 3-4) from knowledge of the child's level of functioning in multiple domains, history, and physical examination.

Parents should be given information about their child's delay as early as possible. Pediatricians serve a critical role in referring children to early intervention or special education programs and in monitoring their progress. Active communication between the providers of early intervention and the physician assists a comprehensive and cohesive approach.

Physicians frequently need the consultation of colleagues in psychology and education to assess the cognitive abilities of their older preschool and school-age patients. A number of methods have been devised for formal assessment of mental achievement, and almost all parents are familiar with the terms *intelligence quotient* or *IQ*. Although not a means of comprehensively assessing all mental capabilities, normal IQ scores are (albeit imperfect) predictors of which children will have the attention, social skills, motivation, and intelligence to perform well in school. Low IQ scores may reflect a child's poor ability to grasp new concepts, or they may indicate poor purposeful attending behaviors, as seen in depression or in attention deficit hyperactivity disorder (ADHD). Low scores may also reflect poor social adjustment or limitations in test-taking capabilities, such as sitting in a chair at a table and applying maximal effort to a task requested by an unfamiliar authority figure. Frequently, low scores result from a combination of difficulties in several areas.

If children with sensory or motor impairments are tested with instruments normalized on able-bodied children, they often obtain low scores. Different assessment techniques have been devised to circumvent specific disabilities while obtaining information about a child's cognitive abilities; these are typically administered by psychologists, child development specialists, or special educators (Table 3-5).

Assessment of a child's abilities to learn must go beyond standardized IQ tests. For example, some children who can score in the normal range on IQ tests are unable to learn to read. A diversified and individualized assessment process should precede any educational recommendation. The pediatrician, in the role of advocate, should ensure that assessments include information about the child's strengths and weaknesses because educational planning should involve attention to all aspects of the child's abilities. Moreover, the pediatrician can encourage families to maintain an active, decision-making role in their children's education.

Language Development

Early Skills in Speech Perception and Production

The use of language is the ability to generate and understand reproducible sounds or gestures that are recognized

---

Table 3-4 Potentially Remediable Disorders Associated with Developmental Delay

FINDINGS SOMETIMES PRESENT ON HISTORY OR EXAMINATION	POSSIBLE DISORDER
Decreased vision or hearing	Specific sensory deficits
Staring spells, motor automatism	Seizure disorders
Lethargy, ataxia	Overmedication with anticonvulsants
Myxedema, delayed return on DTRs, thick skin and tongue, sparse hair, constipation, increased sleep, coarse voice, short stature, goiter	Hypothyroidism
Irritability, cold sweats, tremor, loss of consciousness	Hypoglycemia
Unexplained bruises in varying stages, failure to thrive	Child abuse and neglect
Short stature, weight below third percentile	Malnutrition or systemic illness producing failure to thrive
Poor purposeful attending in multiple settings	ADHD
No specific findings	Environmental deprivation
Anemia	Iron deficiency or lead exposure
Absent venous pulsations or papilledema on funduscopic examination, morning vomiting, headaches, brisk DTRs in lower extremities	Increased intracranial pressure
Vomiting, irritability and seizures, failure to thrive	Some inborn errors of metabolism (e.g., methylmalonicacidemia)
Hepatomegaly, jaundice, hypotonia, susceptibility to infection, cataracts	Galactosemia
Fair hair, blue eyes, "mousy" odor to urine	Phenylketonuria
Ongoing evidence of active or progressive disease	Chronic infection, inflammatory disease, malignancies

ADHD, attention deficit hyperactivity disorder; DTR, deep tendon reflex.

Table 3-5 Tests Used in the Assessment of Cognitive Development

TYPE OF SCALE	TESTS USED	AGE RANGE
Standard intelligence scales	Stanford-Binet Intelligence Scale—IV	2-adult
	Wechsler Intelligence Scale for Children—IV	6-16 years
Nonverbal intelligence scales	Leiter International Performance Scale—R	2-18 years
Infant development tests	Bayley Scales of Infant Development—III	0-3$\frac{1}{2}$ years
	Gesell Developmental Schedules	0-5 years
Developmental scales for the visually impaired	Reynell-Zinkin Developmental Scales for Young Children with Visual Impairments	0-5 years
Adaptive behavior	Vineland Adaptive Behavior Scales—II	0-18 years
	Adaptive Behavior Assessment System—II	0-21 years

by others as representative of concepts. Language development begins slowly and subtly in the first year of life. Language skills are subdivided into two realms: receptive skills—the ability to comprehend communication—and expressive skills—the ability to produce communication.

Neonates demonstrate skills that are useful in the eventual development of receptive language abilities. Even before birth, fetuses detect sounds and show preferences for some sounds over others. Pregnant women report that their unborn children may kick after sudden loud noises and that they may kick harder for rock than classical music. At birth, the newborn is particularly attuned to the human voice and may turn toward a parent who is gently whispering. Children remain interested in sounds as they grow older and turn voluntarily toward the source of a sound by 3 to 4 months of age (Fig. 3-25).

Children can also differentiate speech sounds, even close to birth. Experimental paradigms, using the fact that an infant's heart rate and sucking patterns change when they encounter new environmental stimuli, suggest that infants as young as 1 month of age can differentiate such similar speech sounds as /ba/ and /pa/. Frequent exposure to the native language alters speech perception such that by late infancy it becomes difficult for children to differentiate sounds that are not meaningful distinctions in their own language.

By 2 to 3 months of age, children begin to *coo* or make musical sounds spontaneously. This is the first step toward the development of expressive verbal language. Even in the early stages, children can establish reciprocal patterns, similar to the rhythm of conversation.

By about 6 months of age, children place consonant sounds with vowel sounds, creating what is known as *babble*. In this period the infant says "ma-ma" or "da-da" without necessarily referring to the loving parent. By 9 to 12 months of age, children integrate babble with intonational patterns consistent with the parent's speech. This is called *jargon*.

Later Development

In the second half of the first year the child develops early skills in true receptive language. Milestones are listed in Table 3-6. By 6 months of age, children reliably respond to their names, and at about 9 months, they can follow verbal routines, such as waving bye-bye or showing how big they are. At about the same age, they also learn that pointing shares the focus of attention. The young infant

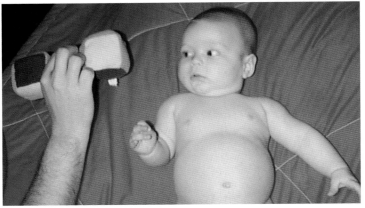

Figure 3-25. Localizing sound. A 3-month-old infant responds to interesting sounds by looking in the direction of the sound.

looks at the point, whereas the older infant looks at the object to which the point is directed.

Receptive language can be demonstrated as children follow increasingly complex commands. For example, children will understand one-step commands such as "throw the ball" by approximately 1 year of age. The labeling of commonplace items in pictures is slightly more complex and begins after 1 year of age. The ability to choose between two pictures when asked "show me the . . ." should be consistent between 18 and 24 months of age.

By 2½ years of age, receptive language skills have advanced beyond the understanding of simple labels. The child is able to identify objects by their use. Continued advances in receptive language occur during the preschool years and are highly susceptible to environmental stimulation or deprivation.

Expressive language skills (see Table 3-6) lag behind receptive skills in the first year of life. But even before word production begins, a child's gestures have communicative intent. Many 9- to 10-month-olds can communicate that their juice or cereal is "all gone" by placing their hands palms up, at shoulder height. Even older children gesture to make themselves understood because gross and fine motor skills develop faster than the oropharyngeal muscle skills used in articulation.

Expressive language at first develops slowly. The child's first meaningful words are produced around the first birthday. Over the next 6 months the child may master only 20 to 50 more words. These early words come and go from the child's vocabulary and tend to be idiosyncratic child-forms. After 18 to 24 months, word usage increases rapidly, standard forms replace baby talk, and word combinations begin.

The child's earliest two-word sentences typically contain important content words but lack prepositions, articles, and verb-tense markings. This two-word phase has been called *telegraphic speech* because, like a telegram, the child leaves out nonessential articles and prepositions. Once the child is capable of three- and four-word utterances, length limitations do not appear to be a significant barrier. By age 3 the child has developed complex language with the use of pronouns and prepositions. The child develops the ability to ask questions. At age 2½ years they usually ask "what?" and by age 3 years they most frequently ask "why?" The child also can use negation within a sentence. By age 5 the child uses all parts of speech, as well as clauses and complex sentences.

The rate of language development appears to be associated with both biological and environmental factors. About half or more of children with first-degree relatives with language and speech delays also show delays. The amount of child-directed speech in the environment is a good predictor of the rate of development for vocabulary and grammar. For this reason, health supervision of infants and toddlers should encourage parents to speak or read to their children.

Mastering Intelligibility and Fluency

Sounds required in language are mastered at different rates. Children who are attempting to say words containing sounds they cannot yet produce have a variety of choices on how to proceed: by omission of the difficult sound (*ba* for bottle), by substitution of a different sound (*fum* for thumb), or by distortion (*goyl* for girl). The infor-

Table 3-6	Receptive and Expressive Language Milestones	
AGE RANGE	**RECEPTIVE RESPONSE**	**EXPRESSIVE RESPONSE**
0-1½ months	Startles or widens eyes to sound	Shows variation in crying (hunger, pain)
1½-4 months	Quiets to voice, blinks eyes to sound	Makes musical sounds; coos; participates in reciprocal exchange
4-9 months	Turns head toward sound; responds with raised arms when parent says "up" and reaches for child; responds appropriately to friendly or angry voices	Babbles; repeats self-initiated sounds
9-12 months	Listens selectively to familiar words; begins to respond to "no"; responds to verbal routine such as wave bye-bye or clap; turns to own name	Uses symbolic gestures and jargon; repeats parent-initiated sounds
12-18 months	Points to three body parts (eyes, nose, mouth); understands up to 50 words; recognizes common objects by name (dog, cat, bottle, ball, book); follows one-step commands accompanied by gestures ("give me the doll," "hug your bear," "open your mouth")	Uses words to express needs; learns 20 to 50 words by 18 months; uses words inconsistently and mixed with jargon, echolalia, or both
18 months-2 years	Points to pictures when asked "show me"; understands *soon, in, on,* and *under;* begins to distinguish *you* from *me;* can formulate negative judgments (a pear is not a cookie)	Uses telegraphic two-word sentences ("go bye-bye," "up daddy," "want cookie")
30 months	Follows two-step commands; can identify objects by use	Uses jargon and echolalia infrequently; makes average sentence of 2½ words; adjectives and adverbs appear; begins to ask questions, asks adults to repeat actions ("do it again")
3 years	Knows several colors; knows what we do when we are hungry, thirsty, or sleepy; is aware of past and future; understands *today* and *not today*	Uses pronouns and plurals; can tell stories that begin to be understood; uses negative ("I can't," "I won't"); verbalizes toilet needs; can tell full name, age, and gender; forms sentences of 3 to 4 words
3½ years	Can answer such questions as "do you have a doggie?", "which is the boy?", and "what toys do you have?"; understands *little, funny,* and *secret*	Can relate experiences in sequential order; can say a nursery rhyme; can ask permission
4 years	Understands same versus different; follows three-step commands; completes opposite analogies (a brother is a boy, a sister is a . . .); understands why we have houses, stoves, and umbrellas	Tells a story; uses past tense; counts to 3; names primary colors; enjoys rhyming nonsense words, enjoys exaggerations; asks many questions a day
5 years	Understands what we do with eyes and ears; understands differences in texture (hard, soft, smooth); understands *if, when,* and *why;* identifies words in terms of use; begins to understand left and right	Indicates "I don't know"; indicates *funny,* and *surprise;* can define in terms of use; asks definition of specific words; makes serious inquiries ("how does this work?" and "what does it mean?"); uses mature sentence structure and form

Table 3-7	Phonemes and Intelligibility	
AGE RANGE*	**SOUNDS MASTERED**	**PERCENT INTELLIGIBILITY (TO A STRANGER)**
2 years	—	50
3 years	14 vowels and *p, b, m*	75
4 years	10 vowel blends and *n, ng, w, h, t, d, k, g*	100
5 years	*f, v, y, th, l, wh*	100
6 years	*r, s, z, ch, j, sh, zh,* and consonant blends	100

*The ages presented here are general guidelines because authorities differ with regard to the specific ages associated with articulation and intelligibility.

mation presented in Table 3-7 provides an estimate of when mastery of particular sounds, along with estimates of overall intelligibility, might be expected.

Assessing Language Development

In the early stages of prelinguistic and linguistic development, direct assessment by the pediatrician may be difficult. Children are likely to remain quiet in new situations, especially in the office where they received an injection. It is usually easy to engage a normally developing child of age 3 in conversation. Before that age the physician may need to rely on parental report. Standard-ized parent reports are available for office use, and parent reports contribute to the assessment of language in screening tests.

The differential diagnosis for delayed expressive language development includes impaired hearing, global developmental delay or mental retardation, environmental deprivation, autism, emotional maladjustment, or specific language impairment. Keeping this in mind, worrisome clinical situations include the 4- to 6-month-old infant who fails to coo responsively, the 9- to 10-month-old child who does not babble or whose cooing and babbling have diminished, and the 18-month-old child whose repertoire of words includes only *mama* or *dada.* Beyond 18 months a convenient rule of thumb is that children 2 years of age should use two-word utterances, at least half of which should be intelligible. By 3 years of age, children should use phrases of three or more words, three quarters of which should be intelligible. Children who fail to achieve these developmental milestones should undergo evaluation for hearing loss, as well as for cognitive and emotional impairment.

Families often attribute language delays in their youngster to superficial and easily remediable physiologic or social factors. "Being tongue-tied," for example, in most cases is not an explanation for delayed speech. However, it may be the effect rather than the cause because the frenulum of the tongue may be tight in some children due to not being sufficiently exercised by early verbal practice. Similarly, children rarely delay language because "they don't need it." Children have tremendous motivation to improve their verbal skills, even if they have older siblings who speak for them. For children who want a particular food, for example, a point toward the cupboard door will not specify precisely what is wanted. The parents must offer the items one at a time and await acceptance or rejection. The use of a verbal label will allow the child to meet needs efficiently.

Delays in the development of intelligibility might include any of the following:
1. Lack of intelligible speech by age 3
2. Frequent omission of initial consonants after age 4
3. Continued substitution of easy sounds for more difficult ones after age 5
4. Persistent articulation errors after age 7

If any of these delays persist for 6 months or more, a referral should be initiated.

During the period in which articulation and vocabulary are being mastered, speech dysfluencies are common. Noticeable stuttering or rapid speech beyond age 4 should prompt further attention. The problems of nasality, inaudibility, and unusual pitch sometimes may be helped by a speech pathologist. Furthermore, children of any age who are embarrassed by their speech are appropriate candidates for referral.

Therapy for speech and language disorders helps improve the communication skills of children with language delays and problems of intelligibility. A child whose unusual language pattern is destined to be outgrown will not suffer from monitoring by a communication disorders specialist; the child whose language impairment will not be outgrown has much to lose when help is delayed.

Social Development

Early Capabilities: Social Responsivity

The earliest social task of newborns is to establish a mutually satisfying relationship with their caregivers. Neonates begin this process by fixing visually on faces in preference to other sights, a skill that is evident during the first few days of life (see Fig. 3-20). The responsive smile develops soon thereafter (Fig. 3-26). The social smile is another innate behavior, although it may not appear until 4 to 6 weeks of life. Smiling appears in infants from all cultures at about the same time. Infants with visual impairment who cannot appreciate a smile on the faces of their caregivers nonetheless smile at ages comparable with sighted children.

Development of Attachment

During the first 6 months of life, infants are rather indiscriminate in their social behavior, smiling and later laughing with anyone willing to play. Infants develop a sense that their parents exist when out of sight sooner than they learn inanimate objects are permanent. By 6 to 8 months of age, children protest when their parents leave the room. As infants begin to recognize faces of familiar caregivers, they may squirm and cling in the company of unfamiliar people, exhibiting stranger awareness. The severity of the reaction varies with the infant's temperament and with previous experiences. Extreme reactions, known as *stranger anxiety,* may occur in children who have not had routine care from alternative caregivers. Pediatricians are advised to refrain from holding the 9- to 12-month-old child at the well-child visit. A child who remains playful and calm while securely in the parent's arms may quickly fret or cry even if gently removed from that security.

By 1 year of age, most children have experienced periods of separation from a parent, whether it be for minutes or hours. Infants who have developed a secure attachment to their parents show signs of recognition and pleasure when they are reunited with them. While progressing in gross motor development, the child initiates separation by walking away independently and exploring at greater distances from parents. Typically, infants return regularly for some verbal encouragement, eye contact, or hugging and then venture farther. In contrast, infants who have not developed secure attachments may show indifference, ambivalence, or disorganization at reunion with their parents. Their exploration of the environment during the toddler years is limited. These children are at risk for troubled social relationships as they become older.

Development of Social Play

Infants and young toddlers tend to line up and engage in similar activities simultaneously. This pattern is called *parallel play.* Although parents often expect their young toddlers to interact or share with peers, success in this age group is unusual. Sharing for a young toddler involves showing or handing a prized toy to another child, only to take it back within seconds.

By 2 years of age, with the development of symbolic capabilities in cognitive development, children begin to pretend. They will seek to engage their parents in activities that satisfy their growing curiosity. They enjoy reading with caregivers and having their labeling questions answered.

Near 3 years of age, children begin to include one another in their pretending games. At first both children may select the same role (e.g., two mothers), whereas later, the roles become more realistic and interactive. The young preschooler is especially interested in imitating the parent of the same gender but shows no preference for same- or opposite-gender playmates.

The child's abilities to share are shaped by social experiences. Children who attend day care may share successfully at an earlier age than children raised at home (Fig.

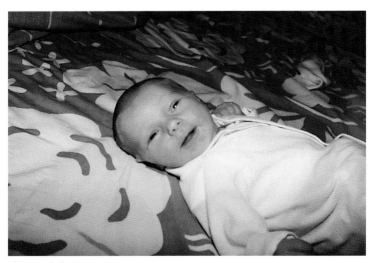

Figure 3-26. Early smiling. A 19-day-old infant smiles for her parents.

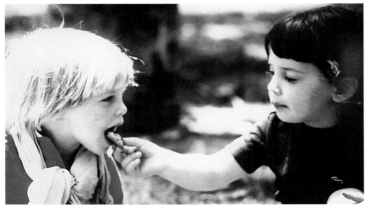

Figure 3-27. Sharing. Two-year-old children with day-care experience share a special treat.

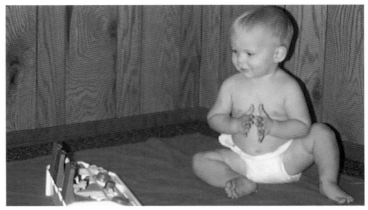

Figure 3-28. Mastery smile. A 15-month-old boy demonstrates that toddlers beyond 1 year of age can take pride in their own accomplishments. This child is applauding his own success at having made the puppets appear.

3-27). Although it can be achieved through consistent experience, taking turns is also a challenge for the preschooler who possesses a limited concept of time. Impulse control is just developing in the preschool years. Active goals for this age group include learning to gain the cooperation of one's peers, learning to communicate ideas to new friends, and learning to handle conflicts.

By 4 to 5 years of age, peer interactions grow increasingly cooperative and complicated; pretend play involves themes requiring greater feats of imagination and experience, such as trips or parties. Older preschoolers enjoy helping with household tasks and frequently are more interested in participating in gender-specific activities than they were at an earlier age. This interest may relate to cognitive and social development. As children understand that they are in the same category as their same-gender parent, they become interested in the implications of category membership. Strict adherence to the rules of category membership reflects the concrete and inflexible thinking of the preschooler.

Preschoolers do not often play games with rules. Rules are seen as variable, to be made and broken at the discretion of the players. Getting through a board game with preschoolers who decide not to follow the rules once they discover that the rules are not working in their favor is often a challenge.

Children become capable of playing by rules when they reach school age. With superior logical capabilities, they realize that rules are invariant and must be followed regardless of the personal implications. As they progress through the elementary school years, board games and sports become preferred activities for groups of peers.

Development of Sense of Self

Self-awareness and independence develop gradually throughout life. The earliest indications of an emerging identity occur at 6 to 9 months of age, when infants display interest in their own mirror images. Some 7- to 8-month-olds may prefer to grab the cups and spoons rather than accept passive roles in eating. These infants may resist pressure to do something that they would prefer not to do (e.g., fussing to stand when placed in a sitting position).

Beyond 1 year of age, toddlers rapidly expand their sense of self. They explore their environment with ease, and they are increasingly able to function independently.

They can feed themselves with a cup and spoon, and they have clear ideas about what they want. Children at 1 to 2 years of age also enjoy their own accomplishments and can clap for their own successes (Fig. 3-28).

An emerging sense of self and the thrust for independence make discipline of the toddler a challenge. Parents may need help in viewing their child's refusals to eat, nap, or be washed as positive steps toward increased independence. They may also need support in setting limits on the child's behaviors.

As the child reaches 2 to 3 years of age, increased independence in verbal abilities, increased awareness of body sensations, and modest skills in donning and doffing clothing combine with the child's desire to imitate adults and to gain parental approval. This combination of accomplishments allows toilet training to begin. In fact, these developmental milestones mentioned may be viewed as readiness signs. The pediatrician can review them with families at the 15- or 18-month visit so that parents can time their toilet-training efforts to the child's developmental rate and style. Children differ substantially in their interest in achieving bladder and bowel control, and parents may benefit from counseling to maintain a relaxed approach.

In other areas as well, children need support in their attempts to initiate and control their own activities. Toward this end, parents can be encouraged to allow their child to practice emerging self-care skills, such as zipping or buttoning a coat, even when the practice costs precious time in a rushed schedule. Should the child become frustrated or disappointed, a response of empathy is likely to soothe more effectively than a response of reason because rational reasoning is limited during this preoperational cognitive period.

By mid to late elementary school, cognitive development has progressed toward abstract and hypothetical thinking such that children are able to reflect self-consciously about themselves and others. First- or second-graders struggle to understand the causes of conflict or their emotional reactions to it. Older elementary-school children and adolescents are able to analyze situations, reasons, and reactions. They begin to understand their own motivations and the environmental triggers of their responses.

Throughout childhood the desire to grow up is in continued conflict with the desire to remain a child. The young preschooler is just beginning to address this issue. Families frequently report that a child's accomplishments in socioemotional functioning backslide when unexpected stresses challenge household equilibrium or when the child becomes ill. As a result, temporary regressions to earlier levels of functioning may occur in some children. Importantly, parents must learn to view these lapses as expected components of development rather than as intentional lapses on the part of the child. However, if the regression is prolonged and significant, the physician may initiate an evaluation of the child's emotional status.

During elementary-school years, at least in Western cultures, the child's self-image is strongly influenced by success or failure in school. Not only do difficulties with learning put additional pressures on the child, they also may damage the child's sense of self-worth. Parents and teachers of children with learning problems should be especially willing to praise the child for effort, accomplishments, and good behavior. Physicians should be particularly sensitive to the higher risk of emotional and behavioral problems in children with learning difficulties so that they can make timely referrals to colleagues in the mental health professions.

Evaluation of Social Development

Subtle indicators of sociodevelopmental status can be gleaned in the course of a routine pediatric visit. The physician has the opportunity to note not only the way the infant behaves but also the style of parental caregiving and the nature of the parent-child relationship. The young infant typically shows social responsiveness to both the parent and the pediatrician, although at 9 months of age, there is a definite preference for the familiar parent. Also at this age, particularly in times of stress, the infant turns to the parent for support and comfort. Children of limited responsiveness, who avoid physical contact, avert their gaze, or in other ways fail to contribute to a mutually satisfying reciprocal exchange are of concern. Of equal concern are parents who are harsh, unresponsive, or threatening in response to the infant's needs.

Given the nature of sociodevelopmental change, the assessment of possible problems must rely largely on history. Parents tend to be frank and open about the nature of their relationship with their child if questions are asked in a direct and nonjudgmental way. Difficulties in social development may relate to constitutional and temperamental characteristics of the child, as well as to philosophy and practices of the parent. By remembering the bidirectional nature of causality in social development, the physician can avoid slipping into criticisms or judgments.

The older preschool or school-age child may be able to give, independently, direct information about social development. For example, the child may be able to name special friends and the activities enjoyed with those friends. Young preschoolers might name both boys and girls and list rough-and-tumble or fantasy play as favorite activities. Older preschoolers might name same-gender friends but similar activities. School-age children might add board games and sports to their list of activities.

Variations in Developmental Patterns

The presence or absence of a single skill at a particular age is rarely sufficient to determine developmental status. Developmental progress is highly dependent on multiple factors: the general health of the child, opportunities for learning, temperamental characteristics, willingness to try new experiences, genetic endowments, coordination and strength, and socioeconomic factors. If delays occur in more than one domain, persist over time, or both, they are considered significant. The challenge for the pediatrician is to differentiate variation from deviation and disorder.

Sometimes the parents raise developmental concerns. These concerns must be addressed freely and openly. Parents are rarely comforted by superficial evaluation and pat reassurance, and although prudent waiting may serve some families well, it may arouse anxiety and anger in others. If a comprehensive evaluation of a given problem is beyond the capabilities of the pediatrician, early referral should be considered.

Evaluation of developmental problems proceeds in the same manner as evaluation of other medical concerns: history, physical examination (including neurologic and developmental evaluation), and laboratory testing. Important in establishing a diagnosis is consideration of the pattern of development across all domains. For example, findings of hypotonia and selective problems in gross motor skills along with normal development in cognition, language, and social skills suggest a neuromuscular disorder or benign congenital hypotonia. In contrast, hypotonia with global developmental delay suggests a central nervous system problem. Differentiating delayed behavior from deviant behavior is also important. For example, because even neonates can make good eye contact with their caregivers, the toddler who avoids eye contact is showing deviancy rather than delay. The combination of sustained deviant social behavior and delayed language development is suggestive of childhood autism.

Cerebral Palsy

Cerebral palsy is a disorder of movement and posture resulting from injury to the brain. The type of cerebral palsy varies according to the location of the injured area. Injury may occur before birth, during labor and delivery, or after birth, up through the preschool years. Affected patients may have a history of perinatal complications. However, in 20% to 30% of cases, no etiology can be established. The key to making the diagnosis is to establish that motor problems are not progressive. Regression of motor skills suggests a different set of diagnostic possibilities including surgically treatable lesions of the brain or spinal cord or inherited neurodegenerative diseases.

Physical Examination

A diagnosis of cerebral palsy and a determination of its subtype can be established through physical examination. However, physical findings over the first year of life are highly variable and nonspecific. Early signs may include decreased passive tone in the presence of brisk deep tendon reflexes (DTRs) without concomitant weakness. Early problems with sucking and swallowing may predate evidence of motor delays.

Because the findings may change, the definitive diagnosis of cerebral palsy should not be made until the child is at least 1 year of age in a child born at term, and 15 to 18 months of age in a child born prematurely. Beyond that point the diagnosis is based on abnormal findings in four of six major motor areas: posture, oromotor functioning, visuomotor functioning, tone, evolution of primitive reflexes, and muscle-stretch reflexes (Table 3-8).

Abnormalities of Tone. Because damage to the central nervous system prevents the inhibition and balance of the inherent tone of the muscles, abnormalities of tone are particularly significant in the diagnosis of cerebral palsy. After initial hypotonia, a child may develop increased tone between 12 and 18 months of age, showing clearly rigid or spastic hypertonia by age 2.

The child who demonstrates increased extensor tone beginning in early infancy is also at risk for cerebral palsy. Under normal circumstances, infants younger than 3 months of age, when supported ventrally, maintain their heads in slight flexion with the trunks mildly convex (Fig. 3-29A). However, with exaggerated tone in the antigravity muscle group, the infant may elevate the head above the horizontally level trunk (Fig. 3-29B). Similarly, the unknowing parents may be pleased by their child's apparent precocious development of head control when the child is prone or rolls belly-to-back in the first 2 months of life, when in fact both of these findings suggest excessive extensor posturing.

Further evidence of abnormally increased tone is found when the supine child is pulled to an upright position and extends at the hips and knees, coming to stand on pointed toes rather than ending up in the appropriate sitting posture. This child, when placed in vertical suspension, will not right the head as expected and will later scissor the lower extremities as a result of hypertonia of the leg adductors and internal rotators (Fig. 3-30). Parents may find it difficult to position these infants for diapering and feeding; knowledge of the Marie-Foix maneuver, used to break up excessive extension in the lower extremities (Fig. 3-31), will help them.

Abnormalities in Development of Primitive Reflexes and Equilibrium Responses. Abnormal persistence of primitive reflexes is helpful in making a diagnosis of cerebral palsy. Damage to the central nervous system prevents high levels of control from superseding and inhibiting the influence of the early reflexes. Thus obligate or persistent primitive reflexes are signs of cerebral palsy. For example, in the normal variant of the ATNR, the infant can move out of the posture if the gaze is directed to the other side of the body. In an obligate ATNR, however, the infant remains in the fencer position until the head is passively moved. This finding is not normal in a child of any age and is highly suggestive of the static encephalopathy and motor deficit characterizing cerebral palsy.

Also strongly suggestive of cerebral palsy is the non-obligate ATNR that persists beyond 6 months of age. This

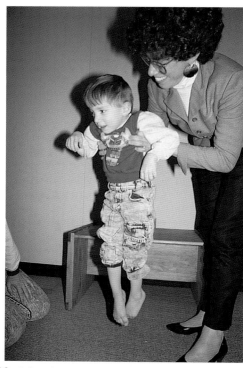

Figure 3-30. Scissoring. Excessive pull of the hip adductors and internal rotators in this child of 3 years results in his legs crossing in a scissor-like pattern while he is supported in vertical suspension.

Table 3-8	The Levine (POSTER) Criteria for Diagnosis of Cerebral Palsy

1. Posturing and abnormal movement patterns—extensor thrusts, blocks
2. Oropharyngeal problems—tongue thrusts, grimacing, swallowing difficulties
3. Strabismus
4. Tone—increased or decreased in muscles
5. Evolutional responses—persistent primitive reflexes or failure to develop equilibrium and protective responses
6. Reflexes—increased deep tendon reflex and extension of the toes during plantar reflexes

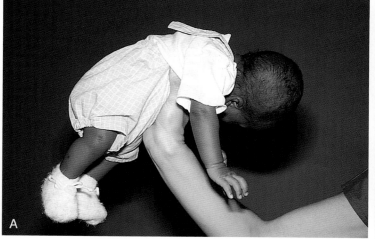
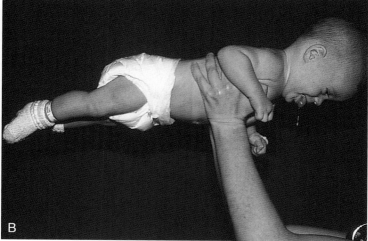

Figure 3-29. Ventral suspension. **A,** This infant's posture is normal for a 1- to 3-month-old child held in ventral suspension. The head, hips, and knees are flexed. **B,** For a child 4 months of age or older held in ventral suspension with normal posture, the head, hips, and knees may be extended. This finding is abnormal in a child younger than 3 months of age.

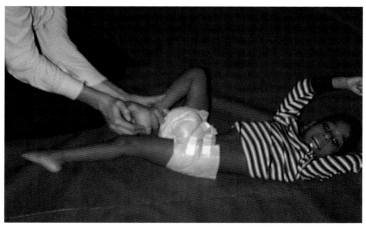

Figure 3-31. Marie-Foix maneuver. By flexing the child's toes, the therapist can reduce extensor tone enough to obtain abduction of the hip and knee flexion in this child with spastic quadriplegia.

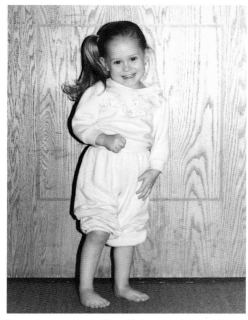

Figure 3-33. Note the arm held in flexion and internal rotation and the leg circumducted on the involved side in this child with hemiplegic cerebral palsy.

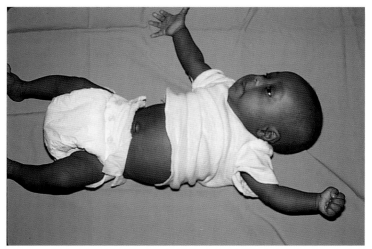

Figure 3-32. Asymmetrical Moro response. Note one hand is fisted and one open. This child warrants a neurologic examination and close follow-up.

is one possible explanation for a consistent preference in a 6- to 12-month-old child to sleep or lie with the head turned in a particular direction. Similarly, persistence of the Moro response beyond 6 months of age is associated with cerebral palsy, as is a lack of development of lateral protective equilibrium reactions by 7 to 8 months or of the parachute reaction by 10 months of age.

Subtypes of Cerebral Palsy

Hemiparesis. Hemiparesis is caused by asymmetrical damage to the motor control areas of the central nervous system. In children with hemiparesis, functional discrepancies often predate asymmetrical changes in tone or reflexes. The upper extremities may be affected more severely than the lower extremities. Asymmetrical use of the upper or lower extremities is rare during the first 4 months of life. When seen in the resting state or when elicited with the ATNR or the Moro response (Fig. 3-32), it is more likely related to lower motor neuron disease than to cerebral injury. At 4 to 6 months, during the development of early reaching and grasping, signs of hemiparesis include the presence of one hand that is fisted, the arm getting caught beneath the body when the child tries to prop up on the elbows or hands, and evidence that the arm is not used in simple tasks. Increased resistance to supination at the wrist, limited flopping of

one wrist when the upper extremities are gently shaken, or extra beats of unilateral clonus at the ankle are other clues.

Later, during the first year of life, abnormal findings include a failure to develop the protective response of lateral propping or the development of an asymmetrical parachute response. In addition, crawling may be uneven, with propulsion coming from one side while the opposite arm and leg are dragged behind.

Children with hemiparesis may have difficulty in compensating for their lack of protective responses, their uneven strength, and poor balance. Walking is typically delayed until 2 to 3 years of age. In mildly affected children, walking may be almost normal, but when asked to run, the child may show posturing of the upper extremity in flexion and internal rotation. Usually, the lower limb rotates internally and the foot may be held in equinus, making it functionally longer on the swing-through part of the gait. To clear the foot from the floor, the child compensates by swinging the leg farther out in abduction or by circumducting the affected side. These patterns, in some cases, also can be observed in standing (Fig. 3-33).

Children with hemiparesis may neglect the visual field on their affected side. Parents should position their infant so that visual stimulation is provided to the intact visual field. Another consideration is that of abnormal bony stresses caused by asymmetrical muscle strength. Unequal spinal stresses predispose children with hemiparesis to scoliosis, especially during growth spurts.

Spastic Diplegia and Quadriplegia. Spastic diplegia implies dysfunction of the lower extremities, with normal or limited involvement of the upper extremities. Spastic quadriplegia implies dysfunction of the upper and lower extremities. The child with spasticity may have presenting symptoms that include delayed sitting, crawling, or walking or toe-walking (Fig. 3-34). In the supine position, children with spastic diplegia may keep their lower extremities in the "frog" position, with the hips and knees flexed and the hips externally rotated. In the erect position the child may internally rotate and adduct the legs, leading to scissoring (see Fig. 3-30). The ankles assume

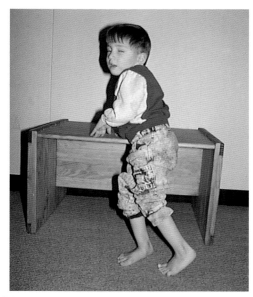

Figure 3-34. Toe-walking. A 4-year-old child with cerebral palsy cruises on furniture. Notice that the child is crouched because of hamstring tightness and is toe-walking because of gastrocnemius tightness.

the equinus position. Children with spastic diplegia who learn to walk often show persistent toe-walking in the presence of brisk DTRs, limited range of ankle motion, Babinski reflexes, and a normally proportioned muscle mass.

The differential diagnosis of toe-walking includes the muscular dystrophies, tethered spinal cords and spinal tumors, peripheral neuropathies, and fixed bony deformities of the feet. Unilateral or asymmetrical toe-walking may indicate leg-length discrepancy or a dislocated hip as an isolated finding or in conjunction with spasticity.

Athetoid or Ataxic Cerebral Palsy. In children with athetoid or ataxic cerebral palsy, involuntary movements do not present until after the first year of life. However, affected infants tend to be hypotonic and normoreflexive from the outset, and motor milestones are delayed. Between 1 and 2 years of age, hypotonia is usually replaced by spasticity, and involuntary movements appear. Exaggerated tone and dyskinetic movements reach maximal intensity around age 3. Athetoid cerebral palsy has been associated with bilirubin encephalopathy and damage to the basal ganglia.

Hypotonic Cerebral Palsy. Some hypotonic infants with exaggerated reflexes do not progress to hypertonicity. The putative explanation is cerebellar dysfunction with pyramidal track involvement. The child with hypotonic cerebral palsy usually exhibits severe motor and intellectual disability. The prognosis for independent functioning is quite poor. Hypotonic cerebral palsy must be differentiated from benign congenital hypotonia, an isolated disorder of tone, which spares other developmental areas.

Associated Findings with Cerebral Palsy

Up to 75% of children with diplegia or quadriplegia have strabismus (see Chapter 19). Refractive errors are found in 25% to 50% of children with cerebral palsy. Clumsiness because of motor imbalance of the lower extremities may be exaggerated by altered depth perception resulting from impaired visual function. Ophthalmologic referral for phorias and tropias that persist beyond 4 months of age is important to prevent amblyopia.

Hearing loss is also associated with cerebral palsy. Although clinical evaluation may suggest hearing loss, a definitive diagnosis requires an audiologic assessment. Brainstem auditory responses can be obtained to assess hearing capabilities in infants younger than 6 months of age and in older children unable to perform in conventional or conditioned play audiometry because of motor or intellectual problems.

Approximately 50% of children with cerebral palsy have cognitive impairment or mental retardation. Learning disabilities and attentional weaknesses are more prevalent in this population than in the general population. Furthermore, behavioral problems may develop as a result of the frustration encountered in trying to adjust to motor disabilities.

Prognosis

Overall, the ability of individuals with cerebral palsy to live and work independently depends on the severity of the motor disability and associated cognitive impairments. If a child is 4 years of age or older and has not achieved sitting balance, independent walking with or without crutches is rarely possible. A child 2 to 4 years of age who cannot sit and has three or more primitive reflexes is also unlikely to walk.

Because cerebral palsy affects multiple systems, children with the disorder are best served by an interdisciplinary team including not only medical professionals but also social workers, psychologists, occupational and physical therapists, speech and communication therapists, and educational and vocational specialists. In many cases, children require educational support for physical and intellectual problems. They may also require behavioral management training or pharmacologic intervention for attentional weaknesses. Some of the behavioral problems can be prevented by matching developmental expectations to the child's functional capacities. These children and their families benefit enormously from the support of a primary care physician who offers routine health care maintenance, diagnostic and preventive procedures such as referrals to audiology and ophthalmology specialists, and advice and counseling on the interpretation of team evaluations.

Mental Retardation

According to the American Association on Mental Retardation, *mental retardation* is a disability characterized by significant limitations both in intellectual functioning and adaptive behavior that arises before age 18 years. *Limitations in intellectual functioning* is generally defined as scores on standardized intelligence tests that are about two or more standard deviations below age-group norms; *adaptive behaviors* refers to the broad areas of conceptual, social, and practical functioning such as learning, communication, self-care, community participation (e.g., riding public transportation, engaging in recreation, voting), and social interactions.

The ability to predict intellectual performance and academic achievement from developmental testing during infancy is quite limited. Only in children falling far behind age expectations should one anticipate permanent intellectual disability. If an infant shows delayed cognitive development, the parents' reasonable concerns can be met with a referral to an early intervention program to increase the probability of improvements over time.

As children with early developmental delays approach school age, particularly if they have had optimal educational support, the ability to predict later difficulties improves. The rate of developmental progress during the preschool years is often a good predictor of later intellectual performance. After initial cognitive developmental delays, if a child can achieve 6 months' progress in 6 months, the prognosis for normal intellectual capacity is good. However, if the child achieves, for example, 4 months' progress in 6 months, the rate of development is 67% of the expected rate and the prognosis for later normal intellectual functioning is poor. By the time a child is 6 to 7 years of age, limitations as measured on an IQ test typically characterize the individual's abilities throughout life. At that point, the term *mental retardation* is more specific and accurate than *developmental delay*.

Physical Examination

Physical examination can be helpful in determining the cause of mental retardation. Most children classified as mentally retarded function in the mild range. These children often have a normal physical examination, with no apparent evidence of major or minor malformations. In contrast to children with severe mental retardation, who are more readily identified, children with mild retardation are likely to have normal motor milestones and delays only in adaptive areas such as self-care, language acquisition, or play. The detection of disability in these mildly affected youngsters may not occur until the child experiences school performance difficulties.

The average IQ of parents of children with mild mental retardation is lower than the population norm. Thus many of these parents also show limitations in intellectual abilities. For this reason the etiology of mild mental retardation is generally felt to be multifactorial, including multiple genetic contributions and limited social enrichment.

The more significant the degree of retardation, the more likely that a specific etiologic factor will be found. Children who score in the moderate, severe, or profound ranges are likely to have congenital malformations of the central nervous system, severe neurologic insults in the prenatal or perinatal period, an inherited disorder, or another specific diagnosis. A systematic approach to the physical examination may reveal clues to the nature of the underlying disorder.

Growth Pattern and Vital Signs. Aberrant growth patterns, which are in and of themselves the cause for assessment, may be associated with developmental delays and mental retardation. Obesity appears as part of a number of syndromes associated with mental deficiency, such as Laurence-Moon syndrome and Prader-Willi syndrome (see Chapter 1). Children who are exceptionally large may have cerebral giantism (Soto syndrome). Small-for-date infants deserve close study for evidence of anomalies or infection; they are also at risk for abnormal development. Extreme to moderate short stature, with or without skeletal dysplasia, is associated with many dysmorphic syndromes that include mental retardation as an associated finding. Growth curves have been prepared for children with various genetic and chromosomal disorders such as Down syndrome because they tend to be shorter than the general population (Fig. 3-35). However, if children are shorter than expected even for the population of children with the disorder or if children fail to maintain their own rate of growth after following a percentile, then endocrine function abnormalities such as hypothyroidism should be investigated.

Skin Findings. Hemangiomas, multiple café-au-lait spots, and sebaceous adenomas may be evidence of an underlying neurocutaneous abnormality, thereby providing a constitutional basis for a developmental delay. Von Recklinghausen disease and tuberous sclerosis, both examples of neurocutaneous disorders, are inherited as autosomal dominant, although there is a high rate of spontaneous mutation. If these disorders are diagnosed or suspected, examination of the immediate family is warranted (see Chapter 15). Hirsutism occurs in fetal alcohol (see Chapter 1) and fetal hydantoin syndromes. Abnormal fingernail formation can signal teratogenic influences or ectodermal dysplasias (see Chapter 20).

Cranial Abnormalities. Head circumference provides an obvious clue to the cause of mental retardation. Undergrowth of the cranium may indicate central nervous system damage or dysgenesis, and overgrowth may indicate hydrocephalus. Abnormal skull shape may indicate that the underlying nervous system has undergone unusual physical stresses.

Transillumination aids in the diagnosis of porencephalic cysts or of other structural defects in young infants. The presence of an intracranial bruit may indicate an arteriovenous malformation, although such bruits are sometimes heard in normal infants. Even in the absence of these signs, children with moderate, severe, and profound mental retardation may warrant an imaging study of the central nervous system because of the high incidence of identifiable abnormalities.

Facial Abnormalities. The presence of certain facial characteristics may suggest a specific etiology of mental retardation. Minor malformations (which include hypotelorism or hypertelorism; epicanthal folds; colobomas; and auricles that are large, abnormally formed, or set low in comparison with the plane of the eyes) are rare in the general population. In isolation, one dysmorphic feature may be insignificant. However, the presence of three or more of these features correlates highly with a major malformation, often of the heart, kidney, or brain. Patterns of dysmorphic features may suggest a specific diagnosis such as a genetic syndrome, chromosomal abnormality, or prenatal exposure. For example, flat facies, upturned palpebral fissures, epicanthal folds, single palmar creases, and clinodactyly are associated with trisomy 21 (Down syndrome) (Fig. 3-36). Likewise, a lengthened philtrum, a thin vermilion border, and microcephaly are clinical features of fetal alcohol syndrome.

Some of these unusual features themselves are clues to the etiology of the intellectual disability or are the result of abnormal functioning, even in prenatal life. For example, aberrant patterning of scalp hair may indicate abnormal cerebral morphology. The pattern of hair growth is affected by pressures from the developing brain on the overlying scalp in early gestation. The absence of a posterior hair whorl or the presence of multiple hair whorls suggests abnormal prenatal brain growth. Small palpebral fissures also result from abnormal brain growth; the eye is an extension of the brain, and small eyes are suggestive of abnormal early brain development. Similarly, a higharched palate may be secondary to abnormal motor activity of the tongue in utero, suggesting a prenatal origin of motor problems.

Other Physical Abnormalities. Hepatosplenomegaly in the neonatal period may suggest congenital infection or in childhood may indicate a heritable storage disease affecting central nervous system and developmental functioning. Large testes are found in youngsters with Fragile X syndrome, whereas hypogonadism is a concomitant of the Prader-Willi syndrome. This syndrome is associated with an abnormality on chromosome 15 (see Chapter 1).

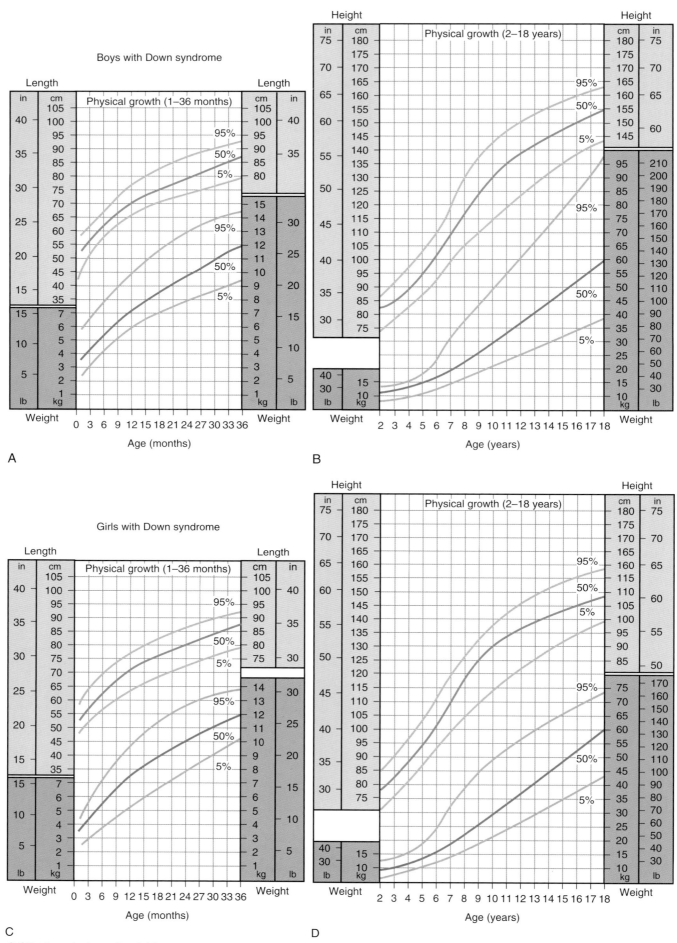

Figure 3-35. Growth charts for children with Down syndrome. (From Cronk C, Crocker AC, Pueschel SM, et al: Growth charts for children with Down syndrome. Pediatrics 81:108, 1988.)

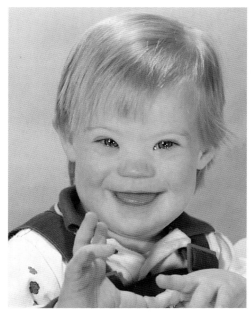

Figure 3-36. Down syndrome. Note the upslanting palpebral fissures, flat nasal bridge, epicanthal folds, small ears, and small hands.

Changes in the long bones of the limbs may show evidence of congenital infection; disproportionate bone length may suggest metabolic disorders such as homocystinuria or the osteochondrodysplasias. Errant toe proportions or changed crease patterns on the hands or soles of the feet may suggest early morphogenetic changes associated with certain defined syndromes. Lethargic or pale children may prompt an examination for iron deficiency or lead intoxication, which also may contribute to subnormal intellectual progress.

Prognosis

Some 3% of newborns are classified as mentally retarded at some point in their lives. In a society that prizes intellectual accomplishment, the identification of a child's cognitive delays is upsetting for a family. Findings of unusual features in any aspect of the physical examination may help provide an explanation for abnormal or delayed cognitive development. In evaluating the cause of developmental delay, the greatest need, beyond that of assessing the possibility of remediation, is that of providing the parents with appropriate genetic, behavioral, and educational counseling. Evidence that a child's lack of developmental progress is related to constitutional factors can help relieve parents of guilt feelings.

In the past, physicians have often underestimated the capabilities of children with mental retardation. Similarly, families often interpret a diagnosis of mental retardation to mean that their child will make no further developmental progress. Estimates of functional abilities for children who are classified as mentally retarded are variable. Children with mild mental retardation (IQ scores two to three standard deviations below the mean [69 to 55]) can learn to read and write and to do simple mathematics. As adults, they often live independently and hold jobs. The extent of their disability is most prominent during the school years or during times of life crisis beyond school age. Children with moderate mental retardation (IQ scores three to four standard deviations below the mean [54 to 40]) probably learn to read and write only to a first- or second-grade level. Nonetheless, their abilities in language, self-care, and adaptation skills may allow them to live and work in semi-independent settings, with supports and supervision as needed. Children with severe and profound mental retardation (four to six standard deviations below the mean [39 to 24 and below]) require substantial lifelong support.

The benefits of early intervention are maximized by early identification. Careful documentation of the child's opportunities for interaction with parents, other children, and stimulating environments helps in determining the type and degree of intervention necessary. The importance of careful screening of infant and preschool development by informed health professionals and of close collaboration between physicians and early intervention personnel cannot be overemphasized.

Autism

Autistic disorder is a disability defined by three core characteristics: qualitative impairment in social interactions including abnormal nonverbal behaviors, such as limited eye-to-eye gaze and unusual facial expressions, and a lack of social and emotional reciprocity; qualitative impairment in communication including a total lack of language or inability to initiate and sustain conversation; and repetitive, restrictive, or stereotyped behaviors including preoccupations with parts of objects, narrow interests, and repetitive hand movements, such as hand flapping. The degree of impairment can vary widely, leading to the current conceptualization of autistic spectrum disorder (ASD). The current diagnostic criteria from the *Diagnostic and Statistical Manual of Mental Disorders,* fourth edition, revised (DSM-IV) describes five conditions on the spectrum. At the mild end are individuals with Asperger syndrome, a disability characterized by impaired social relationships and obsessive interests in a single topic or object, often to the exclusion of other interests. At the severe end of the spectrum are individuals with autistic disorder, who may have extremely limited social contact, no verbal communication, and function in the range of mental retardation on cognitive testing. Autistic disorders appear to have a genetic cause and are most likely caused by multiple genes occurring together. Because the prevalence of autism appears to be rising rapidly in many different countries and societies, environmental triggers are also suspected in the etiology.

Autistic spectrum disorders present in two distinct patterns. Some children show abnormal social and communicative behaviors from early infancy on. Parents often report that these children have low tone when held, fail to look at the human face, and never turn toward the human voice. Some children demonstrate normal development in infancy and then, often in the second year of life, show regression of social and communicative skills, such as loss of early vocabulary and growing disinterest in social interaction. The nature of the presentation is not associated with severity of symptoms and long-term prognosis.

Parent questionnaires have been developed for primary care settings to screen for children at high risk of the condition. Autism-specific interviews and observation protocols are used to establish the diagnosis.

Physical Examination

Children with autistic spectrum disorders generally have a completely normal physical and neurological examination. Increased head circumference in the preschool period is associated with the diagnosis of autism, with or without mental retardation, suggesting that the neurological basis of autism may include overabundant growth of neurons and synapses or failure of normal processes of pruning of synapses.

Autism has been associated with other conditions including Fragile X syndrome, Rett syndrome, and tuberous sclerosis. Therefore the physical examination of children with abnormal social and communicative development should include the following: a survey of dysmorphic features, such as long face, prominent jaw, large or protuberant ears; measurement of head circumference to document relative macrocephaly or microcephaly; the evaluation of facial, truncal, and extremity tone; and careful skin examination looking for hypopigmented lesions. Genetic testing is typically included in the evaluation of children with autistic spectrum disorders. Identifying a specific genetic cause is relevant to counseling about recurrence risk in a family and prognosis for the individual. Children with autistic disorder are at increased risk of seizure disorder. Unusual movements or lapses in consciousness should prompt evaluation with an electroencephalogram.

Prognosis

Children with autistic disorder benefit substantially from intense early intervention services designed to improve their social interactions and communication skills. Some children with such interventions may be able to attend regular education settings without special services by school age. Therefore prompt referral for early intervention and advocacy for intensive programming is appropriate for toddlers and preschoolers on the autistic spectrum. No definitive treatments are currently available for autistic spectrum disorders. Educational and behavioral interventions address the core characteristics. Medication is often used to manage associated findings, such as inattention, hyperactivity, mood lability, and unpredictable outbursts. Addressing the family's challenges in raising a child with autism is central to management and may include referral to family support groups, provision of educational material, and referral for behavior management counseling.

Language and Reading Disorders

Delays and disturbances in language development are most frequently associated with mental retardation, childhood autism, hearing impairment, and environmental deprivation. However, language difficulties may occur in an otherwise normal child; in such cases, they are referred to as specific language impairment, usually of unknown etiology. Some theories stress difficulties with high-level concepts and symbolic capabilities, and others stress auditory perceptual impairments as the root of specific language disorders.

Physical Examination

No specific physical signs are associated with language disorders. The physician's role is in large part to rule out other disorders with different etiologies and prognoses.

Hearing assessment is indicated for any child with delays or deviancies in language development because hearing loss is a treatable condition. Universal newborn hearing screening, now available in most states in the United States and in many other countries, allows identification and treatment of sensorineural hearing loss before it leads to delays in language, speech, and other developmental domains. The screenings use otoacoustic emissions or automated auditory brainstem responses, two inexpensive techniques that assess physiologic responses to sound without requiring voluntary responses from the child. If a newborn does not pass the screen, the definitive testing with the brainstem auditory-evoked response, an electrophysiologic measure that records brain waves as a function of sound exposure, should be performed. Universal newborn hearing screening has successfully lowered the mean age of detection of sensorineural hearing loss. However, in children with language and speech delays, repeating the audiometric assessment is important because hearing loss may be progressive or missed in the newborn period. In older infants and toddlers, conditioning techniques or conventional audiometry assess actual hearing rather than associated physiological markers. The use of earphones allows for evaluation of each ear independently (Fig. 3-37).

Syndromes known to be associated with hearing loss include Treacher Collins, Waardenburg, and osteogenesis imperfecta. Children with abnormalities of the external ear including preauricular tags and pits, the palate, or facial structures may also have sensorineural hearing loss (Table 3-9). Repeated evaluations may be required in congenital rubella or cytomegalovirus infections because of progressive hearing loss. Several genetic causes of congeni-

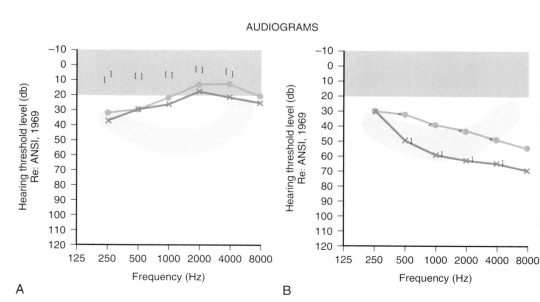

AUDIOGRAMS

Figure 3-37. Audiograms. The red X indicates the threshold for the left ear, and the blue circle indicates the threshold for the right ear. Brackets indicate bone conduction. **A,** This audiogram indicates mild conductive hearing loss in both ears. Notice that more energy is required for detection of sound in the low-frequency range. Bone conduction is normal. **B,** This audiogram demonstrates sensorineural hearing loss. The left ear shows a sloping pattern with mild to moderate loss in the low-frequency range and severe loss in the high-frequency range. The right ear shows mild to moderate loss throughout the frequency range.

A　　　　　　　　　　B

tal hearing loss have been identified. Conditions associated with varying degrees of hearing loss, their disabling effects, and the interventions required for children with these conditions are listed in Table 3-10. Children with congenital hearing loss that is treated with amplification or hearing aids should be evaluated for their responses to spoken words, patterns of vocalization and sound production, visual and verbal attentiveness, social rapport, and development of communication.

Otitis media with effusion is associated with mild, variable, intermittent hearing loss. Randomized clinical trials of otherwise healthy children with prolonged middle ear effusion have compared early insertion of tympanostomy tubes to delayed or no tube insertion if the effusion clears. The results find no short-term or long-term advantages of early tympanostomy tube insertion in terms of levels of speech, language, or cognitive skills.

Prognosis

Many toddlers with speech or language disorders develop adequate speech, language, and communication skills by early elementary school. No variables are consistently associated with a good prognosis; however, the prognosis for communication is clearly improved through early communication therapy. Physicians should not hesitate to refer children with speech and language delays for assessment and treatment.

Many toddlers and preschoolers with selective problems in language acquisition develop reading difficulties during the school-age years. A reading disorder (dyslexia) is a frequent finding in a child with an early history of language delay and a positive family history of language impairment or reading disability. With increasing age, children with reading difficulties tend to improve. However, in many cases, reading remains an area of relative weakness compared with other cognitive and academic skills.

Children with reading disorders show abnormal or inefficient eye movements in the course of reading. This observation has led to visual training as a treatment strategy. However, the literature supports the notion that in most cases, a reading problem is a high-level language difficulty, not a visual or visuomotor problem.

Attention-Deficit Hyperactivity Disorder

Attention-deficit hyperactivity disorder (ADHD) is a syndrome characterized by persistent inattention, hyperactivity, and impulsivity compared with what is expected for a child at a particular developmental level. Judgments about the degree of deviance in these behaviors are based on the degree of interference they cause in the child's social, academic, or other functioning. The diagnosis of ADHD requires that symptoms have been long-standing, that they be present before at least 7 years of age, and that

Table 3-9	Conditions Associated with Sensorineural Hearing Loss

Family history of childhood hearing impairment
Congenital perinatal infection (CMV, rubella, herpes, toxoplasmosis, syphilis)
Anatomic malformations of the head or neck
Birth weight <1500 g
Hyperbilirubinemia above levels indicated for exchange transfusion
Bacterial meningitis
Severe asphyxia
Exposure to ototoxic medications

CMV, cytomegalovirus.

Table 3-10	Disabling Effects of Hearing Loss

AVERAGE HEARING AT 500-2000 HZ (ANSI)	DESCRIPTION	CONDITION	SOUNDS HEARD WITHOUT AMPLIFICATION	DEGREE OF DISABILITY (IF NOT TREATED IN FIRST YEAR OF LIFE)	PROBABLE NEEDS
0-15 dB	Normal range	Serous otitis, perforation, monomeric membrane, tympanosclerosis	All speech sounds	None	None
15-25 dB	Slight hearing loss	Serous otitis, perforation, monomeric membrane, sensorineural loss, tympanosclerosis	Vowel sounds heard clearly; may miss a few consonant sounds	Possible mild auditory dysfunction in language learning	Environmental modifications, such as preferential seating in school and face-to-face communication; auditory training, speech therapy.
25-40 dB	Mild hearing loss	Serous otitis, perforation, tympanosclerosis, monomeric membrane, sensorineural loss	Hears most louder-voiced speech sounds	Possible auditory learning dysfunction, possible mild language retardation, mild speech problems, inattention	Hearing aid, lip reading, auditory training, speech therapy; environmental modifications, such as preferential seating
40-65 dB	Moderate hearing loss	Chronic otitis, middle ear anomaly, sensorineural loss	Misses most speech sounds at normal conversational level	Speech problems, language retardation, learning dysfunction, inattention	All the above, plus consideration of special education services as required
65-90 dB	Severe hearing loss	Sensorineural or mixed loss from sensorineural loss plus middle ear disease	Hears no speech sounds of normal conversation	Severe speech problems, language retardation, learning dysfunction, inattention	All the above, plus probable special education services as required
>90 dB	Profound hearing loss	Sensorineural or mixed loss	Hears no speech or other sounds; candidate for cochlear implantation	Severe speech problems, language retardation, learning dysfunction, inattention	All the above, plus probable special education services as required

ANSI, American National Standards Institute; dB, decibel.
Modified from Stewart JM, Downs MP: Medical management of the hearing-handicapped child. In Northern JL (ed): Hearing Disorders, 2nd ed. Boston, Little, Brown, 1984. Reprinted by permission of Allyn & Bacon.

they occur in multiple settings and not just at either home or school. Multiple genetic, neurologic, toxic, and psychosocial conditions are associated with the presence of ADHD. Among children born prematurely and children with mental retardation, ADHD is more prevalent than in the general population.

Though precise diagnostic criteria have changed over the past 2 decades, certain features have recurred in the lists of defining characteristics. Children with ADHD have difficulty sustaining attention and persisting to task completion. They become easily distracted. Frequently they fail to organize and plan before beginning a task. Because of all these features operating concurrently, these children fail to complete work assignments and eventually may avoid long and demanding tasks. Impulsivity in young children is frequently demonstrated by difficulty waiting for a turn. As children get older, impulsivity is expressed as difficulty delaying responses, blurting out answers, interrupting others, and generally acting before thinking.

The current diagnostic criteria from the *Diagnostic and Statistical Manual of Mental Disorders,* fourth edition, revised (DSM-IV) identify three different subtypes of ADHD. Most children demonstrate ADHD combined type, a variant that includes symptoms of inattention and hyperactivity-impulsivity. However, ADHD predominantly inattentive type is appropriate for children with symptoms of inattention without hyperactivity or impulsivity. An alternative diagnosis is ADHD predominantly hyperactive-impulsive type, in which inattention may be a feature but is less prominent than hyperactivity. The degree of hyperactivity varies in part with the child's age, developmental level, temperament, and style. Young school-age boys with ADHD tend to display excessive fidgetiness and activity, whereas adolescents and girls may be inattentive but not hyperactive.

Most children with ADHD show age-appropriate attention in some highly motivating situations. For example, parents routinely report that their children with ADHD sit for computer games or captivating movies. For this reason, up to 80% of children whose behavior at home and at school meets diagnostic criteria do not show characteristics of the disorder in the physician's office. Diagnosis rests on historical information from parents and confirmatory reports from teachers. Standardized questionnaires are often used in diagnosis to quantify the degree of inattention, hyperactivity, and associated behavioral problems.

Children with ADHD are likely to have other neurobehavioral disorders such as anxiety, depression, conduct disorder, oppositional defiance disorder, and learning disabilities. In conduct disorder, as opposed to ADHD, the child violates the basic rights of others and age-appropriate social norms. In oppositional defiant disorder, the child shows severe and persistent disobedience and hostility directed against authority figures. The evaluation of ADHD should include evaluation for these coexisting conditions.

Physical Findings

On physical examination, it is important to assess the general characteristics of the child to rule out other similar psychiatric disorders such as autism, depression, anxiety, or oppositional disorder. Physical findings in ADHD may be completely noncontributory. However, findings such as short stature or dysmorphic features may suggest an associated genetic or dysmorphic syndrome such as alcohol-related birth defects. Focal neurologic findings may suggest a static or progressive neurologic cause such as periventricular leukomalacia from prematurity. The presence of motor or vocal tics with ADHD raises the diagnostic possibility of a chronic tic disorder or Tourette syndrome.

The physical and neurologic examination of children with suspected ADHD often includes a set of specific maneuvers and tasks referred to as *neurologic soft signs* or *neuromaturational indicators.* Non-normative performance on these specific motor and sensory tasks can be obtained in children who otherwise show no evidence of a localizing neurologic disorder or pathognomonic patterns indicative of generalized encephalopathy. The soft signs are of clinical interest because they serve as an index for cognitive or behavioral dysfunction.

Table 3-11 includes several tasks for eliciting soft signs, the typical ages of acquisition, and indications of immature or positive findings. On rapid alternating pronation-supination of the hands, developing children typically show resolution of dysdiadochochinesia by age 7 years. On the same task and on repeated finger-to-thumb apposition and alternating squeezing and relaxing of handgrip, children usually show a marked decrease in synkinesis after age 9 years.

Including these maneuvers in the physical examination is useful for unmasking a child's inattention, impulsivity, and disorganization that may otherwise go undetected in the clinical setting. Parents may be relieved when the physician observes those traits that have brought the family in for evaluation. In some cases parents have the opportunity to observe the traits that teachers find challenging in the classroom. Difficulty executing discrimination of right and left and particularly crossed commands on themselves and the examiner beyond 8 years of age may be found in children with ADHD. In addition, they may also show problems in executing four or more sequential commands from memory. However, persistence of abnormal findings on these tasks is not diagnostic of ADHD.

Table 3-11	Indicators Associated with Neurologic Immaturity	
TASK	**IMMATURE RESPONSE**	**NORMS**
Rapid pronation-supination	Dysdiadochochinesia	Mature by age 7-8 years
Repeated finger-to-thumb apposition	Synkinesis	Markedly decreased after age 9 years
Alternation of squeezing and relaxation of single handgrip	Synkinesis	Markedly decreased after age 9 years
Sensory integration—tactile recognition from visual presentation	Astereognosis	>90% accurate by age 7 years
Identification of right and left		
On self	Inaccurate	>90% correct by age 7 years
Execution of crossed commands (e.g., touch left eye with right hand [on self])	Inaccurate	>90% correct by age 8 years
On examiner	Inaccurate	>70% correct by age 8 years

Prognosis

Research suggests that ADHD is a lifelong condition. The signs and symptoms of hyperactivity are likely to resolve during adolescence, but relative inattention persists into adulthood. Many individuals with ADHD do better as adolescents and adults than they did as children because they can choose educational programs or occupations that capitalize on their profile. They often prefer vocations that permit frequent shifts in attention and a high energy level and that do not require sustained attention to challenging tasks. Nonetheless, individuals with ADHD have poorer educational attainment, higher rates of automobile accidents, lower job attainment, and greater instability in relationships compared with siblings who do not have the disorder, presumably related to persistent inattention. The prognosis is more favorable in individuals with isolated ADHD, good cognitive skills, no learning disorders, and positive family and peer relationships.

Treatment options for ADHD fall into three categories: behavior management, educational interventions, and psychopharmacology. Combinations of these options often are more effective than a single treatment.

Visual Impairment

Visual experience assists the learning of many important concepts of space and form important in the development of motor skills, perception, cognition, and social skills (Table 3-12). Thus in situations of congenital blindness or visual impairment, developmental patterns may be altered and delayed, demonstrating the close interrelationships that exist among developmental domains. Children with visual impairments can learn to increase the use of residual visual functioning and other sensory modalities. The physician's understanding of the impact of visual impairment is important to evaluate whether developmental progress is being achieved as expected in this population and to ensure that unexpected delays and deviancies are appropriately diagnosed and treated.

Gross and Fine Motor Development

Apparently, much of the motivation for the infant with normal vision to raise the head 90 degrees when in the prone position is to increase the visual field. Without the feedback of interesting sights, the infant with severe visual impairment may not attain this milestone until 11 to 12 months of age. In contrast, rolling occurs in infants who are blind at close to the same age as in infants with normal vision. If sitting independently is an active goal, it can occur by 6 to 7 months of age. However, transitional movements from lying to sitting or from sitting to standing occur several months later in infants without sight than in infants able to see.

Protective reactions develop more slowly in infants with severe visual impairment, and these are expected to appear in the 10- to 12-month age range. This delay, as well as the inability to integrate visual cues in attaining balance and equilibrium, and the lack of a visual impetus to explore distant toys may contribute to a typical delay in crawling or walking. Paired auditory-tactile cues presented to children with severe visual impairment may stimulate their interest in objects beyond their reach, thus accelerating gross motor development.

Regarding fine motor development, information gathering by index finger and manual manipulation may be more accurate in the child who is blind than in the child with normal vision. However, the youngster who is blind may experience a delay in the acquisition of precise prehension, which sometimes never develops, with raking favored as a more efficient means of exploration.

Cognitive Development

The development of cognitive skills in the child with visual impairment must of necessity depend on use of the other sensory modalities. For this reason, careful global evaluation of the child with severe visual impairment should be conducted early in infancy to ensure that the other senses are intact.

A child with normal vision develops the understanding that objects are permanent even when they cannot be seen, felt, heard, sniffed, or tasted. For the child with severe visual impairment, the opportunities for object perception are fewer, and thus the understanding of object permanence typically develops later, stimulated by encouragement of the infant to reach for sound cues. Similarly, this child's understanding of conservation of continuous quantity, that a cup of water contains the same volume of liquid in a tall thin container as it does in a short fat one, also develops later than in the child with normal vision.

Haptic perception, the acquisition of information about objects or spaces by exploration with the hands, appears to be more important in the cognitive development of the child with severe visual impairment than in that of the child with normal vision. For this reason, tactile exploration in the child who is blind cannot be promoted at too early an age. In fact, without such encouragement, these children may be fearful and resistant to unfamiliar new feelings.

Language and Intellectual Development

Verbal imitation and receptive language skills may develop normally in healthy children who are blind. As one might expect, these children may have difficulty with words relating to visual concepts, such as *light*, *dark*, or *color*. They may also have problems with words referring to large things that cannot be touched (*sky* or *stars*), things that change slowly (*age* or *growth*), or the concept "I." However, some children with severe visual impairment show accurate use of all of these concepts and even make the distinction between the words *look* and *see*. In these cases the child probably uses available linguistic information to substitute for visual information.

Table 3-12	Visually Related Behaviors
AGE OF INFANT	**BEHAVIOR**
Term	Focuses on face, briefly tracks vertically and horizontally, turns toward diffuse light source, widens eyes to object or face at 8-12 inches
1 month	Blinks at approaching object, tracks 60 degrees horizontally, 30 degrees vertically
2 months	Tracks across midline, follows movement 6 feet away, smiles to a smiling face, raises head 30 degrees in prone position
3 months	Eyes and head track 180 degrees, looks at hands, looks at objects placed in hands
4-5 months	Reaches for object (12-inch cube) 12 inches away, notices raisins 1 foot away, smiles at familiar adult
5-6 months	Smiles in mirror
7-8 months	Rakes at raisin
8-9 months	Notes visual details, pokes at holes in pegboard and at elevator buttons
9 months	Neat pincer grasp
12-14 months	Stacks blocks, places peg in round hole

Although standard IQ tests cannot be used to assess intellectual capabilities of children with severe visual impairment, standardized instruments have been developed to assess their cognitive development. Receptive and expressive language skills figure prominently in these assessments. In addition, interview schedules of adaptive behavior in communication and self-help skills have been developed specifically for children with visual impairment.

Social Development

Infants who are blind lack the opportunity to benefit from face-to-face contact with their caregivers, from the visual reinforcement of smiling, from the use of facial expressions to assist in the interpretation of voices or actions, and from the experience of tracking parents across the room to know that even when they cannot be heard or felt they are still there. These differences in sensory input affect their social and emotional development. Parents of infants with severe visual impairment frequently need to be coached to use touch and sound to reinforce smiling and other desired behaviors in their child.

At about the same time that children with normal vision smile at familiar faces, children who are blind smile in response to familiar touching and kinesthetic handling. Smiling in response to a familiar voice, however, may occur inconsistently up to 1 year of age. The infant who is blind demonstrates attachment by calming to the tactile exploration of the caregiver's familiar face or hands.

Blind children of about 1 year of age may have stranger awareness, although a greater hurdle will be their reaction to separation. Because these children have a limited capacity to track their caregivers, separations from them may induce panic states even among older ones. Similarly, the development of independent caregiving and play may be delayed and may require specific interventions.

Parents should be advised that, without purposeful stimulation, children who are blind may engage in nonpurposeful motor activities such as eye rubbing or rocking and that these stereotypical behaviors, referred to as *blindisms,* are difficult to extinguish. Blindisms can often be channeled to purposeful stimulation by directing the child's hands to exploration of a toy or by distracting the child with conversation or music. These efforts will serve to channel the child's activities in a more socially adaptive direction.

Summary

The tasks of routine developmental surveillance, identification of children with variations, and referral for appropriate developmental services (especially during infancy and in the preschool years) fall largely, and often exclusively, to the primary care clinician. Although we have provided estimates regarding the expected chronology of development, these developmental milestones are guidelines rather than fixed time frames within which behavior acquisition may be judged as normal or abnormal. In evaluating a child, the physician must use these guidelines, results of screening tests, and clinical judgment, taking into account the child's own personality traits, experiences, and degree of cooperation.

Recommendations for further assessment and treatment should be made in consultation with the family.

Bibliography

Allen MC: Neurodevelopmental assessment of the young child: The state of the art. Ment Retard Dev Disabil Res Rev 11(3):274-275, 2005.

Batshaw ME (ed): Children with Disabilities, 5th ed. Baltimore, Paul H. Brookes, 2002.

Committee on Children with Disabilities: Developmental surveillance and screening of infants and young children. Pediatrics 108:192-195, 2001.

Cooley WC, McAllister JW: Building medical homes: Improvement strategies in primary care for children with special health care needs. Pediatrics 113:1499-1506, 2004.

Dixon SD, Stein MT: Encounters with Children: Pediatric Behavior and Development, 3rd ed. St Louis, Mosby, 2000.

Feldman HM: Evaluation and management of language and speech disorders in preschool children. Pediatr Rev 26:131-142, 2005.

Glascoe FP: Early detection of developmental and behavioral problems. Pediatr Rev 21:272-280, 2000.

Johnson CP, Blasco PA: Infant growth and development. Pediatr Rev 18:224-242, 1997.

Joint Committee on Infant Hearing, American Academy of Audiology, American Academy of Pediatrics, American Speech-Language-Hearing Association, Directors of Speech and Hearing Programs in State Health and Welfare Associations: Year 2000 position statement: Principles and guidelines for early hearing detection and intervention programs. Pediatrics 106:798-817, 2000.

Jones KL: Smith's Recognizable Patterns of Human Malformation, 6th ed. Philadelphia, Elsevier Saunders, 2006.

Levine MD, Carey WB, Crocker AC (eds): Developmental-Behavioral Pediatrics, 3rd ed. Philadelphia, Saunders, 1999.

Lichtenberger EO: General measures of cognition for the preschool child. Ment Retard Dev Disabil Res Rev 11:197-208, 2005.

Perrin E, Stancin T: A continuing dilemma: Whether and how to screen for concerns about children's behavior. Pediatr Rev 23:264-276, 2002.

Vargas C, Prelock PE (eds): Caring for Children with Neurodevelopmental Disabilities and Their Families: An Innovative Approach to Interdisciplinary Practice. Mahwah, NJ, Lawrence Erlbaum, 2004.

CHAPTER 4

Allergy and Immunology

Andrew MacGinnitie and David Nash

Disorders of the immune system are diverse and range from mild to severe in their manifestations and impact on normal function. In this chapter, we review the physical findings and characteristic symptoms of children with hypersensitivity reactions and immune deficiencies, as well as diagnostic techniques and radiographic findings. Topics have been chosen on the basis of their prevalence and importance in the pediatric population and their association with characteristic physical findings.

Immunologic Hypersensitivity Disorders

Hypersensitivity disorders of the human immune system have been classified by Gell and Coombs into four groups (Table 4-1). Type I reactions occur promptly after the sensitized individual is exposed to an antigen and are mediated by specific IgE antibody. Cross-linking of IgE on the surface of mast cells and basophils leads to release of histamine and other inflammatory mediators. This mechanism is responsible for the common disorders of immediate hypersensitivity, such as allergic rhinitis and urticaria. So-called "anaphylactoid" reactions are clinically similar, but are caused by degranulation of mast cells and basophils in the absence of specific IgE. Type II reactions involve antibodies directed against antigenic components of peripheral blood or tissue cells or foreign antigens, resulting in cell destruction. Examples of this type include autoimmune hemolytic anemia and Rh and ABO hemolytic disease of the newborn. In type III reactions, antigen-antibody complexes form and are deposited in the lining of blood vessels, stimulating tissue inflammation mediated by complement or activated white blood cells. Examples of this type of reaction are serum sickness and the immune-complex–mediated renal diseases. Type IV reactions involve T cell–mediated tissue inflammation and typically occur 24 to 48 hours after exposure. Examples of this type are tuberculin (PPD) reactions and contact dermatitis (see Chapter 8).

Type I Disorders

The development of type I hypersensitivity depends on hereditary predisposition, sensitization by exposure to an antigen, and subsequent reexposure to the antigen leading to an allergic reaction. Antigens that stimulate allergic reactions are known as *allergens,* and the mechanism of allergen-induced mediator release in type I hypersensitivity reactions is shown in Figure 4-1. IgE antibodies directed toward specific allergens are bound to the high-affinity IgE receptor on mast cells and basophils. When allergen causes cross-linking of IgE antibodies on the cell surface, the cell becomes activated, leading to the release of preformed mediators and the generation of the early and late mediators of anaphylaxis. The preformed mediators include histamine, tryptase, chymase, heparin, and other proteases that drive the earliest symptoms of anaphylaxis. A serum tryptase level is currently the best biological marker of anaphylaxis, but it is still a relatively insensitive test. Serum tryptase levels should be obtained close to the onset of anaphylaxis because levels peak in 1 hour and only remain elevated for 4 to 24 hours. The early and late mediators generated by mast cell activation include prostaglandins, leukotrienes, and cytokines. These mediators, which are generated over minutes to hours, continue to drive the clinical symptoms of the allergic reaction and initiate an inflammatory cascade that leads to the recruitment of eosinophils, basophils, and lymphocytes.

Type I reactions may occur in one or more target organs including the upper and lower respiratory tracts, cardiovascular system, skin, conjunctivae, and gastrointestinal (GI) tract. Manifestations depend on the systems involved, as shown in Figure 4-2. The most common manifestation of type I reaction is seasonal allergic rhinitis with a prevalence of at least 25%. The most serious manifestation of type I hypersensitivity is anaphylaxis that can simultaneously involve all of the above organ systems.

Type I hypersensitivity has been diagnosed by skin testing for more than 100 years. The percutaneous skin test, also known as either the scratch or prick test, is an in vivo method to detect the presence of IgE antibody to specific allergens. The skin prick test is the safest and most specific test and correlates best with symptoms. The skin prick test is typically performed with a plastic lancet on either the forearm or upper back and involves a superficial disruption of the epidermis that is nearly painless (Fig. 4-3). The test leaves a barely visible mark, and when performed properly, the prick site should not bleed. The test is interpreted after 15 to 20 minutes by measuring the maximum diameter of both the wheal and the flare. Skin test results are compared to a negative control, which is usually saline, and a positive control, which is typically histamine. Historically, intradermal tests have been considered to be more sensitive than prick tests, but the specificity is poor and these tests should only be used when ruling out allergic disease is essential.

Allergy skin testing is contraindicated in four clinical situations: (1) antihistamines have been used in the recent past—this will typically manifest as a negative histamine control; (2) skin disease that limits the area available for testing; (3) during either an asthma exacerbation or episode of anaphylaxis; and (4) when a patient is taking a β-blocking medicine because these can interfere with epinephrine treatment in rare cases of test-induced anaphylaxis. When skin testing is not possible, in vitro testing is a good alternative. The in vitro tests can be accomplished with just a few milliliters of serum and also may be advantageous for some patients who have a difficult time sitting through allergy tests. In vitro allergy tests are more expensive and less sensitive than allergy prick tests (Table 4-2). In vitro tests are especially helpful in the evaluation of patients with possible food allergies. The in vitro test in patients with suspected food allergy can be used to distinguish false-positive from true-positive skin tests for certain foods and can help to identify children who may have outgrown their food allergy.

Table 4-1   Classification of Hypersensitivity Disorders

		INTERVAL BETWEEN EXPOSURE AND REACTION	EFFECTOR CELL OR ANTIBODY	TARGET OR ANTIGEN	EXAMPLES OF MEDIATORS	DISORDER
Type I	Anaphylaxis		IgE	Pollens, foods, drugs, insect venoms		Anaphylaxis
	a. Immediate	<30 minutes			a. Histamine	Allergic rhinitis
	b. Late phase	2-12 hours			b. Leukotrienes	Allergic asthma
Type II	Cytotoxic	Variable (minutes to hours)	IgG, IgM	Red blood cells, lung tissue	Complement	Immune hemolytic anemia Rh hemolytic disease Goodpasture syndrome
Type III	Immune complexes	4-8 hours	Antigen with antibody	Vascular endothelium	Complement Anaphylatoxin	Serum sickness Poststreptococcal glomerulonephritis
Type IV	Delayed type	24-48 hours	Lymphocytes	*Mycobacterium tuberculosis*, chemicals	Cytokines	Contact dermatitis Tuberculin skin test reactions

From Gell PGH, Coombs RRA: Clinical Aspects of Immunology, 2nd ed. Philadelphia, FA Davis, 1968.

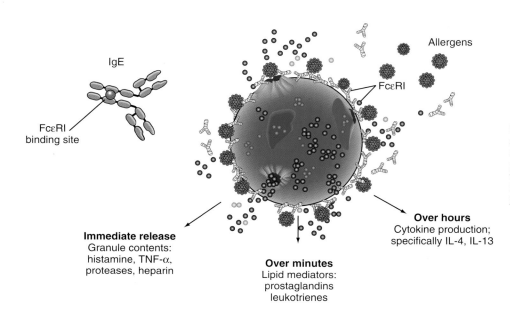

IgE

FcεRI binding site

Allergens

FcεRI

Immediate release
Granule contents: histamine, TNF-α, proteases, heparin

Over minutes
Lipid mediators: prostaglandins leukotrienes

Over hours
Cytokine production; specifically IL-4, IL-13

Figure 4-1. IgE is bound to the mast cell surface, and when cross-linked by antigen, the mast cell becomes activated. The activated mast cell releases preformed mediators and generates additional mediators over minutes to hours. (From Broide DH: Molecular and cellular mechanisms of allergic disease. J Allergy Clin Immunol 108:S65-S71, 2001.)

Systemic Anaphylaxis

Anaphylaxis results from widespread degranulation of mast cells after crosslinking of IgE on the mast cell surface. A clinically similar reaction in which mast cells degranulate without cross-linking of antigen-specific IgE is termed *anaphylactoid*. Onset of anaphylaxis is rapid and often explosive after bee stings, drug administration, or food ingestion (Fig. 4-4). The pattern of organ system involvement can vary based on antigen, dose, and route of exposure and can range from isolated urticaria to cardiovascular collapse (Fig. 4-5). Airway obstruction and hypotension are the most severe manifestations of anaphylaxis. The upper or lower airway, or both, can be affected. Upper airway obstruction is due to laryngeal edema, whereas lower airway involvement is due to edema and bronchospasm. Hypotension is caused by vasodilation, which may be complicated by loss of intravascular volume. Vascular collapse may be aggravated by decreases in myocardial function. In addition to the airway and cardiovascular system, other organ systems are also involved in anaphylaxis. The skin is the most commonly involved organ, with urticaria being nearly universal and angioedema often present. GI involvement can manifest as vomiting, diarrhea, and abdominal pain due to gut edema.

For all reactions but isolated skin symptoms, intramuscular epinephrine is the therapy of choice. Recent studies have demonstrated the superiority of intramuscular injections compared with subcutaneous injections of epinephrine (Fig. 4-6). Patients at risk should carry self-injectable epinephrine and be trained in its use. The EpiPen is the most widely available preparation of self-injectable epinephrine and can be used with three easy steps (Fig. 4-7). Epinephrine is most effective when it is used within 30 to 60 minutes of the onset of anaphylaxis, and other medications should not delay prompt delivery of epinephrine, which is often lifesaving. In cases of hypotension, large-volume fluid resuscitation and intravenous epinephrine may be required. Albuterol inhalation may be useful for lower airway symptoms, and steroids may prevent late-phase reactions. Antihistamines can be used for reactions confined to the skin and as an adjunct to epinephrine in more severe reactions.

Hymenoptera Sensitivity. Contrary to common opinion, life-threatening reactions to Hymenoptera are rare in childhood. The most common reactions are large local reactions or generalized urticaria. Large local reactions represent a late-phase IgE-mediated response to the sting. The swelling associated with large local reactions is contiguous with the sting, begins 12 to 24 hours following

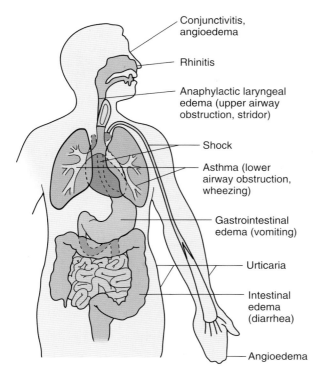

Figure 4-2. Type I hypersensitivity reactions. Note the characteristic physical findings of each affected organ system.

Table 4-2	Skin Testing Versus In Vitro Testing	
VARIABLE	**SKIN TEST**	**IN VITRO**
Risk of allergic reaction	Rare	No
Sensitive	Very	Good*
Affected by antihistamines	Yes	No
Affected by corticosteroids	Not usually	No
Affected by extensive dermatitis or dermatographism	Yes	No
Broad selection of antigens	Yes	Yes
Immediate results	Yes	No
Expensive	No	Yes
Discomfort	Mild	Moderate

*Less sensitive for aeroallergens, drugs, and Hymenoptera.

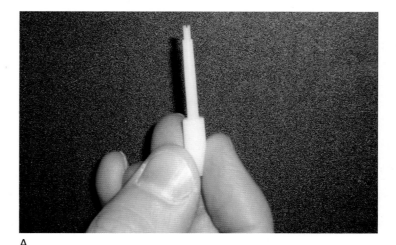

A

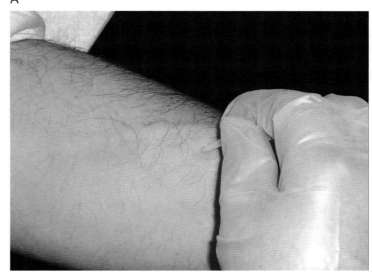

B

the sting, peaks in 2 to 3 days, lasts approximately a week, and should be treated with antihistamines and nonsteroidal anti-inflammatory drugs (NSAIDs). Patients with large local reactions have an excellent long-term prognosis and need neither allergy testing nor to carry epinephrine.

Children 16 years of age or younger who have had generalized urticaria and no respiratory, cardiovascular, or GI symptoms following an insect sting also have a good long-term prognosis. The risk for systemic anaphylaxis from stinging insects in children with symptoms confined to the skin is equal to the risk in the general population. These children do not need allergy testing or desensitization with immunotherapy. At present, consensus among allergists suggests that children with a history of generalized urticaria from stinging insects carry epinephrine.

Children with a history of systemic anaphylaxis following a Hymenoptera sting should undergo allergy testing and, if the test is positive, should receive immunotherapy. Testing should take place 4 weeks or more following the reaction. When testing is done immediately after the reaction, there is an increased rate of false-negative tests. Allergen immunotherapy for Hymenoptera sensitivity is the most effective form of allergen immunotherapy available.

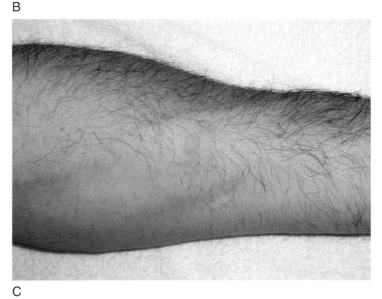

C

Figure 4-3. Allergy prick tests. **A,** The skin prick test is typically performed with a plastic lancet on either the forearm or upper back. **B,** The test leaves a barely visible mark and should be nearly painless. **C,** The test is interpreted after 15 to 20 minutes by measuring the maximum diameter of both the wheal and the flare.

CAUSES OF ANAPHYLAXIS

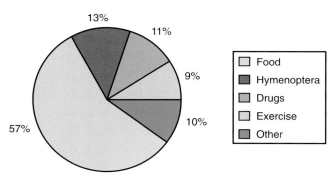

Food
Hymenoptera
Drugs
Exercise
Other

Figure 4-4. Relative frequency of causes of anaphylaxis in children. (From Novembre E, Cianteroni A, Bernardini R, et al: Anaphylaxis in children: Clinical and allergologic features. Pediatrics 101:E8, 1998.)

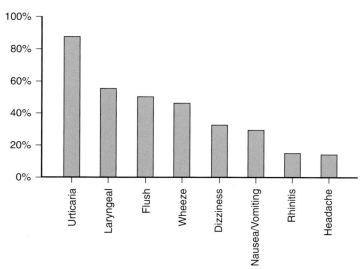

Figure 4-5. Relative frequency of symptoms associated with anaphylaxis. (Modified from Lieberman P: Anaphylaxis: How to quickly narrow the differential diagnosis. J Resp Disease 20:221-232, 1999.)

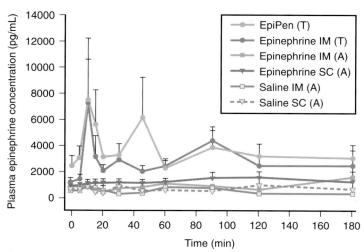

Figure 4-6. During anaphylaxis, intramuscular delivery of epinephrine in the lateral aspect of the thigh produces the highest serum levels of epinephrine. A = anterior deltoid; T = thigh. (From Simons FE: Epinephrine absorption in adults: Intramuscular versus subcutaneous injection. J Allergy Clin Immunol 108:871-873, 2001.)

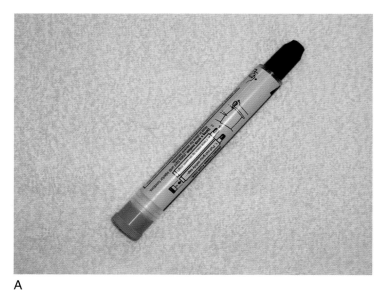

A

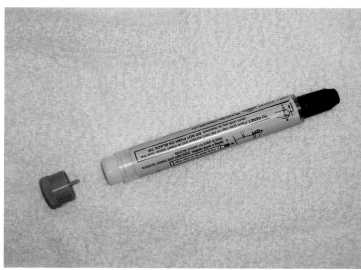

B

Figure 4-7. Anaphylaxis. The EpiPen requires three steps: (1) remove gray cap to activate the device; (2) press black tip firmly against the lateral aspect of the thigh (do not touch the end of the EpiPen); and (3) hold EpiPen in place for 10 seconds.

Venom immunotherapy for wasps, yellow jackets, and hornets provides complete protection from anaphylaxis while on immunotherapy in 95% to 100% of patients. Venom immunotherapy for honeybee is slightly less effective, providing complete protection to 80% of patients while on therapy. Most venom immunotherapy protocols require weekly injections for about 16 weeks and then every 1 to 3 months while on maintenance therapy. The duration of immunotherapy should be 3 to 5 years in most cases.

The Hymenoptera that have been associated with anaphylaxis come from three subfamilies: Apidae (honeybees); Vespidae (yellow jackets, wasps, white- and yellow-faced hornets); and Formicidae (fire ants). In the United States, yellow jackets are the most common cause of Hymenoptera-induced anaphylaxis. Yellow jackets typically nest in the ground; are scavengers for food; and, consequently, are frequently encountered at picnics and around garbage cans. The yellow jacket is small with tight yellow and black bands (Fig. 4-8). The honeybee is the least aggressive of the Hymenoptera family. Stings from honeybees occur most commonly in beekeepers and after accidental contact. The honeybee's stinger is barbed and

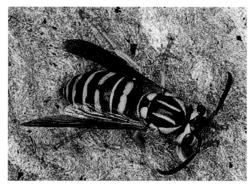

Figure 4-8. Hymenoptera sensitivity. Yellow jacket. Note tight yellow and black bands. Typically nests in the ground and will sting without provocation.

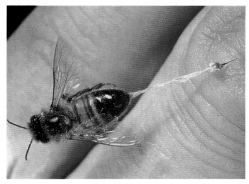

Figure 4-9. Hymenoptera sensitivity. The honeybee is golden brown with black markings. The honeybee has a barbed stinger and leaves the stinger and venom sac after it stings.

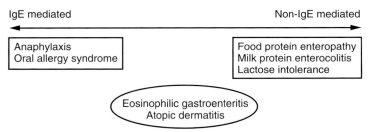

SPECTRUM OF FOOD ALLERGY

Figure 4-10. Reactions to foods can be broadly divided into two mechanistic groups: (1) type I (IgE-mediated) hypersensitivity; and (2) immune (non–IgE-mediated) reactions. Atopic dermatitis and eosinophilic gastroenteritis can be caused by either or both mechanisms.

is retained in the skin after stings (Fig. 4-9). If the stinger is visible, it should be quickly flicked away from the skin with a fingernail. The stinger and venom sac should not be removed by pinching between the thumb and forefinger as this process can express additional venom. Wasps and hornets are very territorial and will sting to protect their nests. The fire ant is an increasingly important cause of Hymenoptera-induced anaphylaxis. Fire ants are found in the southeastern United States, but their natural habitat appears to be expanding.

Food Allergy. Food allergy can be divided into two broad groups on the basis of the mechanism of disease: (1) type I (IgE-mediated) hypersensitivity and (2) other immunologically mediated reactions (Fig. 4-10). Other food reactions (e.g., lactose intolerance) do not have an immune basis and are referred to as *intolerant reactions.* Anaphylaxis is the best described and understood type I

hypersensitivity to food. Milk and egg are the two most common causes of food-induced anaphylaxis in childhood. The onset of type I hypersensitivity to milk and egg is almost always in the first year of life. Fortunately, these two foods rarely cause more than generalized urticaria and the sensitivity is frequently outgrown by 5 years of age. When milk or egg allergy is not outgrown or reactions are more severe, patients should carry epinephrine.

The vast majority of patients with type I hypersensitivity to peanut and tree nut also usually present early in life. In contrast to type I hypersensitivity to milk and egg, less than 25% of patients will outgrow their peanut or tree nut sensitivity. Peanuts and tree nuts cause the majority of life-threatening reactions to foods, and all patients with this hypersensitivity should carry epinephrine. In addition to peanut or tree nut allergy, other risk factors for life-threatening reactions from food-induced anaphylaxis include asthma, adolescence, and the delayed administration of epinephrine. A past history of mild reactions does not rule out the possibility of a future life-threatening episode of food-induced anaphylaxis. A substantial minority of patients with type I hypersensitivity to peanut will develop type I hypersensitivity to one or more tree nuts; and conversely, patients with hypersensitivity to a tree nut have an increased risk of developing peanut hypersensitivity. Most allergists recommend avoiding all nuts if a patient is allergic to either peanuts or tree nuts.

An increasingly common form of type I–mediated hypersensitivity to food is the oral allergy syndrome. Patients with oral allergy syndrome have underlying seasonal allergic rhinitis and develop pruritus and angioedema of the oropharynx when ingesting fresh fruits and vegetables. The reaction is due to cross-reactivity between heat-labile proteins in some fruits and vegetables and outdoor seasonal pollens. The reaction is eliminated by heating the vegetable or fruit. The reaction does not extend beyond the oropharynx, and patients typically do not need to carry epinephrine.

Type I hypersensitivity to foods can be an unrecognized trigger in up to one third of children with severe atopic dermatitis and is an uncommon trigger in children with mild atopic dermatitis. It has rarely been described in adults with atopic dermatitis. The evaluation of type I hypersensitivity to foods in children with atopic dermatitis should be reserved for patients whose disease cannot be managed with good skin care and intermittent use of low- to moderate-potency topical anti-inflammatory medications. When food hypersensitivity plays a role in poorly controlled atopic dermatitis, six foods account for the vast majority of reactions: milk, egg, wheat, soy, peanut, and fish.

One of the challenges with diagnosing type I hypersensitivity to foods is the poor specificity of both the skin prick and the in vitro tests. Over the past decade, research using in vitro allergy tests has identified levels of specific IgE against certain foods that predict with 95% certainty a reaction during a double-blind, placebo-controlled food challenge. The data concerning positive predictive levels depend on the age of the patient and are only available for a few foods: milk, egg, peanut, and fish (Table 4-3). The in vitro allergy test may also be followed over time to try to help with the identification of patients who may have outgrown their sensitivity. The sensitivity of both the skin prick and in vitro test is excellent, but not 100%. If there is a strong clinical history of a type I reaction to a food, it may be necessary to perform an oral challenge in a medically supervised setting before food hypersensitivity can be fully ruled out.

Table 4-3	Food-Specific IgE Concentrations Predictive of Clinical Reactivity				
ALLERGEN	DECISION POINT (kU/L)	SENSITIVITY (%)	SPECIFICITY (%)	POSITIVE PREDICTIVE VALUE (%)	NEGATIVE PREDICTIVE VALUE (%)
Egg	7	61	95	98	38
Infants ≤2 yr*	2			95	
Milk	15	57	94	95	53
Infants ≤2 yr†	5			95	
Peanut	14	57	100	100	36
Fish	20	25	100	100	89
Soybean	30	44	94	73	82
Wheat	26	61	92	74	87
Tree nuts	≈15	—	—	≈95	—

Modified from Sampson HA: Utility of food-specific IgE concentrations in predicting symptomatic food allergy. J Allergy Clin Immunol 107:891-896, 2001.
*Boyano-Martinez T, Garcia-Ara C, Diaz-Pena GM, et al: Validity of specific IgE in children with egg allergy. Clin Exp Allergy 31:1464-1469, 2001.
†Garcia-Ara C, Boyano-Martinez T, Diaz-Pena GM, et al: Specific IgE levels in the diagnosis of immediate hypersensitivity to cow's milk protein in infants. J Allergy Clin Immunol 107:185-190, 2001.

Eosinophilic gastroenteritis is an especially difficult problem to evaluate because eosinophilic infiltration of the gut may be caused by either type I (IgE-mediated) hypersensitivity or other immune pathways. The patients with type I hypersensitivity causing eosinophilic gastroenteritis can be sensitive to either foods or inhaled allergens (pollens/molds) that are inadvertently swallowed. Because eosinophilic gastroenteritis can also be caused by non–IgE-mediated pathways, a negative skin prick or in vitro test does not eliminate the possibility that food allergy may be causing the disease. Recently, patch testing has been studied in patients with eosinophilic gastroenteritis to try to identify foods that are causing eosinophilic inflammation through a non–IgE-mediated pathway. Patients with eosinophilic inflammation of the upper GI tract tend to have problems with dysphagia, food impaction, abdominal pain, and vomiting. Patients with eosinophilic inflammation of the lower GI tract tend to have diarrhea, failure to thrive, and abdominal pain. Eosinophilic gastroenteritis appears to have an increasing incidence, and the long-term prognosis is not well understood.

The term *food allergy* also encompasses the food reactions elicited through non–IgE-mediated immune pathways. The classic example of a non–IgE-mediated hypersensitivity to food is seen in the milk protein enterocolitis of infancy. These children usually present in the first couple of months with bloody diarrhea that improves within days of removing milk proteins from the diet. Milk protein enterocolitis is not IgE mediated, so neither allergy skin prick nor in vitro testing is helpful in the evaluation of this condition. Approximately half of children with milk protein enterocolitis will also experience symptoms with soy protein–based formulas. Almost all infants will outgrow milk protein enterocolitis by 1 to 2 years of age.

Drug Reactions. Reactions to drugs can be mediated through a type I hypersensitivity or any of the other types of Gell and Coombs reactions. Type I hypersensitivity to drugs can range from mild reactions involving only the skin (generalized urticaria and/or angioedema) to multiorgan involvement. Penicillin is the only drug that has been widely studied as a cause of type I hypersensitivity and, consequently, it is the only drug for which well-standardized allergy testing is available. Anaphylaxis from drugs other than penicillin must be diagnosed on the basis of clinical presentation. Patients with type I hypersensitivity to drugs can still receive the drug if a desensitization protocol is used. Desensitization involves slowly delivering increasing doses of the drug over a period of 6 to 12 hours. The mechanism by which desensitization works is not well understood. Patients remain desensitized as long as they are on the medication, but once the drug is discontinued future treatment requires repeated desensitization.

A variety of drugs can cause anaphylactoid reactions. Anaphylactoid reactions are due to generalized mast cell mediator release not caused by cross-linking of specific IgE on mast cell surfaces. The exact mechanism of anaphylactoid reactions is not known, and no diagnostic testing is available. The two most common drug-induced causes of anaphylactoid reactions are radiocontrast media and nonsteroidal anti-inflammatory drugs.

Drugs can also induce type II, III, and IV Gell and Coombs reactions. The classic Gell and Coombs type II reaction is due to IgG antibodies directed against drug bound to cell surfaces causing either hemolytic anemia or thrombocytopenia. Serum sickness represents a Gell and Coombs type III reaction. Serum sickness usually begins 1 to 3 weeks after drug exposure and involves various symptoms including fever, malaise, arthralgias, arthritis, urticaria, and lymphadenopathy. Many patients with serum sickness will develop a characteristic serpiginous, erythematous, or purpuric eruption at the junction of the palmar or plantar and dorsolateral aspects of the hands and feet, respectively (Fig. 4-11). Patients with serum sickness will have reduced levels of complement components C3 and C4 along with the presence of circulating immune complexes. Serum sickness can be treated with antihistamines, and if the patient fails to improve systemic steroids can be used. Erythema multiforme (EM) represents a Gell and Coombs type IV reaction. EM can be caused by drugs or infection or be idiopathic. EM lesions typically begin as dusky, red macules or erythematous papules that evolve into target lesions after 24 to 48 hours (see Chapter 8). The diagnosis is made on the basis of the clinical appearance and the absence of significant mucosal involvement. The symptoms can persist for a few weeks, and if discomfort is significant, either antihistamines or steroids can be used. Patients with EM do not experience long-term sequelae from their disease. Patients with Stevens-Johnson syndrome (SJS) have similar skin symptoms to EM but also have significant mucosal involvement and in rare cases may have long-term complications from their disease. Patients with toxic epidermal necrolysis (TEN) have a greater proportion of their body affected by the disease than patients with SJS and frequently experience long-term complications from the illness.

Allergic Rhinitis

Allergic rhinitis, characterized by inflammation, edema, and weeping of the nasal mucosa, is the most common

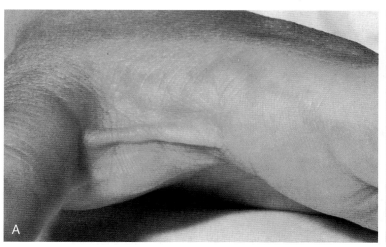
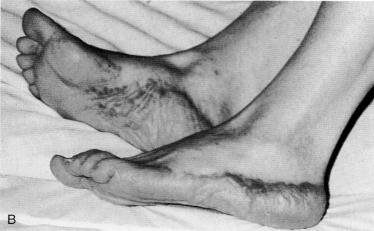

Figure 4-11. Cutaneous eruptions on the sides of the hands and feet of patients with serum sickness. **A,** A scalloped band of erythema can be seen on the side of the finger at the margin of palmar skin. **B,** A band of purpura is seen at the margin of the plantar skin. The purpura was preceded by a band of erythema. (From Lawley TJ, Bielory L, Gascon P, et al: Prospective clinical and immunologic analysis of patients with serum sickness. N Engl J Med 311:1407-1413, 1984. Copyright © 1984 Massachusetts Medical Society. All rights reserved.)

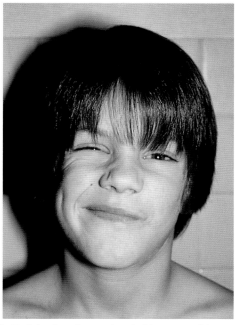

Figure 4-12. Facial grimacing and twitching caused by nasal itching in patient with allergic rhinitis. These are frequently repeated and easily noted during patient evaluation.

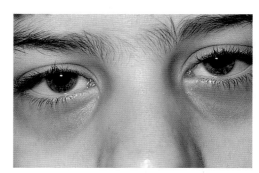

Figure 4-13. Allergic shiners, or dark circles beneath the eyes, in patient with allergic rhinitis.

allergic disorder and occurs in up to 25% of the population. Diagnosis is based on characteristic history, physical findings, and testing for antigen-specific IgE. Common presenting symptoms include nasal congestion and pruritus, clear rhinorrhea, and paroxysms of sneezing. Whereas older children may blow their noses frequently, younger children do not. Instead, they sniff, snort, and repetitively clear their throats. Nasal pruritus stimulates grimacing and twitching (Fig. 4-12) and picking or rubbing the nose (allergic salute). Picking, repetitive sneezing, and blowing along with underlying inflammation may produce enough irritation to cause epistaxis. In the case of allergy to seasonal pollens, the symptoms may be acute, have a sudden onset, and be confined to the period during which the particular airborne pollen is detectable. Trees and grass typically pollinate in the spring, whereas ragweed pollinates in the fall. Interestingly, seasonal allergic rhinitis is often called "hay fever," although hay is not involved and

fever is not a symptom. However, the manifestations can be severe enough to induce flulike symptoms of fatigue and malaise. In contrast, symptoms may be chronic and more indolent in the case of allergy to perennial allergens including molds, house dust mites, and animal dander.

Many patients have prominent itching and watering of the eyes with nasal symptoms, and some experience pruritus of the throat or ears. Associated symptoms include (1) disturbed sleep and snoring; (2) morning dryness and irritation of the throat as a result of mouth breathing; (3) lassitude, fatigue, and irritability from sleep interruption; (4) early nighttime cough; and (5) if the maxillary, frontal, and ethmoidal sinuses are affected, a sensation of pressure over the cheeks, forehead, and bridge of the nose. The extent to which allergic rhinitis affects a patient's quality of life is often underappreciated.

Many children with long-standing allergic rhinitis can be recognized by their facial characteristics. Ocular manifestations of the allergic disposition include cobblestoning of the conjunctivae (see Fig. 4-36), the allergic shiner, and the Dennie sign. Allergic shiners, bluish discolorations or dark circles beneath the eyes, are commonly observed in patients with allergic rhinitis (Fig. 4-13). This finding represents chronic venous congestion secondary to inflammation. The Dennie sign is prominent folds or creases on the lower eyelid (Fig. 4-14) running parallel to the lower lid margin. Although these lines were originally thought to indicate a predisposition to allergy, data suggest that they may be present in any condition associated with periocular pruritus and scratching or chronic nasal con-

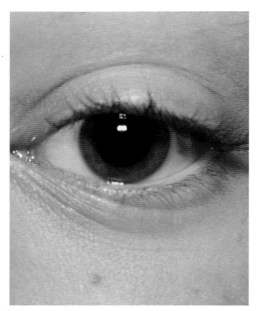

Figure 4-14. Dennie sign. Lines originate in the inner canthus and traverse one half to two thirds the length of the lower lid margin in an arc nearly parallel to it.

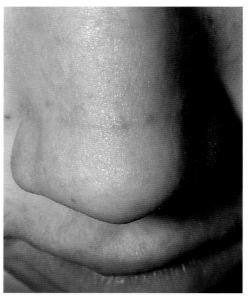

Figure 4-16. Allergic rhinitis. The nasal crease across the lower third of the nose results from chronic upward rubbing of the nose with the hand (allergic salute). (Courtesy Meyer B. Marks, MD, Miami.)

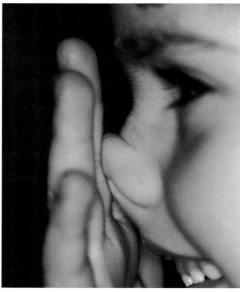

Figure 4-15. Allergic rhinitis. The allergic salute is characteristic of children with allergic rhinitis and nasal itching and is usually noticed by parents.

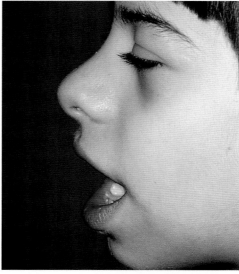

Figure 4-17. Nasal obstruction. Characteristic adenoid-type facies in a patient with long-standing allergic rhinitis. Note the open mouth and gaping habitus.

gestion. Frequent upward rubbing of the nose with the palm of the hand (the allergic salute, Fig. 4-15) promotes development of a transverse nasal crease across the lower third of the nose (Fig. 4-16). Chronic obstruction produced by nasal mucosal edema may result in mouth breathing and a typical open-mouthed, adenoid-type facies (Fig. 4-17).

On nasal examination, attention should be focused on the position of the nasal septum; nasal patency; mucosal appearance; and presence and character of secretions, polyps, or foreign bodies (see Chapter 23). The typical physical examination findings in allergic rhinitis include a marked decrease in nasal patency resulting from swollen inferior turbinates, which appear pale, edematous, and bluish gray (Fig. 4-18). The mucosa appears edematous, and secretions are clear and watery to mucoid in character. Examination of a Wright-stained smear of this discharge typically reveals eosinophils (Fig. 4-19).

Depending on the specific allergens, allergic rhinitis may be acute, recurrent, or chronic and must be distinguished from a number of nonallergic conditions. This necessitates a thorough medical and family history and careful examination. In some instances, response to a trial of medication and/or observations over time may be necessary to confirm the diagnosis. When symptoms are seasonal or regularly associated with exposure to specific allergens, the distinction is generally clear. In evaluating patients with perennial or recurrent but nonseasonal symptoms, allergy, recurrent infection, the nonallergic rhinitis with eosinophilia syndrome (NARES), and vasomotor rhinitis must be considered.

Children with frequent upper respiratory infections and/or persistent nasal congestion can present a diagnostic challenge. In some cases the phenomenon is due to recurrent viral infections, particularly in children in their first year of day care or nursery school. In other patients, tonsillar and adenoidal hypertrophy provides favorable

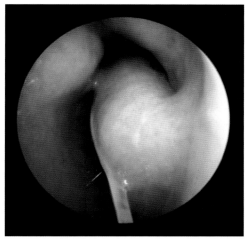

Figure 4-18. Pale, edematous inferior nasal turbinate of patient with allergic rhinitis, as seen through a fiberoptic rhinoscope. Even though this tool is not routinely used in evaluations, the physical findings are well illustrated including watery nasal secretions.

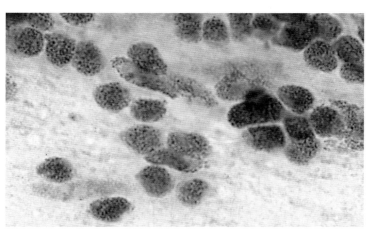

Figure 4-19. Allergic rhinitis. Eosinophilia on nasal smear from a patient with allergic rhinitis.

Table 4-4	Comparison of Allergic and Nonallergic Rhinitis		
		NONALLERGIC	
	ALLERGIC	**NARES**	**Vasomotor**
Usual onset	Childhood	Childhood	Adulthood
Family history of allergy	Usual	Coincidental	Coincidental
Collateral allergy	Common	Unusual	Unusual
Symptoms			
Sneezing	Frequent	Occasional	Occasional
Itching	Common	Unusual	Unusual
Rhinorrhea	Profuse	Profuse	Profuse
Congestion	Moderate to marked	Moderate to marked	Moderate to marked
Physical examination			
Edema	Moderate to marked	Moderate	Moderate
Secretions	Watery	Watery	Mucoid to watery
Nasal eosinophilia	Common	Common	Occasional
Allergic evaluation			
Skin tests	Positive	Coincidental	Coincidental
IgE antibodies	Positive	Coincidental	Coincidental
Therapeutic response			
Antihistamines	Fair to good	Fair	Poor to fair
Decongestants	Fair	Fair	Poor to fair
Corticosteroids	Good	Good	Poor
Cromolyn	Fair	Unknown	Poor
Immunotherapy	Good	None	None

NARES, nonallergic rhinitis with eosinophilia syndrome.
Modified from Fagin J, Friedman R, Fireman P: Allergic rhinitis. Pediatr Clin North Am 28:797-806, 1981.

conditions for recurrent infections (see Chapter 23). Atopic (allergic) children may have increased risk of infection because of impaired flow of secretions due to mucosal edema. Although viral infections tend to produce clear or white discharge and bacterial infections, purulent yellow or green discharge, there is considerable overlap, limiting the value of this distinction.

Other forms of rhinitis that must be distinguished from allergic rhinitis are enumerated in Table 4-4. Although characterized by eosinophilia, NARES does not produce nasal pruritus, and patients lack specific IgE antibodies as measured by skin testing or in vitro serum testing. Patients with vasomotor rhinitis do not complain of pruritus, have a clear discharge without eosinophils, and also lack specific IgE antibodies. Vasomotor rhinitis is thus considered a form of noninflammatory rhinitis, the etiology of which is unknown, although it is often triggered by nonspecific stimuli like cold air exposure or smoke. The condition is diagnosed most frequently in adults but may affect chil-

dren. Congestion or rhinorrhea may predominate in this disorder. Rhinitis medicamentosa is a condition seen in patients who have been using α-adrenergic vasoconstrictor nose drops (phenylephrine or oxymetazoline) as decongestants for prolonged treatment periods. The disorder is characterized by rebound vasodilation that produces an erythematous, edematous mucosa in association with a profuse clear nasal discharge.

Some children with perennial allergic rhinitis have congestion so constant and severe that it produces signs of chronic nasal obstruction. This must be distinguished from other acquired and congenital causes (see Chapter 23). The history, physical findings, and results of allergy tests for specific IgE and nasal smears, along with therapeutic trials of antihistamines and intranasal corticosteroids, will all help lead to a diagnosis.

Many patients with allergic rhinitis have mild symptoms that are adequately controlled by intermittent antihistamine administration and/or environmental controls. In many of these patients the pattern of symptoms suggests the responsible allergens, and testing for specific IgE is not indicated. Those with severe symptoms only partially alleviated by antihistamines, topical anti-inflammatory agents, and environmental controls and those with perennial symptoms who require daily therapy should be referred for specific IgE testing. Desensitization (allergy shots) is an effective treatment for patients who are not well controlled with medications or prefer not to use them regularly.

Respiratory Disease

Respiratory Distress. Respiratory distress in children (tachypnea with or without grunting, flaring, retractions, and cyanosis) should be promptly evaluated and treated. The first step in approaching respiratory distress is to differentiate upper from lower airway disorders. At times, various degrees of upper and lower airway obstruction may coexist, as in laryngotracheobronchitis.

Upper airway obstruction causes difficulty moving air into the chest, whereas lower airway obstruction causes difficulty moving air out of the chest. This difference results in characteristic physical findings. In general, lower airway obstruction produces prolongation of the expiratory phase of respiration and typical expiratory wheezing, whereas upper airway obstruction prolongs the inspiratory phase. *Wheezing* is defined as musical or whistling auscultatory sounds heard more often on expiration than on inspiration, although in severe obstruction both inspiratory and expiratory wheezing is often present. Inspiratory stridor, seen with upper airway obstruction, can mimic wheezing. Both can be detected concomitantly. *Stridor* is defined as a crowing sound usually heard during the inspiratory phase of respiration. It tends to be loud when the obstruction is subglottic and quiet when obstruction is supraglottic. Mild to moderate increases in respiratory and heart rates are common in upper airway obstruction, whereas lower airway disorders such as pneumonitis and asthma often lead to markedly increased respiratory and heart rates. Retractions are often generalized (suprasternal, intracostal, and subcostal) in severe airway obstruction of any etiology.

Asthma. Asthma often, but not invariably, involves type I, IgE-mediated reaction in the large and small airways. The most widely accepted definition of asthma includes the following characteristics: (1) lower airway obstruction that is partially or fully reversible either spontaneously or with bronchodilator or anti-inflammatory treatments, (2) the presence of airway inflammation, and (3) increased lower airway responsiveness (bronchial hyperreactivity). The last is characterized by inherent hyperreactivity of the airways to stimuli including allergens, infections, exercise, chemical agents such as methacholine, cold or dry air, emotions, and weather changes. Many cases of asthma, particularly in children, have an atopic basis. Specific allergens implicated in atopic patients are pollens, molds, house dust mites, and animal danders, whereas drugs, food, and insect venoms typically cause similar symptoms of wheezing and respiratory distress as part of anaphylaxis (see earlier discussion). On exposure, these allergens, via cross-linking specific IgE, produce the characteristic features of asthma: mucosal edema, increased mucus production, and smooth muscle contraction that result in airway inflammation, airway hyperreactivity, and bronchoconstriction. These responses combine to produce a state of reversible obstruction of the large and small airways that is the hallmark of asthma.

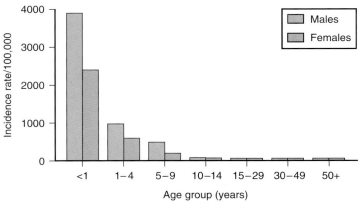

Figure 4-20. Incidence of asthma by age and gender in Rochester, Minn, from 1964 to 1983. Eighty percent of asthma has its onset by 5 years of age. (Modified from Yunginger JW, Reed CE, O'Connell EJ, et al: A community-based study of the epidemiology of asthma: Incidence rates, 1964-1983. Am Rev Respir Dis 146:888-894, 1992.)

Patients with asthma should be evaluated to determine the important triggers for their disease. Affected individuals are often aware of the specific stimuli that trigger exacerbations of their asthma. Viruses are the most common precipitants of acute asthma in children, especially respiratory syncytial virus, parainfluenza viruses, and rhinoviruses. These infections usually affect the upper and lower airways, producing rhinorrhea, nasal congestion, and fever in addition to wheezing, which tends to develop insidiously. In contrast, allergy-triggered episodes typically lack fever and have a more abrupt onset of wheezing.

Asthma is one of the leading causes of pediatric morbidity. Indeed, approximately 5% to 10% of children in the United States show signs and symptoms compatible with asthma at some time during childhood. Peak incidence of onset is before the age of 5 years (Fig. 4-20). In childhood, boys are affected more often than girls and tend to have more severe disease. Beyond puberty, the gender distribution is equal because onset in the teenage years is more common in girls, perhaps due to hormonal factors involved in menarche. Asthmatic children with respiratory allergy and eczema usually have more severe courses than those who wheeze only with upper respiratory infections.

Recently, an unexplained, worldwide increase in asthma-related morbidity and mortality rates has been noted, although these rates have apparently plateaued in the past few years (Fig. 4-21). Indeed, deaths resulting from asthma have now exceeded 5000 per year in the United States, although these occur mostly in adults. In an effort to reverse this trend, a national (National Institutes of Health [NIH]) educational program has resulted in the publication of guidelines on the diagnosis and management of asthma (see Bibliography).

Emergency department visits, hospitalizations, and intensive care unit admissions for asthma usually peak in the late fall or early winter months and, to a lesser extent, in the spring (Fig. 4-22). These seasonal patterns may be related to environmental temperature and humidity changes, allergen exposure, or respiratory infections.

The diagnosis of asthma is frequently based on historical findings alone, indicating the importance of taking a thorough history. Recently published NIH and American Academy of Pediatrics guidelines have stressed the importance of complementing good history taking with the use of objective measurements of lung function (Fig. 4-23). This can include in-office pulmonary function testing and home monitoring of peak expiratory flow rates (PEFR) in children 6 years of age and older. Peak expiratory flow

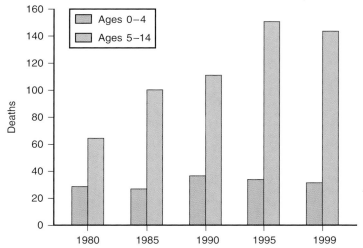

Figure 4-21. Number of pediatric asthma deaths in the United States from 1979 to 1995. (Modified from CDC Surveillance for Asthma—United States, 1960-1999. MMWR Morb Mortal Wkly Rep 51[SS-1]:1-13, 2002.)

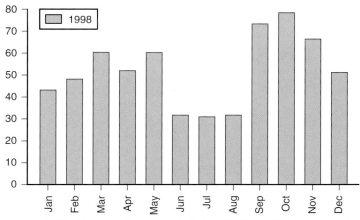

Figure 4-22. Number of asthma admissions (1998) to Children's Hospital of Pittsburgh by month of year. There is a biphasic peak in spring and fall. (Courtesy Eliseo Villalobos, MD, and Gilbert Friday, MD, Children's Hospital of Pittsburgh.)

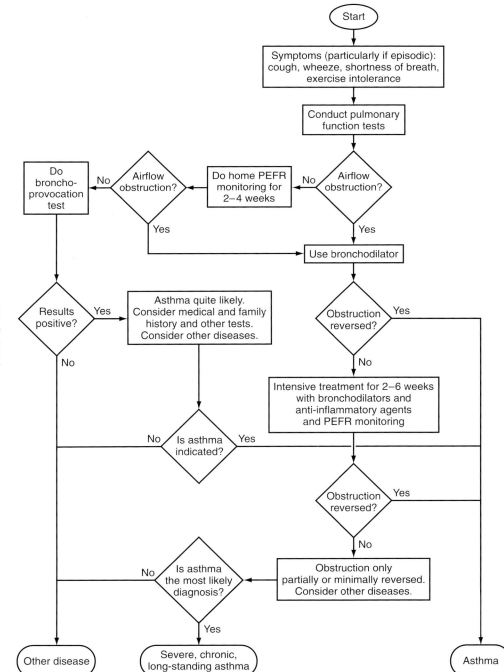

Figure 4-23. Algorithm for diagnosing asthma. PEFR = peak expiratory flow rates. (From National Asthma Education Program: Guidelines for the Diagnosis and Management of Asthma [Publication No. 91-3042]. Bethesda, Md, National Heart, Lung, and Blood Institute, National Institutes of Health, 1997.)

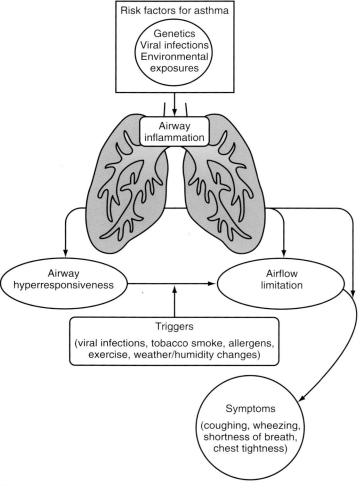

Figure 4-24. An interaction between genetic and environmental factors is involved in the pathogenesis of asthma. (Reprinted with permission from Pediatric Asthma Promoting Best Practice: Guide for Managing Asthma in Children. Milwaukee, Wisc, American Academy of Allergy, Asthma and Immunology, 1999.)

Table 4-5	When Is It Asthma?*

History of recurrent:
Coughing
Wheezing
Shortness of breath or rapid breathing
Chest tightness
Symptoms made worse by:
Viral infection
Tobacco smoke, wood smoke, and other irritants (e.g., strong odors or fumes)
Exercise
Allergens (e.g., house dust mites, pollens, cockroaches, molds, animal dander)
Changes in weather/humidity
Crying, laughing
Symptoms occur/worsen at night, waking the child and/ or parent
Reversible airflow limitation by spirometry in children older than 4 years of age and diurnal variation in peak flow
Wheezing (high-pitched whistling sounds when exhaling) may or may not be present

*No single indicator is diagnostic in itself, but the presence of several increases the probability of asthma. **Objective measures are essential to establish the diagnosis of asthma.** For children younger than 4 years of age or who cannot conduct spirometry, clinical judgment and/or response to asthma treatment may be the only reliable means for diagnosing asthma.

Reprinted with permission from Pediatric Asthma Promoting Best Practice: Guide for Managing Asthma in Children. Milwaukee, Wisc, American Academy of Allergy, Asthma and Immunology, 1999.

rates should be referenced by percentage of the patient's personal best value. Peak flow monitoring is most likely to be helpful in two clinical settings: (1) patients who have poor symptom recognition or (2) patients in whom the diagnosis may be in doubt. The PEFRs add objective data to go along with the patient's subjective appreciation of symptoms. The greatest shortcomings of peak flow monitoring are that it is effort dependent, requires compliance, and does not measure small airway function. When peak flow monitoring is used, patients should be given a written plan with instructions on what to do as their peak flow falls in the setting of increasing symptoms.

As with many common diseases, asthma incidence is influenced by both genes and environment (Fig. 4-24). Family history often reveals affected siblings, parents, or other relatives. An environmental survey can determine possible provocative factors, especially allergens, infections, occupational exposures, smoking, exercise, stress, climate, and medication use (NSAIDs, β-blockers). The history should emphasize the frequency, duration, and intensity of suspected episodes (Table 4-5). A description of symptoms between acute episodes aids in the determination of chronicity (night cough, exercise intolerance, fatigue, school absenteeism, social function). Individuals with asthma commonly present with recurrent episodes of wheezing that, depending on the severity, may require emergency treatment. Episodes may be infrequent and/or seasonal or may occur daily. The spectrum of presenting

complaints, however, is broad, and affected individuals may complain only of mild, occasional wheezing or shortness of breath with exercise and/or colds or a persistent dry, hacking cough. The frequency and severity of acute asthma episodes and the level of symptoms between episodes can be used to grade asthma severity and guide therapy using published guidelines (Table 4-6).

The early stages of an asthma exacerbation in children are characterized by the onset of cough, rhinorrhea, and chest tightness, as well as chest retractions or audible wheezing. The parents should be educated to critically and accurately observe their child for the warning signs and, in collaboration with the managing physician, identify the onset of asthmatic exacerbation at home. As previously mentioned, PEFR provides an objective assessment of lung function that may be useful under these circumstances. A written asthma action plan that details use of rescue medicines such as albuterol can minimize emergency department visits for asthma.

Asthma should be considered part of the differential diagnosis in any child with recurrent or chronic lower respiratory symptoms or signs. Even though a high index of suspicion must be maintained, excessive or erroneous diagnoses may result if they are made hastily without appropriate supportive evidence; normal children or those with potentially more severe disorders may be mistakenly diagnosed with asthma and inappropriately treated. Parents must be instructed that physician assessment is essential during suspected episodes of asthma so that wheezing or other signs of lower airway obstruction and reversibility may be documented. If the diagnosis is unclear on clinical grounds, then specific laboratory studies must be performed to document asthma and rule out disorders that mimic asthma (Table 4-7). Pulmonary function tests in asthmatic children older than 5 years of age show airway obstruction at baseline or after appropriate challenge with methacholine, exercise, or cold air and document reversibility after administration of an aerosolized bronchodilator (Fig. 4-25). In children younger than 5 years of age or those in whom testing is unreliable, the

Table 4-6   Guidelines for Defining Asthma Severity

	CLINICAL FEATURES BEFORE TREATMENT			
CLASSIFICATION *Asthma Severity*	*Symptom Severity*	*Nighttime Symptoms*	*Lung Function in Patients Who Can Use a Spirometer or Peak Flowmeter*	*Short-Acting β_2-Agonist Use*
Severe persistent	• Continual symptoms • Limited physical activity • Frequent exacerbations interfere with normal activities	Frequent	• FEV_1 or PEFR ≤60% predicted • PEFR variability >30%	Use 4 times/day; does *not* completely relieve symptoms
Moderate persistent	• Daily symptoms • Exacerbations ≥2 times/week; may last days; may affect activities	>1 time/week	• FEV_1 or PEFR >60% to <80% predicted • PEFR variability >30%	Daily
Mild persistent	• Symptoms >2 times/week but <1 time/day • Exacerbations may affect activities	>2 times/month	• FEV_1 or PEFR >80% predicted • PEFR variability 20%-30%	>2 times/week but <1 time/day
Mild intermittent	• Symptoms ≤2 times/week • Asymptomatic and normal PEFR between exacerbations • Exacerbations brief (from a few hours to a few days); intensity may vary	≤2 times/month	• FEV_1 or PEFR >80% predicted • PEFR variability <20%	≤2 times/week

FEV_1, forced expiratory volume in 1 second; PEFR, peak expiratory flow rate.
  Reprinted with permission from Pediatric Asthma Promoting Best Practice: Guide for Managing Asthma in Children. Milwaukee, Wisc, American Academy of Allergy, Asthma and Immunology, 1999.

Table 4-7   Children with Asthma May Need Additional Tests to Aid and/or Confirm the Diagnosis

REASONS FOR ADDITIONAL TESTS	SUGGESTED TESTS
Child has symptoms (coughing, wheezing, breathlessness, chest tightness), but spirometry is (near) normal	• Bronchoprovocation with histamine, methacholine, or exercise (if negative, may rule out asthma)
Suspect other factors are contributing to severity of asthma symptoms	• Nasal examination • Allergy tests, gastroesophageal reflux tests, sinus radiology*
Symptoms suggest infection, large airway lesions, heart disease, or obstruction by foreign object	• Routine chest x-ray, high resolution CT scan*
Suspect coexisting chronic obstructive pulmonary disease or restrictive defect	• Additional pulmonary function tests; diffusing capacity test*

*Referral to a specialist is recommended for consultation or co-management.
  CT, computed tomography; PEFR, peak expiratory flow rate.
  Reprinted with permission from Pediatric Asthma Promoting Best Practice: Guide for Managing Asthma in Children. Milwaukee, Wisc, American Academy of Allergy, Asthma and Immunology, 1999.

diagnosis must be made on the basis of historical and physical findings and clinical response to bronchodilator or anti-inflammatory medication. Lack of an immediate response to a bronchodilator does not eliminate asthma as a diagnostic consideration, however.

A thorough physical examination provides valuable information regarding the diagnosis of asthma and its severity and chronicity. The physical findings in asthma vary with the chronicity and state of activity of the disease process at the time of examination. The findings of acute asthma are markedly different from those of chronic and latent or quiescent asthma. Between episodes, the examination is usually entirely normal. Prolongation of the expiratory phase is often noted. Clubbing as a sign of chronic asthma is rare and, if present in a wheezing child, suggests another chronic pulmonary disease.

During acute asthma, the following historical features should be noted: time of onset, possible triggers, present medications, comparison with previous episodes, and presence of complicating factors (e.g., vomiting, fever, chest pain). Examination should document accessory muscle use, retractions, and color. Auscultation should assess air exchange, wheezing, and inspiratory-to-expiratory ratio. The ability to speak (words, phrases, or complete sentences) is a useful measure of dyspnea. Lethargy, decreased air

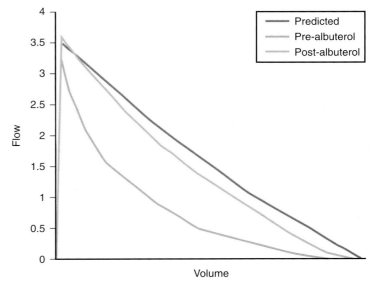

Figure 4-25. Asthma. Flow-volume loop showing predicted values, initial values, and substantial reversibility after albuterol administration. Note downward scooping of curves, which is typical in asthmatics with ongoing obstruction.

Table 4-8	Measurement of Pulsus Paradoxus

	BLOOD PRESSURE IN RELATION TO TIME AND RESPIRATORY PHASE (mm Hg)				
	Expiration	*Inspiration*	*Expiration*	*Inspiration*	*Expiration*
Normal (no airway obstruction)	125/70	120/70	125/70	120/70	125/70
Asthma (airway obstruction)	125/70	100/70	125/70	100/70	125/70

Method
1. Pump sphygmomanometer cuff to occlude the peripheral pulse.
2. As the cuff pressure falls, listen carefully for the onset of the first Korotkoff sound.
3. Note the pressure at which the first Korotkoff sound is detected. This should be heard only during expiration. (In above example, 125 = normal and asthma.)
4. Continue to slowly decrease the cuff pressure until the first sound is detected during inspiration and expiration. Note this pressure. (In above example, 120 = normal; 100 = asthma.)
5. When the difference between the two pressures is greater than or equal to 10, pulsus paradoxus is present.

Table 4-9	Estimation of Severity of Acute Exacerbations of Asthma in Children

SIGN OR SYMPTOM	MILD	MODERATE	SEVERE
PEFR*	70%-90% predicted or personal best	50%-70% predicted or personal best	<50% predicted or personal best
Respiratory rate, resting or sleeping	Normal to 30% increase above the mean	30%-50% increase above the mean	Increase over 50% above the mean
Alertness	Normal	Normal	May be decreased
Dyspnea[†]	Absent or mild; speaks in complete sentences	Speaks in phrases or partial sentences; infant's cry softer and shorter, infant has difficulty suckling and feeding	Speaks only in single words or short phrases; infant's cry softer and shorter, infant stops suckling and feeding
Pulsus paradoxus[‡]	<10 mm Hg	10-20 mm Hg	20-40 mm Hg
Accessory muscle use	No intercostal to mild retractions	Moderate intercostal retraction with tracheosternal retractions; use of sternocleidomastoid muscles; chest hyperinflation	Severe intercostal retractions, tracheosternal retractions with nasal flaring during inspiration; chest hyperinflation
Color	Good	Pale	Possibly cyanotic
Auscultation	End expiratory wheeze only	Wheeze during entire expiration and inspiration	Breath sounds becoming inaudible
Oxygen saturation	>95%	90%-95%	<90%
PCO_2	<35	<40	>40

*Peak expiratory flow rate (PEFR) assessed for children 5 years of age or older.
†Parents' or physicians' impression of degree of child's breathlessness.
‡Pulsus paradoxus does not correlate with phase of respiration in small children.
NOTE: Within each category, the presence of several parameters, but not necessarily all, indicates the general classification of the exacerbation.
From National Asthma Education Program: Guidelines for the Diagnosis and Management of Asthma (Publication No. 91-3042). Bethesda, Md, National Heart, Lung, and Blood Institute, National Institutes of Health, 1991.

exchange, and increased work of breathing are the signs most worrisome for acute deterioration.

In addition, rales are often heard, and pulse, respiratory rate, and blood pressure are frequently elevated. Pulsus paradoxus, an exaggerated decrease in systolic blood pressure during inspiration (Table 4-8), correlates highly with the degree of airway obstruction, although it is rarely measured clinically. This phenomenon may result from physical forces on the pericardium that impede venous return and reduce cardiac output during forced inspiration. Normally, the inspiratory decrease in systolic blood pressure is less than 10 mm Hg and is not discernible during routine sphygmomanometry. In acute asthma, it is usually greater than 10 mm Hg (up to 30 and 40 mm Hg) and is easily detectable.

Individuals with asthma may be distinguished by their characteristic symptoms and signs during acute episodes, which typically change as the degree of airway obstruction increases. Symptoms usually consist of progressively increasing shortness of breath and difficulty breathing with or without rhinorrhea, low-grade fever, and vomiting. On examination, expiratory wheezing or a prolonged expiratory phase may be the only manifestation of mild asthma. However, as the obstructive process progresses, the expiratory phase becomes longer and the wheezing becomes louder and occurs on both inspiration and expiration. Eventually, airways collapse and signs of hyperinflation develop (low diaphragms, decreased lateral excursions of the chest wall with breathing, and hyperresonance to percussion). Visible sternocleidomastoid contractions; increased anteroposterior chest diameter; circumoral cyanosis; and suprasternal, intercostal, and substernal retractions occur. Subjectively, the patient experiences chest tightness and anxiety and works harder to breathe. Accessory muscle use and retractions develop with or without a marked degree of wheezing on auscultation. To maximize air exchange, the child assumes a characteristic sitting posture, bending slightly forward. Frequent examinations are warranted, and any change in sensorium requires prompt evaluation. As respiratory muscles tire, the patient becomes lethargic and cyanotic, even with supplemental oxygen. Decrease in wheezing with increased air entry represents response to therapy. Decreased wheezing with decreased air entry is an ominous sign. With extreme fatigue, respiratory muscles fail, retractions decrease, and respiratory failure is imminent unless appropriate therapy is promptly initiated. After initial examination, serial assessment of the degree of respiratory distress using the parameters outlined in Table 4-9 assists determination of the response to therapy.

A particularly useful aspect of the physical examination is the respiratory rate, which increases as the degree of airway obstruction progresses. Respiratory rates of normal children are shown in Table 4-10.

The underlying pathology of asthma is lung inflammation. Histopathologic features of acute asthma include airway infiltration with inflammatory cells, increased intraluminal mucus with plugging of small airways, edema, bronchoconstriction, and smooth muscle hypertrophy. Because asthma has bronchoconstrictive and inflammatory components, the ideal therapeutic regimen should incorporate a combination of bronchodilator and anti-inflammatory agents. Characteristic features of asthmatic inflammation include mast cell activation, inflammatory cell infiltration, edema, denudation and disruption of the bronchial epithelium, collagen deposition beneath the basement membrane, goblet cell hyperplasia, and smooth muscle thickening. These morphologic changes may not be completely reversible and may contribute to airway remodeling (Fig. 4-26). Education is a key component of asthma therapy, incorporating information about disease pathogenesis; avoidance of environmental triggers (including second-hand tobacco smoke exposure); benefits and risks of medications; and a written, individualized therapeutic plan for chronic and acute management.

The radiographic features of the hyperinflation, peribronchial cuffing, and atelectasis, which are characteristic of uncomplicated acute asthma, are illustrated in Figure 4-27. Complications are generally diagnosed radiographically but may be suggested by symptoms and signs. Pneumothorax (Fig. 4-28) should be suspected in any asthmatic person who develops pleuritic chest pain associated with dyspnea, cyanosis, tachypnea, and occasionally cough. Examination reveals respiratory distress, marked hyperinflation and decreased chest wall excursion, and decreased or absent breath sounds on the affected side. With tension pneumothorax, the trachea, mediastinum, and cardiac landmarks may be shifted to the opposite side. Pneumomediastinum and subcutaneous emphysema (Fig. 4-29), usually involving the neck and supraclavicular areas, are more common than pneumothorax. When mild, they may be asymptomatic and may be detected incidentally on chest or neck radiograph. With more extensive air dissection, the patient may complain of neck and chest

Table 4-10	Respiratory Rates of Normal Children, Sleeping and Awake*					
	SLEEPING			**AWAKE**		
AGE	**No.**	**Mean**	**Range**	**No.**	**Mean**	**Range**
6-12 months	6	27	22-31	3	64	58-75
1-2 years	6	19	17-23	4	35	30-40
2-4 years	16	19	16-25	15	31	23-42
4-6 years	23	18	14-23	22	26	19-36
6-8 years	27	17	13-23	28	23	15-30

*In breaths per minute.
From Waring WW: The history and physical exam. In Kendig E, Chernick V (eds): Disorders of the Respiratory Tract in Children. Philadelphia, WB Saunders, 1983. As appears in National Asthma Education Program: Guidelines for the Diagnosis and Management of Asthma (Publication No. 91-3042). Bethesda, Md, National Heart, Lung, and Blood Institute, National Institutes of Health, 1991.

PROGRESSION TO AIRWAY REMODELING

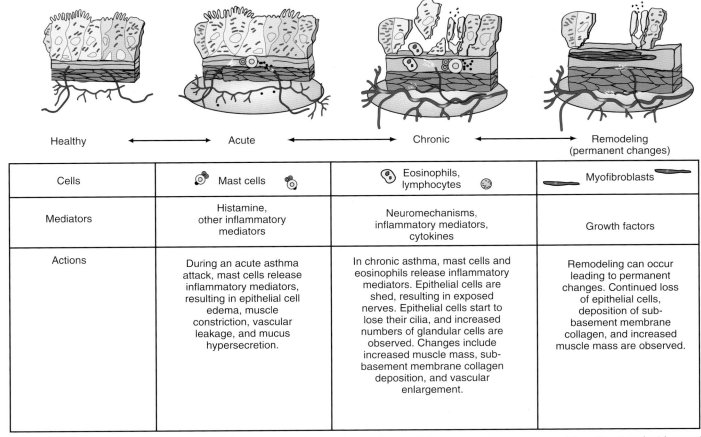

Cells	Mast cells	Eosinophils, lymphocytes	Myofibroblasts
Mediators	Histamine, other inflammatory mediators	Neuromechanisms, inflammatory mediators, cytokines	Growth factors
Actions	During an acute asthma attack, mast cells release inflammatory mediators, resulting in epithelial cell edema, muscle constriction, vascular leakage, and mucus hypersecretion.	In chronic asthma, mast cells and eosinophils release inflammatory mediators. Epithelial cells are shed, resulting in exposed nerves. Epithelial cells start to lose their cilia, and increased numbers of glandular cells are observed. Changes include increased muscle mass, sub-basement membrane collagen deposition, and vascular enlargement.	Remodeling can occur leading to permanent changes. Continued loss of epithelial cells, deposition of sub-basement membrane collagen, and increased muscle mass are observed.

Healthy ← → Acute ← → Chronic ← → Remodeling (permanent changes)

Figure 4-26. Asthmatic inflammation may result in permanent changes in the airways. This process is known as *remodeling*. (Reprinted with permission from The Allergy Report: Diseases of the Atopic Diathesis, vol 2. Milwaukee, Wisc, Task Force on Allergic Disorders, American Academy of Allergy, Asthma and Immunology, 2000.)

pain, and the subcutaneous emphysema may be visibly evident as a soft tissue swelling of the neck and chest that is crepitant (has a crunching sensation) on palpation. Pneumothorax and pneumomediastinum can produce characteristic auscultatory findings including a crackling "mediastinal crunch" at the base of the heart and a systolic crunch or knock. The latter sound has been referred to as *noisy pneumothorax* and is frequently audible to the patient and physician without the aid of a stethoscope.

Other complications diagnosable on physical examination include those induced by chronic systemic steroid use, such as weight gain, "moon-type" facies, hirsutism, polycythemia (red, ruddy complexion) (Fig. 4-30), and short stature (see Chapter 9). The introduction of effective anti-inflammatory therapy, particularly inhaled corticosteroids, has made such sequelae rare.

In children with recent onset of wheezing, asthma must be differentiated from other disorders associated with wheezing. In infants, this differentiation includes bronchiolitis, the features of which are listed in Table 4-11 (see Chapter 16). This differentiation may be difficult because 30% to 50% of children with recurrent bronchiolitis are later diagnosed with asthma, and asthma exacerbations are often triggered by viral infection. However, the distinction remains a clinically useful one for the following reasons: (1) the children with bronchiolitis who do not develop asthma may be inappropriately labeled as asthmatic, and (2) children younger than 2 years of age frequently do not respond to inhaled bronchodilators.

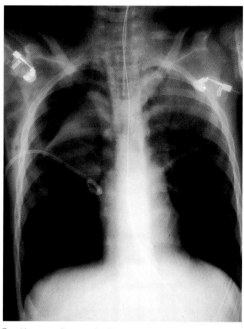

Figure 4-28. Chest radiograph showing right-sided pneumothorax in an intubated patient with acute asthma and respiratory failure. Clinical manifestations include pleuritic chest pain, dyspnea, cyanosis, tachypnea, and cough. Also, note the marked hyperinflation of the lungs, which can result in cardiac compression (narrow cardiac shadow) and compromise of cardiac venous return, as well as extensive right-sided subcutaneous emphysema. (Courtesy Beverly Newman, MD, Pittsburgh, Pa.)

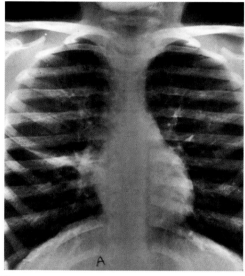

Figure 4-27. Anteroposterior chest radiograph of child with acute asthma. Note the flattened diaphragm, hyperinflation, peribronchial thickening, and right middle lobe atelectasis.

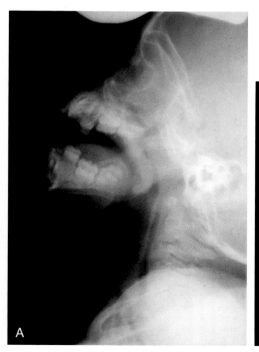

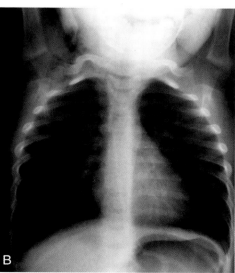

Figure 4-29. Asthma with pneumomediastinum in a 16-month-old child with asthma. Note the dissection of air in the soft tissues just anterior to the vertebrae **(A)** and in the mediastinum and subcutaneous tissues of the right arm **(B).** This highlights the often subtle findings of pneumomediastinum in the chest and the more striking findings in the neck. Also note the hyperinflation **(B).** (Courtesy Beverly Newman, MD, Pittsburgh, Pa.)

| Table 4-11 | Differentiating Features of Asthma and Bronchiolitis in Children |

	ASTHMA	**BRONCHIOLITIS**
Primary etiologies	Viruses, allergens, exercise, and so on	Respiratory syncytial virus, other viruses
Age of onset	50% by 2 years of age	<24 months
	80% by 5 years of age	
Recurrent wheezing	Yes (characteristic)	70% (≤2 episodes)
		30% progress to asthma (≥3 episodes)
Onset of wheezing	Acute if allergic or exercise induced	Insidious
Concomitant symptoms of upper respiratory infection	Yes, if infectious	Yes
Family history of allergy and asthma	Frequent	Infrequent in children with ≤2 episodes
Nasal eosinophilia	With allergic rhinitis	Absent
Chest auscultation	If viral, as in bronchiolitis	Fine, sibilant rales, and coarse inspiratory and
	Nonviral: high-pitched expiratory wheezes	expiratory wheezes
Concomitant allergic manifestations	If allergic asthma	Usually absent
IgE level	Elevated (if allergic)	Normal
Response to bronchodilator	Yes (characteristic)	Unresponsive or partially responsive

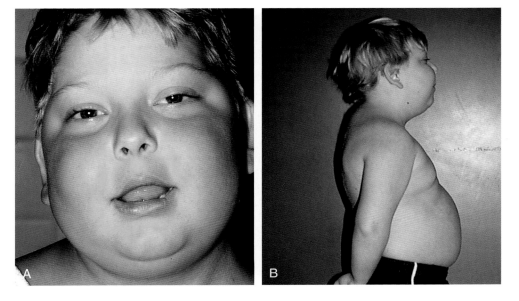

Figure 4-30. Steroid-dependent asthma. Complications of corticosteroid therapy for chronic asthma. Moon-type facies **(A)** and buffalo hump **(B)**, both resulting from abnormal fat distribution.

Depending on the response to a trial dose, ongoing bronchodilator therapy may be indicated in children with bronchiolitis. In infants and young children who wheeze with viral upper respiratory infections, different patterns of illness may emerge over time.

The Tucson Children's Respiratory Study, a large, longitudinal assessment of respiratory illnesses in children, identified different patterns of wheezing illness in children. As summarized in Figure 4-31, 51.5% of children enrolled in this study never wheezed, 19.9% had transient infant wheezing (defined as wheezing during the first 3 years of life but no wheezing at 6 years of age), 13.7% had persistent wheezing (defined as wheezing during the first 3 years of life with wheezing present at 6 years of age), and 15% had late-onset wheezing (defined as no wheezing during the first 3 years of life but wheezing present at 6 years of age). Children with transient wheezing had significantly lower lung function in infancy (before any wheezing illness) than all the other groups (Table 4-12). At the age of 6 years, children with early transient wheezing had significantly lower lung function than those who had never wheezed, and children with persistent wheezing had the lowest levels of lung function of all the groups.

It is hypothesized that children with early transient wheezing have congenitally smaller airways, which predispose to wheezing with viral illnesses in early life. As

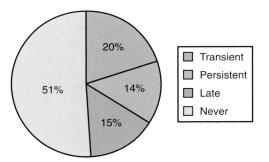

Figure 4-31. Asthma. The Tucson Children's Respiratory Study has shown that in children who wheeze, different patterns of illness may emerge over time. About half the patients in this study had evidence of wheezing before 6 years of age. In the transient group, wheezing occurred during the first 3 years of life but resolved by 6 years of age. In the persistent group, wheezing occurred during the first 3 years of life and persisted to 6 years of age. In the late group, wheezing did not occur during the first 3 years of life but was present by 6 years of age. (Modified from Martinez FD, Wright AL, Taussig LM, et al: Asthma and wheezing in the first 6 years of life. N Engl J Med 332:133-138, 1995.)

their airways grow in absolute size with age, these children outgrow their wheezing during viral infections. In contrast, it is hypothesized that children with persistent wheezing are born with normal airway function, which deteriorates over time, reflecting the effects of the chronic asthmatic disease process. Distinguishing transient versus persistent wheezing during infancy and early childhood remains problematic. Infant pulmonary function testing is still experimental and not widely available, there are currently no reliable genetic markers, and the use of any single biochemical markers is controversial. However, a combination of clinical and biochemical markers may be useful in predicting persistent wheezing (Table 4-13). These include an increased serum IgE level at 9 months of age, atopic dermatitis and rhinitis (unrelated to upper respiratory infection) during the first year of life, severe lower respiratory infections requiring hospitalization, and diminished airway function as measured by spirometry at 6 years. Other factors associated with persistent wheezing include a family history of asthma and/or allergy and perinatal exposure to passive tobacco smoke. A clinical index has been developed to predict which children with recurrent wheezing are at risk for persistent asthma (Table 4-14).

Although children with pneumonia (particularly of viral origin) may wheeze, they are more likely to have rales or normal findings on auscultation, with the diagnosis suggested by tachypnea in association with retractions, nasal flaring, or expiratory grunting. Other causes of wheezing are listed in Table 4-15. Airway compression by anomalous vessels (see Chapter 5) or mass lesions is often distinguishable from bronchiolitis by virtue of absence of signs of infection and from asthma by failure to respond to bronchodilators. The history and presence of infiltrates help in the diagnosis of aspiration, which can mimic asthma closely, often responding to bronchodilator therapy. Radiographic studies such as barium swallow with fluoroscopy can be helpful in distinguishing among these entities (Fig. 4-32). pH-Probe testing may be required to identify gastroesophageal reflux (see Chapter 16), although a trial of antireflux medicines is often attempted.

In older children who have sudden onset of wheezing and respiratory distress, the differential diagnosis includes respiratory infections, left ventricular failure, and aspiration. Respiratory infections such as croup may be distinguished by their characteristic histories and tendencies to involve the upper airways (see Chapter 16). Lower respiratory infections (pneumonia) generally produce fever and more localized findings of rales, a decrease in the number of and change in the quality of breath sounds, and egophony. Left ventricular failure, especially with pulmonary

Table 4-12	Lung Function during Infancy and at 6 Years of Age According to Wheezing History in Patients Enrolled in the Tucson Children's Respiratory Study

	LUNG FUNCTION (V_{max} FRC)		
GROUP	**n (%)**	**Infancy**	**6 Years of Age**
No wheezing	425 (51.5%)	Normal	Normal
Transient wheezing	164 (19.9%)	Diminished	Diminished
Persistent wheezing	113 (13.7%)	Normal	Diminished
Late-onset wheezing	124 (15%)	Normal	Normal

Modified from Martinez FD, Wright AL, Taussig LM, et al: Asthma and wheezing in the first six years of life. N Engl J Med 332:133-138, 1995.

Table 4-13	Factors Predictive of Persistent Asthma

Family history of asthma (maternal > paternal)
- Atopy
  — ↑ IgE or positive allergy skin tests
  — Eczema
  — Rhinitis
- Allergen exposure (dust mites/animals)
- RSV bronchiolitis
- Gender (males > females)
- Environmental smoke exposure
- Severity in childhood

RSV, respiratory syncytial virus.
Modified from Martinez FD, Wright AL, Taussig LM, et al: Asthma and wheezing in the first six years of life. N Engl J Med 332:133-138, 1995.

Table 4-14	Clinical Index to Define Asthma

MAJOR CRITERIA	**MINOR CRITERIA**
1. Physician diagnosis of parental asthma	1. Physician diagnosis of allergic rhinitis
2. Physician diagnosis of atopic dermatitis	2. Wheezing apart from colds
	3. Eosinophilia (≥4%)

The loose index for prediction of asthma consists of early wheezing plus at least one of two major criteria or two of three minor criteria. The stringent index for prediction of asthma consists of early *frequent* wheezing plus at least one of two major criteria or two of three minor criteria.
Modified from Castro-Rodriguez JA, Holberg CJ, Wright AL, et al: A clinical index to define risk of asthma in young children with recurrent wheezing. Am J Respir Crit Care Med 162:1403-1406, 2000.

Table 4-15	Associated Symptoms and Signs in the Wheezing Child That Are Helpful in Differential Diagnosis

	DISEASES ASSOCIATED WITH WHEEZING	
SYMPTOMS AND SIGNS	***In Infants***	***In Older Children***
Positional changes	Anomalies of great vessels, gastroesophageal reflux	Gastroesophageal reflux
Failure to thrive	Cystic fibrosis, tracheoesophageal fistula, bronchopulmonary dysplasia	Cystic fibrosis, chronic hypersensitivity pneumonitis, α_1-antitrypsin deficiency, bronchiectasis
Factors associated with feeding	Tracheoesophageal fistula, gastroesophageal reflux	Gastroesophageal reflux
Environmental triggers	Allergic asthma	Allergic asthma, allergic bronchopulmonary aspergillosis, acute hypersensitivity pneumonitis
Sudden onset	Allergic asthma, croup	Allergic asthma, foreign body aspiration, croup, acute hypersensitivity pneumonitis
Fever	Bronchiolitis, pneumonitis	Infectious asthma, acute hypersensitivity pneumonitis, croup
Rhinorrhea	Bronchiolitis, pneumonitis	Infectious or allergic asthma, croup
Concomitant stridor	Tracheal or bronchial stenosis, anomalies of the great vessels, croup	Foreign body aspiration, croup
Clubbing	—	Cystic fibrosis, bronchiectasis, bronchopulmonary dysplasia

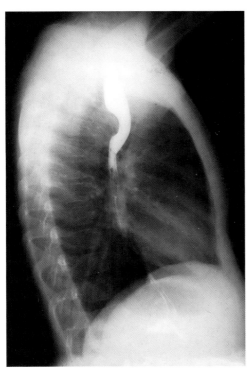

Figure 4-32. Vascular ring/compression. Barium swallow (lateral chest radiograph) shows upper airway compression by a right-sided aortic arch with aberrant left subclavian and diverticulum at the left subclavian origin. Note the round indentation on the posterior wall of the esophagus and the anterior displacement and compression of the trachea, which can cause wheezing and mimic asthma. (Courtesy Beverly Newman, MD, Pittsburgh, Pa. From Fireman P, Slavin RG: Atlas of Allergies. New York, Gower, 1990.)

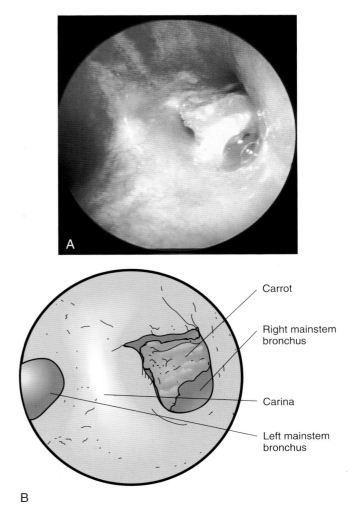

Figure 4-33. Airway foreign body. Piece of carrot lodged in the right stem bronchus just below the carina, as visualized during bronchoscopy. Foreign bodies such as this can cause airway obstruction that is partially responsive to bronchodilator therapy. (Courtesy Dr. Sylvan Stool, Pittsburgh, Pa. From Fireman P, Slavin RG: Atlas of Allergies, New York, Gower, 1990.)

edema, may present with acute respiratory distress and wheezing. A history of cardiac disease, diffuse crackles or basilar rales, and a third heart sound on auscultation help distinguish this condition from asthma. Aspiration of a foreign body that lodges in a mainstem bronchus may produce wheezing (Fig. 4-33). A history of a choking episode and physical findings of unilateral wheezing and hyperresonance aid in distinguishing aspiration from asthma but do not confirm the diagnosis. Remembering that wheezing resulting from foreign body aspiration may respond at least in part to bronchodilator therapy is important.

In the older child with mild, infrequent episodes of wheezing that respond to bronchodilator therapy, asthma is readily diagnosed. However, with daily wheezing, frequent exacerbations, lack of response to bronchodilators, or poor growth, other diagnoses must be considered including chronic obstructive pulmonary disease, cystic fibrosis, α_1-antitrypsin deficiency, carcinoid syndrome, and immunodeficiency. Chronic obstructive pulmonary diseases, which include chronic bronchitis, emphysema, bronchiectasis, and bronchopulmonary dysplasia, are distinguished by their lack of significant reversibility with bronchodilator therapy. Cystic fibrosis may present with chronic cough, wheezing, and recurrent infections. In addition, malabsorption with bulky, foul-smelling stools; failure to thrive; and clubbing of the nail beds are common. α_1-Antitrypsin deficiency, an inherited autosomal recessive disorder, is characterized by the onset of progressive emphysema in a young adult and is one cause of neonatal hepatitis.

Hypersensitivity Pneumonitis. Although IgE-mediated allergic respiratory diseases (allergic rhinitis, asthma) are the most common manifestations of inhalant sensi-

tivities in humans, other immunologic respiratory diseases, involving non-IgE immune mechanisms, may result from the inhalation of antigens from the susceptible individual's environment. A wide variety of inhaled biologic dusts may induce an inflammatory lung disease involving the interstitium, alveoli, and airways. The most common form of hypersensitivity pneumonitis is caused by inhalation of thermophilic actinomycetes *(Micropolyspora faeni)*, antigens present in moldy vegetable compost, and is termed *farmer's lung*. Other forms (and their causative dusts and antigens) include malt-worker's lung (moldy malt, *Aspergillus* species) and bird-breeder's lung (avian dust, avian proteins). The disorder is termed *hypersensitivity pneumonitis* or *extrinsic allergic alveolitis* and appears to be mediated by a complex immune response involving both immune-complexes (type III) and T cells (type IV).

Hypersensitivity pneumonitis is a syndrome with a broad spectrum of presenting symptoms and signs that have been subdivided into acute, subacute, and chronic. The clinical features depend on the following factors: (1) the nature of the inhaled dust, (2) the intensity and frequency of inhalation exposure, and (3) the immunologic responsiveness of the exposed individual. A concomitant upper respiratory infection or another pulmonary insult may be an important factor in induction. Development of sensitization to the inhaled organic dust requires several months to years, although organic dust toxic syndrome

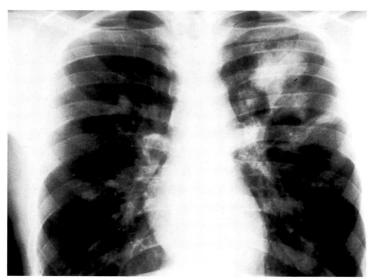

Figure 4-34. Chest radiograph of patient with allergic bronchopulmonary aspergillosis. These patients are frequently asymptomatic despite extensive areas of consolidation. (Courtesy Raymond G. Slavin, MD, St Louis.)

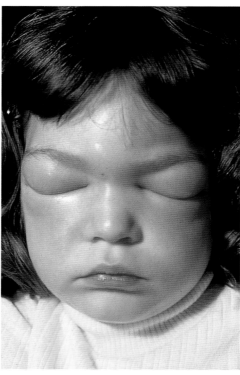

Figure 4-35. Angioedema. Eyelid angioedema in child with a venom allergy. The onset was explosive after exposure to the bee sting. (From Fireman P, Slavin RG: Atlas of Allergies. New York, Gower, 1990.)

can present similarly after a single exposure to a large dose of antigen. The acute form of hypersensitivity pneumonitis is usually readily differentiated from asthma by the lack of wheezing, prominence of rales, and presence of severe systemic symptoms such as high fever and myalgia. Subacute and chronic forms generally present with insidious development of respiratory symptoms.

Allergic Bronchopulmonary Aspergillosis. *Aspergillus* species, in addition to being one cause of hypersensitivity pneumonitis and allergic asthma, cause a disorder termed *allergic bronchopulmonary aspergillosis* (ABPA). This entity is characterized by migrating pulmonary infiltrates and peripheral blood and sputum eosinophilia. Type I and type III hypersensitivity are thought to be involved in the pathogenesis. Affected individuals are usually atopic and have a history of asthma and/or cystic fibrosis. They often present with systemic symptoms and difficulty weaning off systemic corticosteroids. Sputum production is prominent. Physical findings include the general signs of lower airway obstruction (see earlier section on asthma).

Laboratory studies that assist in diagnosis include the following:

1. Peripheral blood examination reveals eosinophilia (generally >1000/mm^3).
2. The serum IgE level is markedly elevated, often greater than 1000 ng/mL, and specific IgE to *Aspergillus fumigatus* is elevated.
3. Skin testing for *A. fumigatus* is positive. Although mold-sensitive asthmatics without ABPA may have a positive reaction, a negative reaction rules out ABPA.
4. Serum precipitating antibody (IgG) to *A. fumigatus* is found in most patients, but the titer has a poor correlation with disease activity.
5. Chest radiography commonly shows infiltrates in active ABPA. The upper lobes are commonly involved, and infiltrates characteristically shift rapidly from one site to the other. Remarkably, radiographic findings do not correlate well with clinical severity, and patients with extensive consolidation may be asymptomatic (Fig. 4-34).
6. High-resolution CT scanning may show bronchiectasis, especially late in the course of the disease.

Diagnosis of ABPA requires a high index of suspicion and should be considered in any asthmatic person who

has pulmonary infiltrates or suddenly uncontrollable disease. Early diagnosis and corticosteroid treatment are necessary to prevent progression to severe, irreversible, end-stage lung disease.

Ocular Allergy

Ocular allergic reactions may involve the eyelid and/or conjunctiva. The eyelids have a rich blood supply and loose connective tissue assisting edema collection from either allergic inflammation or trauma. Immediate hypersensitivity reactions that produce eyelid angioedema may be triggered by a number of stimuli including pollens, dusts, insect stings or bites, foods, or drugs. The most common cause of mild reactions is topical exposure to environmental allergens. These reactions are characterized by periorbital edema, pruritus, and erythema after exposure to an allergen (Fig. 4-35). Severe acute episodes can be distinguished from cellulitis by lack of induration, absence of tenderness and fever, and the fact that involvement is usually bilateral (see Chapter 23).

Allergic conjunctivitis may be acute or chronic and seasonal or perennial, depending on the allergens to which the individual is sensitized. Commonly implicated allergens include weed, tree, and grass pollens; molds; dust; and animal dander. In the acute seasonal form, onset may be rapid and may coincide with the appearance of pollen. This condition frequently accompanies seasonal allergic rhinitis and is commonly due to ragweed, grass, and tree pollens. Itching and excessive tearing are the most prominent symptoms. Pruritus often interferes with sleep, and vision may be impaired by excessive discharge.

Physical findings depend on the degree of chronicity. In the acute form, these findings consist of diffuse bilateral conjunctival edema and hyperemia. Photophobia, profuse tearing, and mild lid swelling are commonly associated. In the chronic form, the conjunctivae appear pale, with mild edema and hyperplasia of the papillae. This

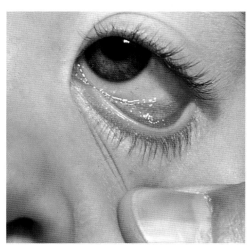

Figure 4-36. Allergic cobblestoning of the conjunctiva in chronic allergic conjunctivitis. This granular appearance is due to edema and hyperplasia of the papillae.

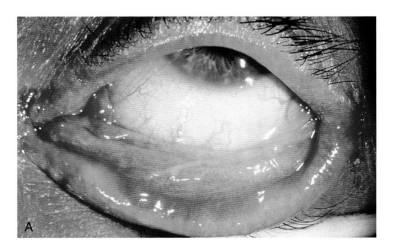

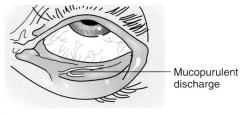

— Mucopurulent discharge

B

Figure 4-37. Atopic keratoconjunctivitis with chronic papillary conjunctivitis. Note the stringy mucopurulent discharge often seen in this disorder. (From Fireman P, Slavin RG: Atlas of Allergies. New York, Gower, 1990.)

may result in a fine, granular appearance of the conjunctivae, which is termed *allergic cobblestoning* (Fig. 4-36). The clinical diagnosis may be confirmed by finding eosinophilia on a smear of conjunctival secretions and skin testing for the suspected allergens.

The differential diagnosis of allergic conjunctivitis includes atopic keratoconjunctivitis, and vernal conjunctivitis. Atopic keratoconjunctivitis occurs in patients with atopic dermatitis and is characterized by erythema and thickening of the conjunctivae (Fig. 4-37). This may progress to scarring and vascularization of the cornea in severe cases. Ocular disease activity parallels that of cutaneous disease. It generally presents in adults.

Vernal conjunctivitis is uncommon and chronic in nature. Young, atopic boys are affected most frequently. Symptoms include severe itching, photophobia, blurring

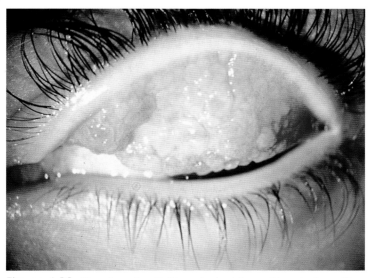

Figure 4-38. Vernal conjunctivitis, palpebral form. The giant papillary elevations are easily seen without magnification. (From Fireman P, Slavin RG: Atlas of Allergies. New York, Gower, 1990.)

of vision, and lacrimation. Physical examination reveals white, ropy secretions containing many eosinophils. A palpebral form manifests hypertrophic nodular papillae that resemble cobblestones on the upper eyelids (Fig. 4-38). The papillae consist of dense fibrous tissue with eosinophilic infiltrates. In the bulbar form, nodules appear as gelatinous masses called *Trantas dots,* usually found at the corneoscleral junction (Fig. 4-39). The symptoms are generally severe and frequently require referral to ophthalmology for topical steroids. This disease usually remits with maturity and is rarely seen in adults. Giant papillary conjunctivitis, which appears clinically and histologically to be a mild form of vernal conjunctivitis, is associated with the use of hard and soft contact lenses (Fig. 4-40). The stimulus is believed to be foreign material that accumulates on the surface of the contact lenses. Whether this material is antigenic and the condition an immune-mediated disease is not known.

Urticaria and Angioedema

Hypersensitivity reactions in which the skin is the major target organ are manifested clinically as diffuse erythema, urticaria, or angioedema. Type I hypersensitivity to inhalants, foods, insect venoms, and drugs is the most common mechanism, but urticaria and angioedema may also accompany type II (transfusion reaction) or type III reactions (cutaneous vasculitis, serum sickness). These disorders result from increased vascular permeability. The resultant edema collects in the dermis in urticaria and primarily in the subcutaneous tissues in angioedema. Although frequently seen in combination, urticaria and angioedema may also appear individually. Urticaria is most frequently an acute disorder that resolves spontaneously. In children it is often secondary to viral illnesses, allergen exposure, or idiopathic in nature. When the duration of recurrences exceeds 6 weeks, the condition is arbitrarily termed *chronic urticaria.* In contrast to acute urticaria, an underlying cause of chronic urticaria is often not found, even with extensive investigation.

Urticarial lesions are well-circumscribed, raised, palpable wheals that blanch with applied pressure (Fig. 4-41). They are usually erythematous but may be pale or white

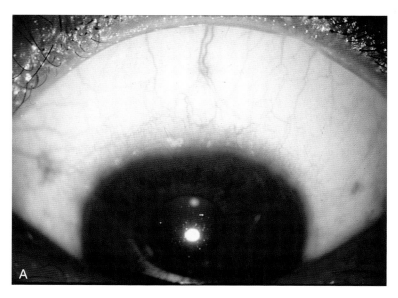

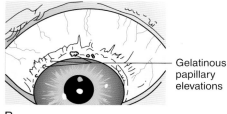

Figure 4-39. Vernal conjunctivitis, limbal form. Note the gelatinous papillary elevations of the limbal tissue. (From Fireman P, Slavin RG: Atlas of Allergies. New York, Gower, 1990.)

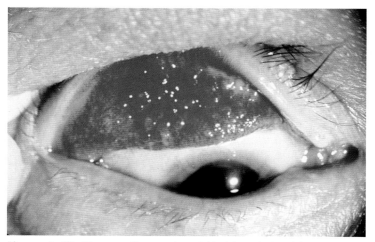

Figure 4-40. Giant papillary conjunctivitis. These hobnail-like elevations of the upper tarsal conjunctiva, evident on eversion of the upper eyelid, occur when the upper lid meets a foreign body such as a contact lens, prosthesis, or exposed suture. (From Fireman P, Slavin RG: Atlas of Allergies. New York, Gower, 1990.)

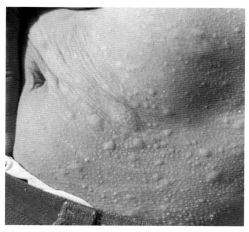

Figure 4-41. Urticarial lesions. Note the well-demarcated borders, redness, elevation, and occasional confluence of the palpable lesions. (Courtesy Michael Sherlock, MD, Bloomfield, NJ.)

with red halos. Typically, the lesions are intensely pruritic; however, in some instances the pruritus is mild. Angioedema is characterized by diffuse subcutaneous tissue swelling with normal or erythematous overlying skin. Angioedema may be more painful than pruritic. The face, hands, feet, and perineum are most commonly involved (Fig. 4-42).

Skin involvement may be generalized or localized to body parts exposed to a provoking stimulus. Careful history taking concerning recent exposures and medications is often rewarding. In cases with associated fever and respiratory and/or GI symptoms, infectious diseases resulting from viruses (including enterovirus, hepatitis B virus, and Epstein-Barr virus), group A β-hemolytic streptococcus, and helminth infestation should be considered. Generalized urticaria with or without angioedema may also be the initial manifestation of erythema multiforme or Henoch-Schönlein purpura. In general, urticaria that is not associated with pain, respiratory or GI symptoms, or residual skin changes, and in which individual lesions are red/pink and last less than 24 hours, is benign and can be managed symptomatically.

A subgroup of urticarial disorders results from hypersensitivity to physical and mechanical factors. These include cold urticaria, pressure-induced urticaria and angioedema, aquagenic and solar urticaria, and exercise-induced urticaria. The history and distribution of lesions often help in identifying the source, which can then be confirmed by challenge (Fig. 4-43).

Dermographism, translated literally as the "ability to write on the skin" (Fig. 4-44), is a form of trauma-induced pressure urticaria. It is elicited by stroking the skin with a fingernail or tongue blade. The initial white line secondary to reflex vasoconstriction is supplanted by pruritic, erythematous linear swelling, as seen in a classic wheal and flare reaction. The condition is chronic and the etiology unclear. Patients with dermographism suspected of having an atopic disorder must be skin tested with caution for specific IgE antibody because all tests appear positive.

Hereditary Angioedema

Hereditary angioedema is an autosomal dominant disorder characterized by the absence or abnormal func-

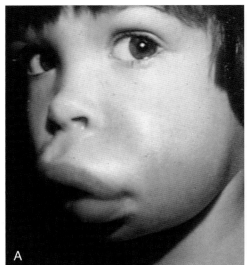
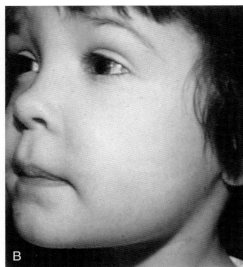

Figure 4-42. Angioedema. **A,** Onset was sudden. **B,** Resolution was complete within 24 hours.

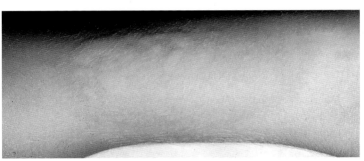

Figure 4-43. Positive ice cube test in child with cold urticaria. An ice cube placed on the arm for 10 minutes results in urticaria of the exposed skin. Onset is usually immediate but may be delayed for up to 4 hours after cold exposure.

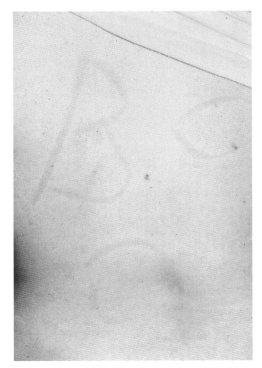

Figure 4-44. Dermographism or writing on the skin is the most common type of urticaria induced by physical or mechanical factors. Firm stroking of the skin with a fingernail or tongue blade results in urticaria of the trau-matized skin.

tion of a protein in the complement cascade known as *C1 esterase inhibitor.* Inhibitors of the complement system are part of the complement pathway and are capable of blocking activated complement components. C1 esterase inhibitor binds to activated C1 and thereby prevents further activation of the classical pathway. It also serves to regulate other blood protein cascades including the bradykinin system. In the absence of C1 inhibitor, these cascades can proceed unchecked. This results in increased vascular permeability and the observed clinical features of angioedema. This disorder is characterized by recurrent bouts of swelling that involve any part of the body with the face, extremities, genitals, and respiratory and GI tracts most frequently involved. The swelling is generally self-limited, episodic, and commonly triggered by minor trauma. The swelling is distinguished from idiopathic angioedema (which is frequently accompanied by urti-caria) by its longer duration (1 to 3 days) and the absence of urticaria. Laryngeal edema is a frightening, life-threatening complication that may result in asphyxiation. Involvement of the GI tract is characterized by severe abdominal pain, bloating, vomiting, and rarely intestinal obstruction resulting from intussusception. C4 levels are persistently depressed while C2 levels decrease during attacks. The diagnosis of hereditary angioedema can be confirmed by measuring C1 esterase level and function. Unfortunately, purified C1 esterase for use during acute attacks or prophylaxis is not available in the United States.

Immunologic Deficiency Disorders

Normal Development of the Immune System

The immune system, which protects against infections, can be divided into innate and adaptive components. The innate immune system starts with mechanical barriers such as skin and also includes cells that cannot generate antigen-specific receptors such as neutrophils, eosino-phils, and monocytes/macrophages. The innate immune system also includes the complement system and other soluble molecules that recognize pathogens. The innate immune system encodes a variety of receptors that recog-

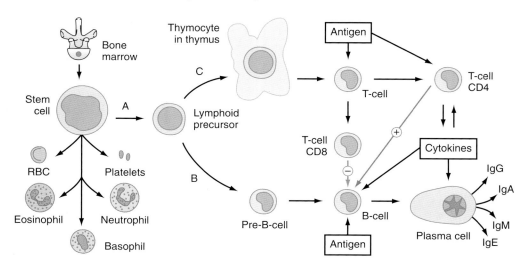

Figure 4-45. Immune development. Schematic representation of T- and B-lymphocyte ontogeny. Defects along pathway A result in combined immunodeficiencies. Pathway B is responsible for normal antibody production, whereas normal cell-mediated immunity requires the integrity of pathway C. Cytokines are soluble products of activated lymphocytes and include interleukins and interferons.

nize pathogen-associated molecular patterns (PAMPs), which are expressed by pathogens.

In contrast, the adaptive immune system is capable of generating a near infinite variety of receptors that can recognize nearly any antigen. The adaptive immune response is composed of B cells, which produce antibodies, and T cells, which, through the T cell receptors, recognize antigens presented by the major histocompatibility complex (MHC) on an antigen-presenting cell. The distinction between the adaptive and innate immune systems is arbitrary, in that there is extensive bidirectional interaction such as the ability of antibodies produced by the adaptive immune system to activate components of the innate immune system, including complement and natural killer cells. Immune deficiencies have been divided broadly into defects in the antibody, cellular, phagocytic, and complement systems, although many cellular defects also have defects in antibody responses and are therefore called *combined deficiencies.*

Adaptive immunity depends on the maturation of two distinct lymphoid cell lines, T lymphocytes and B lymphocytes, both originating from a common bone marrow stem cell. T lymphocytes and B lymphocytes undergo a complex series of maturational changes before arriving at a stage in which they are capable of antigen-stimulated differentiation (Fig. 4-45). The thymus-dependent T lymphocytes are responsible for cell-mediated immune responses directed against viruses, fungi, or less common pathogens, such as *Pneumocystis jiroveci.* Other functions of T lymphocytes include graft rejection and tumor cytotoxicity. Subpopulations of T lymphocytes also collaborate in immunoregulation by the expression of helper and suppressor functional activities. On the other hand, the thymus-independent B lymphocytes are precursors of plasma cells. Plasma cells produce the various classes of immunoglobulins that serve as functional antibodies for antigen recognition. Deficiencies of one or more of the immunoglobulin classes (IgG, IgA, IgM) constitute humoral or serum antibody immunodeficiency. The ability to generate antibodies against specific antigens, as well as total antibody levels, is important for fully effective humoral immunity. Many of the immunodeficiency disorders described in later sections result from an arrest in cell maturation or a defect in the cell interactions necessary for antigen recognition. Abnormalities in the maturation of T lymphocytes result in cellular immunodeficiency, and abnormalities of B lymphocytes result in humoral immunodeficiency.

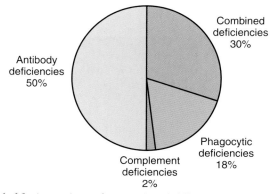

Figure 4-46. Approximate frequencies of different categories of immunodeficiency. (From Stiehm ER: Immunologic Disorders in Infants and Children, 5th ed. Philadelphia, Elsevier Saunders, 2004.)

Presentation of Primary Immunodeficiency

Deficiencies of the immune system can involve lymphocytes (humoral and/or cellular immunodeficiencies), phagocytes (chronic granulomatous disease), the complement system (C3 deficiency), and mucosal barriers (immotile cilia syndrome). Approximate frequencies of the different categories of immunodeficiencies are shown in Figure 4-46. Humoral (antibody) deficiency disorders are characterized by recurrent infections with extracellular encapsulated bacterial pathogens and chronic sinopulmonary infections. In contrast, cellular deficiencies are manifested by recurrent infections with low-grade or opportunistic infectious agents such as fungi, viruses, or *P. jiroveci* and are associated with growth retardation, wasting, and diarrhea. These patients are susceptible to graft-versus-host disease if given nonirradiated blood transfusions and can have severe infection from live virus vaccination. Some immunodeficiencies are associated with an increased risk of malignancy.

Other immune deficiencies, such as mucosal barrier defects, may present in a more subtle fashion, with few life-threatening infections and normal growth. Thus the clinician is frequently confronted with the question of whether a patient should be evaluated for immunodeficiency. A set of warning signals has been widely disseminated (Fig. 4-47). In general, children with infections that are frequent, are recurrent or chronic, and are caused by unusual organisms or respond poorly to therapy should be evaluated for immunodeficiency. Moreover, growth retardation or a family history of early death from infection should raise the clinician's level of suspicion. In the screening for immunodeficiency, quantitative and functional aspects of the components of the immune system are considered (Table 4-16). Laboratory evaluation for immunodeficiency should be guided by the history and physical examination.

Humoral (B-Lymphocyte) Immunodeficiency

Congenital Agammaglobulinemia. Congenital agammaglobulinemia is usually X-linked (Bruton) but can rarely be autosomal recessive. Affected infants are clinically well for the first few months of life because of placentally acquired maternal antibodies but subsequently develop recurrent or chronic infections with virulent bacterial pathogens such as gram-positive cocci and *H. influenzae.* The infections may localize in the upper and lower respiratory tracts, resulting in sinusitis, otitis media, and pneumonia. Sepsis, meningitis, and skin infections are also common. Over time, recurrent lung infections can lead to bronchiectasis. This is characterized clinically by chronic cough with increased sputum production and by abnormal chest radiographs (Fig. 4-48). Treatment consists of gammaglobulin replacement and appropriate antibiotics. In the absence of chronic lung disease, growth is usually unimpaired, and survival to adulthood is common.

The physical findings are those of localized infection, with specific signs depending on the particular structures infected. In addition, these children frequently lack adenoidal, tonsillar, and other lymphoid tissues (Fig. 4-49). The diagnosis of agammaglobulinemia should be considered in any child who has recurrent infections with virulent bacterial pathogens and is confirmed by finding markedly decreased levels of the immunoglobulin classes (IgG, IgA, IgM) in the serum.

Transient Hypogammaglobulinemia of Infancy. As shown in Figure 4-50, term infants are born with high levels of serum IgG because of active placental transport of maternal IgG. The serum IgG level normally declines during the first 7 months of life while the infant progressively attains the ability to actively synthesize IgG. The diagnosis of transient hypogammaglobulinemia is applied to infants and children in whom the low serum IgG concentration observed during the first 7 months of life is prolonged. Serum IgG levels in these infants usually attain age-appropriate values by school age. Despite the low levels of serum IgG, these infants can synthesize specific antibodies to tetanus and other antigens. Gammaglobulin replacement therapy is generally not indicated for this condition, but some may benefit from prophylactic antibiotics.

10 WARNING SIGNS OF PRIMARY IMMUNODEFICIENCY

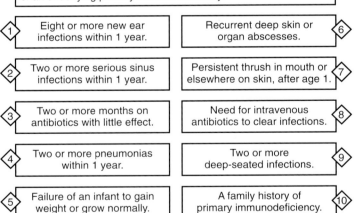

Primary immunodeficiency (PI) causes children and young adults to have infections that come back frequently or are unusually hard to cure. In America alone, up to 1/2 million people suffer from one of the 140 known primary immunodeficiency diseases. If you or someone you know is affected by two or more of the following warning signs, speak to a physician about the possible presence of an underlying primary immunodeficiency.

1. Eight or more new ear infections within 1 year.
2. Two or more serious sinus infections within 1 year.
3. Two or more months on antibiotics with little effect.
4. Two or more pneumonias within 1 year.
5. Failure of an infant to gain weight or grow normally.
6. Recurrent deep skin or organ abscesses.
7. Persistent thrush in mouth or elsewhere on skin, after age 1.
8. Need for intravenous antibiotics to clear infections.
9. Two or more deep-seated infections.
10. A family history of primary immunodeficiency.

Figure 4-47. Ten warning signs of primary immunodeficiency disease. (From the Jeffrey Modell Foundation.)

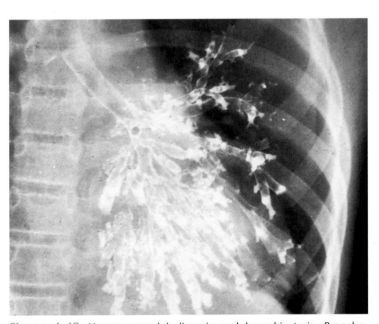

Figure 4-48. Hypogammaglobulinemia and bronchiectasis. Bronchogram reveals bronchiectasis of the left lower lobe in an older child with hypogammaglobulinemia. Symptoms consisted of chronic cough and sputum production.

Table 4-16	Suggested Laboratory Screening Tests for Children with Suspected Immunodeficiency

IMMUNE SYSTEM COMPONENT	EXAMPLE OF IMMUNODEFICIENCY	SCREENING TESTS
B lymphocyte	X-linked agammaglobulinemia	Quantitative immunoglobulin serum levels (IgG, IgA, IgM) Serum antibodies to tetanus, diphtheria, *Pneumococcus*
T lymphocyte	22q11 (DiGeorge) syndrome	T-cell lymphocyte subsets Lymphocyte mitogen stimulation test
Phagocyte	Chronic granulomatous disease	Total neutrophil count Dihydrorodamine assay
Complement	C3 deficiency	CH_{50} (hemolytic complement)

IgG Subclass Deficiency and Selective IgA Deficiency. Serum IgG can be subdivided into four subclasses, each using a different constant region gene. Patients have been identified with low or absent levels of specific IgG subclasses and frequent infections, but whether isolated subclass deficiency represents a true immune deficiency, particularly in the absence of impaired specific antibody responses, is controversial. Many immunologists prefer to assess functional antibody response to immunization rather than to examine IgG subclasses.

Selective IgA deficiency, which affects about 1 in 600 members of the general population, is the most common humoral antibody deficiency. Patients must have a complete absence of IgA. The diagnosis cannot be made until 4 years of age due to the slow development of IgA production in normal children. Even though these patients are deficient in both serum and mucosal secretory IgA, only a minority of affected individuals manifest symptoms of frequent sinopulmonary infections. Synthesis of IgG and IgM is generally normal. Individuals with IgA deficiency have a slightly increased incidence of autoimmune syndromes, atopy, celiac disease, and inflammatory bowel disease.

Common Variable Immunodeficiency (CVID). CVID can occur at any age and requires decreased levels of IgG, as well as IgM and/or IgA. In addition, specific antibody responses are variably depressed. Although defined by decreased antibody responses, many patients with CVID also have evidence of decreased T cell function. Therefore in addition to the expected ear, sinus, and lung infections, patients may have infections with unusual pathogens, as well as autoimmune and granulomatous complications. Several different genetic defects underlying CVID have been identified, but the cause of most cases and the reason for delayed onset, often in midlife, remains unknown.

T-Cell and Combined (B- and T-Lymphocyte) Immunodeficiency

Isolated defects of T-lymphocyte, or cell-mediated, immunity are unusual. Because normal T-lymphocyte function is necessary for regulation of antibody production, many cellular immunodeficiencies are also associated with humoral immunodeficiency. Patients with T-lymphocyte deficiencies experience an increased frequency of severe infections with viral agents such as herpes simplex and cytomegalovirus, certain fungi, intracellular parasites, and other organisms of relatively low virulence. Figure 4-51 demonstrates a severe disseminated varicella infection in a child with congenital cellular immunodeficiency.

22q11 (DiGeorge or Velocardiofacial) Syndrome. 22q11 syndrome is a T-cell immunodeficiency characterized by low to absent T-cell numbers with normal or near-

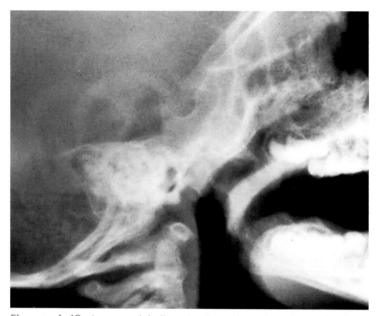

Figure 4-49. Agammaglobulinemia. Lateral neck radiograph shows absent adenoids.

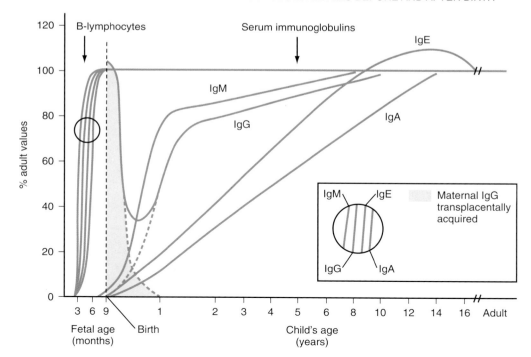

Figure 4-50. Immune development. Serum immunoglobulin levels before and after birth.

normal B-cell numbers and function. Because DiGeorge and velocardiofacial syndrome were applied to specific syndromes that are now recognized to have the same underlying genetic defect, the broad term *22q11 syndrome* is preferred. Thymic hypoplasia, which results from abnormal development of the third and fourth branchial pouches during embryogenesis, is the proximate cause of immunodeficiency in 22q11 syndrome. The thymus provides the necessary microenvironment for the maturation of lymphoid precursors into functioning T lymphocytes. When the thymus is absent, this normal maturation does not proceed, resulting in cellular immunodeficiency. Because major cardiovascular structures and the parathyroid glands are derived from the same branchial pouches, affected children frequently present with signs of congenital heart disease and hypocalcemic tetany or seizures within the first few days of life. Associated abnormalities include unusual facies (Fig. 4-52), esophageal atresia, and hypothyroidism along with a multitude of other reported defects. 22q11 deletion may occur as frequently as 1 in 3000 to 4000 live births, and rare cases with similar phenotype but without 22q11 deletion have been described. It is now recognized that the phenotypic features seen in patients with 22q11 syndrome are much more variable

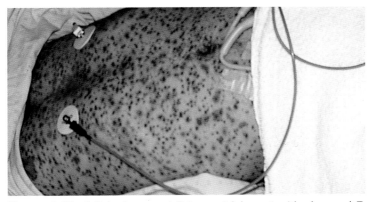

Figure 4-51. Cellular immunodeficiency. Adolescent with abnormal T-lymphocyte function and disseminated varicella, in whom pneumonia resulted in respiratory failure.

and extensive than previously appreciated and include immune, endocrine, cognitive, neurologic, and psychiatric disorders.

Most patients with 22q11 syndrome have some thymic tissue and therefore have present, but reduced, T lymphocyte numbers and avoid infections with low-virulence pathogens. Such patients can often have the sinopulmonary infections typical of antibody deficiency. A minority (<0.5%) of patients with 22q11 syndrome have an absent thymus and present without functional T cells. They act like infants with severe combined immunodeficiency (SCID) and will die of infection unless they receive bone marrow or thymus transplants.

Chronic Mucocutaneous Candidiasis (CMC). CMC is a T-lymphocyte disorder typified by superficial candidal infections of the mucous membranes, skin, and nails. It can be associated with polyendocrinopathy, a disorder linked to deficiency in the AIRE (autoimmune regulator) gene. CMC may be sporadic or familial. Treatment of chronic mucocutaneous candidiasis involves long-term antifungal therapy. Fluconazole given orally has resulted in dramatic clinical improvement and decreased morbidity in affected patients. HIV infection is prominent in the differential of severe or recurrent candidal infections.

Severe Combined Immunodeficiency Disorders (SCID). SCID is a heterogeneous group of disorders with varying etiologies (Table 4-17). The consequent defects in stem cell maturation ultimately result in abnormalities of humoral and cellular immunity (see Fig. 4-45).

Having deficiencies of cell-mediated (T-lymphocyte) and humoral (B-lymphocyte) immunity, these infants have recurrent severe bacterial, viral, fungal, and protozoal infections. Manifestations typically appear in the first few months of life and are often associated with failure to thrive, diarrhea, and candidiasis (Fig. 4-53). Affected infants may be distinguished from normal babies by the frequency and severity of infections and their resistance to appropriate antimicrobial therapy. Presenting symptoms usually involve the respiratory tract, with pneumonia resulting from *P. jiroveci* or virulent bacterial pathogens being common. In addition to the clinical findings of infection, examination discloses hypoplastic or absent tonsils and lymph nodes. Laboratory abnormalities include

Figure 4-52. 22q11 Syndrome. Characteristic facial features, frontal **(A)** and lateral **(B)** views. Note the micrognathia; hypertelorism; low-set, malformed ears; and smooth philtrum. Also note the midline scar from repair of cardiac defect.

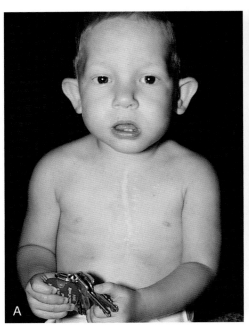

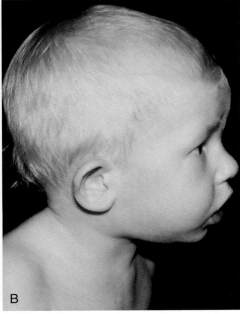

Table 4-17   Classification of Selected Primary Immunodeficiency Diseases

CATEGORY	DESIGNATION	T-CELL LEVELS	B-CELL LEVELS	IMMUNOGLOBULIN LEVELS	GENE DEFECT AND PATHOGENESIS	GENETIC LOCUS
Combined lymphocyte defects	X-linked severe combined immunodeficiency	Low	Normal to high	Low	Defect of γ chain of interleukin-2 (IL-2) receptor and receptors for other cytokines, IL-4, IL-7, IL-9, IL-15	IL2RG (SCIDX1), Xq13.1
	Jak 3 deficiency	Low	Normal to high	Low	Jak 3 intracellular signaling kinase defect	Jak 3, 19p13.1
	Adenosine deaminase deficiency	Progressive decrease	Progressive decrease	Low	Selective lymphocyte toxic effects of purine pathway intermediates	ADA, 20q13.11
	Purine nucleoside phosphorylase deficiency	Progressive decrease	Normal	Normal or low	Lymphocyte toxic effects of purine pathway intermediates	PNP, 14q13
	Major histocompatibility complex class II deficiency	Low CD4	Normal	Normal or low	Mutation in factors controlling major histocompatibility complex II gene expression	CIITA, 16p13, RFX5, 1q
	ZAP-70 kinase deficiency	Low CD8	Normal	Normal	Thymocyte intracellular kinase defect; blocked maturation of T cells	ZAP-70, 2q12
	Recombinase activating gene deficiency	Low	Absent	Absent	No T-cell or B-cell receptor rearrangement; blocked lymphocyte development	RAG1, RAG2, 11p13
	Reticular dysgenesis	Low	Low	Low	Unknown bone marrow stem cell defect	Autosomal recessive
	Omenn syndrome	Low	Low	Low	Unknown	Autosomal recessive
	X-linked hyper-IgM syndrome	Normal	Normal	Normal to high IgM; low IgA, IgG	Defect of CD40 ligand, expressed on T cells: block in B-cell isotype switch	HIGMX, Xq25-q26
	DiGeorge syndrome	Normal to low	Normal	Normal to low	Embryologic defect of thymic development: variable associated defects of heart, parathyroid, face	22q11.2 and other loci
Antibody deficiencies	X-linked agammaglobulinemia	Normal	Very low to absent	Low to absent	Defect of B-cell–specific Bruton tyrosine kinase	XLA, Xq22
	μ Heavy chain deficiency	Normal	Absent	Absent	Defect of cell surface μ chain expression	IGHμ, 14q32.3
	Immunoglobulin deficiency including IgA deficiency and IgG subclass deficiency	Normal	Normal	One or more immunoglobulin types low	Unknown defects in B-cell isotype expression; IgG subclass deficiencies associated with immunoglobulin heavy- or light-chain gene deletions	Complex
	Common variable immunodeficiency	Normal	Normal or low	One or more subtypes low	Unknown late-onset variable defects in B- and T-cell function and regulation	Complex
Other distinctive syndromes	Wiskott-Aldrich syndrome	Normal to low	Normal	Normal (some low IgM)	Defect of WASP gene involved in cytoskeleton; sparse, small platelets; eczema	WASP, Xp11.23
	Ataxia telangiectasia	Normal	Normal	Normal	DNA repair defect in ATM gene; ataxia, progressive neurodegeneration; cancer; radiation sensitivity	ATM, 11q22-q23
	Bloom syndrome	Normal	Normal	Normal	DNA repair defect in BLM gene, progressive neurodegeneration, cancer, radiation sensitivity	BLM, 15q26.1
	Hyper-IgE syndrome (Job syndrome)	Normal	Normal	High IgE	Unknown, susceptibility to cutaneous boils and lung abscess formation	Unknown
	X-linked lymphoproliferative syndrome	Normal	Normal	Normal	Fatal infection or immune compromise on Epstein-Barr virus encounter	XLP, Xq24-q26
	Autoimmune lymphoproliferative syndrome	Normal to high: elevated CD4-/CD8-T cells	High	High	Impaired Fas-mediated apoptosis of B and T cells; lymphadenopathy, autoimmunity	FAS, 10q24; complex
Phagocyte disorders	Chronic granulomatous disease	Normal	Normal	Normal	Impaired killing of ingested organisms due to defects in 4 genes encoding enzymes of cytochrome oxidase system	CYBB, ($gp91^{phox}$), Xp21.1; CYBA ($p22^{phox}$), 16q24.1; NCF1 ($p47^{phox}$), 7q11.23; NCF2 ($p67^{phox}$), 1q25
	Leukocyte adhesion deficiency	Normal	Normal	Normal	Defects of CD18 or other leukocyte surface proteins required for motility, adherence, and endocytosis	CD18, 21q22.3
	Chédiak-Higashi syndrome	Normal	Normal	Normal	Defect of CHM gene causing faulty lysosomal assembly, giant cytoplasmic granules	CHS, 1q42-q44
Complement disorders	Individual component deficiencies	Normal	Normal	Normal	C1, C2, C4, C3 deficiencies associated with autoimmunity and pyogenic infections: C3, C5-9, and properdin deficiencies with neisserial infections	AR: chromosomes 6p, 1q, etc; X: properdin

From Puck JM: Primary immunodeficiency diseases. JAMA 278:1835-1841, 1997. Copyright 1997, American Medical Association.

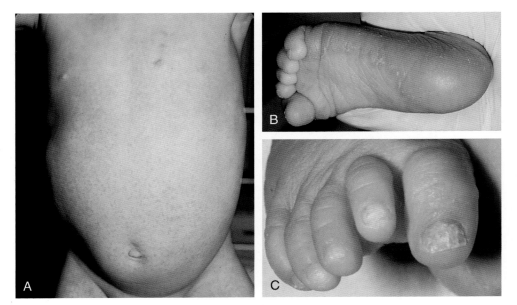

Figure 4-53. Severe combined immunodeficiency. Widespread fungal dermatitis with *Candida albicans* over the trunk **(A)** and foot **(B)** and nails **(C)**.

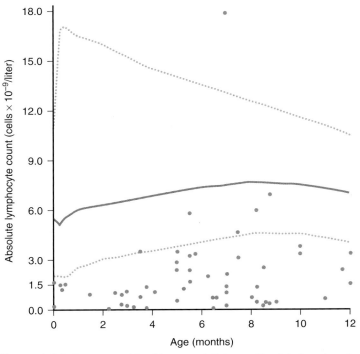

Figure 4-54. Severe combined immunodeficiency. Absolute lymphocyte counts in normal infants and infants with severe combined immunodeficiency disease *(closed circles)*. The heavy line indicates the mean lymphocyte counts in normal infants in relation to age. The light dotted lines indicate the 95% confidence limits. (From Gossage DL, Buckley RH: Prevalence of lymphopenia in severe combined immunodeficiency. N Engl J Med 322:1422-1423, 1990. Copyright © 1990 Massachusetts Medical Society. All rights reserved.)

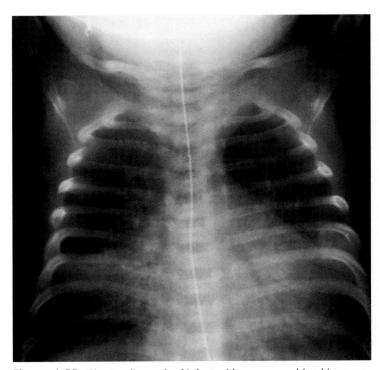

Figure 4-55. Chest radiograph of infant with severe combined immunodeficiency disease. Note the absent thymic shadow and bilateral pulmonary infiltrates.

peripheral blood lymphopenia (Fig. 4-54); decreased serum IgG, IgA, and IgM levels; and defective lymphocyte responses to mitogens such as phytohemagglutinin. Histological examination of tonsillar, adenoidal, and lymph node remnants reveals immature lymphoid tissue. The thymus is typically dysplastic histologically and radiographically (Fig. 4-55); normal lobulation and corticomedullary differentiation are lacking, and the number of lymphocytes is decreased.

Once the diagnosis of SCID is considered, the child must be placed in protective isolation and given appropriate supportive therapy including intravenous gammaglobulin. All administered blood products must be irradiated to prevent the potential development of severe graft-versus-host disease, and live virus vaccines are contraindicated. These patients can be successfully immunologically reconstituted with bone marrow transplants. Children with SCID have been the initial recipients of gene therapy, which is curative but has led to an unexpectedly high incidence of leukemia.

A variety of genetic defects have been identified in patients with SCID, most of which result in a developmental block in T cell maturation. Most common is the X-linked γ common chain that is a component of several cytokine receptors. Lack of IL-7 signaling prevents maturation of functional T cells. Inherited deficiency of the enzyme adenosine deaminase (ADA) is also associated with SCID. The mechanism involves the accumulation of metabolic substrates that are toxic to T and B lympho-

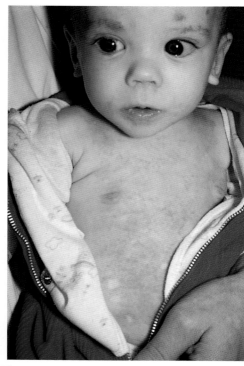

Figure 4-56. Wiskott-Aldrich syndrome. The skin eruptions on the trunk and face are eczematoid and pruritic but not always similar to atopic dermatitis in flexural distribution. (From Fireman P, Slavin RG: Atlas of Allergies. New York, Gower, 1990.)

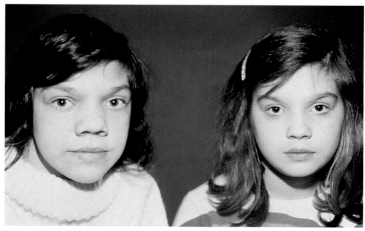

Figure 4-57. Hyper-IgE syndrome. Note coarse facial features in the girl on the left including the broad nasal bridge, fleshy nasal tip, and mild prognathism compared with her unaffected sister.

cytes. ADA deficiency can also lead to other symptoms including skeletal changes, hearing loss, and behavioral issues due to systemic toxicity of adenosine metabolites. Other defects leading to SCID include Jak3, which is responsible for signaling via the γ common chain, and components of the T cell receptor–associated signaling apparatus.

Partial Combined Immunodeficiency Disorders

Wiskott-Aldrich Syndrome (WAS). WAS is an X-linked recessive disorder characterized by eczema, thrombocytopenia and small platelets with cutaneous petechiae, and recurrent infections that begin in infancy (Fig. 4-56). Inability to form antibody to bacterial capsular polysaccharide antigens is the most commonly reported immunologic defect, but some patients also manifest a partial defect in T-lymphocyte responses, which seems to worsen with age. The most common cause of death is intracranial hemorrhage secondary to thrombocytopenia. As boys with Wiskott-Aldrich age, they have an increased risk of malignancy, particularly lymphoma. Bone marrow transplant is curative but has a high mortality rate in the absence of an HLA-matched sibling donor. The defective protein in WAS is termed WASP (Wiskott-Aldrich Syndrome Protein) and serves to link T cell signaling at the cell surface to rearrangements of the cytoskeleton.

Ataxia-Telangiectasia (AT). AT is a complex and intriguing immunodeficiency disorder with autosomal recessive inheritance and an unusually pleiotropic presentation: telangiectasia, progressive ataxia, and variable immunodeficiency. Most patients develop ocular telangiectasia and ataxia during the first 6 years of life (see Chapter 15). The ataxia is cerebellar in nature and characteristically progressive. Neurologic involvement may be extensive including abnormalities of speech, movement,

and gait and mental retardation. The progressive, variable immunodeficiency commonly consists of humoral defects and depressed T-lymphocyte function. Recurrent sinus and pulmonary infections, which may lead to bronchiectasis, are common and may be responsible for early death. These patients have a dramatically higher incidence of neoplasia, consistent with the gene underlying AT, which limits cell division in the presence of DNA damage. Radiation, particularly x-rays, should be avoided as much as possible in ataxia-telangiectasia patients.

Hyper-IgM Syndrome. The hyper-IgM syndrome, although defined on the basis of abnormalities of immunoglobulin production, is actually a combined immune deficiency. The hyper-IgM syndrome is due to an inability of the B cell to class switch from the germ-line encoded IgM heavy chain constant region to other isotypes (e.g., IgA, IgM, IgE). Patients have normal to elevated IgM levels but reduced or absent levels of IgA and IgG. Specific antibody responses are also deficient. The most common form of hyper-IgM syndrome is deficiency of CD154 (CD40 ligand), which is expressed by T lymphocytes and required for B cell class switching. In addition to sinopulmonary infections, *Pneumocystis* pneumonia and *Cryptosporidium* diarrhea are often seen, demonstrating that defects in both humoral and cellular immunity are present. Although CD154 deficiency is X-linked, defects in other, autosomal genes required for class switching can lead to a similar phenotype.

Hyper-IgE Syndrome. The hyper-IgE syndrome is a disorder with both autosomal dominant and autosomal recessive inheritance and is characterized by marked elevation of serum IgE. Clinical features include recurrent staphylococcal infections, a pruritic eczematous dermatitis, and coarse facial features (Fig. 4-57). Recurrent staphylococcal skin infections including impetigo and furuncles are especially common and typically resistant to therapy. Staphylococcal pneumonia complicated by pneumatocele formation (Fig. 4-58) and lung abscesses are frequent. Other organisms of relatively low virulence including *Candida albicans* may cause infection. Immunologic findings include markedly elevated IgE levels (often >2000 IU/μL); eosinophilia; abnormal cell-mediated immunity; and, in certain patients, abnormal polymorphonuclear leukocyte chemotaxis. The autosomal dominant, but not the autosomal recessive, form is also associated with frequent fractures of long bones and delayed eruption of secondary teeth. It should be stressed that many patients with typical

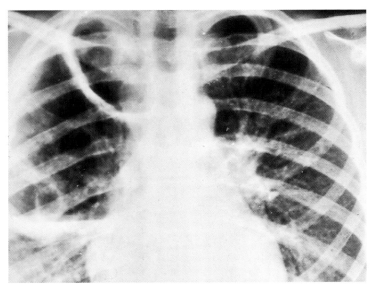

Figure 4-58. Hyper-IgE syndrome. Note clearly outlined pneumatocele in the right lung. This encapsulated lesion frequently complicates *Staphylococcus aureus* pneumonia.

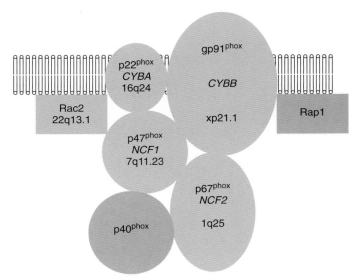

Figure 4-59. Chronic granulomatous disease. The neutrophil NADPH oxidase complex is shown. Components in which mutations have been detected in patients with chronic granulomatous disease are shown in tan. X-linked deficiency of gp91^{phox} is the most common cause of CGD, accounting for about two thirds of cases. (From Bonilla FA, Geha RS: Primary immunodeficiency diseases. J Allergy Clin Immunol 111:S571-581, 2004.)

atopic dermatitis have elevated IgE levels, often markedly so, but do not have the hyper-IgE syndrome.

Phagocytic Disorders

Polymorphonuclear leukocytes and mononuclear cells play vital roles in the defense against acute infections. Normal neutrophil numbers, intact neutrophil chemotaxis, phagocytosis, and killing are necessary for the rapid elimination of microorganisms that invade the skin or mucous membranes. Patients with neutropenia are vulnerable to bacterial infections, as are patients with disorders of phagocyte function. The neutropenias and Chédiak-Higashi syndrome are discussed in Chapter 11.

Chronic granulomatous disease (CGD) is the most common immune deficiency of neutrophil dysfunction. Neutrophil chemotaxis and phagocytosis are intact, but killing of ingested microorganisms is defective. The responsible biochemical defect results in abnormal leukocyte oxidative metabolism and inability to kill microorganisms. Intracellular survival of ingested bacteria, even those not typically associated with granuloma formation, can lead to development of granulomatous lesions. A test of neutrophil oxidative burst is used to diagnose CGD. Historically, a nitroblue tetrazolium (NBT) test has been used for diagnosis, but the NBT has been supplanted by a flow-cytometric assay using reduction of the dye 1,2,3, dihydrorodamine (DHR).

The cytooxidase complex has four subunits (Fig. 4-59). The most common defect is X-linked, but defects in the other subunits are due to an autosomal recessive pattern of inheritance. The X-linked form is generally more severe. Clinically, most children with chronic granulomatous disease become symptomatic early in life with infections with catalase-positive bacteria and fungi. The skin, lungs, liver, and lymph nodes are the most common sites of infections, and five organisms account for the majority of infections: *Staphylococcus aureus, Burkholderia cepacia, Serratia marcescens, Aspergillus* species, and *Nocardia*. Pneumonitis may progress to produce pneumatoceles (see Fig. 4-58), and liver abscesses and invasive *Aspergillus* in the absence of known immunosuppression strongly suggest

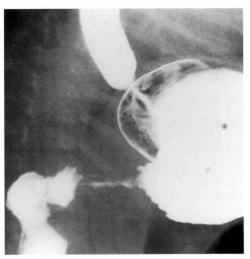

Figure 4-60. Chronic granulomatous disease (CGD). Barium contrast radiogram demonstrating the "string sign," a thin line of barium that represents narrowing of the gastric antrum secondary to granuloma formation. This child had persistent vomiting but none of the usual stigmata of CGD.

CGD. Hepatosplenomegaly is a frequent physical finding and presumably represents involvement of the reticuloendothelial system. Granulomas may also develop in other organs. In the patient whose radiograph is seen in Figure 4-60, the diagnosis of chronic granulomatous disease was suggested by the finding of antral narrowing secondary to granulomatous involvement of the gastric antrum. Effective antimicrobial prophylaxis with trimethoprim-sulfamethoxazole and itraconazole, as well as cytokine therapy with interferon γ, helps minimize infectious complications.

Leukocyte Adhesion Deficiency. Leukocyte adhesion deficiency (LAD) most commonly results from a deficiency in CD18, a component of β₂ integrins, which is required for neutrophils to exit blood vessels and enter tissue. The patients have a variety of symptoms including delayed umbilical cord separation (Fig. 4-61A), persistent peripheral blood granulocytosis (due to lack of vascular margin-

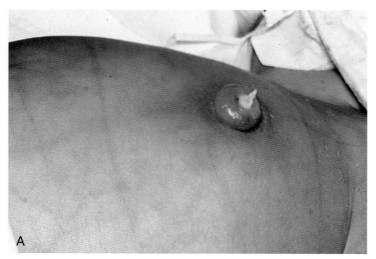

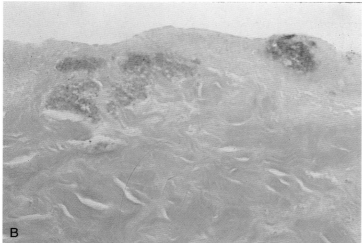

Figure 4-61. Leukocyte adhesion deficiency. **A,** Infection involving and surrounding the umbilical cord. **B,** Histopathologic appearance of a scalp abscess. Note the presence of bacterial colonies (purple staining) and distinct lack of host cellular inflammatory response. (**A,** Courtesy Kenneth Schuit, MD, Pittsburgh, Pa; **B,** courtesy Kenneth Schuit, MD, and William Robichaux, MD, Pittsburgh, Pa.)

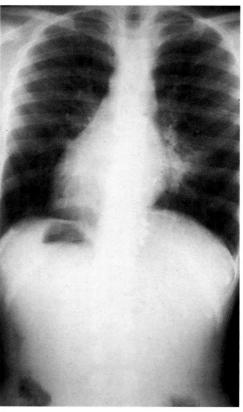

Figure 4-62. Kartagener syndrome. Dextrocardia and situs inversus of abdominal organs. Abnormal ciliary motion is thought to result in malrotation during embryogenesis.

ation), recurrent soft tissue infections, and impaired wound healing. The vast majority of infants with delayed cord separation, however, will not have LAD. Because these patients do not mobilize neutrophils in response to infection, many aspects of the normal inflammatory response are lacking including the formation of pus (Fig. 4-61B). This may confound the diagnosis when infection is suspected. LAD deficiency should be suspected in any infant with periumbilical problems and persistent peripheral blood leukocytosis (frequently >50,000 cells/mm³). Other rare causes of LAD have also been described.

Complement System Disorders

The complement system is a complex system of nine distinct serum proteins, designated C1 through C9, that require serial activation through the classical or alternative complement pathways. Complement mediates and amplifies many of the biologic functions of the immune system. These functions include (1) enhancement of phagocytosis (opsonization) and viral neutralization, (2) mediation of inflammation via chemotaxis and alteration of vascular permeability, (3) cell lysis, and (4) modulation of the immune response. Defects of the complement system result from either absent or nonfunctional components of the complement cascade. Although rare, inherited deficiencies of most complement components have been reported. Clinical presentation varies, depending on the specific complement protein involved. Frequent modes of presentation for complement component deficiencies are collagen vascular diseases for defects in components C1 through C4, disseminated infections with pyogenic bacteria for C3, and disseminated neisserial infections for C5 through C8. The CH50 is a simple screening test for complement deficiency. A normal result effectively rules out complement dysfunction. Defect of C1 esterase results in hereditary angioedema, which is discussed earlier.

Mucosal Barrier Disorders

Intact mucosal barriers are of crucial importance in preventing the entrance of ubiquitous microorganisms into the host. The respiratory and GI mucosa aid in host defense by secreting antibodies (predominantly IgA) into their lumina. Also, physical factors such as saliva flow in the oral cavity, intestinal peristalsis, and the coughing reflex are important in the "washing out" effect on potential pathogens.

Immotile cilia syndrome is characterized by a defect in mucociliary transport, another component of the mucosal barrier. This disorder was first described as Kartagener syndrome, which consists of a triad of situs inversus (Fig. 4-62), chronic sinusitis, and bronchiectasis. These patients were also noted to be infertile because their spermatozoa were poorly motile as a result of lack of dynein arms in their tails. Studies revealed similar defects in mucosal cilia and led to recognition of the fact that the phenomenon

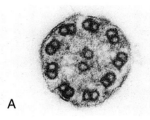 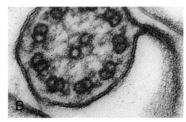

Figure 4-63. Immotile cilia syndrome. **A,** Electron micrograph of cilia from a patient with immotile cilia syndrome. Note the absence of dynein arms from the outer doublets. **B,** Normal cilia with dynein arms. (From Bluestone C, Stool S: Pediatric Otolaryngology, vol 1. Philadelphia, WB Saunders, 1983.)

could exist in the absence of situs inversus. The resultant ciliary dysfunction impedes mucus clearance and produces a combination of the following signs and symptoms: (1) early onset of chronic rhinorrhea, (2) chronic otitis media, (3) chronic sinusitis with opaque sinuses on radiography, (4) chronic productive cough, (5) bronchiectasis, (6) digital clubbing, and (7) nasal polyps. The disorder should be suspected in any child with chronic or recurrent upper or lower respiratory tract infections. When situs inversus is not present, the diagnosis of immotile cilia syndrome requires confirmation by electron microscopic analysis of cilia obtained from a biopsy of the nasal or tracheobronchial mucosa (Fig. 4-63).

Bibliography

Adkinson NF, Yuninger JW, Busse WW, et al: Middleton's Allergy: Principles and Practice, 6th ed. St Louis, Mosby, 2003.

American Academy of Allergy, Asthma and Immunology: The Allergy Report: Diseases of the Atopic Diathesis, vol 2. Milwaukee, Wisc, American Academy of Allergy, Asthma and Immunology, 2000.

Bonilla FA, Bernstein IL, Kahn DA, et al: Practice parameter for the diagnosis and management of primary immunodeficiency. Ann Allergy Asthma Immunol 94:S1-S63, 2005.

Bonilla FA, Geha RS: Primary immunodeficiency diseases. J Allergy Clin Immunol 111:S571-S581, 2004

Borish L: Allergic rhinitis: Systemic inflammation and implication for treatment. J Allergy Clin Immunol 112:1021-1031, 2003.

Castro-Rodriquez JA, Holberg CJ, Wright AL, Martinez FD: A clinical index to define risk of asthma in young children with recurrent wheezing. Am J Respir Crit Care Med 162:1403-1406, 2000.

Global Initiative for Asthma: Global strategy for asthma management and prevention. Web publication, 2005. Available at http://www.ginasthma.com

Gruchella RS: Drug allergy. J Allergy Clin Immunol 111:S548-S559, 2003.

International Consensus Report on the Diagnosis and Management of Rhinitis: International Rhinitis Management Working Group. Allergy (Eur J Allergy Clin Immunol) 49:1-34, 1994.

Laitinen LA, Laitinen A, Haahtela T: Airway mucosal inflammation even in patients with newly diagnosed asthma. Am Rev Respir Dis 147:697-704, 1993.

Lawley TJ, Bielory L, Gascon P, et al: A prospective clinical and immunologic analysis of patients with serum sickness. N Engl J Med 311:1407-1413, 1984.

Martinez FD, Stern DA, Wright AL, et al: Differential immune responses to acute lower respiratory illness in early life and subsequent development of persistent wheezing and asthma. J Allergy Clin Immunol 102:915-209, 1998.

Martinez FD, Wright AL, Taussig LM, et al: Asthma and wheezing in the first six years of life. N Engl J Med 332:133-138, 1995.

Moffet JE, Golden DKB, Reisman RE, et al: Stinging insect hypersensitivity: A practice parameter update. J Allergy Clin Immunol 114:869-886, 2004.

National Institutes of Health: Guidelines for Diagnosis and Management of Asthma (NIH Publication no. 97-4051). Bethesda, Md, NIH, 1997.

National Institutes for Health: Guidelines for Diagnosis and Management of Asthma Update on Selected Topics (NIH Publication no. 02-5075). Bethesda, MD, NIH, 2002.

Ochs HD, Smith CIE, Puck JM, eds. Primary immunodeficiency diseases. New York, Oxford University Press, 1999.

Primer on allergic and immunologic diseases. J Allergy Clin Immunol 111:S441-S778, 2003.

Puck JM: Primary Immunodeficiency diseases. JAMA 278:1835-1841, 1997.

Rachelefsy GS, Shapiro GG, Bergman D, et al: Pediatric asthma: Promoting best practice. Milwaukee, Wisc, American Academy of Allergy, Asthma and Immunology, 1999.

Rosenzweig SD, Holland SM: Phagocyte immunodeficiencies and their infections. J Allergy Clin Immunol 113:620-626, 2004.

Stiehm ER, Ochs HD, Winklestein JA, eds: Immunologic Disorders in Infants and Children, 5th ed. Philadelphia, Elsevier Saunders, 2004.

CHAPTER 5

Cardiology

LEE B. BEERMAN, JACQUELINE KREUTZER,
AND SANG C. PARK

This chapter addresses the initial approach to a patient with suspected or known heart disease with the physical examination, chest x-ray, and electrocardiogram. A proper initial assessment helps to avoid the expense of unnecessary testing. However, the practice of cardiology as a pediatric subspecialty continues to rapidly evolve with expansion and enhancement of imaging technology and therapeutic options. Complex structural congenital anomalies can be precisely defined by a combination of techniques that include echocardiography, cardiac catheterization with angiography, nuclear MRI, and CT angiography. Concomitant with advances in diagnostic capabilities have come remarkable advances in therapy, both surgical and by interventional catheterization. Therefore we have included considerable material on echocardiography and color flow Doppler studies, which remain the preeminent imaging modalities in pediatric cardiology. In addition, we have described the common surgical procedures used and added a section on the expanding array of therapeutic options in the cardiac catheterization laboratory.

The three prerequisites to a good cardiovascular examination are a proper environment, a cooperative child, and the conviction on the part of the physician that the examination is important. A heart murmur is not the only part and often is not even the most important part of the cardiac physical examination. Blood pressure determination, character of the pulse and precordial activity, observation of cyanosis, clubbing of the nail beds of the fingers or toes, and dysmorphic facial or other physical features may provide clues to the diagnosis and nature of congenital heart lesions before auscultation is even performed.

Physical Diagnosis of Congenital Heart Disease

Cyanosis and Clubbing

Even before mild desaturation is detectable, early clubbing and cyanosis may be seen (Figs. 5-1 and 5-2). The base of the nail, especially the thumbnail, may show loss of the angle as early as 3 months of age (see Chapter 16). Elevated hemoglobin and hematocrit and loss of nail angle indicate hypoxemia and the presence of a right-to-left intracardiac shunt (Fig. 5-3).

Observation of the lips and mucous membranes for the presence of cyanosis is best done in good daylight because fluorescent lighting may produce a false cyanotic tinge. In the presence of polycythemia with hemoglobin in the 18% to 20% gm range and hematocrit over 60%, the conjunctival vessels become engorged and plethoric (see Fig. 5-2). Differential cyanosis between the upper and lower extremities is an unusual clinical finding. If the patient has pulmonary vascular disease, reverse flow through a patent ductus arteriosus, and no right-to-left intracardiac shunting, cyanosis and clubbing may be found in the lower extremities but not in the hands (Fig. 5-4).

Blood Pressure and Pulse

Blood pressure determination in infants and children is an integral part of the cardiac physical examination. Attention to proper cuff size prevents the misdiagnosis of systolic hypertension from an undersized cuff. In general, it is better to use an oversized cuff because overestimation in systolic blood pressure can be avoided. Blood pressure can be tracked in children over time, and tables depicting normal blood pressure range for age have been published. Blood pressure determination in both arms and a lower extremity will detect coarctation of the aorta, lend support for the diagnosis of supravalvular aortic stenosis (blood pressure higher in the right arm than in the left arm—Coanda effect), and help to assess the severity of aortic valve disease including aortic valve stenosis (narrow pulse pressure) and aortic regurgitation (wide pulse pressure).

Heart Murmur Evaluation

In the newborn a common innocent heart murmur originates from the branch pulmonary arteries because of their relatively small size compared with the main pulmonary artery resulting from the normal fetal flow pattern, which delivers limited flow to the right and left pulmonary arteries. Characteristically, this murmur is early systolic and loudest over both axillae and the back. The murmur of branch pulmonary artery stenosis has the same distribution as the structural lesions that cause increased pulmonary blood flow. A transient systolic murmur at the middle-low left sternal border in the newborn can be due to tricuspid regurgitation, and a soft systolic ejection murmur at the upper left sternal border may arise from a closing patent ductus arteriosus. A large ventricular septal defect does not produce a murmur in the newborn period because the initially high pulmonary vascular resistance results in minimal shunting across the defect. On the other hand, pathologic systolic murmurs in the newborn are caused by restrictive ventricular septal defects and lesions producing left and right ventricular outflow tract obstruction (i.e., tetralogy of Fallot and valvular aortic or pulmonary stenosis). In the newborn it can be difficult to distinguish the murmur of a small restrictive ventricular septal defect from that of a severe right ventricular outflow tract obstruction in tetralogy of Fallot or left ventricular outflow obstruction. The implications of this differential diagnosis are such that an echocardiogram is recommended for infants with this clinical presentation.

Contrary to popular belief, the presence of a continuous murmur from a patent ductus arteriosus is extremely rare in a full-term newborn. This is because the normal elevation of pulmonary artery pressure at this age minimizes the diastolic gradient between the aorta and pulmonary artery, attenuating or eliminating any diastolic component of the murmur. If a continuous murmur is heard in the newborn, patent ductus–dependent pulmonary blood flow or systemic to pulmonary collateral vessels in association with pulmonary atresia complex should be considered.

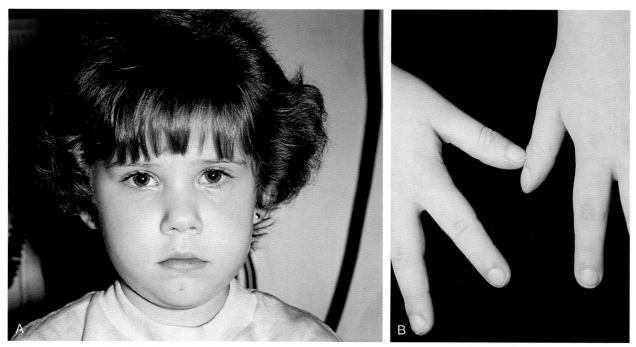

Figure 5-1. Mild cyanosis. **A,** This child shows no obvious cyanosis of the face and lips, although the photograph in **B** demonstrates clubbing; note the loss of nail angle and curvature of nails, especially of the thumb.

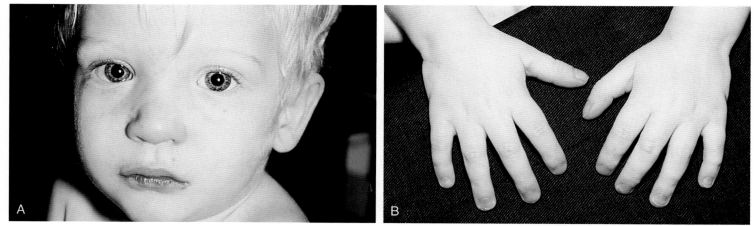

Figure 5-2. Moderate cyanosis. This child demonstrates moderate cyanosis of the lips **(A)** and nails **(B).** Note also the reddish discoloration of the eyes resulting from conjunctival suffusion.

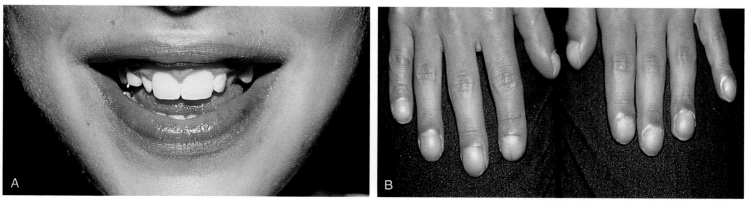

Figure 5-3. Severe cyanosis. Severe cyanosis of the lips, tongue, and mucous membranes can be noted in **A,** associated with marked clubbing and cyanosis of the nails in **B.**

Preschoolers and school-age children are commonly referred for evaluation of a heart murmur. Innocent murmurs of childhood fall into four major categories: systolic ejection murmurs at the base; vibratory, or Still's, murmur; venous hums; and carotid and cranial bruits. In most instances there are associated clinical and laboratory studies that can distinguish the innocent from the pathologic murmur. Table 5-1 summarizes the distinguishing features and differential diagnosis. Figure 5-5 illustrates the sites where murmurs resulting from various cardiovascular lesions are best heard.

Syndrome-Associated Physical Findings

Dysmorphology of the face and habitus suggests certain syndromes associated with congenital heart disease (Table 5-2).

The typical features in *Down syndrome (trisomy 21)* are demonstrated in Chapter 1. About 40% of children with this syndrome have structural lesions such as atrioventricular septal defects, isolated ventricular septal defects,

patent ductus arteriosus, or anomalous origin of the subclavian arteries.

Although many infants with Down syndrome have chronic congestive heart failure and growth failure, there is a subset that grows and develops appropriately. Pulmonary vascular resistance does not decrease in the usual fashion in this group, and these children develop early

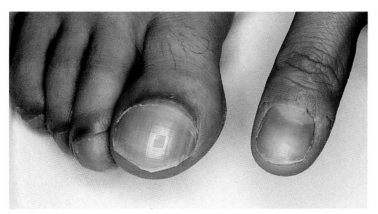

Figure 5-4. Differential cyanosis and clubbing resulting from reverse shunting through a patent ductus arteriosus in a patient with pulmonary vascular disease. Note marked cyanosis and clubbing of the toes, although the finger appears to be normal. (Courtesy J. R. Zuberbuhler, MD, Pittsburgh.)

Table 5-1	Innocent Murmurs Mimicking Congenital Heart Disease
INNOCENT HEART MURMUR	**STRUCTURAL CONGENITAL HEART DISEASE**
Systolic Ejection Murmur at the Base of the Heart	

High left sternal border	Pulmonary valve stenosis
	    Ejection click
	    Transmission to back
	Atrial septal defect
	    *Parasternal lift
	    *S2 wide split
	    *Diastolic murmur of tricuspid
	      flow

High right sternal border	Aortic valve stenosis
	    *Ejection click
	    *Radiation to neck

Still's Murmur	
Vibratory quality	Ventricular septal defect
Location: left midsternal	*Character of murmur

border	Discrete subaortic stenosis
	    *Radiation to aortic area
	Subpulmonic stenosis
	    *Radiation to pulmonic area
	    *Soft P2

Venous Hum	
Continuous	Patent ductus arteriosus
Location: neck and under	*Location under left clavicle
clavicles	*No change with position
Usually loudest when sitting,	Coronary AV malformation
disappears in supine posture	*Accentuated in diastole
Carotid and Cranial Bruits	
Murmur over carotids	Aortic stenosis

and head	AV malformation
	    *Continuous murmur would
	      support AV malformation

*Distinguishing features.
AV, atrioventricular.

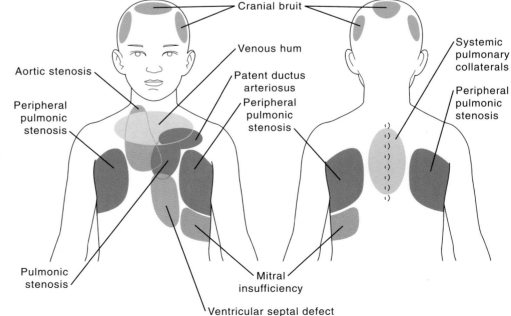

Figure 5-5. Sites where murmurs resulting from various cardiovascular lesions are best heard.

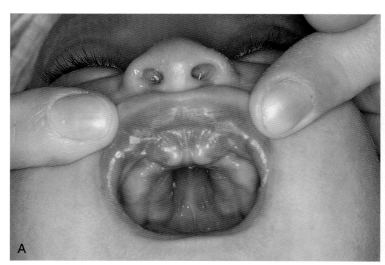
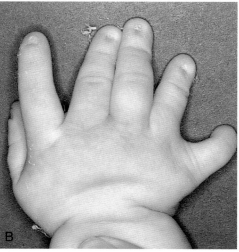

Figure 5-6. Ellis-van Creveld syndrome. Note the gingival frenula and natal teeth **(A)** and multiple digits (polydactyly) **(B)**.

Table 5-2	Syndromes and Trisomies with Associated Cardiovascular Abnormalities

SYNDROME	COMMON CARDIAC DEFECT
DiGeorge/velocardiofacial (22q11 deletion)	Aortic arch abnormalities: interrupted arch (type B), right aortic arch Conotruncal abnormalities: truncus arteriosus, tetralogy of Fallot, pulmonary atresia with ventricular septal defect
Ellis-van Creveld	Atrial septal defect or single atrium
Fetal alcohol	Ventricular septal defect
Holt-Oram	Atrial and ventricular septal defects, arrhythmias
Marfan	Dilation of ascending aorta/aortic sinus, aortic and mitral insufficiency
Noonan	Dysplastic pulmonic valve, atrial septal defect
Turner	Coarctation of the aorta, bicuspid aortic valve
Williams	Supravalvular aortic stenosis, pulmonary artery stenosis
Trisomy	
13	Patent ductus arteriosus, septal defects, pulmonic and aortic stenosis (atresia)
18	Ventricular septal defect, polyvalvular disease, coronary abnormalities
21 (Down)	Atrioventricular septal defects, ventricular septal defect, patent ductus arteriosus, anomalous subclavian artery

pulmonary vascular disease. Because this presentation may be silent, it is important that all children with Down syndrome be thoroughly evaluated during early infancy. The evaluation should include an echocardiogram to rule out congenital heart disease.

DiGeorge and velocardiofacial syndromes are related developmental disorders involving the third and fourth pharyngeal pouches. They have been shown to be caused by deletions within a critical region of chromosome 22q11. Cardiac abnormalities, particularly the conotruncal type and aortic arch anomalies, occur in 75% of patients (see Table 5-2). Other findings include hypocalcemia, cleft palate, renal anomalies, immunologic defects, facial dysmorphisms, and variable developmental delay (see Chapter 4).

Ellis-van Creveld syndrome is an autosomal recessive disorder characterized by multiple gingival frenula, natal teeth, and polydactyly (Fig. 5-6). The patient with this syndrome frequently has an atrial septal defect or a common atrium.

Holt-Oram syndrome, an autosomal dominant disorder, is associated with upper limb deformities consisting of narrow shoulders, hypoplasia of the radius, and phocomelia (Fig. 5-7). Absence of both radius and thumb or proximal displacement of the thumb is the most frequent finding. Commonly associated cardiovascular abnormalities include an atrial septal defect, ventricular septal defect, and arrhythmias (atrial and ventricular ectopy and atrioventricular block).

Marfan syndrome also has an autosomal dominant inheritance; it manifests as a connective tissue disorder in which the elastic fibers are disrupted, causing cystic medial necrosis of the aorta, as well as joint laxity and subluxation of the ocular lens. Affected patients are tall, with increased limb length compared with the trunk. Their arm span exceeds their height. The cardiovascular abnormalities nearly always found in this syndrome include aneurysmal dilation of the aorta and aortic sinuses and mitral valve prolapse. Associated aortic and mitral valve regurgitation are common (Fig. 5-8) (see Chapter 1).

Patients with *Noonan syndrome* have features characteristic of Turner syndrome but possess a defect on chromosome 12 and may be male or female. Clinically, these children have the findings of webbing of the neck, pectus excavatum, shield chest with widely spaced nipples, short stature, epicanthal folds, low-set ears, and increased carrying angle of the arms (Fig. 5-9). Common cardiovascular defects include pulmonary stenosis in association with a dysplastic pulmonary valve, atrial septal defect, and hypertrophic cardiomyopathy. Occasionally, there may be dysplasia of all cardiac valves. The syndrome appears as an autosomal dominant disorder; multiple members of a family are often affected.

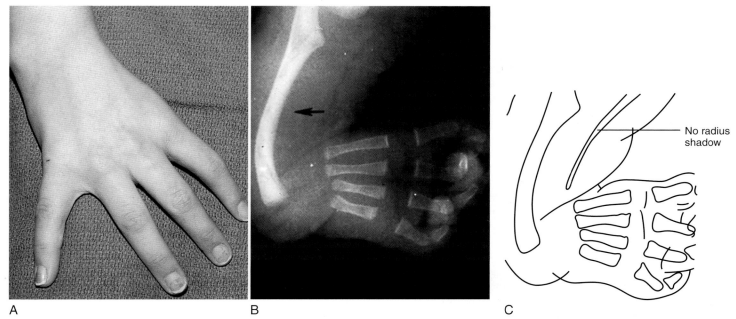

A   B   C

No radius shadow

Figure 5-7. Holt-Oram syndrome. Note the absence of the radius and thumb **(A)**. The associated cardiovascular abnormality is an atrial septal defect. Radiographic examination (**B** and **C**) demonstrates the absence of a radius shadow; the missing thumb is apparent.

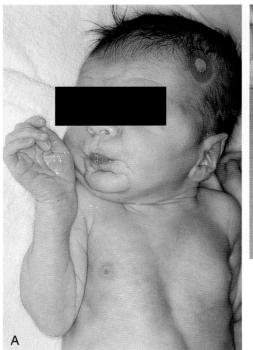

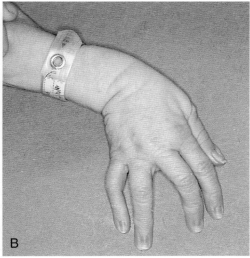

A

B

Figure 5-8. Infant with Marfan syndrome. **A,** Note the narrow elongated face, pectus excavatum, laxity, and long arms and fingers. **B,** A close-up view of the infant's hand.

The most common cardiac defects in *Turner syndrome* are coarctation of the aorta and a bicuspid aortic valve. (See Chapters 1 and 9 for a detailed discussion of Turner syndrome.)

Patients with *Williams syndrome* characteristically have "elfin" facies: a broad maxilla, a small mandible with full mouth and large upper lip (philtrum), upturned nose, and a full forehead (Fig. 5-10). This syndrome has been associated with hypercalcemia in infants and has an identifiable genetic abnormality. Supravalvular aortic stenosis and pulmonary artery branch stenosis are the common cardiovascular abnormalities associated with this syndrome.

In addition, there are many other genetically determined diseases and inborn errors of metabolism with cardiac involvement, the most common of which are listed in Table 5-3.

Visible Clues in Acute Rheumatic Fever

Examination of the skin in a patient with acute rheumatic fever may reveal the typical rash of erythema marginatum, although this rash is not specific for rheumatic fever. It is evanescent, nonpruritic, has sharp serpiginous margins, and is found on the inner aspects of the upper arms and thighs and on the trunk (Fig. 5-11). The differential diagnosis includes (1) drug rash, which is papular and pruritic; (2) erythema multiforme, which has target lesions; (3) rash of juvenile rheumatoid arthritis, which is pink, macular, and lacks wavy margins, and which may be transient; and (4) the cutaneous findings of Kawasaki syndrome (see Chapter 7).

Subcutaneous nodules are rare in chronic rheumatic heart disease, but if found, they are almost always associated with severe carditis. These movable, nontender, cartilage-like swellings vary in size from 2 mm to 1 cm and are never transient. They are seen over the bony prominences of the large joints and external surfaces of the elbows and knuckles of the hands, knees, and ankles. They may also be felt along the spine and over the skull.

Although difficult to photograph, they are easily palpated (Fig. 5-12).

Signs of Bacterial Endocarditis

Although the clinical presentation of bacterial endocarditis varies according to the infecting organism, it should be suspected in any patient with congenital or acquired heart disease who has prolonged fever without apparent cause. The classic skin lesions include petechiae, splinter hemorrhages of the nails, conjunctival hemorrhages, and Janeway lesions (Fig. 5-13), all of which are manifestations of vasculitis. Vegetations occasionally dislodge and embolize in an end artery, which results in hemorrhagic or gangrenous lesions (Fig. 5-14). Osler nodes, which present as small tender erythematous nodules, are found in the intradermal pads of the fingers and toes or in the thenar or hypothenar eminences (Fig. 5-15). All the aforementioned findings are often associated with a new heart

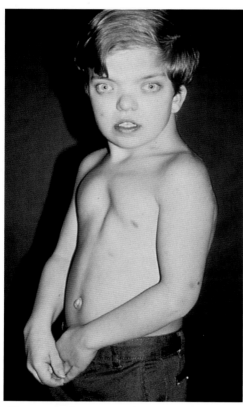

Figure 5-9. Noonan syndrome. Note the widely spaced eyes, low-set ears, webbing of the neck, shield chest, pectus, and increased carrying angle of the arms.

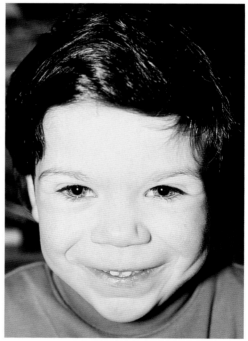

Figure 5-10. Williams syndrome. Note the wide-set eyes, upturned nose, large maxilla, prominent philtrum, and pointed chin. (Courtesy R. A. Mathews, MD, Philadelphia.)

Table 5-3	Genetic Syndromes and Inborn Errors of Metabolism with Associated Cardiovascular Findings

GENETICALLY DETERMINED DISEASES	**CARDIAC FINDINGS**
Metabolic	
Pompe disease (glycogen storage)	Cardiomyopathy (storage of glycogen in myocardium)
MPS	Storage of MPS in arteries, coronaries, and valves with insufficiency and stenosis
	Hurler (MPS I H), Hunter (MPS II), Scheie (I S, I H/S), Morquio (MPS IV)
Hyperlipoproteinemia, familial type II	Premature atherosclerosis of arteries including coronaries
Neurologic	
Friedreich ataxia	Cardiomyopathy (congestive or hypertrophic)
Muscular dystrophies	Myocardial degeneration and fibrosis

INBORN ERROR OF METABOLISM (NO PROVEN GENETIC BASIS)	**CARDIAC FINDINGS**
Progeria	Hypercholesterolemia, atherosclerotic changes in arteries including coronaries

MPS, mucopolysaccharidosis.

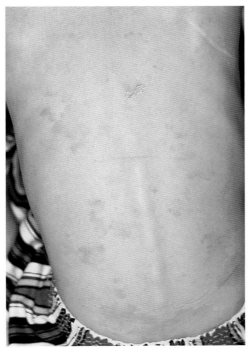

Figure 5-11. Erythema marginatum rash in a child with acute rheumatic fever. Note the wavy margins in the distribution on the trunk.

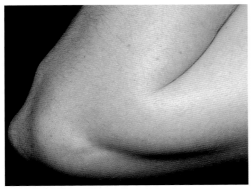

Figure 5-12. Subcutaneous nodules. Note their presence over the bony prominences of the elbow in a patient with chronic rheumatic heart disease.

murmur, splenomegaly, spiking fever, and positive blood culture. Clubbing of the fingers may occur in chronic cases.

Laboratory Aids in the Diagnosis of Congenital Heart Disease

In addition to a comprehensive physical examination, the chest roentgenogram, electrocardiogram, and, most notably, echocardiography provide invaluable information concerning specific congenital heart lesions and have allowed therapeutic decisions to be made without cardiac catheterization.

Chest Roentgenography

The chest x-ray examination is useful to screen patients with suspected congenital heart disease. It is particularly useful in differentiating cardiac from pulmonary pathol-

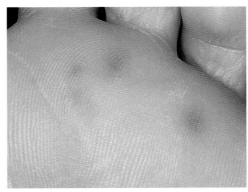

Figure 5-13. Janeway lesions. Note the small (painless) nodules on the sole of a patient with bacterial endocarditis.

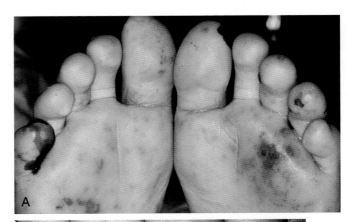

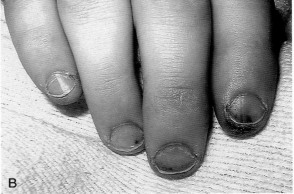

Figure 5-14. Acute bacterial endocarditis. Note the hemorrhagic lesions **(A)** and subungual splinter hemorrhages **(B).**

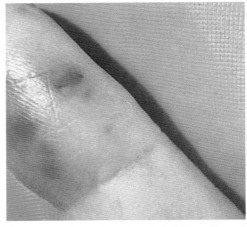

Figure 5-15. Osler nodes. Note the (painful) erythematous nodular lesions resulting from infective endocarditis. (Courtesy J. F. John, Jr., MD.)

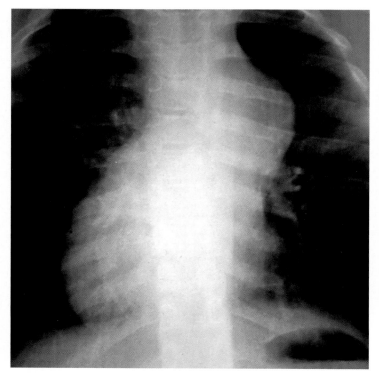

Figure 5-16. Dextrocardia (heart in the right side of the chest) associated with situs solitus. Note the prominent vascular shadow along the left-sided cardiac border that is caused by the aorta. This pattern is commonly associated with ventricular inversion (corrected transposition of the great arteries).

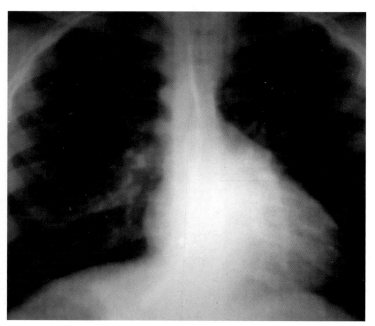

Figure 5-17. Levocardia with situs inversus. Note the prominence of the shadow at the high right-sided cardiac border. Discordance of the apex of the heart and visceral situs is often associated with structural congenital heart defects. The hepatic portion of the inferior vena cava is absent in this patient, and there is azygos vein continuation. Note air in the stomach under the right hemidiaphragm.

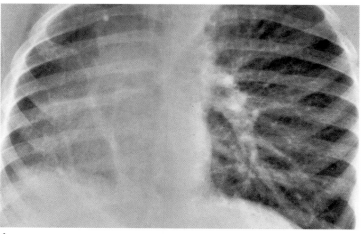

A

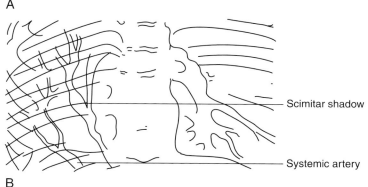

B

Figure 5-18. Scimitar syndrome. **A,** Note the hypoplastic right lung and scimitar-shaped shadow formed by pulmonary veins draining the sequestered segment and connecting to the inferior vena cava. **B,** Note also the systemic artery coursing diagonally upward from the abdominal aorta to the sequestered lobe.

ogy such as pneumonia, pneumothorax, pneumomediastinum, or other parenchymal lung disease that may mimic congenital heart disease. The review of any chest roentgenogram requires a systematic approach.

Cardiac Apex and Visceral Situs

The location of the cardiac apex and visceral situs provides important diagnostic clues. Discordance of the situs and cardiac apex (i.e., apex to the right with situs solitus or apex to the left with situs inversus) is often associated with structural congenital heart disease (Figs. 5-16 and 5-17). Dextrocardia (apex to the right) or mesocardia (apex to the middle) with situs solitus is a frequent presentation of ventricular inversion or corrected transposition of the great arteries (see Fig. 5-16). Dextrocardia can also be seen with primary pulmonary problems. Scimitar syndrome is composed of dextrocardia with hypoplasia of the right lung (Fig. 5-18). In this case a major portion of the right lung (usually the right lower lobe) has its arterial supply by way of a systemic artery from the descending aorta, and the pulmonary venous return from that lung drains abnormally into the inferior vena cava via a vein forming a scimitar (see Fig. 5-18). Patients with levocardia (apex to the left) with either situs inversus or situs ambiguus frequently have complex congenital heart diseases such as transposition of the great arteries, pulmonary atresia, and atrioventricular septal defects. Atrial isomerism is associated with bilateral morphologic right or left lungs and can be recognized as bilateral symmetrical short or long bronchi. This is best demonstrated with a magnified penetrated chest x-ray examination focusing on bronchial anatomy (Fig. 5-19). Almost all patients with this anomaly have complex congenital heart disease.

Shape and Size

Cardiac size is important, but the shape of the cardiac image may provide a clue as to which heart chambers are

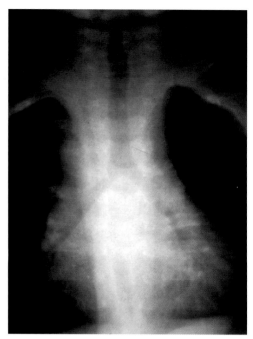

Figure 5-19. Atrial isomerism. Note the symmetric bronchial anatomy. Atrial isomerism should be suspected when the heart is midline on the chest radiograph and situs ambiguous is present. The best radiographic sign of right or left atrial isomerism pertains to the symmetry of bronchial anatomy, with right atrial isomerism being related to bilateral right bronchi and left atrial isomerism to bilateral left bronchi.

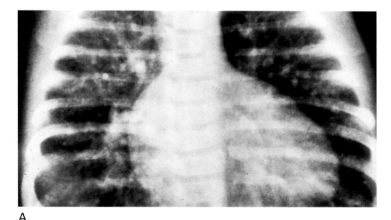

A

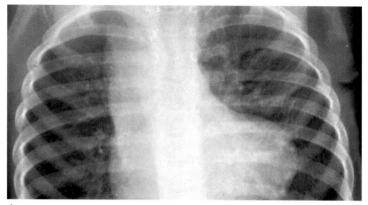

A

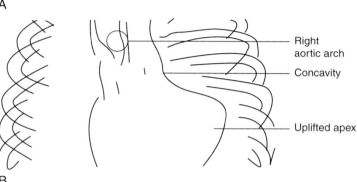

B

Figure 5-21. Tetralogy of Fallot with pulmonic stenosis produces a "boot-shaped" heart, which results from right ventricular hypertrophy, upward tilt of the apex, and the concavity at the left upper heart border caused by a small right ventricular infundibulum and main pulmonary artery. Note also the right aortic arch.

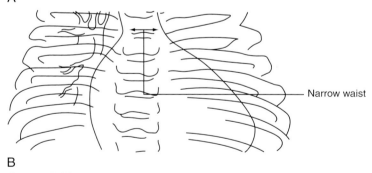

B

Figure 5-20. Transposition of the great arteries. Note the "egg on a string" heart shadow, which results from the position of the main pulmonary artery posterior and slightly to the left of the aorta, contributing to the narrow waist (the "string").

enlarged and the likely structural diagnosis. In the cyanotic newborn with transposition of the great arteries, the cardiac image appears as an "egg on a string" (Fig. 5-20). If the thymic shadow does not obscure it, the mediastinal shadow shows a narrow waist resulting from the postero-medial position of the main pulmonary artery. This

produces the "string." Pulmonary vascular markings are usually increased, although vascularity may be normal in the immediate newborn period.

In tetralogy of Fallot with pulmonic stenosis, the heart appears "boot-shaped" because right ventricular hypertrophy causes the apex (toe of the boot) to turn upward (Fig. 5-21). The concavity of the left upper cardiac border is due to the small right ventricular outflow tract and main pulmonary artery segment.

In tetralogy of Fallot with pulmonary atresia, the heart is shaped like an "egg on its side" (Fig. 5-22). The pulmonary blood flow to the lungs may be supplied by either a patent ductus arteriosus or systemic arterial collateral vessels. The pulmonary vascular markings are decreased if pulmonary blood flow is patent ductus dependent and increased if large systemic collaterals supply pulmonary blood flow.

In corrected transposition of the great arteries, the heart has a "valentine" or "heart" shape with the apex pointing downward just to the left of the midline, as shown in Figure 5-23. The fullness at the left upper border of the cardiac shadow is due to the ascending aorta arising from the left-sided morphologic right ventricle.

Massive cardiac enlargement is typical in patients with Ebstein's anomaly. In this anomaly there is a malformation of the tricuspid valve with downward displacement of the inferior and septal leaflets of the valve into the ventricle, causing severe tricuspid valve regurgitation or stenosis. As a result, the right atrium becomes markedly enlarged and, along with the "atrialized" portion of the right ventricle, contributes significantly to the cardiac image of a large box-shaped heart (Fig. 5-24).

Left-to-right shunt lesions from atrial septal defects, ventricular septal defects, or a patent ductus arteriosus

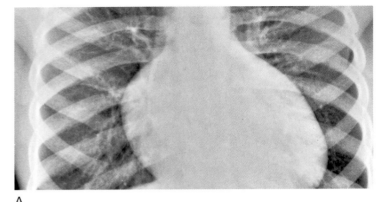

A

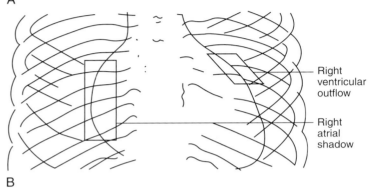

B

Figure 5-22. Tetralogy of Fallot with pulmonary atresia. Note the "egg on its side" appearance of the heart due to the uplifted apex resulting from the right ventricular hypertrophy. The absence of a right ventricular outflow and the diminutive main pulmonary artery segment produce a concavity at the left upper heart border. Note also that a right aortic arch is present.

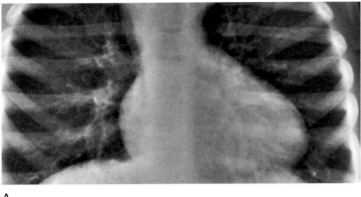

A

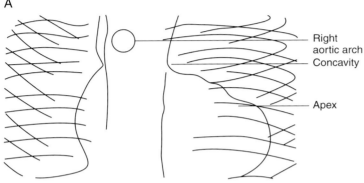

B

Figure 5-24. Ebstein's anomaly of the tricuspid valve. Note the radiograph appearance of a "box-shaped" heart, enlarged right atrium, and prominent right ventricular outflow tract.

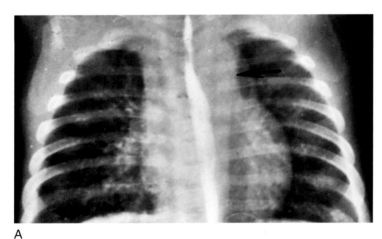

A

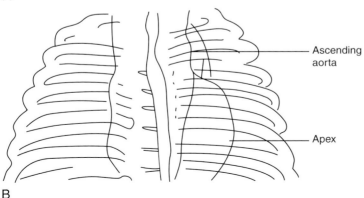

B

Figure 5-23. Corrected transposition of the great arteries. Note the characteristic "valentine-shaped" heart and the left-sided ascending aorta.

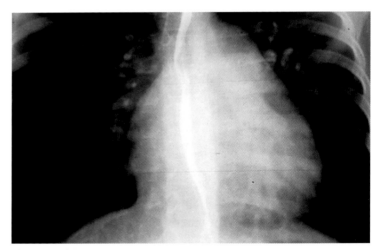

Figure 5-25. Atrial septal defect. Note the enlarged right atrium, right ventricle, and pulmonary artery, as well as the increased pulmonary vascular markings on this radiograph.

demonstrate specific chamber enlargement and increased pulmonary vascular markings. A significant atrial defect shows enlargement of all right-sided cardiac chambers including right atrium, right ventricle, and pulmonary artery (Fig. 5-25). A patent ductus arteriosus shows enlargement of all left-sided cardiac chambers including the aorta. In patients with a ventricular septal defect, the right atrium is the only heart chamber that is not enlarged.

Great Vessels

The radiographic appearance of the great arteries may also suggest a specific structural congenital heart defect. The main and left branch pulmonary arteries are usually enlarged in patients with pulmonary valve stenosis due to poststenotic dilation (Fig. 5-26). The characteristic radio-

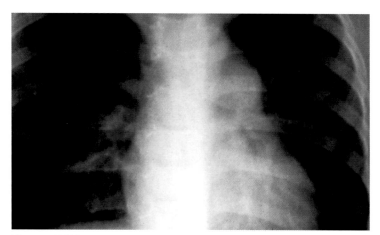

Figure 5-26. Pulmonic valve stenosis. Note the typical radiographic abnormalities of a prominent main and left pulmonary artery.

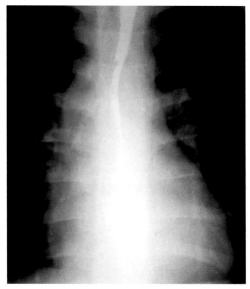

Figure 5-27. Aortic valve stenosis. Note the dilation of the ascending aorta, which is the only radiographic sign in children.

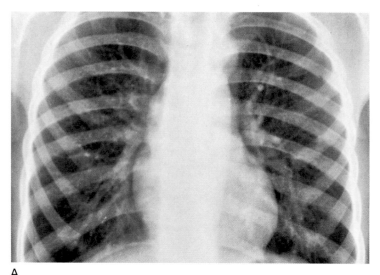

A

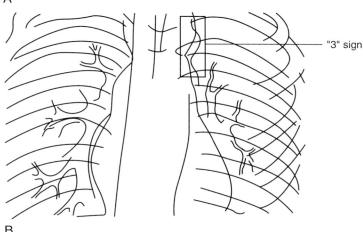

B

Figure 5-28. Coarctation of the aorta. Note that the site of the stenosis can be observed at the center of the "3" sign formed by the prestenotic and poststenotic dilation of the aorta in this characteristic radiograph in a 5-year-old child.

graphic finding of congenital aortic valve stenosis is dilation of the ascending aorta, best seen as an overlapping shadow with the superior vena cava along the right upper cardiac border (Fig. 5-27). Coarctation of the aorta not diagnosed in a timely fashion may show the distinct radiographic finding of a reversed E or 3 sign caused by prestenotic and poststenotic dilation of the descending aorta (Fig. 5-28).

The normal left aortic arch causes a shift of the tracheal air column to the right, whereas a right arch causes a similar deviation to the left (Fig. 5-29). The position of the thoracic descending aorta also helps define the side of the arch and can be determined by noting obscuring of either the left or right side of the vertebral bodies. A right aortic arch should always raise the suspicion of congenital heart disease and is found in approximately 30% of patients with tetralogy of Fallot or truncus arteriosus.

The addition of a barium swallow to the chest x-ray examination has traditionally been an important diagnostic tool in the assessment of patients with upper airway obstruction from vascular rings. If a bilateral indentation is noted on the barium esophagram, a double aortic arch should be suspected (Fig. 5-30). A right aortic arch with distal origin of the left subclavian artery or a left aortic arch with distal origin of the right subclavian artery

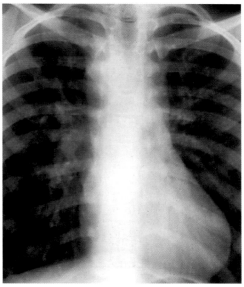

Figure 5-29. Right aortic arch in a child with truncus arteriosus. Note the deviation of the tracheal air column to the left.

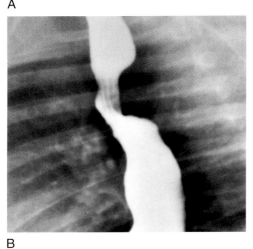

A

B

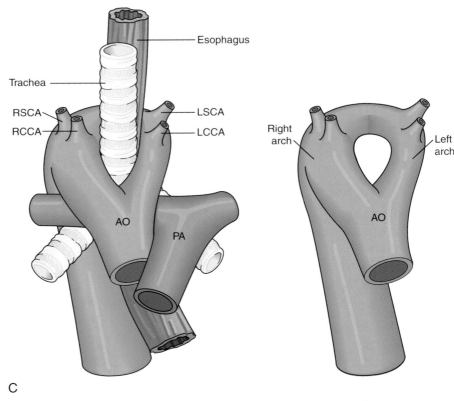

C

Figure 5-30. Barium esophagram with a double aortic arch. **A**, Note the bilateral compressions on the anterior view. **B**, Note the marked retroesophageal indentation on the lateral view. **C**, Schematic of the double aortic arch.

produces a posterior indentation on the barium esophagram, but these anomalies are not associated with airway compromise. An anterior esophageal indentation is almost always caused by distal origin of the left pulmonary artery resulting in this vessel coursing between the trachea and esophagus and causing a pulmonary artery sling (Fig. 5-31). Current practice favors the imaging techniques of MRI or CT scan, which provide clear and precise imaging of aortic arch and great vessel anatomy.

Pulmonary Vascularity

Left-to-right shunt lesions are associated with increased pulmonary blood flow that causes primarily arterial or a combination of arterial and venous markings on the chest radiograph. Hyperinflation seen on the chest x-ray film is a characteristic finding in infants with a large left-to-right shunt associated with pulmonary hypertension (Fig. 5-32). Patients with pulmonary venous obstruction, such as infradiaphragmatic total anomalous pulmonary venous return, show a fine reticular pattern of pulmonary venous obstruction, which may mimic respiratory distress syndrome in the neonate (Fig. 5-33). It should be cautioned that the interpretation of pulmonary vascularity can be quite difficult and should always be interpreted within the context of other clinical findings.

Skeletal Abnormalities

Attention should also be given to the thoracic cage including the spine and ribs. Although abnormal fusions of ribs and hemivertebrae are not pathognomonic for specific congenital heart lesions, there is a higher incidence when these findings are present. Rib notching is a distinct

radiographic finding in patients older than 5 to 10 years of age with coarctation of the aorta (Fig. 5-34). Scoliosis is a common finding in teenage patients with cyanotic congenital heart disease. Pectus excavatum may cause a false impression of cardiac enlargement because of a "pancaking" effect on the heart from a narrow anteroposterior thoracic diameter. Because of its association with chest wall and spine abnormalities, mitral valve prolapse should be considered in this context.

Electrocardiography and Arrhythmias

Electrocardiography

For pediatricians to have a thorough knowledge of detailed electrocardiogram interpretation is impractical and unnecessary; however, it is valuable to be able to recognize certain typical electrocardiographic patterns that yield important diagnostic information. For instance, most normal children have a frontal plane axis that is either normal (0 to 90 degrees) or in the mild right axis deviation range from 90 to 120 degrees. The presence of a *superior axis* (180 to 270 or 0 to −90 degrees) suggests certain specific cardiac defects. A *left axis deviation* that includes an axis in the range of 0 to −90 degrees associated with a QR pattern in leads I and AVL is frequently seen in the following situations: a cyanotic newborn with tricuspid atresia (Fig. 5-35), an atrioventricular septal defect with or without Down syndrome (Fig. 5-36), Noonan syndrome, or some varieties of a single ventricle. When the frontal plane axis falls between 180 and 270 degrees, it is usually referred to as a *northwest axis* and is frequently

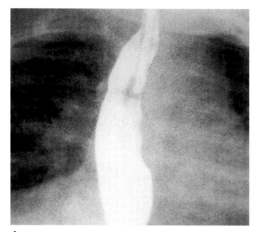

A

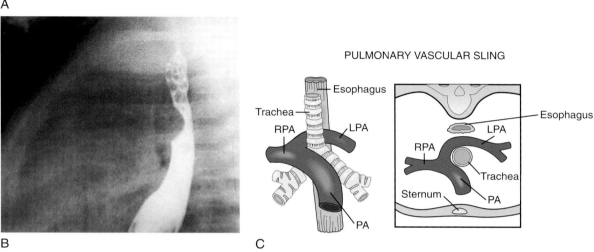

B

Figure 5-31. Anomalous left pulmonary artery (pulmonary artery sling). Note the anterior rounded indentation in the barium-filled esophagus and the posterior bulge into the air-filled trachea anteriorly.

PULMONARY VASCULAR SLING

C

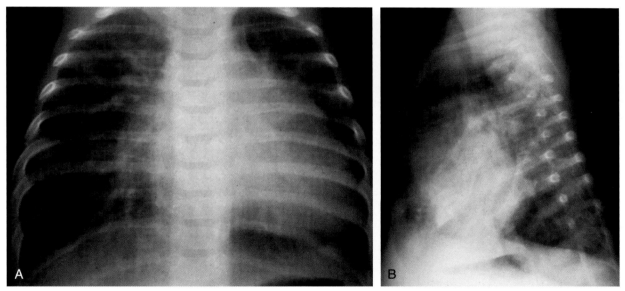

A B

Figure 5-32. Large left-to-right shunt from a ventricular septal defect. Posteroanterior **(A)** and lateral **(B)** radiographs from a 2-month-old infant. Note the increased pulmonary vascular markings and lung hyperinflation. The flattened hemidiaphragms are clearly seen on the lateral projection, a finding predictive of associated pulmonary hypertension.

found in atrioventricular septal defects or other lesions that lead to severe right ventricular hypertrophy.

Being certain about hypertrophy in the pediatric age group is difficult because of the wide range of normal values that vary with age. This is particularly true of right ventricular hypertrophy, which can be a physiologic finding in the first several years of life. On the other hand, left ventricular predominance in the newborn is almost always a pathologic finding and usually indicates one of the hypoplastic right heart syndromes, such as tricuspid atresia or pulmonary atresia with an intact septum.

Conduction abnormalities, such as Wolff-Parkinson-White syndrome, prolonged corrected Q-T interval, and atrioventricular block are readily apparent on the 12-lead electrocardiogram and are discussed further in the following section on arrhythmias.

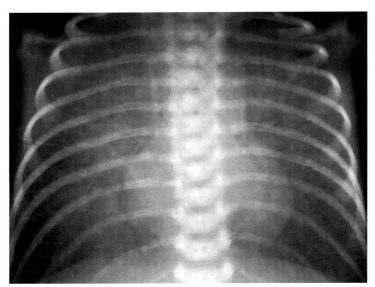

Figure 5-33. Total anomalous pulmonary venous return below the diaphragm. Note the radiographic findings of severe pulmonary venous obstruction and pulmonary edema, mimicking a respiratory distress syndrome.

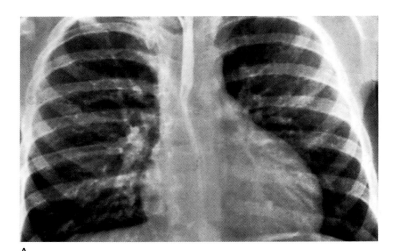

A

Notches

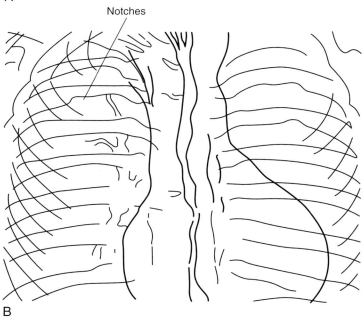

B

Figure 5-34. Coarctation of the aorta. Note the rib notching that can be observed in an older child.

Table 5-4	Pediatric Dysrhythmias
TREATMENT NOT REQUIRED	**TREATMENT REQUIRED**
Sinus arrhythmia	Supraventricular tachycardia
Wandering (ectopic) atrial pacemaker	Ventricular tachycardia
Isolated premature atrial contractions	Third-degree atrioventricular block with symptoms
Isolated premature ventricular contractions	
First-degree atrioventricular block	

Arrhythmias

Disorders of heart rate or rhythm are not nearly as common in childhood as they are in adulthood, but it is vital that pediatricians be familiar with arrhythmias that may occur in otherwise healthy children. An outline of these disorders based on the need for treatment is presented in Table 5-4. For the numerous rhythm disorders not listed, management must be individualized, taking into account the presence or absence of associated heart disease.

Transient arrhythmias may present in the following manner: an asymptomatic child with an irregular heartbeat noted on examination, palpitations, chest pain (a common complaint among children younger than 10 years of age when they sense a tachycardia), dizziness or presyncope, or actual syncope with or without seizure activity. More sustained arrhythmias may lead to congestive heart failure, cardiogenic shock, or even death. The most common irregularity of heart rhythm seen in children is a *sinus arrhythmia*. This is a normal variant that reflects a healthy interaction between autonomic respiratory and cardiac control activity in the central nervous system. Typically the heart rate increases during inspiration and decreases during expiration and may sound wildly irregular on auscultation unless careful attention is paid to the relationship between the heart rate and respirations (Fig. 5-37). Another normal variant occurs when the atrial pacemaker transiently shifts from the sinus node to another atrial site with only minimal variation in the heart rate. This is often referred to as a *wandering atrial pacemaker* (Fig. 5-38). *Premature atrial contractions* are generally benign when they occur in the absence of underlying heart disease. They are particularly common during the newborn period, when they are often associated with aberrant conduction (Fig. 5-39) or apparent pauses (Fig. 5-40) resulting from failure of the premature atrial impulse to conduct to the ventricle. *Isolated premature ventricular beats* are not common but may be seen with an incidence of 0.3% to 2.2% and rarely require treatment as long as there is no associated heart disease. This form of ectopy is recognizable by a wide QRS, a T wave opposite in direction to the QRS in any given lead, dissociation from the P wave, and usually a full compensatory pause (Fig. 5-41). For the above-mentioned abnormalities, an appropriate initial workup includes a 12-lead electrocardiogram and rhythm strip and brief exercise in the office to see if the ectopy is suppressed or becomes more frequent as the heart rate increases. An exacerbation of the arrhythmia with this maneuver would warrant further cardiologic investigation.

By far the most common arrhythmia requiring treatment in the pediatric population is *supraventricular tachycardia* (SVT). The most frequent age of presentation is in the first 3 months of life, with secondary peaks occurring at 8 to 10 years of age and again during adolescence. This rhythm disorder is characterized by a regular, narrow QRS

TRICUSPID ATRESIA

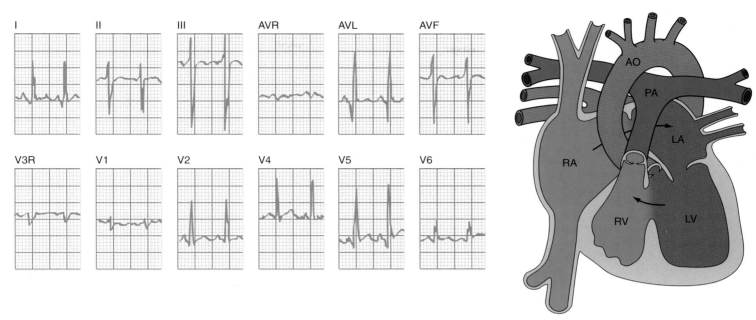

Figure 5-35. Electrocardiogram of a child with tricuspid atresia. Note the left axis deviation, left atrial enlargement, and left ventricular hypertrophy.

ATRIOVENTRICULAR SEPTAL DEFECT

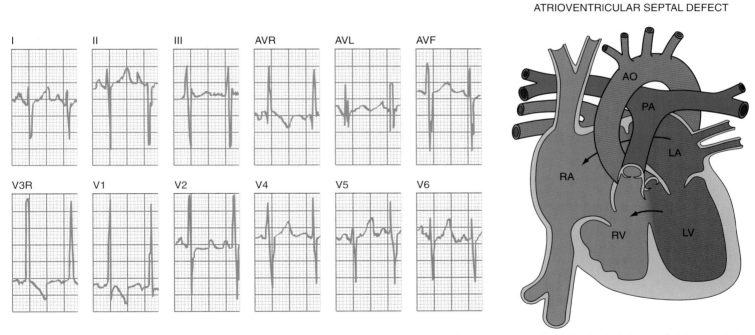

Figure 5-36. Electrocardiogram of a child with an atrioventricular septal defect. Note the superior (northwest) axis deviation and right ventricular hypertrophy.

Figure 5-37. Sinus arrhythmia. Note variable QRS cycle lengths without change in the P wave–QRS relationship.

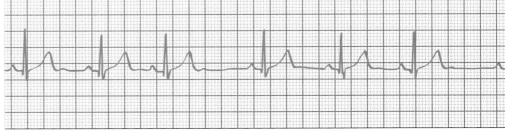

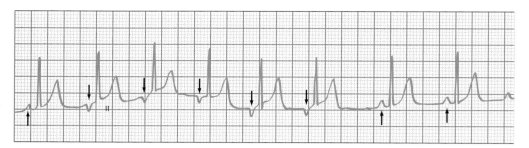

Figure 5-38. Wandering atrial pacemaker. Note the variable morphology of the P wave, indicating origin from either the sinus node *(upward arrows)* or an ectopic atrial site *(downward arrows)*.

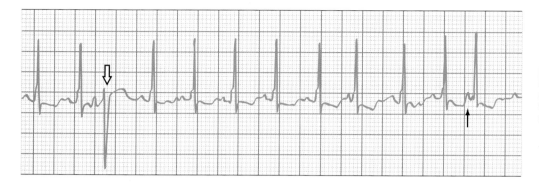

Figure 5-39. Premature atrial contractions. Note these premature complexes may be associated with aberrant conduction of the QRS *(open arrow)* or normal conduction *(solid arrow)*.

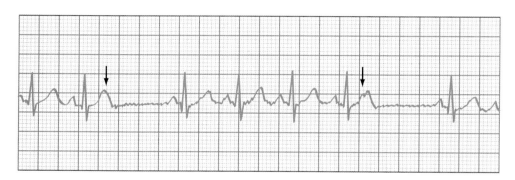

Figure 5-40. Nonconducted premature atrial contractions. Note the premature atrial beats that are not conducted *(arrows)*, resulting in apparent pauses.

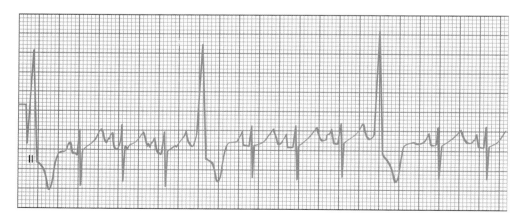

Figure 5-41. Premature ventricular contractions. Note the obvious wide QRS premature complexes with abnormal T waves, a fully compensatory pause, and absence of a preceding P wave.

complex tachycardia with rates that vary with the patient's age. The overall average rate for SVT at all ages is 235 beats/minute; however, in the first 9 months the average is 270 beats/minute compared with 210 beats/minute in older children (Fig. 5-42). Discrete P waves are usually difficult to define, but if present, there is always a one-to-one relationship to the QRS. Dramatic ST segment changes that may occur during tachycardia resolve shortly after conversion to sinus rhythm.

Two important points with regard to SVT include differentiating this arrhythmia from sinus tachycardia in an infant and the value of the 12-lead electrocardiogram after conversion to sinus rhythm. In a child younger than 1 year of age, during periods of severe stress such as sepsis,

dehydration, or high fever, the sinus rate may reach 220 to 250 beats/minute. At this rate the P wave is lost in the T wave. Facial ice water immersion or intravenous adenosine may be invaluable in differentiating rapid sinus tachycardia from SVT: in the latter case the intervention terminates the tachycardia abruptly, whereas in the former it produces only transient slowing and the P waves become evident on the downstroke of the T wave. With regard to the postconversion 12-lead electrocardiogram, it is important to recognize the presence of Wolff-Parkinson-White syndrome, which occurs in 25% of patients with SVT. This syndrome is characterized by a short PR interval, a delta wave, and prolongation of the QRS complex (Fig. 5-43) and is not evident when the tachycardia is present.

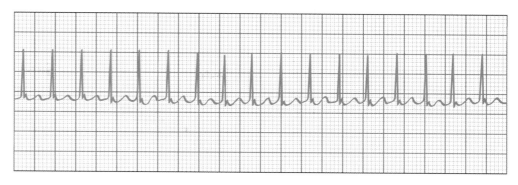

Figure 5-42. Supraventricular tachycardia. Note a normal QRS complex tachycardia at a rate of 214 beats/minute without visible P waves.

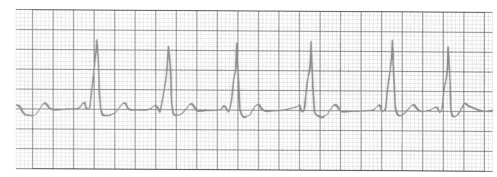

Figure 5-43. Wolff-Parkinson-White syndrome. Note the characteristic findings of a short P-R interval, slurred upstroke of QRS (delta wave), and prolongation of the QRS interval.

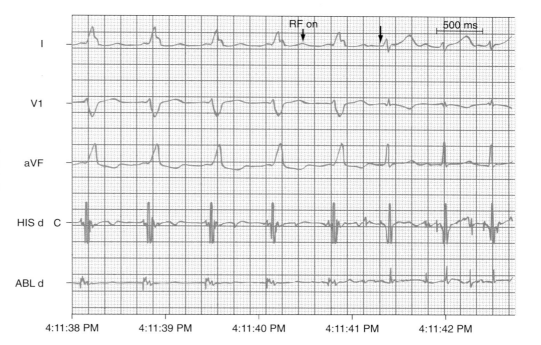

Figure 5-44. Radiofrequency catheter ablation. Note the prompt disappearance of the delta wave (arrow) after radiofrequency ablation of an accessory pathway in a patient with Wolff-Parkinson-White syndrome.

A discussion of the treatment for SVT in the pediatric patient is beyond the scope of this chapter, and detailed algorithms are available in other sources. However, it should be noted that, in recent years, radiofrequency catheter ablation of the common arrhythmia substrates for SVT, accessory atrioventricular connections or dual AV nodal pathways, has become a frontline treatment for older children and adolescents. The abnormal pathway can be accurately mapped during an electrophysiology study, and application of radiofrequency energy at the appropriate site can result in immediate disappearance of the delta wave in a patient with Wolff-Parkinson-White syndrome (Fig. 5-44).

Sustained *ventricular tachycardia* is distinctly uncommon in childhood, and the patient must be thoroughly investigated for underlying heart disease. This arrhythmia is most often associated with hemodynamic compromise and is characterized by a regular wide-complex tachycardia usually with atrioventricular dissociation if P waves are visible (Fig. 5-45). This life-threatening disorder most commonly occurs in children who have had open-heart surgical repair for tetralogy of Fallot or other complex anomalies or who have a cardiomyopathy, myocarditis, or myocardial tumor. Looking for a prolonged corrected Q-T interval (QT_c) is also important because this abnormality of repolarization may lead to recurrent syncope and sudden death secondary to ventricular tachycardia or fibrillation (Fig. 5-46). The QT_c can be calculated using the Bazett formula: the QT interval divided by the square root of the RR interval:

$$QT_c = \frac{QT}{\sqrt{RR}}$$

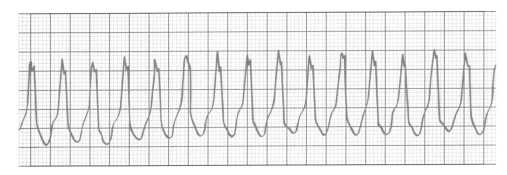

Figure 5-45. Ventricular tachycardia. Note the wide QRS complex tachycardia at a rate of 188 beats/minute.

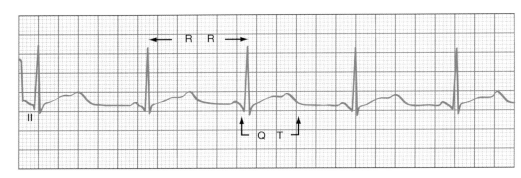

Figure 5-46. Prolonged Q-T syndrome. Note the corrected Q-T interval is prolonged at 0.57 second (upper limit of normal is 0.44 second). The Q-T interval must be corrected for heart rate by using the Bazett formula: measured Q-T interval (0.56 second) divided by the square root of the preceding RR interval (0.96 second).

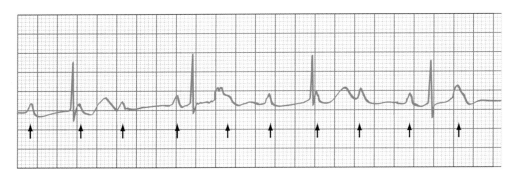

Figure 5-47. Complete heart block. Note that atrial activity *(arrows)* is independent of a slower ventricular rhythm.

Symptomatic bradycardia is rarely encountered in the pediatric age group. One condition that needs to be recognized is congenital *third-degree atrioventricular block* (Fig. 5-47). This may occur with associated structural heart disease, but it occurs more frequently with an otherwise normal heart. The presence of maternal connective tissue disease or antinuclear antibodies should always be sought as a possible cause when congenital atrioventricular block is detected in a newborn.

When a patient is evaluated for a history of syncope or new-onset seizures, it is highly recommended that the physician obtain an electrocardiogram to look for "footprints" of a possible arrhythmic cause. The possibilities include Wolff-Parkinson-White syndrome (providing a substrate for rapid supraventricular tachycardia), prolonged corrected Q-T interval (predisposing to severe ventricular arrhythmias, most often a type known as *torsades de pointes*), or atrioventricular block (leading to Stokes-Adams attacks).

Echocardiography

Cross-sectional echocardiography and color flow mapping first provided remarkable advances in the investigation of congenital heart defects in the early 1980s. Echocardiographic imaging and Doppler and color flow mapping allow accurate anatomic definition of even complex congenital defect, as well as providing a reliable noninvasive hemodynamic assessment of the patient. These tools complement and, in many cases, replace the need for cardiac catheterization and angiography in the management of patients with congenital heart disease.

All types of septal defects can be readily visualized by cross-sectional echocardiography. The atrial septal defects are reliably demonstrated by the subcostal approach. The most common type is the secundum defect, which involves the middle portion of the atrial septum (Fig. 5-48). An ostium primum defect known as a *partial form of an atrioventricular septal defect* is seen in Figure 5-49. The sinus venosus type of atrial septal defect is located in the posterosuperior portion of the atrial septum at the opening of the superior vena cava and is associated with partial anomalous pulmonary venous return of the right upper pulmonary vein (Fig. 5-50).

Ventricular septal defects are well defined by echocardiography and are usually seen clearly using the apical four-chamber view, as shown in Figure 5-51. The most common defect is in the perimembranous septum located in the subaortic area and bordered by the tricuspid valve. Although small defects located in the muscular septum can be difficult to image, particularly if located in the apical trabecular area, they can be readily detected by color flow mapping (Fig. 5-52).

Accurate diagnosis of most structural congenital heart diseases, whether simple or complex, can be made by echocardiography. A systematic approach to define major intracardiac connections is a useful starting point: (1)

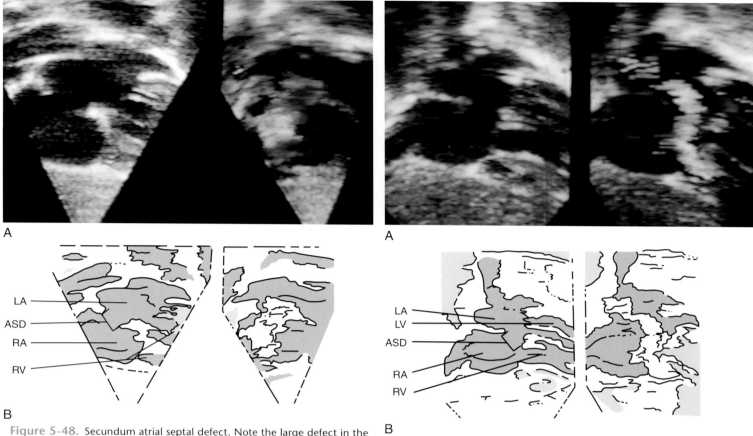

A

B

Figure 5-48. Secundum atrial septal defect. Note the large defect in the fossa ovale area on the subcostal view *(left)*. Color flow mapping *(right)* confirms a prominent left-to-right shunt.

Figure 5-49. Partial form of an atrioventricular septal defect. Note the defect *(left)* is seen in the inferior portion of the atrial septum. A significant left-to-right shunt is shown on color flow mapping *(right)*.

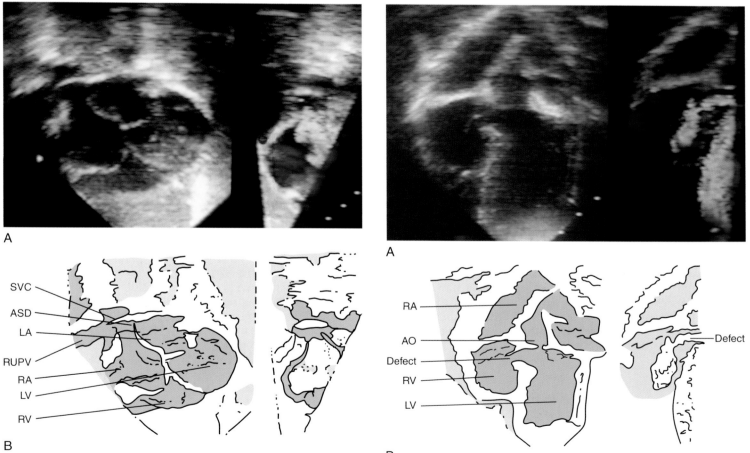

A

B

Figure 5-50. Sinus venosus defect. Note the defect *(left)* in the postero-superior portion of the atrial septum, where the right upper pulmonary vein (RUPV) opens directly into the superior vena cava (SVC). Shunts from the anomalous drainage of the right upper pulmonary vein and from the left atrium are seen on color flow mapping *(right)*.

Figure 5-51. Perimembranous ventricular septal defect. Note the defect in the ventricular septum is well visualized on the apical four-chamber view *(left)*. Significant left-to-right shunting through the defect is confirmed by color flow mapping *(right)*.

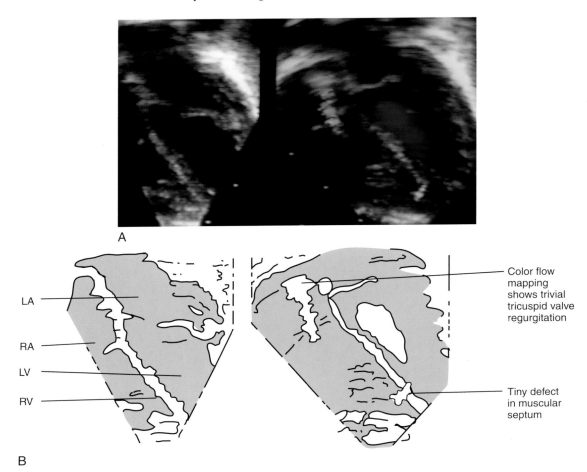

A

B

LA

RA

LV

RV

Color flow
mapping
shows trivial
tricuspid valve
regurgitation

Tiny defect
in muscular
septum

Figure 5-52. Muscular ventricular septal defect. Note that no apparent defect in the ventricular septum could be visualized on two-dimensional imaging (left). However, color flow mapping (right) confirmed a tiny defect in the muscular septum near the apex by showing a jet (yellowish red). In addition, trivial tricuspid valve regurgitation is noted (blue jet).

venoatrial (systemic or pulmonary venous return to the right or left atrium), (2) atrioventricular, and (3) ventriculoarterial (ventricle to the great vessels).

If the pulmonary veins do not communicate with the left atrium, total anomalous pulmonary venous return should be suspected. Congenitally corrected transposition is the most likely diagnosis when the atrioventricular connection is discordant (right atrium to morphologic left ventricle and left atrium to morphologic right ventricle), whereas transposition of the great arteries is suspected when only the ventriculoarterial connection is discordant. The rather characteristic finding of parallel takeoff of the great vessels from both ventricles is seen in transposition of the great arteries, with the aorta arising anteriorly from the right ventricle and the pulmonary artery originating posteriorly from the left ventricle (Fig. 5-53).

Typical findings in another common cyanotic heart lesion, tetralogy of Fallot, are a dilated aortic root that overrides the ventricular septum, a large perimembranous ventricular septal defect, and right ventricular outflow obstruction (Fig. 5-54). The aortic arch is best visualized by a suprasternal approach, and the diagnosis of interrupted aortic arch or coarctation of the aorta can be readily made in most cases (Fig. 5-55).

Cardiac Surgical Procedures

The remarkable progress in treating children with severe congenital heart disease over the past 50 years, progress that has accelerated greatly during the past 2 decades, is largely due to dramatic achievements in the field of pediatric heart surgery. Although the first patent ductus arteriosus ligation was in 1938, the first Blalock-Taussig shunt in 1944, and the initial repair of coarctation in 1945, open-heart repair of complex malformations did not become relatively commonplace until the late 1960s and 1970s. Since then there have been progressive improvements in precise preoperative diagnosis, specialized pediatric heart surgeons have developed stunningly impressive technical skills, and important advances have occurred in the perioperative management of infants with critical heart disease. All of these factors have made it possible to offer successful palliative or corrective surgery for the great majority of even the most severe forms of congenital heart disease.

Although the large number of possible malformations and different operations applied to them may seem bewildering and complex, in reality only a relatively small number of types of surgical procedures are performed. Most of these procedures are associated with an eponym that designates the surgeon who developed a particular technique. The purpose of the following section is to provide schematic diagrams and brief explanations for the commonly used surgical procedures and the types of defects to which they are applied.

Figure 5-56 demonstrates the various types of systemic to pulmonary artery shunt procedures. These are commonly performed palliative operations in newborns and infants with complex congenital heart disease associated with severe obstruction to pulmonary blood flow. These lesions generally have in common either severe subvalvular or valvular pulmonic stenosis or pulmonary atresia leading to inadequate pulmonary blood flow. In the previous era of cardiac surgery, the most common lesion in this category was tetralogy of Fallot. Currently, most children with this entity now have a complete repair in infancy

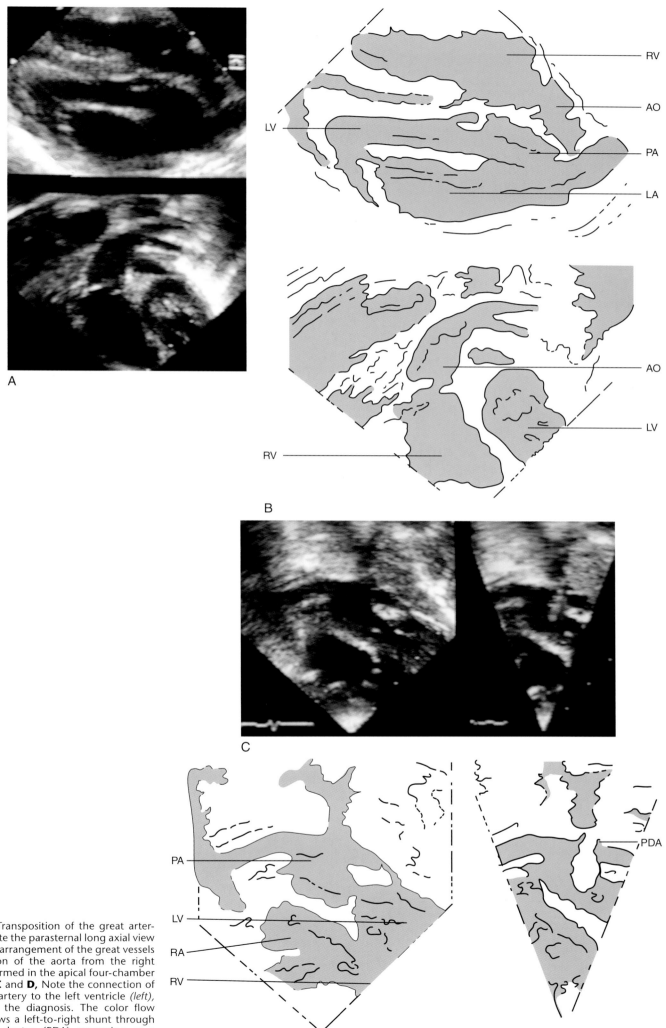

RV

AO

LV — PA

LA

AO

LV

RV

B

C

PA

LV

RA

RV

PDA

D

Figure 5-53. Transposition of the great arteries. **A** and **B,** Note the parasternal long axial view shows a parallel arrangement of the great vessels *(top)*. Origination of the aorta from the right ventricle is confirmed in the apical four-chamber view *(bottom)*. **C** and **D,** Note the connection of the pulmonary artery to the left ventricle *(left)*, which confirms the diagnosis. The color flow map *(right)* shows a left-to-right shunt through a small patent ductus (PDA) appearing as a yellowish red jet.

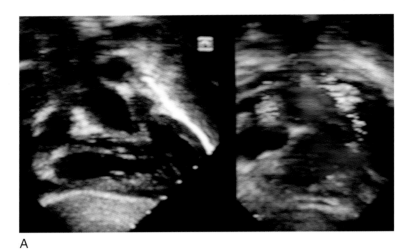

A

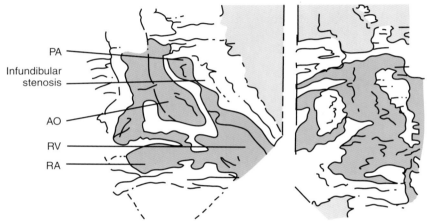

B

Figure 5-54. Tetralogy of Fallot. Note both valvular pulmonic and infundibular stenosis on the subcostal view *(left)*. Color flow map *(right)* confirms turbulent flow *(mosaic color)* across the stenotic area.

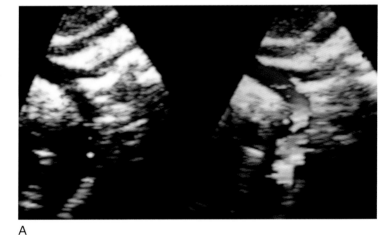

A

Figure 5-55. Coarctation of the aorta. Note the discrete narrowing in the proximal portion of the descending aorta demonstrated on the suprasternal view *(left)*. Color flow map *(right)* confirms a turbulent flow pattern *(aliasing)* across the coarctation. LCCA, left common carotid artery; LSCA, left subclavian artery.

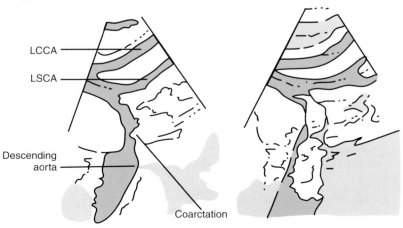

B

TETRALOGY OF FALLOT

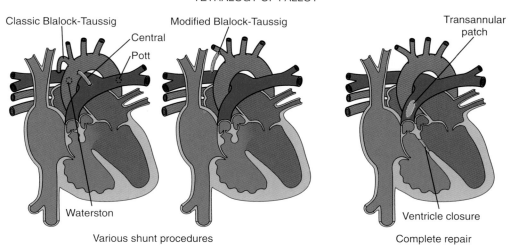

Figure 5-56. Palliative shunt procedures and definitive operative procedure for tetralogy of Fallot.

AORTIC ATRESIA AND
HYPOPLASTIC LEFT HEART SYNDROME

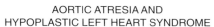

Figure 5-57. Initial palliative (Norwood) procedure for hypoplastic left heart syndrome (aortic atresia complex).

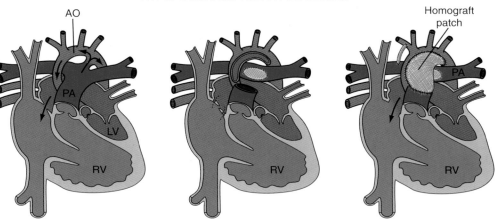

Norwood procedure (first stage)

without prior shunting. The *classic Blalock-Taussig shunt* is performed by dividing the subclavian artery and creating an end-to-side anastomosis of the proximal subclavian artery stump to the ipsilateral pulmonary artery. The most common type of shunt performed in the current era is a *modified Blalock-Taussig shunt,* which uses a Gore-Tex interposition graft between the innominate or subclavian artery and pulmonary artery without dividing the distal subclavian artery. Occasionally, unusual anatomy of the aorta or proximal pulmonary arteries leads to placement of a *central shunt* (placement of a short interposition graft between the ascending aorta and main pulmonary artery). Other procedures, frequently used in the early decades of congenital heart surgery, include a *Waterston shunt* (creation of a window between the ascending aorta and right pulmonary artery) and a *Pott shunt* (creation of a window between the descending aorta and left pulmonary artery).

Figure 5-56 also demonstrates the technique of complete repair for tetralogy of Fallot, which includes closure of the ventricular septal defect, relief of right ventricular outflow tract obstruction with resection of subvalvular muscle, pulmonary valvotomy, and usually a transannular patch.

Figure 5-57 illustrates the initial palliation for aortic atresia and hypoplastic left heart syndrome, which is the most common cause of congestive heart failure in the first

several days of life. A *Norwood procedure* is the first of a three-stage operative approach designed to provide long-term stability for a circulation supported by only one ventricle. In the first stage the aortic atresia is functionally converted to pulmonary atresia. A "neoaortic outflow" for the right ventricle is created by transecting the main pulmonary artery near its bifurcation and anastomosing the proximal root to the hypoplastic ascending aorta, making liberal use of a homograft patch to enlarge the entire aortic arch. Relieving the coarctation that is invariably part of the complex is important. A shunt is subsequently performed to provide pulmonary blood flow, and a large atrial septal defect is created to allow unimpeded flow from the left to the right atrium. A recent modification (Sano procedure) of this operation substitutes a conduit from the right ventricle to the pulmonary artery for the shunt. The second and third stages of this approach are described and shown as follows.

Figures 5-58 and 5-59 show the approach to palliation of hearts with a functional single ventricle. Any malformation that is associated with a hypoplastic right or left ventricle can be treated in this manner, with the two most common examples being tricuspid atresia with a hypoplastic right ventricle and aortic atresia with a hypoplastic left heart, status post–first-stage Norwood procedure. Figure 5-58 demonstrates the first step in separating the systemic and pulmonary circulations in the setting of a

TRICUSPID ATRESIA

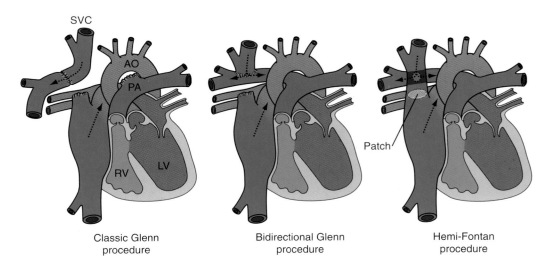

Classic Glenn
procedure

Bidirectional Glenn
procedure

Hemi-Fontan
procedure

Patch

Figure 5-58. Various initial palliative procedures for a functionally single ventricle, such as tricuspid atresia.

TRICUSPID ATRESIA

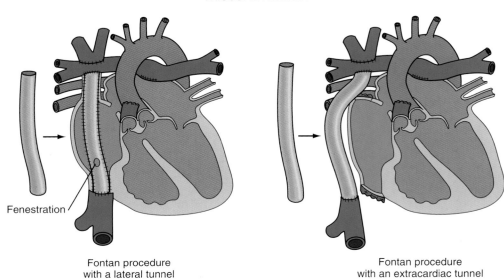

Fenestration

Fontan procedure
with a lateral tunnel

Fontan procedure
with an extracardiac tunnel

Figure 5-59. Completion of palliation for a functionally single ventricle, such as tricuspid atresia.

functional single ventricle. The initial procedure directs approximately one half of systemic venous return directly to the pulmonary artery by creating an anastomosis between the superior vena cava and the right pulmonary artery. In the *classic Glenn procedure,* the right pulmonary artery is divided, the superior vena cava–right atrial junction is closed, and the superior vena cava is anastomosed to the distal right pulmonary artery. This operation has been modified in recent years to a *bidirectional Glenn procedure,* which separates the superior vena cava from the right atrium and creates an end-to-side connection to the pulmonary artery, allowing flow to both the right and left pulmonary arteries. A variation of this latter procedure is the *hemi-Fontan.* In this operation, which produces the identical physiologic results as the bidirectional Glenn, a large superior vena cava–pulmonary artery connection is created, but the superior vena cava–right atrial connection is left intact and the orifice of the superior vena cava is closed with a patch. The *Fontan procedure* completes the process of diverting the entire systemic venous return to the pulmonary artery and is shown in Figure 5-59. This may be done using a *lateral tunnel* approach, in which a tunnel within the right atrium is created with a U-shaped graft attached to the right atrial

wall. The current approach uses an *extracardiac tunnel,* which avoids incorporating right atrial tissue into the connection in the hope of preventing postoperative atrial arrhythmias related to right atrial scarring. In many Fontan operations, a small opening or *fenestration* in the tunnel is created to allow a small amount of right-to-left shunting to decompress the relatively high-pressure systemic venous conduit.

Figures 5-60 and 5-61 depict the various surgical approaches to transposition of the great arteries. The *Mustard* and *Senning procedures* were the original procedures used to correct the circulation in children with transposition. In both of these operations the atrial venous return is "switched" by placing a baffle that directs the superior and inferior vena caval systemic venous return posterior and to the left behind the baffle to the left ventricle, while allowing the pulmonary venous return to flow anteriorly in front of the baffle to the right ventricle. Figure 5-60 demonstrates the preoperative and postoperative flow patterns in transposition in the right and left diagrams, respectively, showing how rerouting systemic venous return allows fully oxygenated blood to go to the aorta. The only difference in the Mustard and Senning operations is the use of more native atrial tissue and less

TRANSPOSITION OF THE GREAT ARTERIES

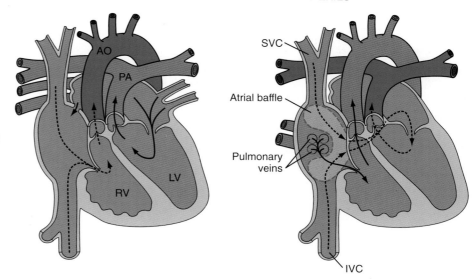

Figure 5-60. Intra-atrial baffle (Mustard or Senning) procedure for transposition of the great arteries.

Mustard or Senning procedure

TRANSPOSITION OF THE GREAT ARTERIES

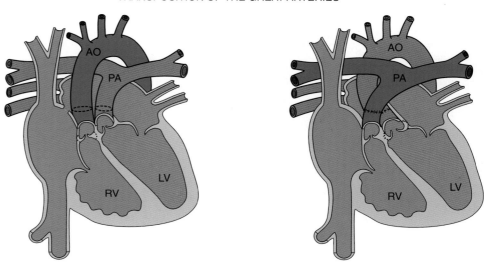

Figure 5-61. Arterial switch (Jatene) procedure for transposition of the great arteries.

Arterial switch
(Jatene procedure)

patch material in the latter operation. In the past 15 years all pediatric cardiology centers have been using the *arterial switch (Jatene) procedure* (see Fig. 5-61) to correct the circulation in transposition of the great arteries. The aortic and pulmonary roots are transected and "switched" to the appropriate ventricles. The most difficult aspect of this operation is the transfer of the right and left coronary arteries from the anterior native aortic root to the posterior pulmonary root that will become the neoaorta.

The key elements of the *Rastelli procedure,* closure of a ventricular septal defect and placement of a conduit to connect the right ventricle to the pulmonary artery, are shown in Figure 5-62. This procedure is used for tetralogy of Fallot with pulmonary atresia, transposition of the great arteries with ventricular septal defect and severe pulmonic stenosis, and truncus arteriosus (pulmonary arteries arising directly from a truncal root that overrides a large ventricular septal defect, as shown in the diagram on the left). The operation for a truncus arteriosus consists of closing of the ventricular septal defect to direct all left

ventricular outflow to the aorta, detachment of the pulmonary arteries from the aorta (truncus), and placement of a homograft conduit between the right ventricle and pulmonary arteries.

Figures 5-63, 5-64, and 5-65 show operations designed to treat aortic valve and systemic outflow tract disease. The *Ross procedure* (see Fig. 5-63) is an ingenious approach to the treatment of severe aortic stenosis or insufficiency when a valve replacement is required. The diseased aortic valve is removed, and the patient's own pulmonary valve is auto-transplanted to the aortic position. The coronary arteries must be reimplanted into the neoaortic root, and a pulmonary homograft is used to reconstruct the right ventricular outflow tract. This operation avoids the life-long anticoagulation that would be required by a prosthetic aortic valve. Aortic stenosis with a small annulus is usually treated with a *Konno procedure* (see Fig. 5-64), which uses patch enlargement of the base of the ventricular septum to increase the size of the aortic annulus, allowing placement of an appropriately sized prosthetic

TRUNCUS ARTERIOSUS

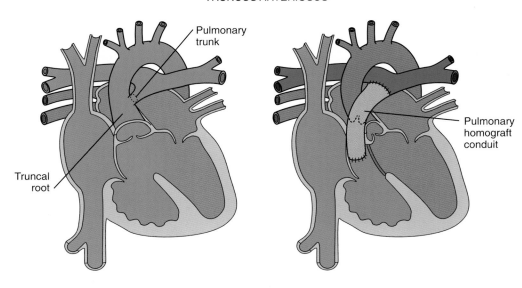

Rastelli procedure

Figure 5-62. Creation of a right ventricle to pulmonary conduit for truncus arteriosus (Rastelli procedure).

AORTIC VALVE DISEASE

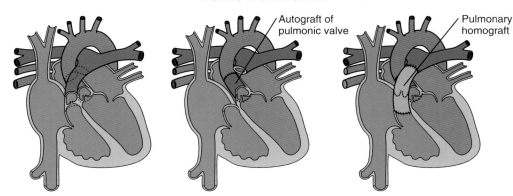

Ross procedure

Figure 5-63. Replacing the diseased aortic valve with the native pulmonary valve (Ross procedure).

AORTIC STENOSIS WITH SMALL AORTIC ANNULUS

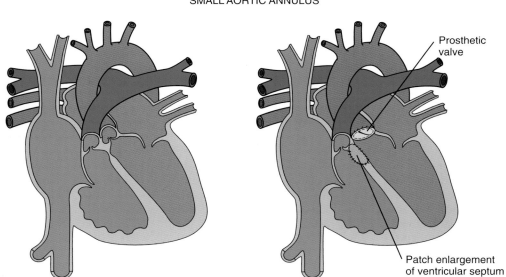

Konno procedure

Figure 5-64. Enlargement of the limited aortic annulus associated with severe aortic valve disease by patch enlargement of ventricular septum and placement of prosthetic valve (Konno procedure).

DIFFUSE SUBAORTIC STENOSIS

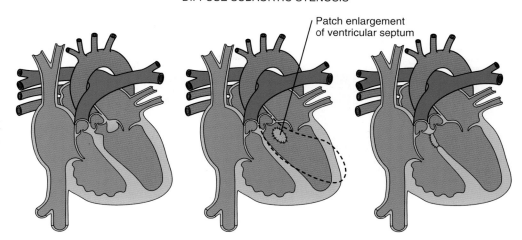

Konno-Rastan procedure

Figure 5-65. Enlargement of diffuse subaortic stenosis by patch enlargement of ventricular septum and resection of subaortic ridge (Konno-Rastan procedure).

DOUBLE INLET LEFT VENTRICLE
WITH RESTRICTIVE VENTRICULAR COMMUNICATION

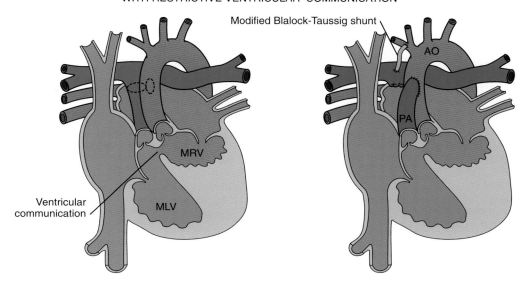

Damus-Stansel-Kaye procedure

Figure 5-66. Bypass of subaortic stenosis by creation of aortopulmonary anastomosis (Damus-Stansel-Kaye procedure).

aortic valve. This procedure may be combined with the Ross procedure. Figure 5-65 shows the *Konno-Rastan procedure*, in which a large patch is used to enlarge the ventricular septum in order to relieve diffuse subaortic stenosis.

Figure 5-66 illustrates the *Damus-Stansel-Kaye* surgical approach, which is used to relieve aortic outflow tract obstruction in the setting of complex heart disease. A double-inlet left ventricle with a restrictive ventricular communication that results in severe "functional" subaortic stenosis is one such example. The main pulmonary artery is transected, and the distal opening is oversewn along with connection of the proximal pulmonary root to the ascending aorta, in essence creating a bypass around the small ventricular communication that leads to the aorta. A modified Blalock-Taussig shunt is created to allow pulmonary blood flow. "MLV" refers to the dominant morphologic left ventricle, which receives both atrioventricular valves. "MRV" refers to the hypoplastic morphologic right ventricle which receives blood only via the ventricular communication and supports the aortic valve.

Interventional Cardiac Catheterization

Interventional cardiology developed as a subspecialty over the past 4 decades after William Rashkind introduced the balloon septostomy to alleviate cyanosis in transposition of the great arteries. In recent years the field has expanded explosively so that currently it plays a role in almost every heart defect. Interventions can be classified according to the purpose to treat:
1. Valvular obstruction
2. Vascular stenosis
3. Creation or enlargement of defects
4. Closure of defects
5. Other

Valvular Obstruction

Pulmonary Valve Stenosis/Atresia
In general, intervention is indicated when peak-to-peak gradients are above 40 mm Hg as measured via cardiac

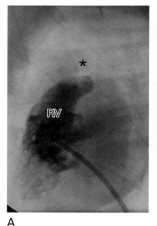
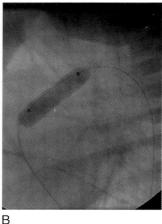
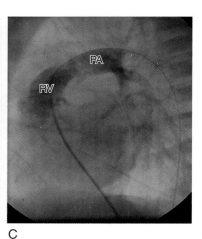

A   B   C

Figure 5-67. Pulmonary valve stenosis or atresia. **A,** A right ventricular angiogram in the lateral projection shows atresia of the pulmonary valve. **B,** After radiofrequency perforation of the pulmonary valve, balloon dilation is performed. **C,** After dilation there is an open pathway between the right ventricle (RV) and pulmonary artery (PA).

catheterization. Balloon dilation has become the standard first-line treatment. In pulmonic stenosis, balloon dilation is highly effective in the large majority of patients. However, the success rate is not as high for the so-called *dysplastic pulmonary valve* (common in Noonan syndrome) where the valve is thick and often has associated supravalvar narrowing. For these valves, high-pressure balloons may be necessary to achieve success. Efficacy is long lasting in most cases, though about 8% of individuals do require repeat dilation for restenosis. A special group of patients are the newborns with critical pulmonary valve stenosis, for which repeat dilation within the first year of life is not uncommon. Though dilation frequently results in regurgitation of the valve because pulmonary artery resistance is normally quite low, the physiologic consequences of the insufficiency are rarely significant. Thus the main long-term issues are observation for the rare case of restenosis and the continued need for endocarditis precautions.

In the newborn period intervention is necessary in those with critical pulmonary stenosis and ductal-dependent circulation, presenting with severe cyanosis. In this setting it is common to see associated variable degrees of right ventricular hypoplasia and even cavitary obliteration. The right ventricle most often remodels over time to allow a biventricular circulation; however, it may take several weeks or months for resolution of right-to-left shunting across the patent foramen ovale. Typically, the prostaglandins that are used to promote ductal patency before the procedure are discontinued following balloon dilation. Some patients may require ongoing prostaglandin therapy for a few days or even weeks, particularly if the severity of the right ventricular hypoplasia is marked. Transcatheter placement of a stent in the ductus arteriosus has become an attractive alternative to surgical palliation for those patients who cannot wean off prostaglandins.

Patients with membranous pulmonary atresia can undergo radiofrequency-assisted valve perforation followed by balloon valvotomy (Fig. 5-67). Although successful perforation has been reported in up 75% to 90% of selected patients, the procedure is definitive for only 35% because they commonly require additional intervention, either transcatheter or surgical.

Aortic Valve Stenosis

Although a few centers in the world continue to perform surgical valvotomies for aortic stenosis, most prefer balloon valvotomy as the procedure of choice. In the newborn, severe aortic stenosis can present as critical with ductal-dependent systemic circulation. Transcatheter balloon dilation can be performed antegrade (femoral vein or

umbilical vein to left ventricle and aorta across foramen ovale) or retrograde (umbilical artery or femoral artery). For premature babies, the carotid artery approach is a good alternative to avoid femoral arterial damage. Currently the procedure can be performed using low-profile balloons, which can be advanced via a 3-French sheath in the femoral artery, with significantly reduced incidence of iliofemoral artery thrombosis.

Natural history data for aortic stenosis have suggested that a peak-to-peak gradient across the valve of more than 50 mm Hg represents obstruction severe enough that intervention is preferable to observation and "medical management." Aortic stenosis represents a very different circumstance with regard to success; all known forms of therapy including balloon dilation, surgical valvotomy, or replacement of the valve are palliative given that further surgery will be necessary at some point in almost all cases. Balloon dilation of the aortic valve creates small tears in the leaflets that result in an increase in the valve orifice size. Some degree of aortic insufficiency is commonly present after the procedure. Attempts to completely alleviate obstruction by using overly large balloons result in an unacceptable amount of regurgitation. Thus even after successful balloon dilation, patients commonly have residual obstruction and/or insufficiency. The benefit achieved after aortic valve dilation is of variable duration. In one report the intervention-free survival was 50% to 60% at 10 years after dilation. The need for subsequent intervention may be due to recurrent obstruction, insufficiency, or both. In the first case repeat valve dilation is an option.

Mitral Stenosis

Isolated congenital mitral valve stenosis is rare, occurring more commonly in association with other left-sided obstructive lesions, as in patients with Shone syndrome or other complex congenital heart disease. Congenital mitral valve stenosis has proven to be a somewhat intractable condition, with a high mortality rate. Given the palliative nature of any intervention for patients with congenital mitral stenosis, newborns that present with a severe form of this condition are typically managed as patients with hypoplastic left heart syndrome.

Mitral balloon valvotomy beyond the newborn period can be effective and may have a lasting beneficial result, especially for rheumatic mitral valve stenosis. However, for congenital mitral valve stenosis, the procedure should be considered palliative and potentially able to delay the need for mitral valve replacement in a small child.

Vascular Stenosis

Pulmonary Artery Stenosis

Peripheral pulmonary artery stenosis can be congenital or acquired after cardiac surgery and constitutes 2% to 3% of congenital heart disease. Congenital pulmonary artery stenosis can occur in isolation or be associated with other congenital heart defects (most commonly, tetralogy of Fallot with or without pulmonary atresia). As a primary lesion, it may be idiopathic or occur in the presence of syndromes, such as congenital rubella, Williams syndrome, and Alagille syndrome. Results of surgery for any of these branch pulmonary artery stenoses have been quite unsatisfactory. In addition, surgery cannot treat peripheral stenoses within the lungs. Thus balloon angioplasty has become the first-line therapy for these patients.

Generally, indications for balloon dilation include an elevated right-to-left ventricular systolic pressure ratio of more than 50%, right ventricular failure, angiographic narrowing, contralateral pulmonary arterial hypertension, and abnormal perfusion by lung scintigraphy. Although there are no contraindications to this procedure by age or size, newborns with severe branch pulmonary artery stenosis should undergo balloon angioplasty only if severely symptomatic. Either discrete stenoses or long diffuse hypoplastic pulmonary arteries can be dilated, with success rates of 50% to 75%. With the use of high-pressure balloons, the success rate is on the order of 75%. Most recently the cutting balloon (Fig. 5-68) has been used for resistant lesions, significantly increasing the success rate of balloon pulmonary angioplasty. In addition, stent implantation allows a significant improvement in success rates to more than 90% (Fig. 5-69). However, not all lesions are amenable to stent implantation. There are theoretical disadvantages to placing stents in infants including more difficult vascular access and the need for subsequent dilations to keep up with somatic growth. Nevertheless, some lesions that have not responded to dilation alone or surgery can be managed successfully with stent implantation, regardless of the age.

Aortic Coarctation

Balloon dilation of native coarctation of the aorta remains a controversial subject. Generally, indications for intervention in infants and children, whether surgical or transcatheter, include the presence of anatomic coarctation associated with a systolic pressure gradient between upper and lower extremities of more than 20 mm Hg or a systolic blood pressure greater than 95% for age or the presence of left ventricular dysfunction. Because of the high restenosis rate during the first month of life, intervention is indicated in this age group only in symptomatic patients with congestive heart failure, failure to thrive, or upper extremity hypertension associated with left ventricular dysfunction. Surgery is considered the management approach of choice for neonates and young infants with severe coarctation, given the unacceptably high incidence of restenosis following balloon angioplasty (at least 50%). However, there are specific clinical conditions in which balloon dilation of a native coarctation in infants can be considered as the procedure of choice: patients with high surgical risks due to severe left ventricular dysfunction and unstable hemodynamic condition, severe pulmonary hypertension or other pulmonary diseases that would significantly increase the risk of thoracotomy, and recent intracranial hemorrhage or other major systemic disorders.

Recurrence of stenosis after balloon dilation decreases as the patient's age increases, reaching about 10% for children older than 2 years of age. The procedure is generally safe, with a mortality of less than 1%[32] and aneurysm formation rates of 7%.

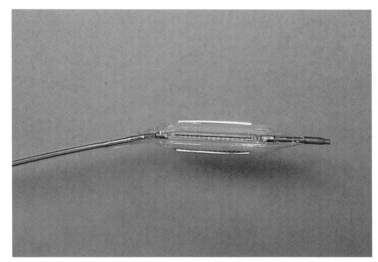

Figure 5-68. Cutting balloon. Note the four tiny blades along the balloon surface.

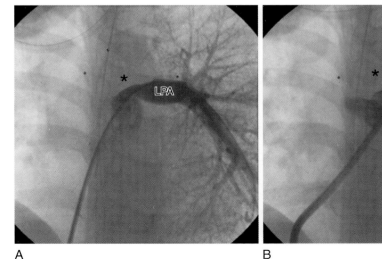

Figure 5-69. Pulmonary artery angioplasty. Note the left pulmonary artery (LPA) stenosis demonstrated on the pulmonary artery angiogram **(A)**; following stent implantation the stenosis has been eliminated **(B).**

A   B

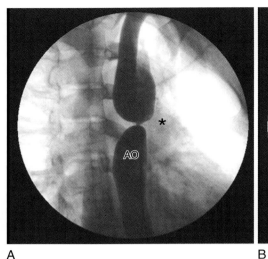
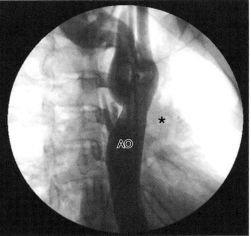

A   B

Figure 5-70. Coarctation angioplasty. Note the severe coarctation of the aorta *(*)* shown by angiography in the descending aorta (AO) **(A);** after balloon angioplasty and stent implantation the coarctation has been eliminated **(B).**

In patients who present after adolescence and into adulthood, transcatheter stenting of the coarctation is widely gaining acceptance as appropriate first-line treatment or at least as an acceptable alternative to surgery (Fig. 5-70). The transcatheter approach is particularly appealing in the absence of any significant collaterals when surgical repair would be of higher risk for spinal cord ischemia. Dilation with stent placement results in effective relief of the obstruction in 92% to 100% of cases.

For patients with postoperative recurrent or residual coarctation, balloon angioplasty is considered the procedure of choice, regardless of the type of previous surgical repair. Success occurs in more than 90% with a restenosis rate of less than 20%. Mortality is 0.7% with a low incidence of aneurysm formation of less than 2%.

Systemic or Pulmonary Vein Stenosis

Symptomatic systemic venous obstruction can occur in infants and children following cardiac surgery or after placement of chronic indwelling lines. Indications for intervention include symptoms of systemic venous hypertension, superior vena cava syndrome, and chronic effusions. Balloon dilation of venous stenoses has been performed since the mid-1980s. Although the immediate success rate is more than 90% for balloon dilation alone, the restenosis rate is more than 50%, suggesting that stent implantation should be considered as first-line therapy.

Pulmonary vein stenosis is generally an intractable disease, occurring either as a congenital lesion or postoperatively. Balloon dilation and stent implantation can only serve as short-term palliation for symptomatic patients awaiting heart lung transplantation. Hemodynamic and angiographic improvement is seen immediately in almost all patients. However, restenosis occurs in virtually all cases within a few months following intervention.

Creation or Enlargement of Defects

Balloon Atrial Septostomy

Following its initial introduction by Rashkind and Miller in 1966, balloon atrial septostomy to improve atrial mixing and increase systemic oxygen saturation has become an essential intervention in the management of most patients with transposition of the great arteries and other forms of congenital heart disease with

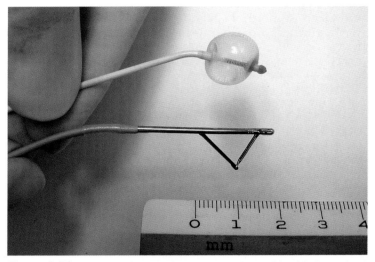

Figure 5-71. Atrial septostomy devices. Note the Rashkind balloon *(top)* and Park blade *(bottom)* septostomy catheters (Cook Incorporated, Bloomington, Ind.).

transposition-like physiology (i.e., some forms of double-outlet right ventricle). At most centers, balloon atrial septostomy is performed routinely on patients with d-transposition of the great arteries and intact ventricular septum, many times in the intensive care unit under echocardiographic guidance. In patients with left-sided obstructive lesions, a thick atrial septum, small left atrium, and restrictive atrial septal defect, balloon atrial septostomy is rarely successful. For these patients, other techniques of atrial septal defect creation and septoplasty are preferred. The success rate of balloon atrial septostomy in newborns is higher than 98%, with a low complication rate.

Atrial Septoplasty/Blade Septostomy

Because balloon atrial septostomy is not feasible in newborns with intact atrial septum or a thick septum, other techniques for septal defect creation are warranted for these patients. Blade atrial septostomy was developed by Sang Park for this purpose (Fig. 5-71). Alternate techniques currently used are a combination of Brockenbrough transseptal puncture followed by serial balloon dilations using angioplasty balloons including the cutting balloon and occasionally stent implantation.

Closure of Defects

Atrial Septal Defects

Now most secundum atrial septal defects are closed via the transcatheter deployment of devices. However, some defects are not amenable to device closure because of the lack of an adequate rim of tissue around the defect to anchor the device. Atrial septal defects of the sinus venosus type or ostium primum defects cannot be closed with devices. Although devices are available to close large holes (up to 40 mm in diameter), the larger devices will only fit in a large adult heart. Two devices are currently approved in the United States for closure of an atrial septal defect, the Amplatzer Septal Occluder (AGA Medical Corporation, Golden Valley, Minn.) (Fig. 5-72) and the Helex Septal Occluder (W.L. Gore & Associates, Inc., Flagstaff, Ariz.). The procedure is performed under transesophageal or intracardiac echocardiographic guidance (Fig. 5-73). Several studies have documented that the efficacy of device closure compares favorably with surgery, with high closure and low complication rates. Late perforations after device closure have been reported to occur up to several years after device implantation; however, these have been rare.

Ventricular Septal Defects

Most ventricular septal defects (VSD) cannot be closed with devices due to the significant size of the defect in relatively small hearts, as well as the proximity to intracardiac valves, particularly tricuspid and aortic valves. An option to overcome the limitations of the technique in a small child is a combined hybrid catheterization-surgical approach. In this method the heart is exposed via a thoracotomy and the device delivery catheter advanced through the free wall of the right ventricle and across the defect. The device is then opened under echocardiographic guidance. This technique has the advantage of avoiding cardiopulmonary bypass and may be particularly useful for ventricular septal defects located in portions of the heart difficult to reach by standard open surgical technique. The CardioSEAL device (NMT Medical, Boston) (Fig. 5-74) is currently approved for closure of muscular ventricular septal defects but requires a large introducer sheath for delivery and cannot be retrieved once opened. The Amplatzer VSD Occluder is still investigational. Although high success rates have been reported with transcatheter closure of ventricular septal defects, in the United States the procedure is currently still reserved for defects that are difficult to close surgically.

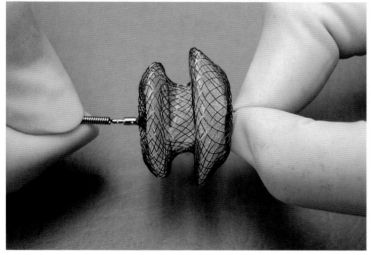

Figure 5-72. Device closure of atrial septal defect. Note the Amplatzer Septal Occluder device held outstretched from each disk to demonstrate its architecture. Two disks and a central waist, which occludes the defect, are shown.

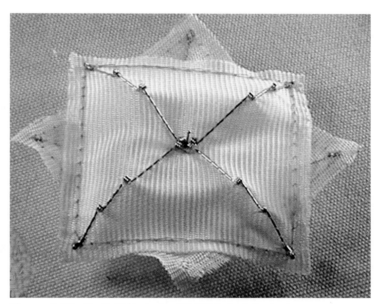

Figure 5-74. CardioSEAL device (NMT Medical, Boston).

Figure 5-73. Illustration of placement of Amplatzer Septal Occluder. Note the delivery sheath is advanced across the defect into the left atrium, and the device is partially extruded out of the sheath with opening the left atrial disk **(A)**; following withdrawal of the sheath the device has been deployed with the right atrial disk opened on the right side of the septum, and the device has been detached from the delivery cable **(B)**.

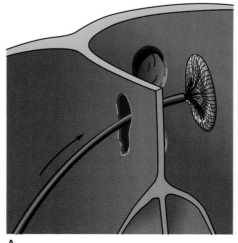
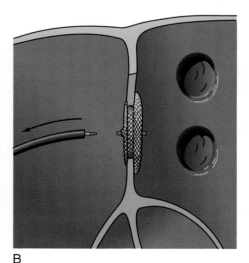

A

B

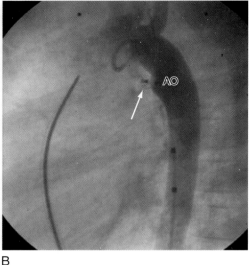

A   B

Figure 5-75. Closure of patent ductus arteriosus. Note the descending aorta (AO) angiogram shows a patent ductus *(arrow)* entering the main pulmonary artery (MPA) **(A)**; a repeat angiogram following placement of an Amplatzer Duct Occluder demonstrates the ductus is completely closed **(B).**

Patent Ductus Arteriosus

Small and moderate patent ducts (PDA) are typically closed in the catheterization laboratory with either embolization coils or the Amplatzer Duct Occluder (Fig. 5-75), while large symptomatic PDAs in the newborn are treated surgically. Transcatheter closure of PDA has been highly successful, with efficacy of more than 97% and a low complication rate.

Other

Closure of Collaterals. Lesions amenable to closure by embolization therapy include systemic venous anomalies (i.e., left superior vena cava to left atrium) or aortopulmonary collaterals, pulmonary sequestration, or congenital arteriovenous malformations. Coil embolization of collaterals is one of the most common procedures in children with congenital heart disease associated with aortopulmonary collateral vessels.

Miscellaneous. Reopening of thrombosed vessels or surgical anastomoses can be performed with good results using transcatheter thrombolysis, although the experience in pediatrics is relatively limited. Other interventions include retrieval of foreign bodies, preservation of ductal patency using stents, coil embolization of coronary artery fistulae, and some novel catheter interventions such as prenatal interventions (for opening of stenotic valves or a restrictive atrial septum) and transcatheter pulmonary valve implantation. These innovative procedures are likely to be only a preview of what will be possible and even commonplace in the next decade as the field of interventional catheterization continues to advance and expand.

Bibliography

Bove EL: Surgical treatment for hypoplastic left heart syndrome. Jpn J Thorac Cardiovasc Surg 47:47-56, 1999.

Bush DM: Evaluating cardiovascular presentations: What does an electrocardiogram have to offer? Pediatr Ann 34:858-869, 2005.

Case CL: Diagnosis and treatment of pediatric arrhythmias. Pediatr Clin North Am 46:347-354, 1999.

Chun TUH, Van Hare GF: Advances in the approach to treatment of supraventricular tachycardia in the pediatric population. Curr Cardiol Rep 6:322-326, 2004.

Du ZD, Hijazi ZM, Kleinman CS, et al: Comparison between transcatheter and surgical closure of secundum atrial septal defect in children and adults: Results of a multicenter nonrandomized trial. J Am Coll Cardiol 39:1836-1844, 2002.

Ettedgui JA, Tersak JM: Cardiological aspects of systemic disease. In Anderson RH, Macartney FJ, Shinebourne EA, et al (eds): Paediatric Cardiology, 2nd ed, vol 2. Edinburgh, Churchill Livingstone, 2002, pp 1777-1808.

Fischer DR, Baker EJ, Anderson RH: Echocardiographic manifestation of ventricular septal defects. In Anderson RH, Neches WH, Park SC, Zuberbuhler JR (eds): Perspectives in Pediatric Cardiology, vol 2, Mount Kisco, NY, Futura Publishing, 1988, pp 25-33.

Fontan F, Baudet E: Surgical repair of tricuspid atresia. Thorax 26:240-248, 1971.

French JW, Guntheroth WG: An explanation of asymmetric upper extremity blood pressures in supravalvular aortic stenosis: The Coanda effect. Circulation 42:31-36, 1970.

Glenn WW, Patino JF: Circulatory bypass of the right heart. Preliminary observations on the direct delivery of vena caval blood into the pulmonary arterial circulation: Azygos vein pulmonary artery shunt. Yale J Biol Med 24:147, 1954.

Greenwood RD: Cardiovascular malformations associated with extracardiac anomalies and malformation syndromes. Clin Pediatr 23:145-151, 1984.

Humpl T, Soderberg B, McCrindle BW, et al: Percutaneous balloon valvotomy in pulmonic atresia with intact ventricular septum: Impact on patient care. Circulation 108:826-832, 2003.

Kirklin JW, Barratt-Boyes BG (eds): Cardiac Surgery, ed 2, vol 1. New York, Churchill Livingstone, 1993, p 546.

Konno S, Imai Y, Iida Y, et al: A new method for prosthetic valve replacement in congenital aortic stenosis associated with hypoplasia of the aortic valve ring. J Thoracic Cardiovasc Surg 70:909-917, 1975.

Kreutzer J, Lock JE, Jonas RA, Keane JF: Transcatheter fenestration dilation and/or creation in postoperative Fontan patients. Am J Cardiol 79:228-232, 1997.

Kreutzer J, Perry SB: Stents. In Lock JE, Keane JF, Perry SB (eds): Diagnostic and Interventional Catheterization in Congenital Heart Disease, 2nd ed. Norwell, Mass, Kluwer Academic Publishers, 2000, pp 221-243.

Kugler JD, Danford DA: Management of infants, children and adolescents with paroxysmal supraventricular tachycardia. J Pediatr 129:324-328, 1996.

National High Blood Pressure Education Program Working Group on Hypertension Control in Children and Adolescents: Update on the 1987 task force on high blood pressure in children and adolescents: A working group report from the National High Blood Pressure Education Program. Pediatrics 98:649-658, 1996.

National Heart, Lung and Blood Institute Task Force on Blood Pressure Control in Children: Report. Pediatrics 59(suppl):797-820, 1977.

Park SC, Neches WH, Zuberbuhler JR, et al: Clinical use of blade atrial septostomy. Circulation 56:600-606, 1978.

Park SC, Zuberbuhler JR: Vascular ring and pulmonary sling. In Anderson RH, Macartney FJ, Shinebourne EA, Tynan M (eds): Paediatric Cardiology, 2nd ed, vol 2. Edinburgh, Churchill Livingstone, 2002, pp 1559-1577.

Pelech AN: Evaluation of the pediatric patient with a cardiac murmur. Pediatr Clin North Am 45:167-188, 1999.

Perry SB, Radtke W, Fellows KE, et al: Coil embolization to occlude aortopulmonary collateral vessels and shunts in patients with congenital heart disease. J Am Coll Cardiol 13:100-108, 1989.

Rashkind WJ, Miller W: Creation of an atrial septal defect without thoracotomy: Palliative approach to complete transposition of the great arteries. JAMA 196:991-992, 1966.

Robinson B, Anisman P, Eshaghpour E: A primer on pediatric ECGs. Contemp Pediatr April:69-94, 1994.

Rome JJ, Kreutzer J: Pediatric interventional catheterization: Reasonable expectations and outcomes. Pediatr Clin North Am 51:1589-1610, 2004.

Rowan S, Adroques H, Mathur A, Kamat D: Pediatric hypertension: A review for the primary care provider. Clin Pediatr 44:289-296, 2005.

Senning A: Surgical correction of transposition of the great vessels. Surgery 45:966-980, 1959.

Sharieff GQ, Rao SO: The pediatric ECG. Emerg Med Clin North Am 24:195-208, 2006.

Spicer RL: Cardiovascular disease in Down syndrome. Pediatr Clin North Am 31:1331-1343, 1984.

Swenson JM, Fischer DR, Miller SA, et al: Are chest radiographs and electrocardiograms still valuable in evaluating new pediatric patients with heart murmurs or chest pain? Pediatrics 99:1-3, 1997.

Tingelstad J: Consultation with the specialist: Cardiac dysrhythmias. Pediatr Rev 22:91-94, 2001.

Yeager SB, Flanagan MF, Keane JF: Catheter intervention: Balloon valvotomy. In Lock JE, Keane JF, Perry SB (eds): Diagnostic and Interventional Catheterization in Congenital Heart Disease, 2nd ed. Norwell, Mass, Kluwer Academic Publishers, 2000, pp 151-178.

Yi MS, Kimball TR, Tsevat J, et al: Evaluation of heart murmurs in children: Cost-effective and practical implications. J Pediatr 141:504-511, 2002.

Zuberbuhler JR: Clinical Diagnosis in Pediatric Cardiology. Edinburgh, Churchill Livingstone, 1981.

CHAPTER 6

Child Abuse and Neglect

HOLLY W. DAVIS AND MARY M. CARRASCO

Child abuse and neglect constitute a pediatric public health problem of enormous magnitude. Their relative contribution to morbidity and mortality in children is likewise huge. In addition to the fact that nearly a million children are identified as victims each year, approximately 140,000 incur serious injuries and nearly 20,000 are left with permanent physical disabilities such as cerebral palsy and blindness. The toll on emotional development may be even more significant.

Although the incidence of abuse and neglect appears to have increased within the past century, improved reporting must also be considered. Caffey in the late 1940s and then Kempe and coworkers in the early 1960s fostered a marked increase in the recognition of the physical manifestations of abuse and of the very real needs and problems of child abuse victims. Subsequent passage of legislation in all 50 states mandating that suspected cases be reported to the proper authorities has further improved the incidence of reporting. Thus although some of the increasing incidence is real, much is probably the result of these developments. Additionally, societal standards have changed, for some of what is currently regarded as abuse was once sanctioned as discipline.

Four major forms of abuse have been delineated: physical abuse, sexual abuse, physical neglect, and emotional abuse. Not infrequently, an individual child is found to be the victim of more than one form and there is some degree of emotional abuse with all forms. For purposes of reporting under child protection laws, the abuse or neglect generally must result from the acts or omissions of a parent, guardian, custodian, or other caretaker of the child.

Statistics (U.S. Dept. of Health and Human Services [HHS] Administration on Children, Youth, and Families) for the United States in 2003 underline the extent of the problem: 2.9 million cases were reported. Thirty-one percent of these reports were classified as indicated or substantiated by child protection authorities. Of these, 60% involved neglect, 19% physical abuse, 9% sexual abuse, and 5% were identified as emotionally maltreated. These figures may significantly underestimate the actual number as it is estimated that for every case reported, at least two go unreported. Clearly, some, perhaps many, reports concerning truly abused children are inaccurately determined to be unfounded. Misleading/deceptive histories, limited investigative resources, lack of witnesses, and inability or unwillingness of victims and family members to attest to the fact that abuse has occurred, all contribute to this phenomenon.

Fatality statistics have also been found to have limited accuracy. The HHS estimates that there were about 1500 deaths in 2003. This is an increase from approximately 1100 cases in each of the preceding several years and is likely due to recent improvements in the reporting of fatality statistics. This in turn probably reflects improved recognition of child abuse–related deaths as a result of the institution of child death review teams in most states. Of fatal victims, 40% to 50% are younger than 1 year of age,

and 85% to 90% are 5 years or younger. Researchers looking at data from additional sources have determined that many, perhaps the majority, of deaths due to abuse are misclassified as due to accident, sudden infant death syndrome (SIDS), or natural or unknown causes. Reasons for misclassification include: incomplete medical evaluation; delay in or inadequate death scene investigation, or no scene investigation; lack of sufficient training of coroners and pathologists regarding child abuse and the techniques and studies necessary to identify abuse at autopsy; failure to require manner of death, as well as cause, on death certificates; and poor communication among investigative agencies. Thus most authorities believe 2000 deaths per year is a more accurate figure, although this, too, may be a significant underestimate. To put this in further perspective, the number of deaths due to abuse of children younger than 5 years is greater than the number due to motor vehicle accidents and fires combined and is more than twice the number of deaths due to accidental choking or suffocation, drowning, and falls combined.

The most common causes of death due to abuse are head trauma, abdominal trauma, and suffocation. Of these, intentional suffocation is most likely to go undetected, as autopsy findings may simulate SIDS. It now appears that a large percentage of cases of SIDS are actually due to accidental suffocation as a result of sleeping prone on a soft surface, of getting the face covered in bed clothing, or of cosleeping with one or more adults whether in bed or on a sofa or easy chair. The "back to sleep campaign" and efforts to educate parents about the risks of cosleeping have dramatically reduced the incidence of these tragic deaths.

All sudden unexpected deaths in infancy warrant thorough investigation to facilitate accurate determination of cause, assess for possible foul play, and aid in future prevention. Certain historical points and physical findings may aid in distinguishing SIDS from intentional suffocation. Infants dying of SIDS are usually younger than 6 months of age, previously well (or have only mild URI symptoms), and found unresponsive in the early morning when their parents awaken. In contrast, those dying of intentional suffocation may range from weeks to 2 or 3 years of age and are more likely to be "found" sometime between midmorning and late afternoon or evening, after a period of being with a single caretaker. In some, subtle bruises or petechiae of the face and/or neck or scant bleeding from the nose or mouth may be noted. Many of these infants have a history of a recent hospitalization for an unexplained illness or for apnea, seizure-like activity, or an apparent life-threatening event (ALTE), for which no cause could be found despite an extensive medical workup. This or a past history of multiple apparent life-threatening events and/or a history of two or more prior sibling deaths attributed to SIDS should raise strong suspicion of intentional smothering.

Epidemiology

Child abuse is a phenomenon found in *all* socioeconomic, cultural, racial, ethnic, and religious subsets of society. The reported incidence per capita is greatest in lower socioeconomic groups. This stems in part from the numerous chronic stresses of living in poverty (Table 6-1), problems of socialization, and different attitudes regarding what constitutes appropriate discipline. It is also clear, and must be recognized by physicians and other professionals, that well-educated parents of higher socioeconomic status can be abusive; however, when they are, they are less likely to be suspected. This is in part due to the fact that they "come across well" as they tend to be well dressed, well spoken, more sophisticated, and have a more confident demeanor than parents who are less well off. Also they are often better able to fabricate a plausible history of how the injury occurred "accidentally." Furthermore, when suspected, they are less likely to be reported, and when reported, they are more likely to have the resources and legal assistance to have the case dropped or dismissed, or to be acquitted of the charges. Hence in evaluating potential abuse victims and their families, it is important *not* to rush to judgment of parents on the basis of appearance, dress, and level of sophistication, and professionals should appreciate that many parents who are poor, unsophisticated, and not well dressed are loving and caring despite their limited means and resources.

The most valuable information is gained using a nonjudgmental approach while keeping an open mind in obtaining a thorough history, making careful behavioral and interactional observations, performing meticulous examination, and ordering a well considered laboratory and imaging evaluation before arriving at a diagnosis.

Parental Risk Factors for Child Abuse and Neglect

1. *Past history of being abused or neglected as a child.* Although this is a big risk factor, it is important to note that not all abused children grow up to become abusive

adults. Those who do not have been found to have had a strong, long-standing, and supportive relationship, from early childhood, with a nurturing and nonabusive adult who loved them unconditionally, helped them recognize their own worth, and taught them how to make good choices. This appears to have enabled them to develop both better self-esteem and trusting relationships and, hence, better social support systems.

2. *Poor socialization and emotional and social isolation.* Inadequately nurtured themselves as children, these parents are poorly equipped or unable to adequately nurture their offspring. Their own mothers may not have bonded well with them, and/or their trust may have been betrayed repeatedly by those they loved unconditionally and should have been able to count on most. They also may have been shuttled back and forth between the parental home and relatives' or foster homes or may have been placed in a series of foster homes over the course of years. As a result, they have trouble with trust and forming close attachments, and hence, are poorly equipped to develop and utilize support systems. They also tend to have little understanding of child development and of children's emotional and other needs and, therefore, of good child-rearing practices and of reasonable expectations of child behavior. Tables 6-2 and 6-3 present common features of many of the families of origin of abusive parents/caretakers, as well as their child-rearing practices, which then tend to be repeated by these younger parents and by ensuing generations. Table 6-4 presents common character traits and historical revelations of many poorly socialized parents/caretakers and of those with character disorders.

3. *Limited ability to deal adaptively with stress and negative emotions such as fear, anger, and frustration, compounded by a tendency to lash out violently, verbally and/or physically, in response to negative feelings.* This behavior is often learned by example in their families of origin.

4. *Alcoholism/substance abuse.* When intoxicated or high, such parents may be "out of it" or may be disinhibited in approaching or dealing with their children. They also may be away for extended periods seeking their substance of choice or the wherewithal to obtain it.

5. *Mental illness* (Table 6-5).

6. *Domestic violence in the parental relationship.*

7. *Being subjected to a sudden spate of major life stresses/crises such as loss of job and financial security; loss of home; loss of parent, spouse, or sibling.*

8. *Membership in certain fringe group cults or sects.*

Table 6-1	Chronic Stresses of Poverty

Financial uncertainty
Poor housing conditions
  General disrepair (lack of attention of landlord or tenants)
  Poor sanitary conditions (plumbing problems, too overwhelmed to keep up with cleaning, does not know where to begin)
  Lack of utilities (unpaid bills)
  Lower level of education/sophistication (less articulate) limits knowledge of and access to services and of how to successfully push for repairs
Sense of hopelessness/helplessness, of having no way to get out
  Greater likelihood of:
    Teenage pregnancy/single parenthood
    Inadequate prenatal care
Greater likelihood of exposure to violence and substance abuse

Table 6-2	Common Characteristics of the Family of Origin of Poorly Socialized Adults Given in Psychosocial History*

HISTORY	POTENTIAL EFFECT ON CHILDREN
Evidence suggestive of impaired bonding:	Failure of bonding in first 6 months results in the following:
Maternal depression postpartum	Inability/impaired ability to truly attach, trust, and, ultimately, to nurture
Mother chose to go right back to work	Inability to feel empathy or remorse
"We were never close"	
Separation/divorce/abandonment	Fracture of parent-child bond, especially in early childhood, can result in long-term anger, distrust, emotional distance, self-doubt, and antisocial behavior
Discord/domestic violence }	These situations all may cause the following:
CPS involvement }	Anxiety, fears for self and siblings, for victimized parent
Alcohol/substance abuse }	Chronic sense of uncertainty
	Difficulty concentrating

*Often repeated in subsequent generations.

Child Risk Factors

1. *Age younger than 3 years.*
2. *Being separated at birth from a mother at high risk for problems with attachment because of illness or prematurity, resulting in impaired bonding.*
3. *Being the product of an unplanned/unwanted pregnancy, with a mother who sought little or no prenatal care.*
4. *Being small for gestational age, born with congenital anomalies, and/or having a chronic illness (possibly due to parental grieving and guilt, compounded by the chronic stress of caring for a handicapped child).*
5. *Being perceived as difficult or different.*
6. *Having attention deficit hyperactivity disorder (ADHD) or being oppositional or defiant.*
7. *Foster children and adopted children.*

Table 6-3	Common Characteristics of Child Rearing Practices of Family of Origin of Poorly Socialized Adults (Often Passed on to Ensuing Generations)

Evidence of limited nurturing/supervision:
Child/children left with multiple caretakers
Children often left alone or in each other's care, or left to watch TV for long periods
Paucity of affection, being held, interaction
Lack of consistent routine/schedule for meals, getting up, naps, bedtime, time together, play

Evidence of problems with discipline:
Inconsistency in limit setting
Paying more attention to misbehavior than good behavior
Giving mixed messages regarding what is or is not allowed
Confusing "bad act" with "bad child"
Confusing discipline with punishment
Harsh discipline often delivered in anger ("You have to beat kids to make them behave")

Evidence of unrealistic expectations of child behavior/capabilities
"She should know better than to cry when I have a headache." (said of a 6-month-old baby)
"He's almost two and should be potty trained by now. He just doesn't want to."
"He should know not to be messy when he eats." (said of an 18-month-old toddler)

Other factors:
Repeated exposure to the following:
　Purposeful lying, deception
　Impulsive or explosive behavior
Criticism for having normal/understandable feelings
Repeated broken promises
Repeated presentation with non-choices: "Do you want to go to bed?" "No." "Well you're going anyway, it's bedtime."
Failure to teach options for behavior in response to different feelings/situations
Failure to teach how to recognize options and make good decisions/choices in life

Two situations place children at particularly high risk for abuse. One involves a couple with an unplanned pregnancy that one parent did not want and then pushed for abortion, and which the other insisted on carrying to term. Following delivery, such infants can be at significant risk when left alone in the care of the parent who opposed the pregnancy. The other involves a common pattern in which a young (often teenage) mother who has trouble with attachment and low self-esteem and who mistakes "attention" and sex for love, and thus, has poor judgment in selection of boyfriends. These young women may then have a revolving door for paramours who opportunistically move in for weeks to months and then leave only to be replaced by another. These men also tend to have attachment issues and often have poor impulse control. Further, they have no vested interest in her offspring by other men and thus may have no compunction about "batting them around" when they become a source of irritation, misbehave, or have accidents while these men are "babysitting."

One common thread connecting all of these risk factors appears to be one of *unmet expectations,* either due to unrealistic parental expectations of the child or to the child's inability to meet realistic expectations as the result of developmental delay, illness, temperament, hyperactivity, or inconsistent disciplining. Typically this stems from lack of parental understanding of normal child behavior and emotional development, and of their children's basic needs for nurturing. The combination can then lead the parent or caretaker to attribute *malicious intent* to an infant who will not stop crying or to a toddler who has had a toilet training accident, is stubborn, or misbehaves. Once "malicious intent" is suspected, this can incite rage in someone with a short fuse.

With this background information, the approach to diagnosis of the major forms of abuse can now be addressed more specifically.

Physical Abuse

Physical abuse is defined as the infliction of bodily injury that causes significant or severe pain, leaves physical evidence, impairs physical functioning, or significantly jeopardizes the child's safety. Individual states have varying definitions of what constitutes abuse reportable to Child Protective Services (CPS) and law enforcement agencies, and practitioners should become familiar with the guidelines in their own states. Many of the methods used by perpetrators are listed in Table 6-6, and weapons commonly employed are detailed in Table 6-7.

Table 6-4	Character Traits and Historical Revelations of Parents/Caretakers Who Are Poorly Socialized or Have Character Disorders

TRAITS	REVELATIONS IN HISTORY
Self-focused	Unable to truly love/care for another and put the other's needs first Everything they recount in the history is in relation to themselves Talk more about themselves than their child
Jealous of spouse's/significant other's attention to the child	"She spends too much time with him/her" "She babies him" "She loves that kid more than me"
Jealous of child's preference for spouse/significant other	"He's a momma's boy, always wants to be with/run to his mother" "He'll come to me but then runs right back to his mother"
Psychopathic/sociopathic tendencies	Little or no conscience/capacity for empathy/remorse No compunction about lying and lie quite convincingly
Poor impulse control, short fuse, bad temper	History of behavior problems—fights, school suspensions
Take little or no responsibility for their own failures, instead blame others	Did not finish school "because the principal had it in for me" Cannot hold a job for more than a few months "because the managers are all nuts"

Table 6-5	Mental Illness Seen in Some Abusive Adults
Severe depression	No energy, often cannot even get out of bed Inability to nurture or relate
Bipolar disease	Cycling of emotional highs and lows Inconsistency (children never know what is going to happen next) Explosive behavior
Schizophrenia/ postpartum psychosis	Hallucinations/delusions including voices saying the infant/child is "evil," "Must be punished," "Must die"

NOTE: Often these parents are resistant to seeking and participating in therapy and to consistently taking their medications.

Table 6-6	Methods Used in Physical Abuse

Hitting—hand, fist, weapon
Grabbing with squeeze, pinch, twist, yank, or snap
Shaking
Throwing
Swinging
Kicking
Stomping
Burning—scalds, contact burns
Biting
Hair pulling
Holding hand over face to stifle crying
Prolonged squeezing of chest
Smothering/strangling
Holding under water

Table 6-7	Weapons Commonly Used in Physical Abuse

Hands/fists/feet
Switch/rod/stick/TV antenna/ruler/broom
Looped extension or cable TV cord
Paddle
Kitchen utensil—wooden spoon/spatula/fork
Hairbrush/comb
Coat hanger
Shoe/slipper
Rope/cord/chain/tourniquet
Hot liquids
Hot objects—iron/curling iron/hair dryer/space heater/cigarette/ match/lighter/stove burner

Infants and toddlers are at greatest risk for physical abuse because they are unable to escape attack, and are developmentally incapable of meeting many expectations and of knowing when to "keep a low profile." Given their small size and physical immaturity, they are also the most vulnerable to severe injury. *Common triggers for abusive behavior* toward infants are *crying,* especially prolonged or inconsolable crying, and *feeding problems.* Crying may be due to hunger; pain with illness such as otitis media and esophagitis with gastroesophageal reflux; gas pain due to aerophagia either precipitated by or induced by respiratory disease or frequent feeding interruptions in avid feeders; pain from prior inflicted trauma (rib or extremity fractures or central nervous system [CNS] irritability from head injury). Feeding problems may stem from neurologic or oral-motor disorders, oropharyngeal deformities (such as cleft palate), or pain on swallowing due to oral lesions or reflux-induced esophagitis. With toddlers, difficulties in toilet training, *toileting accidents,* getting into things they are not supposed to touch, and stubbornness or negativism are common inciting factors. Failure to follow orders or instructions, oppositional or defiant behavior, and getting into trouble at school are notable triggers of abuse of older children.

Table 6-8	Misleading/Deceptive History

1. History given is often vague, incomplete, or even fabricated
2. In the absence of obvious surface injuries, the chief complaint may be one of an unrelated problem (URI or a rash) or may be "peripheral," stemming from nonspecific symptoms following injury, such as irritability, vomiting, decreased use or movement of an extremity or refusal to bear weight on an extremity.
3. When surface injuries are present, the chief complaint is often one of an accidental injury, such as the following:
   A short fall (<4 feet)
   The baby was dropped (<4 feet)
   The parent/caretaker fell with the baby (but the parent is uninjured)
   The baby rolled off the couch
   A sibling or other child injured the child

The spectrum of the severity of injuries caused by physical abuse ranges from isolated surface bruising that may be a product of overzealous discipline to fatal head and abdominal trauma that is the result of extremely violent rage reactions. Important to remember is that relatively unimpressive surface marks or injuries may be associated with far more significant underlying skeletal, abdominal, and CNS trauma (see Fig. 6-13). Additionally, it is well known that physical abuse tends to be repetitive and that the severity of attacks tends to escalate over time and, correspondingly, the severity of injuries. Given this, early recognition, reporting, and intervention are essential in prevention of increased morbidity and mortality. Early recognition can be difficult for a number of reasons. Children with milder injuries generally are not brought to medical attention and may even be kept from those outside the immediate family until visible bruises or other surface injuries fade. Further, when care is sought, a misleading or deceptive history is almost always given (Table 6-8). If a plausible history of accidental injury is provided (as can be the case with more sophisticated abusive parents), abuse may go unsuspected. However, when emergency department physicians make it a general practice to disrobe children and perform a complete surface examination on all those who present with mild or minor trauma, the diagnosis of otherwise unsuspected abuse rises dramatically because of identification of suspicious physical findings on other areas of the body, especially those ordinarily covered by clothing. Because presenting signs and symptoms are often nonspecific (Table 6-9), recognition can be particularly challenging when the victim of mild to moderate inflicted trauma is a young infant and has no surface injuries or ones that are subtle and easily overlooked. Listlessness or lethargy, irritability or fussiness, vomiting (usually without diarrhea), low-grade fever, and vague complaints of trouble with breathing in infants with milder degrees of inflicted head injury can easily be interpreted as being due to early viral infection (Jenny and colleagues). Irritability due to pain from rib and metaphyseal fractures may be mistakenly diagnosed as due to colic or constipation (which may coexist due to stool withholding secondary to pain). Grunting respirations due to rib pain are likely to be attributed to early pulmonary disease such as bronchiolitis or pneumonitis. Relatively rapid dissipation of pain and tenderness (often within 2 to 5 days) in infants with nondisplaced fractures (due to their thick periosteal covering, which resists tearing and promotes prompt healing) can add to the diagnostic difficulty, particularly when presentation is delayed.

Hence diagnosis requires a high index of suspicion when infants, especially young infants, present with unex-

Table 6-9	Nonspecific Symptom Complexes as Modes of Presentation of Physical Abuse

Symptoms
Vomiting—especially without diarrhea
Anorexia, decreased interest in feeding
Irritability, lethargy—singly or alternating, with or without vomiting
Constipation with irritability
Tachypnea with irritability
Grunting respirations with irritability
Fever with irritability
Decreased tone, limpness
Stiffening or staring spells
Apparent life-threatening event
(All easily mistaken for symptoms of acute viral illness, especially in the very young infant)

Key Points in Evaluation
Ask if fussiness increases (or did increase) when baby is picked up, burped, moved, or with diaper change.
Meticulously inspect each square inch of skin and scalp in bright light and under a Wood's lamp.
Palpate each bone with special attention to posterior ribs and long bone metaphyses.
Dilate pupils and check fundi, consider ophthalmology consult.
Consider the following:
  Skeletal survey
  Head CT (unenhanced)
  Bone scan
  Blood work (complete blood cell count and differential with platelets, liver function tests, amylase, lipase, PT/PTT, coagulation profile)
  MRI (T_1 and T_2 weighted conventional or fast spin echo MRI with proton density or FLAIR sequences)

plained irritability and/or lethargy, with or without grunting respirations, and with vomiting without diarrhea. Unusual thoroughness in history taking and physical examination is a must. This includes asking if fussiness or irritability is or was worse with movement, on being picked up, or when held by the chest. The physical examination should include a meticulous surface assessment searching for faint bruises or petechiae including a Wood's lamp examination (see section on bruises); careful palpation of ribs and extremities for tenderness (with particular attention to posterior ribs and long bone metaphyses); and dilated retinoscopy, all of which can be revealing. When a history of pain on motion or bony tenderness is found or when subtle surface injuries are noted, a skeletal survey is indicated, perhaps followed by a bone scan (see sections on fractures later). Presence of metaphyseal and rib fractures and/or retinal hemorrhages mandate a head CT scan (because of their association with subdural hematomas).

Regardless of whether or not abuse is the source of crying and irritability, when presented with an infant with these complaints, physicians should *not* be quick to jump to the diagnosis of colic, constipation, or "normal fussiness." Rather, they should institute a thorough search for a precise cause including inflicted trauma in the differential. Once the cause is found, appropriate measures should be taken and clear recommendations should be given to parents with irritable infants as to what they can do to relieve the baby's symptoms as this may save some from future abuse.

Of note, there is a demonstrated increase in admissions for serious inflicted injury of infants around 6 to 8 weeks of age. This has been attributed to a normal increase in crying from birth to 6 to 8 weeks "unrelated to any underlying pathology." Whether there is an element of truth in the latter claim is unclear. However, given the fact that many, if not most, young infants admitted with serious

inflicted trauma have evidence of prior painful injuries, often of differing ages, it is likely that the true cause of their crying went undetected. This could be due to the fact that no prior care was sought or because when sought, signs of tenderness had abated, symptoms were nonspecific, and the exact cause was not assiduously sought and was therefore missed.

The increasing incidence of severe and fatal cases of physical abuse noted over the past decade by physicians in the field has led to an effort to detect identifiable risk factors that might be predictive of fatal outcome (Starling). The majority of perpetrators of such abuse who have been studied were severely abused themselves as children. Poverty, unemployment, a long history of family violence, drug and alcohol abuse, and adolescent parenthood were common threads. Fathers and paramours are by far the most common perpetrators, responsible for up to 58% of the cases of severe and fatal beatings, followed by babysitters in up to 21% and mothers in up to 13%. Crying and toilet training accidents were the most common triggering events. Victims frequently had histories or evidence of prior suspicious injuries, often of a series of injuries of increasing severity, before the final beating. Mothers are more likely to be the perpetrators of death by suffocation and neglect.

The diagnosis of inflicted injury is established on the basis of a constellation of factors including historical, physical, and behavioral observations. Approaching the case with an open mind, obtaining a thorough present and past medical and psychosocial history, and meticulous physical examination are crucial to ensuring accurate diagnosis of inflicted trauma and in preventing overdiagnosis of abuse. Important elements are detailed in Tables 6-10 and 6-11. Radiographs and laboratory studies are useful, not only in identifying and confirming injuries, but also in detecting evidence of occult trauma and ruling out other differential diagnostic possibilities.

Common Historical Red Flags

In many instances one or more of the following historical red flags may provide the first clue to abuse:
1. *Despite no history of injury, injury is found.*
2. *The history is incompatible with the type or degree of injury.* For example, the distribution of lesions or type of injury does not fit the mechanism reported; the history is consistent with a minor injury, but evidence of major trauma is found; or multiple injuries of differing ages are found for which no prior care has been sought or adequate explanation provided.
3. *The history of the way in which the injury occurred is vague,* or the parent has no idea how it happened.
4. *The history changes* each time it is told to a different health care worker, or even to the same worker who comes back with clarifying questions and asks the parent to remind them of "what you told me about what happened."
5. *The parents, when interviewed separately, give contradictory histories.*
6. *The history is not credible.* The child may be said to have done something developmentally impossible (e.g., having climbed and fallen when he or she cannot even sit).
7. *No history is reported of changes in behavior in an infant or child who has older injuries of differing ages that would have caused severe pain.*

| Table 6-10 | History Guidelines for Suspected Physical Abuse | | | |

GENERAL GUIDELINES	HISTORY OF PRESENT ILLNESS	PAST MEDICAL HISTORY	PSYCHOSOCIAL HISTORY	BEHAVIORAL REVIEW OF SYSTEMS
Start with open-ended questions Follow up with specific clarifying questions If 2 parent figures present, try to take history from each separately and out of child's presence Child should be interviewed alone, if age and condition permit (questions should be nonleading and age appropriate) Where possible, quote questions and answers verbatim	• What brings you to see us? • Onset, course, specific symptoms, pertinent positives and negatives. • Who has been with the child during this time frame? • If irritability reported: Does it increase when picked up, with movement or during diaper changes? • Have bruises or other skin marks been noted? • If injury reported: What happened? When did it occur? Where did it occur? In what circumstances and position was child found? Was incident witnessed, and if so by whom? What kind of forces were involved? If a fall, what precipitated it, from what height, onto what surface, position on landing? If child ambulating, at what speed and what led to fall?	Pregnancy—Planned/ unplanned, wanted/ unwanted Emotional stresses during pregnancy Gravidity, parity, spontaneous/induced abortions Prenatal/perinatal/neonatal course/complications Prior child losses Well-child care—primary care provider(s), visits attended Immunization status If not up to date on visits/ immunizations, why? Growth and development Major medical problems Hospitalizations (where) Surgery (where) Injuries (where treated) Ingestions	Family: Living situation—housing, who lives in household Handling of major developmental hurdles (weaning, toilet training) Methods of discipline Caretakers when parents are not home Support systems Family stresses Parents/parent figures: Duration and quality of relationship History of their families of origin: Parental relationship(s) Quality of interaction/ nurturing of parent as child Methods of discipline Level of education/ employment History of drug or alcohol abuse History of psychiatric illness History of prior CPS involvement History of childhood physical or sexual abuse History of involvement with law enforcement, incarceration History of domestic violence	Nightmares/sleep difficulties Increased aggression Anxiety Depression Low self-esteem Withdrawal from social interaction Regression Increased activity/anxiety PTSD symptoms Phobias Change in appetite Self-abuse Decrease in academic performance/school failure Running away Drug/ETOH use Fire setting Animal abuse Involvement with the law
	MEDICAL REVIEW OF SYSTEMS			

ETOH, ethyl alcohol; PTSD, post-traumatic stress disorder.

| Table 6-11 | Physical Examination for Suspected Physical Abuse |

Vital signs
General appearance, demeanor
Nutritional status and growth parameters
Complete body surface examination
Palpation of each bone
Full general examination including the following:
  Head and scalp, including head circumference in infants
  Ears, nose, mouth (all mucosal surfaces), throat and dentition
  Cardiopulmonary examination
  Palpation of abdomen and serial re-examinations to assess for evolving signs of intra-abdominal injury
  Palpation of regional nodes
  Genitalia including inspection of urethral, vaginal, and anal orifices
Neurologic examination
Ophthalmologic examination including conjunctivae, sclerae, pupils, anterior chamber, and dilated retinoscopy
Developmental assessment

Miscellaneous Historical Red Flags

1. *A history or evidence of repeated visits* necessitated by "accidents" or injuries (often to a number of different facilities).
2. *A history or evidence of repeated fractures or old scars suggestive of prior inflicted injury.*
3. *A history of repeated ingestions.*

4. *Poor compliance with well-child care:* missed visits, immunization delay.

Behavioral/Interactional Red Flags

1. *A significant delay between the time of injury and the time of presentation often exists.*
2. *The parent may not show the degree of concern appropriate to the severity of the child's injury.*
3. *A pathologic parent-child interaction may be observed.* A parent demonstrates unusually rough/angry/impulsive behavior toward the child (yells, yanks, hits). A parent displays inappropriate expectations of child ("sit still," i.e., don't explore, "watch your brother"). A parent is often clearly unaware of the child's needs and insensitive to behavioral cues (crying with hunger, dirty diaper, wants to be held or comforted).

Few victims of physical abuse are brought in with a chief complaint of abuse. Most present with a chief complaint of an accidental injury or of an unrelated (cold, rash) or somewhat peripheral (lethargy, irritability) chief complaint (see Tables 6-8 and 6-9). Whenever the physician's suspicion is aroused by historical or observational findings, he or she (or a designated social worker) should obtain a detailed psychosocial history, seeking more information concerning the family's current living situation, stresses, and emotional support systems. Particular attention should be paid to recent family crises including personal (ill health, job loss, separation) and environmental (pending eviction, heat or utilities discontinued) crises; degree of isolation (no family or social supports, no phone); and prior problems with family violence, mental health, alcohol, or drugs. Answers to questions about methods of discipline and parental reactions to common triggering events such as prolonged crying, toilet training accidents, and stubborn behavior can be most illuminating, as can answers to questions about how they felt when they learned of the baby's pregnancy, when they first saw the baby, and what the baby is like (see Table 6-10). Although a detailed history takes time, it can be invaluable in facilitating accurate diagnosis, individualizing care, arranging appropriate family supports, and assisting CPS and law enforcement in their investigations. This and the medical history should be obtained in a supportive, nonjudgmental manner because aggressive interrogation will only serve to alienate the parent, limiting the value of the data obtained.

During the evaluation one should bear in mind that the person who has brought the child in for care may not be the abuser, and that many parents of abused children truly want help, whether they have been directly abusive or unable to protect their child from abuse. In many cases a parent may have been unaware that abuse was occurring, had suspicions but no confirmation, suspected on some level but did not want to believe that abuse could be occurring, or was too fearful of an abusive mate to come in earlier. In some cases an abusive parent accompanies the child and the nonabusive parent in an effort to keep up a good front and to prevent disclosure. In occasional instances the nonabusive parent may actually be supportive of the abuser's "harsh discipline."

Table 6-12 presents additional historical and behavioral clues that may become apparent in the course of interviewing the parents/caretakers of an abused child.

In approaching abused children, one must recognize that their parents are the only ones they know; that they love them and, usually, their other caretakers; and that at times, they may even feel in some way deserving of abuse. Young children rarely acknowledge that a parent or other caretaker has injured them, especially when questioned directly, often because they have been threatened or sworn to secrecy. If they can be interviewed alone (when old enough to give a history) in pleasant, nonthreatening surroundings, helpful historical information can often be obtained by means of nonleading questions and through drawings or play. In some cases in which the perpetrator

is a paramour of the mother who has not been around long, the child may be more willing to disclose, especially when he or she can honestly be reassured that they will have no further contact with him and is, therefore, safe from further assault.

It is also important to remember is that siblings, especially older siblings, can often provide useful historical information. Strong consideration should be given to interviewing them as soon as possible after abuse is identified. Their histories can be quite helpful, and they may prove to be good witnesses in subsequent hearings.

Physical Findings and Patterns of Injury

Surface Marks

The most obvious manifestations of physical abuse are those visible on the surface of the skin. They include bruises, welts, scars, abrasions, lacerations, tourniquet and bite marks, and burns. Despite differing opinions on the appropriateness or inappropriateness of physical methods of discipline, there is a good rule of thumb in distinguishing the boundary between discipline and abuse: Discipline does not inflict significant pain and does *not* cause physical injury or leave marks.

All external signs of trauma found should be carefully documented in writing, on body diagrams, and in photographs (preferably with a ruler and color wheel in the frame).

Bruises, Welts, and Scars
Bruises are the most common clinical finding in cases of physical abuse, seen in up to 75% of victims, and their presence should prompt a search for other deeper injuries. Inflicted bruises and welts may be the result of direct blows or of impacts with firm objects when pushed, shoved, thrown, or swung into them. They frequently involve more than one plane of an extremity, the torso, and/or head, and are often found in places that are unusual sites for accidental injury (see "Differential Diagnosis of Inflicted Injuries versus Findings Caused by Accident or Illness" later). These include the back, buttocks, upper arms, thighs, abdomen, perineum, and feet, all of which are typically covered by clothing and, thereby, hidden from public view (Figs. 6-1 and 6-2). When due to slaps or blows, these locations suggest some forethought in site selection. Among other unusual sites are the face (including the periorbital area and eyelids, cheeks, sides of the forehead, lateral aspects of the chin and mouth); ears; neck; hands; calves; and volar or ulnar (defensive posture) aspects of the forearms. Being more exposed, bruises in these areas may reflect greater impulsivity on the part of the perpetrator.

Bruises involving the head, face, mouth, neck, and ears (Fig. 6-3) are seen in a substantial percentage of physical abuse victims: approximately 50% of infants and 38% of toddlers. Subgaleal hematomas and contusions and petechiae involving the scalp may be the result of direct blows or impacts against hard surfaces. On occasion they are caused by forceful hair pulling (Fig. 6-4). Slaps of moderate force may produce diffuse bruising with petechiae (Fig. 6-5). More forceful slaps leave handprint marks, consisting of petechial outlines of the fingers of the perpetrator as maximal capillary distortion occurs at the margins of the fingers on impact (Fig. 6-6). Periorbital and eyelid

Table 6-12	Historical and Behavioral Clues from Caretakers' Demeanor during Interview

Lack of affect in describing the baby (does not glow, even when asked about when he or she first saw the baby following delivery)
Relative lack of concern regarding severity/extent of injury
Negative comments regarding the child's (especially an infant's) behavior, appearance, or personality:
   "She has a bad temper." "She's mean." "He's fussy, cries all the time." "She's greedy, eats like a pig, is never satisfied," "He likes to irritate me."
Betrayal of unrealistic expectations:
   "She should know better than to cry when I have a headache," "when I want to watch NASCAR"
Openly more invested in spouse/significant other.

NOTE: Perpetrators often disclose a watered-down version of what they did when abusing the child when asked what they think might have happened to cause the injuries found.

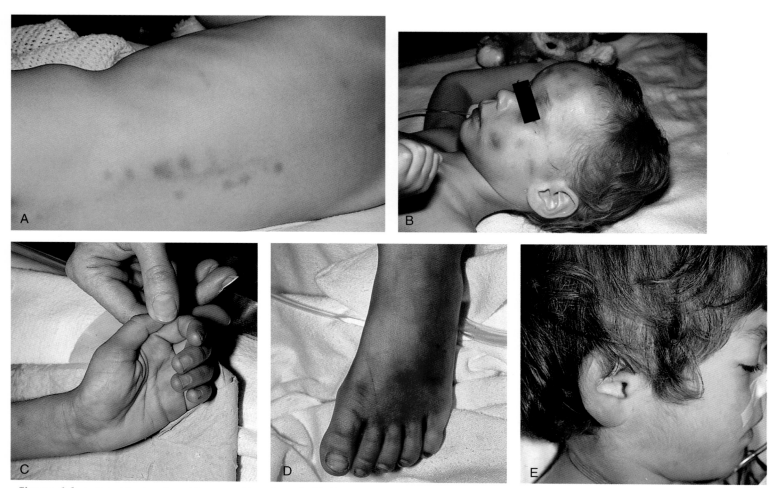

Figure 6-1. Inflicted bruises found in unusual locations. **A,** Multiple ecchymoses are evident over the back and upper chest of this child who presented in a poorly nourished condition. **B,** The same patient with multiple bruises involving differing planes of the face and forehead. Note the fingerprint bruise on the cheek. **C** and **D,** This child had severe contusions over the hands and feet, which were inflicted with a ruler. **E,** He also had a markedly swollen and contused ear and patches of hair loss where the perpetrator had pulled out hanks of hair. Both boys had been removed from abusive mothers and placed with maternal grandmothers who had physically abused their daughters in the past.

bruises in the absence of evidence of an overlying fore-head hematoma or an accidentally incurred frontal skull fracture are likely to be inflicted and caused by direct blows to the face (Fig. 6-7A and B).

Surface injuries involving more than one plane of the head or face are highly suspicious for abuse. It is also important to recognize that contusions of the head, face, and ears are often associated with underlying intracranial injury, especially in infants. Such injuries are indicative of severe loss of control and intent to harm on the part of the perpetrating caregiver and have serious implications for the child's future safety unless he or she is removed from contact with the offender.

Round impressions of the thumb and forefinger may be seen on the cheeks, sides of the forehead, or sides of the chin in infants and young children who have been grasped and forcefully squeezed (see Fig. 6-1B). Similar fingerprint bruises may be noted on the upper arms, trunk, abdomen, or extremities where the infant has been grasped and held tightly while being shaken or forcibly restrained (see Fig. 6-13). More elongated grab marks may also be found on the extremities (Fig. 6-8). When round bruises similar to fingerprint marks are found in a linear pattern, they may be fingertip impressions or knuckle marks from punching (see Fig. 6-2C and D). In the latter instance, one may note partial central clearing of the rounded contusions. Finger-prints or grab marks located on the thighs, especially the medial surfaces, should prompt careful examination for

signs of concurrent sexual abuse. Pinching produces apposed fingerprint marks with a shape that may be reminiscent of a butterfly or figure-of-eight. These may be seen singly or in rows, usually on clothing-covered areas (Fig. 6-9).

Attempted smothering, choking, or severe and pro-longed thoracic compression may produce showers of petechiae over the shoulders, neck, and face (Fig. 6-10 A-D). The oral and conjunctival mucosa may be involved as well and should be carefully inspected. If a hand or other object is held forcefully over the nose and mouth of a child with erupted teeth, imprint bruises, abrasions, or lacerations left by the teeth on the labial mucosa may be noted in addition to facial petechiae (see Fig. 6-10E). When strangulation is the mechanism, neck bruises are usually visible (see Fig. 6-10B). These petechiae may range from florid to faint and may be especially subtle when there has been a delay in seeking care. They can be mis-taken for a rash if the examiner fails to check for blanch-ing. Failure to detect such lesions has resulted in a number of subsequent deaths.

Bruises are often seen over the curvature of the buttocks and across the lower back following severe spankings, whether with a hand or an object such as a paddle, belt, or hairbrush (Fig. 6-11). When linear marks from fingers, belt, or brush edges are seen, these tend to be horizontally or diagonally oriented (see Fig. 6-11B). However, in some cases a linear pattern of petechiae may be noted on either

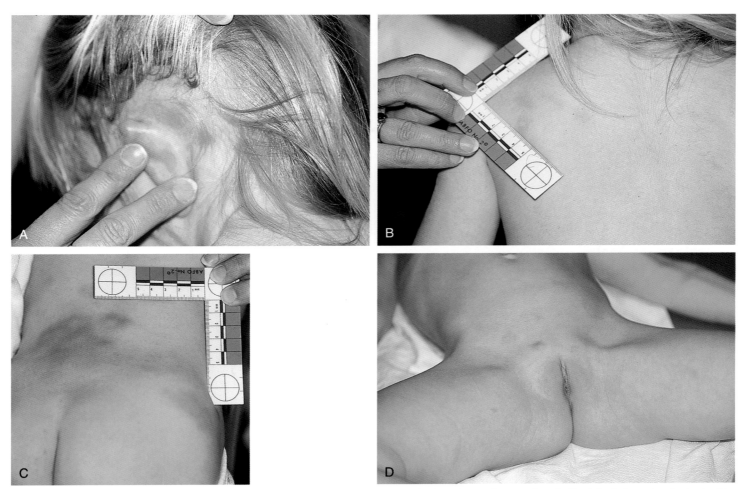

Figure 6-2. This toddler, the victim of repetitive beatings by her mother's boyfriend while the mother was hospitalized, had **A,** postauricular bruising, **B,** a line of fingerprint or knuckle bruises over the posterior left shoulder, and **C,** extensive bruising over the lower back in a pattern suggestive of knuckle marks, along with a large contusion over the right iliac crest. **D,** Rounded bruises over the lower abdomen and mons pubis may represent grab or punch marks. Some of her injuries were due to impacts against stairs and furniture when thrown forcibly by the perpetrator. Other injuries included a healing left radius fracture, refracture through a healing distal clavicle fracture, and evidence of old central nervous system trauma (see Figs. 6-26, 6-39B, and 6-55).

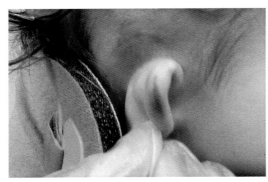

Figure 6-3. Ear bruising. This infant was hit so forcibly on the side of his head that he has an impression bruise on his scalp in the shape of his external ear. The linear bruise over the top rim of his ear is the result of capillary distortion caused by compression between the impacting hand and the child's skull.

side of the gluteal crease (see Fig. 6-11C). Despite their vertical orientation, these are also the result of forceful horizontal blows across tightly tensed glutei, as when the blows are delivered, the involved sites are closely apposed along the crease and thus are subject to maximal capillary distortion on impact.

Bruises involving the abdominal wall below the rib cage and above or anterior to the pelvic girdle are rarely seen with accidental injury and are relatively unusual in cases of abuse (see Figs. 6-2D and 6-13). This is because of the great flexibility of the abdominal wall and its padding with adipose tissue. In fact, many children with inflicted intra-abdominal injuries have little or no cutaneous evidence of trauma over the abdomen, although in some cases their absence may be due to delayed presentation. When abdominal bruises are present, they are indicative of forceful grabbing or pinching or of forceful blunt impact (such as a punch or kick). In these cases, abuse should be strongly suspected and evidence of internal injury should be sought (see Abdominal and Intrathoracic Injuries, later, and Fig. 6-57).

In many instances the surface marks are recognizable imprints of the edge of a weapon used to inflict the injury because the edge causes maximum capillary deformation on impact. Those most commonly seen are looped-cord marks, caused by whipping the child with a looped electrical cord (Fig. 6-12A and B), belt and belt-buckle marks (see Fig. 6-12C, D, and F; see also Fig. 6-11B), and switch marks (see Fig. 6-10E and F); but almost any implement can be used including hairbrushes (see Fig. 6-11B), shoes (see Fig. 6-12G and H), kitchen utensils (see Fig. 6-12I), and chains (see Fig. 6-12J).

The size, nature, and rate of healing of bruises depend on the amount of force applied; the firmness and shape of the impacting object or surface; and the duration of

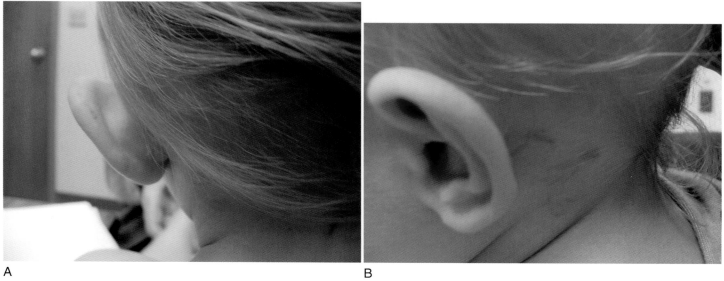

A   B

Figure 6-4. Subgaleal hematomas. This toddler, in the care of mother's paramour, was reportedly well until about 45 minutes after being put to bed, when she "woke up screaming." On being picked up, she was noted to have a "mushy head." At the hospital, she was found to have large bilateral sub-galeal hematomas, with surface bruising and petechiae over the occipito-parietal scalp. She also had semicircular bruises behind her left ear consistent with fingernail marks. Skull radiographs and a head CT scan showed no evidence of skull fracture or intracranial injury. Further examination revealed extensive bruising and lacerations of the introitus consistent with sexual assault (see Fig. 6-90B). The perpetrator apparently grabbed her by her hair and by her head, leaving fingernail marks while in the process of assaulting her. Her hair was pulled so forcibly that the scalp was pulled away from the skull, leading to the extensive subgaleal bleeding, which continued to expand over the ensuing 72 hours. **A,** Thinning of the hair from hair loss and bruising of the scalp are evident, and the subgaleal hematoma over her left temporal area is so large that it is pushing her external ear out laterally. **B,** Curvilinear marks behind her left ear are fingernail impressions.

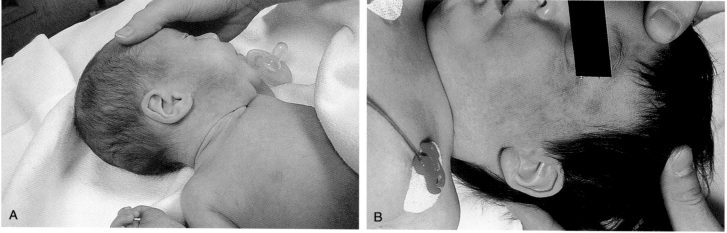

A   B

Figure 6-5. Facial slap marks. **A,** Diffuse facial bruising and petechiae seen over the side of the face and head of this 3-week-old infant were the result of repeated slaps by his father, a paranoid schizophrenic who had stopped taking his medication. He acknowledged slapping his son to make him cry, after which he would give him his bottle, the purpose being to teach him to cry when hungry. The baby also had metaphyseal chip fractures due to forced hyperextension of the knees to the point of screaming because "his muscles were tight" and "needed to be loosened up." **B,** This older infant has even more extensive petechiae and bruises that were tender on palpation.

impact, as well as on the degree of skin thickness, its vascularity and depth, elasticity, and adipose padding of the underlying subcutaneous tissue. Hence the initial appearance of bruises and the time it takes for them to resolve vary widely. Superficial bruises appear almost immediately and resolve more quickly than deeper contusions. The latter may not discolor the overlying skin for days and may take up to 2 weeks to resolve. Bruises of the face and perineum, where the skin is more loosely attached to underlying soft tissues and where blood vessels are less well supported, also appear early. Furthermore, the evolution of bruises in terms of color change is also variable. Although red, blue, and purple are more typical of fresh bruises, these colors can persist in some cases until resolution. Yellow, green, and brown are more characteristic of older bruises but can be seen relatively early in superficial

bruises. Hence it is difficult to determine precisely the ages of ecchymotic lesions and to be certain that bruises of differing colors are truly of different ages. One can only say that they appear fresh or old. However, if tenderness, swelling, and/or fresh overlying abrasions are present, one can be more confident that the lesions are new.

Some additional considerations regarding inflicted bruises warrant mention. In many cases of abuse, surface bruises and petechiae are faint or even imperceptible to the naked eye. This may be because they are early in their evolution or it may be the result of fading due to delay in seeking care. *In cases in which blows or impacts involving surface tissues also cause severe internal bleeding in the head, chest, or abdomen, bruises may be delayed in forming, may never appear, or may be subtle in their appearance.* This stems from the intense cutaneous vasoconstriction that occurs

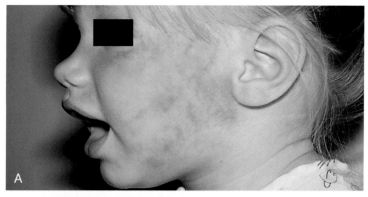

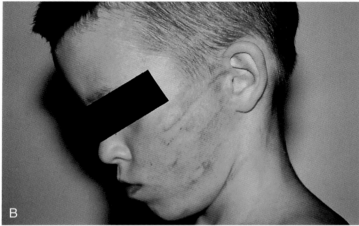

Figure 6-6. Hand prints. **A** and **B**, These children were slapped so forcefully that the outlines of their abuser's fingers are clearly evident.

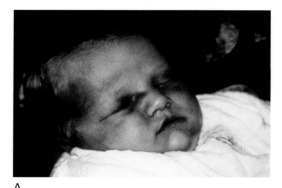

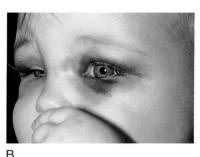

Figure 6-7. **A,** Bilateral black eyes are seen in this 12-day-old baby. His father, who was well-to-do, well dressed and sophisticated, reported that he had fallen on the stairs while holding the baby in a football hold and that, in the fall, the baby hit the steps face first with father landing on top of him. Bruises involving multiple planes of the face, the absence of an associated forehead hematoma or frontal fracture, and the presence of an occipital fracture consistent with impact against a hard surface (not the father's chest) belied this story. Nevertheless, abuse was not suspected, and the baby was sent home. He returned 6 weeks later in extremis with massive intracranial injury and died. On this occasion, the father said he had found the infant choking and gasping for breath and had picked him up and shaken him to revive him. **B,** This infant's bilateral black eyes are the result of direct blows to the periorbital areas bilaterally.

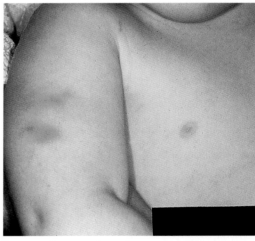

Figure 6-8. Linear finger grab marks are seen on the outer aspect of this infant's upper arm. A thumb print bruise was present medially. (Courtesy Dr. Kent Hymel, INOVA Fairfax Hospital for Children, Falls Church, Va.)

in response to shock, which severely restricts the flow of red blood cells to injured surface capillaries, thus minimizing their extravasation. Appreciation of the potential subtlety of bruises and petechial lesions (which may provide the only clinical clue that abuse has occurred and that other injuries may be present) enhances recognition of the importance of taking special care in performing the surface examination and checking the oral mucosa. It is also important to remember that petechiae may be mistaken for a fine macular rash if the clinician does not check to see if the lesions blanch or not. Recent research (Vogeley) has demonstrated that Wood's lamp examination may increase the visibility of faint or subtle bruises and can reveal bruising that is invisible under regular light (Fig. 6-13).

When bruising is severe, deep, and extensive, underlying muscle breakdown may occur, resulting in myoglobinuria (Fig. 6-14). When severe, this may precipitate renal failure unless the risk is recognized, appropriate tests performed, and aggressive treatment measures are instituted.

Although bruises are relatively easy to see in victims with fair skin, they can be difficult to appreciate in children with darkly pigmented skin unless extra care is taken. Bruises may be further obscured when such children have dry skin with a fine surface scale, sometimes termed "ashy skin." Application of baby oil or a moisturizing cream clears the "ashy" surface, making lesions more readily visible. Small scalp lesions in children with thick dark hair can easily elude detection unless the scalp is inspected inch by inch for evidence of contusions, abrasions, and sometimes hair loss. Finally, all infants with bruises and all children between 1 and 2 to 3 years of age with multiple bruises suspicious for abuse should have a skeletal survey to search for clinically occult fractures and blood work to screen for occult intra-abdominal injury.

Clearly documenting the size, color, and configuration of bruises is important in potential abuse cases. This is best done with photographs that have a ruler and a standard color wheel in the frame, thereby ensuring that the lesion's true dimensions and color can be determined even

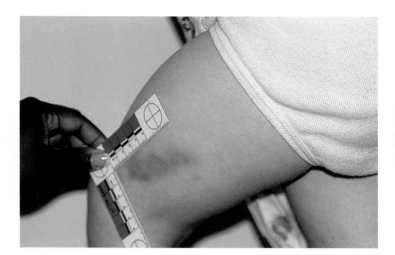

Figure 6-9. Pinch marks. A row of fading bruises secondary to pinching, used as a method of discipline by his mother, is seen on the lateral aspect of the thigh of this preschool-age boy. More than a year later, his sister nearly died of multiple stab wounds also inflicted by their psychotic and delusional mother (see Fig. 6-16).

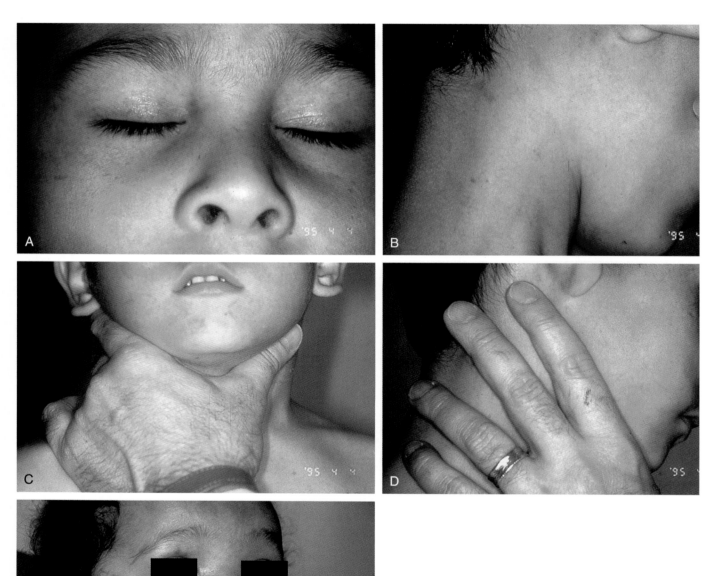

Figure 6-10. **A-D,** Petechial lesions secondary to choking. **A,** Numerous petechiae are seen over this boy's face. **B,** Linear marks noted on the side of his neck correspond with the hand and finger placement demonstrated in **C** and **D.** The boy was choked to a point of near-unconsciousness by his mother's boyfriend for tracking grass onto a freshly vacuumed carpet. **E,** Central facial petechiae were present bilaterally in this infant. The perpetrator confessed to holding his hand over her mouth and nose and squeezing her cheeks with thumb and forefinger to stop her crying. (Courtesy Dr. Kent Hymel, INOVA Fairfax Hospital for Children, Falls Church, Va.)

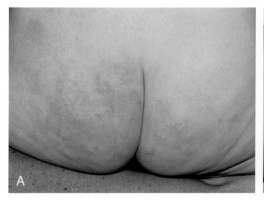
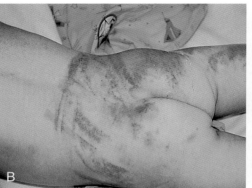
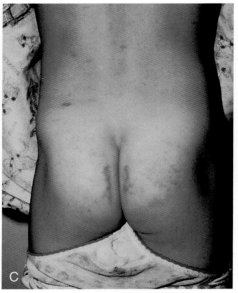

Figure 6-11. Buttock bruises. **A,** At first glance, this toddler appeared to have a diaper rash, but on closer inspection the lesions were found to be petechiae produced by a severe spanking. **B,** The severe contusions of the buttocks and lower back seen in this child were inflicted by hand, hairbrush, and belt. **C,** A linear pattern of petechial hemorrhages is seen on either side of the gluteal cleft in this boy who was subjected to repeated rapid-fire blows across the gluteal crease.

if there are problems with exposure or photographic technique. Despite the difficulties in determining the ages of bruises, finding old scars that reflect prior use of a weapon in a child with acute injuries can be helpful in identifying abuse or confirming prior abuse (see Fig. 6-12B).

To avoid errors in diagnosis, children who present with multiple bruises in unusual locations that do not reflect use of a weapon should be thoroughly examined to check for evidence of an underlying coagulopathy, and screening coagulation studies should be performed before arriving at a final diagnosis.

Abrasions and Superficial Lacerations. Abrasions are also seen in abuse victims, though less commonly than bruises. In some cases outline bruises of forcefully applied weapons have an overlying abraded or even lacerated surface (see Fig. 6-14). Abrasions also may result from friction on impact with a hard surface or from being dragged across a carpet or other rough surface (Fig. 6-15A). Fingernails can be dug into the skin on grabbing the child or holding him or her down, or they can be used to poke at the skin, leaving small straight or arc-shaped abrasions or superficial lacerations (Fig. 6-15B and see Fig. 6-4B). They can also be raked across the skin, leaving parallel linear abrasions. Simple lacerations, especially of the scalp, face, and upper extremities, while usually accidental in origin, can be the result of inflicted blows or impacts. Child abuse experts suspect that in many such cases a plausible history is provided, and the injury is classed as accidental. Here again, the practice of performing a complete surface examination on all children with minor wounds can provide clues that abuse may be the actual cause.

Slashing knife wounds and deep stab-induced lacerations are fortunately rare and are usually inflicted by caretakers with severe mental disorders (Fig. 6-16).

Strangulation, Restraint, and Tourniquet Injuries. Strangulation and restraint marks result from attempts to hang; choke; or, in some instances, tie the child to a crib, bed, or chair. Abraded or blistered circumferential ligature marks, often reflecting the surface pattern of the type of restraint used, are seen in these cases, due to friction either in forceful tightening or in the child's struggle to get free (Fig. 6-17). When extremities are involved, distal edema and often early signs of skin breakdown are seen

(see Fig. 6-17B). On rare occasions involving tight and prolonged tourniquet application, severe ischemia results in gangrene (see Fig. 6-16C). In these unusual cases the perpetrator is likely to be psychotic, a drug addict, or both.

Bite Marks. Bite marks can be another manifestation of physical abuse. Lesions tend to be oval or semicircular. The impressions of the incisal surfaces may be variably clear, depending on the force applied and the age of the bite. Suction petechiae may be noted centrally in some fresh lesions. In children in whom the resulting imprint is distinct, it is as identifiable as a fingerprint, and its size enables the examiner to clearly distinguish between the bite of another child and that of an adult, the latter being greater than 3 cm in diameter (Fig. 6-18A-C). Each bite mark should be carefully photographed in its entirety, and then photos should be taken perpendicular to the plane of the imprint of each arch, with a ruler or measuring tape in each photo. Such evidence can enable a forensic dentist to make a model of the perpetrator's dentition, which can specifically reveal his or her identity. Ultraviolet photography can disclose a clear image of bite marks weeks or months after all surface marks have disappeared (Fig. 6-18D). This has proved highly useful in identifying abusers of children who have a past history of being bitten but who have no acute lesions. Finally, if the patient has not bathed or washed the bite wound since it was inflicted, swabbing the area with a saline-soaked, cotton-tipped applicator is indicated to obtain a sample of the perpetrator's saliva. Crime laboratory analysis of this material can positively identify the perpetrator.

Burns. Burns are generally accidental, but they are also a fairly common mode of abusive injury. Although there is no one pattern that is absolutely pathognomonic for abuse, dip burns, back and buttock burns in infants and toddlers, burns over the dorsum of the hand, and deep contact burns with a clear imprint of the hot surface are highly suspect. Here, too, inconsistency of history, the pattern of injury, and the delay in seeking medical attention are valuable clues.

Immersion scalds or dip burns are among the most common forms of inflicted burns. Typical patterns include symmetrical burns of both hands or both feet in a

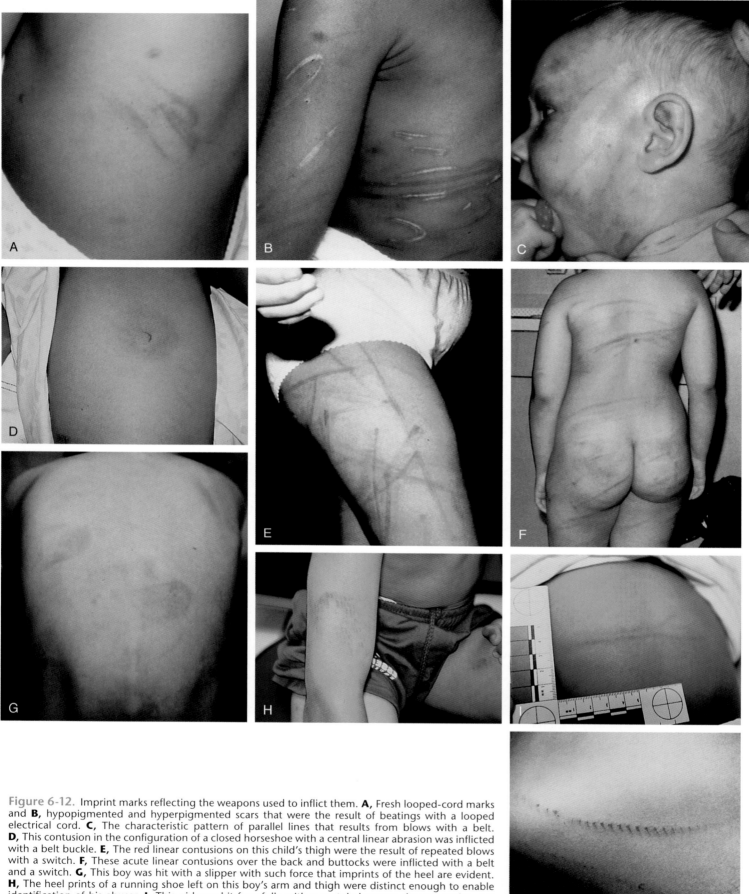

Figure 6-12. Imprint marks reflecting the weapons used to inflict them. **A,** Fresh looped-cord marks and **B,** hypopigmented and hyperpigmented scars that were the result of beatings with a looped electrical cord. **C,** The characteristic pattern of parallel lines that results from blows with a belt. **D,** This contusion in the configuration of a closed horseshoe with a central linear abrasion was inflicted with a belt buckle. **E,** The red linear contusions on this child's thigh were the result of repeated blows with a switch. **F,** These acute linear contusions over the back and buttocks were inflicted with a belt and a switch. **G,** This boy was hit with a slipper with such force that imprints of the heel are evident. **H,** The heel prints of a running shoe left on this boy's arm and thigh were distinct enough to enable identification of his abuser. **I,** This girl was hit forcefully with a spatula because she was acting out while her mother was trying to prepare dinner. **J,** This boy was struck with a chain, leaving a clear imprint of the links.

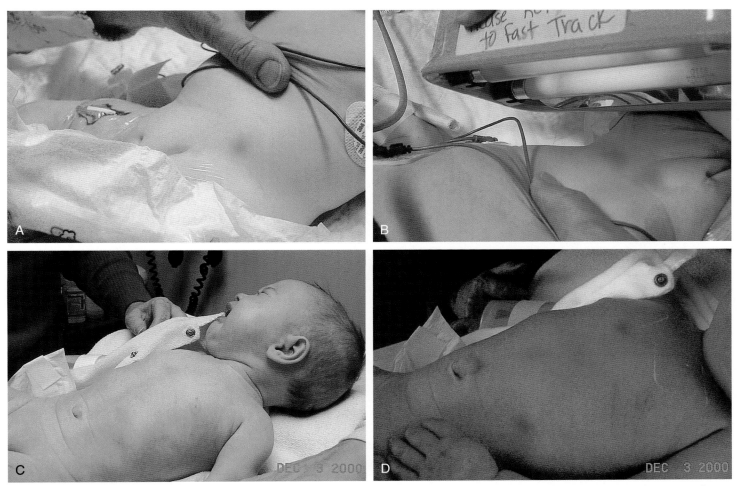

Figure 6-13. Wood's lamp enhancement of visualization of bruises. **A,** Medics were called to the home of this 2-month-old baby with a report of apnea. Examination and CT revealed bilateral retinal hemorrhages, subdural hematoma with edema, and loss of gray/white matter differentiation. The only external signs of trauma were three fingerprint-like bruises, two on the back and one on the lower abdomen seen here. **B,** Viewed from the opposite side under Wood's lamp, the lower abdominal bruise is seen to be even larger in extent, and a suprapubic bruise that was invisible in regular light is revealed. **C,** This 5-month-old baby presented with a history of decreased responsiveness following a crying/choking spell after which she vomited. Subtle surface bruises were missed, and she was discharged with a diagnosis of gastroesophageal reflux. She returned a few hours later with persistent vomiting and increasing lethargy. At the second visit, multiple faint bruises were noticed over the chest, abdomen, back, buttocks, thighs, and scalp. Bruises over the chest and abdomen are barely visible in regular light. **D,** Under Wood's lamp they are seen with much greater clarity. Other injuries included an occipital fracture with diastasis of the lambdoid suture, a posterior interhemispheric subdural hematoma (see Fig. 6-44), and a metaphyseal fracture of the distal radius seen in Figure 6-28B. (Courtesy Dr. Eva Vogeley, Children's Hospital of Pittsburgh, Pa.)

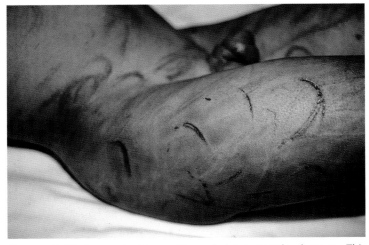

Figure 6-14. Severe bruising with underlying muscle damage. This toddler was covered from head to toe with severe looped cord contusions and lacerations. He had secondary myoglobinuria necessitating intensive care management to prevent renal failure.

stocking-glove distribution, with a sharp line of demarcation at the level of the water line (Fig. 6-19A); circumferential burns of the feet and lower legs along with burns of the perineum and flexor surfaces of the thighs are seen in children who are held under the axillae and knees and have their legs and bottoms dipped in scalding water (see Fig. 6-19B and C). If the child is forcibly held down in a sink or tub as it fills with scalding water, partial sparing of the palms, soles, and buttocks may be noted because these sites were pressed against the cooler sink or tub surface. Sparing of apposed skin surfaces in flexor creases may also be noted in these cases. Lower extremity/perineal burns and tub burns are typically inflicted following toileting accidents.

Despite claims to the contrary, immersion burns are rarely accidental. Table 6-13 shows the time required to produce a full-thickness burn in adult skin at different water temperatures. Although the time may be slightly shorter for a child, normal children would, if they accidentally put a hand or foot into water higher than 120° F, withdraw it in a fraction of a second after the tips of their fingers or toes made contact with the water,

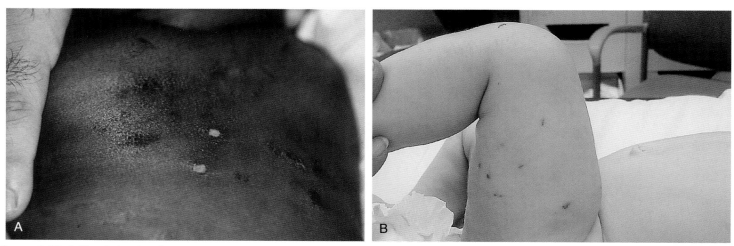

Figure 6-15. Inflicted abrasions/lacerations. **A,** A pattern of parallel abrasions that overlie ribs and vertebral bodies is seen on the back of this infant who was dragged over a carpet. The lesions are at least one to a few days old, and surface scabs have separated from two areas. A displaced spiral fracture of the right humerus, with marked soft tissue swelling and pain on motion, was also detected. **B,** This 3-month-old had numerous small linear and arc-shaped abrasions and superficial lacerations over both legs, consistent with fingernail marks. She also had many other bruises of varying hues, an occipital skull fracture, a posterior interhemispheric subdural hematoma, multiple metaphyseal chip fractures, and an abscessed nasal septal hematoma (see Fig. 6-25).

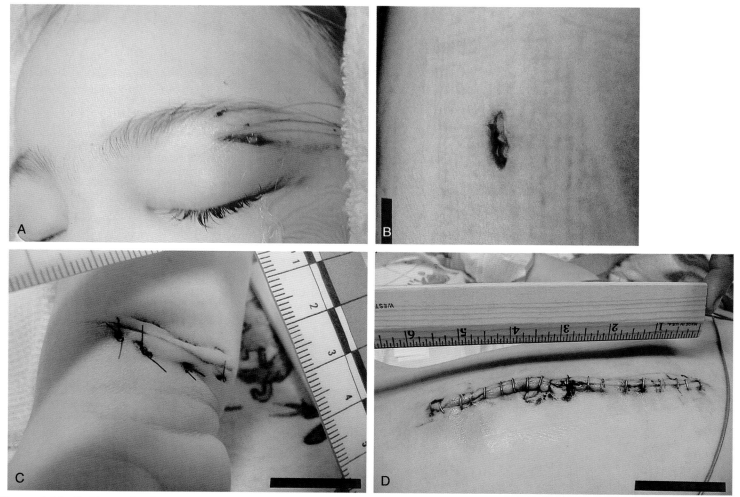

Figure 6-16. Slashing and stab wounds. This 22-month-old toddler was viciously and repeatedly attacked by her psychotic mother wielding a carving knife. She was left to die outside in the snow and, on rescue, was severely hypothermic and in shock. **A,** A superficial laceration is seen over the left eyelid. **B,** A deeper stab wound over the right flank penetrated into the subcutaneous tissue. **C,** A 3-cm wrist laceration sutured in the operating room had partially severed the median nerve. **D,** Eviscerated bowel projected through this 13-cm midabdominal laceration, which did not need to be extended for exploration. A through-and-through stomach laceration and a tear of the colonic mesentery were the only internal injuries found. Her throat had also been slit. Her brother is seen in Figure 6-9 a year earlier.

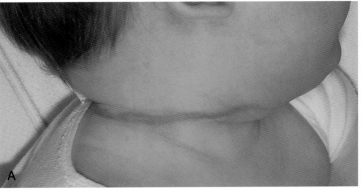

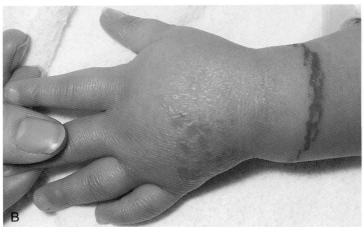

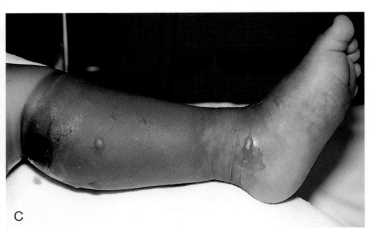

Figure 6-17. Strangulation, restraint, and tourniquet injuries. **A,** This circumferential cord burn was the result of an attempted strangulation. **B,** A deep, circumferential rope burn of the wrist with considerable edema and early skin breakdown of the hand is seen in this infant, who had been tied to the side rails of her crib. **C,** This toddler was brought in with severe skin, soft tissue, and muscle necrosis of his entire lower leg. His mother, a paranoid schizophrenic and heroin addict, reported finding a strap wrapped tightly around the leg below the knee on checking him in the morning. She did not know how it had gotten there and denied hearing his cries of pain, which surely lasted for hours.

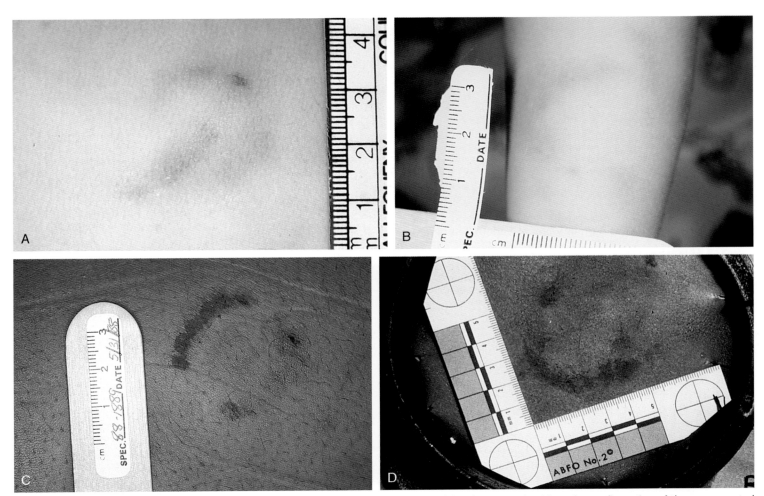

Figure 6-18. Bite marks. **A,** In this bite mark inflicted on a toddler by a much older child with mature dentition, the configuration of the upper central incisors is clearly seen (note the diastema or wide spacing between them). **B,** At first glance this fading bite mark could be mistaken for a bruise; however, on close inspection, the outline of the dental arch becomes evident. The size of the arch is clearly that of an adult or adolescent. **C,** A child-size bite inflicted on adolescent baby sitter illustrates difference in size of dental arch between children and adults. **D,** Viewed under ultraviolet light, bite marks that are weeks to months old can still be identified, even though the skin overlying the site has returned to normal. (**A, B,** and **C,** Courtesy Dr. Michael N. Sobel, Pittsburgh, Pa.; **D,** courtesy Dr. Thomas J. David, Atlanta.)

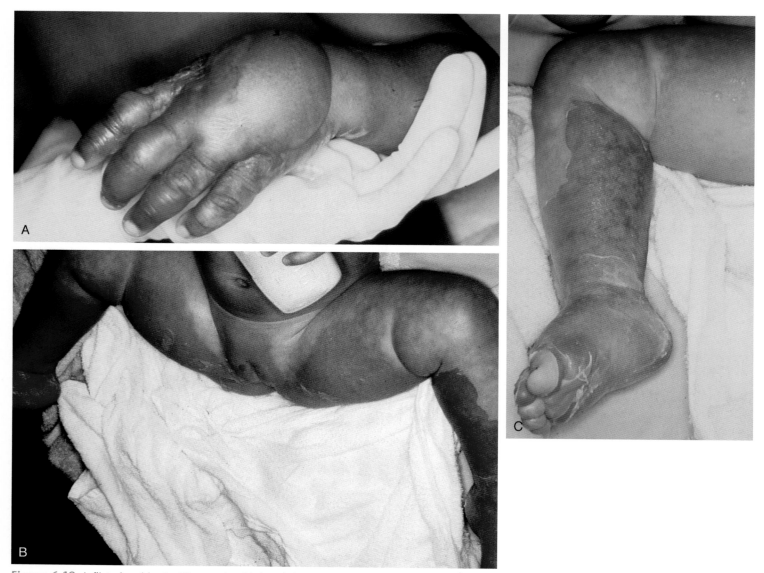

Figure 6-19. Inflicted scalds. **A,** After getting his hands into something he was not allowed to touch and making a mess, this child's hands were held down in hot water, resulting in severe second-degree dip burns. Note the sharp line of demarcation just above the wrist joint and the uniform depth of the burn. **B,** This toddler was dipped in a tub of scalding water while being held under the arms and knees, as an object lesson following a toileting accident. **C,** Close-up of severe second-degree burns of the foot and lower leg of the same child. (Courtesy Dr. Thomas Layton.)

Table 6-13	Duration of Exposure Required to Produce Full-Thickness Burn in Water at Various Temperatures

WATER TEMPERATURE	DURATION OF EXPOSURE
120°F	10 minutes
130°F	30 seconds
140°F	5 seconds
150°F	2 seconds
158°F	1 second

leaving them with only superficial burns of the tips of their fingers or toes.

Contact burns, sometimes termed *branding injuries,* show the imprint of the instruments used to inflict them and have a depth or degree of burn that is relatively even throughout. For example, one may see the full-thickness imprint of a hot iron or of the grill of a space heater or radiator cover (Fig. 6-20A to D). No child with normal sensation would remain in contact with these objects long enough to incur such a burn. Burns caused by holding a

hot hair dryer next to the skin leave an imprint of the screen that covers the heating element (see Fig. 6-20E), and those inflicted with a curling iron produce cigar-shaped, deep partial- or full-thickness imprints (see Fig. 6-20F). Most of these burns are found in unusual locations for accidental burns or over areas such as the extensor surfaces of the upper arms or legs, the back, chest, abdomen, or buttocks that are usually covered by clothing.

Inflicted *cigarette burns* usually leave sharply circumscribed, full-thickness imprints approximately 7 to 8 mm in diameter (5 mm if a slim cigarette is used). These are surrounded by a deep, partial-thickness halo blister and then a rim of superficial erythema (Fig. 6-21A). A thick, black eschar soon forms over the central, full-thickness burn. If this eschar is removed, one sees full-thickness skin loss. Subacutely, these lesions fill in with granulation tissue (see Fig. 6-21B), and on completion of healing the child is left with a deep, punched-out scar (see Fig. 6-21C). When a lit cigarette is held on the skin for only a fraction of a second, the resulting partial-thickness burn heals to form a uniform macular scar (see Fig. 6-21D).

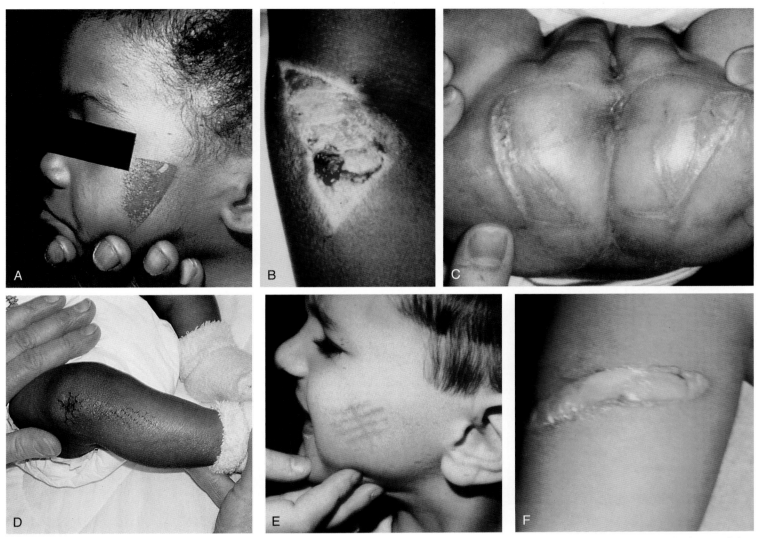

Figure 6-20. Contact burns or branding injuries. **A,** This child, who was acting out while his mother ironed, was punished when she held the tip of the iron against his cheek. **B,** A healing full-thickness burn in the shape of an iron was found when this boy's shirt was removed prior to his being given vaccine injections. He had been sent home after his first day in kindergarten with instructions not to return until he was caught up on his immunizations. **C,** These linear full-thickness burns were incurred when this 6-week-old infant was forced to sit on the hot grille of a space heater. The history given was that she had crawled over to the space heater, knocked it over, and then sat on it. **D,** Another infant presented with a history of irritability and a rash. The "rash" has a honeycomb configuration that matched that of a radiator cover in her home. She also had multiple fractures. **E,** These facial burns are the result of being branded with the grill of a hair dryer. The boy had been acting out while he was supposed to be getting ready for school and his mother was drying her hair. **F,** The hot wand of a curling iron leaves a cigar-shaped, partial- to full-thickness burn.

An unusual pattern of serrated first- and second-degree burns in parallel lines is made when the wheels of a butane lighter are heated and then pressed or run over the child's skin (Fig. 6-22).

Oral and Nasal Injuries

Occasionally, child abuse results in oral bruises and lacerations. One of the most typical patterns is bruising of the mucosa of the upper lip or the maxillary gingiva associated with tearing of the frenulum (Fig. 6-23). This can be produced when the perpetrator holds a hand tightly over the child's mouth to silence screaming and can be associated with facial petechiae (see Fig. 6-10E). Attempts to force a bottle or pacifier into a crying infant's mouth can also produce semicircular central gingival bruising or ulcerations. Force-feeding with a spoon may produce contusions or lacerations of the lips, floor of the mouth, and tongue. Gag marks at the corners of the mouth can be mistaken for cheilosis or for impetiginous or candidal

lesions. On rare occasions, bizarre intraoral lacerations are found (Fig. 6-24). Their usual mode of presentation is a complaint of spitting or vomiting up blood.

Even more rarely, oral injuries inflicted with fingers or utensils can result in penetration of the posterior pharynx. Most of these cases involve infants who may present with subcutaneous emphysema or with fever, drooling, and respiratory distress caused by a secondary retropharyngeal abscess (see Chapter 23).

In older children, punches; forceful slaps, especially with the back of a hand; or kicks can cause lip lacerations and contusions, frenulum and gingival tears (see Fig. 6-23), dental fractures, displacement injuries and avulsions, chin lacerations, and even mandibular fractures. These injuries can also stem from impact with hard surfaces when the child is violently pushed or thrown (see Chapter 20). Often these older victims present with a plausible history of accidental trauma and are not recognized as abuse victims. Sometimes the only clue that the injuries are abuse related is that the lesion is more severe than would be expected from the reported mechanism,

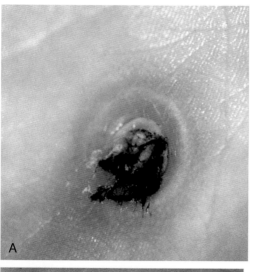

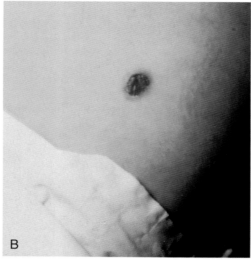

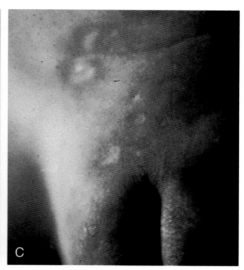

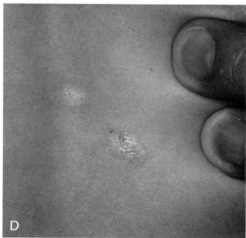

Figure 6-21. Cigarette burns. **A,** This sharply circumscribed burn was inflicted through the child's sock. The burn is perfectly circular with a blistered rim and a full-thickness punched-out center to which charred fabric adheres. The configuration did not fit the history that he had accidentally stepped on a cigarette. **B,** The eschar has separated from this older burn, revealing underlying granulation tissue. **C,** Punched-out scars of healed full-thickness cigarette burns. **D,** These uniform macular scars are the result of cigarette burns in which the coal is held against the skin for only a fraction of a second. (**D,** Courtesy Dr. Kent Hymel, INOVA Fairfax Hospital for Children, Falls Church, Va.)

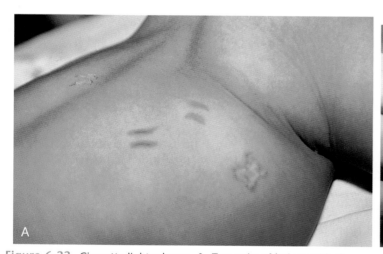

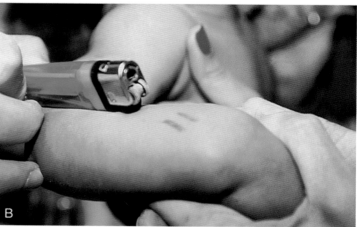

Figure 6-22. Cigarette lighter burns. **A,** Two pairs of lesions with the appearance of parallel serrated lines and a deep burn in the shape of a butterfly were found on examining this infant, who was brought to the emergency department for treatment of a rash. **B,** Astute deduction by a resident and social worker led to the discovery that heated cigarette lighter wheels had been used to inflict the burns. The full-thickness butterfly is the result of repeated application.

unusual reticence on the part of the child in providing the history, or a parent who appears determined not to let the child talk.

Nasal injuries may be due to direct blows or impacts. When mild, epistaxis may be the only manifestation. More severe injuries can result in fractures of the nasal bone or cartilage, septal deviation, and septal hematoma. The abused child with a septal hematoma is especially vulnerable to developing a septal abscess due to delay in

presentation, and affected infants tend to present with external nasal swelling, fever, and respiratory distress due to nasal obstruction (Fig. 6-25 and see Chapter 23).

Skeletal Injuries

Skeletal injuries are second only to bruises in terms of frequency in abused infants and children. Depending on

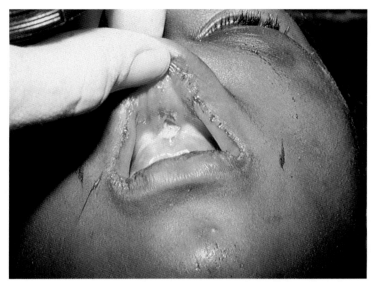

Figure 6-23. Frenulum tear. This badly beaten boy incurred a torn frenulum when his abuser tried to muffle his cries by forcibly holding his hand over the child's mouth. Note the facial bruises. (Courtesy Dr. Robert Hickey, Children's Hospital of Pittsburgh, Pa.)

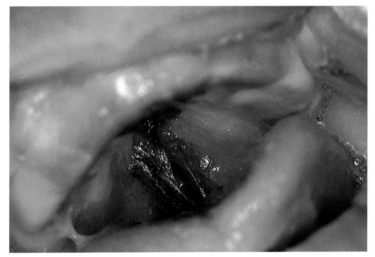

Figure 6-24. Inflicted palatal lacerations. This infant's soft palate was shredded by repeated stabs with a sharp object. He presented with a complaint of spitting up blood and no history of trauma.

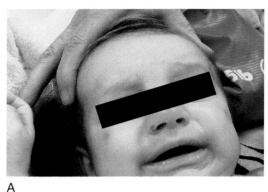

A

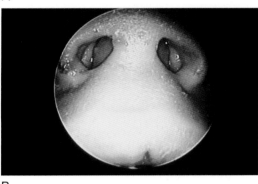

B

Fig. 6-25. Abscessed nasal septal hematoma. This 3-month-old baby brought to the emergency department with complaints of fever and difficulty breathing was found to have **A,** a red swollen nose and **B,** erythematous bulging of the nasal septum bilaterally, obstructing her nasal passages. Note the small central lip laceration. She also had multiple bruises, fingernail abrasions (see Fig. 6-15B), an occipital skull fracture, a subdural hematoma, and multiple metaphyseal chip fractures.

the series reported, anywhere from 11% to 55% of abused children have fractures. Most involve infants younger than 1 year of age. Approximately 60% of inflicted fractures are seen in children younger than 18 months, and the vast majority occur before age 3 years. This contrasts sharply with the low incidence of accidental fractures in infants and toddlers. Often, fractures are clinically occult and in many, if not most, cases no history of trauma is provided. When a history of injury is given, it is often one of a minor mechanism (fall off a couch) that does not fit with radiographic findings. Furthermore, parents of abused children tend to minimize reports of pain, discomfort, and loss of function. The high frequency of inflicted fractures in the very young and their potential for clinical subtlety necessitate that examination of suspected abuse victims include careful palpation of all bones for tenderness, crepitus, or palpable callus, and that all children younger than 2 to 3 years of age (sometimes up to 5 years) undergo skeletal survey.

Diagnosis of inflicted fractures can be especially challenging in infants because nondisplaced rib and spiral

fractures, metaphyseal chip and buckle fractures, and periosteal stripping injuries have minimal swelling, even acutely, and heal with great rapidity, as is detailed later. Further, in infants a history of trauma is especially unlikely to be reported. Rather, the chief complaint may be of unexplained irritability or grunting respirations (due to rib pain) or the child may be brought in with a totally unrelated complaint such as a cold or a rash (see Table 6-9, Nonspecific Symptom Complexes as Modes of Presentation of Physical Abuse). Some present with a history of minor accidental injury (often when the infant has surface bruises), usually with a reported mechanism that does not fit the fracture pattern or severity. Furthermore, as healing is faster in the infant or young child (due to the thickness of the periosteum, which resists tearing, reducing risk of displacement, and due to its being richly invested with osteoblasts that facilitate healing), tenderness and pain on being picked up, or on motion, may abate within a few days. This is particularly true of rib and metaphyseal fractures, periosteal stripping injuries, and other nondisplaced fractures.

When presentation occurs after tenderness has disappeared but before radiographically visible signs of healing have developed, the diagnosis is likely to be missed. In these cases, when other findings raise suspicion, it is wise to obtain a second skeletal survey in 10 to 14 days. Fortunately, delay in presentation in many cases is great enough that signs of healing are noted. These include medullary sclerosis (Fig. 6-26), callus formation (Fig. 6-27, and see Figs. 6-29 and 6-31), and the presence of subperiosteal new bone (Fig. 6-27 and see Fig. 6-32). It should be noted that symmetrical thin rims of subperiosteal new bone (<2 cm in width) can be a normal finding in the long

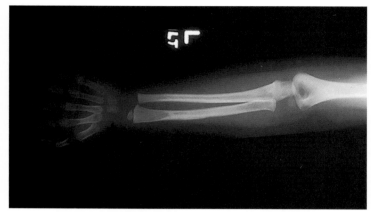

Figure 6-26. Medullary sclerosis seen in the left radius reflects the latter stages of healing. The fracture line is no longer visible, and the bone has remodeled. This is the child whose surface injuries are shown in Figure 6-2. She also had a refracture of an old clavicle fracture (see Fig. 6-39B) and evidence of prior head trauma on MRI (see Fig. 6-55).

bones in infants younger than 3 to 6 months of age. Because many fractures are often not brought to medical attention and are thus not immobilized, and given abuse tends to be repetitive, reinjury at sites of prior injury is not uncommon. When this occurs, it can result in unusually "exuberant" callus formation (Fig. 6-27 and see Fig. 6-31).

In evaluating skeletal injuries, one must bear in mind the child's developmental capabilities because accidental skeletal fractures are rare in infants who are not crawling or cruising and are quite uncommon in children younger than 3 years. Likewise, being knowledgeable regarding the mechanisms of injury and the magnitude of the forces that result in different fracture patterns makes it less likely to be misled by deceptive histories.

A paradigm of child abuse, since Caffey's first report in the late 1940s, is the finding of multiple, unexplained, often symmetrical fractures of varying ages involving the ribs and/or long bones of an infant or young child who has otherwise normal bones (see Fig. 6-27). Many of these fractures are clinically inapparent and therefore unsuspected. Metaphyseal fractures in infants and toddlers and rib fractures are also findings highly specific for abuse.

Metaphyseal Fractures

In infancy the cartilage of the chondro-osseous junctions adjacent to the metaphyses of long bones is poorly mineralized, making these structures the weakest points in long bones and predisposing to planar fractures through these sites when the bones are subjected to shearing forces. The periosteum overlying the epiphyseal cartilage is firmly adherent and extends close to the diaphysis to cover the subperiosteal bony collar. Thus when fractures do occur, their peripheral segments are thicker. In toddlers and older children, who have slower growth rates and a much greater amount of chondro-osseous mineralization, the same forces that produce metaphyseal fractures in infants are more likely to result in fractures through the physeal cartilage.

Metaphyseal fractures can be produced by the application of torsional or tractional forces, delivered when an extremity is grabbed and yanked. Frequently, they are caused by rapid, repetitive acceleration and deceleration as the extremities flail back and forth in the process of violent shaking. They also result from forced hyperextension of the knees. Metaphyseal fractures can be found in any long bone but are most commonly seen in the distal femur, proximal and distal tibias, and proximal humerus.

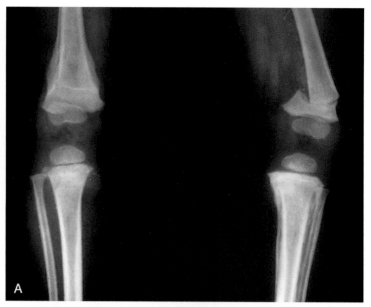

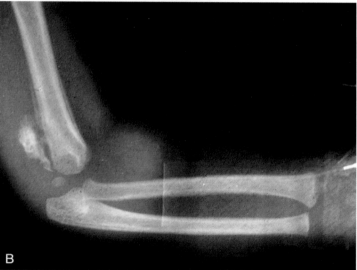

Figure 6-27. Multiple fractures of varying ages. This boy was seen with a chief complaint of refusing to bear weight. On examination, he was found to have marked swelling, tenderness, and crepitance over the distal left femur. **A,** Radiographic examination confirmed the presence of an acute transverse fracture and also revealed multiple additional fractures in various stages of healing. These include an old transverse fracture of the distal right femur with callus and subperiosteal new-bone formation that is in the process of remodeling. Relatively new metaphyseal chip fractures are seen involving the right proximal tibia, and vigorous subperiosteal new-bone formation encompasses the left tibia. **B,** On skeletal survey he was also found to have a healing fracture of the distal humerus with vigorous callus and subperiosteal new-bone formation and considerable soft tissue swelling. Note that the cortices of his long bones are of normal thickness. No care had ever been sought for the older fractures. (Courtesy Department of Radiology, Children's Hospital of Pittsburgh, Pa.)

They are often bilateral. They may traverse the entire metaphysis or only a portion of it. Clinically, they are not associated with any significant soft-tissue swelling, and pain and tenderness (which can be quite localized) tend to abate within 2 to 5 days.

Radiographic manifestations of metaphyseal fractures have led to the terms "metaphyseal chip" or "corner" fractures and "bucket handle" fractures. The first derives from the fact that in the anteroposterior (AP) view the central portion of the fracture is often invisible and only a chip of bone is seen on either the lateral or medial aspect of the metaphysis, or both (Fig. 6-28 and see Fig. 6-27). Chips may also be seen on lateral projections. In some

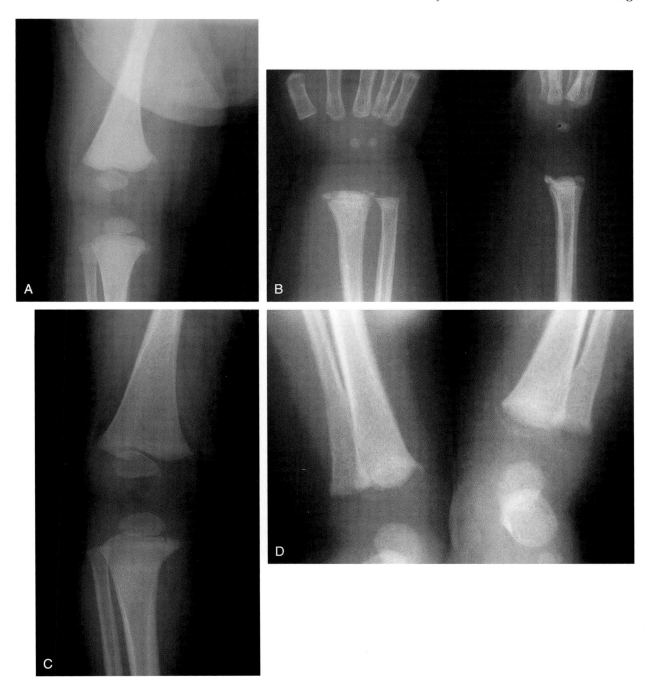

Figure 6-28. Metaphyseal fractures. **A,** Metaphyseal chip fractures involving the medial aspects of the distal right femur and proximal tibia were found in this infant whose mother confessed to repeated episodes of shaking, after which she would throw the baby down onto a bed or couch. Note the subperiosteal new bone along the lateral aspect of the femur and medial margins of the tibia. The baby had presented with a large subgaleal hematoma and a history of having been hit on the head with a plastic nursing bottle by a toddler. Bilateral skull fractures (see Fig. 6-47), a distal right clavicle fracture (see Fig. 6-39A), and a healing radius fracture were also found. **B,** In another child, metaphyseal chips are seen on either side of the radial metaphysis in the AP view along with a faint central metaphyseal lucency. In the lateral projection, metaphyseal chips of both radius and ulna are evident. Subtle rims of subperiosteal new bone can be seen along the diaphyses of both bones. This is the same 5-month-old whose faint surface bruises are shown in Figure 6-13C and D. Her skull radiograph is presented in Figure 6-44B. **C,** A prominent diagonal metaphyseal fracture of the medial aspect of the proximal right tibia was found on a skeletal survey obtained of this 10-month-old infant, who presented with an unexplained supracondylar fracture (see Fig. 6-38). His proximal tibia was nontender clinically, yet no evidence of healing is seen, suggesting that the fracture is older than a few days and newer than 10 days old. Failure to detect this rib and metacarpal fractures (see Fig. 6-40A) on films obtained because of hand swelling and decreased movement of the right leg noted during an admission for gastroenteritis and dehydration (vomiting without diarrhea) had subjected him to this further trauma a month later (see Fig. 6-38). **D,** In the oblique projection the planar nature of metaphyseal fractures is more easily appreciated. Fracture lines traverse the entire metaphysis of each tibia, and the disc-shaped distal fragments appear offset, giving rise to the term "bucket handle fracture." (**D,** Courtesy Dr. Bruce Rosenthal, Children's Hospital of Pittsburgh, Pa.)

cases a thin central metaphyseal lucency can be detected (Fig. 6-28B). Special oblique views are necessary to reveal the true extent of the fracture, as in this projection the separation of the metaphyseal disk becomes readily evident, resembling a bucket handle (Fig. 6-28D). Healing of metaphyseal fractures is not usually accompanied by prominent callus or extensive subperiosteal new-

bone formation. Reinjuries, however, can result in prominent fragmentation and sclerosis at the metaphyseal margins.

Rib Fractures

Rib fractures are also relatively unique to abused infants. Because of the plasticity and pliability of the thoracic cage

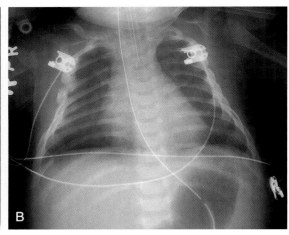

Figure 6-29. Rib fractures due to shaking. **A,** This 3-month-old infant has bilateral and nearly symmetrical posterior rib fractures with fairly mature callus involving the 2nd through 8th ribs on the left and the 3rd through 6th on the right. The latter are partially obscured by the mediastinal shadow and the right heart border. **B,** This 10-week-old, who presented with "shaking spells" and no history of trauma, has healing posterior rib fractures of the 2nd through 5th ribs on the right and 2nd through 7th on the left. Those of the right 2nd and 3rd and the left 7th appear newer than the others with less well-defined margins. He also has lateral rib fractures on the right involving the 3rd and 4th and possibly the 7th ribs. Additional fractures "appeared" during his hospital stay as healing proceeded. His central nervous system findings are shown in Figures 6-51 and 6-52.

in infancy, application of major forces is required to break ribs, and accidental rib fractures are rarely seen short of major motor vehicle accidents. Causative mechanisms include violent shaking while holding the child by the chest. This is done with the attacker's palms to the sides, thumbs in front, and fingers over the back. In the process of shaking, the ribs are subjected to marked AP compression forces and the posterior ribs are levered against the fulcrum of the vertebral bodies and their transverse processes. This often produces rows of multiple, often bilateral ("mirror image") posterior rib fractures, located near the costovertebral articulations (Fig. 6-29). Extreme squeezing of the chest with or without shaking can produce fractures at multiple sites along the rib arcs, as can stomping on the chest. Direct blows with the edge of a hand or blunt instrument, kicks, and slamming or hurling resulting in chest wall impact against the edge of a table or door jamb produce fractures at the site of impact. Stomping and slamming usually produce fractures that are more severe and extensive, more likely to be displaced, and associated with intrathoracic and intra-abdominal injuries (see Fig. 6-59).

Like metaphyseal fractures, rib fractures tend not to be associated with soft tissue swelling, and tenderness often resolves in 3 to 5 days, the exception being unusually severe and displaced fractures as shown in Figure 6-59. In some cases of repetitive injury with unusually florid callus, lumps can be palpated at healing fracture sites.

Radiographically, rib fractures tend to be invisible before the appearance of callus and/or subperiosteal new bone. This is because the periosteum is only partially disrupted, and it and the arc of the rib cage keep the fracture ends apposed. These breaks can, however, be detected by bone scan at this early stage. Hence this procedure should be strongly considered when there are no visible fractures but examination reveals thoracic bruises or tenderness; when one or a few rib fractures are seen and others are suspected, or when other injuries associated with shaking—metaphyseal chip fractures, retinal hemorrhages, central nervous system findings—are found in the absence of visible rib fractures. Bone scans often reveal multiple fractures not visible in standard radiographs (Fig. 6-30B). Alternatively, one can wait and obtain a repeat skeletal survey 10 days to 2 weeks later, if assured that the infant can be protected in the interim. These follow-up films can

reveal fractures invisible on the first study. An early sign of healing, seen 5 to 10 days postinjury on standard radiographs, consists of a vertical lucency at the site of the fracture surrounded by soft callus with indistinct margins (Fig. 6-31A). Subsequently (at 14 to 21 days), callus takes on a more nodular appearance with sharper margins and is then termed *hard callus* (Figs. 6-30A and 6-31B). Reinjury can result in florid callus formation (Fig. 6-31B). Complete remodeling and radiographic disappearance occur within a few months in the absence of reinjury.

The frequent association of rib and metaphyseal fractures with head injury in infants is so great (≈70%) that when these fractures are discovered, a CT scan of the head should be obtained, even when neurologic status appears normal. Not infrequently, this study will reveal evidence of prior intracranial injury that is subclinical or nonspecific in its manifestations at the time of presentation.

Long Bone Fractures

The high incidence of long bone fractures in abused children has been attributed to the fact that the extremities serve as "convenient handles" for inflicting trauma. Formation of subperiosteal new bone is seen commonly in infants and toddlers with healing diaphyseal fractures (see Figs. 6-27A and B and 6-32A and B). In infancy, it can also be seen in the absence of cortical fractures when a long bone is subjected to twisting or torsional forces short of those required to produce cortical breaks. These result in separation of the periosteum from the outer cortex and subperiosteal hemorrhage. Termed *periosteal stripping injuries*, they are relatively specific to infants, for although the epiphyseal segment of the periosteum is firmly attached, the diaphyseal portion is more loosely adherent because of sparseness of the Sharpey fibers that anchor it. As the complement of Sharpey fibers increases in early childhood, periosteal separation becomes less and less likely. Because of the attendant subperiosteal hemorrhage, the formation of subperiosteal new bone following periosteal stripping tends to be prominent and greater than 2 mm in width. This, too, becomes visible on radiographs in about 5 to 10 days in infants (10 to 14 days in toddlers). Initially, it is seen as periosteal haziness, and subsequently increasing calcification becomes evident (Fig. 6-32). These findings are easy to miss unless the physician inspects diaphyseal margins with great care. Like metaphyseal

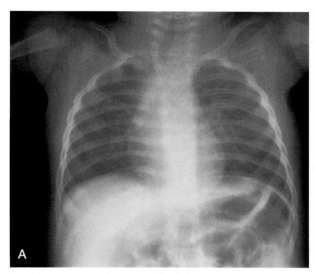
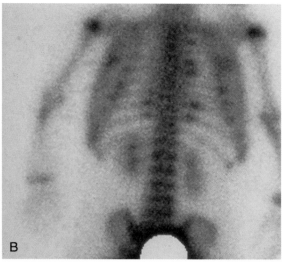

Figure 6-30. Use of bone scan to detect occult rib fractures. **A,** At 3 months of age, this infant presented with low-grade fever, nasal congestion, cough, tachypnea, and intermittent grunting respirations. Pneumonia was suspected, and a chest radiograph was obtained. On review of the films, a subtle, nearly completely remodeled fracture of the posterolateral aspect of the right 3rd rib was detected. In addition to his tachypnea, he was noted to cry when picked up by the chest. **B,** Bone scan revealed occult posterior fractures of the 2nd through 5th ribs on the left and the 8th and 9th ribs bilaterally, as well as the one fracture seen on the chest film. The occult fractures became visible radiographically over the ensuing 2 weeks.

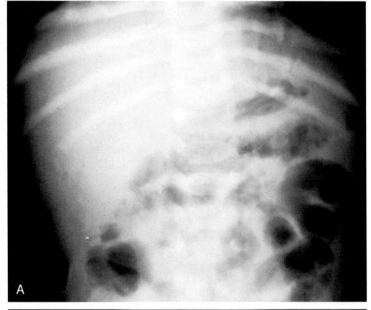
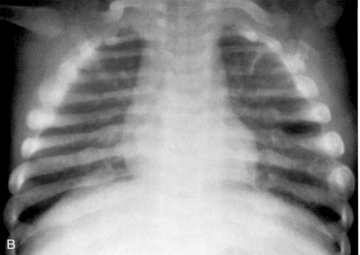

Figure 6-31. Healing rib fractures. **A,** This infant was seen because of a history of vomiting and irritability. An abdominal film obtained to rule out intestinal obstruction showed a normal bowel gas pattern but revealed posterior rib fractures in the early stages of healing. Note the vertical lucencies surrounded by soft callus. The fractures were missed. **B,** When the infant was finally tracked down 2 months later, her chest radiograph showed in excess of 20 healing rib fractures, some posterior and others lateral and anterolateral. The exuberance of the callus in many places reflects repetitive reinjury. Some of these were palpable clinically. (Courtesy Department of Radiology, Children's Hospital of Pittsburgh, Pa.)

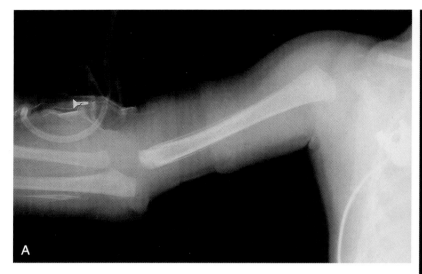

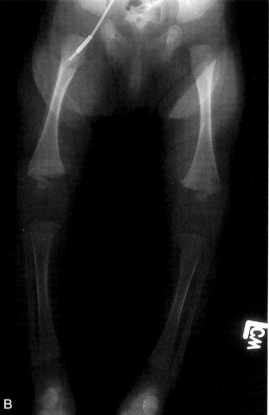

Figure 6-32. Periosteal stripping injuries. Wide strips of subperiosteal new bone were noted along the diaphyses of both humeri **(A)** and both femurs **(B)** of this infant. Their width was too great to be considered physiologic. She also had severe intracranial injury and multiple healing rib fractures. Dating of the periosteal stripping and rib fractures coincided with a 3- to 4-day period of nearly constant crying, "even when we picked her up," that had occurred more than 2 weeks earlier and was attributed to constipation.

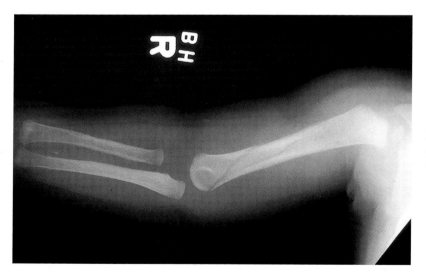

Figure 6-33. Spiral fracture. This 8-month-old presented with unexplained swelling of his right upper arm and decreased use of the extremity. He had no history of trauma. A spiral fracture courses from the distal portion to the upper third of the diaphysis. Moderate associated soft tissue swelling is also seen.

fractures, periosteal stripping injuries are clinically subtle even acutely because they are not associated with any significant degree of soft tissue swelling, and associated tenderness may disappear in as little as 2 to 5 days.

Although metaphyseal and periosteal stripping injuries are more common in young infants, diaphyseal or shaft fractures are not at all unusual and become even more common in older infants and toddlers who are victims of abuse. Although not specific for inflicted injury, diaphyseal fractures are highly suspect when found in infants who are not yet crawling or walking, especially when seen in the absence of a history of significant trauma; as noted, accidental fractures are also relatively uncommon in toddlers as compared with older children. Spiral, oblique, torus, transverse, and compression/distraction (or three-point bending) fractures may all be seen. An understand-ing of the direction and magnitude of force required to produce a given type of diaphyseal fracture and a comparison of that with the history given often enable the clinician to distinguish between accidental and inflicted injury.

Spiral fractures (Fig. 6-33), which, in cases of abuse, are usually the result of grabbing an extremity and rapidly twisting it, are relatively low-energy injuries in comparison with other fracture types and are not uncommonly seen as a result of accidents. However, when these injuries are caused by abuse, fracture edges are more likely to be widely separated, suggesting somewhat greater force application than is true of most accidental spiral fractures. *Oblique fractures* can also be the product of torsional forces or of slowly applied bending forces. They appear to require application of significantly greater energy than with spiral

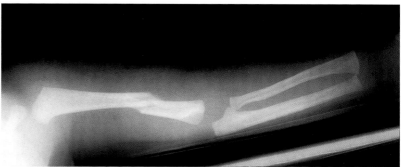

Figure 6-34. This partially displaced oblique fracture of the left humerus has faint evidence of early callus formation. The persistence of soft tissue swelling may be due to lack of proper immobilization and/or reinjury. (Courtesy Dr. Robert Hickey, Children's Hospital of Pittsburgh, Pa.)

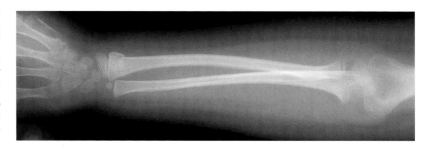

Figure 6-35. Torus or buckle fracture. This 5-year-old girl with mild cerebral palsy presented with a history of unresponsiveness lasting greater than an hour, following a possible seizure, and was found to have a hyperacute subdural hematoma similar to the one shown in Figure 6-48. Subsequent skeletal survey found a previously unrecognized and clinically silent torus fracture of the left distal radius. After an initial history reporting two falls on stairs, her mother's live-in boyfriend, who was frustrated with her slowness at toilet training, confessed to having pushed her down forcibly and to slamming her into an entertainment cabinet. When buckle fractures are displaced to this extent, they are perhaps more accurately described as compression/distraction injuries.

fractures, especially when the fracture is complete and displaced (Fig. 6-34).

Though more commonly accidental in origin, *torus or buckle fractures* can be the result of abuse, especially in very young children. When mild with only slight cortical buckling, they are the result of mild-to-moderate compression forces delivered in a direction parallel or nearly parallel to the axis of a long bone. When higher energy forces are delivered, whether accidental or inflicted, there is usually some degree of angulation; in such cases it may be more accurate to classify them as a form of compression/distraction injury. Milder fractures tend to have little associated soft tissue swelling and often only mild discomfort on motion. As degree of severity of angulation increases, so do swelling and pain. As is true of accidental fractures, they most commonly involve the distal radius and ulna, but volar angulation is more common in inflicted fractures, and dorsal angulation is more typical of those incurred accidentally. The usual scenario is that of a child who is thrown or forcefully pushed and lands on a outstretched arm (Fig. 6-35 and see Fig. 21-27 for the appearance of an accidental buckle fracture). Another involves grabbing by the wrist and bending it forcefully. More severe forms involving the femur or tibia can be caused by throwing or slamming a child feet first or onto the knees on a hard surface.

Transverse and three-point bending fractures are high-energy injuries that are much more likely to be accompanied by acute soft tissue swelling and deformity. Severe pain on motion with secondary splinting and limitation of motion are the rule. *Transverse fractures* are often the result of a rapidly delivered direct blow perpendicular to the long axis of a bone, such as "karate chop" or "night stick" injury (Fig. 6-36). They can also occur when a child is thrown or swung and, in the process, hits an extremity against a hard edge such as that of a table, as a result of falls of greater than 6 feet, and when half of an extremity is held with both hands and snapped.

Violently yanking a child up from his crib while holding an extremity and grabbing an arm and yanking it upward or sideways when the child is fixed in position by the belt of a high chair or infant seat are common scenarios for

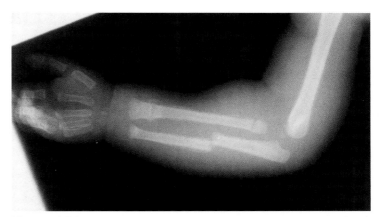

Figure 6-36. Transverse fractures. An acute transverse fracture of the proximal radius with associated soft tissue swelling is seen in this toddler who has another nondisplaced transverse fracture with early callus formation distally and a healing displaced transverse fracture of the mid-ulna with subperiosteal new-bone formation.

compression/distraction or three-point bending fractures (Fig. 6-37), as is the snapping mechanism described earlier. Inflicted supracondylar humerus fractures of the compression/distraction type are the result of grabbing an arm and yanking it into hyperextension (Fig. 6-38 and see Fig. 6-27B).

Other Fractures

Fractures of the clavicle as a result of abuse are fairly unusual. Like accidental fractures, they can be located at the junction of the outer third with the middle two thirds. When they involve the very distal portion (Fig. 6-39), they are highly suspect for abuse and are often associated with chip fractures of the acromion process and fractures of the proximal humerus and the upper ribs. Direct impact when thrown or slammed down and forceful yanking or pulling of the arm upward are common mechanisms. Medial clavicular and sternal fractures are extremely rare and reflect massive impacting forces. The same is true for fractures of the first rib and scapular body.

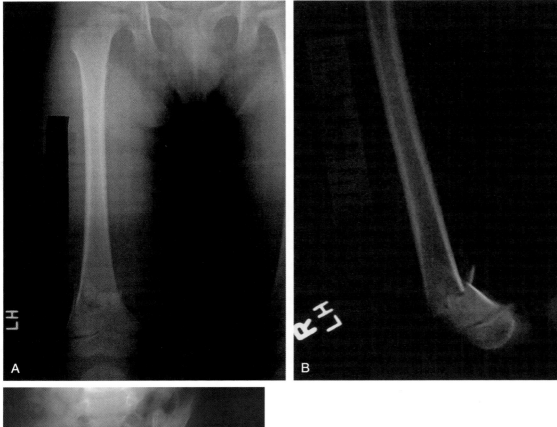

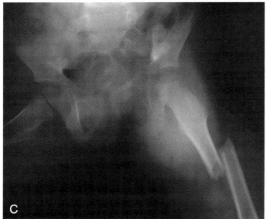

Figure 6-37. Compression/distraction (three-point bending) fracture. **A,** A comminuted and angulated fracture of the distal femur with irregular margins is seen in this child who was brought in for refusal to bear weight, after a "fall" down wooden steps. **B,** The degree of angulation is better appreciated in the lateral view. The nature of the fracture indicates a high-energy mechanism inconsistent with the history. The father later confessed to throwing the child at a coffee table, which broke on impact. **C,** A more typical example of a completely displaced three-point bending fracture is seen in another child.

Fractures of the hands and feet are relatively uncommon but have a strong likelihood of being inflicted and tend to be clinically inapparent when first seen. Grabbing and yanking, twisting, or bending the hand or foot tend to produce metacarpal/metatarsal fractures, most commonly the second and third in the hand and the first in the foot. Subtle subperiosteal new-bone formation and/or medullary sclerosis are common radiographic findings (Fig. 6-40A). Repetitive knuckle raps with a ruler or other hard object produce radiographic changes that consist of widening and sclerosis of the distal metaphyses of the metacarpals. Forced hyperextension of the phalanges can cause buckle fractures at their bases (see Fig. 6-40B).

Vertebral fractures are reported infrequently, although it is thought that many may be missed. In most cases, compression of a vertebral body is found. Cervical fractures are usually the result of violent hyperflexion or hyperextension (hangman's fracture). More rarely, the child may be held by the head and the neck twisted or the head is used as a handle while the assailant violently swings or shakes the child, usually resulting in catastrophic cervical cord injury. Below the cervical spine, most fractures occur near the thoracolumbar junction. Axial loading (slamming the buttocks onto a hard surface) and violent hyperflexion are the major mechanisms reported. Forced hyperflexion can also result in multiple avulsion fractures of the spinous processes as they are torn from their ligamentous attachments.

Diagnostic Imaging of Skeletal Injuries

Radiographic examination of infants and children for reasons other than suspected fractures (e.g., chest and abdominal films) may provide the first clue to inflicted trauma if clinicians and radiologists follow the maxim of carefully looking at each structure on the film (see Figs. 6-30A and 6-31A). Too often, fractures are missed because complaints of respiratory distress or vomiting lead clinicians to focus exclusively on lungs and heart or the abdominal gas pattern. This results in missed diagnoses, especially when bony abnormalities are subtle, and return of the child to the family with major risk of even more severe subsequent injury.

When evaluating an infant or child younger than 2 or 3 years of age who is found to have multiple bruises and/or fractures, fractures of differing ages and fractures with high (metaphyseal, rib) or moderate (vertebral body, hand, foot, and complex skull fractures) specificity for abuse, it is essential to obtain a skeletal survey because of the greater probability of finding multiple clinically occult fractures. Surveys may also yield valuable additional information in selected cases of children 3 to 5 years of age,

especially if they are developmentally delayed or have other evidence of severe abuse and/or neglect. After age 5 years, careful history and physical examination should point to areas that warrant radiographic evaluation.

We cannot emphasize enough the importance of optimal imaging techniques in identification of inflicted skeletal trauma. High-detail skeletal surveys with two views of each bone and additional oblique views of the hands and feet maximize the potential for detection but have to be specifically ordered because many surveys show only one view of each bone plus two views of the head. We also advocate four views (AP, Townes, left, and right) of the skull. These radiographs should be examined with meticulous care, comparing paired structures from left to right and comparing adjacent structures. This is important in order to avoid missing subtle metaphyseal fractures and early collections of subperiosteal new bone. Given that some occult fractures may be invisible at the time of initial evaluation, consideration should be given to obtaining a bone scan or a repeat skeletal survey with oblique views of the ribs 2 weeks later when callus will be evident.

Although bone scans are not ideal as a primary imaging modality in detecting inflicted fractures, they can serve as a good complementary adjunct to skeletal surveys, especially in infants who have multiple bruises (highly suspicious for abuse) but no visible fractures, rib or metaphyseal fractures, retinal hemorrhages, or obvious CNS findings consistent with shaking (see Fig. 6-30), when further evidence is needed to ensure the child's protection. Scans are particularly helpful in detecting occult rib fractures and periosteal stripping injuries that are no longer tender on examination but have not yet formed radiographically visible callus or subperiosteal new bone (Fig. 6-41A). There is some evidence that bone scans may be able to detect fractures that have already remodeled (see Fig. 6-41B). They are not good at detecting metaphyseal injuries because the adjacent growth centers have high uptake. They are also poor at detecting skull fractures. Ultrasound, CT, or MRI examination may be useful when injuries of unossified growth centers or epiphyseal separation injuries are suspected in toddlers or older children.

Strong consideration should be given to obtaining a head CT, a complete blood cell count and differential with platelets, prothrombin and partial thromboplastin times,

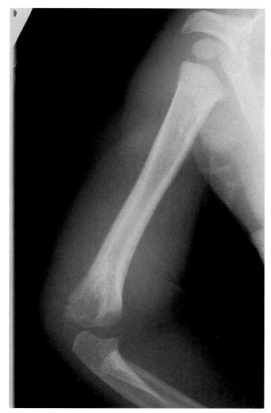

Figure 6-38. Supracondylar fracture. An inflicted supracondylar humerus fracture caused by forced hyperextension is seen in a 9-month-old infant who was brought to his local emergency department for unexplained arm swelling. Note the diagonal linear lucency over the posterior aspect of the distal humerus and the prominent soft tissue swelling. Early signs of callus formation distal to the new fracture indicate that this is a repeat injury. He had been seen a month earlier with irritability, vomiting, hand swelling, and decreased movement of his right leg. Though chest, leg, and hand films were obtained at that time, his tibial and metacarpal fractures were missed (see Figs. 6-28C and 6-40A).

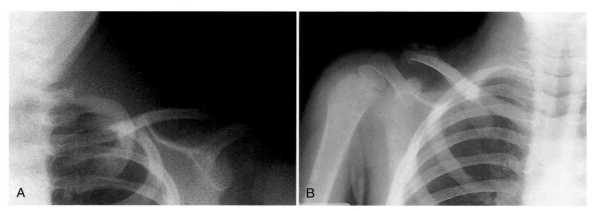

Figure 6-39. Inflicted distal clavicle fractures. **A,** Fracture of the distal right clavicle is seen in this infant victim of shaken impact syndrome. Lack of associated soft tissue swelling and absence of callus suggests the fracture is between 3 and 10 days old. Her metaphyseal fractures are shown in Figure 6-28A, and her skull fractures in Figure 6-47. **B,** A refracture through the callus of a healing distal right clavicle fracture is seen in the toddler whose surface injuries are shown in Figure 6-2. She had been repeatedly thrown or shoved down stairs and into furniture.

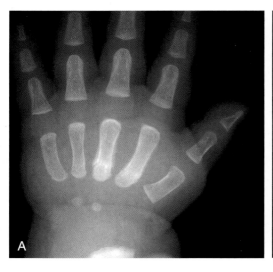
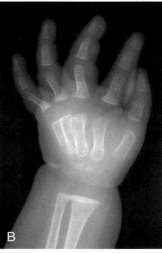

Figure 6-40. Hand fractures. **A,** A healing fracture of the left third metacarpal is seen in this 9-month-old infant who was brought to his local emergency department with a 2-day history of marked irritability, vomiting, and hand swelling. Subperiosteal new bone is evident along the shaft of his left middle metacarpal along with slight medullary sclerosis proximally. This, rib, and proximal tibial fractures were missed until the films were reread when he returned a month later with an unexplained distal humerus fracture (see Fig. 6-28C). **B,** Buckle fractures of the proximal phalanges due to forced hyperextension of the fingers are seen in this infant, who presented with redness and swelling of his hand and no history of trauma. He returned 6 weeks later in extremis with a hyperacute subdural hematoma (see Fig. 6-48).

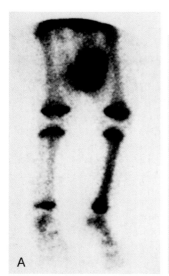
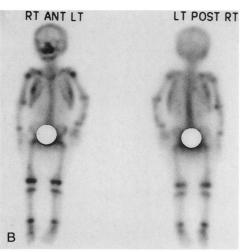

Figure 6-41. Usefulness of bone scans in detecting both acute and chronic occult injuries. **A,** This 14-month-old was seen for low-grade fever and refusal to walk. Initial standard radiographs were normal. The scan, obtained because of suspicion of infection, revealed increased uptake throughout the entire left tibia. Work-up for infection was negative. Repeat radiographs obtained 2 weeks later revealed a healing fracture and extensive subperiosteal new-bone formation. **B,** This 21-month-old toddler reportedly collapsed at home after falling from her crib. She had a right frontal hematoma, multiple abrasions, and a cigarette burn scar. On head CT, subdural blood and cerebral edema were found. An abdominal CT obtained because of elevated liver function tests revealed the bilateral adrenal hemorrhages shown in Figure 6-58. This bone scan obtained after a negative skeletal survey shows increased tracer uptake in the left distal ulna, right proximal femur, and right clavicle and over the lateral aspects of the rib cage bilaterally. As callus over the distal right clavicle was the only positive finding on a repeat skeletal survey 2 weeks postinjury, it was postulated that the other areas of increased uptake represented healed and fully remodeled old fractures.

liver function tests, and amylase lipase when evaluating children, especially infants, with multiple fractures and those with injuries of moderate to high specificity for abuse because clinically inapparent CNS and intra-abdominal injuries can be associated findings.

Finally, we cannot give enough emphasis to the importance of considering fractures in the differential diagnosis of unexplained irritability or of grunting respirations in infants who have no pulmonary findings. Failure to identify the cause of irritability has the potential to subject previously abused babies to further, often more severe, trauma and to place infants from high-risk families who have not yet been abused at risk for future inflicted injury.

Central Nervous System Injuries

The incidence of recognized head injury in child abuse victims ranges from 7% to 19% as reported in various large case studies. Up to 80% of victims are younger than 1 year of age, and the majority of the remaining 20% are toddlers. Numbers have risen over the past decade because more infants with subtle or subclinical intracranial injuries are imaged and abnormalities are detected because of greater recognition of associated surface and/or skeletal injuries. To put inflicted head trauma in infants in per-

spective, findings reported in recent literature (Billmire) reveal that approximately 65% of all head injuries (excluding uncomplicated calvarial fractures) and 95% of all serious intracranial injuries in infants younger than 1 year of age are inflicted. Further, 60% to 80% of head injury deaths in children younger than 2 years are due to abuse.

Head injuries are also the major source of morbidity and mortality due to abuse. From 20% to 25% of known victims of inflicted head trauma die, and they account for up to 80% of fatal abuse cases. Survivors are often left with sequelae, ranging from microcephaly with neurodevastation to mild cognitive deficits. In long-term follow-up studies of former victims of physical abuse (not selected for head injury), Martin found 5% were microcephalic, 31% were in less than the fifth percentile for height and/or weight, and 53% had abnormalities on neurologic examination, nearly one third of which were moderate to severe. Although only 30% of the previously abused children studied in follow-up by Elmer and Gregg had known CNS injury at the time of their initial identification, 57% had IQs lower than 80, and 32%, known to have been abused before 13 months of age, had evidence of significant developmental delay. Given the fact that some head injuries go undetected because they are relatively mild and/or associated with nonspecific symptoms, and given that many victims of abuse are never recognized as such, it is probable that a fair percentage of infants and children with milder degrees of "idiopathic" developmental delay, cognitive deficits, learning disabilities, attention deficit hyperactivity disorder, and behavioral problems are former victims of inflicted injury that went undiagnosed.

Pathophysiology and Biomechanics

An infant's head is uniquely vulnerable to injury, whether from impact or from shaking, for several reasons:

1. It is relatively large, accounting for up to 10% of body weight, as opposed to 2% in the adult. This weight adds to the momentum of acceleration and deceleration forces with shaking and accounts for the fact that infants who are dropped, thrown, or bodily ejected from motor vehicles tend to land on their heads.
2. Highly elastic, underdeveloped cervical ligaments; relatively weak neck muscles; shallow, horizontally oriented cervical facet joints; and incompletely ossified and anteriorly wedged cervical vertebrae hinder an infant's ability to protect against whiplash forces. Together they make the infant susceptible to extreme hyperflexion and hyperextension of the neck and greater head motion when subjected to acceleration/deceleration (A/D) forces.
3. The soft calvarium, which elongates with acceleration and deceleration, and the relatively large subarachnoid space place the bridging veins between the dura mater and cerebral cortex at greater risk of tearing. In addition, with impact, the pliable skull is more likely to transfer force to the underlying brain rather than fracturing and thereby absorbing some of the force along the fracture line. Even when fractures do occur on impact, greater inbending of the pliable calvarial bones still transfers much of the impacting force to the adjacent cortex.
4. Because of its higher water content, minimal myelination, and paucity of dendritic and glial connections, the brain of a young infant is far more gelatinous than that of an older child or adult. As a result, it is much more deformable when subjected to impact and/or A/D forces, and its thin unmyelinated axons are much more vulnerable to shearing injuries, especially at the gray/white matter interfaces.
5. The relatively flat calvarial base assists rotation of the brain about the brainstem when subjected to rotational acceleration.

In terms of biomechanics, the majority of head injuries in children, whether accidental or inflicted, are the result of rapidly applied dynamic blunt forces. Some are caused by direct contact forces, and some are caused by indirect inertial forces that result from A/D of the head. The distinction is somewhat arbitrary because in most cases of "contact" injury there is some degree of A/D, and most cases of "indirect" injury involve some impact or contact.

In direct contact injuries the calvarium, its overlying soft tissues, and potentially its underlying intracranial contents are subjected to focal strains or distortions. When applied forces are mild, they may result in abrasion, bruising, or laceration of the scalp, and when more moderate they tend to result in calvarial fracture. Because the amount of force applied rises beyond mild to moderate, skull fractures are more likely to be diastatic or complex, and transmission of impacting forces inward to intracranial structures increases, producing focal injuries ranging from epidural hematomas to focal subdural hematomas and ultimately to cerebral contusions or parenchymal shearing.

The three main scenarios for contact injury are as follows:

1. A moving object such as a hand, fist, thrown missile, swung baseball bat or golf club strikes a stationary head, which, on impact, is accelerated in the same direction as the applied force. If the head is resting against a surface (e.g., mattress or wall), it then incurs a second impact. In most cases the impacting force is linear, but if delivered with a spin, a rotational component is added.
2. A moving and thus accelerated head (in a fall while running, or as a result of being thrown, pushed, slammed, or swung and slammed) strikes a stationary object (e.g., floor, furniture, wall, lamp post). In such cases there is initial acceleration followed by deceleration on impact and then a bounce back.
3. A head in motion strikes another object in motion (e.g., two children running or backing up in opposite directions butt heads, child riding bicycle hits moving car), in which case there is acceleration in two different directions.

The degree of force involved in impact injury depends on the rate of acceleration (which, in a fall, depends on the child's weight and the distance of the fall); the type of surface struck; and the duration of impact. When an impacted or impacting surface is hard, greater focal calvarial deformation is likely to occur on impact and external signs of injury are typical. This is ameliorated to some extent by the fact that, when striking a firm or hard surface, the head tends to bounce back, reducing the duration of impact. When an infant's or child's head strikes a soft surface such as a pillow or mattress, it tends to sink into it. This increases the surface area of contact and, as a consequence, focal deformation is reduced, along with the risk of surface injuries; however, duration of contact is prolonged, and thus the duration of force application.

Indirect trauma due to A/D forces results in inertial loading and, depending on velocity and direction, subjects the intracranial contents to shearing strains. When great enough (e.g., forceful to violent), these can result in tearing at interfaces between differing structures (e.g., bridging veins) or at the interface of tissues of differing density (e.g., gray and white matter). A/D forces can be translational or linear, as from anterior to posterior in the sagittal plane (whiplash), or they can have a rotational component, as when forces are applied from two different directions (auto in motion is broadsided) or when the force is delivered with spin (blow delivered to side of head with "english"). Because A/D forces are more likely to produce shearing strains, they are more apt to cause diffuse intracranial injury, as opposed to contact forces, which are more apt to result in focal trauma. However, in the case of young infant abuse victims, impact trauma may also produce shearing strains, especially when the victim is thrown.

Injuries caused by linear A/D forces, in the sagittal plane, may include shearing of the bridging veins between the dura and cerebral cortex, along with veins in their thin arachnoid sheaths, as well as contact injuries of frontal and occipital lobes incurred in striking their respective calvarial bones. They can be diffuse and severe, especially when the head is subjected to the to-and-fro motion of violent repetitive shaking. In this scenario, the brain and calvaria have a greater propensity to get "out of sync" in their motion, increasing shearing strains. This is further magnified by the greater deformability of the gelatinous infant brain. Application of rotational forces tends to cause even more severe injury because these are more likely to induce shearing of neuronal axons at the gray/white matter interfaces. This is because more peripheral brain structures rotate more rapidly and through a wider arc than deeper, more fixed structures.

To summarize, most head injures are caused by some combination of acceleration and/or deceleration forces and contact or impact forces. In the majority of cases of accidental trauma, especially in infants or toddlers, the forces involved are mild and the resulting injuries minor. In most cases of abusive head trauma, the forces are moderate to major and the injuries are correspondingly more severe. A chronicle of advances in recognition of the differing magnitude of applied forces and severity of injury in accidental versus inflicted impact trauma can be found in the literature on fall-related head injuries. For many years it was believed that short falls (3 to 4 feet or less) could cause severe injury. This changed on publication of a series of studies of victims of falls witnessed by people other than caretakers, and of children who had fallen from beds and examining tables in hospitals. These studies demonstrated that indoor falls of less than 10 feet (3 meters), even onto hard surfaces, did not cause serious, let alone life-threatening, head injuries. Simple linear skull fractures tended to be the most severe injuries seen, and these were associated with mild focal underlying intracranial injury only in rare instances. Furthermore, in cases of outdoor falls, injuries tended to be mild unless the activity preceding the fall added angular momentum to the forces incurred because of the height of the fall (e.g., swinging on a swing, trapeze, or jungle gym). These findings led to the recognition that study populations described in earlier literature on pediatric head trauma had included many unrecognized child abuse victims, and to refutation of the conclusions of earlier investigators that short falls and other minor mechanisms of injury could result in

serious, even fatal, head trauma. Research has also found that accidental falls down stairs consist of a series of short falls and do not result in serious head injury unless the infant is in a walker.

The major identified mechanisms of inflicted head trauma include violent shaking; throwing or slamming against a hard object or a soft surface; hitting with a hand, fist, or other object; and kicking. Each is associated with application of varying degrees of impact forces and acceleration and/or deceleration. It must also be noted that many victims of inflicted CNS trauma are subjected to injury on more than one occasion. In fact, 45% of infants confirmed as victims of inflicted head trauma had evidence of prior intracranial injury on initial neuroimaging (Jenny).

Evolution of Understanding of the Pathophysiology of Shaking

Our current understanding of the forces involved and of mechanisms, including the role of shaking in inflicted head trauma, derives from much questioning and research over the past several decades, during which time theories have been proposed and investigated, some verified, some disproved, and others modified.

In the late 1940s Caffey first described the association of subdural hematomas with multiple fractures in infants. Subsequently, the question of intentional injury was raised, and shaking was postulated as the probable mechanism, leading to the concept of the *shaken baby syndrome*, characterized by a constellation of findings that included subdural hematomas (Fig. 6-42), retinal hemorrhages (Fig. 6-43), and posterior rib and metaphyseal fractures (see Figs. 6-27A, 6-28, and 6-29 through 6-31).

For many years thereafter, it was believed that these injuries were due solely to shaking. Indeed, studies using

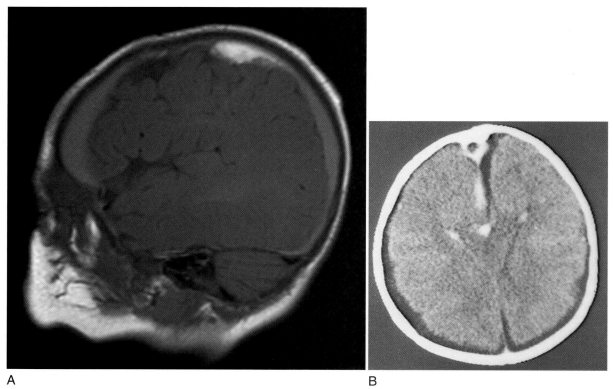

A   B

Figure 6-42. Diffuse subdural hematomas in the shaken-baby syndrome. **A,** Acute on chronic subdural hematomas are evident on this sagittal MRI view of an infant with shaken baby syndrome. **B,** This CT scan of another infant reveals chronic subdural hematomas along the falx and over the cerebral convexities. These are seen as a dark rim along the falx and between the bony calvaria and the brain substance. (**A,** Courtesy Lynda Flom, MD, department of pediatric radiology, Children's Hospital of Pittsburgh, Pa; **B,** courtesy division of neuroradiology, University Health Center of Pittsburgh, Pa.)

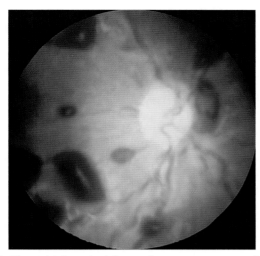

Figure 6-43. Multiple retinal hemorrhages are seen on funduscopic examination of this infant who was a victim of the shaken-baby syndrome. Subdural hematoma and multiple metaphyseal "shake" fractures are typical associated findings. (Courtesy Dr. Stephen Ludwig, Children's Hospital of Philadelphia.)

monkeys, conducted in the late 1960s (Ommaya), showed that violent shaking generates rapid A/D forces, with both linear and rotational components, and that either the rotational forces or the combination of forces were necessary for producing the subdural, subarachnoid, and retinal hemorrhages seen in the animals.

Subsequent advances in neuroimaging and forensic examination, together with improvements in the identification of inflicted head trauma, have expanded our knowledge of the spectrum of CNS injuries seen in abuse victims. In addition to subdural hematomas (seen particularly in the interhemispheric fissure along the falx, as well as over the cerebral convexities), subarachnoid hemorrhages, cerebral contusions, diffuse axonal injury with shearing at gray/white matter interfaces, and white matter tears have been reported. Epidural and subdural hematomas at the cervicomedullary junction in association with ventral cord contusions at high cervical levels have also been linked to shaking.

In 1987 the role of shaking in producing these injuries was called into question by a group of investigators (Duhaime and colleagues) who developed an infant model using a life-size doll with a rubber neck and weighted head. They concluded that shaking alone failed to generate sufficient G forces to cause the CNS injuries attributed to shaking in human infants and noted that, on close examination, many of their victims showed signs of impact injury. Thus they postulated that some form of impact was necessary, in addition to shaking, and suggested that the impact in patients with no external evidence of injury may have been on a soft surface such as a mattress. In reviewing old autopsy cases and carefully examining new victims, subsequent investigators have found that a majority of victims of abusive head trauma do indeed have evidence of associated impact injury, albeit at times subtle, and in some instances, seen only in the form of petechiae and contusions over the internal surface of the galea at surgery or on postmortem examination. However, a significant percentage (ranging from 11% to 50%, depending on the series), especially of very young infants, do not have any evidence of impact. Furthermore, on the basis of confessions, it does appear that severe CNS injury can result from violent shaking alone. The validity of the Duhaime infant model has also been questioned

because its neck was stiffer than an actual infant's and, therefore, capable of less hyperflexion, and further, the forces required were derived from adult primates with mature brains. Thus some victims' injuries appear to be due solely to shaking; others result from a combination of shaking and impact trauma; and still others from impact alone.

In addition to the unique vulnerability of the young infant brain to deformation, there are two major explanations for the presence of severe injury in shaken babies who have no physical evidence of impact. One is that when the child's head strikes a soft surface, no external marker of impact may be left. The other relates to the fact that *repetitive impacts actually do occur with shaking alone,* especially when a very young infant with poor head control is violently shaken back and forth over and over again. These impacts consist of the chin hitting the chest and the occiput hitting the vertebral column at opposite ends of the arc of head motion. In the process, impacts of the frontal lobes against the frontal bone and the occipital lobes against the occipital bone occur with attendant brain deformation, on both impact and rebound. Further, in the course of violent shaking, the perpetrator's motion may not be consistently linear, the baby may turn its head to avert its gaze from the perpetrator, or the infant may lose consciousness (and therefore tone) in the process of being shaken, the head then lolling down and slightly sideways, thereby introducing rotational momentum to the A/D forces.

Most victims of suspected shaking are less than 1 year of age, frequently under 6 months, and most have no external signs of injury, although careful inspection may reveal faint finger impression bruises (see Fig. 6-13). On the basis of confessions and videotapes obtained with hidden cameras, it is now known that the infant is subjected to repetitive, violent shakes usually while being held by the trunk facing the perpetrator, less often when grasped by arms and shoulders or by hands or feet.

Metaphyseal fractures, posterior rib fractures, and retinal hemorrhages appear to be highly specific for shaking, especially when seen in combination. Retinal hemorrhages, typically numerous, diffuse, often extending out to the periphery, and located in multiple layers of the retina, are found in 70% to 90% of infants and children with inflicted head injury and in nearly 100% of those who suffer serious sequelae and death (see Fig. 6-43). Although the uniqueness of their association with shaking has been the subject of some controversy, studies of infants and children whose accidental severe head trauma was witnessed have shown that the incidence of retinal hemorrhages is vanishingly small and is largely limited to children who incurred severe crush injuries to the head; who suffered high-velocity, lateral-impact rotational injuries; or who incurred injuries outdoors in falls while swinging on playground equipment or jumping on a trampoline, which involved significant angular momentum. In the rare reports of accidental in-home falls resulting in subdural hematomas with retinal hemorrhages, each case involved significant momentum from being swung, falling down stairs while on the move in a walker, or a straight fall of 8 to 10 feet onto concrete. Each child was brought promptly for care and had no associated injuries or history of injury. Subdural hemorrhages were small and resolved in 24 to 48 hours. Furthermore, in these accidental scenarios retinal hemorrhages seen were fewer in number and tended to be localized over the posterior pole. Similarly, research on children who have undergone prolonged cardiopulmonary resuscitation has revealed a very low incidence of retinal hemorrhages, and the majority of cases in which they were found involved victims of abuse or massive accidental head injury. A small minority were suffering from malignant hypertension, coagulopathy, or septic shock. Similarly, posterior and lateral rib fractures have not been found following prolonged cardiopulmonary resuscitation in either infants or animal models. Thus when cardiopulmonary resuscitation is given as an explanation for head trauma with retinal hemorrhages and rib fractures, it is false.

Clinical Picture of Inflicted Head Trauma

Modes of presentation of inflicted head trauma vary, depending on the age of the victim and severity of injury. When signs and symptoms are mild, no care may be sought, and if it is, there is often a significant delay between the time of the injury and time of presentation. When there are no external signs (which is often the case), a history of trauma is almost never reported. An unrelated chief complaint or a history of nonspecific symptoms such as vomiting, lethargy, irritability, or trouble breathing is likely to be given when neurologic abnormalities are not blatant. When injuries are more severe, complaints of unresponsiveness, shaking or stiffening spells, and apnea or choking are more likely to be reported. In patients with significant contact injuries and obvious surface bruising, a chief complaint of a bump on the head may be given with a history of a minor mechanism of injury such as rolling off a couch and falling 15 to 18 inches to a carpeted floor, or the caretaker may report having dropped the baby a short distance (usually <3 or 4 feet). In some cases another young child has been reported to have hit the baby on the head. These mechanisms do not explain intracranial injury (see Table 6-8).

In cases of more severe injury, presentation is more likely to be prompt, but delays in seeking care still occur. Often, when an infant loses consciousness as a result of shaking and/or impact, the perpetrator becomes frightened and delays seeking medical attention for fear of being caught. He or she then leaves the baby to rest for a while, hoping that the infant will revive on its own. During the ensuing interval, intracranial pressure may rise as a consequence of increasing cerebral edema and/or the mass effect of intracranial hemorrhage, compromising cerebral perfusion and resulting in varying amounts of cerebral ischemia. Associated alteration in level of consciousness and/or seizures can result in hypoventilation,

apnea, or respiratory arrest, resulting in hypoxia. Hence hypoxic/ischemic injury may be added to that of the physical trauma (see Fig. 6-53). (Note: Studies have shown that the person alone with the child at the time worrisome symptoms are first noted is usually the perpetrator.)

Infants with milder degrees of injury may have nonspecific lethargy and/or irritability without focal neurologic signs. Some may have subtle surface bruises or petechiae evident only on close inspection, and some (but by no means all) may cry when picked up by the chest or moved because of new fractures. Funduscopic examination may reveal retinal hemorrhages. In other, more severely injured infants, physical findings may include lethargy, increased or decreased tone, rhythmic eye opening, eye deviation, extremity twitching or bicycling movements of the extremities, and sometimes posturing. Decreased ability to follow the examiner's face, decreased responsiveness to pain, and poor suck and grasp are important findings. The fontanelle is often full but may or may not be tense. On occasion, infants may present in shock resulting from massive subgaleal or intracranial hemorrhage. Diffuse retinal hemorrhages (see Fig. 6-43) are more likely to be found in these sicker babies, and dilated ophthalmoscopy should be performed in all infants seen for altered levels of consciousness. These infants should also undergo meticulous inspection of the skin and mucous membranes.

Inflicted impact injuries are seen in infants and children who have been thrown to the floor, against a wall, or into other objects or who have received direct blows to the head with a fist or other blunt object. Surface injuries are likely in these cases and may range from subtle bruising or a small patch of petechiae on the scalp to large subgaleal hematomas. Surface injuries of the face and other sites are also common (Fig. 6-44A and see Fig. 6-7A). In these cases, skull fractures are frequently present. Simple linear fractures (Fig. 6-45), diastatic linear fractures with or without diastatic sutures (see Fig. 6-44B), and more complex T-shaped and eggshell fractures (Fig. 6-46) have all been reported in cases of inflicted trauma. Given the greater magnitude of injury forces involved in most cases of abuse (as opposed to those in the majority of accidental injuries), diastatic and complex fractures, and bilateral fractures (Fig. 6-47) are more likely to be the result of abuse and are inconsistent with histories of minor mechanisms of injury. Conversely, when these types of skull fractures are seen and no major mechanism of injury is found, abuse should be strongly suspected. Associated

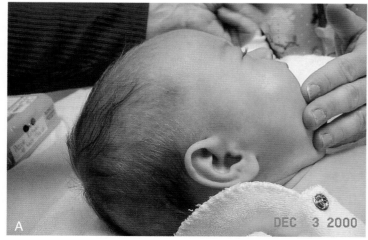
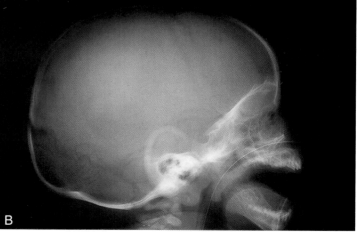

Figure 6-44. Shaken impact syndrome. **A,** Subtle bruising is seen over the right fronto-temporal area in this infant. **B,** Her skull radiograph reveals an occipital fracture with diastasis of the lambdoid suture. On CT scan, a posterior interhemispheric subdural hematoma was found. Other bruises are shown in Fig. 6-13.

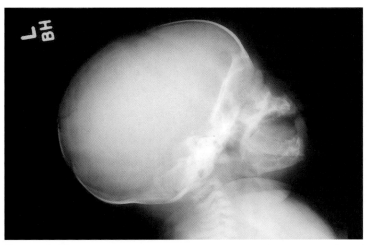

Figure 6-45. Linear skull fracture. This linear occipital fracture was found in the infant with bilateral black eyes shown in Figure 6-7A.

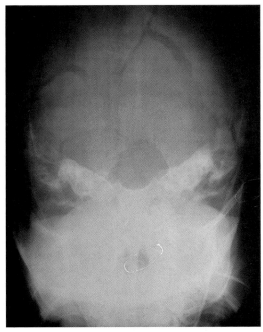

Figure 6-46. Eggshell fracture. Multiple occipital fractures are seen in a child who presented with a history of a minor fall and scalp swelling. It was later acknowledged that he had been thrown against a brick wall. (Courtesy Department of Radiology, Children's Hospital of Pittsburgh, Pa.)

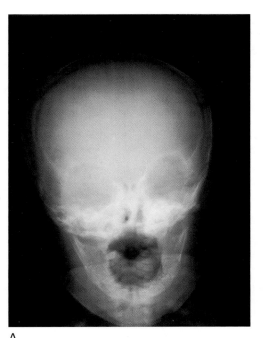

A

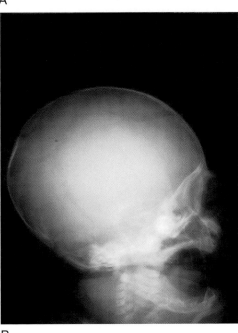

B

Figure 6-47. Shaken impact syndrome. **A** and **B**, These bilateral, diastatic, parieto-occipital skull fractures, shown in anteroposterior and oblique views, were the result of impacts on the arm of a couch after bouts of shaking. Her metaphyseal fractures are shown in Figure 6-28A, and her clavicle fracture is shown in Figure 6-39A.

intracranial injuries may include focal subdural hematomas (Fig. 6-48 and see Fig. 6-50) and focal cerebral contusions (Fig. 6-49) with adjacent edema, which, when severe, produces a midline shift and may be associated with focal shearing injury.

In cases due to shaking alone or shaking plus impact, diffuse subdural hematomas may be found over the convexities and along the falx (see Fig. 6-42). A combination of focal and interhemispheric subdurals is another common finding (Fig. 6-50), again often accompanied by varying amounts of cerebral edema. Extreme A/D forces with a rotational component produce loss of gray/white matter differentiation due to axonal shearing (Fig. 6-51A), which on occasion is further highlighted by arc-shaped hemorrhages (see Fig. 6-51B). Severe cerebral edema and ventricular effacement are typical in these cases. In the ensuing days the magnitude of neuronal loss can be appreciated, and the full extent of loss is seen in the ensuing months (Fig. 6-52). In cases of severe hypoxic or ischemic injury, the cortex appears hypodense in comparison with the basal ganglia, termed a *reversal sign* (Fig. 6-53), which is often seen when there is a long delay in seeking care.

Occasionally, patients who have incurred milder trauma and are not seen acutely may present weeks later with one or more of the following symptoms: intermittent vomiting and irritability, rapidly increasing head circumference with split sutures and a full fontanelle, failure to thrive, and developmental delay typically affecting social more than motor development. Some of these patients are found to have *chronic subdural hematomas*.

Neuroimaging
Routine skull radiographs are best for detecting most skull fractures, and when abuse is suspected, four views

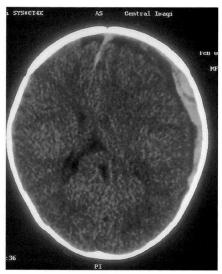

Figure 6-48. A focal subdural hematoma, caused by severe impact forces, is seen in the left frontal area of this 6-month-old infant who presented with decreased responsiveness after "rolling off a bed." The layering of the subdural blood was due to rapid collection and at surgery was found to consist of newly clotted blood and fresh hemorrhage, classified as a *hyperacute subdural hematoma.* Note also the acute subdural blood along the anterior interhemispheric fissure and the midline shift. Multiple phalangeal fractures found 6 weeks earlier, but not recognized as inflicted, are shown in Fig. 6-40B.

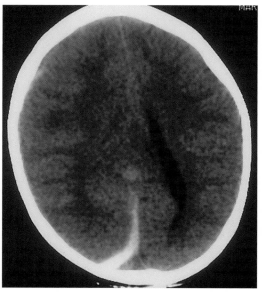

Figure 6-50. Focal occipital and interhemispheric subdural blood are seen in this toddler who "collapsed at home after a fall from her crib." Note the effacement of the right lateral ventricle and slight anterior midline shift due to cerebral edema. Her bone scan is shown in Figure 6-41B and her abdominal CT in Figure 6-58.

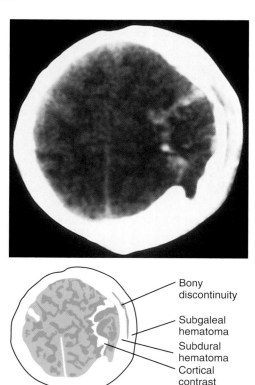

Bony discontinuity

Subgaleal hematoma

Subdural hematoma

Cortical contrast enhancement

Figure 6-49. Cerebral contusion. CT scan from a 4-week-old infant who allegedly rolled out of his crib while the side rails were up shows a large subgaleal hematoma obscuring an underlying fracture, severe cerebral swelling with a shift of the midline, and cortical contrast enhancement indicative of a cerebral contusion. (Courtesy Division of Neuroradiology, University Health Center of Pittsburgh, Pa.)

(AP, Townes, right, and left) should be obtained. CT has proved highly valuable in the acute assessment of CNS injuries, and an unenhanced head CT with brain and bone windows is indicated whenever there is any suspicion of intracranial injury, whether due to abnormal neurologic signs and symptoms, presence of metaphyseal and/or rib fractures, multiple bruises, or

retinal hemorrhages. It clearly delineates most intracranial hemorrhages and cerebral edema, as well as the majority of subdural hematomas and many fractures. CT is especially good at revealing interhemispheric subdural hematomas along the falx and in the parietooccipital area, which are seen frequently in victims of shaking (see Fig. 6-42). It is also good at detecting cerebral edema (see Figs. 6-48 to 6-51), loss of gray/white matter differentiation due to axonal shearing (see Fig. 6-51A and B), and subsequent cortical necrosis (see Fig. 6-52), as well as cortical hypodensity as a result of hypoxic/ischemic injury (see Fig. 6-53).

CT does have limitations, however. It may not reveal the full extent of injuries and may fail to detect thin subdural hemorrhages (especially over the convexities) and subtle cerebral contusions or hemorrhages. CT is also unable to distinguish between the layering of subdural blood as a result of rapid or hyperacute bleeds from layering of hemorrhages of differing ages (see Fig. 6-48). It should be noted that most acute subdurals appear bright white on CT, whereas older and chronic subdurals appear light gray or black.

MRI is up to 50% more sensitive in detecting small subdural hematomas over the convexities (Fig. 6-54A and B). MRI can also identify subdural hemorrhages of differing ages because the imaging intensity changes as blood begins to break down (Fig. 6-54C). However, subdural hematomas of varying ages may be the result of repetitive injury or spontaneous rebleeding. MRI is far superior to CT in detecting subtle contusions and small parenchymal hemorrhages, in identifying diffuse axonal injury, and in detecting abnormalities of posterior fossa structures, the brainstem, and the cervical cord. It is good at detecting signs of prior or old injuries (Fig. 6-55) and is far superior to CT at differentiating subdural from subarachnoid fluid collections and in distinguishing between cerebrospinal fluid and old blood. Its usefulness in child abuse cases is often greatest 5 to 7 days postinjury. For optimal results a T_1 and T_2 weighted conventional or fast spin echo MRI should be ordered with proton density or fluid attenuated inversion recovery (FLAIR) sequences.

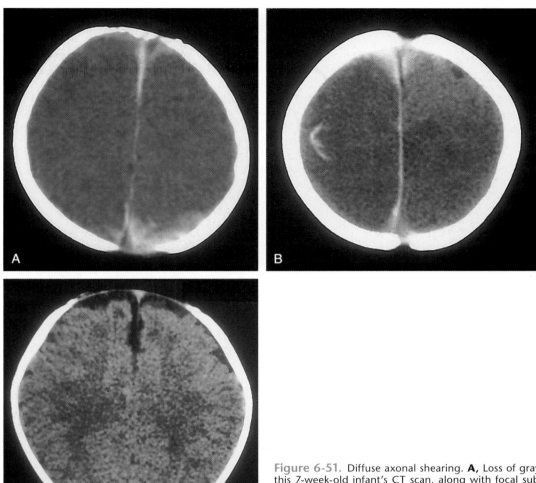

Figure 6-51. Diffuse axonal shearing. **A,** Loss of gray/white matter differentiation is evident on this 7-week-old infant's CT scan, along with focal subdural blood around the left occipital lobe and an interhemispheric subdural hematoma. **B,** This arc-shaped hemorrhage seen in a 2-month-old infant, who also has loss of gray/white matter differentiation, is located at the gray/white interface. This is a sign found occasionally with diffuse axonal shearing injuries. Note the frontal subdural hematoma. **C,** This CT scan of a normal 2-month-old shows normal gray/white matter differentiation.

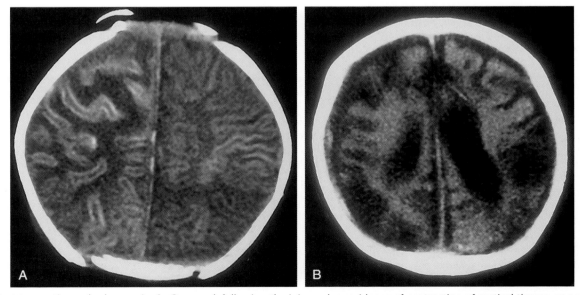

Figure 6-52. Post-traumatic cerebral necrosis. **A,** One week following the injury, clear evidence of contraction of cortical tissues, as a result of extensive neuronal death, can be appreciated. **B,** Six months later, extensive cerebral atrophy is present. This is the same child shown in Figure 6-51B.

Abdominal and Intrathoracic Injuries

Although less common than inflicted surface, skeletal, and head injuries, abdominal and intrathoracic injuries have been found in up to 2% of victims of physical abuse, with a mortality rate of up to 50%. Intra-abdominal injuries predominate over intrathoracic injuries and range in severity from subclinical to catastrophic, with the majority identified as being moderate to severe. They are second only to head injury and suffocation as a cause of abuse-related deaths.

Intraabdominal Injuries

Young children are more vulnerable to internal abdominal injury with blunt trauma than adolescents or adults for three major reasons: their abdominal muscles are relatively weak, allowing impacting forces to be transmitted inward more easily; the distance between the abdominal wall and the vertebral column is relatively short; and their costal margins are more horizontally oriented, affording less protection to underlying viscera. Midabdominal struc-

tures that are fixed in place by pedicles or overlying ligaments (small intestines, liver, and pancreas) are particularly vulnerable. Typically, inflicted abdominal trauma is caused by blunt force injury and is the result of violent kicks or punches or of being thrown or slammed against hard objects. Penetrating injuries, fortunately, are rare (see Fig. 6-16D). External findings are often minimal or absent (see Figs. 6-13 and 6-57A).

As is the case with skeletal and CNS injuries, it is uncommon for caretakers to provide a history of trauma and the severity of attendant symptoms is often minimized. When a history of trauma is reported (usually when bruises are prominent), it is one of a minor mechanism that does not correspond with the type and severity of clinical findings. Presentation is often delayed but may be prompt if signs and symptoms are severe.

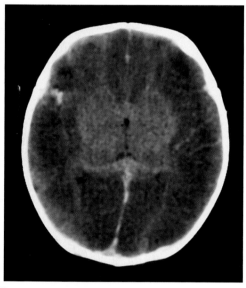

Figure 6-53. Hypoxic injury. This infant, who was found unresponsive in his crib, has a pattern of diffuse cortical hypodensity on CT scan, indicative of extensive cerebral infarction caused by hypoxia.

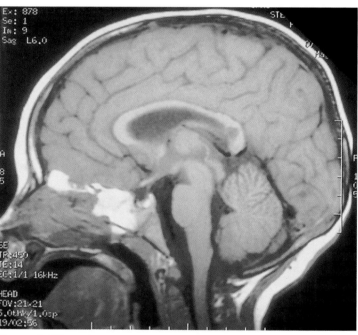

Figure 6-55. Evidence of prior intracranial injury. An MRI obtained of the child whose external injuries are shown in Figure 6-2 shows evidence of prior shearing injury. Note the thinning of the corpus callosum posteriorly and the cyst, both of which reflect degeneration following axonal tearing and subsequent neuronal death.

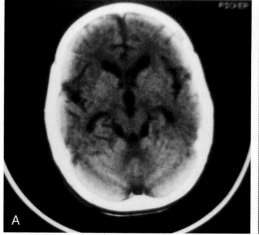
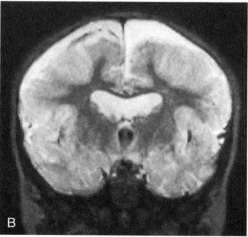
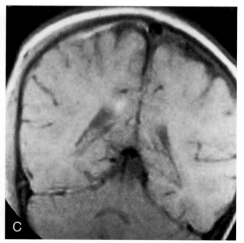

Figure 6-54. **A** and **B,** This 3-year-old abuse victim presented with lethargy, vomiting, hyporeflexia, and the acute onset of blindness. The CT scan reveals ventricular enlargement and cortical atrophy, which were the result of severe shaking 1 year earlier, but no hemorrhage. His MRI shows small, bilateral subdural hemorrhages that were missed on CT. **C,** This 5-month-old infant with head and facial bruises, bilateral retinal hemorrhages, and multiple rib fractures was found to have subdural hemorrhages of differing ages on MRI. The white subdural hematoma is between 0 and 14 days old, and the gray subdural hematoma is more than 14 days old. (Courtesy Dr. Randall Alexander, Moorehead School of Medicine, Atlanta.)

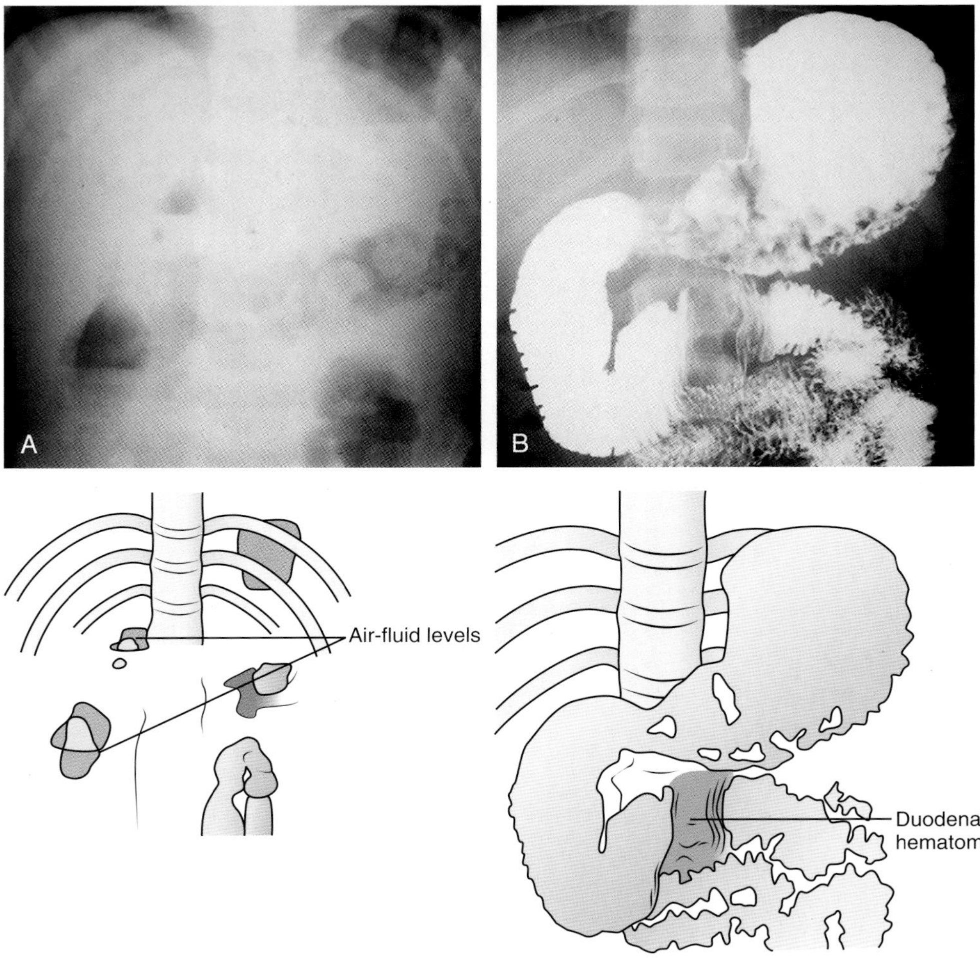

Figure 6-56. Duodenal hematoma. **A,** Abdominal film reveals an air-fluid level in a dilated duodenal loop proximal to a duodenal hematoma. **B,** This upper gastrointestinal series shows narrowing of the duodenal lumen and widening of the duodenal wall at the site of a hematoma. The obstruction is partial because some barium has passed through the narrowed segment. This latency-aged boy was from a wealthy family, and although the victim told physicians that his father had punched him in the stomach 3 days before admission, the father, who was granted access to his son after discharge, made him recant his story and was acquitted. (Courtesy Department of Radiology, Children's Hospital of Pittsburgh, Pa.)

The major types of abdominal pathology seen are duodenal hematomas, small intestinal tears at sites of supporting ligaments, mesenteric tears, contusions or lacerations of the liver or spleen, and pancreatic and renal contusions.

Patients with duodenal hematomas present with signs and symptoms of high intestinal obstruction (e.g., vomiting and abdominal pain without abdominal distention). Plain radiographs may reveal an air-fluid level in a dilated duodenal loop (Fig. 6-56A) proximal to the hematoma, and upper gastrointestinal series and ultrasound studies reveal narrowing of the lumen and thickening of the duodenal wall, respectively (see Fig. 6-56B).

Because spillage of intestinal contents into the peritoneal cavity results in intense peritoneal irritation and rapid onset of infection, children with acute small intestinal tears generally have severe abdominal pain within an hour or two of injury. In most cases this is diffuse at time of presentation and is associated with marked abdominal distention, due to third spacing of fluid by the inflamed peritoneum (Fig. 6-57A) along with diffuse, direct, and rebound tenderness, and signs of sepsis and shock. In cases in which the rent or tear is small and the child can wall off the infection, signs and symptoms will be more localized, less marked, and similar to those of a youngster with an appendiceal abscess.

At a minimum, small tears of the mesentery, which carries the vascular supply to the large and small bowel, result in some bleeding with secondary, often localized, irritation and pain because bowel integrity tends to be preserved by collateral circulation. In the absence of prominent peritoneal signs and surface injuries, pain may be attributed to another cause. When rents are large (Fig. 6-57B), however, interruption of the vascular supply to the

adjacent bowel occurs, and as the involved segment gradually loses viability, it undergoes necrosis and ultimately perforates (Fig. 6-57C). This process can take days, in part because of collateral circulation and in part because of evolution of the inflammatory process that thins the bowel wall before perforation ultimately occurs. During this time the child is likely to have significant abdominal pain, anorexia, vomiting, and markedly decreased activity. Parents, however, are unlikely to report these symptoms. Once perforation occurs, the clinical picture of diffuse peritonitis and sepsis, described earlier, rapidly evolves.

Abuse victims with hepatic and splenic injuries may have minimal symptomatology when these viscera are merely contused. Localized pain and peritoneal irritation are likely with small lacerations. With large lacerations, intense abdominal pain and often pain referred to the ipsilateral shoulder tend to develop within an hour because extravasated blood stimulates peritoneal and diaphragmatic irritation. In addition, signs of pallor and hypovolemia are likely to evolve with comparable rapidity. Sudden "unexplained" collapse is the rule when inflicted blows shatter one or both of these organs.

In the majority of cases of inflicted abdominal trauma, abuse is not confirmed until an abdominal CT scan is obtained, whether because of elevated liver function tests or findings on examination. In some instances the true origin of the problem is not identified until surgery is performed.

Findings from Coant's study in 1992 indicate that the true incidence of intra-abdominal injury in abuse victims may be significantly underestimated. Using transaminase levels as screening tests, the investigators found evidence of hepatic injury including three small liver lacerations in 4 of 49 patients with multiple bruises being evaluated for

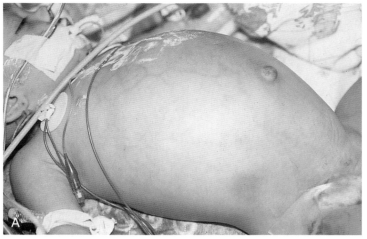

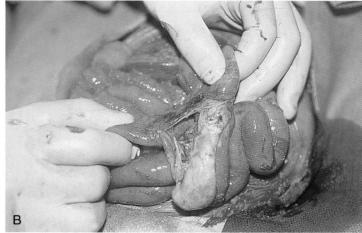

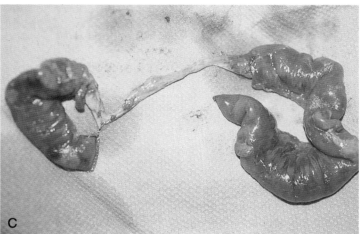

Figure 6-57. Mesenteric tears with secondary bowel necrosis. The mother of this 13-month-old infant (who was described as previously well) reported finding her unarousable in the morning, with bilious vomitus on her sheets. She was rushed to the hospital, where she was in profound shock. Her abdomen was markedly distended and tense and was noted to be exquisitely tender when her level of consciousness improved. **A,** A round, fading bruise is seen in this view over the right lower abdominal wall; a few even fainter bruises were seen around the umbilicus. Note the marked abdominal distention. **B,** At surgery she was found to have diffuse peritonitis, and two large rents were discovered in the jejunal mesentery. **C,** A long segment, found to be necrotic with a perforation, and adjacent bowel that appeared nonviable were resected. Inflammatory infiltrates on pathologic examination suggested that the inciting injury had occurred 5 to 7 days earlier.

possible physical abuse. Although some patients had clinical evidence of head injury and some had facial or thoracic bruises, none had any external evidence of abdominal trauma or any abdominal tenderness. All were younger than 5 years of age. This indicates that serum transaminase levels should be checked in suspected victims of physical abuse who are younger than 5 years of age, much as a skeletal survey is recommended for those younger than 2 years. If levels are elevated, an abdominal CT scan should be obtained.

Renal and adrenal injuries (Fig. 6-58) are considerably less common than those involving other intra-abdominal organs, probably because of their relatively protected location. Associated symptoms may be subtle and overshadowed by other injuries, unless there is extravasation of blood into the peritoneal cavity.

Thoracic Injuries

Because of the great plasticity of the thoracic cage in infants and young children, inflicted intrathoracic injuries are relatively uncommon, despite the frequency of rib fractures. They have high morbidity and mortality rates, however, because they are the result of application of massive forces to the chest such as stomping, slamming, or violent throws. When they are seen, they are usually associated with multiple, often displaced rib fractures (Fig. 6-59). Associated intrathoracic findings may include hemothorax, pleural effusion in response to smaller subpleural bleeds, pulmonary and myocardial contusions, and parenchymal lacerations. On rare occasions a pleural effusion may be seen on chest radiographs in the absence of visible rib fractures. In such cases a bone scan may reveal the true extent of the associated skeletal injuries.

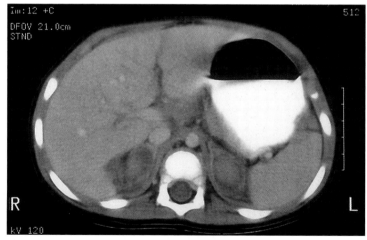

Figure 6-58. Bilateral adrenal hemorrhages. This 21-month-old girl was admitted with a history of altered level of consciousness after falling from her crib. She had multiple bruises, a clavicle fracture, bilateral retinal hemorrhages, subdural hematomas with cerebral edema, and a midline shift (see Fig. 6-50). Her abdominal CT scan, performed when liver function tests were found to be elevated, reveals bilateral adrenal hemorrhages.

The major mode of presentation of inflicted intrathoracic chest trauma is likely to be one of significant respiratory distress, with complaints of severe chest pain in victims old enough to speak. Less often, sudden collapse is reported. Typically, no history of injury is provided or one of a minor mechanism is given. Clinical findings may include dyspnea, tachypnea, grunting respirations, and anxiety, often with evident pain on movement and chest wall tenderness. When associated blood loss is significant, pallor, weak pulses, and hypotension are seen.

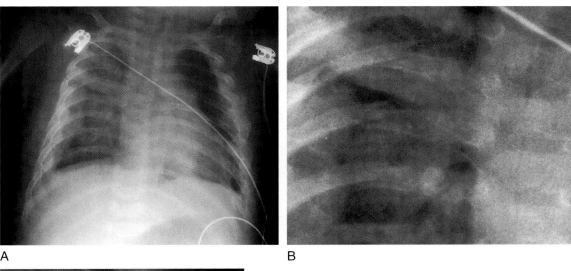

A

B

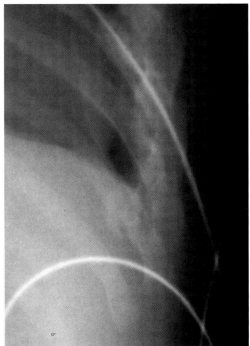

C

Figure 6-59. Intrathoracic trauma. This 4-month-old boy was brought in with severe respiratory distress and found to have paradoxical chest wall movement, caused by flail chest, and respiratory failure. **A,** His chest radiograph reveals bilateral rib fractures, with multiple fractures along many of the rib arcs, some with and some without callus. Three of the posterior fractures on the right are badly displaced. He has bilateral pleural effusions and bilateral soft tissue swelling over the chest wall, along with multiple pulmonary contusions seen as patchy infiltrates. **B,** Close-up of fresh, displaced fractures of the fifth to seventh ribs posteriorly. **C,** Close-up of left lateral rib fractures shows refracture through the callus of the ninth rib.

Differential Diagnosis of Inflicted Injuries versus Findings Caused by Accident or Illness

Although it is highly important to detect injuries resulting from abuse in order to protect children from future and potentially more serious trauma, it is also important to avoid diagnosing abuse erroneously because this subjects innocent families to the ordeal of a CPS investigation and sometimes results in removal of the child to foster care, causing tremendous emotional stress. Accurate diagnosis requires clear knowledge, not only of patterns of injury seen following abuse, but also of mechanisms of injury and their resulting findings, of the types of accidental injuries commonly seen at various ages, and of the diseases and congenital disorders that predispose to bleeding or increased bony fragility. In the vast majority of cases of significant accidental injury, the patient is brought in promptly for care by appropriately concerned parents who give a clear history of a mechanism that fits the findings. Typically there are no associated injuries unless the mechanism involves a motor vehicle accident or major fall, and there is no history or evidence of multiple prior injuries. These families usually have been compliant with well-child care and although interviews may reveal an occasional risk factor, there is no worrisome pattern of risk factors and red flags, and parent-child interactions demonstrate warmth, caring, attentiveness, and affection. If doubt exists the services of experienced physicians with expertise in the fields of child abuse, orthopedics, pediatric surgery, and neurosurgery should be sought. In addition valuable information and insight may be gained in conferring with the child's primary care physician.

Differential Diagnosis of Surface Bruises

Accidental Bruises
Ordinary, play-related bruises can be distinguished from those resulting from abuse by virtue of the fact that they tend to be small and nonspecific in configuration. They are typically located over the bony prominences of the

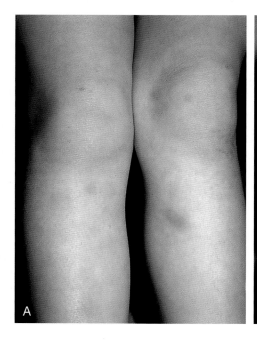

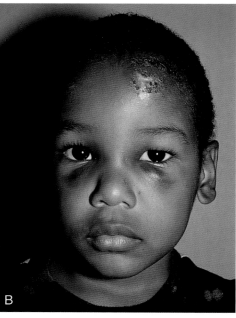

Figure 6-60. Normal bruises. **A,** Numerous small, nonspecific bruises are present over the knees and shins of this active youngster. **B,** Black eyes occurring after a forehead contusion. This boy had fallen from the ladder of a slide 3 days before. Blood from his forehead hematoma had tracked down through the facial soft tissues, creating these shiners, which were nontender.

shins, knees, elbows, extensor forearms, midchin, or mid-forehead (Fig. 6-60A). Larger bruises and even those with configurations suggesting they were inflicted by an object can also be accidental or the result of an altercation with another child. In such cases, however, presentation for care is prompt, the mechanism of injury is consistent with the findings, and in most instances the incident was witnessed.

Black eyes following forehead contusions may be mistaken for inflicted bruises. If the initial injury produces a large forehead hematoma, subsequent tracking of blood through the soft tissue planes of the face is likely to occur over the ensuing 24 to 72 hours, producing ecchymotic discoloration along the sides of the nose and under the lower eyelids (Fig. 6-60B). This gives the illusion of an injury resulting from direct periorbital trauma. The history, presence of residual forehead contusion, and absence of tenderness in the infraorbital area help confirm the true origin of these findings.

Bruises Caused by Subcultural Healing Practices
The influx of immigrants from Southeast Asia to the United States and Canada since the late 1970s has made it important to be aware of nonabusive healing practices that produce unusual bruising patterns. The most common of these is coin rubbing, in which the skin of the trunk and back is rubbed vigorously with the edge of a coin as a means of treating fever. This leaves a pattern of bruises resembling the branches of a fir tree (Fig. 6-61). In another practice termed *cupping,* a candle is lit and placed under a small glass cup or the inner surface of the cup is coated with alcohol that is then burned off. The cup is then applied to the forehead or trunk. As oxygen is consumed by the flame, or as the cup cools, a vacuum is created, and the cup adheres to the skin. On removal, a round imprint is left on the skin. As the indentation resolves, a characteristic circular ecchymosis remains that encircles central petechiae (Fig. 6-62).

Purpura Due to Bleeding Disorders or Vasculitis
Purpuric lesions associated with coagulopathies and acute vasculitic disorders must also be recognized and

distinguished from inflicted bruises. It is also important to recognize that children with disorders that predispose to easy bruising may on occasion be victims of abuse.

Thrombocytopenia
Patients with acute idiopathic thrombocytopenic purpura (ITP) and acute leukemia can have multiple purpuric lesions located anywhere on the body. Because they reflect thrombocytopenia, they are usually associated with petechiae (Fig. 6-63). Children with ITP commonly have a history of an antecedent viral illness, and those with leukemia may have a history of fatigue, anorexia, and weight loss, sometimes accompanied by bone pain. They usually have adenopathy and splenomegaly. Patients with aplastic anemia can have bruises with round, thick, indurated centers similar to those seen in children with clotting factor deficiencies, but typically their bruises are surrounded by petechiae (Fig. 6-64). These hematologic abnormalities are usually readily detected by a complete blood cell count with differential and platelet count.

Clotting Factor Deficiencies
Children with clotting factor deficiencies—the hemophilias and von Willebrand disease—tend to bruise easily, and their bruises are often much more impressive than one would ordinarily expect from the reported mechanism of injury. Those with factor VIII or IX deficiencies tend to have bruises with round, thick, indurated centers as are seen in aplastic anemia (see Fig. 6-64) but without the satellite petechiae. Although severe X-linked hemophilia is diagnosed prenatally in most males because of known family history or in early infancy (frequently following circumcision), those with milder forms of the disease who are uncircumcised may not be identified until they start crawling and develop prominent ecchymoses over their knees and palms, along with other evidence of easy bruising.

Von Willebrand disease, which occurs in both males and females, is characterized by partial factor VIII deficiency and platelet dysfunction and may escape detection for years. The disorder is diagnosed in some patients when they suffer unexpectedly severe bleeding postoperatively. In many girls or young women, it is identified when they

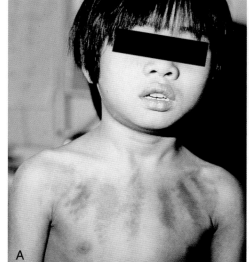
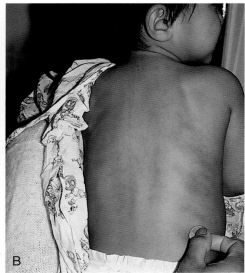

Figure 6-61. Coin rubbing. **A,** Vigorous stroking of the skin of a febrile child with a coin produces a peculiar bruising pattern. **B,** Here the father of another child demonstrates the technique. (**A,** Courtesy Dr. Thomas Daley, St. Joseph's Hospital, Paterson, N.J.)

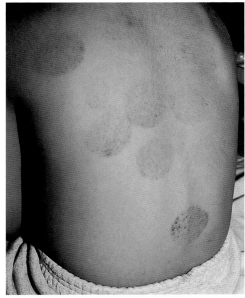
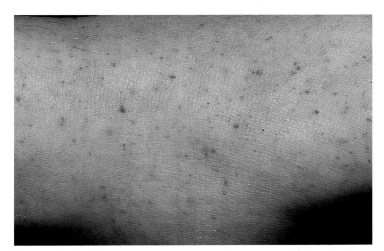

Figure 6-62. Cupping. These circular bruises with central petechiae are the sequelae of the Southeast Asian practice of cupping. (Courtesy Dr. Robert Hickey, Children's Hospital of Pittsburgh, Pa.)

Figure 6-63. Idiopathic thrombocytopenic purpura. This school-age child was seen with a chief complaint of a rash after a viral upper respiratory tract infection. Examination revealed diffuse petechiae, shown here over her ankle, and scattered purpuric lesions. Her hemoglobin and white blood cell count and differential were normal, but her platelet count was markedly reduced.

develop menorrhagia during adolescence or have severe bleeding following childbirth. Suspicion of abuse may arise when an affected child presents with an unusually florid bruise following relatively mild accidental trauma. Clues to an underlying factor deficiency include (1) bruises with round, thick, indurated centers (see Fig. 6-64); (2) a clear mechanism of injury consistent with the configuration but not the severity of the bruise; and (3) a family and child who seem well adjusted and interact appropriately. A positive family history for bleeding problems, especially after surgery or the birth of a baby, may also exist. Whenever any question exists about a possible factor deficiency, a full coagulation profile is recommended because platelet counts are normal and many patients with von Willebrand disease have normal prothrombin and partial thromboplastin times.

Vasculitis

Patients with vasculitic disorders may develop diffuse purpuric lesions that can be mistaken for inflicted bruises. In the pediatric population, *Henoch-Schönlein purpura* is by

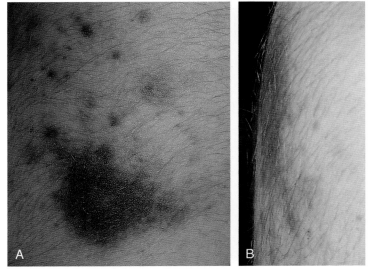

Figure 6-64. **A,** Bruises with thick round centers can be seen in children with aplastic anemia or with clotting factor deficiencies. **B,** This view from the side shows the elevation of the indurated central portion of the ecchymosis in a patient with chronic aplastic anemia.

far the most common of these. Knowledge of the pattern and course of evolution of its exanthem can help prevent misdiagnosis. Affected children often have a history of antecedent viral or streptococcal infection, followed by the appearance of the exanthem. In many children the initial lesions are urticarial, although pruritus is mild or absent. The purpuric lesions appear in crops, with the first distributed below the waist. Subsequent crops tend to involve the extensor forearms, cheeks, and ears. Periarticular swelling and stocking-glove angioedema, which wax and wane, are common, as is crampy or colicky abdominal pain (see Chapters 7 and 8 and Fig. 8-63).

Ehlers-Danlos Syndrome

Children with various forms of Ehlers-Danlos syndrome tend to not only have hyperextensible skin but also bruise easily and thus often have multiple bruises of varying ages that are usually located over their extremities. This has been mistaken in some cases for child abuse but can be distinguished by careful assessment for skin distensibility, joint hypermobility, and thin atrophic scars that are typical associated findings (see Chapter 1 and Fig. 1-30).

Hyperpigmentation

Mongolian Spots. Most infants of African, Mediterranean, and Asian descent have patchy areas of hyperpigmentation, termed "mongolian spots", in which the epithelial cells contain increased amounts of melanin. These are most commonly located over the sacrum and buttocks, although they may be found elsewhere on the trunk and extremities. These areas are flat, nontender, and typically a bit more blue or green than true acute ecchymotic lesions (Fig. 6-65; see also Chapter 8 and Fig. 8-87).

Postinflammatory Hyperpigmentation. Following resolution of the acute phase of an inflammatory exanthem, many children with darkly pigmented skin are left with patchy hyperpigmentation at the sites affected (see Fig. 8-124). These patches can be mistaken for bruises on occasion, particularly when the initial rash involved the buttocks or back. Lesions are brown to dark brown, nontender, and do not change in hue over a period of days or even

weeks, as do bruises. A history of antecedent dermatitis helps in distinguishing the true nature of the problem.

The bites of blood-sucking insects, especially fleas and bed bugs, can induce a hypersensitivity reaction in some children, known as *papular urticaria* (see Fig. 8-68). This is manifest clinically by symmetric chronic/recurrent eruptions of highly pruritic papules and wheals that tend to vesiculate centrally Because itching is intense, scratching to the point of excoriation is typical. On resolution the child is left with target-shaped macular scars that are hyperpigmented peripherally and hypopigmented centrally (see Fig. 6-73). These may be mistaken for bruises or healed cigarette burns (see Fig. 6-21C and D).

One particular type of postinflammatory hyperpigmentation is more often confused with bruising than others, *phytophotodermatitis*. In this disorder, plant-derived photosensitizers (psoralens) found in the juices of lemons, limes, figs, dill, parsley, parsnips, carrots, and celery are inadvertently wiped or spilled on the skin. Subsequent exposure to sunlight can then induce an exaggerated sunburn reaction. Initially, lesions are erythematous macules. In some cases, surface blistering occurs. Lesions then become hyperpigmented, and because the juice is often wiped on by the hands of a parent who was in the process of cutting one of the fruits, herbs, or vegetables when approached by the child, the patches often have bizarre or hand- or finger-shaped patterns that can be mistaken for grab or slap marks (Fig. 6-66). Again, the history of a preceding erythematous rash and the persistence of the same coloration over days or weeks can help in identifying the true source.

Patterned Tanning. Although not commonly mistaken for bruises, patterned tanning, resulting from sun exposure while wearing articles of clothing (often bathing

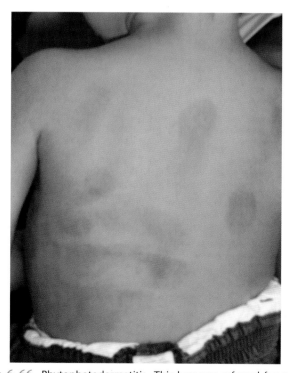

Figure 6-66. Phytophotodermatitis. This boy was referred for concerns regarding possible inflicted bruises. The bizarre hand/finger marks are actually due to hyperpigmentation caused by a phototoxic reaction to psoralens. More than 2 weeks earlier, while his family was on vacation at the shore, he had been picked up by his father, who had just been cutting limes for a party. The family then went to the beach for the afternoon. Subsequently the child developed erythematous patches in the distribution seen, which then became hyperpigmented.

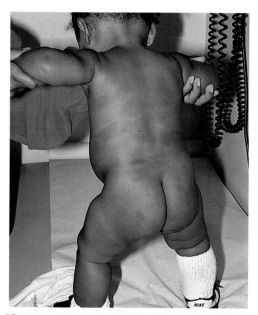

Figure 6-65. Mongolian spots. This toddler, referred from a day care center because of "multiple bruises," actually had an unusual number of hyperpigmented mongolian spots.

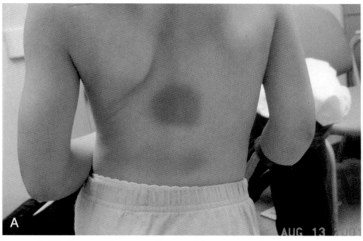
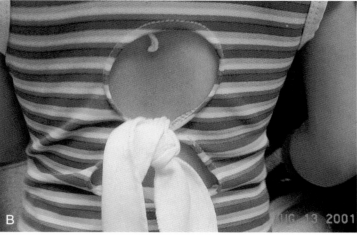

Figure 6-67. Patterned tan marks. **A,** This young girl, a former victim of abuse and neglect, was noted to have an odd, perfectly round patch of dark brown skin over her back seen during a visit for a mild acute injury. Despite its perfect shape, which was unlike common weapons of discipline, bruising was suspected. Neither mother nor child could think of a related incident. **B,** Then, her new shirt was remembered.

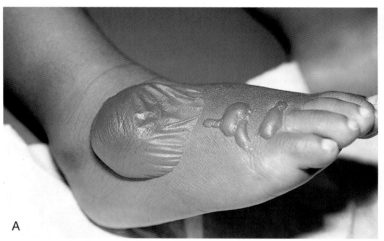
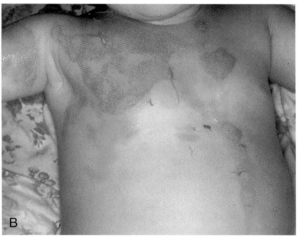

Figure 6-68. Accidental scalds. **A,** The splash-and-droplet pattern of an accidental scald is evident on the foot of a toddler who grabbed a hot cup of tea from the table while sitting on his grandmother's lap. **B,** This toddler grabbed a pot handle projecting out over the edge of a stove, spilling hot soup over her chest and shoulder. Cooling of the hot liquid as it flowed downward produced the inverted arrowhead pattern, the burn being wider and of greater depth proximally and narrowing and becoming more superficial distally. There is also a descending droplet and splash pattern to the left of the midline.

suits) that have cut-out designs (Fig. 6-67), can be a source of confusion. The mistake is more likely when the cut-outs are round or linear, when different apparel is being worn at the time the child is seen, and when clinicians fail to recognize that children who have naturally dark skin tan with sun exposure, just as do those with fair complexions.

Differential Diagnosis of Accidental versus Inflicted Burns

All children incur accidental burns in the course of growing up, and it is important to be able to distinguish these from inflicted burns. Many are so small and minor that no medical care is sought. Children with more significant accidental burns usually present soon after the incident, and the history is consistent with the physical findings. Presentation may be delayed, however, if a minor burn being treated at home becomes secondarily infected.

Accidental Scalds
Accidental scalds typically occur when a hot liquid is spilled, producing a splash-and-droplet pattern in the case

of a small spill (Fig. 6-68A) or an inverted arrowhead in cases of larger spills over the chest (Fig. 6-68B). The child usually presents with a history of having grabbed a cup of hot coffee, tea, or cocoa from the table while sitting on someone's lap, or of having reached up and grabbed the projecting handle of a pot on the stove. In some instances a parent or older sibling has stumbled while carrying a pan of hot liquid or food, and resulting burns commonly involve the chest, a hand, a foot, or occasionally the head. As noted earlier, presentation is prompt and parents/ grandparents are appropriately concerned, and often feeling very guilty about this happening. Accidental spill scalds cannot be distinguished clinically from purposeful spills, unless there is a clear delay in seeking care for large burns.

Vesicular Reactions to Insect Bites
Some mites when biting inject a blistering agent that causes vesiculation. Such vesicles and blisters have been mistakenly attributed to sprinkling the child with scalding water. On close inspection, however, the lesions (which are pruritic rather than painful) are found to be almost perfectly round with no evidence of splash, and the roof of each blister or vesicle is noted to have a thicker wall

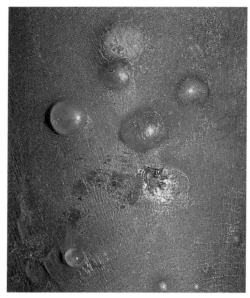

Figure 6-69. Vesiculation due to mite bites. These vesicles initially thought to be due to burns are relatively thick walled and almost perfectly round, and they show no evidence of splash. Furthermore, the lesions were pruritic, not painful.

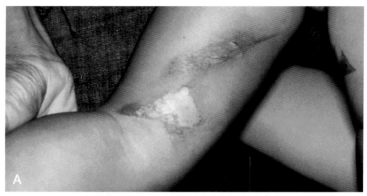

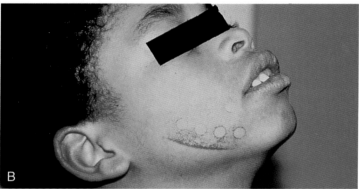

Figure 6-70. Accidental iron burns. **A,** These linear and patchy burns are characteristic of an accidental iron burn. In this case the patient's brother pulled the iron down by grabbing the cord while she had her back turned. **B,** This hyperactive boy decided to test the iron on his cheek while his mother went to answer the phone. Though the imprint of the iron is clear, the superficial depth of the burn is more consistent with an accidental than with an inflicted burn.

than that of the blisters of a second-degree burn (Fig. 6-69).

Accidental Iron Burns

Pulling an iron down from the ironing board by yanking on its cord is the classic scenario for an accidental iron burn in a young child. The iron, being heavier at one end, falls end over end, producing a configuration of two or three linear or patchy first- or second-degree burns separated by gaps (Fig. 6-70A). On rare occasions the flat surface of the iron may land on the leg of a child seated on the floor, but the child's immediate reflex action to get the hot object off will result in at most a superficial pattern burn (see Fig. 6-70B). In older children and adolescents, burns are more often acquired in the course of ironing and usually consist of small, superficial, linear burns of the hand or fingers. Occasionally, impulsive behavior results in accidentally self-inflicted burns, which also tend to be superficial (Fig. 6-70B).

Accidental Curling Iron Burns

Accidental curling iron injuries occur most commonly when an older infant, toddler, or preschool-age child grabs the hot wand of a curling iron that has been left unattended by a parent or older sibling. The resulting first- and second-degree burns thus involve the palm and flexor surfaces of the fingers of one hand and are of varying depths (Fig. 6-71). Preadolescent and adolescent girls may incur superficial burns of the ears or nape of the neck if they are not careful when curling their hair.

Accidental Space Heater Burns

During winter months, accidental burns can be incurred as a result of brushing up against the grid of a space heater while walking or running by it or when engaging in wrestling or horseplay near it. The lesions produced tend to be superficial and tangential and usually involve the dorsum of a hand or occasionally the lateral aspect of the lower leg or forearm. Less commonly, crawling infants and toddlers engaged in exploration may grab the grid, incurring palmar burns, or may fall against it.

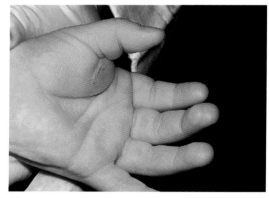

Figure 6-71. Accidental curling iron burn. First- and second-degree burns are seen over the palm and flexor surfaces of the fingers of this toddler who grabbed her mother's curling iron.

Blistering Distal Dactylitis

This acute infection, usually caused by group A streptococci (less often by group B streptococci or *Staphylococcus aureus*), is characterized by formation of 0.5- to 1-cm blisters of the tips and distal pads of the fingers or toes (see Fig. 8-50). Because of their location, they are sometimes mistaken for fingertip burns. The fact that the vesicular fluid is cloudy, in contrast to the clear fluid of acute partial-thickness burn blisters, distinguishes these lesions from burns, and Gram stain of the fluid is positive for organisms. It should also be noted that fingertip burns are more likely to be accidental than inflicted.

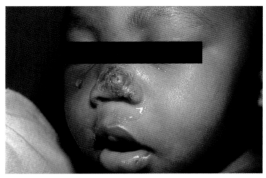

Figure 6-72. Impetigo. This infant was initially suspected of having a cigar burn, but close inspection revealed a new peripheral bullous rim. This and the presence of another early impetiginous lesion on the cheek enabled the correct diagnosis to be made.

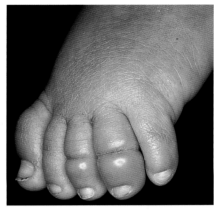

Figure 6-74. Hair tourniquet. The erythema and edema of the third and fourth toes seen here are the result of constriction by hairs that accidentally became wrapped around them. (Courtesy Dr. Thomas J. Daley, St. Joseph's Hospital, Paterson, N.J.)

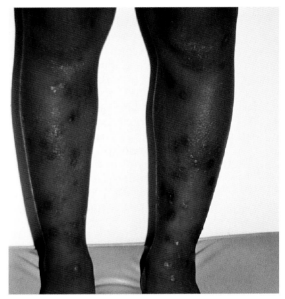

Figure 6-73. Postinflammatory hyperpigmentation following insect bites or papular urticaria. When this child was seen at a follow-up visit for the treatment of flea bites, he was found to have a multitude of round, hyperpigmented spots at the sites of the original bites. Their macular appearance, distribution, and target configuration distinguish them from cigarette burn scars. (Courtesy Dr. Michael Sherlock, Lutherville, Md.)

Accidental Cigarette Burns

Unintentional cigarette burns usually occur when a child accidentally brushes against the lit end of an adult's cigarette. They tend to be single superficial, tangential burns and usually involve one hand, a forearm, or the cheek.

Lesions Often Mistaken for Cigarette Burns

On occasion, impetiginous lesions have been mistaken for cigarette or cigar burns. This is often the case with bullous impetigo, after the initial central bulla has ruptured and crusted over. On careful inspection, one can detect the formation of bullous rims around the more central crusts, and other lesions can usually be found nearby (Fig. 6-72). Removal of the crust will reveal that the lesion is superficial, in contrast to the full-thickness depression seen on removal of the eschar from most inflicted cigarette or cigar burns.

On resolution of the acute inflammatory phase of insect bites or papular urticaria, children are often left with round target-shaped macular scars that are hyperpigmented peripherally and hypopigmented centrally. These have been mistaken for healed cigarette burns (Fig. 6-73).

However, their usual distribution is over the lower legs above the sock line in older children, or over the arms, legs, face, neck, and scalp in crawling infants and toddlers. The fact that these are macular and not punched-out scars should enable the clinician to distinguish between these and the scars left by full-thickness cigarette burns (see Fig. 6-21C). Flea bite scars also tend to have a target pattern, probably because of the central punctum within the wheal of the acute bite. This differs from the uniform surface of most macular cigarette burn scars (see Fig. 6-21D).

Accidental Tourniquet Injuries

Perhaps the most common form of accidental tourniquet injury is that caused by a hair that becomes tightly wrapped around the toe of an infant (Fig. 6-74). The constriction causes pain and irritability, which prompts the parent to seek the cause. Hence such patients are brought in promptly before circulatory compromise occurs. If they are not and the toe is gangrenous, neglect should be suspected. We have also seen young children with mild hand edema as a result of putting colored rubber bands that are too small and tight around their wrists for bracelets.

Differentiation of Accidental and Pathologic Fractures from Inflicted Fractures

Accidental Fractures

In most instances it is relatively easy to recognize a truly accidental fracture: the incident is usually witnessed, and the mechanism of injury is clearly reported and fits the findings unless it is the result of an unwitnessed fall or fall down stairs. Care is typically sought promptly, although occasional exceptions occur, especially if the patient is a stoic athlete with a mild buckle fracture of the radius, who avoids complaining in order not to miss an important game. Families are appropriately concerned and interact well with the child. Accidental fractures are usually single or isolated or involve both bones of the forearm or lower leg, and typically there are no associated injuries and no history or evidence of prior injuries.

A thorough history and knowledge of the types of fractures produced by various mechanisms of injury assist accurate diagnosis. Some of the most common fractures and their mechanisms include buckle (torus) and greenstick fractures of the radius and ulna (see Figs. 21-26 and 21-27) due to a fall forward onto an outstretched arm; midclavicular fractures caused by a direct blow to the clavicle or a fall sideways onto the shoulder or outstretched arm (see Fig. 21-20); supracondylar humerus fractures (see Figs. 21-34 and 21-18) due to a fall backward onto a hyperextended outstretched arm; toddler's fractures or spiral fractures of distal to midtibia (see Fig. 21-43) resulting from a fall with a twist while trying to extricate a caught foot, following a sudden turn while running, or on landing from a jump; and transverse diaphyseal fractures (see Fig. 21-28) following a vertical fall of greater than 6 to 10 feet or the result of getting the thigh caught against a firm surface (e.g., having the leg slip between the mattress and outer slat of a bunk bed) and having the upper body fall in the opposite direction.

One type of accidental humerus fracture described fairly recently can easily be mistaken for an inflicted injury. This spiral fracture of the humeral shaft can occur unintentionally when someone turns an infant from prone to supine position without completely lifting the trunk from the surface on which the baby is lying. This occurs when an infant, lying prone, has one arm extended out from the body, palm down and, while held by the opposite arm or axilla, is rolled over to the supine position. Being unable to adduct the extended arm as he is turned, the upper arm is subjected to a twisting force, which produces the spiral fracture.

Conditions Associated with Pathologic Fractures

Three relatively unusual conditions account for most pathologic fractures seen in the pediatric population: osteogenesis imperfecta (OI), demineralization from disuse, and bone cysts.

Osteogenesis Imperfecta. OI is a family of disorders characterized most notably by brittle bones. Nearly 90% of identified cases have been determined to be the result of mutations of either the COL1A1 or COL1A2 genes, which code for the pro-chains of type I collagen, the major structural protein of bone and other connective tissues. Hundreds of different mutations have been identified thus far, nearly all autosomal dominant. Four main types of OI exist, and numerous different mutations have been found causative in each, resulting in significant phenotypic variability, and thereby, range of severity within each type. In mutations causative of OI type I, the synthesized mRNA or its resulting pro-chain are so abnormal that they are destroyed. Hence the abnormal gene is *unexpressed*, and only 50% of the expected amount of collagen is produced, although it is structurally normal. In types II, III, and IV, causative mutations result in synthesis of collagen that is structurally abnormal (see Chapters 1 and 21).

Structural abnormalities are greatest in types II and III, and affected children have severe disease and are born with obvious fractures and deformities (see Chapter 21 and Figs. 21-115 and 21-116). In these cases there should be no confusion with abuse. In contrast, types I and IV are milder, and on occasion, fractures incurred accidentally can be mistaken for inflicted trauma. In this section we focus on the clinical features of types I and IV and how to distinguish affected children from abuse victims with normal bones. It should be emphasized from the outset that infants with these two types are not so brittle that they suffer fractures in the course of normal handling. It should further be noted that, although many, if not most, children with these milder forms of OI have positive family histories for brittle bones and other char-

acteristic features, children with new mutations are not uncommon. Type I is by far the more common of the two, accounting for more than 60% to 80% of all cases of OI, whereas type IV is much rarer, accounting for only about 5% to 6% of all cases.

The vast majority of infants with OI type I are born with distinctly blue or grayish-blue sclerae (see Fig. 21-114A), although the degree varies somewhat and tends to lessen with age. Bony fragility is mild to moderate, and while an occasional patient incurs a fracture during delivery, most do not experience their first break until they have begun to cruise or walk. The most common sites involve the diaphyses of the long bones of the extremities. Radiographically, wormian bones are evident on skull films in infants and toddlers (see Figs. 15-28 and 21-114B), but otherwise bones tend to appear normal in infancy. Then, over the ensuing few years, osteopenia and thinning of the cortices become increasingly evident (see Fig. 21-114C). Other common clinical features include femoral bowing at birth and generalized ligamentous laxity that persists. Teeth are normal except for a small subset who have dentinogenesis imperfecta. Easy bruising and slight thinning of the skin are seen in some but are not striking. Approximately 50% of affected individuals develop progressive hearing loss in their late teens or twenties.

In type IV OI the sclerae are normal in color or slightly gray or bluish gray. The vast majority have dentinogenesis imperfecta, which becomes readily apparent when teeth erupt. This is characterized by dental discoloration, which may be yellowish brown, pinkish brown, or blue with an opalescent sheen (see Chapter 20 and Fig. 20-35). Degree of bony fragility ranges from mild to moderate, less commonly moderately severe. Occasionally, fractures of long bones occur in utero or during delivery, but most affected children do not experience their first break until later in infancy, typically after they have begun to cruise or walk. By far, the majority of fractures involve the diaphyses of long bones. Radiographically, wormian bones are usually apparent on skull films but other bones tend to appear normal in infancy. Thereafter, as in type I, osteopenia and cortical thinning become increasingly evident.

Linear growth tends to be mildly impaired, and by age 2 to 3 years most children with type IV OI are at or below the third percentile in height. Femoral bowing is seen in newborns, and subsequently bowing and/or valgus deformity of the lower extremities becomes evident in the majority during the toddler and preschool years.

Differentiating Osteogenesis Imperfecta and Abuse.

Distinguishing infants and children with mild OI who incur accidental fractures from normal children with inflicted injuries is usually quite feasible. Those with OI typically are brought promptly to medical attention by appropriately concerned parents who interact warmly with their child. Unless the fracture is the result of an unwitnessed fall, they give a clear history of a mechanism of injury that fits the fracture pattern found, although the amount of force involved may be somewhat less than that usually required to cause a fracture. Generally, a single fracture of the diaphysis of a long bone, or both bone diaphyseal fractures of a forearm or lower leg are found. Furthermore, one does not see evidence of multiple fractures of differing ages for which no prior care has been sought (especially not fractures in close succession). Instead, when the child has suffered prior fractures, care for these also has been sought promptly, and parents readily report this in the history along with details of the treatment prescribed. Further, if OI has not previously been diagnosed and there is no positive family history, they may even ask if anything can be done to determine why their child is so prone to fractures.

Several other points warrant emphasis. Blue sclerae are evident in the vast majority of children with type I disease, as are the findings of short stature, bowing or valgus deformities of the lower extremities, and the dental discoloration of dentinogenesis imperfecta, once teeth have erupted, in children with type IV OI. Furthermore, the "classical metaphyseal lesions," rib and skull fractures so common in young abuse victims, are rare in infants and children with mild forms of OI. The same is true of subdural hematomas and retinal hemorrhages (see "Differential Diagnosis of Accidental versus Inflicted Head Injuries" later), and visceral injuries have not been reported. When these findings are present, one must seriously consider the possibility of abuse of a child with OI.

The major potential source of confusion involves a young infant with type IV OI or the rare baby with type I OI whose sclerae are not noticeably blue and who has incurred one or more nondisplaced fractures in utero or during delivery that went undiagnosed in the newborn period. If this infant then has an accidental fracture in the ensuing few months, radiographs may reveal old, "unexplained" healing fractures. Even in this situation, careful clinical evaluation with close attention to timeliness of presentation with the acute fracture, consistency of reported mechanism with fracture type, and parental demeanor, combined with lack of evidence of other signs of injury and family and psychosocial history, can aid in making the correct diagnosis. Reviewing radiographs including skull films with an experienced pediatric radiologist is also useful to check for wormian bones and any signs of osteopenia. Finally, it can be most helpful to confer with the child's primary care physician regarding prior experience with the family and older siblings and the family's compliance with care.

Another scenario that can be a source of concern may occur when an older child with mild OI who has a high pain threshold incurs a mild nondisplaced fracture. In such instances the child may experience pain or an aching sensation that seems "not worth complaining about," until it persists, thereby resulting in a delay in seeking care. Again, using the same principles of careful and open-minded evaluation, as described earlier, can assist correct diagnosis. Furthermore, in older children, osteopenia is more likely to be evident radiographically.

In the rare case in which a clinical diagnosis cannot be made with any degree of assurance, and where an exact diagnosis is necessary, a skin biopsy can be obtained for analysis of collagen synthesis by cultured fibroblasts. However, this procedure takes 3 to 4 months and will be negative in 12% to 14% of cases (see later).

Three other types of OI (V through VII) that have no detectable defect of type I collagen have been described more recently. All are rare, and each has distinct clinical and/or radiographic findings that help distinguish affected from normal infants and children (see Chapter 21). These likely account for many, if not most, of the negative findings on analysis of collagen synthesis.

Temporary Brittle Bone Disease. "Temporary brittle bone disease" is a disorder that has been proposed by Patterson and Miller as a transient phenomenon seen only in the first year of life, in which affected infants are unusually vulnerable to fractures with minimal trauma. On review, the few articles published on the subject are not only not peer reviewed but have poor methodology. Cases presented are not well documented and include

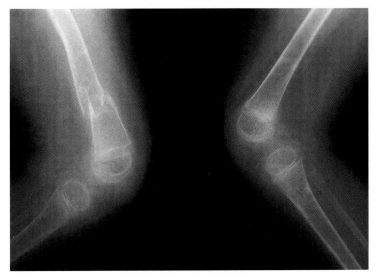

Figure 6-75. Demineralization from disuse. Severe osteopenia and a femur fracture incurred during physical therapy are evident in this child who was left quadriplegic as the result of an earlier injury. Note the lack of muscle mass. (Courtesy Department of Radiology, Children's Hospital of Pittsburgh, Pa.)

infants with unequivocal findings of inflicted trauma. Among these are cases in which signs of callus formation became apparent during the course of hospitalization for suspected abuse, which the authors describe as having "occurred in hospital." This is a clear misinterpretation of a well-known phenomenon seen especially in abused infants who are admitted with inflicted head trauma, as many of these babies have at least some nondisplaced fractures less than 10 days old when admitted. Initially invisible radiographically, these fractures then become apparent as healing progresses, often being seen on repeat chest films in intubated infants or on follow-up skeletal surveys. There are no scientific data, and there is no corroborative evidence to support the existence of this "disorder" or the hypotheses of transient metabolic defects proposed to explain it.

Demineralization from Disuse. Children with severe cerebral palsy, myelodysplasia, advanced neuromuscular diseases, paraplegia, or quadriplegia that essentially leaves them confined to bed or a wheelchair develop muscular atrophy and bony demineralization as the result of disuse. Cortical thinning is marked (Fig. 6-75) and makes the patient vulnerable to fractures after the application of mild forces, whether in minor falls or in the process of manipulation during physical therapy.

Bone Cysts. Benign bone cysts in pediatric patients are usually seen near the metaphyseal ends of long bones. As they enlarge, they cause cortical thinning, leaving the bone vulnerable to fracture (Fig. 6-76). Similar pathologic fractures may occur at sites of osteomyelitis or in portions of bone replaced by tumor.

Conditions Associated with or Mimicking Fractures

Congenital Pseudarthrosis of the Clavicle. Congenital pseudarthrosis of the clavicle is a rare congenital anomaly that usually involves the right clavicle and probably results from failed maturation of an ossification center. The clavicle appears foreshortened and has a visible bulbous deformity near its midportion (see Fig. 21-82). Hypermobility and crepitance are felt on palpation over the bump. This is distinguishable from a fracture because the site is nontender and the patient has full range of motion of the shoulder without pain. On radiography the

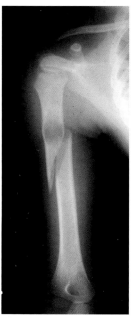

Figure 6-76. Fracture through a unicameral bone cyst. This boy was seen because of intense pain and swelling of his upper arm after a relatively minor fall (due to slipping on wet grass while running to get out of the rain). The radiograph reveals a pathologic fracture through a unicameral bone cyst, which has caused considerable cortical thinning. (Courtesy Department of Radiology, Children's Hospital of Pittsburgh, Pa.)

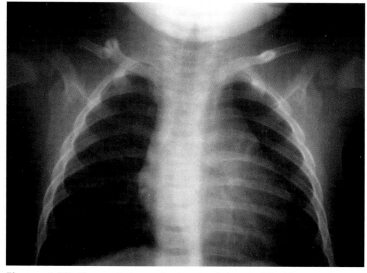

Figure 6-77. Congenital pseudarthrosis of the clavicle. The overlapping ends of bone near the midpoint of this infant's clavicle are smooth, rounded, and well corticated, distinguishing this congenital anomaly from a fracture.

two ends of the clavicle at the point of deformity are seen to be smooth and rounded and covered with a well-formed bony cortex (Fig. 6-77). Pseudarthroses of the tibia, fibula, femur, or clavicle can also be seen in children with neurofibromatosis type 1 (see Chapter 15 and Fig. 8-131B). Hence NF1 should be considered whenever a pseudarthrosis is detected.

Rickets. Because of poor mineralization, the bones of infants and young children with rickets are prone to bending and fracture. Radiographic changes include metaphyseal cupping and fraying, cortical thinning, and periosteal reaction (Fig. 6-78A and B; see also Fig. 10-11). Clinically, widened metaphyses (Fig. 6-78C) and costochondral beading also help to establish the diagnosis (see Fig. 10-10).

A significant rise in the incidence of nutritional rickets has been noted in the past few years in breast-fed African American infants who are not given supplemental vitamin D. Limited sunlight absorption by their dark skin and the fact that breast milk does not contain added vitamin D combine to produce vitamin D deficiency and hence rickets.

Premature infants who are born before much of the mineralization of bone that occurs in utero is complete and who, because of severe illness or lung disease, have prolonged nutritional problems necessitating total parenteral nutrition are particularly vulnerable to developing rickets with attendant bony fragility. Because they often require chest physiotherapy, they may incur multiple rib fractures. When these are detected on chest radiographs obtained during evaluation of a respiratory illness following discharge from the nursery, abuse is often suspected. Given a history of prematurity and prolonged hospitalization, it is wise to contact the hospital where the child was cared for and review prior films before diagnosing abuse. Careful inspection of the current films often shows residual metaphyseal and costal changes characteristic of rickets.

Copper Deficiency. Copper deficiency is an exceptionally rare phenomenon that should be readily distinguishable from abuse. It occurs in nutritional and inherited forms. Prematurity; a change in early infancy to whole, powdered, or evaporated milk; severe malabsorption syndromes; and prolonged total parenteral nutrition without copper supplementation are the major predisposing factors. Clinically, affected infants have pale skin, hypopigmented hair, edema, enlarged scalp veins, and seborrhea, with or without failure to thrive or developmental delay. All have neutropenia and a hypochromic microcytic anemia that is resistant to iron therapy; radiographically, their bones are grossly abnormal. Findings include overt osteoporosis; cupped metaphyses; metaphyseal spurs; widened anterior ribs; periosteal reaction; and, at times, soft tissue calcification (see Fig. 10-12).

Menkes' kinky hair syndrome is the inherited form and results from an X-linked recessive defect in copper absorption. These children are markedly pale and have a characteristic facies with pudgy cheeks; horizontal, twisted eyebrows; and little facial expression. Their hair is dull or lusterless, sparse, and kinky with pili torti (see Fig. 8-142). Affected infants are also grossly abnormal neurologically, with hypertonia, decreased movement, lethargy, myoclonic seizures, and difficulty maintaining normothermia being major findings.

Scurvy. Children with vitamin C deficiency (now exceedingly rare) tend to bruise easily because of vascular fragility, but scurvy should be readily distinguishable from abuse on the basis of radiographic findings. Although a periosteal reaction resulting from subperiosteal hemorrhage is seen and there may be fractures through the zone of provisional calcification and through metaphyseal spurs, their cortices are thin and the ends of the long bones show characteristic changes consisting of increased density of the zone of provisional calcification and increased lucency of the underlying spongiosa (Fig. 6-79). These infants are irritable, tend to move little because of bone pain, and often have gingival bleeding.

Hypervitaminosis A. Chronic vitamin A intoxication produces a thick, wavy periosteal reaction that most commonly involves the ulnas and metatarsals, although other long bones can be affected. Hard, tender swellings may be evident on palpation. Absence of fractures and metaphyseal abnormalities should help distinguish this from abuse. The history and findings of papilledema or split sutures

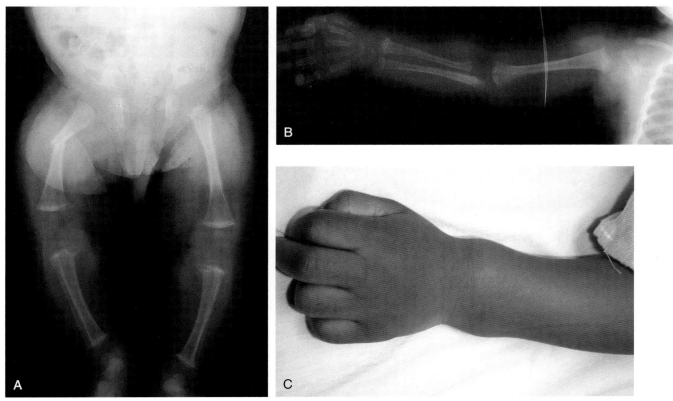

Figure 6-78. Rickets. This 3-month-old African American infant presented with pain and decreased movement of his right leg. Symptoms had appeared after playtime with his much older brother, who was bouncing him up and down. **A,** A skeletal survey revealed a greenstick fracture of the right femur and **B,** the fraying and cupping of the metaphyses characteristic of rickets. Reduced sunlight absorption due to his darkly pigmented skin and prenatal and postnatal factors appear to have contributed etiologically. The baby's mother had not taken vitamins for the last half of her pregnancy and did not eat dairy products. The baby was small for gestational age and had more than doubled his birth weight; hence his need for vitamin D outstripped the amount provided by his formula. **C,** In this older child who developed rickets after being placed on a vegan diet by his mother, the wrist is nearly as wide as his hand due to underlying metaphyseal widening and fraying of the radius and ulna.

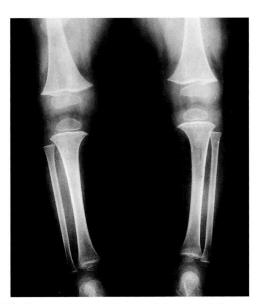

Figure 6-79. Scurvy. Note the increased density of the zones of provisional calcification and the lucency of the underlying spongiosa. The metaphyses are also widened, and early spur formation is seen medially. (Courtesy Department of Radiology, Children's Hospital of Pittsburgh, Pa.)

on skull radiograph resulting from concomitant pseudotumor cerebri also aid in differentiation.

Leukemia. Children with acute leukemia may develop diffuse demineralization, periosteal reactions, and osteolytic lesions. Lucent metaphyseal bands, termed *leukemic lines,* are also seen (Fig. 6-80). The relative osteopenia and typical absence of fractures, combined with the antecedent history, often of fatigue, anorexia, and weight loss; physical findings that may include adenopathy, visceromegaly, and sternal tenderness; and the results of hematologic tests should distinguish these findings from those of abuse.

Caffey's Disease. A rare disorder of unknown etiology, Caffey's disease is characterized by cortical thickening and a painful periosteal reaction (Fig. 6-81). Bones are otherwise normally mineralized, and fractures are not seen. Involvement of the mandible, seen in 75% of affected patients, results in dramatic thickening. The clavicle and ulna are also common sites, although other bones can be involved. Most patients are younger than 6 months of age, and all have fever, anorexia, and marked irritability. The skin overlying affected areas is neither warm nor discolored. There is no soft tissue swelling, and palpation reveals bony-hard thickening below the subcutaneous tissues, which are adherent to the underlying bone.

Differential Diagnosis of Accidental versus Inflicted Head Injuries

Accidental head injuries are common in childhood as a result of falls and other accidents, and the majority are minor. Presentation is usually prompt because a head injury, no matter how minor, tends to provoke considerable parental anxiety. Again, the history is usually clear, and the mechanism reported is consistent with the physical findings observed. Mild forehead and scalp contusions with or without small lacerations or abrasions are by far the most common injuries. Simple (usually nondiastatic) linear skull fractures often involving the parietal bones can result from falls of greater than 4 feet onto hard surfaces (as from a changing table or a shopping cart), but these do not tend to be associated with significant changes in level of consciousness or with intracranial injury. More severe injuries are incurred as a result of more serious mechanisms including major falls (>10 feet and falls with angular momentum as from swings, trapezes, or trampolines), bicycle and sports accidents, and motor vehicle accidents.

In evaluating an infant or toddler who presents with a history of minor trauma but is found to have intracranial bleeding, especially one with subdural hematomas and retinal hemorrhages, it is important to rule out coagulopathy or the presence of an underlying disorder that makes the child unusually susceptible to development of subdural bleeding. A coagulopathy can be ruled in or out by obtaining a complete blood cell count with differential and platelet count, prothrombin and partial thromboplastin times, and, if necessary based on family history, a von Willebrand or full coagulation profile.

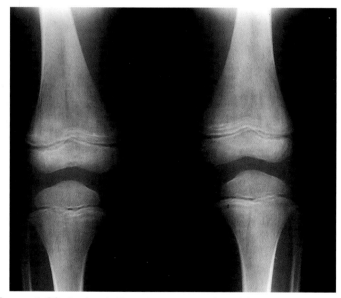

Figure 6-80. Leukemic lines. Lucent metaphyseal bands can be seen in some children with acute leukemia or other severe systemic illnesses. However, they are rarely associated with fractures. (Courtesy Department of Radiology, Children's Hospital of Pittsburgh, Pa.)

In two disorders, subdural hematomas and retinal hemorrhages can be seen following minimal trauma. These must be considered in the evaluation and distinguished from abuse. They are benign extra-axial fluid collections (BEAFCs) and glutaric aciduria type 1 (GA1).

Disorders Simulating or Predisposing to Subdural Hemorrhage

Benign Extra-axial Fluid Collections

In BEAFCs, also known as *benign external hydrocephalus*, macrocephaly is associated with bilateral symmetric widening of the subarachnoid space (SAS), most prominently in the frontal and fronto-parietal areas and along the anterior interhemispheric fissure and the Sylvian fissures. This expanded space is filled with cerebrospinal fluid. Usually the ventricles are normal in size or only slightly enlarged, and there is no evidence of increased intracranial pressure (ICP). The condition is thought to be due to transient mild impairment of cerebrospinal fluid (CSF) resorption by the arachnoid villi. Widening of the SAS results in significant stretching of the bridging veins that run from the cerebral cortex to the dural venous sinuses, and it is thought that being stretched makes them more vulnerable to tearing in the face of minimal or minor trauma.

Infants with BEAFCs are usually diagnosed as a result of imaging performed as part of an evaluation for macrocephaly or enlarging head circumference. Most are neurodevelopmentally normal, although some may have mild delays and hypotonia. Many have a family history of macrocephaly that suggests autosomal dominant transmission. Usually the abnormality resolves spontaneously with normalization of findings on imaging by 2 to 5 years of age.

Approximately 10% of infants followed with BEAFCs develop subdural hematomas in association with retinal hemorrhages, either "spontaneously" or following a minor head bump. Although some of these infants have had associated seizures and/or mild transient alterations in consciousness, most appear relatively normal neurologically even on presentation with subdurals. On MRI the subdural hemorrhages are usually small, and diffuse enlargement of the subarachnoid space (occupied by cerebrospinal fluid) is easily appreciated. Importantly, these infants tend to be brought in promptly for care

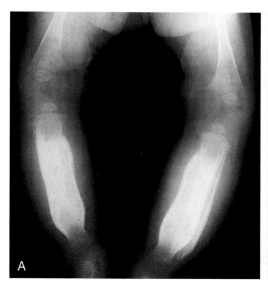
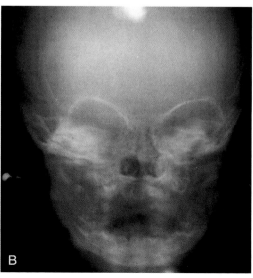

Figure 6-81. Caffey's disease. **A,** Intense periosteal reaction and cortical thickening are seen in the lower extremities. **B,** Mandibular involvement has resulted in dramatic thickening. These findings, associated symptoms, and absence of fractures distinguish this condition from the skeletal changes characteristic of abuse. (Courtesy Department of Radiology, Children's Hospital of Pittsburgh, Pa.)

when symptomatic or following falls, are accompanied by appropriately concerned parents, and have no associated injuries.

BEAFCs can be distinguished from cerebral atrophy as the sulci are not widened and because of the greater prominence of SAS widening frontally. In communicating hydrocephalus ventricular enlargement is much more prominent, and symptoms of increased intracranial pressure (ICP) may be present.

Glutaric Aciduria

Glutaric aciduria type 1 (GA1) is an autosomal recessive disorder resulting in deficiency of glutaryl-CoA dehydrogenase. Affected infants appear relatively normal at birth, although approximately 40% are born with mild macrocephaly, and over ensuing months, these infants gradually cross toward the 97th percentile. Nonspecific neurologic signs consisting of irritability, jitteriness, mild hypotonia, and feeding problems are common in the first 6 months, then improve, and by a year most appear normal except for slight gross motor delays. If undiagnosed and untreated, most affected infants develop an acute encephalopathy between 12 and 18 months of age usually in association with an acute upper respiratory or gastrointestinal infection. Subsequently, they are left with severe dystonias and dyskinesias and suffer major regression in milestones.

Findings on neuroimaging, whether performed before or after the severe encephalopathic event, include marked bilateral frontotemporal atrophy along with prominent widening of the Sylvian fissures and delayed myelination. Twenty to thirty percent have associated chronic subdural effusions and/or hematomas. Following the encephalopathy, basal ganglia atrophy also becomes evident. As in children with BEAFCs, it is thought that the marked widening of the subarachnoid space due to cortical atrophy results in stretching of the bridging veins, making them more vulnerable to shearing with minimal trauma. When subdurals are present, retinal hemorrhages are also seen. Interestingly, the subdurals may or may not be associated with symptoms. The presence of marked cerebral atrophy in association with subdural hematomas (Fig. 6-82) helps distinguish GA1 from both inflicted head trauma and BEAFCs. No skeletal abnormalities are associated with GA1, and usually no other evident injuries exist unless irritability has provoked abuse.

Strong evidence indicates that diagnosis and institution of treatment before an encephalopathic event can prevent the encephalopathy and subsequent movement disorder. Hence neuroimaging and testing for GA1 should be strongly considered in the evaluation of infants with mild macrocephaly, especially if they are fussy, jittery, and/or hypotonic.

Subdural Hematomas and Osteogenesis Imperfecta

There have been scattered reports regarding a small number of children with OI who have presented with subdural hematomas and retinal hemorrhages. On close review the numbers are small, the histories given often incomplete, and presence of associated injuries (i.e., femur fracture in a child with mild OI who was not yet walking, and 3 spiral fractures in 3 different long bones in another) raises suspicion of inflicted injuries. Hence, it is not clear and probably unlikely that infants with OI are more susceptible to developing subdural hematomas than normal children.

Differentiation of Accidental from Inflicted Oral Injuries

Falls and sporting and bicycle accidents are the usual sources of accidental oral injuries. These include lip and chin lacerations (see Fig. 20-55); fractured, loosened, or avulsed teeth (see Figs. 20-59 through 20-64); and gingival, lingual, palatal, or retropharyngeal lacerations, the latter resulting from falls with an object in the mouth (see Figs. 20-54, 20-56, and 23-73). These injuries, like head injuries, provoke considerable parental anxiety and result in prompt presentation for care, with a clear history and consistent mechanism of injury.

Differential Diagnosis of Accidental versus Inflicted Chest and Abdominal Injuries

Accidental chest and abdominal injuries in children are predominantly the result of major blunt force trauma and may be similar in nature to those caused by abuse. However, victims of accidental injuries have a clear history of a major mechanism of injury, such as a major motor vehicle accident, that was often witnessed. Immediate care is sought, and findings are consistent with the history.

Sexual Abuse

Sexual abuse is defined as the misuse of a child for the sexual gratification of an adult. In sexual abuse the perpetrator misuses his or her power over a child, involving her or him in sexual activities that may or may not involve physical contact. The best available data indicate that in the 1980s there was a significant rise in the number of reports of sexual abuse, stemming in part from increased public and professional awareness, and in part as a consequence of a greater willingness of victims to disclose the abuse. This trend appears to have reversed since 1992, and data from 2000 indicate that approximately 87,900 cases of sexual abuse were substantiated by child protection agencies and court systems, representing a further decline. Given the fact that 20% of adult women and 5% to 10% of adult men report having been sexually abused before 18 years of age, it appears that sexual abuse still continues to be underreported, especially among males, and it is estimated that substantiated cases constitute less than one third of all cases of sexual abuse.

Extrapolating current prevalence data to a pediatric practice of 1500 children, it is likely that 12 of them will be abused each year, only 8 of whom will disclose their abuse to a professional, not necessarily a pediatrician. It is of concern that only 40% of cases disclosed to professionals are then reported to authorities, despite mandatory reporting laws in all 50 states. Also worrisome is the fact that CPS will be able to substantiate only half of the cases disclosed and reported to them, for a variety of reasons, sometimes unrelated to the veracity of allegations.

Forms of sexual abuse may include visual exposure to exhibitionistic, masturbatory, or copulatory behavior; fondling, masturbation, and digital manipulation; oral/genital contact; and direct genital contact including penetration or attempted penetration of the vagina, anus, or mouth. Twenty to twenty-five percent of cases reported retrospectively by women involve vaginal or orogenital penetration. Data regarding perpetrators indicate that approximately 40% are parents or step-parents, and 25% are other relatives. Strangers probably constitute no more

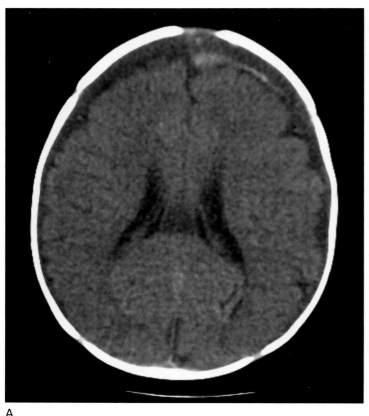

A

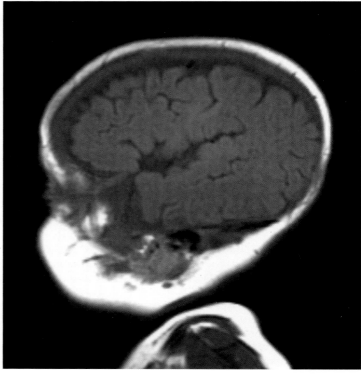

B

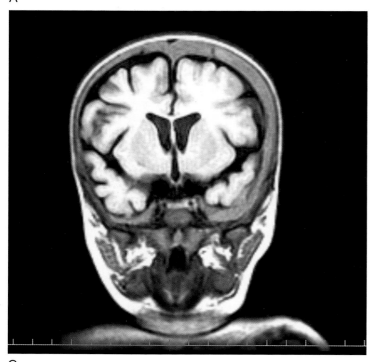

C

Figure 6-82. Glutaric aciduria type 1. This 3-month-old infant was brought to the emergency department with complaints of being limp and unresponsive with a recent history of pneumonia. The initial history given was that, while alone with father, he had suddenly become lethargic, his eyes had rolled back, and he had stopped breathing for a few seconds. Lethargy resolved soon after arrival. **A,** A head CT obtained because retinal hemorrhages were found revealed diffuse acute and subacute/chronic subdural hemorrhages over the convexities in the fronto-temporal areas, as well as more acute collections along the posterior interhemispheric fissure and over the right frontal area. **B** and **C,** On MRI large acute on chronic subdural hemorrhages were confirmed, along with early signs of atrophy including mild flattening of the gyri, sulcal widening, and mild ventricular enlargement. This prompted testing for possible glutaric aciduria, which was positive in results obtained a week later. Interestingly, in the interim, the father acknowledged having shaken the baby after he didn't feed well whereupon he went limp.

than 10% of perpetrators. The rest are people who are known by but unrelated to the victim. By far, the majority of perpetrators are male. Adult females, who are responsible for 20% of abusive sexual contact with prepubescent boys and 5% of such contact with prepubescent girls, are much less likely to be reported.

Adults who prefer children and young adolescents for physical sexual gratification are *pedophiles*. They should not be confused with homosexuals who mutually prefer same sex partners in their own age range. Although some pedophiles may be more restrained than others, many tend to be compulsive in seeking their victims. It is also

important to recognize that they often marry or cohabit with an opposite sex partner, in part as cover and in part so as to victimize their children.

Of increasing concern is the fact that more and more children are disclosing that they have been exposed to pornography and have been used as subjects in pornographic photographs and videotapes, which have ever more sophisticated distribution over the Internet. Furthermore, the Internet, through use of chat rooms, has become a major vehicle for pedophiles to seek, find, and entice victims.

The issue of "sexually reactive" children is another concern, and it is important to distinguish this behavior from normal sexual play. Children who entice or coerce other children into sexual behavior, simulate intercourse, or try to insert foreign objects into themselves or other children may be evincing "sexualized behavior" because they themselves have been victims of sexual abuse. Hence they too should be evaluated in addition to their victims.

Rape, which by legal definition is "forced sexual intercourse" and may involve penetration, however slight, may occur with the use of physical force or coercion and the misuse of a power relationship. Adolescents have the highest rates of rape of any age group and, in general, tend to delay or avoid seeking care after being assaulted. Male victims are even less likely to report the assault or seek care. Not infrequently, adolescents who are raped have been using drugs or alcohol or have been given drugs surreptitiously before the event. The "date rape drug" flunitrazepam (not legally available in the United States), which is colorless and tasteless and usually administered in a drink or beverage, is reported to have increased the incidence of rape, despite the fact that *reported* rapes have been decreasing in frequency since 1992.

If the perpetrator of sexual abuse is a family member or acquaintance, the encounter is more likely to be physically nonviolent, with persuasion, bribery, or threats used to enlist the victim's cooperation. Not infrequently, these experiences are repetitive and occur over long periods of time. There is a well-described pattern of escalating levels of involvement, with initial fondling and digital manipulation progressing to actual penetration. The victim's cooperation and subsequent silence may be ensured by various means including persuasion, bribes, gifts, praise, fear of the perpetrator's power, and threats of dire consequences if the child discloses the abuse. Thus the victim bears both the guilt of engaging in unwanted sexual activity and the pressure of keeping it secret. Absence of physical violence or injury *does not* imply consent, as the offender is usually in a position of power over the victim, making it difficult for the child both to refuse to engage in the activity and to disclose it. Children abused by family members or family friends have also disclosed fears of being harmed or of having other loved ones or pets injured, or even killed, by the abuser. Episodes perpetrated by strangers are more likely to be isolated incidents and involve physical violence, adding the emotional stress of being in a potentially life-threatening situation.

Forensic requirements for a detailed history, physical examination, and multiple laboratory specimens (all carefully documented) necessitate a lengthy evaluation that, if not sensitively handled, can compound existing emotional trauma. This can be minimized if the physician approaches the patient and family with patience, gentleness, and tact. If the disclosed sexual abuse does not involve allegations requiring collection of evidence of ejaculate and/or if there is no bleeding or significant discomfort, the physical examination may be postponed; conducted in stages; or, if necessary, performed under anesthesia or conscious sedation.

Since physical findings are normal in up to 80% to 96% of cases, and, even if abnormal, are frequently nonspecific, the history is the most important aspect of the evaluation. Hence it is essential that historical information be documented meticulously, if possible verbatim, because many of these cases have the potential for legal prosecution (usually months to years later). Ideally, this history is obtained by an experienced clinician, using forensic interviewing principles. Clinicians should avoid asking leading questions, although in certain situations, after all other

avenues have been exhausted, such questions may be necessary in order to elicit enough information to ensure protection of the child. When possible, the parent or persons accompanying the child should be interviewed first, apart from each other and separately from the child. During this interview one can obtain information about the youngster's emotional status and recent behavior; present and past history; family psychosocial situation; household members or other persons caring for the child; people who share or visit the home frequently who might have unwitnessed access to the child; the events that appear to have led to the disclosure or suspicion of abuse; and terms used by the child for body parts. When the chief complaint is not sexual abuse, but findings on examination point to molestation, this information should be sought in a further interview with the parent, or parents, after the examination, with the child out of the room.

In approaching the child, it is essential for the clinician to show kindness, empathy, and gentleness. Importantly, one should not convey shock or disgust or to presume what the child's reactions to the abuse may have been. If the child is willing and able to give a history, it, as well as the exact phrasing of the questions asked, should be documented verbatim. In the initial portion of the interview, talking about favorite subjects such as friends, favorite toys, games, and activities can help reduce the child's anxiety and establish rapport between him or her and clinician. Thereafter, it is best to begin with general questions, reserving more specific questions for clarification. If the child is unwilling or unable to discuss the episode or episodes, and there is a strong suspicion that sexual abuse has occurred, a return visit or referral for a session with a forensically trained clinician is recommended. In such interviews a variety of alternative techniques can be used if the child still has difficulty disclosing verbally. These include having the child try to draw what happened (Fig. 6-83), demonstrate what happened with anatomically correct dolls, or write about the incidents.

Documentation of the manner in which disclosure occurs is important. When children give spontaneous detailed descriptions of sexual experiences in language appropriate to their developmental level, these are usually accurate and not imagined. Asking nondirective questions to ascertain the site where the activity occurred and the number of times it happened, as well as questions related to such things as clothing worn, can be useful in documenting the child's credibility. Also important is determining the patient's understanding of the need for accuracy in relating the history and of the difference between telling the truth and telling a lie. This further aids in determining not only the child's credibility but also his or her ability to testify in court.

Recognition of the problem of false accusations of sexual abuse made in the heat of child custody battles has raised questions regarding the veracity of many such claims. Findings from ongoing research suggest that if the child's disclosure is made without benefit of leading questions and is reported with feeling and often some hesitancy, and in age-appropriate terms, the report is more likely to be accurate. In contrast, children coached to make false claims tend to relate the history in a rote manner and often use adult-oriented words.

Other problems have arisen when the child has been required to repeat the history to multiple authorities—family members, physicians, CPS workers, psychologists, attorneys, and detectives. When this occurs, many victims begin to sound robotic in their reports (raising questions regarding their truthfulness) and others become so trau-

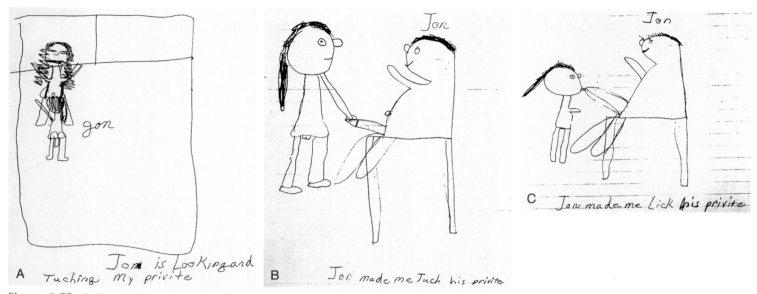

Figure 6-83. A, B, and **C,** Drawings of a school-age sexual abuse victim. Though the child had difficulty verbalizing a description of the abuse, she was able to clearly depict the acts in her drawings.

matized by the repetition and the impact on their family that they recant their story to avoid further painful questioning. In an effort to address this, many centers have developed a team approach in which an experienced clinician trained in forensic interviewing techniques conducts the interview while being observed by members of law enforcement and CPS, thereby reducing the number of interviews the child must undergo. These programs have also called attention to the importance of cautioning distraught or unbelieving parents and family members against asking the child repeated questions about the abuse.

Before proceeding with the physical examination, one should convey to the child that the purpose is not to determine the veracity of the history but to ensure his or her continuing health. Sharing details of the examination process with the adults accompanying a young child and providing reassurance that a speculum will not be used is also helpful as many fear that the examination will be invasive. This can allay much parental anxiety, which in turn helps them to reassure the child during the process. Following physical assessment, it is important to convey that there is no permanent damage related to physical function because that is another common parental concern.

Giving the child some feeling of control over the examination process in a number of small ways helps avoid further trauma and may aid in starting the child along the process of recovery. This can be accomplished with a surprisingly high proportion of children by an examiner who is comfortable with the process. Letting the child look at familiar objects such as an item of clothing through the colposcope or demonstrating to a young child, in a playful way, that the light on the colposcope is not hurtful may help. Allowing the child to choose the order in which various nonessential areas are examined can be calming, as well.

A thorough and complete physical examination is warranted for all patients suspected of having been sexually abused, with inspection of the genitalia and rectum deferred until last. Each part of the process should be explained as the examiner proceeds. If possible, and the child so chooses, a parent or supportive adult should be present. In our experience with prepubescent patients,

external inspection of the genitalia suffices in the majority of cases and the insertion of a speculum is almost never indicated.

If the attempt to examine the perineum provokes anxiety that cannot be allayed and there is gross bleeding, pain, discharge, or evidence of sexually transmitted disease, the examination and specimen collection should be performed with the patient under general anesthesia or deep conscious sedation. When the patient is too anxious to proceed and is asymptomatic with no evidence of trauma, bleeding, discomfort, or discharge, the procedure can be deferred and performed at a follow-up visit. The child *must not* be made to feel that he or she is being assaulted yet again during the examination and interview process.

Modes of Presentation

Because the majority of cases of sexual abuse do not involve physical violence, most patients have no signs of injury. In most instances (up to 80% to 96%) there are either no physical findings specific for sexual abuse or the examination is completely normal. Many reasons for the absence of physical findings exist even when there is a confession of vaginal penetration by the perpetrator. These include the delay in disclosure so common in young victims; the rapid healing of injuries involving the mucosa; the fact that hymenal tissue is capable of regrowth and that, with the onset of puberty and increased estrogen production, the hymen becomes more elastic; the fact that the anal sphincter can distend considerably; and the possibility that perpetrators of sexual abuse may have erectile and/or ejaculatory dysfunction, as do many adult rapists.

In cases of sexual assault involving violence and resulting in major injury, a significant proportion of victims seek medical care promptly. Most acknowledge the nature of the problem at the time of presentation, and physical findings are more often positive. However, even in some of these cases a history of an accidental mechanism of injury that does not fit the physical findings is given.

Although there has been a significant increase in the percentage of patients who have disclosed inappropriate

Table 6-14	Most Common Substitute Chief Complaints in Sexual Abuse Cases*		
ANY AGE	**PRESCHOOL AGE**	**SCHOOL AGE**	**ADOLESCENCE**
Abdominal pain	Excessive clinging	Decreased school performance	Same as school age plus:
Anorexia	Sudden onset of excessive thumb sucking	Truancy	Runaway behavior
Vomiting	Speech disorder	Lying, stealing	Suicide attempts
Constipation	Encopresis/enuresis	Tics	Commission of sexual offenses[†]
Sleep disorders	Excessive masturbation[†]	Anxiety reaction	
Dysuria		Phobic and obsessional states	
Vaginal discharge[‡]		Depression	
Vaginal bleeding[‡]		Conversion reaction	
Rectal bleeding		Encopresis/enuresis	

*Most of these complaints are also symptomatic of disorders more prevalent than sexual abuse.
[†]Symptoms highly suggestive of sexual abuse.
[‡]Symptoms somewhat suggestive of sexual abuse.

touching prior to presentation, it continues to be true that some victims of long-term sexual abuse may present with vulvovaginitis with vaginal discharge caused by a sexually transmitted pathogen or with substitute chief complaints generated by physical or emotional sequelae (Table 6-14). There are many such complaints that are somewhat age dependent, and each of which has many potential causes other than sexual abuse. Although there is a wide range of differential diagnostic possibilities in patients presenting with many of these problems, sexual abuse should be considered and addressed among the differential diagnostic considerations, and not merely after all other causes have been ruled out. When a child presents with a substitute chief complaint and/or has a history of compulsive masturbation, witnessed self-insertion of foreign objects into the vagina, and unusually sexualized behavior, the likelihood that he or she has been a victim of sexual abuse is high.

During the evaluation of children presenting with substitute chief complaints, it is appropriate to ask questions of parent and child separately about the possibility of inappropriate touching, and if there is any suspicion of this, a more detailed psychological assessment performed by a specially trained clinician is warranted. Even with skilled evaluation, a significant proportion of these victims do not disclose immediately. This, in our experience, seems to be particularly true of children seen for signs and symptoms of a sexually transmitted disease. However, after repeated visits with a single clinician during a stepwise evaluation for the underlying cause of their problem, many are able develop enough trust to disclose sexual abuse or another source of their stress. A team approach may be particularly valuable in such cases.

Examination Techniques

Perineal Examination

Several techniques may be used for examination of the genital and perianal areas in different age groups. In the *postpubescent age group,* a standard gynecologic examination can usually be performed with the patient in the lithotomy position (see Chapter 18). When an estrogenized hymen is redundant, a saline-moistened swab may be inserted through the orifice and then used to spread out the membrane segment by segment in order to better assess for presence of contusions, tears, notches, or scars. This is not painful and is therefore possible in adolescents and peripubertal children because, once estrogenized, the hymen is not nearly as sensitive as it is before puberty. Alternatively, a Foley catheter may be inserted, the balloon

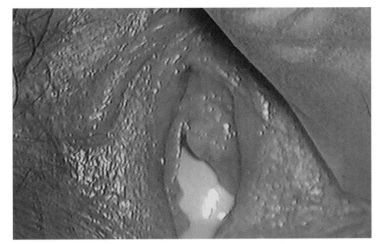

Figure 6-84. Use of Foley catheter to enhance visualization of the full extent and margins of the hymenal membrane. The catheter is inserted through the hymenal orifice, and the balloon inflated while in the vagina and then gently pulled forward. It can then be angled to the left or right or downward to ensure a full view of all segments. (Courtesy Dr. Earl Greenwald, Harrisburg, Pa.)

inflated within the vagina, and then gently pulled forward as a means of spreading out the hymenal tissue for better visualization (Fig. 6-84). In cases of acute injury, consideration must be given to the severity and extent of the injuries before proceeding. If examination and specimen collection are likely to cause severe physical pain or emotional distress to an adolescent patient, or if internal injuries are likely, strong consideration should be given to examination under conscious sedation or even general anesthesia.

In the *prepubescent child* the purposes of the perineal examination are (1) to obtain full visualization of the patient's perineal and perianal anatomy; (2) to detect any evidence of acute injury, infection, distortion of anatomy, or scarring indicative of prior injury; (3) to assess the amount and appearance of hymenal tissue and determine the size and configuration of the hymenal orifice; and (4) to collect specimens as indicated. If abnormalities of the hymen are seen, the membrane may be "floated" up by inserting saline into the vaginal area. As noted earlier, internal examination is not necessary unless there is evidence of internal extension of injury, and, in such cases, the examination, specimen collection, and repair should be done in the operating room under general anesthesia.

In examining prepubescent patients, a number of positions may be used to achieve visualization of the genital area. The one most commonly used is the *supine frog-leg*

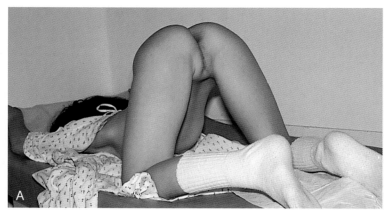

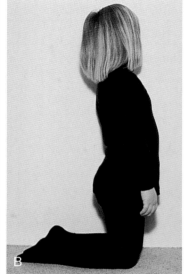

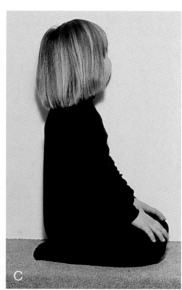

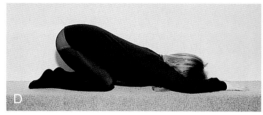

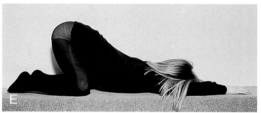

Figure 6-85. Knee-chest position. **A,** The sway-back position with knees widely separated assists examination and provides the best visualization of anatomic structures and abnormalities. **B-E,** After looking at enlargements of this series of photographs, the patient practices getting into position while still fully clothed. The steps are **(B)** kneel, **(C)** sit back, **(D)** stretch arms out and place arms and chest on table, and **(E)** move forward. This helps children become more comfortable with being examined from behind.

position, with the patient lying supine on the examining table. This position can also be achieved with the child semireclining on the parent's lap—*semisupine frog-leg position.* We have also had good success with the *semisupine lithotomy position* (see Figs. 18-5A and B). The latter is accomplished by having the parent sit on the examining table and lean back. The child sits on her lap, with the buttocks resting just above the parent's knees, and leans back. The parent then places her hands under the patient's knees, flexing them and abducting the hips. The *knee-chest position* (Fig. 6-85A) provides the best exposure of perineal structures and generally a clearer picture of anatomic features and abnormalities (Fig. 6-86; see also Fig. 6-92). Therefore experts prefer it in sexual abuse evaluation. The child's shoulders and chest must touch the table, achieving a swayback posture. The knee-chest position is difficult for children younger than 2 years of age, however, and some older children object to it. Nevertheless, most children can be made comfortable with the knee-chest position and helped to relax by engaging them in an ongoing conversation about an unrelated subject, having the child count as high as she can, or using a variety of visually interesting toys (e.g., kaleidoscopes, oil-based timers) held by an assistant at eye level. We also have the child practice the position while fully clothed before the examination (Fig. 6-85B to E).

To assist visualization of the introitus in the supine or semisupine frog-leg or lithotomy positions, the labia must be separated manually. In the *labial separation* method, the examiner places the index fingers over the lower portion of the labia majora and gently presses downward and laterally. In the *labial traction* technique, the labia majora are grasped between the thumbs and index fingers and gently pulled down and toward the examiner. The latter usually achieves better visualization of the hymen and its orifice

and the greatest hymenal opening with the child in these positions, and it is often possible to see the posterior aspect of the lower third of the vagina using this technique (see Figs. 18-2 and 18-6). It is important to bear in mind that one should be careful not to use undue force when applying labial traction so as to avoid tearing any labial adhesions present or causing undue discomfort.

In the knee-chest position, exposure of the introitus is assisted by placing the thumbs over the edge of the gluteus muscles at the level of the introitus and lifting them upward. As the hymen drops down with gravity in the knee-chest position, its width and margins are more easily assessed. Transverse diameter of the hymenal orifice varies with position and amount of relaxation and by itself is no longer considered a useful measurement in assessing for signs of sexual abuse (see Figs. 6-86 and 18-6). Rather, assessment of the appearance of the hymen and surrounding tissues is far more valuable.

Good lighting and magnification are also important. Use of a colposcope is ideal, but most practitioners do not have access to this device. Alternatively, a magnifying halogen lamp or an otoscope may be used. The latter device is most readily available, but the child must be reassured that this is only being used to get a good view with the light and that no speculum will be used as it is for ear examinations.

A complete description of the appearance of the genitalia using anatomically correct terms must be documented in the chart (Fig. 6-87). If at all possible, magnified photographs of the genital area should be taken, as these may obviate the need for reexamination if a second opinion is requested. Documentation should include (1) Tanner staging; (2) the presence or absence of an abnormal degree of erythema or of discharge; (3) the presence or absence and location of bruises, abrasions, or lacerations of the

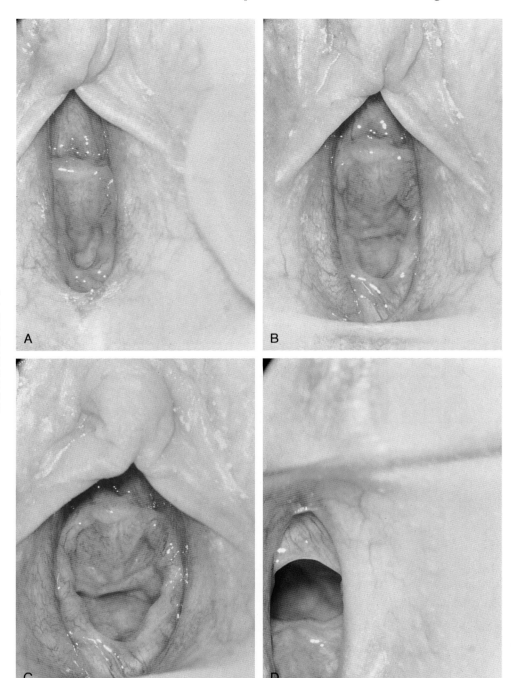

Figure 6-86. Variation in the transverse or horizontal hymenal diameter with position and technique. **A,** Supine with labial separation. **B,** Supine with labial traction. **C,** Lithotomy with more labial traction. **D,** Knee-chest position. Note that the hymenal orifice is widest with good traction and that the hymen appears wrinkled and thickened in **B** and **C**. This is due to a mild redundancy. In the knee-chest position, the hymen unfolds and drops down with gravity and is seen to be thin with smooth, sharp edges having fully stretched out.

labia majora and perineum; (4) the appearance of the vestibule and (5) of the labia minora; (6) the presence, extent, and character of labial adhesions (thin and translucent or thickened); (7) the appearance of the posterior fourchette and presence or absence of scarring; (8) the configuration of the hymen (annular, crescentic, redundant), and the appearance of its edges (e.g., thin and sharp, thickened or rolled, notched); and (9) the width of hymenal tissue from its attachment to its margin, and its regularity. Also important is recording the patient's position and method used to separate the labia. Such documentation requires knowledge of basic gynecologic anatomy and terminology, which are shown in Figure 6-88 and given in Table 6-15 (see also "Differential Diagnosis of Sexual Abuse" later and "Normal Female Genitalia" in Chapter 18).

If acute external contusions or tears are seen, internal injury must be suspected. The prepubescent girl is particu-larly vulnerable to severe internal trauma as a result of forceful penetration of either the vagina or rectum (see Fig. 6-90). This stems from the fact that the structures are relatively small and the tissues more delicate and rigid than is the case following estrogenization. Young children with relatively mild external injuries may, in fact, have major internal tears including perforation of the peritoneum and damage to pelvic vessels, mesentery, and intestine (see Figs. 18-16 to 18-19). Signs of internal injury may be subtle, but such patients will have evidence of vaginal bleeding or of a vaginal hematoma, and some may have lower abdominal tenderness or evidence of occult blood loss. Therefore when such findings are present, an examination under anesthesia is indicated. In contrast, the postpubescent female can usually be adequately assessed by careful pelvic examination sometimes, with use of a Foley catheter to enhance visualization of the hymenal surface and margins (see Fig. 6-84). However, if, despite good

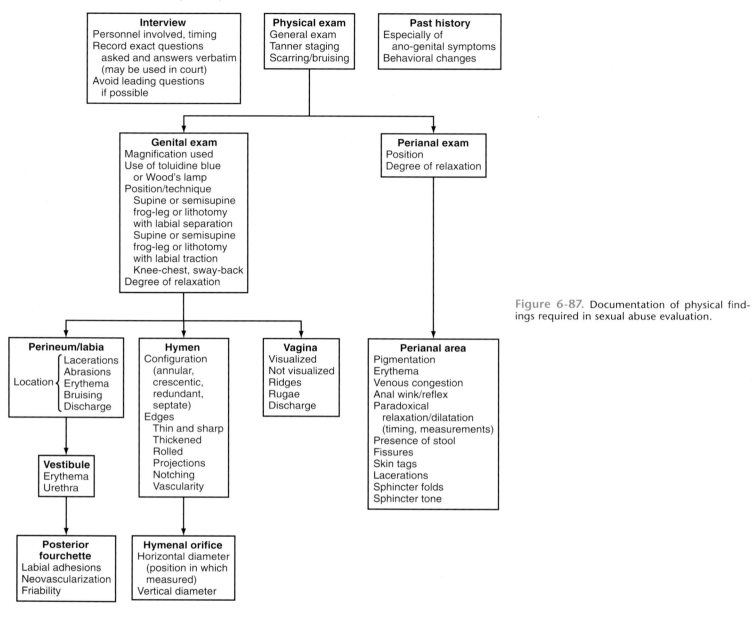

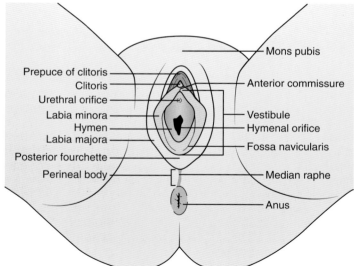

Figure 6-88. Normal anatomy. Location of the genital structures of the prepubescent female.

emotional support, reassurance, and careful preparation, she is emotionally unable to tolerate the procedure, an examination under anesthesia is also advisable.

Perianal Examination

Rectal penetration (sodomy) is a common form of sexual abuse in both boys and girls. To achieve optimal visualization, the perianal examination should be conducted in the knee-chest position. Care should be taken to look for evidence of abrasions, tears, fissures, other lesions, or immediate dilation of the sphincter to greater than 2 cm on adopting the knee-chest position when there is no visible stool in the rectum. Venous congestion of the perianal area occurs within minutes of the child being placed in the knee-chest position and does not indicate evidence of abuse. The absence of physical findings is the norm and does not make the history any less credible. In most cases of sexual abuse, external inspection of the perianal area with spreading of the anal folds is sufficient; however, following specimen collection, rectal examination is necessary in cases of acute anorectal injury in order to assess for internal rectal tears, pelvic tenderness, and sphincter tone and for bimanual palpation. When there is evidence of forceful penetration (marked bruising or lacerations) or

Table 6-15	Gynecologic Anatomic Terminology
Anal verge	The tissue overlying the subcutaneous external anal sphincter at the most distal portion of the anal canal, extending exteriorly to the margin of the anal skin.
Anterior commissure	The union of the two labia minora anteriorly.
Clitoris	A cylindrical, erectile body situated at the superior portion of the vulva, covered by a sheath of skin called the *clitoral hood* or *prepuce*.
Fossa navicularis/ posterior fossa	Concavity of the lower part of the vaginal vestibule situated inferiorly to the vaginal orifice and extending to the posterior fourchette (posterior commissure).
Hymen	A thin membrane located at the junction of the vestibular floor and the vaginal canal that partially covers the vaginal orifice.
Labia majora	Rounded folds of skin forming the lateral boundaries of the vulva.
Labia minora	Thin longitudinal folds of tissue enclosed within the labia majora; in the prepubertal child they extend from the clitoral hood to the midpoint of the lateral wall of the vestibule. After puberty they lengthen and join posteriorly (inferiorly), thereby enclosing the structures of the vestibule.
Median raphe	Ridge or furrow that marks the line of union of the two halves of the perineum.
Mons pubis	Rounded, fleshy prominence, created by the underlying fat pad, which overlies the symphysis pubis.
Perianal folds	Wrinkles or folds of the skin of the anal verge that radiate from the anus.
Perineal body	The central tendon of the perineum located between the vulva and the anus in the female and between the scrotum and anus in the male.
Perineum	The pelvic floor and associated structures bounded anteriorly by the symphysis pubis, laterally by the ischial tuberosities, and posteriorly by the coccyx.
Posterior fourchette	The junction of the two labia minora inferiorly (posteriorly). This is termed the *posterior commissure* in the prepubertal child, as the labia minora are not completely developed and have not extended and joined posteriorly or inferiorly as they do after puberty.
Vagina	The uterovaginal canal extending from the inner aspect of the hymen to the uterine cervix.
Vaginal vestibule	Anatomic cavity containing the opening of the vagina, the urethra, and the ducts of Bartholin glands; bordered by the clitoris superiorly, the labia laterally, and the posterior commissure (fourchette) inferiorly, and encompassing the fossa navicularis immediately inferior to the vaginal introitus.
Vulva	The external genitalia or pudendum of the female; includes the clitoris, labia majora, labia minora, vaginal vestibule, urethral orifice, vaginal orifice, hymen; and posterior fourchette (or commissure).

Modified from the American Professional Society on the Abuse of Children.

if perineal findings suggest possible internal extension of other injuries, thereby necessitating an examination under anesthesia, the rectal examination should be deferred and performed in the operating room with the patient heavily sedated but not yet fully anesthetized. This is important because complete sphincter relaxation and anal dilation occur with full anesthesia.

Physical Findings

The changes in appearance of the female genitalia with age are described in Chapter 18. Practitioners must become familiar with the normal anatomy at different ages and with normal variations. Extensive, carefully done studies (McCann, Berenson) have documented in detail numerous normal variants, some of which have been mistaken for abnormal findings in the past (see "Differential Diagnosis of Sexual Abuse" later). One example is apparent enlargement of the hymenal orifice. Although once thought significant, it is now known that the appearance of increased transverse diameter, in the absence of other abnormal findings, should not be used in isolation as evidence for sexual abuse. Also, for unknown reasons, obese children may have an increased anteroposterior hymenal diameter, the significance of which is unclear. Thanks to McCann's and Berenson's work, we now have a much better understanding of what is normal and what is abnormal.

Perineal Abnormalities
Abnormal and Suspicious Findings in Cases of Sexual Abuse. As noted earlier, findings on examination in victims of molestation or incest are totally normal in up to 80% to 96% of cases. In the remainder, abnormal or suspicious findings can be detected with careful examination. Marked enlargement of the hymenal orifice, with a thickened, rolled hymenal rim and little remaining

hymenal tissue, is suspicious for sexual abuse (Fig. 6-89A and B, and see Fig. 6-92C), as is deep notching of the rim through greater than 50% of hymenal width, especially when located between 3 and 9 o'clock (Fig. 6-89A-C). Presence of bumps or mounds (not associated with an intravaginal ridge) along the rim of the posterior portion of the hymenal membrane between 3 and 5 o'clock and 7 and 9 o'clock in patients with loss of hymenal tissue (Fig. 6-89A and B), and scarring of the perineal body (Fig. 6-89D) are abnormal findings that also may be seen as a result of prior sexual abuse. In addition, we have observed lichenification of the labial skin of the medial surfaces of the labia majora and marked thickening of labial adhesions due to chronic abrasive action (Fig. 6-89E and see Fig. 18-23). It should be noted that acute perineal injuries often heal quickly and, at times, completely with no residual scarring. Hence patients who have incurred injuries in the past may have no abnormal findings.

Acute Traumatic Findings of Sexual Assault and Sexual Abuse. Important to recognize is that victims of sexual assault who present acutely may show evidence of physical trauma other than genital injuries. Bruises and abrasions of the head, face, neck, chest, abdomen forearms, knees, and thighs are common (see Fig. 6-4). Occasionally, even more severe nongenital injuries are encountered.

Genital and perianal examination may reveal contusions, erythema, abrasions, or lacerations (Fig. 6-90; see also Figs. 18-14 to 18-19). Perineal lesions due to sexual abuse tend to be located in the posterior portion of the introitus, as opposed to those caused by straddle injury, which are usually more anterior, are often unilateral, and rarely involve the hymen in isolation (see Figs. 6-101, 18-14A and B, and 18-16).

Erythema is a common but totally nonspecific finding that may be significant within the context of a specific history. However, it is more likely to be a normal finding or one resulting from nonsexual irritation or scratching

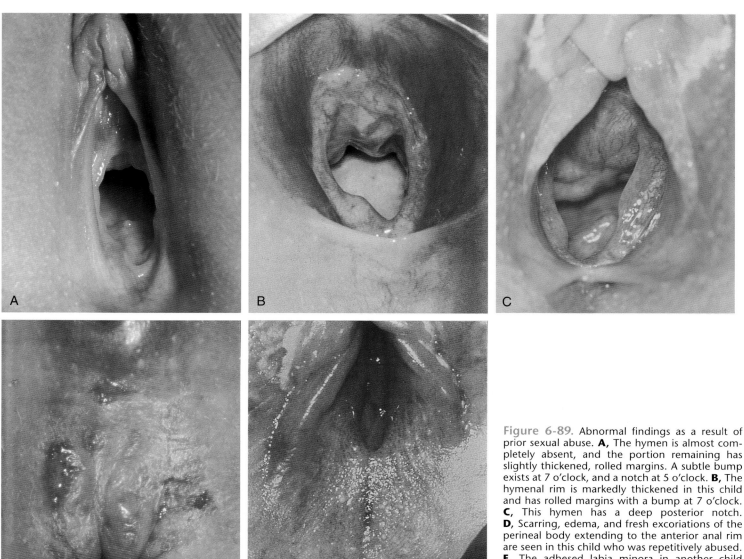

Figure 6-89. Abnormal findings as a result of prior sexual abuse. **A,** The hymen is almost completely absent, and the portion remaining has slightly thickened, rolled margins. A subtle bump exists at 7 o'clock, and a notch at 5 o'clock. **B,** The hymenal rim is markedly thickened in this child and has rolled margins with a bump at 7 o'clock. **C,** This hymen has a deep posterior notch. **D,** Scarring, edema, and fresh excoriations of the perineal body extending to the anterior anal rim are seen in this child who was repetitively abused. **E,** The adhesed labia minora in another child are markedly thickened secondary to chronic frictional trauma incurred during sexual abuse. (**B** and **D,** Courtesy Dr. Pat Bruno, Sunbury, Pa.; **E,** courtesy Dr. John McCann, University of California at Davis.)

(see Table 18-8) and should not be interpreted as specific for abuse when it is the sole finding.

At times, evidence of seminal products in the form of a vaginal discharge may be observed if the patient is seen within 24 hours of the latest incident and has not bathed in the interim (Fig. 6-91). Seminal fluid has been reported to fluoresce under Wood's lamp, but in our tests we have found only weak fluorescence when fluid has been wet and none when dry. Urine may also fluoresce, although it is reported to fluoresce differently from semen. Under normal light, dried seminal products are practically invisible. If a history of ejaculation is obtained and the area has not been washed, swabbing the perineum and inner thighs with saline-moistened cotton swabs *may* yield a sample of dried seminal fluid that can be identified by the crime laboratory. Swabs should be air-dried after the collection process. Clinicians should note, however, that seminal products are rarely found in the prepubertal child, in part because disclosure tends to occur long after the event.

In some cases, when labial separation or traction is performed with the victim in the supine or semisupine frog-leg or lithotomy position, findings can be obscured by redundant hymenal tissue that has folded over on itself.

Hence when suspected abuse victims appear to have posterior hymenal narrowing in a supine position, an assessment in knee-chest position is indicated. If the posterior portion of the hymen was indeed folded over when supine, it will tend to unfold because of gravity in the knee-chest position, revealing the true hymenal edge (see Fig. 6-86). Application of a few drops of saline can assist this. Examination with the child in the knee-chest position, with its superior visualization, also assists recognition of abnormal findings (Fig. 6-92A to C).

Male victims may have evidence of urethral discharge and mild abrasions and contusions of the penis, scrotum, or median raphe (see Fig. 6-90D and E).

Oral Abnormalities

Although most children forced to perform oral sex have no physical findings, forceful orogenital contact may result in perioral and intraoral injuries. These may include fissuring or tears at the corner of the mouth, as well as gingival and palatal contusions. Rarely, forceful oral penetration and thrusting can cause lacerations of posterior pharyngeal tissues, with potential complications of subcutaneous air dissection and abscess formation. While

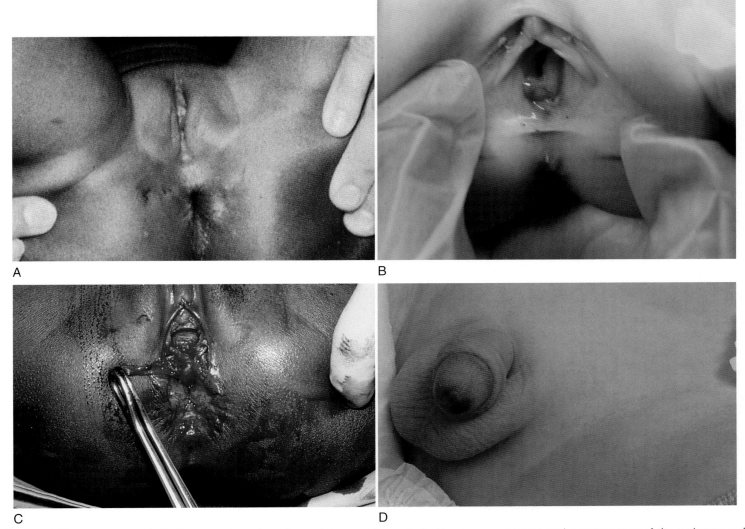

Figure 6-90. Acute traumatic findings seen in victims of sexual abuse and assault. **A,** Abrasions, contusions, and punctate tears of the perineum and perianal areas can be seen in this prepubescent girl. **B,** In this 21-month-old infant, raped by her mother's paramour, erythema and edema of the entire hymen are evident, along with bruising of its inferior aspect and of the posterior fourchette. A laceration is at 5 o'clock. **C,** Severe genital trauma in a prepubescent girl after rape. Inspection reveals a hymenal tear at 6 o'clock, extending posteriorly through the perineal body to the rectum. With the patient under anesthesia, a 1-inch (2.5-cm) vaginal tear was discovered, along with a rectal tear and complete disruption of the external anal sphincter. **D,** Acute bruising of the glans is seen in this baby, who also had a femur fracture. *(Figure continues on next page.)*

oral lesions are unusual, asymptomatic gonococcal infection of the pharynx is relatively common.

Anal and Perianal Abnormalities

Patients who have been repetitively sodomized may have normal findings or may manifest paradoxical anal sphincter relaxation in response to gluteal stroking done to assess for an anal wink reflex. They also may exhibit immediate dilation of the anal sphincter to greater than 2 cm when placed in the knee-chest position. If the latter phenomenon is seen in the absence of stool in the rectal vault, the findings are considered suspicious. The presence of tears in the perianal area and fissures is also suspicious. However, fissures are not specific to sexual abuse, as they are seen frequently in children with chronic or recurrent constipation, whereas tears that extend beyond the hair follicle-bearing areas are thought to be more characteristic of abuse. Burns may be inflicted in an attempt to obscure injuries resulting from sodomy. Hence evidence of perianal burns is strongly suggestive of abuse, as is perianal bruising (see Fig. 6-90F and G). Thickening and irregularity of the rectal folds may be suspicious (see Fig. 6-89D); however, wedge-shaped smooth areas in the midline and

skin tags are commonly seen without abuse (see Figs. 6-104 and 6-105). The observation of venous congestion after the child has been in the knee-chest position for a few minutes is a normal finding.

Evidence of Sexually Transmitted Disease

The presence of sexually transmitted diseases in the prepubescent child is strongly suggestive of sexual abuse, except in occasional instances in which other modes of transmission can be documented. In fact, many victims are identified on presenting with a vaginal or urethral discharge that is positive for a venereal pathogen. In females, this is usually manifest as vulvovaginitis with a vaginal discharge, with *Neisseria gonorrhoeae* and *Chlamydia trachomatis* the most commonly identified pathogens (see Chapter 18 and Fig. 18-36). Although asymptomatic vulvovaginal infection is quite unusual prior to puberty, oral and rectal gonococcal infections are typically subclinical. Males may have overt urethritis or asymptomatic urethral infection.

Gonococcal vulvovaginal, urethral, oral, and rectal infections are almost always acquired through sexual contact, as are vulvovaginal *Chlamydia* infection in the

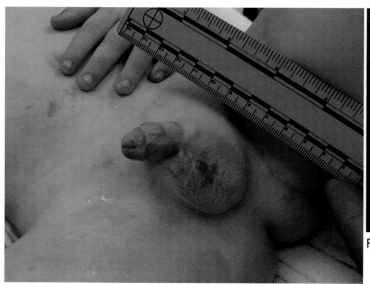

E

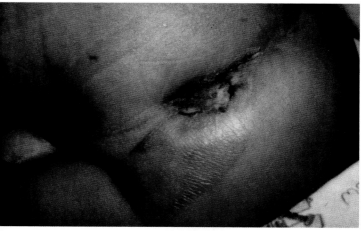

F

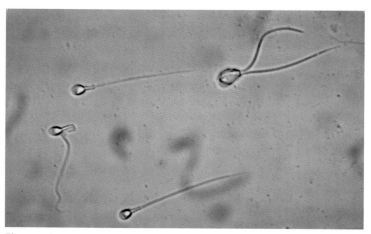

G

Figure 6-90, cont'd **E,** In this older boy, penile and scrotal bruising are evident along with multiple small bruises over the lower abdomen. **F,** Perianal lacerations, abrasions, and burns are apparent in this prepubescent boy. The examiner suspected that the burns were inflicted to obscure the evidence of sodomy. **G,** Prominent, perianal ecchymoses were found in this 3-year-old boy who had been sodomized. (**C,** Courtesy Kamthorn Sukarochana, MD; **D** and **E,** courtesy Janet Squires, MD, Children's Hospital of Pittsburgh, Pa.)

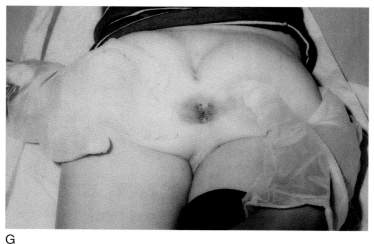

Figure 6-91. Microscopic appearance of seminal fluid removed from a young rape victim. If a vaginal discharge is found in a patient presenting within 24 hours of sexual abuse, a wet mount may reveal sperm. A portion of the discharge should also be collected for acid phosphatase, blood grouping, and enzyme studies.

child older than 2 to 3 years (see later discussion) and *Trichomonas* infection in the peripubescent child.

Development of condylomata acuminata caused by *human papillomavirus* (HPV) during infancy can be due to transmission from the mother during delivery. Because the latency period can be as long as 9 to 12 months,

lesions having their onset in the first year cannot be considered as likely due to abuse. When lesions appear thereafter they are suspicious, though not diagnostic, for abuse (Fig. 6-93) as it is now thought that many of these cases are the result of nonsexual transmission from warts on the hand of a parent or caretaker of a child who still needs assistance with toileting. However, when the warts are restricted to the hymen in a prepubertal child, sexual abuse is the likely source. When human papillomavirus is strongly suspected but no lesions are visible, application of a 3% to 5% solution of acetic acid will impart an "aceto-white" appearance to any lesions present.

In the very young child, *genital herpes* infections may be acquired through sexual contact but are more often the result of spread from oral or hand lesions from the patient, or from a parent with a cold sore, as a result of poor attention to hand washing (see Fig. 18-33A). In the latency-aged child, however, sexual contact is the more likely source. Nonspecific vaginal discharges that are culture-negative for sexually transmitted, respiratory, and enteric pathogens, especially if chronic or recurrent, are also suspect, and testing for seminal fluid should be considered.

Nonsexual transmission of gonococci, *Chlamydia, Trichomonas,* and human papillomavirus occurs primarily during vaginal delivery. Gonococcal infections tend to produce symptoms early in the neonatal period. Perinatally acquired *Trichomonas* infection causes a copious vaginal discharge in the neonate, which abates even without treatment,

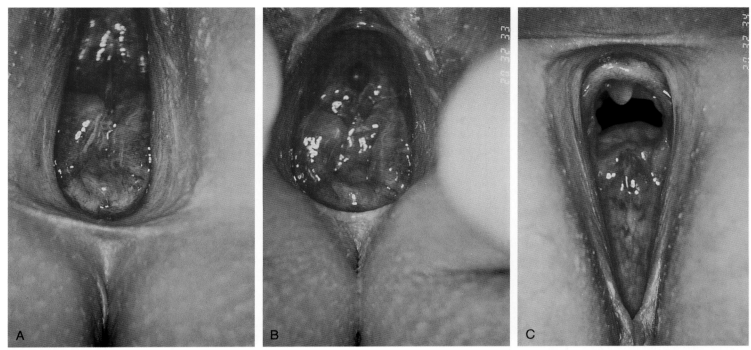

Figure 6-92. The superiority of visualization using the knee-chest position is demonstrated in this sexual abuse victim whose redundant tissues made it difficult to see the true configuration of her hymen when she was supine with labial separation **(A)** or labial traction **(B). C,** In the knee-chest position, narrowing and thickening of the hymenal rim can be seen clearly. (Courtesy Dr. John McCann, University of California at Davis.)

although the organism can persist for months. In contrast, *Chlamydia* infection acquired neonatally may persist for 18 months to 3 years. Hence finding this organism in the very young child cannot be considered diagnostic of sexual abuse. As noted earlier, because of its prolonged incubation period, the human papillomavirus acquired during delivery may not produce lesions until several months later.

Finally, it must be noted that in some instances children acquire sexually transmitted diseases as the result of sexual contact with other infected children. In such cases aggressive case finding can result in identification of the index child who is highly likely to be a victim of sexual abuse.

Specimen Collection

Laboratory studies are designed to augment the physical assessment of injury, identify sexually transmitted pathogens, and document the presence or absence of seminal fluid. Data confirm clinical experience that the yield for evidence of ejaculate on the body of a prepubertal patient presenting more than 24 hours after the abuse is low. Hence studies to detect semen can be omitted if the patient seeks attention later than this. However, it is particularly important to collect articles of unlaundered clothing and bed linens that may have evidence of ejaculate on them because semen may be retrieved from these items even 12 months (or more) later. Unfortunately, this is often overlooked in the process of evidence collection in sexual abuse cases. Because the yield of positive results from vaginal cultures obtained from asymptomatic prepubertal victims is so low, the collection of specimens sometimes uncomfortable, and the cost high, many centers are advocating a more selective approach in obtaining cultures in this age group on the basis of the level of risk. However, oral and rectal cultures should be strongly considered because oral and rectal gonococcal infections are typically asymptomatic.

In the prepubescent child with vaginal discharge, all cultures, except for *Chlamydia,* may be obtained from discharge present on the perineum. *Chlamydia* cultures necessitate swabbing the vaginal wall. (Note: ELISA, Chlamydiazyme, and Gen-Probe tests are not indicated in prepubescent patients because of potential inaccuracy in this age group and because in court their results do not constitute adequate legal evidence of infection.) This requires great care in specimen collection because the hymen, prior to puberty and estrogenization, is extremely sensitive, and touching it with a swab induces a significant amount of pain in most patients. Although usually unnecessary, application of topical anesthetic cream or ointment to the hymenal area prior to collection of specimens can help to reduce discomfort and may be a wise measure for girls with small hymenal openings or redundant hymenal tissue. Because topical lidocaine can produce transient discomfort before taking effect, use of EMLA cream may be preferable, although its onset of action takes more time. Saline-moistened calcium alginate swabs on thin metal wires are the easiest to insert atraumatically. As the knee-chest position produces maximal hymenal opening, this is the optimal position for vaginal specimen collection, if the child will tolerate it.

Cultures should be considered in the adolescent, regardless of time of presentation or of presence or absence of symptoms, because STDs may be asymptomatic in postpubertal girls, and may have been acquired earlier as a result of consensual sexual activity. Cervical cultures for gonorrhea and *Chlamydia* infection in addition to cultures of the vaginal pool are indicated. The possibility of pregnancy must also be considered in all such patients, and a pregnancy test must be performed.

In obtaining rectal specimens for gonorrhea and *Chlamydia* cultures, the swab should be inserted no more than 1 to 2 cm to avoid fecal contamination, which interferes with culture results.

Patients with evidence of trauma need urinalysis and rectal examination to check for evidence of bleeding and

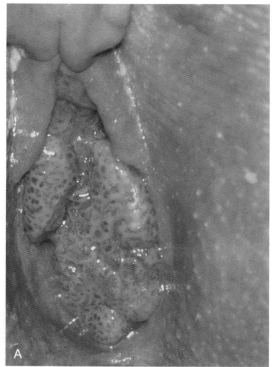

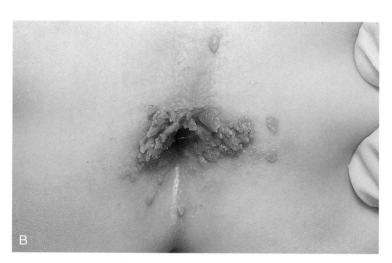

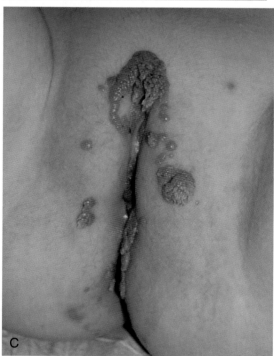

Figure 6-93. Condylomata acuminata. **A,** Although human papillomavirus infection is not specific for abuse and is perhaps more commonly transmitted nonsexually, when condylomata are restricted to the hymen, as seen in this child, sexual abuse is the likely source. In this case the victim reported that the perpetrator had visible genital warts. **B,** Coalescent and discrete condylomata are seen in the perianal area of this 4-year-old boy with a history of being sodomized. **C,** More extensive lesions involving the mons, the introitus, the labia, and perianal area developed in another child. (**C,** Courtesy Robin Gehris, MD, Children's Hospital of Pittsburgh, Pa.)

may require sonography or CT if physical findings are suggestive of internal extension of injury. However, if anal rape is reported or if anal inspection suggests evidence of forceful anal penetration with marked bruising or lacerations, especially in a prepubertal child who has clearly been traumatized emotionally and physically, rectal examination should be deferred until the patient is sedated prior to full anesthetic administration in the operating room. Loss of sphincter tone and anal dilation occur normally when a child is fully anesthetized and should not be mistaken for abnormal findings. Prepubescent girls with evidence of vaginal bleeding or a vaginal hematoma must have an internal examination performed under anesthesia to check for internal extension of injury. In

such instances, specimen collection is deferred until that time.

Table 6-16 presents guidelines for specimen collection in sexual abuse cases, and Table 6-17 enumerates the additional specimens required by law enforcement authorities in rape cases. Note that, given the extremely low yield in prepubertal children presenting after 24 hours, a full rape kit is not indicated in such situations. Because the examination is for the purpose of gathering forensic evidence, in addition to assessing the patient's physical status, procedure must be meticulous. Each specimen for the crime laboratory should be packaged and labeled immediately on collection. All evidence should then be kept together and must remain under the direct supervision of the

Table 6-16	Documentation Required in Sexual Abuse Evaluation: Guidelines for Specimen Collection in Sexual Abuse Examination at Children's Hospital, Pittsburgh, Pa.

	GENITAL CONTACT		
OROGENITAL CONTACT	**No Evidence of Penetration**	**Evidence Consistent with Vaginal Penetration**	**ANAL CONTACT**

1. Swabs: use two at a time*
  a. For wet mount for sperm[†]
  b. For two air-dried slides[†]
  c. For GC culture
  d. Consider *Chlamydia* culture if patient older than 3 years
2. Consider baseline RPR (repeat in 4-6 weeks if initial test result is negative)[§]
3. Consider HIV testing with repeat test in 3-6 months[§]
	1. Urinalysis for occult blood
	2. Vaginal swabs or aspirate*[‡]
	  a. For wet mount for sperm[†], *Trichomonas,* and *Candida*
	  b. For two air-dried slides[†]
	  c. For GC and routine culture[‡]
	  d. For *Chlamydia* culture if patient older than 3 years[‡]
	  e. For Gram stain if vaginal discharge is present[‡]
	3. Consider baseline RPR (repeat in 4-6 weeks if initial result is negative)[§]
	4. Consider HIV testing with repeat test in 3-6 months[§]
		1. Urinalysis for occult blood
		2. If vaginal bleeding or hematoma seen in prepubertal child:
		  a. Consult pediatric surgeon or gynecologist for possible EUA
		  b. If EUA done, collect specimens, then
		3. Vaginal swabs or aspirate*[‡]
		  a. For wet mount for sperm,[†] *Trichomonas,* and *Candida*
		  b. For two air-dried slides[†]
		  c. For GC and routine cultures[‡]
		  d. For *Chlamydia* culture if patient older than 3 years[‡]
		  e. For Gram stain if vaginal discharge present[‡]
		4. Consider RPR (repeat in 4-6 weeks if initial result is negative)[§]
		5. Consider HIV testing with repeat test in 3-6 months[§]
			1. If marked bruising or external tears seen:
			  a. Consult pediatric surgeon or gynecologist for possible EUA
			  b. If EUA done, collect specimens, then
			2. Swabs: Use two at a time and insert no more than 1 cm* (must be done before rectal examination)
			  a. For wet mount for sperm[†]
			  b. For two air-dried slides[†]
			  c. For GC and routine cultures
			  d. For *Chlamydia* culture if patient older than 3 years
			3. If no major bruising or tears:
			  a. Rectal examination
			  b. Stool guaiac: if positive, consult general surgeon
			4. Consider baseline RPR (repeat in 4-6 weeks if initial result is negative)[§]
			5. Consider HIV testing with repeat test in 3-6 months[§]

*Two of the swabs used to obtain specimens should be air dried and placed in a sterile test tube for acid phosphatase, blood group, DNA, and enzyme studies. When specimens are obtained by vaginal aspirate, a small amount of aspirate should be applied to two swabs, which should then be processed in the same manner.
[†]Omit if seen >24 hours after the last incident, except in patients with vaginal discharge.
[‡]In postpubescent patients, cervical swabs must be obtained for GC and *Chlamydia* cultures and for Gram stain.
[§]These studies are indicated in cases of abuse by an unknown stranger or by a perpetrator known to be at high risk for these diseases (IV drug user), especially in areas where these diseases are endemic.
NOTE: **Follow-up in 2-4 weeks is recommended, with additional specimen collection as needed.**
EUA, examination under anesthesia; GC, gonococcal; RPR, rapid plasma reagin test.

Table 6-17	Additional Specimens Needed in Rape Cases (Seen within 72 Hours*)

SPECIMENS MAY BE OBTAINED BY THE PHYSICIAN OR NURSE. ALL CONTAINERS USED IN EVIDENCE COLLECTION SHOULD BE PAPER AND MUST BE LABELED WITH:

Patient's name	Body site	Initials of collector
Type of specimen	Date and time	

Clothing	If the patient is wearing the same clothes, they should be collected along with any debris because this may provide valuable clues regarding the assailant. The patient should disrobe while standing on a towel or sheet. Each article including the towel or sheet should then be placed in a separate paper bag. Avoid shaking the articles. Each bag is then labeled and sealed.
Fingernail scrapings[†]	These may provide bits of skin, fiber, and debris from the assailant. Scrapings from beneath the nails or nail clippings should be obtained. Specimens from each hand should be collected over separate sheets of paper and placed in separate paper envelopes, sealed, and labeled.
Hair samples[†]	Any loose or suspected foreign hairs should be collected, placed in an envelope, and labeled. If patient is postpubescent, comb pubic hairs onto a sheet of clean paper, fold, place in an envelope with the comb, label "combed pubic hair," and seal. Then, gently pull pubic hairs from the patient (12 hairs are needed), place on clean paper, fold, put in envelope, label "standard pubic hair," and seal. Then, comb and pull head hairs in this same manner.
Blood sample	5 mL of blood should be drawn for blood grouping and enzyme typing and placed in a purple-top tube.
Saliva sample	This enables testing of the patient's secretory status. The specimen should be obtained either by wiping the patient's oral mucosa with a gauze pad or by having the patient expectorate onto a gauze pad. The pad is then placed in an envelope, sealed, and labeled.

Destination of Specimens
The following specimens are handled by the hospital laboratories or performed in the emergency department:

Urinalysis	Gram stains	RPR
Wet preps	Stool guaiac	Cultures

All other specimens are to be signed over to police custody for transport to the crime laboratory.

Maintaining an Unbroken Chain of Evidence
Evidence should be packaged and labeled on collection. All evidence should be kept together and must remain under the direct supervision of the collecting physician or nurse until signed over to hospital security or the police. Receipt for release of evidence to law enforcement should be signed before evidence is given over to security or the police.

*The yield is very low after 24 hours and almost zero if the child is prepubertal.
[†]Omit if patient has already bathed and shampooed.
RPR, rapid plasma reagin (test).

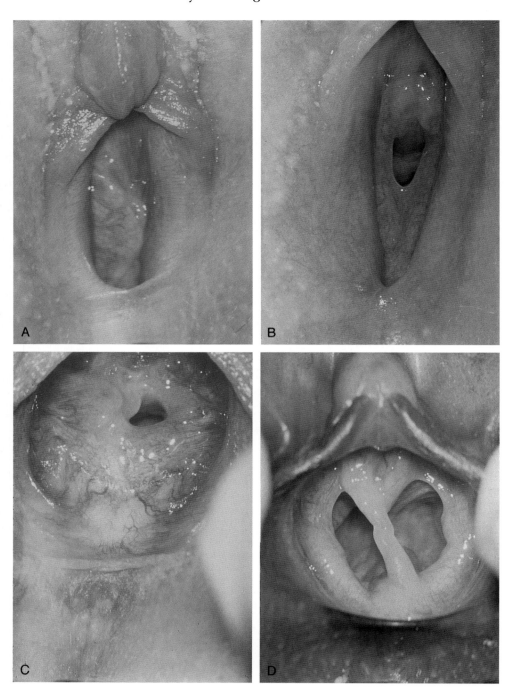

Figure 6-94. Variations in normal hymenal configuration. **A,** A redundant hymen. **B,** A crescentic hymen with thin smooth edges. **C,** A somewhat redundant hymen with an annular orifice. **D,** A septate hymen resulting from failure of lysis of the embryonic hymenal septum.

physician or nurse who was present at the time of collection until it is signed over to hospital security or law enforcement. Finally, police should sign a receipt for release of evidence on accepting the specimens. Commercially available rape assessment kits greatly assist this process. Failure to adhere to these procedures breaks the chain of evidence and invalidates its use in legal proceedings. If the assault or rape has been perpetrated by a stranger (e.g., not a caretaker), the patient or parent usually must sign a consent form before collection of evidence.

Differential Diagnosis of Sexual Abuse

Not only is there a wide range of nonabusive causes of the physical and behavioral symptoms that serve as presenting complaints of many sexual abuse victims, but physical findings, when present, are also variable and often nonspecific and many have a variety of other potential causes. Furthermore, as a result of McCann's pioneering work, the wide range of normal anatomic variations is being increasingly appreciated.

Normal Anatomic Variations

A wide variation in normal hymenal configuration and shape of orifice exists (Fig. 6-94; see also Figs. 18-3 and 18-6), as well as some amount of variation in diameter that must be appreciated by the examining physician (see Fig. 18-3). Several normal anatomic variants are now recognized as well. *Septal remnants* (Fig. 6-95), seen as tags near the midline on either the anterior or posterior portion of the hymenal membrane (see Chapter 18) and even anterolateral *hymenal flaps* (Fig. 6-96) are normal findings, as are periurethral bands. These and *intravaginal ridges* (Fig. 6-97) were once erroneously thought to be the

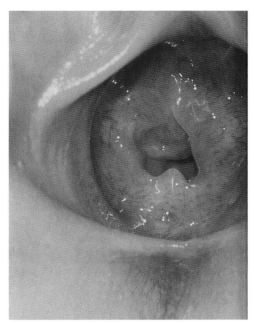

Figure 6-95. Septal remnant. This skin tag at 6 o'clock is a remnant of the vaginal septum present earlier in fetal development and constitutes a normal finding seen in about 5% of girls.

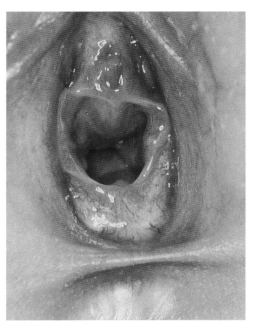

Figure 6-97. Intravaginal ridges. The bands of tissue along the vaginal walls that appear here to extend medially and downward from the 11 and 2 o'clock positions are normal features of the vaginal walls, which in the past were erroneously thought to be the result of scarring. (Courtesy Dr. John McCann, University of California at Davis.)

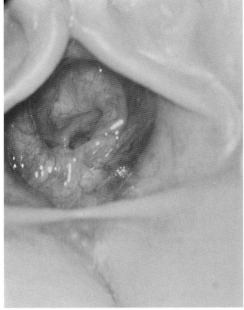

Figure 6-96. Hymenal flap. This child has a redundant hymen with an everted anterolateral flap, another normal variant.

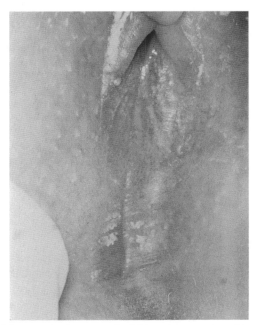

Figure 6-98. Labial adhesions. The labia minora are fused in the midline as a consequence of prior inflammation. They are separated by a thin lucent line, and the epithelium of the labia is normal.

result of scarring. Thin *labial adhesions* are a common finding in normal children as well (Fig. 6-98 and see Fig. 18-11).

Vulvar Erythema and Inflammation

Erythema of the vaginal vestibule is common in asymptomatic, nonabused, prepubescent girls. It can also be seen in abuse victims and in children with irritant and other forms of vulvovaginitis (see Figs. 18-21, 18-22, 18-27, 18-33, and Table 18-8). *Vulvovaginitis* has a wide variety of causes, many of which are noninfectious, including chemical irritation, poor perineal hygiene or aeration, nonabusive frictional trauma, contact dermatitis, or itching and scratching due to pinworms or other sources of irritation. These conditions may be associated with nonspecific erythema, maceration, or superficial abrasions/excoriations (see Figs. 18-20 to 18-22). Many infectious cases are caused by respiratory or gastrointestinal pathogens (the former transmitted from nose or throat by the child's hands, the latter often due to perineal contact with infected stool) or are seen concurrently with urinary tract infections (see Chapter 18). Thus vulvovaginitis resulting from sexually transmitted disease probably constitutes a minority of vulvovaginal complaints in prepubescent children. To avoid misdiagnosis of abuse, it is wise to defer diagnosis until definitive culture results are obtained.

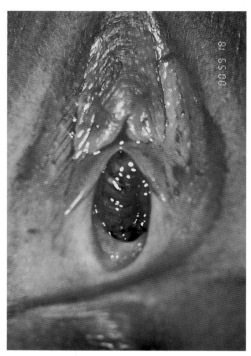

Figure 6-99. Urethral prolapse. This child was referred for evaluation for possible sexual abuse when blood was noted on her underwear, and "traumatized tissue" was seen on examination. On close inspection, this was found to be edematous, friable prolapsed urethral mucosa.

Urethral Prolapse

The clinical findings of *urethral prolapse* (Fig. 6-99) have been mistakenly attributed to sexual abuse because the purplish-red prolapsed mucosal tissue that protrudes between the labia minora bleeds easily and often overlies the vaginal orifice, simulating edematous, traumatized, redundant hymenal folds. The condition is often first discovered when blood or a serosanguineous discharge is found on the diaper or underwear, because associated dysuria is unusual and urination is not impeded. With magnification, the urethral orifice can be seen at the center of the mass, which is soft and markedly tender to touch. After application of topical anesthetic, the prolapse can be lifted, revealing the hymen underneath. The condition is unusual and tends to occur only in children younger than 12 years of age; two thirds of affected girls are African American. The cause is unknown, although many affected girls have a history of constipation.

Lichen Sclerosus

Lichen sclerosus et atrophicus has often been mistakenly attributed to sexual abuse. The involved perineal skin is paper-thin and tends to be hypopigmented. During periods of acute inflammation, hypopigmentation may be partially obscured by erythema and areas of superficial ulceration that bleed easily (Fig. 6-100; and see Fig. 18-26 and accompanying text). Its cause remains unknown.

Accidental Trauma

As noted earlier, trauma inflicted in the course of attempted or actual sexual penetration generally results in contusions and tears of the posterior portion of the hymen and introitus. In contrast, *straddle injuries* produce lesions of the anterior and anterolateral portions because these are tissues most likely to be crushed between the pubic ramus and the object on which the child falls. Findings include contusions, abrasions, and superficial lacerations, the latter being frequently found at the junction

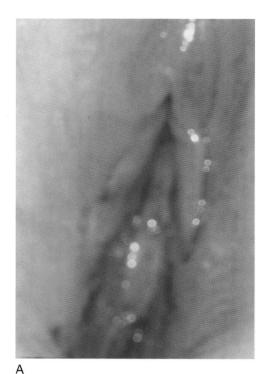

A

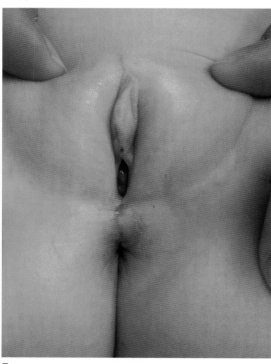

B

Figure 6-100. Lichen sclerosus et atrophicus. **A,** Multiple small points of bleeding dot the atrophic mucosa in this child. **B,** In another girl, acute inflammation has largely subsided, leaving an hourglass pattern of hypopigmentation extending from the mons to below the anal folds. (**B,** Courtesy Robin Gehris, MD, Children's Hospital of Pittsburgh, Pa.)

of the labia majora and minora (Fig. 6-101 and see Fig. 18-14).

Vaginal Foreign Bodies

The presence of foreign objects within the vaginal canal sometimes precipitates an inflammatory response with production of a copious brown, sometimes blood-tinged, discharge with a foul odor. The discharge and its odor generally prompt presentation. Foreign bodies may or may not suggest abuse. Whereas finding firm objects within

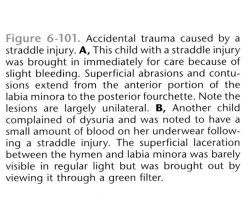
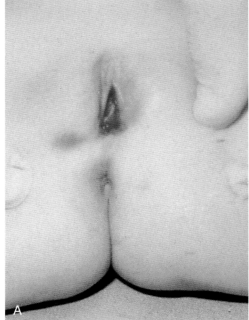
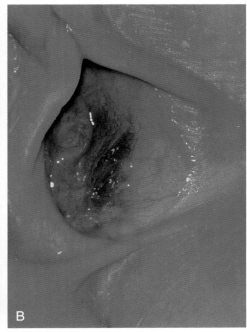

Figure 6-101. Accidental trauma caused by a straddle injury. **A,** This child with a straddle injury was brought in immediately for care because of slight bleeding. Superficial abrasions and contusions extend from the anterior portion of the labia minora to the posterior fourchette. Note the lesions are largely unilateral. **B,** Another child complained of dysuria and was noted to have a small amount of blood on her underwear following a straddle injury. The superficial laceration between the hymen and labia minora was barely visible in regular light but was brought out by viewing it through a green filter.

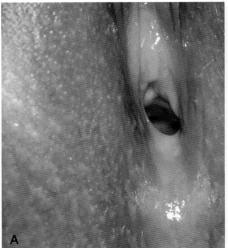
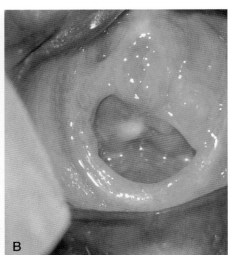

Figure 6-102. Vaginal foreign body. **A,** A white object is noted within the vagina on perineal inspection. **B,** This was better visualized with labial traction. Toilet paper had become enlodged in the process of wiping after toileting.

the vagina and witnessing a child stroking herself with crayons or similar objects and then inserting them are suspicious for prior sexual abuse, the not uncommon finding of a small wad of toilet tissue lodged within the vagina is more likely an inadvertent consequence of vigorous wiping (Fig. 6-102).

Midline Defects

Perineal midline fusion defects are an unusual phenomenon in which a small portion of the median raphe adjacent to the anus fails to fuse in utero. The anomaly, seen only in female infants, is present at birth and may be located anteriorly or posteriorly to the anus. When the unfused edges of the median raphe are spread apart they reveal an underlying pink or reddish mucosal-like surface (Fig. 6-103). The defect often goes unnoticed until days or weeks after delivery during a diaper change, bathing, or a well-child care visit. When first detected by a parent or physician unfamiliar with the problem, findings may be mistaken for a laceration due to sexual abuse. Medical recognition of the true nature of the abnormality is enhanced by knowledge of its existence, and by the fact that the edges of the outer layer of tissue and of the underlying "mucosal" surface are smooth and intact. Other

features that help distinguish midline defects from abuse-related injury are the absence of associated introital and anal abnormalities and of bleeding.

Normal Anal and Perianal Variants

Anal fissures and *perianal skin tags* (Fig. 6-104) are common sequelae of constipation. The fissures caused by the passage of hard or large-caliber stools are superficial and usually do not extend beyond the perianal skin bearing hair follicles, whereas tears produced by sodomy usually exceed this limit.

Infantile perianal pyramidal protrusion consists of a single benign papule with a pyramidal shape located in the midline of the perineal raphe, usually just anterior to the anus (occasionally just posterior). It is smooth, soft, pink, and totally asymptomatic (Fig. 6-105). The protrusion is either present at birth or noted shortly thereafter, and there is no association with antecedent fissures or fistulas. The "lesion" usually resolves spontaneously over weeks to months. Exact etiology is as yet unclear, although an association with lichen sclerosis et atrophicus has been noted.

Spontaneous anal sphincter relaxation occurring 30 seconds to 3 or 4 minutes after adopting the knee-chest position is normal. Immediate sphincter dilation when there is

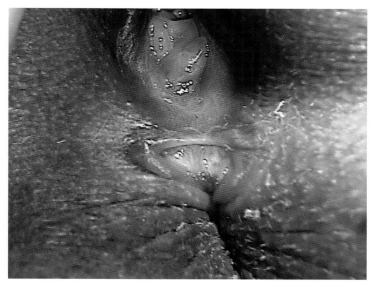

Figure 6-103. Perineal midline fusion defect. This toddler was referred for concern of sexual abuse when this defect was noticed by her new foster mother during a diaper change. The unfused edges of the median raphe are spread apart to reveal an underlying mucosal-like surface. Both are smooth and intact with no evidence of inflammation or bleeding. Note that she has another congenital anomaly, an anteriorly displaced anus. A normal redundant hymen is also seen. (Courtesy Carol Byers, CRNP, Children's Hospital of Pittsburgh, Pa.)

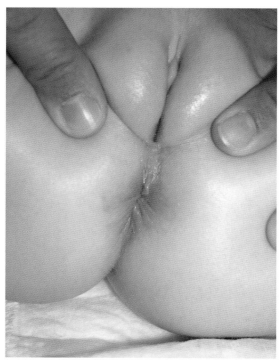

Figure 6-105. Infantile perianal pyramidal protrusion. This smooth, soft, pink papule, located in the midline just anterior to the anus, has a pyramidal shape. It was noted by the mother shortly after birth and was totally asymptomatic.

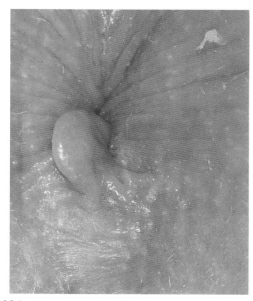

Figure 6-104. Perianal skin tag. This is a common finding, particularly in children with a history of constipation and prior problems with anal fissures.

stool present in the rectal vault is also considered normal, as is anal dilation in the fully anesthetized child. However, reproducible immediate sphincter dilation to greater than 2 cm on adopting the knee-chest position is considered to be suspicious for repetitive prior anal penetration. Perianal erythema, hyperpigmentation, and venous engorgement are other common findings seen in normal children.

Passive Abuse or Neglect

Passive abuse or neglect is by far the most commonly reported type of child abuse, accounting for more than 50% of cases each year. In its mildest form, this may consist of a pattern of lack of vigilance and safeguarding of young children, who are thereby at greater risk for accidents and ingestions. This may include leaving them unattended for long periods, placing them in a hazardous environment, or leaving an older child in charge who is too young and/or unprepared to take on responsibility for the care of younger siblings. In its most severe form, the patient presents with severe growth failure and developmental delay as a result of inadequate provision of calories and minimal or ineffective nurturing.

Typically, in severe cases, the patient has been fed irregularly, offered insufficient volumes of formula and food, given little interactional attention, and received minimal basic care. In some cases it appears that an infant may have picked up on maternal anxiety and/or depression and developed secondary anorexia and autonomic disturbances of intestinal motility. Some affected infants actually begin to resist contact and become difficult to feed. In addition, as malnutrition worsens, babies tend to become listless and irritable, making care more difficult and less rewarding. Furthermore, secondary malabsorption worsens nutrient utilization.

Risk factors are similar to those seen in cases of active physical abuse, with a few additions. More of these infants were *unplanned* and *unwanted*. Often *little or no prenatal care* was sought. In numerous cases there is a history of the father having abandoned the mother after learning of the pregnancy. Mothers of these babies are more likely to be frankly depressed or cognitively limited and to have had difficulty caring for the children they already have. In some cases the mother appears to have been coping reasonably well with the children she'd already had, but this last baby has proved one too many. The incidence of maternal *drug abuse* as a predisposing factor has increased substantially over the past few decades.

Infants born to a *teenage mother* have twice the risk of suffering neglect as those born to older women, often because of the deprivation of nurturing, love, attention, and affection they suffered themselves as infants and children. As a consequence, these young women are emotionally needy yet have difficulty with attachment and bonding, not only to their infants but also to friends and family who might be of support. Further, they have neither the emotional wherewithal nor the experience necessary to nurture their offspring. Some fantasize that the unconditional love of a child will meet their unmet needs for love. Often emotionally immature and self-focused, the teenage mothers may have little concept of what is involved in caring for a child, thinking it not much different from caring for a doll. Once the demands are evident, they may become disenchanted and lose interest. Disinterest may be manifested by bottle propping; talking on the phone during feedings; leaving the baby in a crib much of the time; leaving the baby home alone; or frequently dropping the baby off with relatives, friends, acquaintances, or neighbors (often with dubious child care skills) so that they can go out when they want. A challenging subset of adolescent mothers are those who are pseudoindependent with "attitude." Despite limited knowledge and experience, these girls are convinced they know all they need to know about caring for their baby and are resistant to and often suspicious of suggestions, advice, and offers of help.

Economic situation and lack of education also play a role. *Poverty* with its stresses and pressures, its association with poor housing conditions (nonfunctioning appliances, poor sanitary conditions, and general disrepair); lack of utilities because of unpaid bills; or homelessness is another common thread. This is further complicated by social isolation, lack of transportation, and mental health problems that can interfere with a mother's ability to mobilize herself to sign up for food stamps and the Women, Infants, and Children program to which she is entitled (see Table 6-1).

Limitations in knowledge and understanding of the importance of nutrition and children's needs are also common and, when combined with ill-informed dietary beliefs (juice is as good as formula because the Women, Infants, and Children program gives it out) or fears (regarding obesity, cholesterol or animal products [vegans], and milk/food allergy), contribute to inappropriate feeding practices.

Major *infant risk factors* are prematurity; being born small for gestational age; being the last of a large sibship or the latest of three or four born in rapid succession; being passive and undemanding; or being perceived as difficult.

Psychosocial Failure to Thrive

On presentation, the mother of an infant with *psychosocial failure to thrive* often appears relatively unconcerned about her baby's state of nutrition, even when this has reached the point of emaciation. When asked about it, she may report not having noticed it or may state that all her babies are small. Typically, she has brought the child for treatment of a minor unrelated problem, such as a cold, rash, vomiting, or constipation. Some present with a history of colic, crying "all the time," or a feeding problem. In many cases there are glaring inconsistencies in the feeding history (e.g., "he takes 6 oz. every 4 hours," yet "he takes 16 oz. in 24 hours"). Many mothers readily

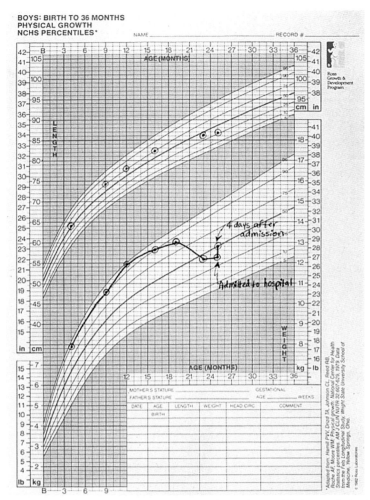

Figure 6-106. Growth chart of a child with psychosocial failure to thrive. This boy's growth was normal until he was 15 months of age, when his mother became addicted to crack. His weight gain slowed between 15 and 19 months, after which he showed a precipitous weight loss and slowing of height growth. He showed rapid catch-up growth within a week of removal from the home. (Courtesy Robin Gehris, MD, Children's Hospital of Pittsburgh, Pa.)

acknowledge that they often do not hold the baby for feedings but instead prop the bottle on a towel or against the side of the crib. When observed, even when they do hold the infant during a feeding, they often do not make good eye contact and tend to put him or her down immediately afterward. A high percentage of these infants have received little or no professional well-child care and are behind on their immunizations.

On examination, the infant or child with *psychosocial failure to thrive* is usually found to be significantly undergrown. Weight may be below the third percentile, or there may be evidence of plateauing of weight gain. In long-standing cases, height and head circumference are abnormally low as well. Comparison with birth parameters and measurements made at prior visits (if any) reveal that the child has "fallen off the growth curve" (Fig. 6-106). In the more severe case the child presents with decreased subcutaneous tissue (most notably over the buttocks, thighs, and upper arms); a pinched face; and sunken prominent eyes. In some there are frank physical findings of multiple vitamin deficiencies, which include a nonspecific or seborrhea-like dermatitis that can progress to skin breakdown, cheilosis, glossitis and stomatitis, and erythema and thinning of the skin over the palms and soles (Fig. 6-107A-E).

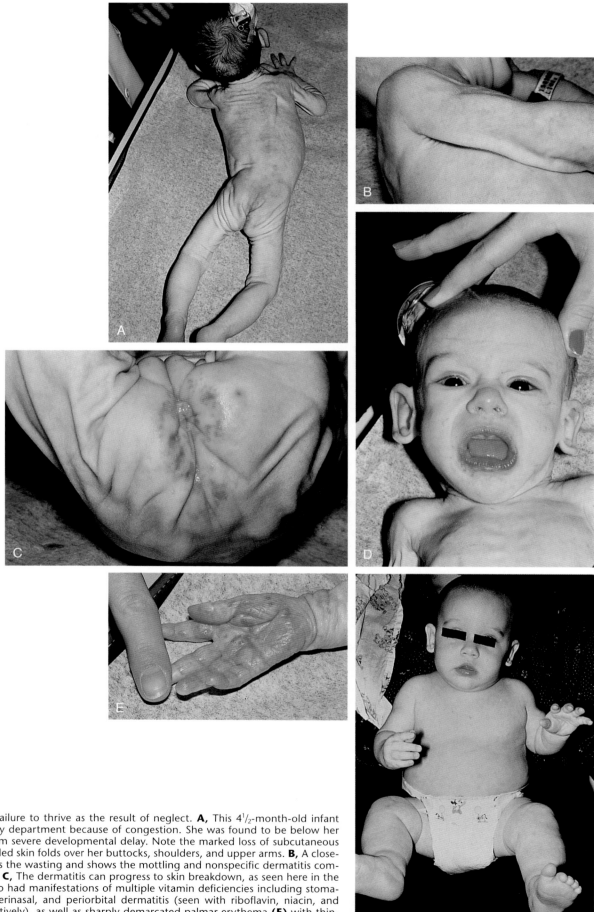

Figure 6-107. Psychosocial failure to thrive as the result of neglect. **A,** This 4½-month-old infant was brought to the emergency department because of congestion. She was found to be below her birth weight and suffering from severe developmental delay. Note the marked loss of subcutaneous tissue manifested by the wrinkled skin folds over her buttocks, shoulders, and upper arms. **B,** A close-up of her upper arm highlights the wasting and shows the mottling and nonspecific dermatitis commonly seen with malnutrition. **C,** The dermatitis can progress to skin breakdown, as seen here in the perianal area. **D,** The baby also had manifestations of multiple vitamin deficiencies including stomatitis, glossitis, and perioral, perinasal, and periorbital dermatitis (seen with riboflavin, niacin, and vitamin B₆ deficiencies, respectively), as well as sharply demarcated palmar erythema **(E)** with thinning of the skin (niacin deficiency). **F,** Three and a half months after removal from the home, she was well nourished and had caught up developmentally.

Affected infants tend to look serious, smile infrequently, appear apathetic and withdrawn when left alone, and often lie on their backs with their arms up beside their heads. They show more interest in inanimate objects than in people, and although they appear vigilant toward people at a distance, they tend to become upset when someone approaches and avoid making eye contact. They often object to being touched, held, or cuddled. When health care personnel persist in trying to get them to interact, they find they must work hard to get the baby to calm down and sit in their lap; when put back in the crib, the child cries only briefly, if at all. Vocalization is sparse, and development is delayed and uneven, with social milestones being farther behind than motor development. We have seen some who have had abnormal tone, scissoring, and posturing suggestive of a neurologic problem, which promptly abated within a few days of hospitalization.

Poor hygiene, dirty clothes, badly neglected diaper rashes, and severe baby-bottle caries are common additional findings suggestive of neglect (Fig. 6-108).

The easiest, least traumatic way to confirm the diagnosis of psychosocial failure to thrive is to remove the infant from its home and observe its growth in a nurturing environment. Infants and children with milder cases will gain weight promptly, whereas marasmic infants may take 1 to 2 weeks before resuming growth (see Fig. 6-107F).

Although pure psychosocial failure to thrive is the most common form of growth failure in infancy, accounting for between 33% and 50% of cases, up to 25% of cases are of purely organic origin; in another 25%, growth failure is due to a combination of organic and psychosocial factors. In the latter instances, affected infants often have suffered prenatal or perinatal insults that have resulted in growth retardation and/or physical conditions that make them difficult to feed and care for.

Organic Causes of Failure to Thrive

Of cases of *organic failure to thrive,* CNS, gastrointestinal, cardiac, genetic, pulmonary, renal, and endocrine disorders account for organically based growth failure, in descending order of frequency. The majority of such disorders can be recognized during physical examination because of the obvious abnormalities seen. The remainder tend to be revealed by history or can be readily diagnosed on the basis of a few simple screening laboratory tests.

Neurologic Disorders

Severe cerebral palsy, neuromuscular disorders, encephalopathies, and neurodegenerative diseases are the major CNS problems associated with failure to thrive. Poor suck; problems coordinating sucking and swallowing; and lethargy, irritability, and altered level of consciousness are the more common factors that impede adequate intake in these infants. Some also have excess losses because of vomiting. Neurologic dysfunction may also impair an infant's ability to provide interactive feedback to the mother.

Gastrointestinal Disorders

A variety of gastrointestinal problems cause growth failure, and numerous mechanisms are responsible. Oral malformations including cleft lip and palate, severe micrognathia, and macroglossia interfere with sucking and swallowing. Many of these conditions are also associated with chronic or recurrent ear and nasopharyngeal infections. Esophageal and gastric disorders can interfere with

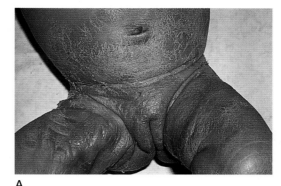

A

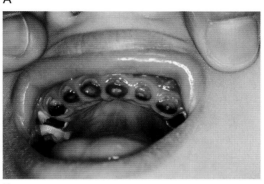

B

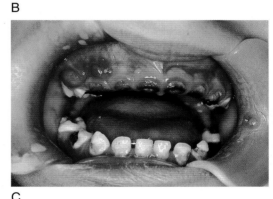

C

Figure 6-108. Neglect. **A,** Another infant with severe failure to thrive has a badly neglected case of irritant diaper dermatitis. **B** and **C,** Severely neglected baby bottle caries were among the findings noted on evaluation of a toddler with failure to thrive. She was examined after her marasmic baby brother was referred by Women, Infants, and Children personnel. Their mother was suffering from immobilizing depression. In **B,** one can see that the upper teeth are markedly discolored by decay and have eroded down to the gingiva. In **C,** note the abscesses over the upper left gingiva.

growth by causing pain on swallowing, resulting in decreased intake, or by causing repetitive vomiting (abnormal losses), with or without aspiration. These include gastroesophageal reflux (GER), esophageal stricture, stenosis, or atresia; external esophageal compression by abnormal vessels, an enlarged heart, or mass lesions; chalasia; and achalasia. Among these, GER predominates, and it must be remembered that this disorder has varied manifestations. Although vomiting or repetitive spitting are common modes of presentation, they are not uniformly present. Other symptoms include crying after every few swallows during feedings (with or without writhing or arching) and/or feeding refusal due to esophagitis. In some cases snoring, coughing, wheezing, and even apnea are prominent and tend to worsen during sleep or while recumbent (see Chapters 10 and 23).

With the exception of pyloric stenosis, which can cause FTT due to repeated vomiting when diagnosis is delayed, malabsorption is the major mechanism of growth failure in patients with small or large intestinal disorders and pancreatic disease. These infants may also experience pain associated with eating caused by gas, hyperperistalsis, or inflammation, each of which may also cause anorexia. Further, they typically have a history of excessive stool losses, and stool examination may suggest the underlying cause. Carbohydrate malabsorption is characterized by large, watery stools, which are positive for reducing substances, have a low pH, and are accompanied by considerable gas. Fat malabsorption results in large, bulky, greasy stools, and protein malabsorption in foul-smelling stools. Infants with blind-loop syndromes resulting from webs, bands, or stenoses have large, watery stools as a result of bacterial overgrowth in the gut lumen proximal to the site of partial obstruction. Short-gut syndrome following surgical resection and parasitic infections with *Giardia* or *Strongyloides* organisms are other causes of malabsorption.

Impaired bile acid metabolism results in fat malabsorption in infants with severe liver disease. Associated anorexia, malaise, and fatigue further impede intake in these children, and vomiting contributes to caloric losses. It must also be remembered that malnutrition itself causes malabsorption.

Infants and toddlers with symptomatic *celiac disease* or gluten-sensitive enteropathy may present between 6 months and 2 years of age with failure to thrive. In the "textbook case" the child has diarrhea with foul-smelling stools, vomiting, abdominal distension, anorexia, and pallor, and has an irritable, unhappy demeanor. A wide range of symptomatology exists, however. Some patients may only have vomiting and growth retardation, others only short stature, and a majority of affected children are probably asymptomatic. The disorder and its symptoms stem from a genetic susceptibility to intolerance to the gliadin fraction of gluten, which then sets off a T cell–mediated immunologic response. This results in chronic inflammation of the mucosa of the small intestine, impairing its absorption and digestive functions. Because gluten is found in wheat, rye, barley and, to a lesser extent, oats, symptoms cannot develop until the infant or child has been exposed to cereals, breads, or crackers containing these grains for some period of time.

Cardiac Disease

Severe cardiac disorders including those characterized by chronic congestive heart failure, large shunts, or pulmonary hypertension appear to result in growth failure primarily as a result of dyspnea with feeding and secondarily decreased intake. Slow feeding and a history of diaphoresis with feeding and during sleep are commonly noted. The role of hypoxia and malabsorption (resulting from impaired intestinal lymphatic drainage in children with congestive heart failure) remains unclear. Many of these patients also have recurrent pulmonary infections, and in some, intrauterine growth retardation, congenital infections, and genetic disorders play a role.

Genetic Disorders

The genetic disorders associated with impaired growth include chromosomal disorders, storage diseases, skeletal disorders and dysplasias, inborn errors of metabolism, idiopathic hypercalcemia, and heritable CNS defects. Nearly all are characterized by obvious physical stigmata.

Pulmonary Disease

Of the pulmonary disorders associated with failure to thrive, bronchopulmonary dysplasia and persistent viral infections are the two main sources. Dyspnea with feeding and secondarily decreased intake appear to be the major underlying mechanisms, often compounded by recurrent infection. *Cystic fibrosis* can be put in this category, but it is malabsorption due to pancreatic enzyme deficiency more than pulmonary dysfunction that appears to affect the growth of these patients.

Renal Disease

Renal diseases that involve the interstitium and tubular structures are the major nephric sources of growth failure. These include dysplasia; multicystic or polycystic kidney disease; severe hydronephrosis with azotemia; chronic obstructive uropathy; renal tubular acidosis; nephrogenic diabetes insipidus; chronic or recurrent urinary tract infections with severe reflux or other anatomic abnormalities; and chronic renal failure. Inability to concentrate the urine, abnormalities of urinary sediment, or abnormal serum chemistry values are found on screening tests in these patients. Inadequate intake stemming from anorexia and protein restriction; malabsorption; abnormal vitamin D absorption and secondary hyperparathyroidism with renal osteodystrophy; decreased somatomedin levels; and abnormal peripheral utilization and degradation of insulin may contribute to growth failure in these children.

Endocrine Disease

Among the endocrine disorders, *diabetes mellitus* and pituitary, thyroid, and adrenal disorders can all be associated with growth impairment. Urinary losses of glucose, dehydration, and excessive protein catabolism result in weight loss in children with diabetes mellitus. A history of polyuria, polydipsia, or polyphagia and tests for serum and urine glucose readily enable diagnosis. The growth curves of children with *isolated growth hormone deficiency* and *panhypopituitarism* level off between 9 and 12 months of age, with height affected more than weight. Such patients appear well nourished for height but often have an elfin physiognomy. *Congenital hypothyroidism* is characterized by an open posterior fontanelle, umbilical hernia, macroglossia, mottled skin, prolonged physiologic jaundice, and severe constipation. Although height is short and bone age markedly delayed, weight is normal or increased for height. Characteristic physical stigmata assist diagnosis. *Congenital hyperthyroidism* results in failure to thrive because of poor feeding and frequent loose stools. Affected infants are irritable and hyperactive and have tachypnea, tachycardia, and diaphoresis. The presence of goiter makes this condition obvious. Patients with *adrenocortical insufficiency* grow poorly because of anorexia, vomiting, and diarrhea, which also predisposes them to dehydration. Basic serum chemistry tests reveal hyponatremia and hyperkalemia.

Other Organic Factors

In late infancy and early childhood, severe tonsillar and adenoidal hypertrophy with secondary sleep apnea assumes significance as a cause of impaired growth. Difficulty swallowing, whether mechanical (due to mass effect) or secondary due to tonsillopharyngeal pain; immune stress from chronic or recurrent adenotonsillar and middle ear infection; and the effect of sleep interruptions on nocturnal growth hormone secretion are contributing factors.

Nursing or baby bottle syndrome secondary to being put to bed with a bottle of milk or juice at night and poor dental hygienic practices (little or no brushing) tends to develop in late infancy or during the second year. When severe, numerous deep caries, enamel erosion, and abscesses make sucking and chewing painful (see Fig. 6-108B and C), and the chronic infection adds immune stress, which also can contribute to inadequate intake and secondary growth impairment. This age group is also the most likely to be given large quantities of juice throughout the day, damping their hunger for more nutritious foods and milk.

Of all the organic causes of or contributors to failure to thrive, gastroesophageal reflux, whether with decreased feeding due to esophagitis or increased losses from vomiting, or both, and chronic nonspecific diarrhea are the major contributors. The latter may stem from diet (high juice, sorbitol intake), recurrent infection with its combination of immune stress and cycles of antibiotic administration, or malabsorption due to malnutrition, among other factors.

Whether of psychosocial, organic, or combined origin, growth failure in infancy and early childhood is the result of insufficient provision, retention and/or absorption of nutrients—protein, fat, carbohydrates (and often micronutrients and vitamins)—to meet the needs for protein and energy required for normal growth and development of the child. This insufficiency can result from failure of the mother to offer adequate amounts of breast milk, formula, and, later, foods and milk or from inappropriate feeding (psychosocial); inadequate intake by the infant (anorexia, feeding refusal, feeding/swallowing difficulty); inability to retain adequate nutrition (vomiting/malabsorption); growth inefficiency (chronic infection, cardiopulmonary disease, hypothyroidism); or unusually high caloric needs (malignancy, chronic illness, hyperthyroidism).

Once undernutrition reaches a significant level (generally when weight, height, and head circumference growth are all impaired), the infant tends to become caught up in a vicious cycle: with malnutrition impairing immune function, which increases frequency/chronicity/severity of infection, which causes anorexia with decreased intake and decreased nutrient absorption while adding to caloric needs, thereby further exacerbating the malnutrition. In addition to this cycle there is another involving maternal/child interaction: the malnourished infant, regardless of cause, tends to become progressively more irritable and listless; less engaging and engageable; and, therefore, less rewarding to care for. Hence a combination of physical and psychosocial factors comes into play in all cases of severe failure to thrive.

Evaluation and Management of Failure to Thrive

Given the vicious cycles described earlier; given the prevalence of undernutrition, variably estimated at between 2% and 10% in the United States; given the high percentage of cases in which psychosocial factors are the primary cause or a prime contributor in an infant with organic disease; and given the stresses of caring for infants with severe organic disorders, it is essential in evaluating the infant with poor growth to obtain a thorough psychosocial and family history, as well as a detailed medical history (see Table 6-18). The latter should include information regarding duration of the problem, mode of onset, and pattern of growth. Asking the parents how easy or difficult it is to take care of this child is also helpful. A complete review of systems—gastrointestinal, cardiorespiratory, neurologic, genitourinary, and endocrine—emphasizing intake and output is often helpful. A thorough, specific, and concrete feeding and dietary history is essential, including the following:

1. Specific items offered and amounts taken at each feeding, with calorie counts
2. Times fed—regular or erratic, of sufficient frequency?
3. Feeding situation—place in home, fed by whom, held for feeding or bottle-propped
4. Feeding atmosphere—noise level, calm or chaotic, discord
5. Feeding method:
   - Breast—time at each breast, sufficient to empty?
     - Child's positioning
     - Milk production
     - Adequacy of mother's diet
   - Bottle—type of formula
     - How mixed?
     - How much fed, how often?
     - Total volume per 24 hours
6. Infant's demeanor/behavior during feedings:
   - Disinterest/anorexia
   - Refusal
7. Mother's dietary beliefs/concerns/fears
8. Home facilities for food storage/preparation

It is also highly important to observe the maternal/child interaction, especially during feedings, to assess the behavior and demeanor of each and their degree of mutuality, cueing, and attentiveness to cues. A thorough general physical examination will reveal gross abnormalities in patients with underlying CNS, cardiopulmonary, or genetic problems.

A few basic screening tests (complete blood count and differential; urinalysis and culture; stool pH, reducing substance, and fat stain; and urea nitrogen, electrolytes, and creatinine) can serve to rule out most other organic causes of failure to thrive. If onset of poor growth follows introduction of wheat into the diet, a celiac panel should be obtained. Table 6-18 summarizes the most common causes of infantile growth failure and their major findings on evaluation.

The earlier that growth impairment/undernutrition is recognized, evaluated as to cause(s), and treatment instituted, the better, because the more long-standing the problem, the more difficult it is to treat, and the greater the risk of long-term sequelae, especially in cases of neglect and primary psychosocial failure to thrive. The latter include developmental delay and cognitive deficits secondary to impaired brain growth and inadequate stimulation that may not be fully reversible with therapy and early intervention. There is evidence that even if good nutrition is reestablished and catch-up growth achieved, failure to improve emotional nurturing perpetuates developmental delays. An increased incidence of behavior problems and of affective and motivational disorders has also been found later in childhood in children who had psychosocial failure to thrive as infants and toddlers.

Effective treatment depends on helping the mother (in a supportive and nonthreatening manner) understand the nature of the problem, her child's nutritional needs, and the need for increased caloric density to accomplish catch-up growth (1.5 to 2 times normal requirements), thereby enlisting her as part of the treatment team and the process. This must be supplemented by education regarding her baby's emotional and developmental needs and the importance of warm, consistent nurturing. The process may also necessitate helping her to get and accept help with feeding support, early intervention services, housing, and mental health issues. This is often best accomplished by a specialized multidisciplinary team.

| Table 6-18 | Findings in Failure to Thrive in Infancy | | | |

CAUSE	APPROXIMATE PERCENTAGE OF ALL CASES	HISTORY	SYSTEM-SPECIFIC PHYSICAL FINDINGS	SYSTEM-SPECIFIC LABORATORY STUDIES
Psychosocial	Up to 50% or more	Vague, inconsistent feeding history, history of bottle propping	None, may have soft neurologic signs	None
Central nervous system	13%	Poor feeding, gross developmental delay, vomiting	Grossly abnormal neurologic findings	Frequent gross abnormalities on EEG and CT scan or grossly abnormal tests of neuromuscular function
Gastrointestinal	10%	Chronic vomiting and/or diarrhea, abnormal stools, crying with feedings, nocturnal cough/snoring	Often negative, may have abdominal distention	Abnormal barium, pH probe or endoscopic study; abnormal stool findings (pH, reducing substances, fat stain, Wright stain)
Cardiac	9%	Slow feeding, dyspnea and diaphoresis with feeding, restlessness and diaphoresis during sleep	Often cyanotic or have signs of congestive heart failure	Abnormal echocardiogram, ECG, catheterization findings
Genetic	8%	May have positive family history or a history of developmental delay	Often have facies typical of a syndrome, skeletal abnormalities, neurologic abnormalities, or visceromegaly	May have typical radiographic findings, chromosomal abnormalities, abnormal metabolic screens
Pulmonary	3.5%	Chronic or recurrent dyspnea with feedings, tachypnea	Grossly abnormal chest examination findings	Abnormal chest radiographs
Renal	3.5%	May be negative or may have history of polyuria	Often negative, may have flank masses	Abnormal urinalysis, frequently elevated BUN and creatinine, signs of renal osteodystrophy on radiographs
Endocrine	3.5%	With hypothyroidism, constipation and decreased activity level; with diabetes, polyuria, polydipsia	With hypothyroidism, no wasting but mottling, umbilical hernia, often open posterior fontanelle. With diabetes, often without specific abnormality, but may have signs of dehydration, ketotic breath, and hyperpnea. With hypopituitarism and isolated growth hormone deficiency, growth normal until 9 months or later, then plateaus, but normal weight for height; delayed tooth eruption	Decreased T_4, increased TSH; glucosuria and hyperglycemia; abnormal pituitary function study results

ECG, electrocardiogram; EEG, electroencephalogram; TSH, thyroid-stimulating hormone.

Emotional Abuse

It must be emphasized that emotional abuse accompanies *all* of the other forms of abuse described previously. It can also occur in isolation and can range from inattentiveness to frank rejection, scapegoating, or even terrorizing. Because isolated emotional abuse is difficult to document, leaving no visible stigmata, it accounts for the smallest proportion of reported cases. Victims may present with chronic severe anxiety, hyperactivity, depression, agitation, or frank psychotic reactions. Many victims are socially withdrawn, have trouble relating to peers, and generally perform poorly in school. Low self-esteem is the rule. If emotional abuse is suspected, psychological testing and psychiatric examination may prove helpful in confirming its existence and directing treatment.

Reporting

Each state has regulations requiring health care providers, hospitals, and professionals involved in child care to report suspected cases of abuse and neglect to CPS agencies. Although these regulations are similar, they vary from state to state, and clinicians should become familiar with the regulations in their respective states. The suspected abuse or neglect must result from the acts or omissions of a parent, step-parent, or other person in a caretaking role. For abuse to be reported, reasonable grounds for suspicion are required, not clinical certainty. There is no penalty for reporting in good faith after careful evaluation, but there can be severe penalties for failure to report.

Many states require physicians and hospitals to notify police regarding cases involving severe abuse (potentially life-threatening or threatening a vital sense organ or limb), as well as sexual abuse. This can be done by the clinician evaluating the patient or by CPS, but, unfortunately, the latter often do not notify police promptly. Cases of stranger rape, physical assault, or abuse perpetrated by a person in a noncaretaking role must be reported to law enforcement and not CPS because such situations usually do not involve caretakers. CPS should be notified, however, if it is suspected that parental negligence was also contributory.

Pediatricians may be unaware of the definition of statutory rape, which varies by state. In these cases a child may "consent" to intercourse but may, by legal definition, not be considered old enough to give consent. These laws usually specify the age difference between the sexual partners. Particularly when dealing with adolescents, who may hesitate to disclose either consensual activity or sexual assault for fear of mandatory reporting to the police and having to testify, one must consider what, in the clinician's best judgment, is in the best interest of the patient, given the information at hand. In rare instances the child may be at further risk if the physician reports the abuse (e.g., believable threats of suicide by the patient). In those instances one must document reasons for failure to report the event to the authorities and try to ensure follow-up with the patient.

Conclusion

Although treatment and follow-up are beyond the scope of an atlas of physical diagnosis, a few additional points bear emphasis. Use of a team approach including physicians, nurses, and social workers or psychologists greatly assists evaluation of victims of abuse and their families, and it reduces the burden on any one health care worker. Reporting requirements necessitate only *reasonable* grounds for suspicion and place the onus of full investigation on state agencies. Unfortunately, close follow-up, though highly important, is often neglected, especially when patients get caught up in large bureaucratic systems. Having improved our performance on identification and documentation of cases, we must increasingly apply ourselves to assisting better long-term follow-up to ensure that victims are not only safe from harm but also have access to medical, educational, and mental health services to help them cope with, and when possible, overcome physical and emotional sequelae, thereby improving outcomes.

In memory of
Elizabeth Elmer, MSW
1911-2007
Pioneer in the field of child abuse and neglect

Bibliography

Ablin DS, Greenspan A, Reinhart M, Grix A: Differentiation of child abuse from osteogenesis imperfecta. Am J Radiol 154:1035-1046, 1990.

Ablin S, Sane SM: Nonaccidental injury: Confusion with temporary brittle bone disease and mild osteogenesis imperfecta. Pediatr Radiol 27:111-113, 1997.

Alexander R, Crabbe L, Sato Y, et al: Serial abuse in children who are shaken. AJDC 144:58-60, 1990.

Alexander R, Sato Y, Smith W, Bennett T: Incidence of impact trauma with cranial injuries ascribed to shaking. Am J Dis Child 144:724-726, 1990.

Alexander RC, Schor DP, Smith WL: Magnetic resonance imaging of intracranial injuries for child abuse. J Pediatr 109:975-979, 1986.

American Academy of Pediatrics, Committee on Child Abuse and Neglect: Distinguishing sudden infant death syndrome from child abuse fatalities. Pediatrics 107:437-441, 2001.

Amodio J, Spektor V, Pramanik B, et al: Spontaneous development of bilateral subdural hematomas in an infant with benign infantile hydrocephalus: Color Doppler assessment of vessels traversing extra-axial spaces. Pediatr Radiol 35:1113-1117, 2005.

Bauer CH (ed): Failure to thrive. Pediatr Ann 7:737-795, 1978.

Case ME, Graham MA, Corey Handy T, et al: National Association of Medical Examiners Ad Hoc Committee on Shaken Baby Syndrome: Position paper on fatal abusive head injuries in infants and young children. Am J Forens Med Pathol 22:112-122, 2001.

Chadwick DL: The diagnosis of inflicted injury in infants and young children. Pediatr Ann 21:477-483, 1992.

Chadwick DL, Berkowitz CD, Kerns DL, et al: Color Atlas of Child Sexual Abuse. Chicago, Year Book, 1989.

Chadwick DL, Chin S, Salerno C, et al: Deaths from falls in children: How far is fatal? J Trauma 31:1353-1355, 1991.

Christian CW, Lavelle JM, DeJong AR, et al: Forensic evidence findings in prepubertal victims of sexual assault. Pediatrics 106:100-104, 2000.

Coant PN, Kornberg AE, Brody AS, Edwards-Holmes K: Markers for occult liver injury in cases of physical abuse in children. Pediatrics 89:274-278, 1992.

Dubowitz H, Bross DC: The pediatrician's documentation of child maltreatment. AJDC 146:596-599, 1992.

Duhaime AC, Gennarelli TA, Thibault LE, et al: The shaken baby syndrome: A clinical, pathological and biomechanical study. J Neurosurg 66:409-415, 1987.

Ewing-Cobbs L, Prasad M, Kramer L, et al: Acute neuroradiologic findings in young children with inflicted or noninflicted traumatic brain injury. Childs Nerv Syst 16:25-34, 2000.

Finkelhor D: Current information on the scope and nature of child sexual abuse. Future Child 4, Summer/Fall 1994.

Finkelhor D: Improving research, policy, and practice to understand child sexual abuse. JAMA 280:1864-1865, 1998.

Gilliand MGF, Folberg R: Shaken babies—some have no impact injuries. J Forens Sci 41:114-116, 1996.

Green FC (ed): Incest and sexual abuse. Pediatr Ann 8:1-103, 1979.

Hadley MN, Sonntag VKH, Rekate HL, Murphy A: The infant whiplash-shake injury syndrome: A clinical and pathological study. Neurosurgery 24:536-540, 1989.

Heger A, Emans SJ, Muram D: Evaluation of the Sexually Abused Child, 2nd ed. New York, Oxford University Press, 2000.

Helfer RE: The neglect of our children. Pediatr Clin North Am 37:923-942, 1990.

Helfer RE, Kempe HC (eds): The Battered Child, 5th ed. Chicago, University of Chicago Press, 1997.

Herman-Giddens ME, Brown G, Verbiest S, et al: Underascertainment of child abuse mortality in the United States. JAMA 282:463-467, 1999.

Hodge D, Ludwig S: Child homicide: Emergency department recognition. Pediatr Emerg Care 1:3-6, 1985.

Hoffman GF, Athanossopoulos S, Burlina AB, et al. Clinical course, early diagnosis, treatment and prevention of disease in glutaryl-CoA dehydrogenase deficiency. Neuropediatrics 27:115-123, 1996.

Homer MD, Ludwig S: Categorization of etiology of failure to thrive. Am J Dis Child 135:848-851, 1981.

Hymel KP, Jenny C: Abusive spiral fractures of the humerus: A videotaped exception. Arch Pediatr Adolesc Med 150:226-227, 1996.

Hymel KP, Hall CA: Diagnosing pediatric head injury. Pediatr Ann 34:358-370, 2005.

Jenny C, Hymel KP, Ritzen A, et al: Analysis of missed cases of abusive head trauma. JAMA 281:621-627, 1999.

Jenny C for the Committee on Child Abuse and Neglect: Evaluating infants and young children with multiple fractures. Pediatrics 118:1299-1303, 2006.

Johnson CF: Inflicted injury versus accidental injury. Pediatr Clin North Am 37:791-814, 1990.

Kessler DB, Dawson P (eds): Failure to Thrive and Pediatric Undernutrition, a Transdisciplinary Approach. Baltimore, Paul H Brookes, 1999.

Kleinman P: Diagnostic Imaging of Child Abuse, 2nd ed. St Louis, Mosby, 1998.

Kleinman PK, Blackbourne BD, Marks SC, et al: Radiologic contributions to the investigation and prosecution of cases of fatal infant abuse. N Engl J Med 320:507-511, 1989.

Krugman RD: Recognition of sexual abuse in children. Pediatr Rev 8:25, 1986.

Lavy U, Bauer CH: Pathophysiology of failure to thrive and gastrointestinal disorders. Pediatr Ann 7:10-33, 1978.

Levin AV, Magnusson MR, Rafto SE, Zimmerman RA: Shaken baby syndrome diagnosed by magnetic resonance imaging. Pediatr Emerg Care 5:181-186, 1989.

McCann J, Voris J, Simon M, Wells R: Perianal findings in prepubertal children selected for non-abuse: A descriptive study. Child Abuse Negl 13:179-193, 1989.

McCann JJ, Kerns DL: The Anatomy of Child and Adolescent Sexual Abuse: A CD-ROM Atlas/Reference. St Louis, InterCorp, 1999.

Morris AAM, Hoffmann GF, Naughton ER, et al: Glutaric aciduria and suspected child abuse. Arch Dis Childhood 80:404-405, 1999.

Ophthalmology Child Abuse Working Party, Royal College of Ophthalmologists: Child abuse and the eye. Eye 13:3-10, 1999.

Paradise JE: The medical evaluation of the sexually abused child. Pediatr Clin North Am 37:839-862, 1990.

Piatt JH Jr: A pitfall in the diagnosis of child abuse, external hydrocephalus, subdural hematomas and retinal hemorrhages. Neurosurg Focus 7:4, 1999. Available at http://www.aans.org/education/journal/neurosurgical/oct99/7-4-4.asp

Pierce MC, Bertocci GE, Janosky JE, et al: Femur fractures resulting from stair falls among children: An injury plausibility model. Pediatrics 115:1712-1722, 2005.

Pierce MC, Bertocci GE, Vogeley E, Moreland MS: Evaluating long bone fractures in children: A biomechanical approach with illustrative cases. Child Abuse and Neglect 38:505-524, 2004.

Reece RM: Unusual manifestations of child abuse. Pediatr Clin North Am 37:905-922, 1990.

Reece RM, Ludwig S (eds): Child Abuse: Medical Diagnosis and Management, 2nd ed. Philadelphia, Lippincott Williams & Wilkins, 2001.

Reece RM, Sege R: Childhood head injuries, accidental or inflicted? Arch Pediatr Adolesc Med 154:11-22, 2000.

Reiber GD: Fatal falls in childhood: How far must children fall to sustain fatal head injury? Report of cases and review of the literature. Am J Forens Med Pathol 14:201-207, 1993.

Rosenberg NM, Marino D: Frequency of suspected abuse/neglect in burn patients. Pediatr Emerg Care 5:219-221, 1989.

Rosenn DW, Loeb LS, Jura MB: Differentiation of organic from non-organic failure to thrive syndrome in infancy. Pediatrics 66:698-704, 1980.

Schwartz ID: Failure to thrive: An old nemesis in the new millennium. Pediatr Rev 21:257-264, 2000.

Sills RH: Failure to thrive. Am J Dis Child 132:967-969, 1978.

Starling SP, Holden JR, Jenny C: Abusive head trauma: The relationship of perpetrators to their victims. Pediatrics 95:259-262, 1995.

Stephenson T, Bialas Y: Estimation of the age of bruising. Arch Dis Child 74:53-55, 1996.

Sugar NF, Taylor JA, Feldman KW: Bruises in infants and toddlers: Those who don't cruise rarely bruise. Arch Pediatr Adolesc Med 153:399-403, 1999.

Vogeley E, Pierce M, Bertocci G: Experience with Wood lamp illumination and digital photography in the documentation of bruises on human skin. Arch Pediatr Adolesc Med 156:265-268, 2002.

West MH, Billings JD, Frair J: Ultraviolet photography: Bite marks on human skin and suggested technique for exposure and development of reflective ultraviolet photography. J Forensic Sci 32:1204-1213, 1987.

Woodlong BA, Kossosis PD: Sexual misuse. Pediatr Clin North Am 28:481-499, 1981.

CHAPTER 7

Rheumatology

PAUL ROSEN AND SARA C. MCINTIRE

The rheumatic diseases of childhood are a heterogeneous group of disorders usually manifested by signs and symptoms of inflammation. Although significant progress has been made in the understanding of the pathophysiology of these disorders, their etiologies remain largely unknown. Despite available laboratory markers, the cornerstones of diagnosis remain the history and physical examination. Knowledge of the natural history of these disorders is also helpful for diagnosis and management.

The majority of the common rheumatic diseases that occur during childhood are classified as inflammatory arthritis or enthesitis syndromes, connective tissue disorders, and vasculitides, although overlap does occur. Noninflammatory disorders that cause musculoskeletal pain include joint hypermobility syndromes and idiopathic musculoskeletal pain syndromes. This chapter illustrates the more distinctive clinical features of these unique disorders.

Musculoskeletal History

A meticulous rheumatologic history is the foundation of accurate diagnosis (Table 7-1). The exact location that the patient complains about should be given careful attention. Muscle, bone, and tendon or ligament insertion pain (enthesitis) may be interpreted as joint pain unless the clinician asks specifically for the parent or child to describe the symptoms. Often it is helpful for the clinician to ask the child to point with one finger to the site of maximum discomfort.

The patient's age and gender serve as initial guides to a possible etiology. The clinician must then try to discern whether musculoskeletal symptoms are inflammatory or mechanical. Pain that involves swelling, morning stiffness, warmth, redness, and improvement with movement is indicative of inflammation. Pain that is worse at the end of the day, worse with activity, and lacking persistent swelling is more mechanical in nature.

A history of prior illnesses, medications, immunizations, trauma, bites, and the acuteness of symptoms can be a clue to diagnosis. Joint pain (arthralgia) is a common symptom of childhood. However, the symptoms associated with inflammatory joint pain (arthritis) are uncommon in the pediatric population. In children with arthritis, the duration and pattern of the symptoms can be telling. Acute migratory arthritis affecting large and small joints is seen in acute rheumatic fever (ARF). Arthritis resolving within a few weeks is consistent with a reactive arthritis (i.e., *Streptococcus*, Epstein-Barr virus, parvovirus B19). An additive arthritis persisting for more than 6 weeks is consistent with a chronic form of arthritis (i.e., juvenile rheumatoid arthritis [JRA] or a juvenile spondyloarthropathy). The chronic arthritides cause indolent and persistent joint changes. Joint stiffness, or gel phenomenon, can be seen not only in the morning, but also after a child has napped or been immobile in a vehicle. As the day progresses, the child with chronic arthritis may become more limber and may even appear normal.

Differences in the quality and duration of arthritis exist among the various rheumatoid diseases. The arthritis in patients with systemic lupus erythematosus (SLE) may feature less swelling with more intense pain, whereas the arthritis of children with JRA is characterized by more stiffness and swelling and less pain. The joint pain of the patient with SLE may be intermittent in nature. The joint stiffness of JRA is usually a daily occurrence without treatment. The joints of ARF can also be distinguished from those of JRA by the presence of exquisite pain that is out of proportion to physical findings. A rapid response to nonsteroidal anti-inflammatory drugs further supports a diagnosis of ARF.

A careful family history can be helpful. Children with an extensive family history of autoimmune diseases in their first-degree relatives are at slightly greater risk for developing a rheumatologic condition. Because these diseases are complex genetic traits, there is often little direct genetic linkage. Some diseases such as psoriasis, SLE, acute rheumatic fever, and autoimmune thyroiditis have a stronger genetic penetrance than other rheumatic diseases. Other conditions have little or no penetrance. A child with first-degree relatives with adult rheumatoid arthritis is not at increased risk for developing juvenile rheumatoid arthritis.

Physical Examination of the Musculoskeletal System

The only way of confirming the diagnosis of JRA is to demonstrate arthritis by physical examination of the joints. The elucidation of joint inflammation by examination may be the only indication of a rheumatic disease. Because most joints are near the surface of the body, the examiner has an excellent opportunity to obtain significant information about many diseases. A rheumatologic diagnosis requires a thorough joint examination and meticulous general physical examination with special attention to the skin, mucous membranes, nail beds, and muscles.

The physical examination begins with observation of the child and parents walking from the waiting area to the examination room. The physician notes the general appearance of the patient and interactions among family members. Nutritional status and an incremental graph of height and weight must be carefully documented. Certain skin and mucous membrane changes provide valuable information (Table 7-2). Muscle strength must be evaluated first by attempting to elicit a Gower sign (Fig. 7-1) and then by testing resistance capacity of individual muscle groups and grading them on a standard scale (Table 7-3).

The hallmark of a good physical examination of the musculoskeletal system is a careful examination of the joints, consisting of inspection, palpation, and measurement of each joint's range of motion. The examiner should develop a standard order for examining joints and follow the same pattern so that no joints are missed. Large effusions are easily felt and often ballotable; synovial hypertrophy may be more subtle and has a doughy, spongy, boggy feel. Synovial outpouchings are common in children with arthritis and can resemble ganglion cysts, especially in the wrists and ankles. A ganglion cyst does not cause pain. In children with arthritis the findings may be

Table 7-1	Distinguishing Features of the Rheumatologic History

1. Musculoskeletal pain
2. Joint swelling
3. Morning stiffness that improves with activity
4. Constitutional symptoms (e.g., recurrent fevers, fatigue, weight loss, growth disturbance)
5. Ocular symptoms (e.g., eye redness, visual change)
6. Cardiopulmonary symptoms (e.g., dyspnea, chest pain, hemoptysis)
7. Gastrointestinal symptoms (e.g., dysphagia, abdominal pain, melena)
8. Neurologic symptoms (e.g., vascular headache, weakness, seizure, altered mental status)
9. Cutaneous and mucous membrane symptoms (e.g., photosensitive rash, Raynaud's phenomenon, oral, nasal, or genital ulcerations, xerostomia, and keratoconjunctivitis sicca)
10. Psychosocial history (e.g., family dysfunction, fibromyalgia, depression, chronic pain)
11. Family history (e.g., psoriasis, rheumatic fever, systemic lupus erythematosus)

Table 7-2	Mucocutaneous Signs of the Rheumatic Diseases

1. Malar rash
2. Discoid rash—rare in childhood; often heals with atrophy and scarring
3. Periungual erythema
4. Telangiectasias
5. Fingertip ulcers
6. Alopecia and fracturing of frontal hair
7. Heliotrope-violaceous eyelid edema
8. Gottron papules—scaly, symmetrical, erythematous papules over MCP and PIP joints
9. Skin thickening, contractures, calcinosis
10. Palpable purpura
11. Livedo reticularis—lacy, fishnet appearance of skin
12. Evanescent salmon-pink rash
13. Erythema nodosum—panniculitis with septal inflammation
14. Rheumatoid extensor nodules
15. Psoriasis
16. Onycholysis (lifting up of the distal portion of the nail), nail pits
17. Balanitis circinata—small, shallow, painless ulcers of the glans penis and urethral meatus
18. Keratoderma blennorrhagicum—clear vesicles on erythematous bases that progress to macules, papules, and keratotic nodules

MCP, metacarpophalangeal; PIP, proximal interphalangeal.

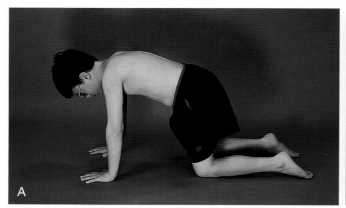
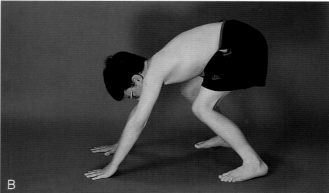
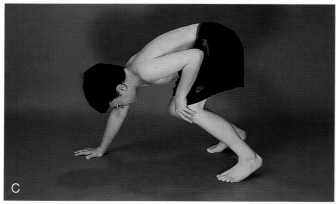
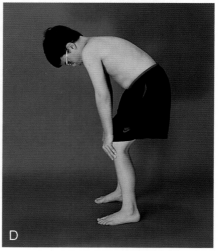

Figure 7-1. Gower sign. The child begins in a supine position and is asked to stand. The child is unable to rise without rolling over and progressively pushing to the knees and using hands to push up to a standing position.

subtle and often appreciated only because of pain or decreased range of motion.

Temporomandibular Joint

The temporomandibular joint (TMJ) permits three types of motion: (1) opening and closing of the jaw, (2) anterior and posterior motion, and (3) lateral or side-to-side motion; each type should be carefully measured. Careful observa-

tion of the TMJ may reveal micrognathia, a clue to the diagnosis of JRA (Fig. 7-2).

Cricoarytenoid Joint

The cricoarytenoid joint is rarely involved in JRA but can present a life-threatening complication if edema and scarring interfere with respiration. An early symptom is

Table 7-3 Standard Muscle Strength Grading

MUSCLE GRADE	DESCRIPTION
5	Complete range of motion against gravity with full resistance
4	Complete range of motion against gravity with some resistance
3	Complete range of motion against gravity
2	Complete range of motion with gravity eliminated
1	Evidence of slight contractility; no joint motion
0	No evidence of contractility

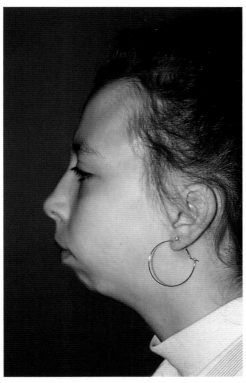

Figure 7-2. Micrognathia. Note the underdevelopment of the jaw and retracted chin. This occurs in patients with juvenile rheumatoid arthritis.

hoarseness because arytenoid movement is important to phonation.

Acromioclavicular Joint

The acromioclavicular (AC) joint is formed by the lateral end of the clavicle and the medial margin of the acromial process of the scapula; it allows for "shrugging" of the shoulders.

Sternoclavicular Joint

The two sternoclavicular (SC) joints are the only points of articulation between the shoulder girdle and trunk; they move with any motion of the shoulders. The SC joints can be involved in the spondyloarthropathies and rarely in JRA, in which they become ankylosed (fused).

Shoulder

The shoulder is usually involved only in severe polyarticular JRA. It is an extremely complicated joint, but range of active motion can be conveniently tested by having the child perform three simple maneuvers (Fig. 7-3). These maneuvers require 180 degrees of abduction, 45 degrees of adduction, 90 degrees of flexion, and 45 degrees of external rotation of the glenohumeral joint and related articulations.

Elbow

The examiner must distinguish swelling in the olecranon bursa from involvement of the true elbow joint. The elbow is frequently affected in all forms of JRA and is the most common upper extremity joint affected in spondyloarthropathy. Range of motion of the elbow is easily tested (Figs. 7-4 and 7-5).

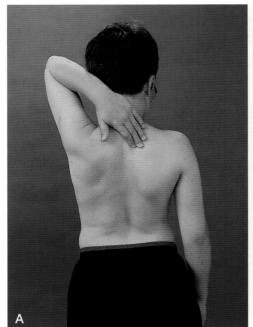
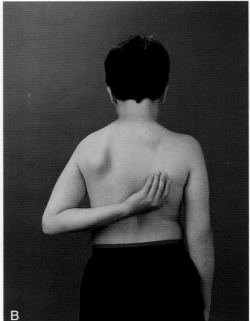
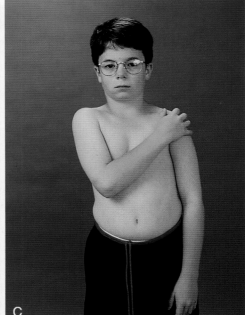

Figure 7-3. A, Place hand behind head on opposite shoulder (external rotation and abduction). **B,** Place back of hand behind the back and touch opposite scapula. **C,** Place hand on opposite shoulder. (**B** and **C** test internal rotation and adduction.)

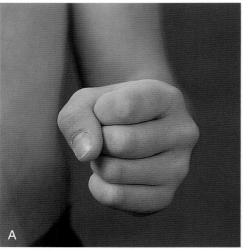
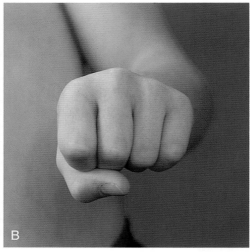
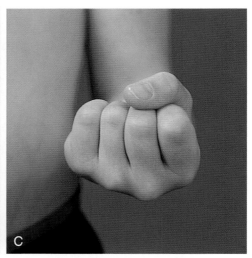

Figure 7-4. Supination and pronation of the elbow. The elbow should be held flexed at 90 degrees and against the body. The fist is held in a neutral vertical position **(A)**, then rotated 90 degrees in pronation **(B)**, and 90 degrees in supination **(C)**.

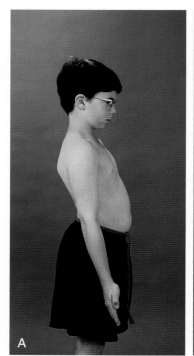
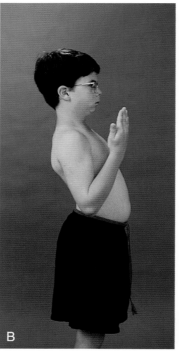

Figure 7-5. A, The elbow should extend from 0 degrees with the arm held down and **B,** flex to 150 degrees.

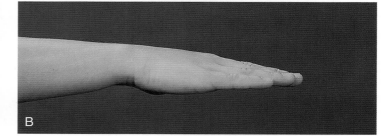
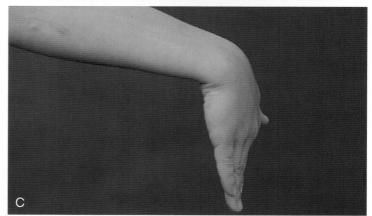

Figure 7-6. The wrist should extend to 70 degrees **(A)** from neutral position **(B)** and flex to 80 degrees **(C).**

Wrist and Hand

Children do not require much extension to perform most activities of daily living and thus can lose strength and mobility in the wrist, which may go unnoticed. The wrist is frequently affected in childhood arthritis, and thus a careful range of motion examination is essential. Normal is 70 degrees of extension, 80 degrees of flexion (Fig. 7-6), 20 degrees radially, and 30 degrees to the ulnar side.

Metacarpophalangeal (MCP) joints extend 30 degrees and flex 90 degrees. Normal range of motion for the proximal interphalangeal (PIP) joints is illustrated in Figure 7-7.

Spinal Column

In children the neck can be extended so that the head can touch the back and flexed so that the chin touches the chest; 90-degree rotation and 45-degree lateral bending in each direction is also normal (Fig. 7-8).

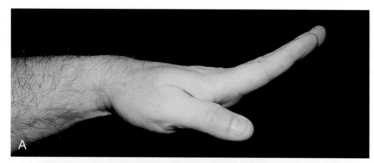

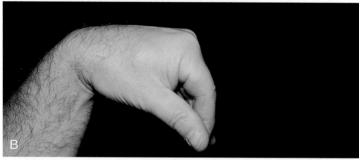

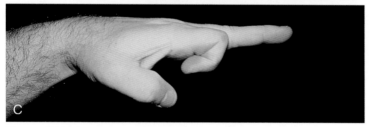

Figure 7-7. The metacarpophalangeal joints can extend 30 degrees **(A)** and flex 90 degrees **(B)**. Note the normal range of motion for the proximal interphalangeal joints **(C)**.

The entire spine including all spinous processes should be carefully palpated to elicit tenderness. Flexion, extension, and lateral motion of the spine should be measured using S1 as the focal point. Thirty degrees of extension and 50 degrees of lateral motion are normal. Careful examination of the sacroiliac joints (Fig. 7-9) may give an important clue to the diagnosis of a spondyloarthropathy in an adolescent. Chest expansion, occiput to wall, and finger-to-floor measurements (Fig. 7-10) are useful in following patients with inflammatory back disease. To detect limitation of forward flexion of the lumbar spine, the Schober test is quite useful. The patient is asked to stand erect, and the skin overlying the spinous process of the fifth lumbar vertebra (usually at the level of the "dimples of Venus") and another point 10 cm above in the midline is marked. The patient is asked to maximally bend the spine forward without bending the knees. If the lumbar spine is mobile, the distance between the two points increases by 5 cm or more; that is, the distance between the two points becomes equal to or greater than 15 cm. An increase of 4 cm or less indicates decreased mobility of the lumbar spine.

Hip

The normal hip examination consists of 45 degrees of abduction and 20 degrees of adduction (Fig. 7-11) with the knee bent 20 degrees. The hip can extend 30 degrees, externally rotate to 45 degrees, and internally rotate to 35 degrees. An increase in lumbar lordosis may be the first sign of decreased hip flexion. Normally, hip flexion reaches to about 135 degrees (Fig. 7-12).

Knee

The knee is the joint most commonly involved in childhood arthritis. Swelling of the knee may be diffuse or localized to the suprapatellar bursa, which communicates with the true knee joint, or to the gastrocnemius-semimembranosus bursa (Baker cyst) (Fig. 7-13), which

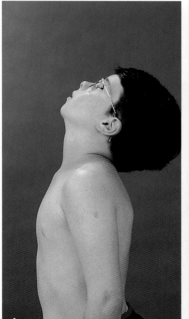
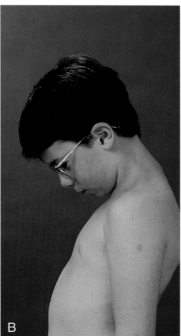
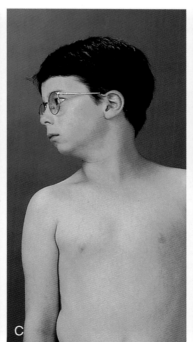
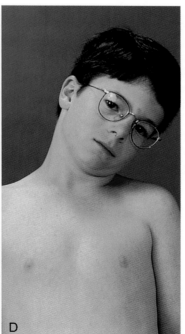

Figure 7-8. The neck normally can be extended so that the head touches the back **(A)**, flexed so that the chin touches the chest **(B)**, rotated 90 degrees **(C)**, and tilted laterally 45 degrees **(D)**.

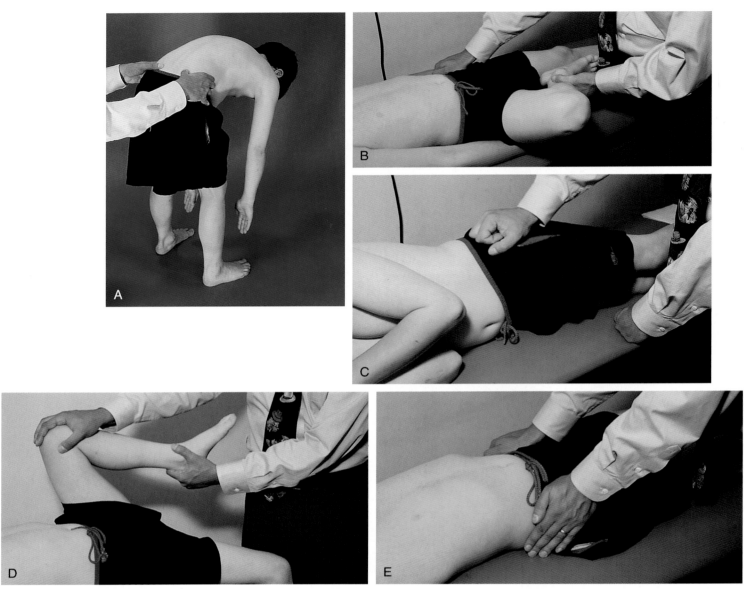

Figure 7-9. Clinical tests for sacroiliitis. **A,** Application of direct pressure by thumbs over the sacroiliac joints to elicit tenderness. **B,** With knee flexed and hip flexed, abducted, and externally rotated, downward pressure is applied on the flexed knee and the contralateral anterosuperior iliac spine. **C,** Compression of the pelvis with patient lying on side. **D,** Patient lying supine, with flexed knee pushed maximally toward the opposite shoulder. **E,** Anterosuperior iliac spines forced laterally apart.

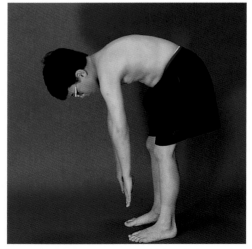

Figure 7-10. With feet together, the child bends forward. The measurement from floor to fingertip is recorded and compared with subsequent examination.

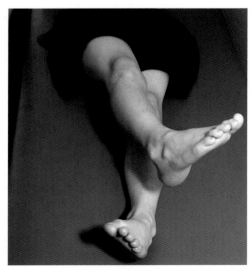

Figure 7-11. The normal hip can be adducted 20 degrees.

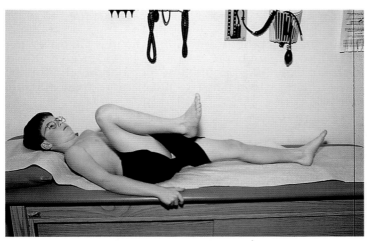

Figure 7-12. The normal hip can be flexed 135 degrees.

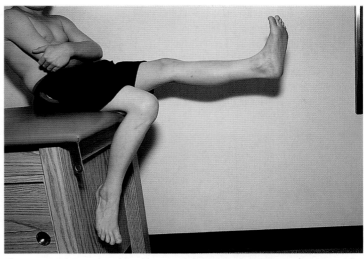

Figure 7-14. Normal knee range of motion extends from 10 degrees hyperextension *(left knee)* to 130 degrees of flexion *(right knee)*.

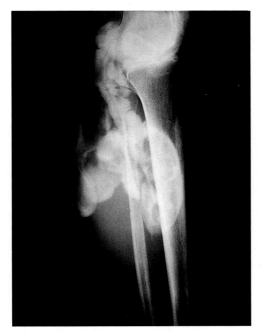

Figure 7-13. Arthrogram demonstrates communication of Baker cyst with synovial cavity of knee joint.

may dissect down the leg. The patella must be carefully evaluated for "roughening of the undersurface" indicative of chondromalacia patellae, which is not uncommon in teenage girls. Normal knee range of motion is illustrated in Figure 7-14.

Foot and Ankle

The foot and ankle can offer valuable clues to the diagnosis of arthritis in childhood. Evidence of Achilles tendonitis or plantar fasciitis can suggest a spondyloarthropathy. First metatarsophalangeal (MTP) joint involvement is also a strong clue to the diagnosis of a spondyloarthropathy. Normal ranges of motion of the true ankle joint and subtalar joint are illustrated in Figure 7-15, and decreased range of motion is common in pauciarticular JRA.

Careful flexion and extension of all interphalangeal joints of the feet must be evaluated, especially the first MTP (80 degrees extension to 35 degrees flexion). The MTP joints should be squeezed enough to wrinkle the skin.

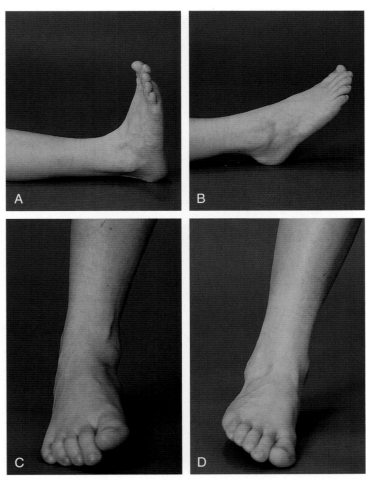

Figure 7-15. The ankle normally can flex to 20 degrees **(A)** and extend to 45 degrees **(B)**. Inversion occurs to 30 degrees **(C)** and eversion to 20 degrees **(D)**.

Leg Length

Leg-length discrepancy (Fig. 7-16) is common in JRA because of hyperemia of an affected joint and subsequent overgrowth. Compensatory scoliosis may also develop.

Juvenile Rheumatoid Arthritis

Juvenile rheumatoid arthritis (JRA) is the most common rheumatic disease in children. The American College of Rheumatology criteria for the diagnosis of JRA are the most frequently used in North America (Table 7-4). Of note, there are no laboratory tests, such as a positive anti-nuclear antibody or rheumatoid factor, required to make a diagnosis of JRA.

The incidence of JRA is approximately 10 cases per 100,000 population per year. The prevalence of JRA is approximately 100 per 100,000 population. JRA in the United States is estimated to affect more than 300,000 persons.

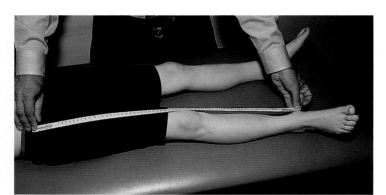

Figure 7-16. Leg length is measured from the anterosuperior iliac spine to the medial malleolus.

Table 7-4	Criteria for the Diagnosis of Juvenile Rheumatoid Arthritis

1. Age at onset younger than 16 years
2. Arthritis (swelling, effusion, or presence of two or more of the following signs: limited range of motion, tenderness or pain on motion, and increased heat) in one or more joints
3. Duration of disease 6 weeks or longer
4. Onset type defined by type of disease in first 6 months:
   (a) Polyarticular arthritis: 5 or more inflamed joints
   (b) Pauciarticular arthritis: <5 inflamed joints
   (c) Systemic arthritis with characteristic fever
5. Exclusion of other forms of juvenile arthritis

Modified from Cassidy JT, Levinson JE, Bass JC, et al: A study of classification for a diagnosis of juvenile rheumatoid arthritis. Arthritis Rheum 29:274-281, 1986.

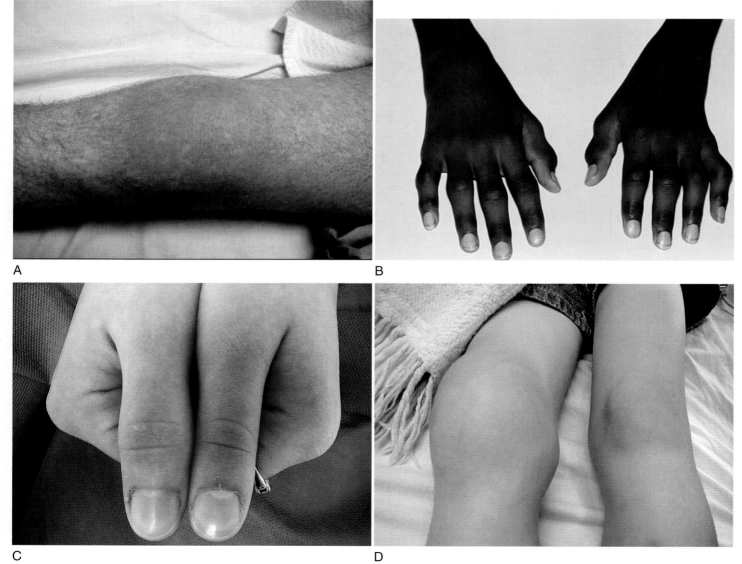

A

B

C

D

Figure 7-17. Juvenile rheumatoid arthritis (JRA). **A,** Erythema of the knee in a patient with systemic-onset JRA (Still's disease). **B,** Swelling and inflammation of the small joints of the hands in a patient with polyarticular JRA. Note the inability to fully extend the fingers. **C,** Swelling of the right thumb interphalangeal joint. **D,** Right knee swelling in a patient with pauciarticular JRA.

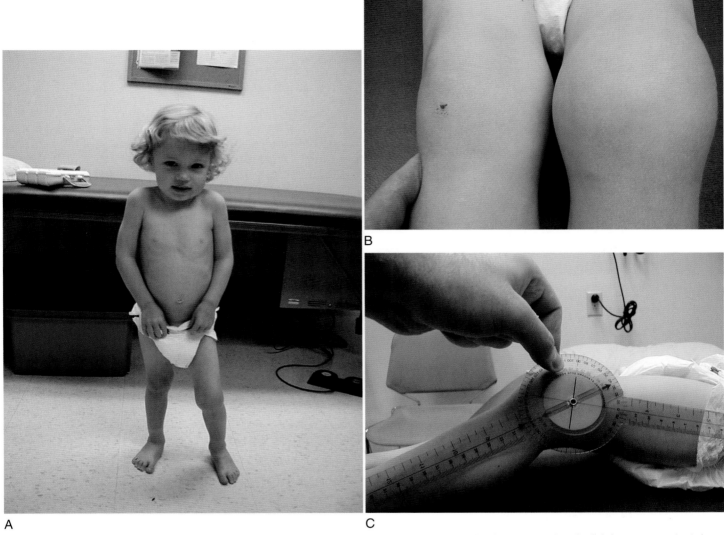

A   C

Figure 7-18. Pauciarticular juvenile rheumatoid arthritis. **A,** Two-year-old girl with arthritis of the left knee. Note that the left lower extremity is bent at the knee as she bears weight on the extended right lower extremity. **B,** A closer look at the knees reveals left knee swelling. **C,** The left knee can only be extended to 35 degrees (secondary to a flexion contracture).

The first clear description of these entities was presented by George Still in 1897. He postulated multiple etiologies for JRA, and this concept is still supported today. JRA can be a systemic, polyarticular, or pauciarticular disease, all having inflammation of the synovial tissue as one of their cardinal features. Synovium is usually hypertrophied, and joint effusions may occur. On physical examination (Fig. 7-17), joint swelling, loss of normal anatomic landmarks, tenderness, decreased joint mobility (Fig. 7-18), warmth, erythema, and joint deformity may be noted. It is typical for the child with JRA to have more joint stiffness than pain. Symptoms often develop gradually over a period of weeks or months before evaluation. Morning stiffness is often reported. The duration of morning stiffness correlates well with the degree of inflammation in children with JRA. Immobility and weather changes may exacerbate symptoms, although they have no impact on the underlying inflammatory component of the disease. Although arthralgia alone can be the initial presentation of JRA, the diagnosis cannot be confirmed without the presence of arthritis on physical examination.

Despite objective signs of arthritis, the JRA patient may not experience pain. When inflammation persists for a long enough period of time, destruction of the articular surface and bony structures may occur (Fig. 7-19). Because of the poor regenerative properties of articular cartilage, these deformities are usually permanent. Fortunately, most cases of JRA are not associated with permanent joint deformity.

The group of diseases placed under the JRA rubric combines diverse entities, generally divided into three categories: (1) systemic-onset disease, (2) polyarticular disease (rheumatoid factor negative or rheumatoid factor positive), and (3) pauciarticular disease. The JRA onset type is based on the disease presentation during the first 6 months of illness (Table 7-5). The presenting subtype of JRA may differ from the child's ultimate disease course.

Systemic Onset

Systemic-onset JRA (Still's disease) accounts for approximately 10% of all children with JRA. Fever, rash, irritability, arthritis, and visceral involvement dominate the clinical presentation. The patient's temperature usually rises to greater than 39° C, and this often occurs twice daily in a double quotidian pattern. Chills are associated with fever, but rigors rarely occur. Though the late

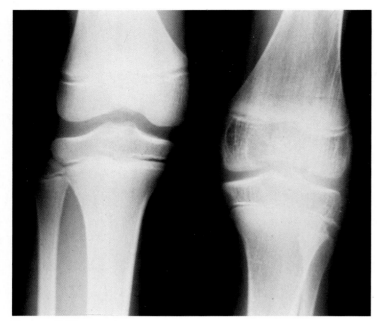

Figure 7-19. Juvenile rheumatoid arthritis. Demineralization of the left femur and tibia with soft tissue swelling and hypertrophy of the epiphyses secondary to hyperemia.

afternoon is a typical time for a temperature rise, many other patterns may occur. Other manifestations of systemic-onset JRA, such as rash and joint symptoms, may wax and wane during febrile periods. A helpful clinical feature during the febrile phase is one subnormal temperature during every 24-hour period, which suggests JRA.

The rash of JRA is macular, 2 to 6 mm in diameter, evanescent, and salmon or red in color, with slightly irregular margins (Fig. 7-20). An area of central clearing often exists. The rash usually occurs on the trunk and proximal extremities, but it may also be distal in distribution, with palms and soles affected. Although the rash generally does not produce discomfort, some older patients report pruritus. Superficial mild trauma to the skin, exposure to warmth, and emotional upset may precipitate the rash (Koebner phenomenon). Although the rash is seen with polyarticular JRA, it does not occur with pauciarticular disease. Arthritis may not occur invariably at the onset of systemic-onset JRA, and thus the diagnosis may not be readily apparent. When fever of unknown origin is the sole initial presentation of systemic-onset JRA, it must remain a diagnosis of exclusion until the clinician observes inflammatory arthritis on the physical examination. Arthralgia and myalgia can be prominent early, as can hepatosplenomegaly and lymphadenopathy. Serositis, pleuritis, pericarditis, hyperbilirubinemia, liver enzyme elevation, leukocytosis, and anemia are supporting clinical features. About 50% of systemic-onset JRA patients progress to have a chronic inflammatory arthritis (Fig. 7-21).

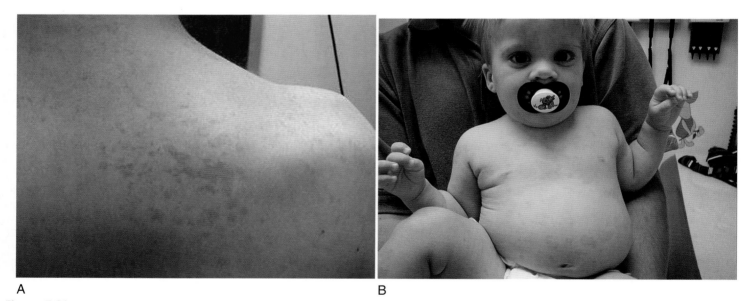

A   B

Figure 7-20. Systemic-onset juvenile rheumatoid arthritis. **A** and **B,** The rash is erythematous, macular, and often evanescent. It can be more prominent during periods of fever.

Table 7-5	Characteristics of Juvenile Rheumatoid Arthritis by Onset Type					
TYPE	**PERCENT OF CASES**	**NUMBER OF JOINTS INVOLVED**	**GENDER RATIO (F:M)**	**FREQUENCY OF RF/ANA POSITIVITY**	**IRIDOCYCLITIS RISK**	**PROGNOSIS**
Systemic	10	Variable	1:1	Rare/10%	Minimal	Guarded
Polyarticular	30	≥5	3:1	10%/50%	5%	Guarded in RF+ patients
Pauciarticular	60	≤4	5:1	Rare/80% (girls with uveitis)	20%	Excellent if uveitis not present

ANA, antinuclear antibody; F, female; M, male; RF, rheumatoid factor.
Modified from Cassidy JT, Petty RE: Textbook of Pediatric Rheumatology, 4th ed. Philadelphia, WB Saunders, 2001.

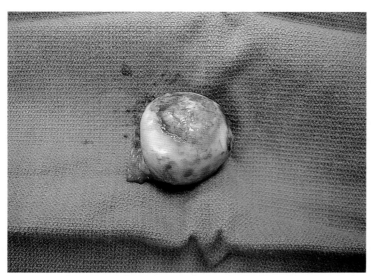

Figure 7-21. Systemic-onset juvenile rheumatoid arthritis (JRA). The femoral head from a 13-year-old girl shows bony erosion. Patients with systemic and polyarticular JRA are more likely to suffer joint destruction than patients with pauciarticular JRA.

Table 7-6	Characteristics of Macrophage Activation Syndrome in Patients with Systemic-onset Juvenile Rheumatoid Arthritis

Acutely ill with bruising, purpura, mucosal bleeding
Hepatosplenomegaly
Lymphadenopathy
Decrease in white blood cell count, hemoglobin, and platelet count
Decrease in erythrocyte sedimentation rate
Elevation of alanine aminotransferase, aspartate aminotransferase, prothrombin time, partial thromboplastin time, fibrin split-products, ferritin, and triglycerides
Decrease in fibrinogen, clotting factors
Tissue biopsy (i.e., bone marrow, liver) may demonstrate active phagocytosis by macrophages.

Modified from Cassidy JT, Petty RE: Textbook of Pediatric Rheumatology, 4th ed. Philadelphia, WB Saunders, 2001.

Patients with systemic-onset JRA are at risk for developing a potentially fatal disorder called *macrophage activation syndrome* (MAS). Patients present with a toxic appearance, fever, hepatosplenomegaly, lymphadenopathy, and mucosal bleeding. If not recognized early, MAS can progress to hepatic failure, encephalopathy, and disseminated intravascular coagulation. Laboratory testing that supports a diagnosis of MAS includes evidence of hepatitis and coagulopathy. In addition, the white blood cell count, hemoglobin, and platelet counts are depressed with a normal or low sedimentation rate (Table 7-6). Diagnosis is confirmed by bone marrow aspiration demonstrating activated macrophages engulfing surrounding cells (Fig. 7-22).

Polyarticular Onset

Polyarticular onset of disease accounts for approximately 30% of all children with JRA. To make the diagnosis, five or more joints must be involved in the absence of prominent systemic signs and symptoms. There appear to be two subgroups within this category—rheumatoid factor negative and rheumatoid factor positive. The seropositive group is believed to be nearly identical to the adult entity

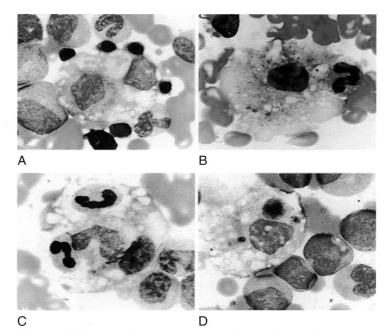

Figure 7-22. Macrophage activation syndrome (MAS). Bone marrow aspirate shows activated macrophages with foamy cytoplasm engulfing surrounding erythrocytes and neutrophils. (Courtesy Alexi Grom, MD, Cincinnati, Ohio.)

of rheumatoid arthritis (RA). Although onset of rheumatoid factor–positive polyarticular JRA can occur as early as 8 years of age, it usually occurs in the early teens and girls predominate. Rheumatoid factor–negative polyarticular JRA can occur at age 1 year with a peak incidence at age 2 years. Although 80% of all adult patients are seropositive, only 5% of children have a positive rheumatoid factor.

In addition to the joint findings of warmth, swelling, erythema, and tenderness seen in both subgroups, seropositive disease provides some additional clues to diagnosis. The subcutaneous nodules that occur in seropositive disease are firm, nontender nodules on the skin surface with a predilection for pressure points or extensor areas. The most common location is the elbow, but the nodules also occur on the heels, hands, knees, ears, scapula, sacrum, and buttocks. Other features of seropositive disease may include cutaneous vasculitis, Felty syndrome (leukopenia and splenomegaly), and Sjögren syndrome (keratoconjunctivitis sicca and xerostomia with or without parotid swelling).

The onset of polyarthritis may be insidious or acute. The seropositive subgroup tends to progress to destructive synovitis and a prolonged chronic course. Children with seronegative disease generally have a better prognosis, but a subset can progress to joint destruction and flexion contractures. Any synovial joint may be involved in the inflammatory process including the knees, wrists, elbows, ankles, small joints of the feet, and PIP and MCP joints. The lumbosacral spine is usually spared.

Pauciarticular Onset

Pauciarticular-onset JRA is strictly defined as onset of disease in fewer than five joints. The large joints (knees, ankles, and elbows) are often asymmetrically involved. Systemic symptoms do not dominate the clinical picture. If the disease does not progress to polyarticular involvement within the first 6 to 12 months of illness, the patient often maintains the pauciarticular pattern. Patients with this form of JRA are at increased risk of developing iridocyclitis (or uveitis). Although photophobia, eye pain, and erythema can occur, uveitis is often asymptomatic. For that reason, children with pauciarticular JRA must receive slit lamp examinations more frequently than those with other JRA subtypes.

The first clinical sign of uveitis is cellular exudate in the anterior chamber. If the uveitis is left untreated, synechiae (adhesions) between the iris and lens may develop, leading to an irregular and poorly functioning pupil (Fig. 7-23). Further along in the clinical course, band keratopathy (calcium deposits in the cornea) (Fig. 7-24) may occur, as well as cataracts or glaucoma. For these reasons, strict adherence to the recommendations for eye examination outlined in Table 7-7 is necessary to help prevent visual loss in these children. Ophthalmologic complications do not parallel the activity of the arthritis.

Extra-articular Manifestations

Many extra-articular features of JRA have been reported. The more common ones are listed in Table 7-8. Linear growth retardation is common in the child with active JRA, especially with systemic-onset JRA or polyarticular disease. The degree of retardation and the ultimate prognosis for reaching adult height are related to the severity and duration of inflammation and the use of corticosteroids. Pauciarticular arthritis, however, can present with bizarre growth abnormalities, usually confined to leg-length discrepancy or an enlarged hand or foot related to refractory ankle or wrist involvement. Leg-length measurements must be recorded on a regular basis because a compensatory scoliosis can develop in these children. During early illness, bony development may be advanced;

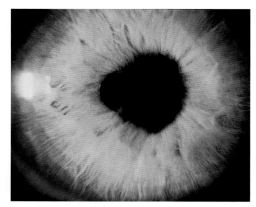

Figure 7-23. Iridocyclitis. An irregular pupil in a patient with pauciarticular juvenile rheumatoid arthritis. Note synechiae projecting posteriorly toward the lens.

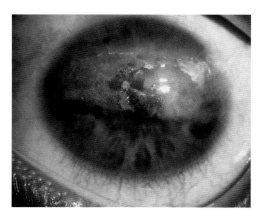

Figure 7-24. Band keratopathy. Note the calcium deposits in the Bowman layer in this patient with juvenile rheumatoid arthritis.

Table 7-7   Recommended Frequency of Ophthalmologic Examinations in Juvenile Rheumatoid Arthritis

TYPE	ANA	AGE AT ONSET	DURATION OF DISEASE, YEARS	RISK CATEGORY	EYE EXAMINATION FREQUENCY, MOS
Oligoarthritis or polyarthritis	+	≤6	≤4	High	3
	+	≤6	>4	Moderate	6
	+	≤6	>7	Low	12
	+	>6	≤4	Moderate	6
	+	>6	>4	Low	12
	−	≤6	≤4	Moderate	6
	−	≤6	>4	Low	12
	−	>6	NA	Low	12
Systemic disease (fever, rash)	NA	NA	NA	Low	12

ANA, antinuclear antibodies; NA, not applicable.
Recommendations for follow-up continue through childhood and adolescence.
From Cassidy J, Kivlin J, Lindsley C, Nocton J: Ophthalmologic examinations in children with juvenile rheumatoid arthritis. Pediatrics 117:1843-1845, 2006.

Table 7-8   Extra-articular Manifestations of Juvenile Rheumatoid Arthritis

	POLYARTICULAR (%)	PAUCIARTICULAR (%)	SYSTEMIC DISEASE (%)
Fever	30	0	100
Rheumatoid rash	2	0	95
Rheumatoid nodules	10	0	5
Hepatosplenomegaly	10	0	85
Lymphadenopathy	5	0	70
Chronic uveitis	5	20	1
Pericarditis	5	0	35
Pleuritis	1	0	20
Abdominal pain	1	0	10

Modified from Cassidy JT, Petty RE: Textbook of Pediatric Rheumatology, 4th ed. Philadelphia, WB Saunders, 2001.

Table 7-9	Differential Diagnosis of Juvenile Rheumatoid Arthritis

Systemic Onset	**Polyarticular Onset**
Systemic lupus erythematosus	Systemic lupus erythematosus
Kawasaki syndrome	Psoriatic arthritis
Acute rheumatic fever	Hypermobility syndrome
Henoch-Schönlein purpura	Enthesitis syndrome
Polyarteritis nodosa	Reactive arthritis
Dermatomyositis	**Pauciarticular Onset**
Systemic sclerosis	Septic joint (monoarthritis)
Inflammatory bowel disease	Reiter syndrome
Malignancy (leukemia,	Juvenile ankylosing spondylitis
neuroblastoma)	Pigmented villonodular
Lyme disease	synovitis
Viral syndrome	Psoriatic arthritis
Familial Mediterranean fever	Lyme disease

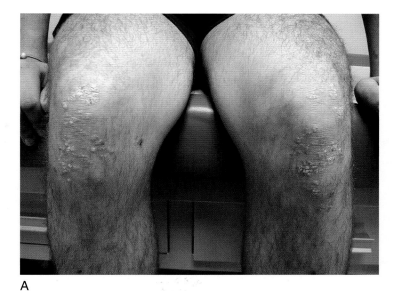

A

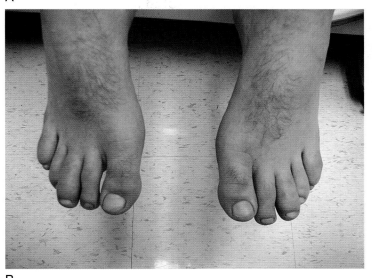

B

Figure 7-25. Psoriatic arthritis. **A,** Erythematous plaques with silver scale. **B,** Dactylitis (sausage toe) of the bilateral third and fifth toes.

later in the course of the illness the opposite may be true. Premature epiphyseal fusion may occur. Careful use of standardized growth curves assists in the early detection of growth failure. This may in turn guide the long-term therapeutic approach.

Cardiac involvement occurs in more than one third of systemic-onset JRA patients. Pericarditis, myocarditis, and endocarditis occur, with pericarditis being the most common. Chest pain, a friction rub, tachycardia, dyspnea, and supportive x-ray, electrocardiogram, and echocardiographic findings may occur. These episodes may last for weeks to months and are usually associated with a generalized flare of disease. Various other extra-articular manifestations including hepatosplenomegaly and lymphadenopathy are particularly common in systemic-onset JRA.

Differential Diagnosis

Because JRA is a clinical diagnosis, strict clinical criteria have been established to make the diagnosis. Most authors suggest the presence of objective joint findings (arthritis) for a minimum of 6 consecutive weeks coupled with the exclusion of other causes of arthritis in children (Table 7-9).

The differential diagnosis of JRA includes the juvenile spondyloarthropathies. These forms of chronic arthritis involve the axial skeleton and cause arthritis of the spine and sacroiliac joints in addition to the peripheral joints. They include ankylosing spondylitis, psoriatic arthritis (Fig. 7-25), arthritis of inflammatory bowel disease, and Reiter syndrome. A unique clinical feature of the juvenile spondyloarthropathies is enthesitis. Enthesitis refers to inflammation of the sites of attachment of ligament, tendon, fascia, or capsule to bone. JRA and the juvenile spondyloarthropathies are not distinguished in some classification systems and are categorized together as *juvenile idiopathic arthritis* (JIA).

Because of its destructive nature, pyogenic arthritis (e.g., staphylococci, streptococci, *Haemophilus influenzae*) must be ruled out in any child with active joint disease, especially monoarthritis. The intensely red and tender joint should raise suspicions of a bacterial pathogen. This combined with systemic symptoms of infection (fever, chills, malaise, rigors) should prompt the clinician to perform an arthrocentesis early in the course of the illness. If the joint in question is the hip, suspicion should be even higher because of the rarity with which the hip is the first affected joint in JRA.

Lyme arthritis can mimic pauciarticular JRA. This spirochetal form of arthritis is tickborne and usually affects the knee, elbow, or wrist in a monoarthritic pattern with spontaneous exacerbations and remissions. Malaise, fever, myalgia, lymphadenopathy, headache, meningismus, and weakness also may occur in the first phase of the illness. The distinctive rash, known as *erythema migrans* (Fig. 7-26), begins as an erythematous macule or papule. After this clears, the borders of the lesion expand to form an erythematous circular lesion that can be as large as 30 cm in diameter. These lesions can initially occur singly but can progress to multiple lesions over the legs, arms, and trunk. Other manifestations of Lyme disease include neurologic complications such as seventh nerve palsy, meningitis, radiculoneuritis, and the cardiac manifestations of heart block and myopericarditis. Bilateral Bell palsy or seventh nerve paralysis even more strongly suggests the diagnosis of Lyme disease.

Other infections cause a reactive arthritis that dissipates in less than 6 weeks. *Salmonella, Shigella, Yersinia,* and *Campylobacter* organisms should also be considered. A multitude of viruses cause arthritis. These include rubella; hepatitis B; adenovirus; and herpesviruses including Epstein-Barr virus, cytomegalovirus, varicella zoster, and

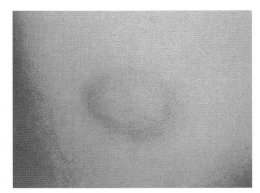

Figure 7-26. Lyme disease. The lesion of erythema migrans may be a large erythematous macule with central clearing, occurring singly or multiply.

herpes simplex. Parvoviruses, mumps, and enteroviruses including echovirus and coxsackievirus are associated with acute polyarthritis and occasionally have been recovered from joints. Other viruses result in reactive arthritis and may not infect the joint directly.

Malignancies such as neuroblastoma and leukemia may present with musculoskeletal pain. More careful evaluation generally reveals bone pain. Sickle cell disease, particularly in the form of dactylitis, can have prominent digital involvement. Inflammatory bowel disease, acute rheumatic fever, hemophilia, trauma, hypermobility syndrome, psoriasis, Henoch-Schönlein purpura, and autoimmune thyroiditis must also be considered in the patient with arthritis. All of the connective tissue diseases can have significant joint disease; however, their clinical features and laboratory tests usually distinguish them from JRA. Differential diagnoses of JRA are proposed in Table 7-9 with respect to disease onset, as outlined in Table 7-5.

Systemic Lupus Erythematosus

Systemic lupus erythematosus (SLE) is a complex autoimmune disease with a myriad of clinical presentations. SLE is a syndrome composed of multiple disease subsets, which may be identified by particular antibodies that may define particular disease types. SLE may present in an insidious fashion and hence escape early diagnosis, or it may present acutely and progress rapidly, leading to the patient's demise. As with other collagen vascular diseases, the etiology of SLE is unknown. The disease may involve just one organ system or, more commonly, it may be a multisystem disease. Because of the large number of serologic markers known to occur in SLE, it is considered by many to be the prototype of autoimmune diseases. To increase diagnostic accuracy, the American College of Rheumatology revised its classification criteria of lupus (Table 7-10). This classification is highly sensitive and specific for the diagnosis of this disease; however, the criteria are not meant for the clinical application of diagnosis and, although 4 of the 11 criteria must be present to make the diagnosis, they should be used as a study guide rather than applied to the clinical arena.

The word *lupus,* which means wolf, alludes to the erosive nature of the rash of SLE ("wolf bite") (Fig. 7-27). This feature of the disease was critical to the diagnosis of SLE until the discovery of the lupus erythematosus (LE) cell in 1948. The LE cell represents a healthy neutrophil that has phagocytosed the nuclear debris of a nonliving cell that has been coated with antibody. The antibody is

Table 7-10	Criteria for the Classification of Systemic Lupus Erythematosus*

Malar (butterfly) rash
Discoid-lupus rash
Photosensitivity
Oral or nasal mucocutaneous ulcerations
Nonerosive arthritis
Nephritis[†]
   Proteinuria >0.5 g/day
   Cellular casts
Encephalopathy[†]
   Seizures
   Psychosis
Pleuritis or pericarditis
Cytopenia
Positive immunoserology[†]
Antibodies to double-stranded DNA
Antibodies to Smith antigen
Positive antiphospholipid antibodies based on:
   1. IgG or IgM anticardiolipin antibodies or
   2. Lupus anticoagulant or
   3. Biologic false-positive test for syphilis
Positive antinuclear antibody test

*Four of 11 criteria provide a sensitivity of 96% and a specificity of 96%.
[†]Any one item satisfies this criterion.
Modified from Hochberg MC: Updating the American College of Rheumatology revised criteria for the classification of systemic lupus erythematosus. Arthritis Rheum 40:1725, 1997.

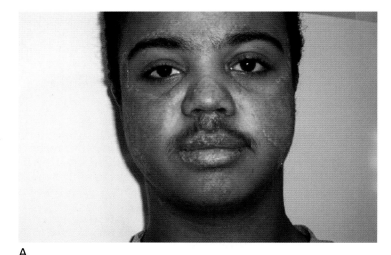

A

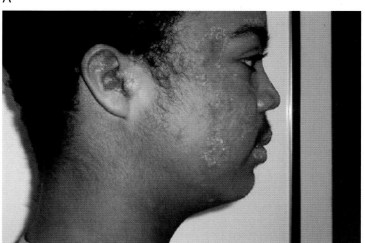

B

Figure 7-27. Systemic lupus erythematosus. **A,** Malar rash of systemic lupus erythematosus. Erythema, erosion, and atrophy are present. Note sparing of nasolabial folds. This patient also has rash involving the forehead and chin. **B,** Lateral view shows ear involvement.

directed against deoxyribonucleoprotein (DNP), which is made up of both DNA and histones. The presence of this serologic marker for lupus greatly expanded the recognized clinical entity of SLE. Although the LE preparation has proved to be of historical interest, time has shown that it is a nonspecific immunologic phenomenon and has no specificity with respect to the diagnosis of SLE.

SLE accounts for 10% of patients with rheumatic diseases and less than 5% of children seen in pediatric rheumatology practices. The incidence is estimated at 0.5 per 100,000 children per year. From prevalence data, it has been inferred that there are between 5000 and 10,000 children with SLE in the United States. The disease is rare in children younger than the age of 5 years. Before menarche, the boy-to-girl ratio is equal. After menarche, the ratio of affected girls to boys is about 8:1. African Americans and Asians are more commonly affected than whites.

The incidence of other connective tissue diseases is higher among family members of patients with SLE. Hematologic malignancies and immunodeficiencies are also reported in increased frequency among SLE relatives. These well-described phenomena may reflect a genetic alteration of immunity or, as some researchers suggest, the effects of a transmissible agent. The high incidence of disease in girls supports the role of hormonal factors as contributing or modulating agents to the pathogenesis of SLE. Other investigators suggest the influence of viruses, sunlight, and emotional stress on those developing lupus.

Although immunologic markers contribute to making the diagnosis of SLE, a high index of suspicion is necessary to obtain these studies. The early symptoms are often nonspecific and sometimes go unrecognized as harbingers of serious disease. Fever, fatigue, malaise, anorexia, and weight loss may be the only symptoms. In the adolescent population these symptoms may be all the more difficult to interpret. Conversely, this multisystem disease may present with a plethora of physical findings and the presentation may be so dramatic that the diagnosis is readily apparent. Among the more commonly involved areas are the skin, joints, muscles, liver, spleen, lymph nodes, kidneys, heart, and lungs.

Cutaneous manifestations of SLE occur at some time during the course of the disease in 80% of affected individuals. The classic butterfly rash in the malar distribution is seen in about one third of cases (see Fig. 7-27). In contrast to patients with dermatomyositis, the nasolabial folds of patients with SLE are spared. The rash of lupus is often reddish purple and raised with a whitish scale (Fig. 7-28). When the scale is removed, the underlying skin often shows "carpet-tack–like" fingers on the unexposed side of the scale itself. Carpet tacking is caused by the contouring of the scale into the skin follicles. These fingerlike projections on a scale strongly suggest the diagnosis of lupus. Purplish red urticarial lesions also occur, but these do not produce scales and do not cause atrophy as other lupus lesions do. If the skin manifestations are left untreated, the patient's appearance will be marred by hypopigmentation and hyperpigmentation. Mucosal erosions and ulcers of the oral cavity and nasal mucosa are part of lupus as well (Fig. 7-29). Alopecia (Fig. 7-30) occurs in 20% of patients and may present as broken hair shafts or patchy, red, scaling areas on the scalp, which may eventually scar and cause permanent hair loss. Other reported mucocutaneous findings are livedo reticularis (lacy, fishnet appearance of the skin); urticaria; atrophy; and telangiectasia. The presence of livedo reticularis may be the clinician's only clue to an associated hypercoagulable state mani-

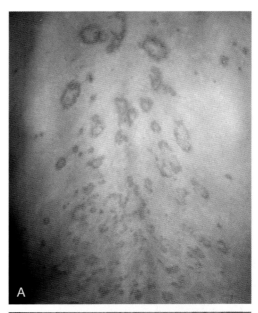

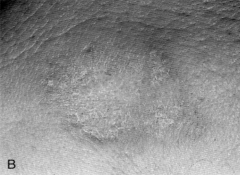

Figure 7-28. Systemic lupus erythematosus (SLE). **A,** Note the localized erythematous rash in a nonmalar distribution. **B,** The rash of SLE often has a slight white scale.

fested by antiphospholipid antibodies. This tendency can be diagnosed by obtaining a partial thromboplastin time (PTT) and anticardiolipin antibodies of the IgG and IgM classes. Although the antiphospholipid antibody syndrome can occur as an entity alone, it is commonly associated with SLE, a hypercoagulable state, and a tendency toward venous and arterial thrombosis.

The vasculitis of lupus, a small vessel vasculitis, is responsible for a number of easily recognizable clinical findings. The skin may be purpuric, or in more severe instances necrotic lesions may result (Fig. 7-31). The vasculitic component of lupus may also present with full-blown Raynaud phenomenon. With repeated tissue injury, glossy, atrophic, ulcerated skin and distorted nail architecture may be present.

The heart is often significantly involved in patients with lupus. Although the pericardium is involved most commonly, the myocardium and the endocardium may also be of clinical importance. Pericarditis can be painless and may present only as cardiomegaly on a chest radiograph or as pericardial effusion on an echocardiogram. However, chest pain may be noted or a friction rub auscultated. Although pericarditis is usually mild, it can progress to life-threatening cardiac tamponade. If the myocardium is affected, life-threatening complications including dysrhythmia, heart failure, and infarction can result. *Libman-Sacks endocarditis* is the term given to the verrucous projections of fibrinoid necrosis in the endocardium. These lesions rarely cause clinical symptoms, though the presence of a murmur raises suspicion of endocardial

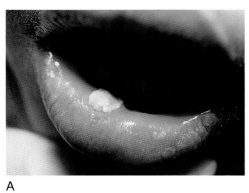

A

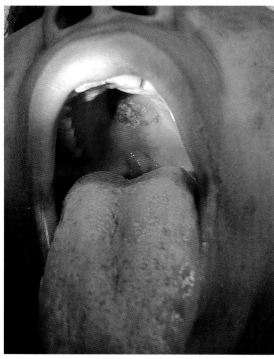

B

Figure 7-29. Systemic lupus erythematosus (SLE). **A,** Mucosal ulceration of the lip as evidence of vasculitis in SLE. **B,** Ulceration of the hard palate.

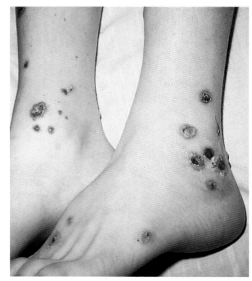

Figure 7-31. Systemic lupus erythematosus. Purpuric, ulcerative, and necrotic skin lesions of cutaneous vasculitis.

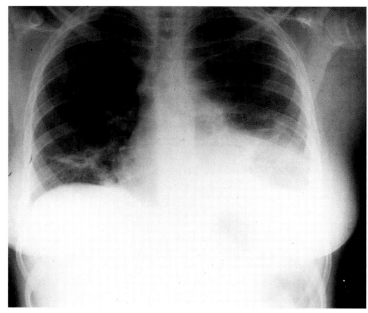

Figure 7-32. Systemic lupus erythematosus. Atelectasis, pleural effusions, and pulmonary infiltrates in a teenage girl.

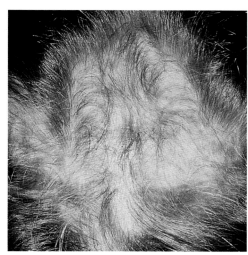

Figure 7-30. Systemic lupus erythematosus. Scarring alopecia.

disease. The mitral valve is most commonly involved, although aortic and tricuspid valves may be similarly infected. The presence of Libman-Sacks endocarditis should also alert the clinician to the possibility of an underlying antiphospholipid antibody syndrome.

Pulmonary manifestations of lupus are particularly difficult to diagnose noninvasively. Migrating pneumonitis, particularly involving the lung bases, suggests "lupus lung"; however, distinguishing these entities from infection may be impossible without invasive procedures. Typically, patients have atelectasis, pleural effusions, interstitial pneumonitis, or hemorrhage (Fig. 7-32). These sequelae may present as cyanosis, dyspnea, or almost any other form of respiratory distress. Patients with SLE can also develop a "shrinking lung" syndrome. This is manifested by diaphragmatic involvement and progressively smaller lung volumes recorded by pulmonary function testing. Also, the clinician should always be suspicious of the diagnosis of SLE in the setting of hematuria and hemoptysis and must rule out other entities such as Wegener granulomatosis, hemolytic uremic syndrome, Goodpasture syndrome, and infective endocarditis.

Unlike the destructive arthritis of JRA, lupus arthritis is more transient and episodic and rarely results in loss of function. Jaccoud arthropathy, which is a nondeforming, easily reversible, soft tissue arthritis that can mimic the boutonnière (flexion of PIP and hyperextension of distal interphalangeal [DIP] joints) and swan-neck (hyperextension of PIP and flexion of DIP joints) deformities associated with JRA, is strongly associated with the diagnosis of SLE. The fact that arthralgia is more predominant than arthritis has been noted consistently. Any joint may be involved, but the fingers are particularly susceptible. Myalgia and weakness also occur as features of lupus but do not dominate the clinical picture as they do in dermatomyositis.

Central nervous system (CNS) signs and symptoms of lupus are a great challenge to physicians. A wide range of neurologic and psychiatric manifestations of the disease have been described. Further complicating the spectrum of CNS lupus is the difficulty in distinguishing the disease itself from side effects of therapy such as corticosteroid psychosis, emotional response to disease, and a non-CNS etiology of CNS pathology such as hypertensive encephalopathy. Chorea is a neurologic manifestation of lupus that must be distinguished from the chorea of rheumatic fever. Altered mental status and focal neurologic defects occurring in lupus also suggest the possibility of cerebral vascular accident and again alert the clinician to diagnose the antiphospholipid antibody syndrome. Approximately one quarter of all lupus patients have some form of CNS disease. The findings range from mononeuritis multiplex (inflammatory lesions of multiple nerves located in anatomically unrelated parts of the body) to ataxia, peripheral neuropathy, seizures, headaches, psychosis, pseudotumor cerebri, and intellectual impairment. The thorough investigation of a large number of neurologic signs and symptoms mandates screening serologies for lupus. As a direct extension of the brain, the retina may also show evidence of disease (i.e., retinal vasculitis). The best-known ocular manifestation is the cotton-wool spot, an exudative, whitish lesion of the retina. Hemorrhage and papilledema are also seen (Fig. 7-33). The CNS effects of lupus are responsible for much morbidity and mortality.

At least as important as CNS disease in determining ultimate prognosis is the degree of renal involvement. Approximately 75% of all children with SLE have some degree of clinically apparent renal disease. This often manifests itself in the first 2 years of illness but can also appear many years after the initial diagnosis. The type of pathology largely relates to the nature of immune complex deposition at various sites in the kidney (i.e., size and electrical charge of the immune complexes). At a histologic level, renal involvement is classified using the World Health Organization classification of lupus nephritis (Table 7-11). A pathologic diagnosis must be made in children with rapidly progressive renal problems or change in their renal disease to rule out diffuse proliferative glomerulonephritis with the presence of subendothelial deposits on electron microscopy. Other than the glomeruli, the tubules, interstitium, and blood vessels can be involved. From the clinician's point of view, these lesions are difficult to distinguish. More importantly, renal involvement must be monitored at frequent intervals because of the possible development of diffuse proliferative glomerulonephritis. This is best accomplished by urinalysis for protein, hematuria, red cell casts, and abnormalities in the specific gravity patterns over time. The clinician must also obtain blood urea nitrogen and creatinine levels, 24-hour urine for creatinine clearance, and protein levels at periodic intervals. Hypertension may also direct the clinician to the presence of renal disease, and control of hypertension is as important as any other therapeutic maneuver in delaying the progression to renal failure. To complicate the clinical picture, histologic evidence of renal pathology may be present even when all of the clinical parameters are normal. Patients with SLE require careful serologic and clinical monitoring. Renal biopsies should be obtained when kidney involvement is suspected.

Additional clinical findings in SLE include lymphadenopathy with or without hepatosplenomegaly, hepatitis, anemia, leukopenia, thrombocytopenia, disorders of esophageal motility, pancreatitis, malabsorption, diarrhea, and abdominal pain.

Perhaps more than in any other rheumatic disease, the clinical diagnosis of lupus can be confirmed serologically.

Table 7-11	World Health Organization Classification of Lupus Nephritis
CLASS	**CHARACTERISTIC**
I	Normal
II	Mesangial
IIA	Minimal alteration
IIB	Mesangial glomerulitis
III	Focal and segmental proliferative glomerulonephritis
IV	Diffuse proliferative glomerulonephritis
V	Membranous glomerulonephritis
VI	Glomerular sclerosis

Modified from Cassidy JT, Petty RE: Textbook of Pediatric Rheumatology. Philadelphia, WB Saunders, 2001.

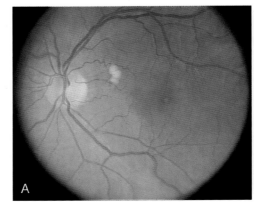 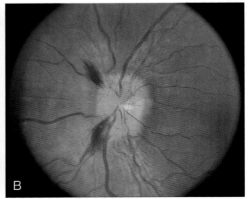

Figure 7-33. Systemic lupus erythematosus. **A,** A white exudate (cotton-wool spot) between the disk and macula. **B,** Papilledema with flame hemorrhages.

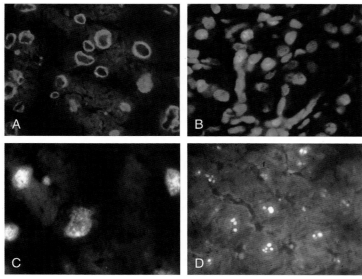

Figure 7-34. Antinuclear antibody patterns in systemic lupus erythematosus (SLE). **A,** Peripheral; correlates with anti-dsDNA-active renal disease. **B,** Homogeneous; nonspecific for SLE. **C,** Speckled; seen with SLE and mixed connective tissue disease (MCTD). To further delineate a diagnosis, anti-RNP is present in MCTD, and Smith (Sm) antibody is present in SLE. **D,** Nucleolar; suggests scleroderma.

Table 7-12	Antibodies Found in Systemic Lupus Erythematosus Patients	
ANTIBODY		**PATIENTS (%)**
Native DNA (double-stranded)		50-60
DNP (DNA and histone protein)		Up to 70 (usually high titer)
RNP (RNA and nonhistone protein)		30-40
Histones		
All SLE patients		60
Drug-induced lupus patients		95
anti-SS-A (anti-Ro)		30-40
anti-SS-B (anti-La)		15
Smith		30

DNP, deoxyribonucleoprotein; RNP, ribonucleoprotein.
Modified from Tan EM: Antinuclear antibodies in diagnosis and management. Hosp Pract 18:74-79, 1983.

The ANAs represent a group of antibodies found in serum and are directed against antigens within the cellular nuclei of lupus patients. ANAs are usually reported with a titer and a pattern. The patterns are either peripheral, homogeneous, speckled, or nucleolar (Fig. 7-34).

Other antibodies found in SLE patients are listed in Table 7-12. Anti–double-stranded DNA antibodies are detected in 50% to 60% of lupus patients and are specific for the diagnosis of SLE. It also should be noted that anti–double-stranded DNA antibody levels correlate with disease activity, especially renal and CNS disease. Ribonucleoprotein (RNP), though better known for its presence in high titers in mixed connective tissue disease, is also seen in low titers in 30% to 40% of lupus patients. Other SLE antibodies include anti-SS-A and anti-SS-B, also known as anti-Ro and anti-La, respectively. Lastly, the clinician may find antibodies to Smith antigen (Sm), a nonhistone antigen that also appears to be specific for the diagnosis of lupus.

In summary, SLE is a chronic disease with a variable course and with periods of varying activity. Although the mortality and morbidity remain high, marked improvement in prognosis has occurred in recent years.

Though rare in children, discoid lupus refers to the absence of systemic disease in the presence of typical

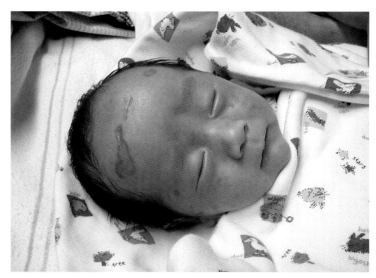

Figure 7-35. Neonatal lupus erythematosus. Note the annular rash in a sun-exposed area.

lupus dermatologic pathology. Another entity, referred to as *subacute cutaneous lupus,* in which the traditional ANA is sometimes negative but the SS-A (anti-Ro) is positive, has been described. This syndrome can occur in an annular pattern or psoriasiform pattern and can progress to full-blown SLE.

Lupus also occurs in infants whose mothers have the disease. SS-A antibody of the IgG class is passed via the placenta to the fetus, leading to positive serologies and the diagnosis of neonatal lupus. The presence of rash (Fig. 7-35), thrombocytopenia, Coombs-positive hemolytic anemia, liver function abnormalities, and congenital heart block should suggest the diagnosis of neonatal lupus. The majority of infants with congenital heart block and neonatal lupus have entirely asymptomatic mothers, although a percentage of these women develop Sjögren syndrome rather than SLE. Fortunately, neonatal lupus is transient, lasting only a few months until the disappearance of passively transferred maternal antibody; however, the congenital heart block is permanent.

Drugs induce a lupus-like reaction, and their withdrawal leads to a resolution of this syndrome usually within 6 months. Many patients on certain drugs such as minocycline, hydralazine, procainamide, isoniazid (INH), chlorpromazine, or certain anticonvulsants develop a positive ANA without developing a lupus syndrome, and this is not an absolute reason to discontinue the medication. Oral contraceptives have also been shown in some studies to be associated with a lupus-like syndrome.

Scleroderma

Scleroderma, or "tight skin," remains an enigmatic entity with no known etiology and no consistently effective therapy. The estimated annual incidence of scleroderma is from 4.5 to 14 per million, but childhood onset is extremely rare. In children, the localized forms of scleroderma (Fig. 7-36) are much more common than systemic sclerosis (SSc), although the exact numbers are unknown. Systemic sclerosis occurs with equal frequency in boys and girls younger than the age of 8, whereas girls outnumber boys 3:1 when disease onset is after the eighth birthday.

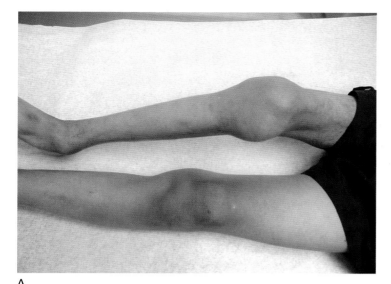

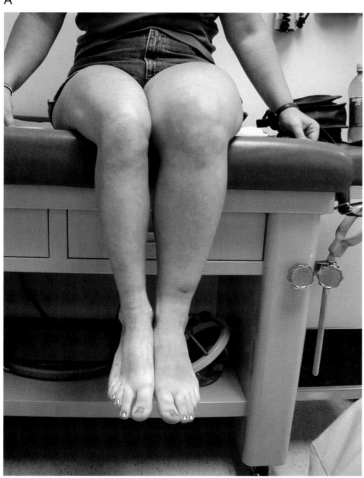

B

Figure 7-36. Scleroderma. **A** and **B,** Linear form of scleroderma affecting the right lower extremity of two children. Note the extensive atrophy.

Table 7-13	Classification of Scleroderma and Related Disorders

Primary	Secondary
Systemic Sclerosis	**Graft-versus-Host Disease**
Diffuse scleroderma	Drug or chemical induced
Limited scleroderma (CREST syndrome)	Vinyl chloride
	Bleomycin
Localized Scleroderma	Pentazocine
Morphea	Tryptophan
Linear scleroderma and *en coup de sabre*	Silicone
	Toxic oil syndrome
Eosinophilic fasciitis	**Scleroderma-Like Illnesses**
	Phenylketonuria
	Progeria
	Werner syndrome
	Scleredema
	Porphyria cutanea tarda
	Diabetic cheiroarthropathy*

*Arthropathy of the hand.
CREST, calcinosis cutis, Raynaud's phenomenon, esophageal dysfunction, sclerodactyly, and telangiectasia; PSS, progressive systemic sclerosis.

Table 7-14	Clinical and Laboratory Characteristics of Patients with Systemic Sclerosis According to Serum Autoantibody Type

AUTOANTIBODY	PATTERN	CLINICAL ASSOCIATION
Centromere	Centromere	Limited
Th	Nucleolar	—
U1RNP	Speckled	Overlap
PM-Scl	Nucleolar	Overlap with myositis
U3RNP	Nucleolar	Pulmonary hypertension
RNA polymerase, I, III	Speckled nucleolar	Diffuse
Scl-70	Speckled nucleolar	Diffuse

PM-Scl, polymyositis-scleroderma; RNP, ribonucleoprotein; Scl, scleroderma; Scl-70, antitopoisomerase.

derma features absent or nonprogressive skin thickening (distal extremities) and late visceral disease (pulmonary arterial hypertension, malabsorption). Patients with the CREST syndrome (calcinosis, Raynaud's phenomenon, esophageal dysmotility, sclerodactyly, and telangiectasia) are considered to have systemic disease with limited scleroderma (see Fig. 7-39). Systemic sclerosis with overlap is diffuse or limited skin thickening associated with another connective tissue disease such as dermatomyositis or SLE. The antibody picture is also helpful in defining subsets of systemic sclerosis (Table 7-14).

Localized scleroderma includes plaque morphea, generalized morphea, bullous morphea, linear morphea, and deep morphea. The group of disorders is characterized by fibrosis that is confined to skin, subcutaneous tissue, or muscle. Early active lesions are characterized by a violaceous inflammatory border. Morphea may present in the form of plaques or drops (the "guttate" variety) or with diffuse cutaneous involvement (Fig. 7-37). Linear scleroderma affects a single dermatome and can cause severe deformity and growth arrest in an affected limb. When this lesion occurs on the face or scalp, it is referred to as *scleroderma en coup de sabre* because of its resemblance to a scar from a dueling sword (Fig. 7-38). Parry-Romberg syndrome is a rare form of linear scleroderma with en coup de sabre that causes hemifacial dysplasia and neurologic disease consisting of headache, seizure, and transient ischemic attacks. Eosinophilic fasciitis is a form of deep morphea. No laboratory test exists to diagnose linear scleroderma. Rheumatoid factor is present in one third of patients. Antinuclear antibody may also be positive. Sedimentation rate and serum immunoglobulin levels

Scleroderma can be a primary idiopathic disease or a secondary phenomenon (Table 7-13). The classification of idiopathic scleroderma consists of systemic disease (systemic sclerosis) and localized disease. Systemic disease may be associated with diffuse scleroderma, with limited scleroderma, or with an overlap syndrome. Systemic sclerosis associated with diffuse scleroderma involves widespread and rapidly progressive skin thickening (proximal to elbows and knees) and early visceral disease (lung, heart, and kidney). Systemic disease with limited sclero-

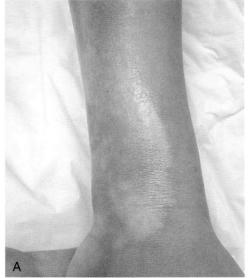

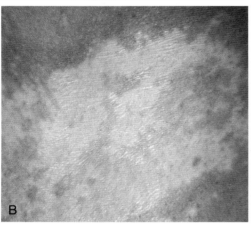

Figure 7-37. Morphea. **A,** Hypopigmented plaque of scleroderma with surrounding erythema. **B,** "Salt-and-pepper" appearance of a plaque in a patient with scleroderma. Note the hyperpigmentation within the hypopigmented lesion.

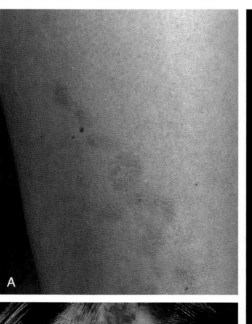

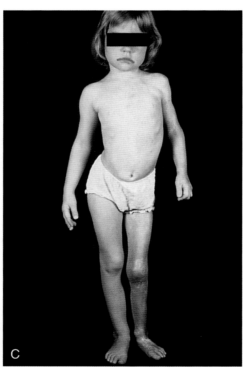

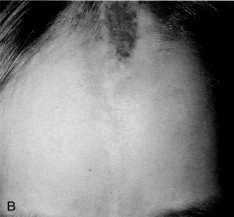

Figure 7-38. Linear scleroderma. **A,** Localized involvement of a dermatome with hyperpigmentation. **B,** An unusual form of localized scleroderma affecting the scalp, termed *en coup de sabre* (stroke of the saber). **C,** Linear scleroderma affecting the left side of the body.

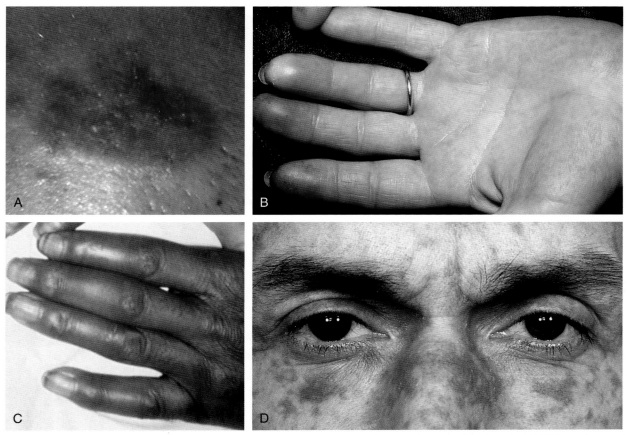

Figure 7-39. Patient with calcinosis, Raynaud's phenomenon, esophageal dysmotility, sclerodactyly, and telangiectasia (CREST) syndrome. **A,** Cutaneous calcinosis. **B,** Raynaud's phenomenon (note cyanosis and pallor of the fingertips). **C,** Sclerodactyly. **D,** Telangiectasia. Esophageal dysmotility may also occur.

may be useful markers of disease activity in localized scleroderma.

The ultimate prognosis of children with systemic sclerosis depends on the nature and extent of visceral involvement. American College of Rheumatology criteria for the clinical diagnosis of scleroderma consist of one major and three minor criteria. The single major criterion is the presence of proximal scleroderma (tightness, thickening, and nonpitting induration involving areas proximal to the metacarpophalangeal or metatarsophalangeal joints). The three minor criteria are sclerodactyly (Fig. 7-39C), digital pitting scars (Fig. 7-40), and bilateral basilar pulmonary fibrosis (Fig. 7-41).

Children with systemic sclerosis almost always have Raynaud's phenomenon (see Fig. 7-39B), which is a triphasic color change of the hands (first white because of vasoconstriction, then blue secondary to cyanosis, and finally red because of reperfusion with subsequent swelling and pain). This phenomenon can occur in response to cold or stressful stimuli. In its most severe form, fixed vasospasm can lead to gangrene and autoamputation.

The presence of Raynaud's phenomenon can be helpful in distinguishing systemic sclerosis from localized forms of scleroderma. Healthy individuals can also experience the color changes of Raynaud's without being at risk for developing an underlying connective tissue disease.

Many organ systems can be involved in the child afflicted with scleroderma. Cutaneous manifestations frequently bring children to medical attention, but because of the insidious and subtle onset of skin lesions, there is often a delay in diagnosis. Early in the clinical course, the skin is edematous with particular predilection for the distal extremities; rarely, more proximal limb, face, and

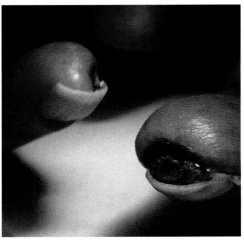

Figure 7-40. Scleroderma. Digital pitting ulcers, one of the three minor diagnostic criteria for scleroderma.

trunk involvement is present. The induration phase, for which scleroderma is named, is characterized by loss of the natural pliability of the skin and the presence of a palpable skin thickness. The skin takes on a shiny, tense appearance, with distal tapering of the fingers (see Fig. 7-39C). The visual impression that movement might be impaired is supported by the lack of flexibility in the hands (Fig. 7-42). The typical scleroderma facies of tight skin and skin atrophy produces the appearance of a fixed stare, pinched nose, thin pursed lips, small mouth, prominent teeth, and characteristic grimace (Fig. 7-43).

Subcutaneous calcium deposits (calcinosis cutis) may occur at pressure points and may occasionally extrude

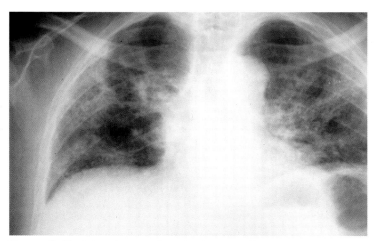

Figure 7-41. Scleroderma. Bilateral pulmonary fibrosis.

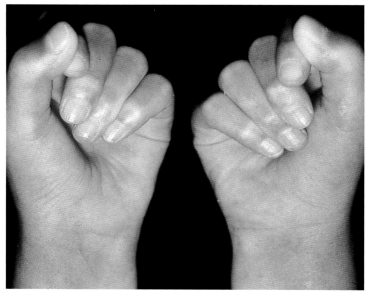

Figure 7-42. Scleroderma. Lack of flexibility in the hands is another characteristic of scleroderma.

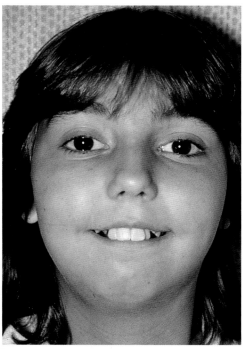

Figure 7-43. Scleroderma. Facial features show that the skin appears tight and drawn, without evidence of wrinkles. (Courtesy J. Jeffrey Malatack, MD, Philadelphia.)

Whereas morbidity and mortality in adults with scleroderma is usually related to hypertension and renal failure, sick children with scleroderma suffer from pulmonary arterial hypertension and pulmonary fibrosis. Other cardiac involvement includes heart block, congestive heart failure, electrocardiographic changes, and pericardial effusion. These abnormalities appear to be a result of myocardial fibrosis, vascular insufficiency, and inflammation.

Mixed Connective Tissue Disease

A syndrome characterized by features of rheumatoid arthritis, scleroderma, SLE, and dermatomyositis and associated with high-titer anti-RNP antibodies was first described in 1972 and termed *mixed connective tissue disease* (MCTD). Clinical characteristics of MCTD in children are summarized in Table 7-15.

Cardiopulmonary disease and esophageal dysmotility are common in MCTD; nephritis occurs but is less common and usually less severe than in SLE. Anti-RNP antibodies are strongly associated with the diagnosis of MCTD. High-titer positive antinuclear antibody (ANA) is common. Rheumatoid factor (RF) may also be present.

The outcome and course of children with MCTD is variable. Sick children with MCTD suffer from cardiopulmonary or renal complications.

Juvenile Dermatomyositis

Juvenile dermatomyositis (JDM) is a rare but distinctive disease that accounts for approximately 5% of all rheumatic disease in childhood. Though it was first described in 1887, its etiology remains unknown. The hallmarks of this entity are various skin manifestations coupled with nonsuppurative inflammation of muscle. Dermatomyositis affecting the adult generally carries a worse prognosis

through the skin in a fashion similar to dermatomyositis (Fig. 7-44). These lesions may be painful and may ulcerate. Often, generalized hyperpigmentation occurs with punctated areas of hypopigmentation or vitiligo (complete depigmentation) (see Figs. 7-37 and 7-38). Telangiectases of three varieties are known to occur: (1) linear telangiectasia of the cuticles, (2) well-defined macules of various sizes and shapes, and (3) the reddish purple papules typical of Osler-Weber-Rendu disease (tiny circular lesions positioned eccentrically from their telangiectatic spokes) (see Fig. 7-39D).

Gastrointestinal symptoms occur in approximately half of the children. More detailed investigation often indicates the presence of abnormalities in a larger percentage. Esophageal dysmotility associated with gastroesophageal reflux often leads to dysphagia and symptoms of esophagitis. In some affected individuals, aspiration or cough may occur and esophageal strictures can develop if the process of reflux is chronic. If the small bowel is involved, cramps, diarrhea, and constipation may result from peristaltic dysfunction. Bacterial overgrowth, steatorrhea, weight loss, volvulus, and even perforation can occur. Colonic disease occurs in the form of wide-mouth diverticula and a loss of the normal colonic architecture.

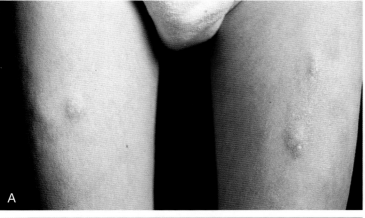

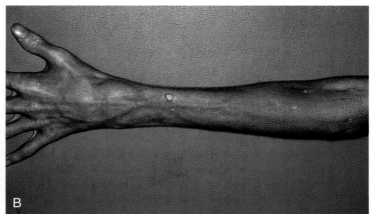

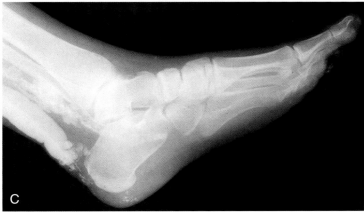

Figure 7-44. Juvenile dermatomyositis. **A,** Nodular calcific densities in the thighs. **B,** Atrophy, hyperpigmentation, and subcutaneous calcium deposits in the arm of a patient with "burned-out" JDM. **C,** Radiologic evidence of soft tissue calcification.

Table 7-15	Clinical Characteristics of Children with Mixed Connective Tissue Disease

CHARACTERISTIC	PATIENTS (%)
Arthritis	93
Raynaud's phenomenon	85
Scleroderma skin	49
Rash of SLE	33
Rash of DM	33
Fever	56
Abnormal esophageal motility	41
Cardiac	30
Pericarditis	27
Myositis	61
CNS disease	23
Pulmonary	43
Renal	26

CNS, central nervous system; DM, dermatomyositis; SLE, systemic lupus erythematosus.
Modified from Cassidy JT, Petty RE: Textbook of Pediatric Rheumatology. Philadelphia, WB Saunders, 2001.

than that encountered in the pediatric age group. There is no association with malignancy in JDM patients, although it appears to be a paraneoplastic syndrome in certain adult populations. Nevertheless, vasculitis of varying severity is often seen earlier in the course of the illness in children, and there is the possibility of calcinosis (nodular calcium deposits) in nonvisceral tissues such as muscle and subcutaneous tissue (see Fig. 7-44). Pressure points and severely affected soft tissue are particularly susceptible.

Although the age range for JDM is broad, presentation of the disease is usually between ages 4 and 10 years. Girls predominate by a 2:1 ratio. No racial bias exists, nor is there any evidence of a familial predisposition.

Clinically, patients usually have fatigue and symmetric, proximal muscle weakness, particularly affecting the hip girdle and legs. Although weakness is the hallmark of the disease, muscle pain can exist. Though shoulders and arms are often involved, this may not be detected as easily in the child. The first complaints are often inability to climb stairs and disturbances of gait. Dysphagia, dysphonia, and dyspnea may occur if the respective muscles for these functions are affected. The involved muscles may be tender and indurated, with a superficially edematous appearance. A pathognomonic rash found in three quarters of JDM patients can confirm the diagnosis. Even in the absence of this distinctive rash, all patients have some degree of cutaneous disease. The rash is symmetric and erythematous, with atrophic changes located over the extensor surfaces of the knees and elbows. Such changes over the PIP and MCP joints are called *Gottron's papules* (Fig. 7-45). JDM can exist with skin involvement only, and skin involvement can antedate muscle involvement for months to years. Other features of the rash include a violaceous discoloration of the eyelids, eyelid edema, a scaly red rash in a malar distribution, periungual erythema, telangiectasia (Fig. 7-46), and the characteristic dystrophic skin changes. As opposed to SLE, which also has a malar rash, the nasolabial folds are not spared in JDM. Nail bed telangiectasia (Fig. 7-47), digital ulceration, and hyperpigmentation or hypopigmentation of the skin also occur. The rash of JDM, similar to that of SLE, may be extremely photosensitive. However, because of the pathognomonic features of the rash, the diagnosis of JDM can often be suspected before overt symptoms occur. Constitutional symptoms such as anorexia, malaise, weight loss, and fever may be present. The illness may progress at variable rates in different patients; however, the majority of patients have a more insidious rather than acute course.

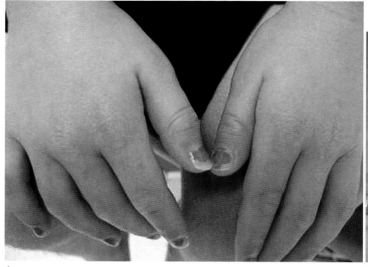

A

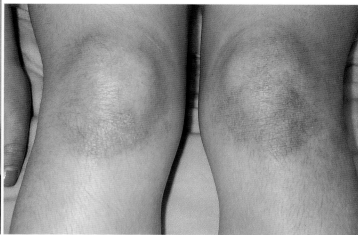

B

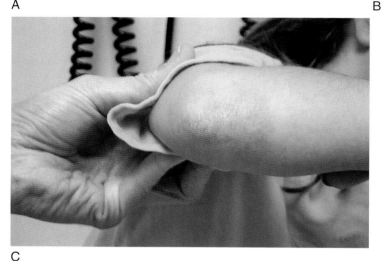

C

Figure 7-45. Juvenile dermatomyositis (JDM). **A,** Gottron's papules: Erythematous, atrophic skin changes overlying the metacarpophalangeal and proximal interphalangeal joints. **B** and **C,** Typical rash of JDM, as seen on the knees **(B)** and the elbow **(C).**

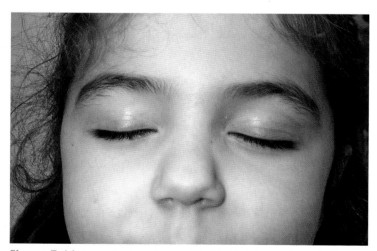

Figure 7-46. Juvenile dermatomyositis. The facial rash shows heliotrope discoloration and violaceous suffusion with edema of the eyelids. Note the faint malar blush.

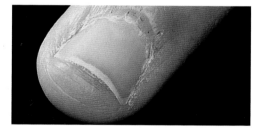

Figure 7-47. Juvenile dermatomyositis. Nail bed telangiectasia. Erythema can be seen around the nail edge. The pinpoint telangiectasia may require a magnifying lens to identify.

Unfortunately, long delays in diagnosis can occur, particularly in the insidious group. Other more uncommon findings are mouth ulcers, retinitis, hepatosplenomegaly, pulmonary infiltrates, myocarditis, and pericarditis. Although calcinosis may occur in children with JDM, it does not occur during the acute phase of the illness. In chronic, indolent disease it may be the presenting com-

plaint and may often be the most difficult feature of the disease to control, causing significant morbidity.

Elevated muscle enzymes may be the first clue to the diagnosis of inflammatory muscle disease; the creatine kinase, aspartate transaminase, alanine aminotransferase, aldolase, and lactate dehydrogenase should be checked serially because they can be useful in following disease activity. Not all of the aforementioned muscle enzymes may be elevated in the setting of floridly active myositis. Serum neopterin is another marker of disease activity in dermatomyositis. An elevated serum von Willebrand factor antigen level is thought to be a measure of endothelial cell damage due to vasculitis.

An abnormal magnetic resonance image (T2-weighted image with fat suppression) can show edema and active

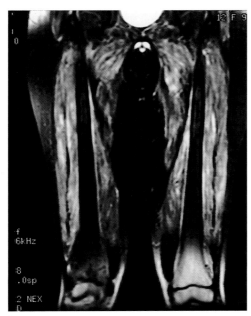

Figure 7-48. Juvenile dermatomyositis. Magnetic resonance image of the thigh (T2 fat-suppressed image) illustrates marked diffuse muscle edema and inflammation. Note patchy white area in muscle similar in appearance to fluid in bladder.

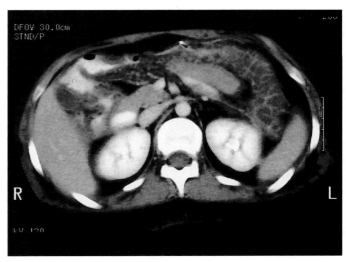

Figure 7-49. Juvenile dermatomyositis. CT scan of the abdomen demonstrates bowel wall thickening and edema in the transverse colon. The patient's bowel eventually perforated because of active vasculitis.

Table 7-16	Classification of Vasculitis by Vessel Size

Large-Vessel Vasculitis
Giant cell arteritis (seen in adults only)
Takayasu arteritis

Medium-Vessel Vasculitis
Kawasaki syndrome
Polyarteritis nodosa (PAN)
Primary granulomatous central nervous system vasculitis

Small-Vessel Vasculitis (ANCA Associated)
Microscopic polyangiitis
Wegener granulomatosis
Churg-Strauss syndrome
Drug-induced

Small-Vessel Vasculitis (Immune Complex Associated)
Henoch-Schönlein purpura
Essential cryoglobulinemic vasculitis
Hypocomplementemic urticarial vasculitis
Vasculitis with lupus, rheumatoid arthritis, or Sjögren syndrome
Behçet syndrome
Goodpasture syndrome
Serum sickness
Drug-associated
Infection-associated

Small-Vessel Vasculitis (Paraneoplastic)
Lymphoproliferative
Myeloproliferative
Carcinoma

Small-Vessel Vasculitis (Inflammatory Bowel Disease)

From Jennette JC, Falk RJ: Small-vessel vasculitis. N Engl J Med 337:1512, 1997.

inflammation in the case of myositis (Fig. 7-48). A muscle biopsy, usually taken from the lateral thigh, will confirm the diagnosis. Some clinicians, faced with a child with muscle weakness, Gottron's papules, elevated muscle enzymes, and abnormal muscle MRI, choose to make the diagnosis of JDM and initiate therapy without a muscle biopsy.

Corticosteroids are the mainstay of therapy. Their early use often preserves muscle function and minimizes the potentially destructive nature of this disease, and corticosteroids may prevent the development of calcinosis universalis. One of the most dreaded and potentially lethal complications of JDM in childhood is perforation of the intestines secondary to active vasculitis. The clinician must maintain a high index of suspicion because many of the classic signs of an acute condition in the abdomen may not be present in the setting of high-dose corticosteroid therapy. Pneumatosis intestinalis may be visualized on abdominal plain film or CT. This complication of JDM may be an indication for cytotoxic therapy (Fig. 7-49).

Systemic Vasculitides

The vasculitides are a broad group of disorders with a common pathology characterized by blood vessel inflammation. The type of inflammation, organ system affected, and size of the vessels vary with each disease entity. A classification of the systemic vasculitides based on the size of the blood vessel involved is noted in Table 7-16. Kawasaki syndrome (KS) is a common form of vasculitis affecting children and is discussed later in this chapter. Polyarteritis nodosa (PAN), the prototype of the medium-sized vessel vasculitis, can occur in older children and is occasionally noted in the setting of poststreptococcal infection. The major clues to the diagnosis of PAN are hematuria, hypertension, abdominal pain, arthritis, and fever. Wegener granulomatosis and Churg-Strauss vasculitis are systemic necrotizing vasculitides with a granulomatous component. They frequently present with pulmonary and upper respiratory manifestations, can have neurologic involvement in the form of a mononeuritis multiplex, and are extremely unusual in childhood. The most common forms of vasculitis are the hypersensitivity, or leukocytoclastic, vasculitides. Hypersensitivity, or leukocytoclastic, vasculitis is characterized by inflammation of small vessels such as arterioles, capillaries, and venules. Henoch-Schönlein purpura is the prototype of these illnesses and is discussed in the following section.

Henoch-Schönlein Purpura

Henoch-Schönlein purpura (HSP) consists of nonthrombocytopenic palpable purpura, arthritis, bowel angina, and renal abnormalities. Ninety percent of cases occur in children younger than 10 years of age with the median

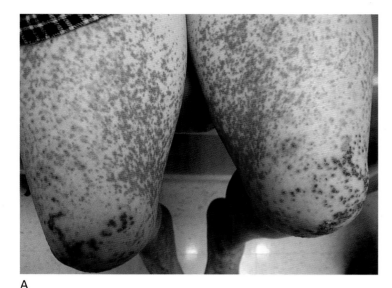

A

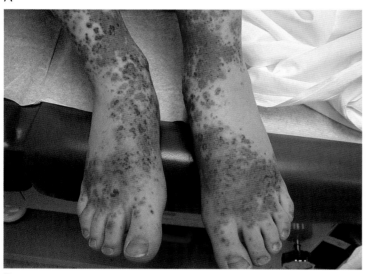

B

Figure 7-50. Henoch-Schönlein purpura. **A** and **B,** Rash characteristically involves the lower extremities, with purpuric coalescent lesions.

age being 5 years. Children younger than 2 years of age generally develop milder disease with less frequent gastrointestinal and renal involvement. This syndrome may or may not occur after an identifiable trigger such as viral illness, bacterial infection, insect bite, dietary allergen, immunization, or medication usage. A familial predilection does not appear to exist, and all races have been affected. Seasonal peaks occur in fall and winter, but a definite etiology remains elusive.

The clinical picture of HSP is that of a previously well child who acutely develops a distinctive skin rash, arthritis, and abdominal pain. The skin rash allows for definitive diagnosis, and hence it is said to occur in all patients with HSP. Fifty percent of patients present with rash, which usually involves the buttocks and lower extremities (waist-down distribution) (Fig. 7-50). The lesions begin as petechiae that coalesce and become confluent with nearby lesions. They begin as red macules or papules and progress with time to purplish and then brownish areas. Early in the course of the disease the rash may blanch with pressure, but with time this feature disappears. Typically, varying stages of eruption are simultaneously present. Some patients have lesions that mimic urticaria. Pruritus can be a feature of the rash, and about 25% have sub-

cutaneous edema (Fig. 7-51). The edema is nonpitting, painless, evanescent, and most commonly affects the hands (see Fig. 7-51B) and feet. The child younger than 2 years of age is most likely to have edema as a feature of this illness. The younger child is also more likely to display facial involvement (Fig. 7-51A and C).

Approximately 85% of patients display some gastrointestinal symptoms. Simple colicky abdominal pain can be the only symptom, but its severity can raise physician concerns about more threatening abdominal complications. Massive gastrointestinal hemorrhage or intussusception is seen in less than 5% of patients, and complete perforation rarely occurs. Melanotic stools, vomiting, ileus, and hematemesis may be present as well. In rare circumstances abdominal pain can precede the other features of HSP, making diagnosis difficult until the characteristic rash appears.

The periarticular swelling that occurs presents as arthritis or arthralgia and is a part of HSP in three quarters of reported cases. Knees and ankles are the most common sites of involvement (Fig. 7-52). Warmth and erythema are not usually associated with the pain and swelling that occur. The joints are never affected permanently, and this feature of HSP generally resolves in several days. As with the gastrointestinal symptoms, arthritis can precede the rash. For this reason, HSP should be considered in the child with acute onset of arthritis.

Renal involvement is detected in about half of HSP patients. The degree of renal pathology generally affects the patient's ultimate prognosis. Renal manifestations can range from mild hematuria or proteinuria to end-stage renal disease (less than 1% of patients). Patients usually declare themselves within several months, but cases of renal failure and hypertension have occurred years after the initial illness. Berger disease (IgA glomerulonephritis) is believed by many to be HSP without rash and hence an alternative manifestation of the same pathologic process.

Other features of HSP include low-grade fever, malaise, scrotal swelling with pain, periorbital and scalp edema, headache, cerebral vasculitis, CNS bleeding, seizures, nosebleeds, parotitis, pancreatitis, hydrops of the gallbladder, and cardiopulmonary disease.

The course of the illness varies with age. The majority of patients are over their initial illness in 4 weeks; however, 50% have at least one recurrence. Recurrences are generally limited to cutaneous and mild abdominal symptomatology.

Clotting functions are generally normal, and platelet counts are normal or elevated. The presence of IgA complexes in the glomeruli, skin, and serum of affected individuals may be a clue to diagnosis. Skin biopsy documents leukocytoclastic vasculitis with IgA deposits in dermal capillaries and postcapillary venules. Elevated serum IgA and IgM levels are found in about half of HSP patients. Because there are no diagnostic laboratory examinations for this syndrome, the history and physical examination provide clues to the successful recognition of HSP.

Kawasaki Syndrome

Although the etiology of KS has eluded investigators, the clinical features and natural history of this distinctive vasculitic entity are well described. The need to rapidly recognize the presentation of this disease is heightened by its potentially devastating cardiac sequelae. The early recognition of KS favorably affects morbidity and mortality.

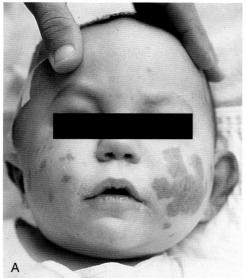

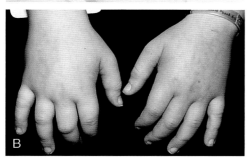

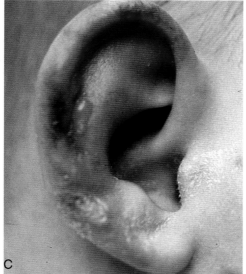

Figure 7-51. Infant with Henoch-Schönlein purpura (HSP). **A,** The rash may occur on the face along with edema. **B,** Rash and edema may be present in the extremities. **C,** Ulceration and vesicles are an unusual manifestation of HSP.

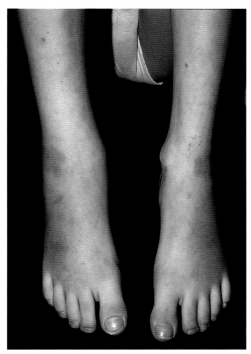

Figure 7-52. Henoch-Schönlein purpura with arthritis. Note the swelling of the right ankle in addition to the purpuric rash.

Table 7-17	Kawasaki Syndrome: Diagnostic Criteria

1. Fever for 5 or more days
2. Conjunctivitis (bilateral, bulbar, nonsuppurative)
3. Lymphadenopathy
4. Rash (polymorphous, no vesicles or crusts)
5. Change(s)* in the mucous membranes of the oropharynx, such as:
   Injected pharynx
   Injected lips
   Dry, fissured lips
   "Strawberry" tongue
6. Change(s)* of the peripheral extremities, such as:
   Hand or foot edema (acute)
   Hand or foot erythema (acute)
   Fingertip desquamation (convalescent)

*One is sufficient to establish criterion.
Diagnosis requires 5 of 6 criteria, or 4 criteria plus coronary artery aneurysms shown on echocardiography.
It has been suggested that, in the presence of classic features, the diagnosis of KS can be made (and treatment initiated) before the fifth day of fever.
Modified from Centers for Disease Control: Multiple outbreaks of Kawasaki syndrome—United States. MMWR 34:33, 1985.

and Japanese and Korean children have a particularly high incidence. The risk to African American children is greater than the risk to white children. Boys are more commonly affected than girls by a ratio of approximately 1.5:1. The peak age of KS patients in the United States is 18 months to 2 years, with 80% of cases occurring in children younger than 4 years. Middle and upper socioeconomic classes are overrepresented. A variety of etiologies have been suggested as the cause of KS, but all have fallen short of complete acceptance.

The clinical features of typical KS are remarkably constant (Table 7-17). However, incomplete KS adds uncertainty to the clinician's approach to diagnosis. The diagnosis must be considered when a child has fever for

KS, first described in 1967 in Japan by Tomisaku Kawasaki, consists of a unique constellation of clinical findings initially labeled as *mucocutaneous lymph node syndrome.* This multisystem syndrome was independently described by Melish in 1976 in Hawaii. Since that time the syndrome has been recognized in all racial groups worldwide. Individuals of Asian ancestry are most commonly affected,

more than 4 days and has two other clinical criteria. Children younger than 1 year of age are at highest risk of developing KS without fulfilling criteria. The importance of appropriate clinical suspicion in the *forme fruste* of the disease cannot be overemphasized.

The course of the illness is triphasic: acute (lasting 7 to 14 days), subacute (days 10 to 25), and convalescent (days 21 to 60). The acute phase is characterized by fever, irritability, conjunctivitis, oropharyngeal erythema, rash, lymphadenopathy, and distal extremity edema and erythema. The onset of fever is sudden, often spiking as high as 40° C. It is remitting in character, with a mean duration of 12 days in the untreated individual. Some patients may continue to be febrile for 30 days or more without therapy. Fever generally precedes other clinical signs and symptoms by 1 to 2 days. The conjunctivitis appears early in the progression of the illness. The conjunctivitis is nonexudative and nonulcerative with bulbar predominance, and it usually persists for 1 to 2 weeks in the untreated patient. Limbic sparing is a common feature (Fig. 7-53). Additional eye findings include a transient anterior uveitis in most patients during the first 2 weeks of illness. Because these findings are not seen in many entities in the differential diagnosis of KS, their presence may be a helpful diagnostic tool. Oral findings include red, cracked, fissured lips; "strawberry tongue"; and diffuse mouth erythema (Fig. 7-54). These findings may last for several weeks as well. The rash of KS may manifest itself in many forms: scarlatiniform, morbilliform (Fig. 7-55), macular and papular erythema, multiforme-like with target lesions,

urticarial plaques, or even pustular. It can be pruritic, but the presence of vesicles, erythroderma, petechiae, or purpura suggests another diagnosis. A predilection for involvement of intertriginous areas, particularly the perineum, has been noted (Fig. 7-56). Peeling of the perineum generally occurs several days before the desquamation of fingers and toes. A particularly striking feature of the acute phase of the syndrome is erythema and edema of the hands (Fig. 7-57) and feet, often associated with refusal to walk. The characteristic desquamation of fingers and toes beginning at the nail-fingertip junction occurs between 10 and 21 days during the subacute phase (Fig. 7-58). The toes are involved later and to a lesser degree than the fingers. In the syndrome's most dramatic form, the entire distal extremity can peel. Months after the acute phase of illness, transverse grooves called *Beau lines* are noted in the fingernails (Fig. 7-59). Although the initial syndrome was named mucocutaneous lymph node syndrome, the presence of a 1.5-cm or greater cervical lymph node is the least consistent feature, occurring in about 50% to 75% of children. The other five features are each found in the majority of patients. The "lymphadenopathic" presentation of KS strongly mimics pyogenic lymphadenitis.

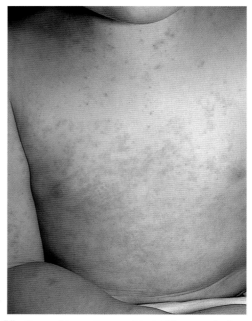

Figure 7-55. Kawasaki syndrome. Morbilliform rash is one possible manifestation.

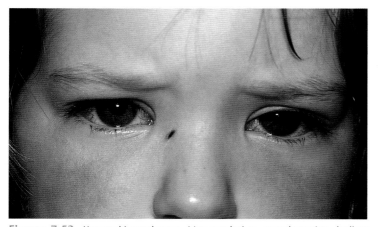

Figure 7-53. Kawasaki syndrome. Nonexudative, nonulcerative, bulbar conjunctivitis. Note sparing of the limbus.

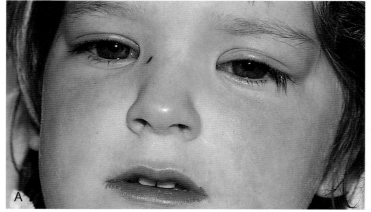

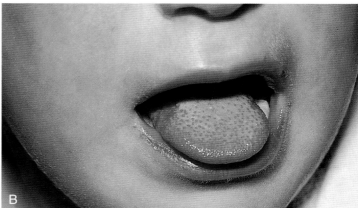

Figure 7-54. Kawasaki syndrome. **A,** Erythematous, cracked lips. **B,** "Strawberry tongue."

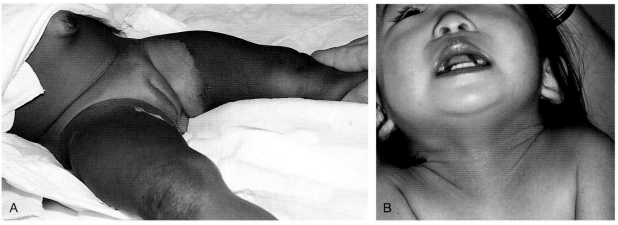

Figure 7-56. Kawasaki syndrome. **A,** Perineal rash with peeling. **B,** Neck rash with peeling. Note that peeling of intertriginous rash occurs before extremity peeling.

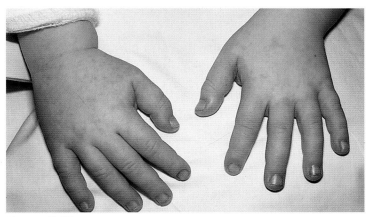

Figure 7-57. Kawasaki syndrome. Swollen, erythematous hands. Note fusiform appearance.

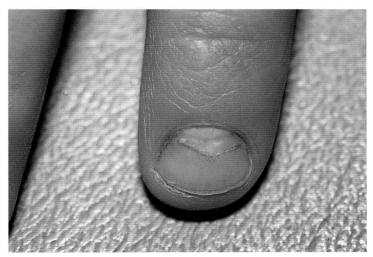

Figure 7-59. Kawasaki syndrome. Beau lines of fingernails in the convalescent phase.

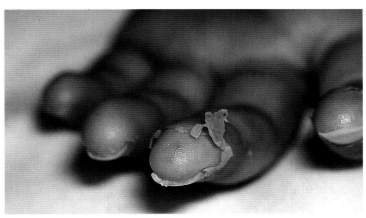

Figure 7-58. Kawasaki syndrome. Fingertip and toe tip peeling in subacute phase.

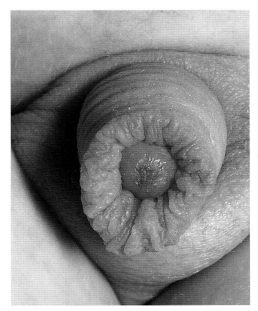

Figure 7-60. Kawasaki syndrome. Inflammation of the urethral meatus (often associated with sterile pyuria).

Although many of the aforementioned features are considered central to the diagnosis of KS, it is often the associated features of the disease that add credence to the diagnosis. Both an "early" and a "late" form of arthritis and arthralgia occur. The small and large joints may be affected. Urethritis and inflammation of the urethral meatus occur and generally are accompanied by sterile pyuria (Fig. 7-60). Central nervous system findings such as lethargy, meningismus, aseptic meningitis, facial nerve palsy, and paralysis of extremities have been described. Sensorineural hearing loss has been reported as well. Diarrhea, vomiting, abdominal pain, and hepatitis are frequent gastrointestinal features seen early in the illness. During the acute phase cardiac features include tachycardia, dysrhythmias, pericarditis, pericardial effusion, myocarditis, mitral or aortic insufficiency, and congestive heart failure. Because of the dynamic nature of this syndrome, meticulous and frequent physical examinations are essential.

Additionally, pancreatitis, transient gallbladder dilation (Fig. 7-61), and arthritis may occur. Thrombocytosis occurs more frequently than thrombocytopenia. Arterial aneurysms occur in axillary; iliac; renal; hepatic; cerebral; brachial; femoral; and, most notably, coronary arteries.

The combination of coronary artery aneurysms (Fig. 7-62) and thrombocytosis places patients in the subacute phase at particular risk for myocardial infarction. Approximately 20% of untreated patients develop coronary artery aneurysms. Although many regress spontaneously, less than 1% of affected individuals die from related complications. Of these deaths, 85% occur during the first 10 to 40 days of illness. The natural history of these aneurysms includes thromboembolism and vessel occlusion and leads to myocardial infarction in a small group of patients. Others develop coronary artery stenosis or persistent asymptomatic aneurysms of varying sizes. Giant aneurysms of 8 mm or greater are most likely to result in stenosis, thrombosis, and myocardial infarction. Particularly worrisome indicators for the development of aneurysms include male gender, age younger than 1 year, fever lasting more than 2 weeks, recurrent fever after defervescence, recurrence of rash, exaggerated leukocytosis and elevated sedimentation rate, and cardiac rhythm disturbances other than first-degree heart block. Current therapeutic interventions with aspirin and particularly intravenous immunoglobulin have significantly decreased the risk of cardiac complications.

The late convalescent phase is a period of relatively low risk for the development of aneurysms, although the long-term impact of coronary artery vasculitis on vessel function and on the incidence and severity of atherosclerotic heart disease remains a concern.

In addition to the clinical features described, laboratory studies such as acute-phase reactants; complete blood cell count (differential, platelets); urinalysis; liver enzymes; electrocardiography; echocardiography; chest radiography; and slit lamp ophthalmologic examination may also be helpful in the diagnosis of KS.

Differential diagnosis includes scarlet fever (both streptococcal and staphylococcal), staphylococcal scalded skin syndrome, toxic shock syndrome, leptospirosis, disseminated yersiniosis, Rocky Mountain spotted fever, rubeola, enteroviral infection, reactive arthritis, JRA, PAN, and SLE. Cultures, serologic tests, patient age, and clinical course of disease help in distinguishing these other disorders (Table 7-18).

Behçet's Disease

Behçet's disease (BD) is a rare systemic vasculitis with no known etiology. BD is extremely uncommon in children, and the exact incidence is unknown. The majority

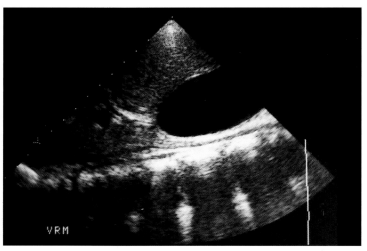

Figure 7-61. Kawasaki syndrome. Transient dilation of the gallbladder noted by ultrasonography.

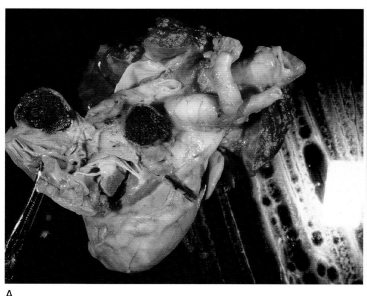

A

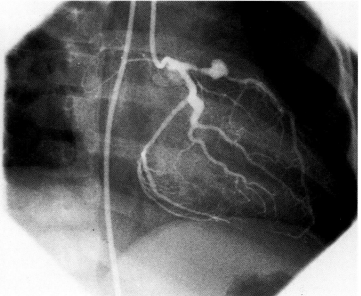

B

Figure 7-62. Kawasaki syndrome. Coronary artery aneurysms. **A,** The autopsy specimen of this infant heart shows a dilated right coronary artery filled with thrombus (dissected in cross-section). The inferior portion of the heart demonstrates a dilated left coronary artery. (Courtesy David Witte, MD, Cincinnati, Ohio). **B,** Selective left coronary angiogram in the right anterior oblique view demonstrating coronary artery aneurysms.

Table 7-18 Differential Diagnosis of Kawasaki Syndrome

AGENT	DISEASE	DISTINGUISHING CHARACTERISTICS
Bacteria	Streptococcal	Positive culture and serology, palatal petechiae, no anterior uveitis
	Staphylococcal Scalded skin syndrome	Positive culture, bullous lesions, Nikolsky sign, earlier desquamation, no anterior uveitis
	Toxic shock syndrome*	Primarily females, older age predilection, toxin detection, positive culture
Rickettsia	Rocky Mountain spotted fever*	Petechial rash, positive serology, regional geography, no anterior uveitis
Spirochetes	Leptospirosis*	Positive culture and serology, muscle pain and tenderness, rigid abdominal muscles
Toxins	Acrodynia (mercury poisoning)	Photophobia, no conjunctivitis, slow onset, diaphoresis, severe pain in hands and feet, pruritus
Autoimmune/allergic	Stevens-Johnson syndrome	History of drug or infection exposure, no predominant lymph node, corneal ulcers, blisters, more severe mucous membrane involvement
	Systemic-onset JRA Polyarteritis nodosa	Nondesquamating evanescent rash, hepatosplenomegaly, generalized adenopathy, vasculopathy
	Reiter syndrome	HLA-B27 positive, not toxic appearing
Viral infection	Epstein-Barr virus*	Positive serology, splenomegaly, atypical lymphocytes
	Rubella	Minimal enanthem, distal extremities not affected, not toxic appearing
	Rubeola	Cough, catarrh more prominent, lips not cracked, fewer oral changes, distal extremities generally not affected
	Roseola	As fever ends rash begins, shorter course
	Enterovirus*	Seasonal, epidemic, not toxic appearing

*May fulfill diagnostic criteria for Kawasaki syndrome.
JRA, juvenile rheumatoid arthritis.
Modified from Lohr JA, Rheuban KS: Kawasaki syndrome. Infect Dis Clin North Am 1:559-574, 1987.

of affected patients live in Japan and the Mediterranean area. In the United States the disease is more likely to affect males than females. The onset of the disease generally occurs in the second or third decade of life, but cases do occur in infancy and childhood. Presence of the HLA-B51 allele is associated with susceptibility to the disease.

BD may affect virtually any organ in the body. It classically presents as a triad of findings: recurrent oral and genital ulcers and uveitis. The International Study Group (ISG) for Behçet disease proposed diagnostic criteria. The criteria are the presence of recurrent oral ulceration plus two of the following (in the absence of another clinical explanation): recurrent genital ulceration (aphthous ulceration or scarring observed by the patient or physician); eye lesions (anterior or posterior uveitis, cells in the vitreous, or retinal vasculitis observed by an ophthalmologist); skin lesions (erythema nodosum, pustular lesions, palpable purpura, pseudofolliculitis); or a positive pathergy test read by a physician at 24 to 48 hours. Oral ulcers include minor aphthous, major aphthous, or herpetiform ulcers that have been observed by the patient or physician and that have recurred at least three times over a 12-month period. A positive pathergy test occurs when a sterile needle prick into the skin produces a sterile erythematous papule greater than 2 mm in diameter by 24 to 48 hours (Fig. 7-63). The pathergy test is sensitive but not specific and may be seen in patients with other disorders such as Sweet syndrome.

The most well-recognized feature of Behçet disease in childhood is recurrent aphthous stomatitis. Ulcers occur on the lips, buccal mucosa, tongue, and tonsils and may involve the larynx. Genital ulcers occur frequently; the penis and scrotum are affected in the male patient (Fig. 7-64), and the vulva and vagina are affected in the female patient. Ocular involvement is important to recognize because visual loss and other complications may result if untreated.

All organ systems may be affected in patients with BD. The skin, joints, CNS, and blood vessels are important and frequent targets of the disease. Erythema nodosum is the most frequent skin finding followed by pseudofolliculitis and nodular acneiform lesions. Recurrent arthralgia and

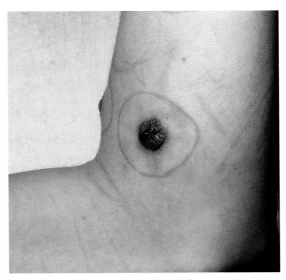

Figure 7-63. Behçet's disease. A positive pathergy test.

peripheral arthritis may be seen; the number of joints affected may vary from a single joint to multiple joints. Arthritis may be symmetrical or asymmetrical and most commonly affects the knees. CNS manifestations include headaches, meningoencephalitis, pyramidal tract and brainstem lesions, seizures, and memory loss. Vascular lesions include thrombosis of deep and superficial veins, arterial occlusion, aneurysms, and varices. Organ involvement occurs, albeit less frequently, in the heart, lungs, gastrointestinal tract, and genitourinary tract. Symptoms may be vague and nonspecific; thus the clinician must maintain a high index of suspicion that even minor symptoms could be clues to the diagnosis.

The diagnosis of Behçet's disease may be quite challenging in view of the spectrum of symptoms. No specific diagnostic tests exist, and the diagnosis is made on clinical grounds in the absence of other clinical explanations. Skin biopsy does not distinguish erythema nodosum in BD from that in other rheumatologic diseases. Inflammatory markers, such as the erythrocyte sedimentation rate

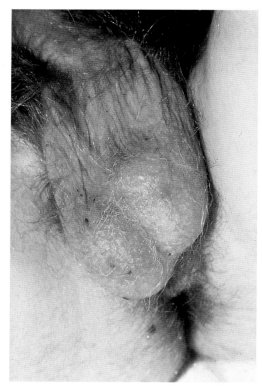

Figure 7-64. Behçet's disease. Ulcers on the scrotum.

(ESR) and C-reactive protein (CRP), tend to be elevated in patients with BD. Treatment is directed at the relief of symptoms, and close monitoring of eye involvement is imperative. The prognosis is variable; remissions and exacerbations are typical. Patients with vascular complications, in general, do more poorly than those patients without vascular lesions.

Periodic Fever Syndromes

The periodic fever syndromes are a group of disorders characterized by febrile attacks that occur in a predictable, periodic fashion. The fevers may reach a peak of 107 degrees and last several days before subsiding. Often the pattern is a few weeks without symptoms before the next episode of fever begins. The parents can often predict the start of the next attack on the basis of the child's pattern of fever. During the febrile illness, the child may also suffer abdominal pain, rash, arthralgia, arthritis, loss of appetite, pleuritis, and peritonitis. Markers of inflammation such as white blood cell count, platelet count, sedimentation rate, and C-reactive protein will be elevated during the attacks. The varying phenotypes of the periodic fever syndromes depend on the genetic mutations involved. Thus far, the identified syndromes include familial Mediterranean fever (FMF); hyperimmunoglobulinemia D syndrome (HIDS); PFAPA syndrome (Periodic Fever, Aphthous stomatitis, Pharyngitis, and cervical Adenitis); and TRAPS (Tumor necrosis factor Receptor-Associated Periodic Syndromes).

Familial Mediterranean fever is an autosomal recessive disorder affecting people of Eastern Mediterranean descent. The defect is the MEFV gene on the short arm of chromosome 16, and several mutations have been identified. Attacks are characterized by fever, abdominal pain, pleuropericardial pain, arthritis, myalgia, and erysipelas-like erythema. Episodes occur at intervals of days to months. Laboratory findings are nonspecific. Colchicine is the recommended treatment.

The hyper-IgD syndrome is an autosomal recessive disorder resulting from a mutation in the MVK gene on chromosome 12, which encodes for mevalonate kinase. Ancestry is usually Dutch, French, or other European descent. Symptoms may start in the first year of life and can include periodic fever, vomiting, diarrhea, arthritis, lymphadenopathy, splenomegaly, and maculopapular rash. Other cutaneous findings in HIDS may include urticaria, erythematous nodules, morbilliform rash, annular erythema, purpura, and petechiae. Serum IgD level may be elevated during an acute attack.

PFAPA syndrome is characterized by high periodic fevers, pharyngitis, lymphadenopathy, and splenomegaly. Attacks last 4 to 5 days with a symptom-free period of 4 to 7 weeks. All patients with the syndrome have periodic fever and at least one of the following: aphthous stomatitis, pharyngitis, or splenomegaly. Growth and development are normal in this syndrome. Corticosteroids or cimetidine have been beneficial in PFAPA patients.

TRAPS includes the dominantly inherited periodic fever syndromes such as familial Hibernian fever. The affected gene is TNFRSF1A, which encodes for a tumor necrosis factor receptor. Clinical manifestations include periodic attacks of fever, abdominal pain, and myalgias. Other features include episodic erythematous patches, conjunctivitis, and unilateral periorbital edema. Unlike FMF and HIDS, the febrile attacks in TRAPS can last for weeks. Effective treatments have included corticosteroids and TNF antagonists.

In summary, the periodic fever syndromes are a heterogeneous group of disorders characterized by episodic fevers and other systemic systemic sequelae. Because of the combination of fever and abdominal pain, an acute attack can masquerade as acute appendicitis. Cyclic neutropenia must also be ruled out when considering periodic fever. The syndromes may be difficult to distinguish clinically but can often be diagnosed with genetic testing. Aggressive treatment with potentially toxic medications is warranted when there are disturbances of growth, development, or function.

Idiopathic Musculoskeletal Pain Syndromes

The idiopathic musculoskeletal pain syndromes are characterized by intense chronic pain in light of an essentially healthy physical examination. The nomenclature can be confusing, and it includes syndromes such as fibromyalgia, reflex sympathetic dystrophy, reflex neurovascular dystrophy, complex regional pain syndrome, myofascial pain, causalgia, pain amplification, and neuropathic pain.

Children with chronic pain present with a mean age of onset of 12 years. Female-to-male ratio is 4:1. In the history, a triggering event may sometimes be identified. For example, the pain may begin after a minor sprain or fall. In other cases, the pain begins after the onset of a stressful event in the child's life such as a divorce or a death in the family. Children can present with marked pain and disability. Limp, dependence on crutches or a wheelchair, or bracing of a limb have all been observed. The pain can be described as intense, burning, sharp, and numbing, and the severity is often a 10 on a 1 to 10 scale. The pain may be exacerbated by bizarre triggers, such as the wind blowing on the skin, putting on a sock, or light touch. Pain-relieving medications offer little or no relief.

A complete psychosocial history must be obtained in families with suspected idiopathic musculoskeletal pain syndrome. In some families there is a model for pain—adult family members may have fibromyalgia, chronic back pain, migraines, or other forms of chronic pain. Patients are often described as high achievers, perfectionistic, and having a desire to please. Many are straight-A students, successful athletes, or talented musicians. In witnessing the interaction between the mother and the patient, the examiner may note *enmeshment,* in which a child is directly asked a question and the mother acts as the spokesperson.

Children with localized idiopathic musculoskeletal pain may report changes in color, temperature, or perspiration in an affected part of the body. The body part, such as a hand or a foot, may be guarded and braced by the child. The pain usually follows a nonanatomical distribution. On physical examination, light touch by the examiner may elicit a wince-and-withdraw reaction. The allodynia has a variable border, such that successive examinations will feature different areas of pain distribution.

In generalized idiopathic musculoskeletal pain, patients often present with the triad of disorganized sleep, lack of exercise, and widespread body pain. Fatigue is a common symptom. Teenage patients often enter a cycle of sleeping irregularly with daytime napping, reducing aerobic exercise, and developing muscle and joint pain. On physical examination there may be tender points as in adult fibromyalgia patients.

Patients who present with idiopathic musculoskeletal pain syndromes often undergo extensive medical testing. Repeated phlebotomy, radiographs, nuclear scintigraphy, magnetic resonance imaging, endoscopy, and surgical biopsy have been performed in these patients to try to identify the etiology of pain. Testing is normal or noncontributory.

Treatment begins by making the diagnosis on clinical grounds and ceasing medical testing. The patient's pain should be acknowledged without judgment. Therapy involves intensive desensitization physical therapy, aerobic exercise, normalization of sleep pattern, and psychological counseling. Comorbidities include anxiety, depression, eating disorders, and family dysfunction. When a child presents with chronic idiopathic musculoskeletal pain, the syndrome often envelops the entire family. Delay in diagnosis can increase the frustration and anxiety. With physical therapy, psychology, and sometimes family therapy, the child can be returned to normal function.

Acknowledgments

We extend our deepest thanks to the original author of this chapter—Dr. Aldo V. Londino. Dr. Londino, until the time of his passing in 2000, was the sole pediatric rheumatologist in Western Pennsylvania and was widely recognized for his superb teaching and clinical skills. We are also grateful for the contributions of Drs. Andrew H. Urbach; Bernard Cohen; John Zitelli; A'Delbert Bowen; Basil Zitelli; J. Carlton Gartner, Jr.; J. Jeffrey Malatack; Joseph McGuire; Holly Davis; Virginia Steen; Joseph Warnicki; Albert Biglan; Cora Lennox; Sang Park; Chester Oddis; Alexi Grom; David Witte; and Susan Gelnett for their valuable assistance with photographs and text.

Bibliography

Cassidy JT, Petty RE: Textbook of Pediatric Rheumatology, 4th ed. Philadelphia, WB Saunders, 2001.

Emery H: Pediatric scleroderma. Semin Cutan Med Surg 17:41-47, 1998.

Hsieh Y, Wu M, Wang J, et al: Clinical features of atypical Kawasaki disease. J Microbiol Immunol Infect 35:57-60, 2002.

Kakalamani VG, Vaiopoulos G, Kaklamanis PG: Behçet's disease. Semin Arthritis Rheum 27:197-217, 1998.

Kone-Paut I, Yurdakul S, Bahabri SA, et al: Clinical features of Behçet's disease in children: An international collaborative study of 86 cases. J Peds 132:721-725, 1998.

Lee W, Yang M, Lee K, et al: PFAPA syndrome (periodic fever, aphthous stomatitis, pharyngitis, adenitis). Clin Rheum 18:207-213, 1999.

Narchi H: Risk of long term renal impairment and duration of follow up recommended for Henoch-Schönlein purpura with normal or minimal urinary findings: A systematic review. Arch Dis Child 90:916-920, 2005.

Newburger JW, Takahashi M, Gerber MA, et al: Committee on Rheumatic Fever, Endocarditis, and Kawasaki Disease, Council on Cardiovascular Disease in the Young, American Heart Association: Diagnosis, treatment, and long-term management of Kawasaki disease: A statement for health professionals from the Committee on Rheumatic Fever, Endocarditis, and Kawasaki Disease, Council on Cardiovascular Disease in the Young, American Heart Association. Pediatrics 114:1708-1733, 2004.

Petri M: Hopkins Lupus Cohort. 1999 update. Rheum Dis Clin N Am 26:199-213, 2000.

Oen K, Malleson PN, Cabral DA, et al: Disease course and outcome of juvenile rheumatoid arthritis in a multicenter cohort. J Rheum 29:9, 2002.

Ramanan AV, Feldman BM: Clinical features and outcomes of juvenile dermatomyositis and other childhood onset myositis syndromes. Rheum Dis Clin N Am 28:833-857, 2002.

Reed AM, Mason T: Recent advances in juvenile dermatomyositis. Curr Rheum Reports 7:94-98, 2005.

Saulsbury FT: Henoch-Schönlein purpura: Report of 100 patients and review of the literature. Medicine 78:395-409, 1999.

Schneider R, Passo MH: Juvenile rheumatoid arthritis. Rheum Dis Clin N Am 28:503-530, 2002.

Sherry DD: An overview of amplified musculoskeletal pain syndromes. J Rheum Suppl 58:44-48, 2000.

Thomas KT, Feder HM Jr, Lawton AR, Edwards K: Periodic fever syndrome in children. J Pediatr 135:15-21, 1999.

Vierra E, Cunningham BB: Morphea and localized scleroderma in children. Semin Cutan Med Surg 18:210-225, 1999.

CHAPTER 8

Dermatology

*BERNARD A. COHEN, HOLLY W. DAVIS,
AND ROBIN P. GEHRIS*

Most of us think of our skin as a simple durable covering for our skeleton, muscles, and internal organs. However, the skin is a complex organ, consisting of many parts and appendages (Fig. 8-1). The outermost layer, the stratum corneum, is an effective barrier to irritants, toxins, and organisms, as well as a membrane that holds in body fluids. The remainder of the epidermis manufactures this protective layer. Melanocytes within the epidermis help protect us from the harmful effects of ultraviolet light, and Langerhans cells are one of the body's first lines of immunologic defense.

The dermis, consisting largely of fibroblasts and collagen, is a tough, leathery, mechanical barrier against cuts, bites, and bruises. Its collagenous matrix also provides structural support for a number of cutaneous appendages. Hair, which grows from follicles deep within the dermis, is important for cosmesis and protection from sunlight and particulate matter. Sebaceous glands are outgrowths of the hair follicles. Oil produced by these glands helps to lubricate the skin and contributes to the protective epidermal barrier. The nails are specialized organs of manipulation that also protect the sensitive digits. Thermoregulation of the skin is accomplished by eccrine sweat glands and changes in cutaneous blood flow, which is regulated by glomus cells. The skin also contains specialized receptors for heat, pain, touch, and pressure. Sensory input from these structures helps to protect the skin surface against environmental trauma. Beneath the dermis, in the subcutaneous tissue, fat acts as stored energy and as a soft, protective cushion.

Defects or alterations in any component of the skin may result in serious systemic disease or death. Each and every part of the skin can be affected by congenital, inflammatory, infectious, and degenerative disorders and tumors. For example, an altered stratum corneum is seen in ichthyosis, melanocytes are selectively destroyed in vitiligo, the epidermis proliferates in psoriasis, excess collagen is produced in the connective tissue nevus of tuberous sclerosis, hair is preferentially infested by certain fungi, and so on. In addition, the skin is affected by many systemic diseases and thus may provide visible markers for internal disorders. A skin examination may demonstrate lesions of vasculitis, explaining a child's hematuria. The white macules of tuberous sclerosis may give insight into the cause of seizures.

Examination and Assessment of the Skin

The skin is the largest, most accessible, and most easily examined organ of the body and is the organ of most frequent concern to patients. Therefore physicians should be able to recognize basic skin diseases and dermatologic clues to systemic disease.

Optimal examination of the skin is performed in a well-lit room. The physician should inspect the entire skin surface including hair, nails, scalp, and mucous membranes. This may be particularly problematic with infants and teenagers because it may be necessary to examine the skin in small segments to prevent cooling or embarrassment. Although no special equipment is required, a hand lens and side lighting aid in the assessment of skin texture and small, discrete lesions. A Wood's lamp can improve precision in distinguishing hypopigmented from depigmented patches of skin.

Despite the myriad conditions affecting the skin, a systematic approach to the evaluation of a rash or exanthem assists and simplifies the process of developing a manageable differential diagnosis. After assessing the patient's general health, the practitioner should obtain a detailed history of the skin symptoms including the date of onset, inciting factors, evolution of lesions, and

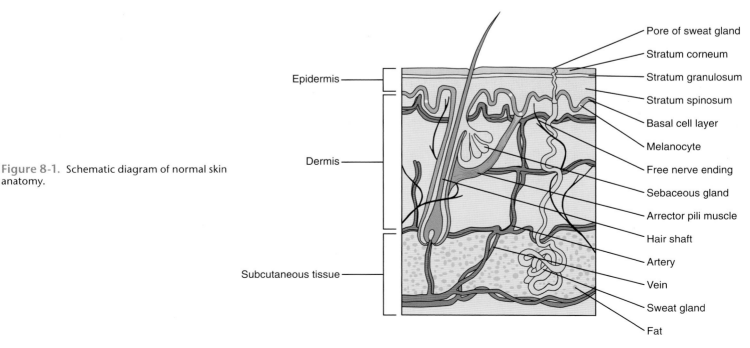

Figure 8-1. Schematic diagram of normal skin anatomy.

Epidermis

Dermis

Subcutaneous tissue

Pore of sweat gland
Stratum corneum
Stratum granulosum
Stratum spinosum
Basal cell layer
Melanocyte
Free nerve ending
Sebaceous gland
Arrector pili muscle
Hair shaft
Artery
Vein
Sweat gland
Fat

presence or absence of pruritus. Recent immunizations, infections, drugs, and allergies may be directly related to new rashes. The family history may suggest a hereditary or contagious process, and the clinician may need to examine other members of the family. Review of nursery records and photographs helps to document the presence of congenital lesions. Attention should then turn to the distribution and pattern of the rash. The term *distribution* refers to the location of the skin findings, whereas the term *pattern* defines a specific anatomic or physiologic arrangement (e.g., the distribution of a rash may include

the extremities, face, or trunk, and the pattern could be flexural or intertriginous). Identification of a pattern can assist in the development of a differential diagnosis even before the detailed morphology of the skin lesions is studied. Other common patterns include sun-exposed sites, acrodermatitis (involvement primarily of the distal extremities), pityriasis rosea, clothing-covered sites, acneiform rashes (Fig. 8-2), and dermatomal configurations.

Next, the clinician should consider the local *organization* of the lesions, defining the relationship of primary and secondary lesions to one another in a given location.

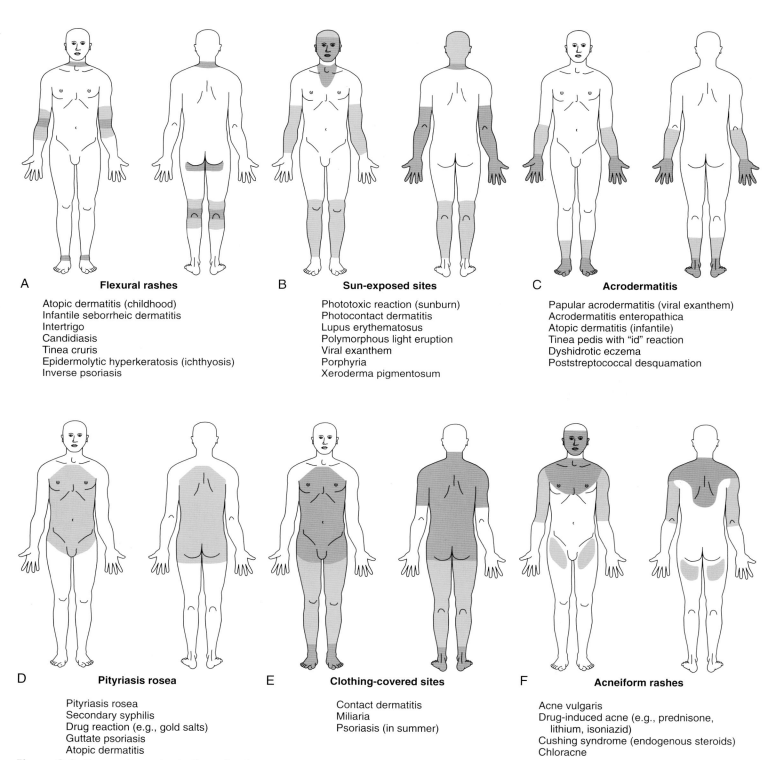

A   Flexural rashes

Atopic dermatitis (childhood)
Infantile seborrheic dermatitis
Intertrigo
Candidiasis
Tinea cruris
Epidermolytic hyperkeratosis (ichthyosis)
Inverse psoriasis

B   Sun-exposed sites

Phototoxic reaction (sunburn)
Photocontact dermatitis
Lupus erythematosus
Polymorphous light eruption
Viral exanthem
Porphyria
Xeroderma pigmentosum

C   Acrodermatitis

Papular acrodermatitis (viral exanthem)
Acrodermatitis enteropathica
Atopic dermatitis (infantile)
Tinea pedis with "id" reaction
Dyshidrotic eczema
Poststreptococcal desquamation

D   Pityriasis rosea

Pityriasis rosea
Secondary syphilis
Drug reaction (e.g., gold salts)
Guttate psoriasis
Atopic dermatitis

E   Clothing-covered sites

Contact dermatitis
Miliaria
Psoriasis (in summer)

F   Acneiform rashes

Acne vulgaris
Drug-induced acne (e.g., prednisone,
   lithium, isoniazid)
Cushing syndrome (endogenous steroids)
Chloracne

Figure 8-2. Pattern diagnosis. **A,** Flexural rashes. **B,** Sun-exposed sites. **C,** Acrodermatitis. **D,** Pityriasis rosea. **E,** Clothing-covered sites. **F,** Acneiform rashes.

Table 8-1	Anatomic Depth of Lesions	
CUTANEOUS STRUCTURE	**PHYSICAL FINDINGS**	**SPECIFIC SKIN DISORDERS**
Epidermis	Altered surface markings Scale, vesicle, crust Color changes (black, brown, white)	Impetigo Café-au-lait spot Atopic dermatitis Vitiligo Freckle
Epidermis + dermis	Altered surface markings Scale, vesicle, crust Distinct borders Color changes (black, brown, white, and/or red) Edema	Psoriasis Atopic dermatitis Contact dermatitis Cutaneous lupus erythematosus
Dermis	Normal surface markings Color changes Altered dermal firmness	Urticaria Granuloma annulare Hemangioma Blue nevus
Subcutaneous tissue	Normal surface markings Normal or red skin color Altered skin firmness	Hematoma Cold panniculitis Erythema nodosum

From Cohen BA: Pediatric Dermatology, 2nd ed. London, Mosby, 1999.

Are the lesions scattered or clustered (herpetiform)? Are they linear, serpiginous, confluent, or discrete?

Finally, the practitioner should identify the *morphology* of the cutaneous lesions. *Primary lesions* (macules, papules, wheals, plaques, vesicles, bullae, nodules, and tumors) arise de novo in the skin. *Secondary lesions* (pustules, erosions, ulcers, crusts, excoriations, fissures, lichenification, atrophy, and scars) evolve from primary lesions or result from the patient's manipulation (e.g., scratching, picking, or popping) of primary lesions. Delineation of the primary and secondary lesions allows the clinician to develop a differential diagnosis on the basis of the *anatomic level* of the skin lesions (Table 8-1). Disorders restricted to the epidermis may be associated with macular color changes, such as in vascular telangiectasias, freckles, and vitiligo. In *epidermal disorders,* surface markings are commonly altered by scales, vesicles, pustules, crusts, and erosions. Bullous impetigo, atopic dermatitis, and ichthyosis are primarily epidermal disorders. When the dermis is also involved, lesions usually display distinct borders because of dermal inflammation and edema. Disorders with both epidermal and dermal changes include psoriasis, lichen planus, and erythema multiforme. Inflammatory disorders or tumors restricted to the dermis do not usually alter the surface markings. Lesional borders are distinct, and color changes and edema may be present. Examples of *dermal disorders* include granuloma annulare, intradermal nevi, urticaria, and hemangiomas. The diagnosis of *subcutaneous disorders* is made by careful palpation. The surface markings are normal, and the color of the skin may be normal or red. There is altered skin firmness, and tenderness may be present. Subcutaneous lesions include lipomas, deep hemangiomas, hematomas, subcutaneous fat necrosis, and erythema nodosum.

Because an outline of specific pediatric dermatoses defies any one scheme of organization, this text follows a clinically practical format. First, this chapter covers common papulosquamous and vesiculopustular eruptions, which account for a majority of rashes seen in children. This is followed by sections covering reactive erythemas, insect bites and infestations, tumors and infiltrations of the skin, neonatal dermatology, vascular lesions, congenital and acquired nevi, and disorders of pigmentation. The chapter concludes with a discussion of disorders of the hair and nails and complications of topical therapy.

Papulosquamous Disorders

Papulosquamous eruptions share the morphologic features of papules and scales. However, the clinician must understand that the papulosquamous disorders, which are quite diverse, are produced by a variety of different mechanisms. In psoriasis, increased production of keratinocytes by the basal cell layer results in a markedly thickened epidermis and stratum corneum (scaly surface layer). In dermatitic processes such as atopic dermatitis, contact dermatitis, seborrheic dermatitis, pityriasis rosea, and fungal infections, inflammation results in increased production and abnormal maturation of epidermal cells, with subsequent scale production. Increased adherence of cells in the stratum corneum may result in the retention hyperkeratosis characteristic of ichthyosis vulgaris, which is frequently found in association with atopic dermatitis.

Psoriasis

Psoriasis is a common disorder characterized by red, well-demarcated plaques covered with dry, thick, silvery scales. These tend to be located on the extensor surfaces of the extremities, the scalp, and the buttocks). In some patients, the distribution consists of large lesions over the pressure points of the knees and elbows (Fig. 8-3A-D). Thickening and fissuring of the skin of the palms may also be seen (Fig. 8-3E). In some children, numerous droplike (guttate) lesions are found scattered over the body (Fig. 8-4), often after a bout of group-A β-hemolytic streptococcal infection (which may have been recognized or have been subclinical). In infants, psoriasis may present as a persistent diaper dermatitis (see Fig. 8-45). Lesions of psoriasis are often induced at sites of local injury such as scratches, surgical scars, or sunburn, a response termed the *Koebner phenomenon* (Fig. 8-5). Nail changes include reddish-brown psoriatic plaques in the nail bed (oil drop changes), surface pitting, and distal hyperkeratosis (see Fig. 8-148).

The factors that initiate the rapid turnover in epidermal cells that produce the psoriatic plaques are unknown, although an inherited predisposition is suspected and upper respiratory tract and streptococcal infections may precipitate lesions, especially in cases of guttate psoriasis.

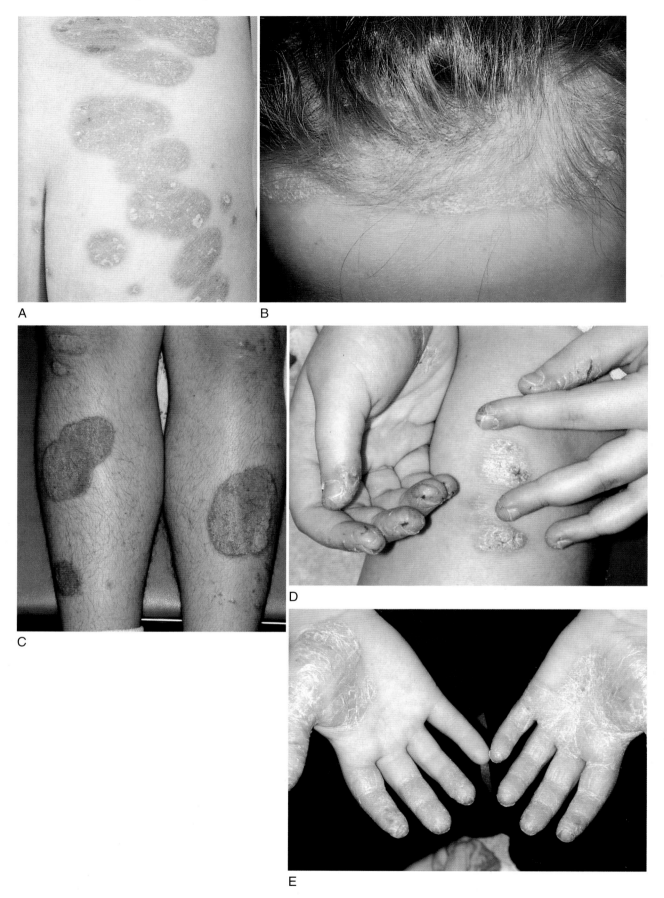

Figure 8-3. Psoriasis. **A,** Typical erythematous plaques are topped by a silver scale. **B,** Thick tenacious scale on a red base extends from the forehead to the scalp of this 10-year-old girl. **C,** Large plaques are located over the shins and right knee. **D,** In this child lesions are prominent over the pressure point of the knee and the distal fingers. **E,** The skin of the palms is markedly thickened, with silvery fissuring of the palmar creases.

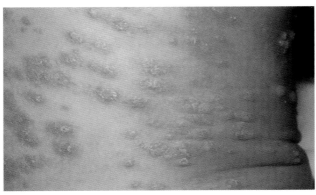

Figure 8-4. Guttate psoriasis. Small droplike plaques with typical scales quickly developed in a generalized distribution in this child following strep-tococcal pharyngitis. (From Cohen BA: Atlas of Pediatric Dermatology. London, Mosby-Wolfe, 1993.)

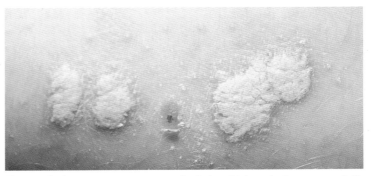

Figure 8-6. Auspitz sign. Removal of the thick scale from a psoriatic plaque produces small points of bleeding from tortuous capillaries.

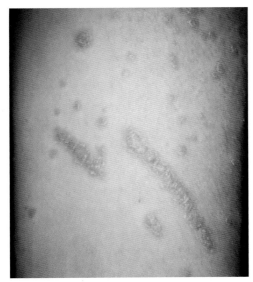

Figure 8-5. Koebner phenomenon in psoriasis. Lesions are often induced in areas of local trauma such as these scratches.

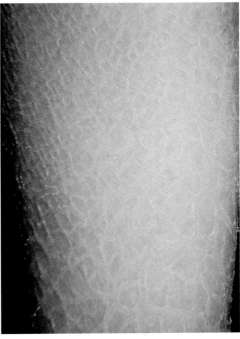

Figure 8-7. Ichthyosis vulgaris. The typical fish scale appearance is seen in this closeup of a fair-skinned patient's shin.

Although the increased epidermal growth causes a thickening of the skin in the psoriatic plaque, there are also areas between the epidermal ridges where the skin is thin and the scale is close to the subepidermal vessels. Thus when the scale is removed, small bleeding points are often seen. This is called the *Auspitz sign,* and it is the hallmark of psoriasis (Fig. 8-6).

Except in cases of guttate psoriasis, which are usually self-limited, the course of psoriasis is chronic and unpredictable, marked by remissions and exacerbations. Although psoriasis is thought to be rare in childhood, 37% of adults with the disorder first develop lesions before the age of 20.

The Ichthyoses

Ichthyosis refers to a group of genodermatoses characterized by dry, scaly skin. Various types have been identified according to clinical course; histopathology; biochemical markers; and, in some cases, specific genetic mutations.

Ichthyosis Vulgaris

Ichthyosis vulgaris is transmitted as an autosomal dominant trait and affects about 0.5% of the population. Although the rash is not present at birth, by 3 months of age thick, fishlike scales may be apparent on the shins and extensor surfaces of the arms (Fig. 8-7). Occasionally, scales become more generalized, involving the trunk, but the flexures are usually spared. Lesions tend to flare during the winter (because of the drying effect of central heating) and improve during the summer, particularly with increasing age. Biopsy of involved skin shows retention hyperkeratosis and a thinned granular layer in the epidermis. Liberal use of topical emollients usually keeps pruritus and scaling under control.

X-Linked Ichthyosis

X-linked ichthyosis occurs in 1 in 6000 males, although findings are occasionally present in hemizygous female carriers. Affected newborns may have a collodion membrane at birth (see Fig. 8-93) but more commonly present between 3 and 12 months of age with generalized "dirty" brown scales, particularly on the abdomen, back, and anterior legs and feet (Fig. 8-8). The central face and flexures are spared. Skin biopsy demonstrates an increased granular layer and stratum corneum, and biochemical studies demonstrate decreased or absent steroid sulfatase in the serum and skin.

Lamellar Ichthyosis

Lamellar ichthyosis is a rare autosomal dominant disorder occurring in less than 1 in 250,000 births. Infants are usually born with a collodion membrane (see Fig. 8-93). During the first month of life, thick, brownish gray, sheet-like scales with raised edges appear. Scaling is prominent over the face, trunk, and extremities (Fig. 8-9). In contrast to ichthyosis vulgaris, the flexural areas are involved in the lamellar form (Fig. 8-9B). Eversion and fissuring of the eyelid margins (ectropion) and lips (eclabium) are common

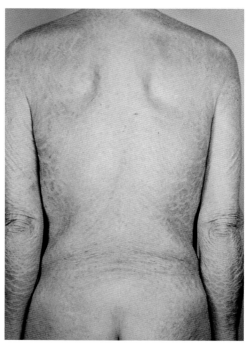

Figure 8-8. X-linked ichthyosis. "Dirty" brown scales persist on the flanks, elbows, and shoulders despite the use of topical lubricants.

complications (Fig. 8-9C). The palms and soles show thick keratoderma with fissuring. Some improvement of the scaling occurs with age, and topical keratolytics such as lactic acid and salicylic acid may provide some benefit. Severe cases may respond to oral administration of retinoids such as 13-*cis*-retinoic acid.

Epidermolytic Hyperkeratosis

Epidermolytic hyperkeratosis is a rare autosomal dominant form of ichthyosis characterized by the development of generalized, thick, warty scales and intermittent blistering with severe involvement of the flexures (Fig. 8-10). In newborns, blisters may be widespread, suggesting a diagnosis of herpes simplex or epidermolysis bullosa. Histologically, massive hyperkeratosis is associated with ballooning of squamous cells and formation of microvesicles. Epidermal turnover is also markedly increased. The mainstay of treatment includes use of keratolytics, lubricants, and antibiotics for secondary infection, which is common and usually caused by *Staphylococcus aureus*. Oral retinoids may also significantly decrease scaling.

The Dermatitides

Depending on duration of involvement, the dermatitides are characterized clinically by acute changes (including redness, edema, and vesiculation) and/or chronic changes (such as scaling, lichenification, and increased or decreased pigmentation) in the skin. Microscopically, these disorders are characterized by infiltration of the dermis with inflammatory cells, variable thickening of the epidermis, and scaling.

Atopic Dermatitis (Eczema)

Atopic dermatitis, or eczema, is one of the most common and stressful of all chronic skin disorders in children. This

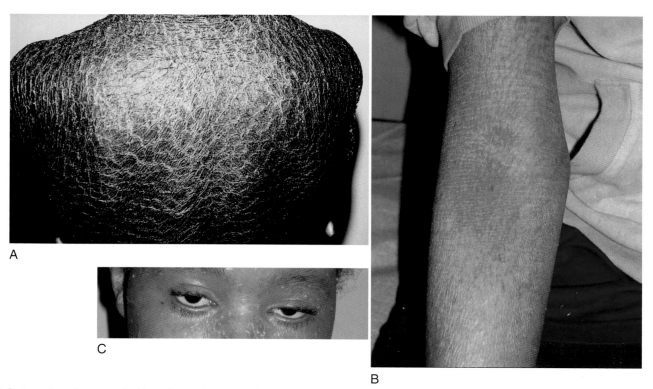

Figure 8-9. Lamellar ichthyosis. **A,** Note the thick, brownish-black scales covering the entire skin surface. **B,** Flexural involvement helps differentiate lamellar ichthyosis from ichthyosis vulgaris. **C,** Ectropion (note the exsersion of the lower lids) is a unique finding in this form of the disorder.

entity is divided into three phases on the basis of the age of the patient, each having a different distribution.

The *infantile phase* of atopic dermatitis begins between 1 and 6 months of age and lasts about 2 or 3 years. Characteristically, the rash is manifest by red, itchy papules and plaques that ooze and crust. Lesions are distributed over the cheeks, forehead, scalp, trunk, and extensor surfaces of the extremities, and patches are often symmetrical (Fig. 8-11).

The *childhood phase* of atopic dermatitis occurs between ages 4 and 10 years. The dermatitis is typically dry, papular, and intensely pruritic. Circumscribed scaly patches are distributed on the wrists, ankles, and antecubital and popliteal fossae (Fig. 8-12); these patches frequently become secondarily infected, probably as a result of organisms introduced by intense scratching. Cracking, dryness, and scaling of the palmar and plantar surfaces of the hands and feet are also common (Fig. 8-13). Remission may occur at any time, or the disorder may evolve into a more chronic type of adult dermatitis. Of children with atopic dermatitis, 75% improve between the ages of 10 and 14; the remaining children may go on to develop chronic dermatitis.

The *adult phase* of atopic dermatitis begins around age 12 and continues indefinitely. Major areas of involvement include the flexural areas of the arms, neck, and legs (Fig. 8-14). Eruptions are sometimes seen on the dorsal surfaces of the hands and feet and between the fingers and toes. Lichenification may be marked (Fig. 8-15).

Other associated findings include xerosis (dryness); ichthyosis vulgaris (see Fig. 8-7); **keratosis pilaris**, keratin plugging of hair follicles and formation of perifollicular scales over the extensor surfaces of the extremities and sometimes the trunk and abdomen (Fig. 8-16 and see also Fig. 8-25D); hyperlinearity of the palms; Dennie-Morgan lines (double skin creases under the lower eyelid [see Chapter 4]); and hyperpigmentation and hypopigmentation, which may be marked and at times may be the predominant findings (see Figs. 8-124 and 8-125). There is also some evidence that patients with atopic dermatitis may have altered cellular immunity. More than 90% are colonized with *Staphylococcus aureus* at the time of a flare; and many appear to be unusually susceptible to other cutaneous infections including warts, herpes simplex, and molluscum contagiosum. Patients with eczema should be warned to avoid people with cold sores because they are at great risk for developing generalized eczema herpeticum (see Fig. 12-13). Parents of children with eczema who themselves have recurrent herpes simplex lesions should be taught hygienic techniques that reduce the risk of transmitting the virus to their children.

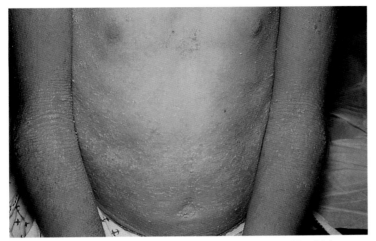

Figure 8-10. Epidermolytic hyperkeratosis is characterized by thick, warty scales and intermittent blistering. The flexural creases are particular sites of involvement.

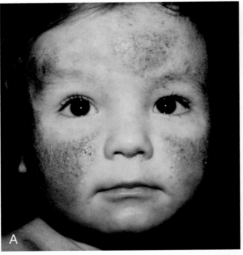
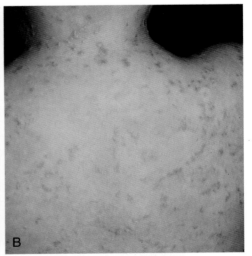
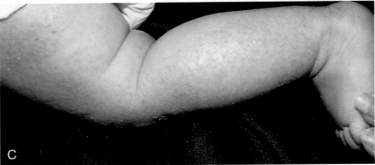

Figure 8-11. Infantile atopic dermatitis or eczema. **A,** This infant has an acute, weeping dermatitis on the cheeks and forehead. **B** and **C,** Involvement of the trunk and the extremities, with erythema, scaling, and crusting, are evident. Usually the diaper area is the only portion of the skin surface that is spared. (**B** and **C,** From Fireman P, Slavin RG: Atlas of Allergies. New York, Gower, 1991.)

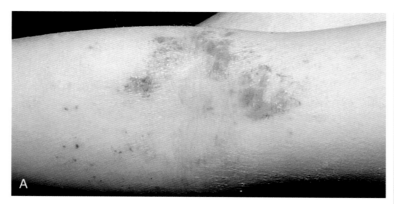

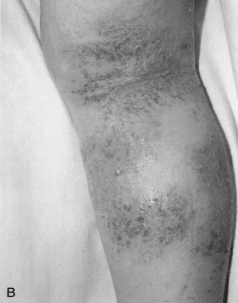

Figure 8-12. Childhood atopic dermatitis with lesions on the arms **(A)** and the legs **(B).** In childhood, eczema involves the flexural surfaces of the upper and lower extremities. The neck, ankles, wrists, and posterior thighs also may be severely affected. (**A,** From Fireman P, Slavin RG: Atlas of Allergies. New York, Gower, 1991; **B,** Courtesy Michael Sherlock, MD, Lutherville, Md.)

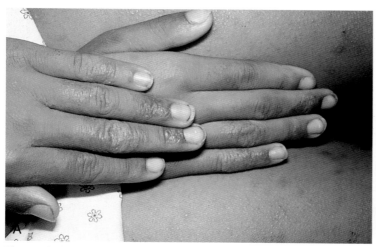

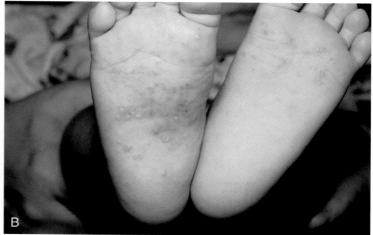

Figure 8-13. Involvement of the hands and feet in eczema. **A,** A 10-year-old atopic child has lichenification of the skin over the dorsum of his fingers and "buff" nails from chronic rubbing. **B,** This infant has numerous red excoriated lesions over the soles of his feet.

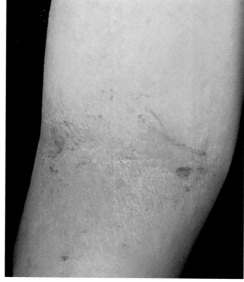

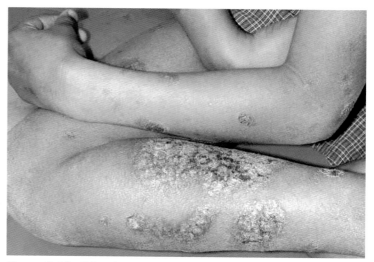

Figure 8-15. Lichenification refers to marked thickening of the skin seen in areas of atopic dermatitis that have been subject to chronic scratching. In addition, this patient demonstrates significant postinflammatory hyperpigmentation.

Figure 8-14. Adult atopic dermatitis. Erythematous excoriated plaques with indistinct borders are seen in the antecubital areas. Note the dried blood from recent excoriation.

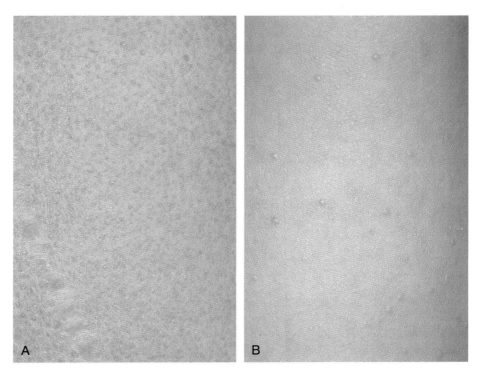

Figure 8-16. Keratosis pilaris. **A,** Diffuse fine follicular papules and sandpaper scaling are seen on the extensor surface of the arm of this adolescent. **B,** In this 5-year-old boy, characteristic white follicular papules are more widely spaced and more prominently seen on the extensor surface of his thighs and upper arms. His mother had similar lesions. (Courtesy Cohen BA, Lehman CU [eds]: Johns Hopkins University Dermatlas. Available at http://www.dermatlas.org.)

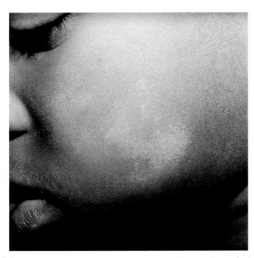

Figure 8-17. Pityriasis alba. In some atopic individuals, subtle inflammation may result in development of poorly demarcated, hypopigmented patches that are covered by a fine superficial scale.

In the rash of *pityriasis alba,* which is common in patients with atopic dermatitis, inflammatory changes are minimal. Poorly defined, hypopigmented, round or oval scaly patches measuring 2 to 4 cm in diameter are noted most commonly on the face and extremities (Fig. 8-17), although they may involve the trunk as well. Lesions are more prominent in children with dark skin and are more noticeable during spring and summer because they do not tan like surrounding skin. Surface scaling is more evident when the skin is dry (especially in winter). Etiology is unknown. Because the disorder is usually asymptomatic and spontaneously resolves in several months to a few years, treatment is usually unnecessary, although moisturizers may help reduce surface scaling.

The cause of atopic dermatitis remains elusive. An immunologic etiology is suggested by the chronic elevation of IgE seen in a majority of patients. Some investigators propose an aberrant cutaneous response to histamine and other mediators of inflammation as a primary mechanism. However, laboratory findings vary from patient to patient and in the same patient at different times in the course of the disease. Atopic dermatitis does seem to occur in families and in association with other atopic conditions including asthma, allergic rhinitis, and food allergies, suggesting some degree of genetic predisposition. Pathophysiologically, a number of external factors including dry skin, soaps, wool fabrics, foods, infectious agents, and environmental antigens may act individually or in concert to produce pruritus, which is universal in atopic individuals. The resultant scratching leads to the acute and chronic changes typical of atopic dermatitis.

The differential diagnosis of atopic dermatitis includes seborrhea, contact dermatitis, pityriasis rosea, psoriasis, fungal infections, Langerhans cell histiocytosis, and acrodermatitis enteropathica. It can be distinguished from seborrhea on the basis of the distribution of lesions and associated pruritus; atopic dermatitis spares moist, intertriginous areas such as the axillae and perineum, where seborrhea is prominent. Exposure history and distribution help differentiate it from contact dermatitis, as does the discreteness of lesions and their distribution in pityriasis rosea. The thick, silvery scale and Koebner phenomenon help distinguish psoriasis, and central clearing with an active border of red papules, vesicles, and/or pustules helps differentiate tinea corporis. The rash of histiocytosis is crusted, atrophic and may be more generalized. It is associated with petechiae and often accompanied by chronically draining ears, hepatosplenomegaly, and lymphadenopathy (see Fig. 8-85 and Chapter 11). The acral and periorificial distribution of lesions and gastrointestinal symptoms help in distinguishing eczema from acrodermatitis enteropathica.

The mainstays of atopic dermatitis treatment are elimination or avoidance of predisposing factors, hydration and lubrication of the skin, use of antipruritic agents to relieve itching and break the itch-scratch cycle, and the use of topical steroids to further relieve itching and decrease inflammation. Pimecrolimus cream and tacrolimus ointment are two agents in the new class of nonsteroidal topical immunomodulators that may also dramatically interrupt the itch-scratch cycle. They have been approved as second-line therapy for the management of atopic dermatitis in children older than 2 years of age. Use of these agents should be accompanied by an explanation of the boxed warning regarding the theoretical risk of lymphoma and skin cancer. However, these tumors have only been seen with systemic use.

All children with atopic dermatitis should be monitored closely for secondary bacterial infection, which must be treated promptly with topical or systemic antibiotics to prevent progression to cellulitis. Herpes simplex can also rapidly disseminate in patients with active atopic dermatitis, resulting in the severe disorder known as *eczema herpeticum* (see Fig. 12-13). Hence, patients' families should be warned to have their children avoid contact with people with cold sores, and if parents have recurrent herpes labialis, they should be instructed in strict hand washing precautions. Further, patients should be treated with antiviral agents at the first sign of infection with herpes simplex.

Dyshidrotic eczema and *nummular eczema* are manifestations of atopic dermatitis, whereas *juvenile plantar-palmar dermatosis* and *lip-licking* and *thumb-sucking eczema* represent irritant dermatitides that may be associated with atopic dermatitis.

Dyshidrotic Eczema
Dyshidrosis is a severely pruritic, chronic, recurrent, vesicular eruption affecting the palms, soles, and lateral aspects of the fingers and toes. Characteristically, the vesicles are symmetrical, multilocular, and 1 to 3 mm in diameter. These lesions rupture, leaving scales and crust on an erythematous base (Fig. 8-18). Pathologically, this eruption demonstrates spongiotic vesicles and normal eccrine sweat glands. The cause is unknown; however, frequent exposure to water, wet or sweat-soaked shoes, or chemicals (on the hands) may trigger or exacerbate the condition. Hyperhidrosis, or excessive sweating of the palms and soles, may also play a role. Treatment is similar to that for acute atopic dermatitis. Use of charcoal-

impregnated foam insoles can significantly improve conditions affecting the foot.

Nummular Eczema
Nummular eczema is an acute papulovesicular eruption named for its coin-shaped configuration. Lesions are intensely pruritic, well-circumscribed, round to oval, red, scaly patches studded with 1- to 3-mm vesicles (Fig. 8-19A). They are usually located on the extensor thighs or abdomen of children who also may have atopic dermatitis. Vigorous scratching causes excoriation and crusting (Fig. 8-19B). Lack of central clearing helps distinguish these lesions from tinea corporis (see Fig. 8-35). Although the rash is often resistant to therapy, it may respond to the treatment for acute dermatitis outlined previously. Treatment with oral antibiotics that cover *S. aureus* may hasten resolution.

Juvenile Plantar-Palmar Dermatosis
Juvenile plantar-palmar dermatosis ("sweaty sock syndrome") is common in toddlers and school-age children. Chronic, red scaly patches with cracking and fissuring

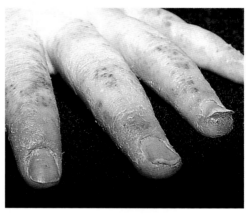

Figure 8-18. Dyshidrosis. Chronic cracking, oozing, and scaling develop after the initial tiny pruritic vesicles have been scratched.

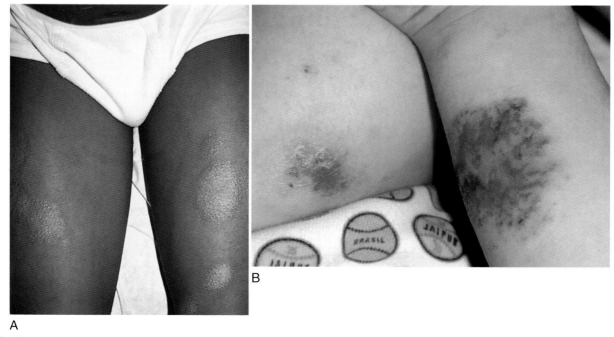

A

B

Figure 8-19. Nummular eczema. **A,** Round- to oval-shaped lesions studded with tiny vesicles are typically located over the extensor thighs or abdomen. They do not show central clearing. **B,** Vigorous scratching results in excoriation with weeping and crusting. (**A,** Courtesy Michael Sherlock, MD, Lutherville, Md.)

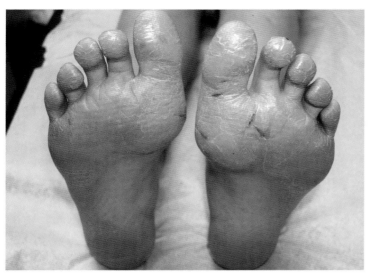

Figure 8-20. Juvenile plantar dermatosis. This variant of atopic dermatosis is usually localized to the plantar surfaces of the toes and feet. Note the glistening erythema, scaling, and fissuring. In some patients the palms may be affected as well.

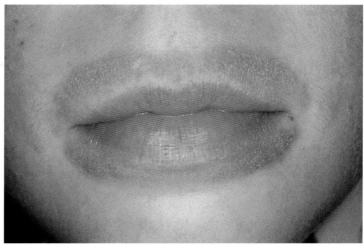

Figure 8-21. Lip-licking eczema. The perioral skin is inflamed, scaly, and thickened as a result of repetitive licking of the lips. (Courtesy Douglas W. Kress, MD, University of Pittsburgh Medical Center.)

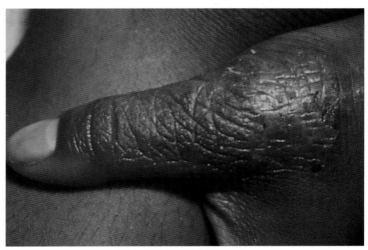

Figure 8-22. Thumb-sucking eczema. Repeated wetting and drying from persistent thumb sucking result in eczematoid changes with cracking, fissuring, and lichenification. (Courtesy Michael Sherlock, MD, Lutherville, Md.)

typically begin in the fall or winter on the anterior plantar surfaces of the feet and big toes (Fig. 8-20).The palms may be involved as well, though less severely. Although the cause is unknown, the condition is triggered by excessive sweating and/or repeated wetting of the skin inside the child's shoes (especially those made of synthetic materials that do not breathe), followed by drying of the skin at night. Consequently, the mainstay of treatment consists of lubricating and covering the feet at night. Topical steroids may be necessary in severe cases. The eruption tends to subside in the summer, and resolution in adolescence is common. Use of charcoal-impregnated foam insoles is also helpful.

Lip-Licking and Thumb-Sucking Eczema
The repeated wetting and drying from persistent lip licking (especially in winter) or thumb sucking can produce eczematoid changes of the perioral skin (Fig. 8-21) or the skin of the involved thumb (Fig. 8-22). Lip-licking eczema can be the result of a habit or can be a manifestation of anxiety, and sources of stress should be explored on history taking. Once the process begins, it can become a vicious cycle as the child licks with increasing frequency to moisten the dry skin.

Seborrhea
Seborrheic dermatitis is characterized by a red scaling eruption that occurs predominantly on hair-bearing and intertriginous areas such as the scalp, eyebrows, eyelashes, perinasal, presternal, and postauricular areas and the neck, axillae, and groin. Lesions often involve the intertriginous areas of the arms, legs, neck and trunk, and occasionally become generalized (Fig. 8-23A-D). In affected infants, scalp lesions consist of a thick, tenacious, scaly dermatitis that is often salmon colored and is commonly known as *cradle cap* (Fig. 8-24A and B). In adolescents the dermatitis may manifest as dandruff or flaking of the eyebrows, postauricular areas, or flexural areas.

Although the pathogenesis of seborrheic dermatitis is unknown, *Pityrosporum* and *Candida* species have been implicated as causative agents. A role for neurologic dysfunction is suggested by the increased incidence and severity in neurologically impaired individuals.

The dermatitis of seborrhea is usually nonpruritic and mild in nature. Most cases respond to topical steroids, and many clear spontaneously, although residual postinflammatory hypopigmentation may persist for weeks or months thereafter (see Fig. 8-125). Some practitioners find that use of a topical antifungal cream, as well as a low-potency topical steroid, hastens resolution. Antiseborrheic shampoos may also be helpful for patients with scalp involvement. In infants and young children, atopic dermatitis can have a greasy, scaly appearance and may be confused with seborrhea. However, infantile atopic dermatitis produces intense pruritus and invariably spares moist sites such as the diaper area and axillae. The differential diagnosis of seborrhea also includes Langerhans cell histiocytosis (in which the rash is generalized, in part petechial, and usually associated with chronic draining ears and hepatosplenomegaly) and tinea corporis (in which lesions usually are more circumscribed, with an active border and central clearing). Scalp lesions may be difficult to differentiate from psoriasis.

Hyper-IgE (Job) Syndrome
Job syndrome is a rare genetic disorder with prominent cutaneous manifestations. It has been linked to a muta-

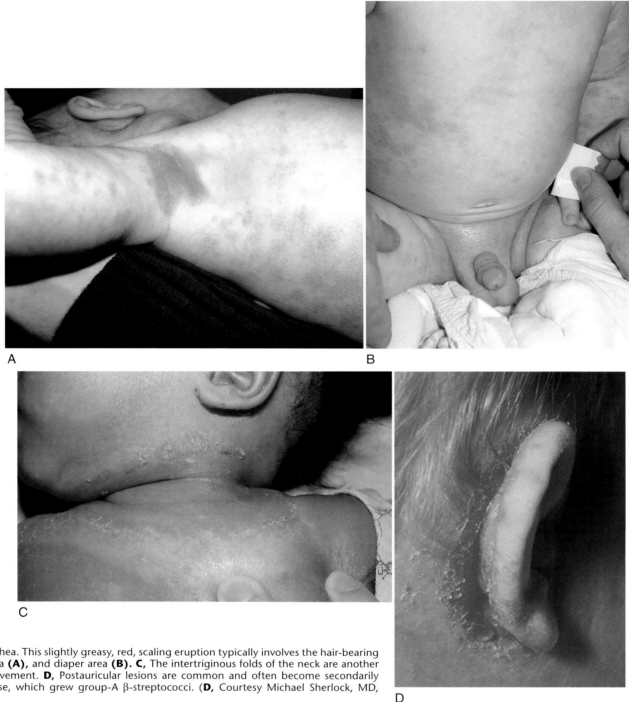

Figure 8-23. Seborrhea. This slightly greasy, red, scaling eruption typically involves the hair-bearing areas of the face, axilla **(A)**, and diaper area **(B)**. **C,** The intertriginous folds of the neck are another common site of involvement. **D,** Postauricular lesions are common and often become secondarily infected as in this case, which grew group-A β-streptococci. (**D,** Courtesy Michael Sherlock, MD, Lutherville, Md.)

tion on chromosome 4q and is usually inherited as an autosomal dominant trait with variable severity of expression. Affected patients have abnormalities of the immune response involving T-lymphocytes, neutrophils, cytokines, and interleukins. They also have variably but significantly elevated levels of serum IgE and circulating eosinophils.

Dermatologic features include a pruritic dermatitic rash that shares features with both atopic dermatitis and seborrhea, and which tends to develop shortly after birth (earlier than seborrhea and atopic dermatitis). It rapidly becomes superinfected with *S. aureus,* which results in formation of weeping, crusting, and folliculitic lesions, as well as cutaneous abscesses (Fig. 8-25A-D). In contrast to furuncles in patients with a normal immune response, the abscesses in children with Job syndrome cause little pain and show few signs of inflammation. Development of

mucocutaneous candidiasis is also common. Other clinical manifestations include recurrent/chronic infections such as bronchitis, pneumonia (with pneumatoceles), sinusitis, otitis, gingivitis, dental abscesses, septic arthritis, and osteomyelitis. Decreased bone density is the source of multiple fractures, which cause remarkably little pain. With age and growth, facial features tend to coarsen (see Fig. 4-57) and scoliosis is common.

Treatment is aimed at controlling infections and ameliorating symptoms. The major differential diagnostic consideration is Langerhans histiocytosis (see Fig. 8-85).

Pityriasis Rosea

Pityriasis rosea is a benign, self-limited disorder that can occur at any age but is more common in adolescents and young adults. A prodrome of malaise, headache, and mild

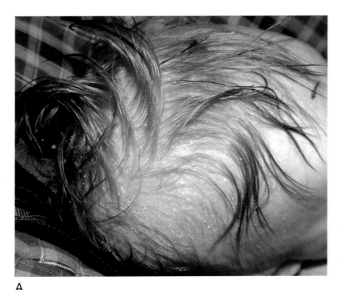

A

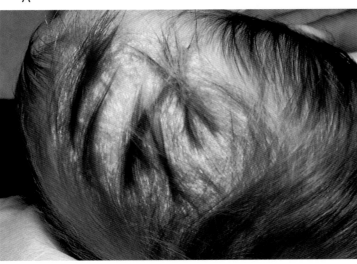

B

Figure 8-24. Seborrhea of the scalp. **A,** Note the oily appearance and salmon-pink hue. Numerous scales, some adherent to the scalp and many interlaced through the baby's hair, are present. **B,** In this infant the scales have formed a thick crust, and erythema is less evident.

constitutional symptoms occasionally precedes the rash. The typical eruption begins with the appearance of a "herald patch" (Fig. 8-26A), which is a large, isolated, oval lesion, usually pink in color and slightly scaly; it may occur anywhere on the body. Occasionally, it clears centrally, simulating tinea corporis. From 5 to 10 days later, other smaller lesions appear on the body, frequently concentrated over the trunk but also seen on the proximal extremities, especially the thighs (see Fig. 8-26B-G). On occasion, lesions predominate on the face and distal extremities including the palms and soles, a phenomenon known as *inverse pityriasis,* which is more common in African-American boys. Pityriasis lesions begin as small, round papules that enlarge to ovals up to 1 to 2 cm in size, with a scaly surface. They are usually somewhat raised but can be macular, and they can be erythematous, hyperpigmented, or hypopigmented. The long axes of the ovals tend to run parallel to the lines of the cleavage of the skin, creating a "Christmas tree" pattern over the thorax (Fig. 8-26C and D). The rash reaches its peak in several weeks, then slowly fades over 4 to 6 weeks. The average total duration is 2 to 3 months. Oral erythromycin and ultra-

violet light may hasten the disappearance of the eruption. Although the cause is unknown, the peak incidence in late winter and the low recurrence rate favor an infectious etiology.

Other eruptions that can resemble pityriasis rosea include guttate psoriasis, benign parapsoriasis, viral exanthems, measle-like (morbilliform) drug eruptions, and secondary syphilis (see Fig. 18-32). As noted earlier, the appearance of the herald patch may simulate tinea corporis, but a potassium hydroxide (KOH) preparation is negative.

Contact Dermatitis

Contact dermatitis refers to a group of conditions in which a dermatitic or inflammatory reaction in the skin is triggered by direct contact with environmental agents. In the most common form, *irritant contact dermatitis,* changes in the skin are induced by caustic agents such as acids and alkalis, hydrocarbons, and other primary irritants. Anyone exposed to these agents in a high enough concentration for a long enough period will ultimately develop a contact dermatitis. The rash is usually acute, with well-demarcated erythema, crusting, and/or blister formation.

In contrast, allergic contact dermatitis is a T-lymphocyte–mediated immune reaction to an antigen coming into contact with the skin. Although patients typically present with acute onset of erythema, vesiculation, and pruritus, in some cases they delay seeking care until after the rash has become chronic with scaling, lichenification, and pigmentary changes. Often, the allergen is obvious, as is the case with poison ivy or nickel jewelry. However, in other cases, careful questioning may be required to detect the inciting agent.

The initial reaction occurs after a 7- to 14-day period of sensitization in susceptible individuals. Once sensitization has occurred, reexposure to the allergen provokes a more rapid reaction, sometimes within hours. This is a classic example of type IV (delayed) hypersensitivity (see Chapter 4).

Rhus Dermatitis (Poison Ivy). The most common type of allergic contact dermatitis in the United States is poison ivy, or rhus dermatitis. This typically presents as linear streaks of erythematous papules and vesicles (Fig. 8-27A); however, with heavy exposure, the rash may appear in relatively large patches (Fig. 8-27B and C). When lesions involve the skin of the face or genitalia, impressive swelling can occur (Fig. 8-27D).

Direct contact with the sap of poison ivy, poison oak, or poison sumac from leaves, stems, or roots (whether the plant is alive or dead) produces the dermatitis (Fig. 8-28). Contact with clothing that has brushed against the plant, with logs or railroad ties on which the vine has been growing, or with smoke from a fire in which the plant is being burned are other means of exposure. Areas of skin exposed to the highest concentration of plant oil develop changes first. Other sites that received lower doses then vesiculate in succession, giving the illusion of spreading. This is not the case however, as within about 20 minutes of initial contact, the rhus oil becomes tissue-fixed to the epithelial cells and cannot be spread farther. Thorough washing within minutes of exposure can prevent fixation, and hence, the eruption.

Other Common Causes of Contact Dermatitis. Other common offending agents are nickel (Fig. 8-29), rubber (Fig. 8-30), glues and/or dyes in shoes (Fig. 8-31), ethylenediamine in topical lotions, neomycin, and topical anesthetics (Fig. 8-32). Paraphenylenediamine dye used in amateur henna tattoos is an increasingly common cause

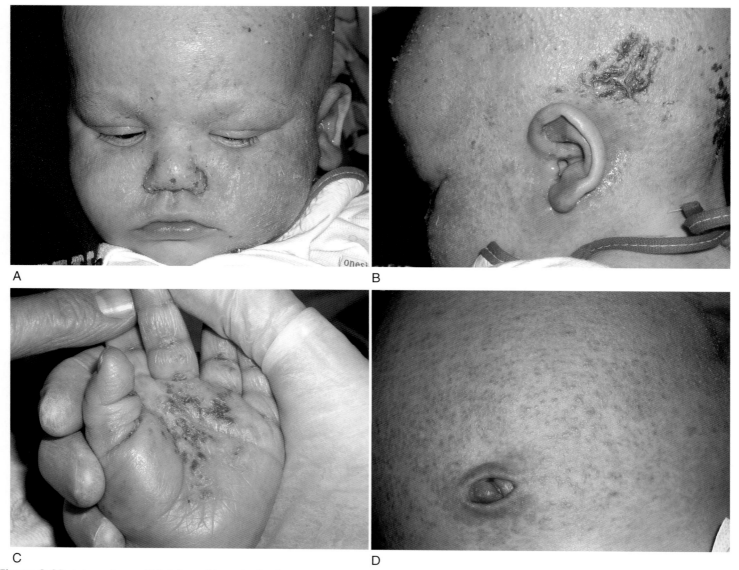

Figure 8-25. Job syndrome. This infant with markedly elevated IgE experienced early onset of a pruritic dermatitis that shared clinical features with both seborrhea and atopic dermatitis. **A,** Note the erythema and scaliness, the evidence of excoriation from scratching, and the perinasal crusting due to *Staphylococcus aureus* infection. **B,** In this view, in addition to the erythema, scaling, and thickening of the skin, there are weeping areas around the ear and crusts and scabs over the scalp. Note also the purulent ear drainage. **C,** He also had crusted palmar lesions. **D,** The skin over his abdomen had the classic features of keratosis pilaris.

of contact dermatitis among adolescents, and the pattern reflects the image of the original tattoo (Fig. 8-33).

Photocontact Dermatitis and Phototoxic Reactions. Photocontact or photoallergic dermatitis is a true cell-mediated delayed hypersensitivity reaction and necessitates a 7- to 10-day period of sensitization, after which sun exposure may precipitate development of a dermatitic or urticarial eruption. When caused by systemically administered drugs, it characteristically erupts in a symmetrical distribution on the face, the V of the neck, and the arms and legs distal to the end of shirt sleeves and shorts. Potentially causative agents include the tetracyclines, sulfonylureas, thiazides, nonsteroidal anti-inflammatory drugs, fluoroquinolones, and griseofulvin. Topical photosensitizers (sunscreens with PABA esters or oxybenzone; fragrances in soaps, creams, lotions or cosmetics; coal tar; furocoumarins; and halogenated salicylanilides in germicidal soaps) produce localized patches of dermatitis when used on sun-exposed sites (Fig. 8-34).

Phototoxins, when applied to the skin, are the source of a non-immunologic exaggerated sunburn reaction in which the initial erythema progresses to hyperpigmenta-tion. Of these, phytophotodermatitis is the most common. In this form, plant-derived photosensitizers, psoralens, found in the juice of lemons, limes, figs, dill, parsley, parsnips, carrots, and celery, are responsible for the reaction. Typically a child is touched by a parent who has been cutting the fruit, herbs, or vegetables, thereby getting the juice on the child's skin. Subsequent exposure to sunlight then results in the appearance of erythematous macules, with or without accompanying bullae, which then go on to become hyperpigmented. These patches often have bizarre or hand/finger-shaped patterns that can mimic child abuse (see Fig. 6-66).

"Id" Reaction. Occasionally, the local reaction of a contact dermatitis is so severe that the patient develops a widespread secondary eczematous dermatitis. When the dermatitis appears at sites that have not been in contact with the offending agent, the reaction is referred to as autoeczematization or an "id" reaction. Id reactions can also occur in patients with tinea, especially coincident with the start of oral therapy.

Basic Principles of Management. Although localized patches of contact dermatitis are best treated topically,

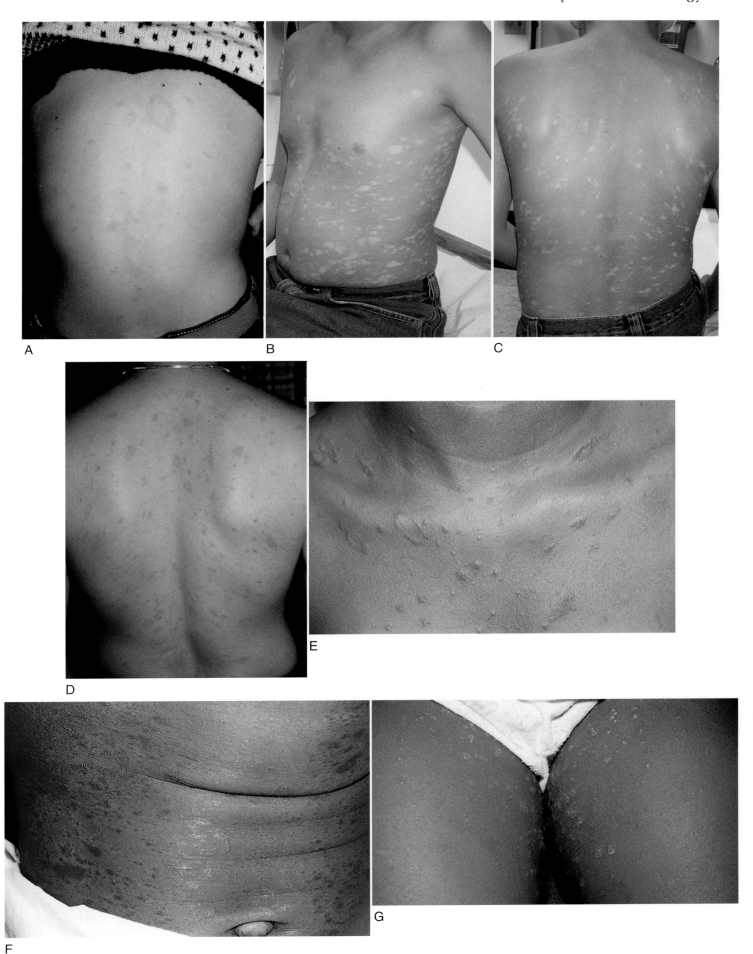

Figure 8-26. Pityriasis rosea. **A,** The large herald patch on this boy's back shows evidence of central clearing, mimicking tinea corporis. **B,** Numerous oval lesions with their long axes oriented along lines of skin cleavage are seen over the trunk of this adolescent. **C** and **D,** This feature creates the appearance of a fir tree distribution on the back. **E-G,** Lesions can be raised, macular, or scaly and can be erythematous, or hyper- or hypopigmented. (**A** and **C,** Courtesy Douglas W. Kress, MD, University of Pittsburgh Medical Center; **E** and **F,** Courtesy Michael Sherlock, MD, Lutherville, Md.)

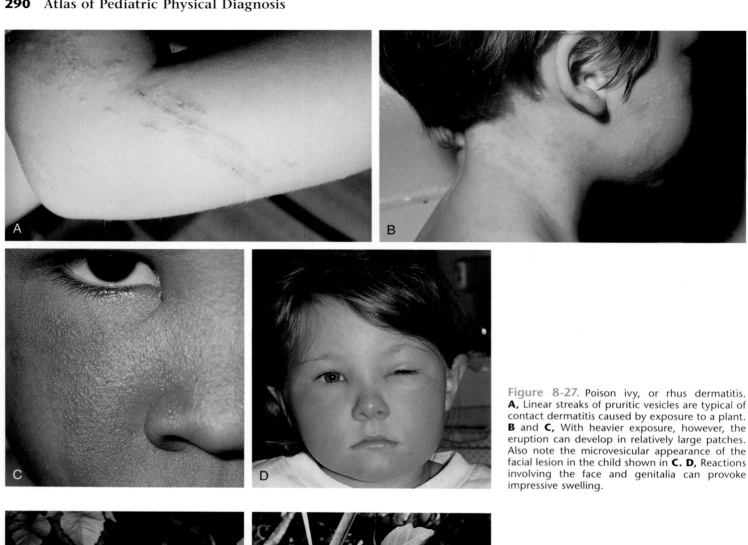

Figure 8-27. Poison ivy, or rhus dermatitis. **A,** Linear streaks of pruritic vesicles are typical of contact dermatitis caused by exposure to a plant. **B** and **C,** With heavier exposure, however, the eruption can develop in relatively large patches. Also note the microvesicular appearance of the facial lesion in the child shown in **C. D,** Reactions involving the face and genitalia can provoke impressive swelling.

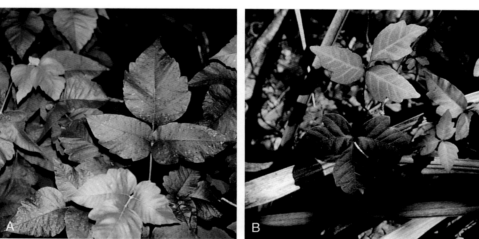

Figure 8-28. **A,** Poison ivy. The plant has characteristic shiny leaves in groups of three. It may resemble a vine, a low shrub, or a bush. **B,** Poison oak. This also has leaves in groups of three, although the edges tend to be more scalloped than those of poison ivy. (**B,** Courtesy Mary Jelks, MD.)

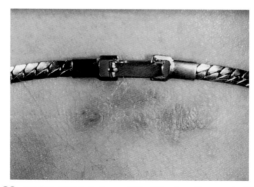

Figure 8-29. Nickel contact dermatitis. The location and distribution of the rash is often helpful in determining the cause of a contact dermatitis. In this case wrist lesions were triggered by the nickel in her bracelet clasp.

widespread reactions require a 2-week tapering course of systemic corticosteroids beginning at 0.5 to 1 mg/kg/day. Patients may experience rebound of the rash if treated with a shorter course. Response usually occurs within 48 hours. Oral steroids may also be indicated in localized reactions involving the eyelids, extensive areas of the face, genitals, and/or hands, where swelling and pruritus may become incapacitating.

Prevention requires identification of the offending agent and then its avoidance. Children with rhus dermatitis should be shown pictures of the causative plants and taught where they are commonly found. Patients sensitive to nickel must ensure that jewelry, particularly earring posts, are made of 24-karat gold, stainless steel, or sterling silver. However, painting watchband buckles with clear nail polish every several weeks can obviate the difficult

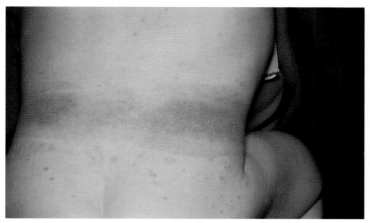

Figure 8-30. Rubber contact dermatitis. This child had become sensitized to the elasticized waist bands of his underpants.

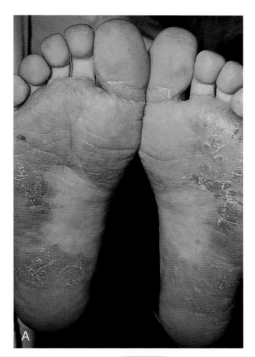

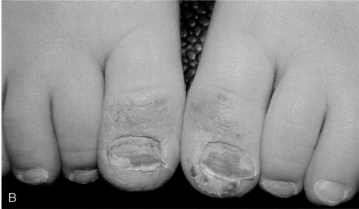

Figure 8-31. Contact dermatitis of the foot due to glues/dyes in shoes. **A,** This adolescent became sensitized to the glue under the insoles of his shoes. Note the sparing of the instep. **B,** Another child had a similar problem with the toe reinforcers in his shoes. Note that the web spaces are spared. (**A,** Courtesy Michael Sherlock, MD, Lutherville, Md.; **B,** Courtesy Douglas W. Kress, MD, University of Pittsburgh Medical Center.)

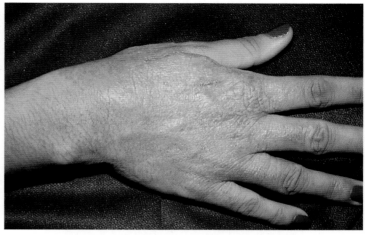

Figure 8-32. Contact dermatitis due to topical anesthetics. This adolescent became sensitized to the topical anesthetic Lanacaine in a moisturizing cream that she applied to her hands daily. Note the line of demarcation at the wrist.

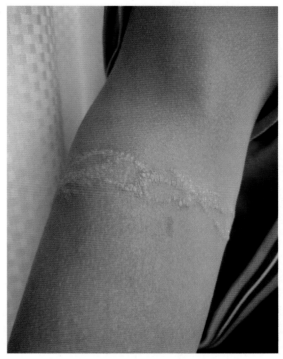

Figure 8-33. Contact dermatitis due to henna dye. This young teenager developed vesicular lesions in the precise pattern of a henna tattoo she had had applied 2 weeks earlier.

task of trying to find watchbands with pure gold or silver buckles.

Fungal Infections

Two types of fungal organisms produce clinical cutaneous disease: dermatophytes and yeasts. Dermatophytes include the tinea or ringworm fungi, and yeasts include *Candida* species, which are associated with diaper dermatitis and *Pityrosporum* species, which cause tinea versicolor. Both *Candida* and *Pityrosporum* have been implicated as partially causative in seborrhea.

Tinea Corporis

Tinea corporis is a superficial fungal infection of the nonhairy or glabrous skin. It has been labeled "ringworm"

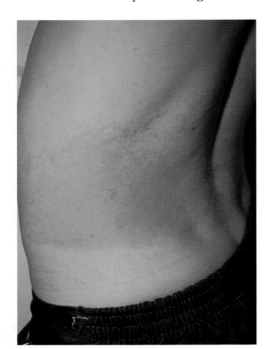

Figure 8-34. Photocontact dermatitis. This boy developed contact dermatitis after sun exposure while outside for a day of swimming. The offending agent was found to be in his soap. (Courtesy Michael Sherlock, MD, Lutherville, Md.)

because of its characteristic configuration consisting of pruritic, annular lesions with central clearing and an active border made up of microvesicles that rupture and then scale (Fig. 8-35A-C). Lesions, which may be single or multiple, typically begin as pruritic red papules or pustules that rupture and evolve to form papulosquamous lesions, which are also pruritic. These then spread out from the periphery as new vesicles form at their outer margins, and at the same time begin to clear centrally (see Fig. 8-35D and E). Over a period of several weeks, the patches may expand up to 5 cm in diameter. Tinea corporis can be found in any age group and is usually acquired through direct human contact (*Trichophyton tonsurans*) or from an infected kitten.

Clinically, tinea may be differentiated from atopic dermatitis by the propensity for autoinoculation from the primary patch to other sites on the patient's skin, by the spread to close contacts, and by the central clearing noted in many lesions. Moreover, the rash of atopic dermatitis tends to be symmetrical, chronic, and recurrent in a flexural distribution. Unlike tinea, patches of nummular eczema are self-limited and do not clear centrally. The herald patch of pityriasis rosea is often mistaken for tinea. However, it is KOH negative, and the subsequent development of the generalized rash with its characteristic truncal distribution is distinctive (see Fig. 8-26). The clinical pattern, findings, and chronic nature of psoriasis and seborrhea help differentiate them from tinea. Although granuloma annulare produces a characteristic ringed eruption, on palpation the lesions are firm and usually asymptomatic. They tend not to show epidermal changes other than occasional slight scaling (see Fig. 8-86).

The diagnosis of tinea corporis is confirmed by KOH examination of skin scrapings. The first step is to obtain material by scraping the loose scales at the margin of a lesion (Fig. 8-36A). These should be mounted onto the center of a glass slide, with one or two drops of 20% KOH solution added. Next, a glass coverslip is applied and gently pressed down with the eraser end of a pencil to crush the scales (Fig. 8-36B). The clinician then heats the slide, taking care not to boil the KOH solution, and again the coverslip is pressed down. When viewing the slide under the microscope, the clinician sets the condenser and light source at low levels to maximize contrast, with the objective at ×10. On focusing up and down, true hyphae are seen as long, branching, often septate rods of uniform width that cross the borders of epidermal cells (Fig. 8-37). Cotton fibers, cell borders, or other artifacts may be falsely interpreted as positive findings.

Tinea infections on glabrous skin readily respond to topical antifungal creams such as miconazole, clotrimazole, econazole, naftifine, ketoconazole, and ciclopirox. When lesions are multiple and widespread, oral therapy with griseofulvin is indicated. Although not yet approved by the Food and Drug Administration for the treatment of dermatophytoses in children, itraconazole, terbinafine, and fluconazole are good alternatives for systemic antifungal therapy. Like griseofulvin, they are effective against most ringworm organisms, but unlike griseofulvin, these medications are concentrated in skin, hair, and nails for weeks to months after they are discontinued.

Tinea Pedis

Commonly referred to as *athlete's foot*, tinea pedis is a fungal infection of the feet with a predilection for the web spaces between the toes. Tinea pedis is quite common in adolescence, somewhat less so in prepubertal children. The infecting organisms are acquired from contaminated shower, bathroom, locker room, and gym floors, and their growth is fostered by the warm, moist environment of shoes.

In some cases, scaling and fissuring predominate; in others, vesiculopustular lesions and maceration are found. The infection begins between and along the sides of the toes, where it may remain (Fig. 8-38A). However, lesions can extend over the dorsum of the foot (see Fig. 8-38B) and may involve the plantar surface as well, particularly the instep and ball of the foot. Patients complain of a combination of burning and itching, which is frequently intense.

This diagnosis often can be made on clinical grounds and is confirmed by KOH preparation of skin scrapings. The mainstays of treatment are topical antifungal creams or powders, as well as measures designed to reduce foot moisture. The latter include careful drying of the feet after bathing, wearing cotton rather than synthetic socks, and wearing shoes that do not promote sweating or, better still, sandals. In patients with severe inflammatory lesions, oral antifungal agents may be required. Onychomycosis (see Fig. 8-144) responds well only to oral agents and requires treatment for 4 months, occasionally longer (see later, "Disorders Affecting the Nails"). Secondary bacterial infection (particularly with gram-negative organisms) may be a problem.

Tinea pedis is distinguished from contact dermatitis of the feet by virtue of the fact that the latter spares the interdigital web spaces (see Fig. 8-31). Dyshidrosis can have a similar distribution, but KOH preparation is negative (see Fig. 8-18).

Tinea Versicolor

Tinea versicolor is a common dermatosis characterized by multiple small, oval, scaly patches measuring 1 to 3 cm in diameter, usually located in a guttate or raindrop pattern on the upper chest, back, and proximal portions of the upper extremities of adolescents and young adults (Fig. 8-39A and B). However, all ages may be affected,

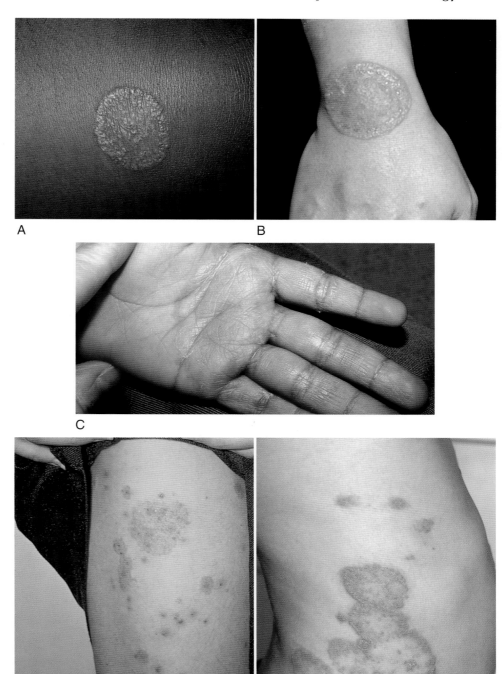

Figure 8-35. Tinea corporis. The characteristic annular lesions show many variations in appearance. **A,** This lesion has a raised, active border and shows partial central clearing. **B,** In another case the inflammatory response is intense, and only a little central clearing is seen. **C,** The lesion shown here involving the palm and flexor surfaces of the fingers is macular and scaly and has a sharply circumscribed proximal border. **D,** The evolution of lesions from papules and pustules into larger papulosquamous patches is seen on this girl's leg. **E,** In another child, small papules, plaques that have not cleared centrally, and larger lesions with varying degrees of central clearing are seen. (**B,** Courtesy Douglas W. Kress, MD, University of Pittsburgh Medical Center; **D,** Courtesy Michael Sherlock, MD, Lutherville, Md.)

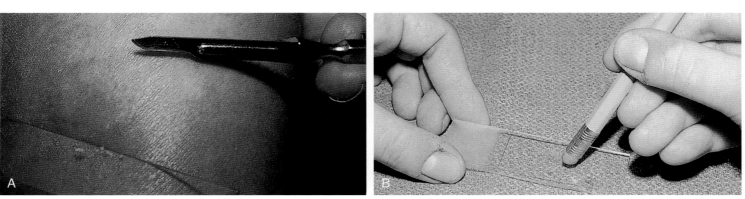

Figure 8-36. Potassium hydroxide (KOH) preparation. **A,** Small scales should be scraped from the edge of the lesion onto a microscope slide. **B,** To more easily visualize the fungus, the scales should be crushed, making a thin layer of cells.

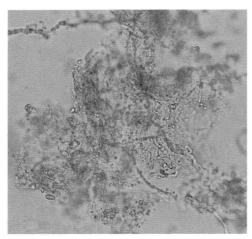

Figure 8-37. Positive KOH preparation of skin scrapings. Fungal hyphae are seen as long septate branching rods at the margins and center of the scales.

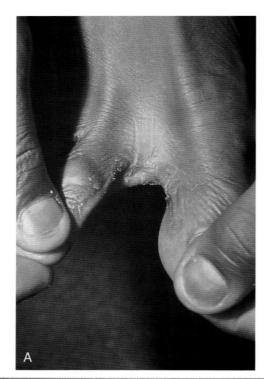

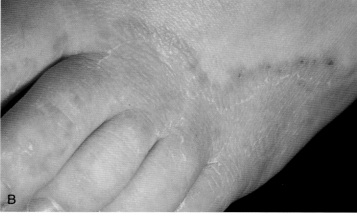

Figure 8-38. Tinea pedis. **A,** Cracking and scaling are seen in the web space. **B,** In this patient the lesions began in the web spaces but then extended onto the dorsum of the foot. Note the active border. (**B,** Courtesy Douglas W. Kress, MD, University of Pittsburgh Medical Center.)

including infants. Facial involvement occurs occasionally. The eruption is caused by a dimorphous form of *Pityrosporum*. Warm, moist climates, pregnancy, immunodeficiency, and genetic factors predispose people to the development of infection.

The rash is usually asymptomatic, although some patients complain of mild pruritus. Typically, patients go to the physician because they are bothered by the cosmetic appearance of the lesions. Lesions may be light tan, reddish, or white in color, giving rise to the term *versicolor*. They are darker than surrounding skin in non–sun-exposed areas (Fig. 8-39C) and lighter in areas that have tanned on exposure to sunlight (see Fig. 8-39A and B).

The diagnosis of tinea versicolor can generally be made on the basis of the clinical appearance of lesions and their distribution. It can be confirmed by examining the lesions under a Wood's lamp, which reveals a characteristic tan to salmon-pink glow. Although pathogenesis of the color change under a Wood's lamp is not fully understood, the fungus is known to produce a substance that interferes with tyrosinase activity and subsequent melanin synthesis. A KOH preparation of the surface scale demonstrates short hyphal and yeast forms that resemble spaghetti and meatballs (Fig. 8-40).

The differential diagnosis of tinea versicolor includes postinflammatory hypopigmentation and vitiligo. The history and distribution help to distinguish tinea versicolor from postinflammatory hypopigmentation; the presence of fine superficial scaling and some residual pigmentation (even in hypopigmented areas) help rule out vitiligo.

Topical desquamating agents such as selenium sulfide and propylene glycol produce rapid clearing of the superficial lesions. Localized eruptions may be treated with topical antifungal creams such as miconazole, clotrimazole, or econazole, and recalcitrant cases respond to oral fluconazole or itraconazole. Patients must be counseled about the high risk of recurrence, which often necessitates ongoing prophylactic selenium sulfide washes for several days each month. They should also be reminded that pigmentary changes may take months to clear, even after eradication of the fungus.

Diaper Dermatitis

Because the diaper area is warm, often moist, and frequently contaminated by feces laden with organisms, diaper dermatitis is one of the most common skin disorders of infancy and early childhood.

Irritant Diaper Dermatitis

The diaper area is a prime target for irritant dermatitis because it is bathed in urine and stool and occluded by plastic diaper covers. Failure to change diapers frequently is a major predisposing factor because it provides time for fecal bacteria to form ammonia by splitting the urea in urine. Harsh soaps, irritant chemicals, and detergents can contribute to the process. Moderate to severe diarrhea is another predisposing condition. The erythema; scaling; and, at times, maceration characteristic of irritant diaper dermatitis are usually confined to the convex surfaces of the perineum, lower abdomen, buttocks, and proximal thighs, sparing intertriginous areas (Fig. 8-41). When neglected, this may progress, with further skin breakdown and ulceration. Frequent diaper changes; gentle, thorough cleansing of the area; and application of lubricants and barrier pastes usually result in clearing of the dermatitis.

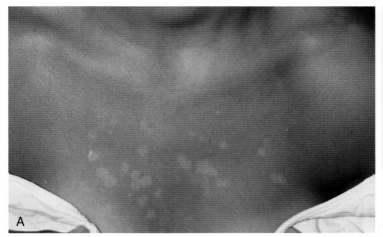

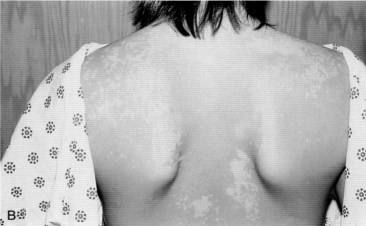

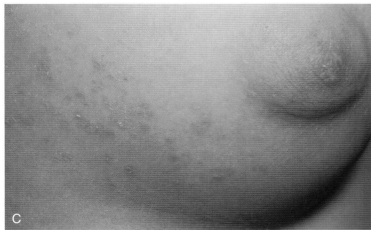

Figure 8-39. Tinea versicolor. **A** and **B,** Multiple oval patches are seen in a guttate or raindrop pattern over the upper chest and back of two patients. **C,** In areas not exposed to sunlight, lesions are darker than surrounding skin, whereas in **A** and **B** sun-exposed lesions fail to tan, remaining lighter than surrounding skin. (Courtesy Michael Sherlock, MD, Lutherville, Md.)

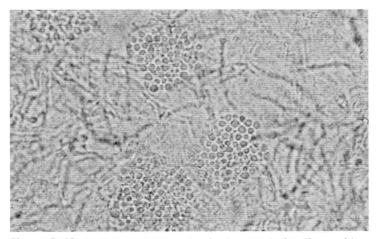

Figure 8-40. Positive KOH preparation for tinea versicolor. The combination of hyphal and yeast forms of the fungus simulates the appearance of spaghetti and meatballs.

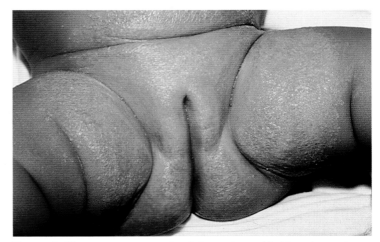

Figure 8-41. Irritant or ammoniacal diaper dermatitis. Note the erythema and scaling involving the convex surfaces and sparing the intertriginous creases.

A short course of low-potency steroids may hasten resolution.

Persistent diaper dermatitis that does not resolve with conservative therapy may be due to other disorders such as candidiasis, seborrheic dermatitis, and psoriasis. These should be suspected particularly when intertriginous areas are involved.

Candidal Diaper Dermatitis

Candidal diaper dermatitis appears as a bright red eruption, with sharp borders and pinpoint satellite papules and pustules (Fig. 8-42A and B). Examination of pustule contents by KOH preparation reveals the typical budding

yeasts and pseudohyphae of *Candida* organisms (Fig. 8-43). Candidal diaper dermatitis is occasionally associated with oral thrush, and it is a common sequela of oral or parenteral antibiotic therapy. One should suspect a secondary invasion by *Candida albicans* whenever intertriginous areas are involved or when a diaper rash fails to respond to symptomatic treatment. Most cases respond well to topical antifungal therapy, but the occasional resistant case may require a brief course of oral medication.

Staphylococcal Diaper Dermatitis

Irritant diaper dermatitis is frequently complicated by secondary staphylococcal infection, or pustules may

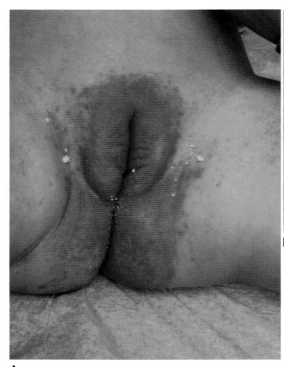

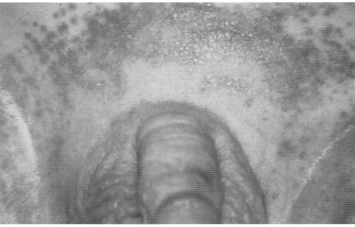

A

B

Figure 8-42. Candidal diaper dermatitis. **A** and **B,** The eruption is bright red with numerous pinpoint satellite papules and pustules. Intertriginous areas are prominently involved.

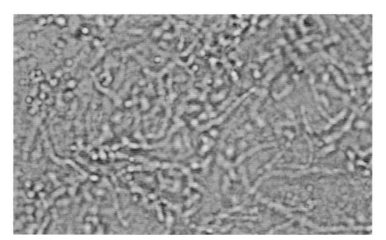

Figure 8-43. KOH preparation of skin scrapings from an infant with candidal diaper dermatitis demonstrating pseudohyphae and spores.

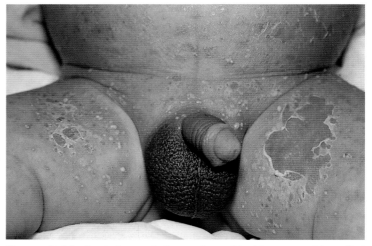

Figure 8-44. Staphylococcal diaper dermatitis. Numerous thin-walled pustules are surrounded by erythematous halos, as well as multiple areas in which pustules have ruptured, leaving a collarette of scale around a denuded erythematous base.

appear as primary lesions, especially in the first few weeks of life. The presence of thin-walled pustules on an erythematous base (larger than those seen with candidiasis) alert the clinician to the diagnosis. Typically, these rupture rapidly and dry, producing a collarette of scaling around the denuded red base (Fig. 8-44). A Gram stain of pustule contents demonstrates neutrophils and clusters of gram-positive cocci. Bacterial cultures are confirmatory but are rarely necessary. Early diagnosis and treatment with oral and topical antibiotics result in rapid resolution.

Seborrheic Diaper Dermatitis
Seborrheic diaper dermatitis is characterized by salmon-colored lesions with a yellowish scale. The rash is particularly prominent in the intertriginous areas (see Fig. 8-23B). Although concurrent infection with *Candida* or *Pityrosporum* is likely, satellite lesions are usually not seen. Typically, seborrheic dermatitis of the scalp, face, and postauricular areas is seen in association with this form of diaper dermatitis.

Psoriatic Diaper Dermatitis
Psoriasis occasionally begins as an erythematous, scaling eruption in the diaper area (Fig. 8-45A and B), which is clinically indistinguishable from seborrheic diaper dermatitis. Perhaps because the diaper area tends to be moist, the thick silvery scale typical of psoriatic lesions at other sites is not seen. Although lesions may develop subsequently on the trunk and extremities, the rash may persist for months in the diaper area alone. Failure of a seborrheic-like diaper rash to respond to empiric therapy over several weeks or months should raise psoriasis as a diagnostic possibility. Skin biopsy is the only way to confirm the diagnosis.

Tinea Diaper Dermatitis
Although less common than the other dermatitides in the differential diagnosis of diaper dermatitis, tinea must

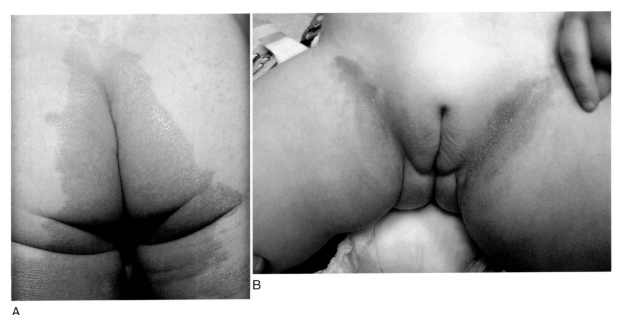

B

A

Figure 8-45. Psoriatic diaper dermatitis. **A,** This child had a persistent diaper rash that did not respond to routine therapy. Note that scaling is not as intense as in psoriatic lesions seen elsewhere on the body. **B,** Another infant with inverse psoriasis involving the inguinal creases had also failed to improve despite multiple courses of topical antifungal treatment.

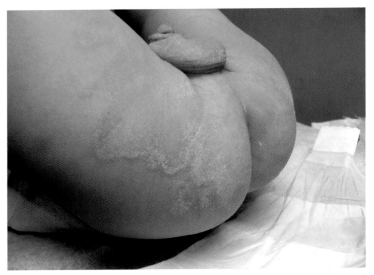

Figure 8-46. Tinea diaper dermatitis. Note the prominent scaling and the elevated active border.

be kept in mind when examining a scaly perineal rash. Its characteristic features are those of a recalcitrant scaly eruption with an elevated or "active" scaly border (Fig. 8-46), from which scales can be scraped and tinea demonstrated on KOH preparation. It responds well to topical antifungals alone and should not be treated with topical steroids.

Lichenoid Eruptions

Lichen Planus

Lichen planus is the prototypic lichenoid inflammatory eruption in that it displays flat-topped pruritic polygonal violaceous papules and plaques, which have a fine lacy pattern (Wickham's striae) over their outer surfaces. They are often noted first over the dorsal surfaces of the extremities and can display koebnerization at sites of prior trauma (Fig. 8-47). The disorder may involve the nails (leading to dystrophy), as well as the oral mucosa where lesions appear as lacy white plaques. Topical steroids are the mainstay of

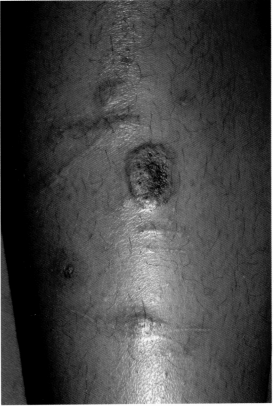

Figure 8-47. Lichen planus. These flat-topped violaceous papules of varying sizes and shapes overlying the anterior shin are typical. Note the linear lesions that formed after scratching, examples of the Koebner phenomenon.

initial treatment. Following resolution of primary lesions, a prolonged period of postinflammatory hyperpigmentation can be expected (see Fig. 8-124).

Lichen Striatus

Lichen striatus is one of the more common and distinctive lichenoid papulosquamous eruptions. Lesions consist-

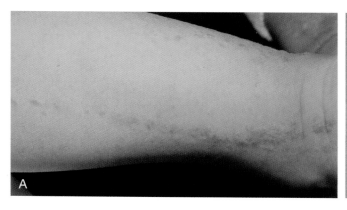

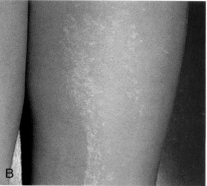

Figure 8-48. Lichen striatus. **A,** In this school-age child, mildly erythematous scaly flat-topped papules are seen in a linear distribution on the lower leg. **B,** Another child with darker skin has lesions that are hypopigmented on the posterior thigh. (**A,** From Cohen BA: Atlas of Pediatric Dermatology. London, Mosby-Wolfe, 1993; **B,** from Cohen BA: Pediatric Dermatology, 2nd ed. London, Mosby, 1999.)

ing of flat-topped papules appear fairly abruptly, usually in a linear or sometimes swirled distribution along the lines of Blaschko. Although they may involve any portion of the skin, they are more typically located on the extremities, neck, or upper back. They may be slightly erythematous or hypopigmented, and their surfaces are covered with fine scale (Fig. 8-48A and B). When lesions form on a digit, lichen striatus can lead to temporary linear nail dystrophy. The cause of this otherwise asymptomatic disorder, which has its peak incidence in school-age children, is unknown. Spontaneous resolution within 1 to 2 years is the norm.

Vesiculopustular Disorders

Vesiculopustular eruptions range from benign, self-limited conditions to life-threatening diseases. Early diagnosis, especially in the young child, is mandatory. Systematic evaluation of the clinical findings and a few rapid diagnostic techniques allow these various disorders to be readily differentiated from one another.

Viral Infections

Viral infections including herpes simplex and varicella-zoster produce characteristic vesiculopustular exanthems, which are discussed in Chapter 12. However, the technique of confirming the suspicion of a herpetic lesion by preparing a Tzanck test is discussed here.

The Tzanck smear is obtained by removing the roof of a vesicle with a scalpel or scissors and scraping its base to obtain the moist, cloudy debris. This is then spread onto a glass slide with the scalpel blade, air dried, and stained with Giemsa or Wright stain. The diagnostic finding in viral blisters is the multinucleated giant cell (Fig. 8-49). This is a syncytium of epidermal cells with multiple, overlapping nuclei; hence it is much larger than other inflammatory cells. Unfortunately, a positive Tzanck test cannot be used to differentiate one blistering viral exanthem from another, and a viral culture, or the more rapid direct fluorescent antibody test, should be obtained when the clinical situation mandates precise identification.

Bacterial Infections

Several common cutaneous bacterial infections present with vesiculopustular reactions as well. In impetigo, the eruption tends to be discrete and localized, whereas in staphylococcal scalded skin syndrome (SSSS) it tends to

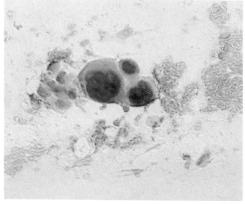

Figure 8-49. Tzanck preparation. Note the multinucleated giant cell characteristic of viral infection with herpes simplex and varicella-zoster.

be associated with a diffuse erythroderma. Gram stain of material aspirated from bullae or removed from the base of an impetiginous lesion is positive for organisms. However, in patients with SSSS, the organism must be sought from noncutaneous sources (nasopharynx, conjunctivae, sinuses) because the diffuse cutaneous blistering is due to elaboration of the toxin epidermolysin by the infecting organism and not to the organism's direct action within individual lesions (see Chapter 12 and Fig. 12-18).

Blistering Distal Dactylitis
Blistering distal dactylitis is a superficial bacterial infection involving the tips of the pads of fingers or toes. Lesions consist of tense blisters 0.5 to 1 cm in diameter that are filled with thin purulent fluid and surrounded by a narrow erythematous rim. With evolution, they may coalesce and extend proximally along the lateral aspect of the nail fold. On rupture, a thick crust forms (Fig. 8-50). Group-A β-streptococci are the usual causative organisms and are detected by Gram stain and culture of vesicular fluid. Occasionally, group-B streptococci and *S. aureus* are isolated. The disorder can be distinguished from a paronychia by the distal location of initial lesions; from a herpetic whitlow by the larger size of the initial vesicles and Gram stain of the purulent fluid; and from burns by the purulence of the vesicular fluid and Gram stain revealing white blood cells and bacteria.

Erythema Multiforme

Erythema multiforme (EM) is a distinctive, acute hypersensitivity syndrome that may be caused by many different types of agents including drugs, viruses, bacteria, foods, and immunizations. It may also arise in association with connective tissue disorders. In children, infections are the most common cause, and recurrent EM, in both children and adults, is invariably triggered by recurrent herpes simplex virus (HSV) infection. EM should not be confused with either *Stevens-Johnson syndrome* (SJS) or *toxic epidermal necrolysis* (TEN), which are severe potentially life-threatening eruptions characterized by variably widespread cutaneous blistering and sloughing, and by involvement of multiple mucous membranes.

The classic eruption of EM is symmetrical and may occur on any part of the body. However, the dorsum of the hands and feet and the extensor surfaces of the arms and legs are affected most commonly. Involvement of the palms and soles also is typical. The initial lesions are dusky red macules or erythematous wheals that evolve into iris- or target-shaped lesions, the hallmark of EM (Fig. 8-51A). In many instances the initial crop of lesions simulates diffuse urticaria, although EM lesions are typically much less pruritic, if at all, and ultimately they become painful and persistent, in contrast to true urticarial lesions, which remain pruritic and tend to migrate over a 24-hour period. The target configuration is due to formation of a central depression that may be blue, violaceous, or white, whereas the elevated periphery tends to remain erythematous. In some cases, vesicles or bullae develop centrally, and in others the peripheral rings may vesiculate or become bullous (Fig. 8-51B and C). The eruption continues in crops that last from 1 to 3 weeks. In most patients the disease is self-limited, and systemic manifestations are relatively mild, consisting of low-grade fever, malaise, and myalgia. Mucous membranes tend to be spared, although, on occasion, the oral mucosa may be mildly involved.

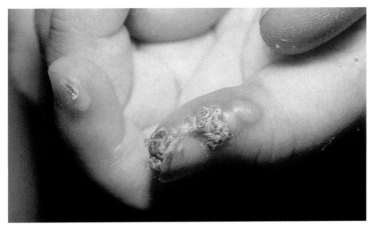

Figure 8-50. Blistering distal dactylitis. A tense blister filled with purulent fluid first developed at the tip of the thumb pad of this child. Subsequently, the lesion ruptured and crusted and newer lesions formed more proximally along the nail fold and at the tip of the index finger. (From Cohen BA: Pediatric Dermatology, 2nd ed. London, Mosby, 1999.)

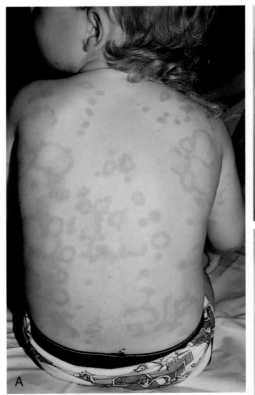

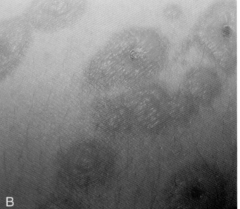

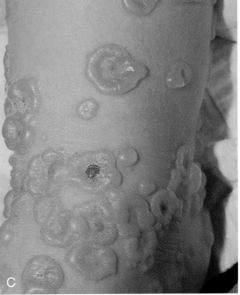

Figure 8-51. Erythema multiforme. **A,** The characteristic target lesions are symmetrically distributed. **B,** These lesions are dusky centrally and their peripheral rims are beginning to vesiculate. **C,** In this case, the peripheral rims have become frankly bullous. (**C,** Courtesy Michael Sherlock, MD, Lutherville, Md.)

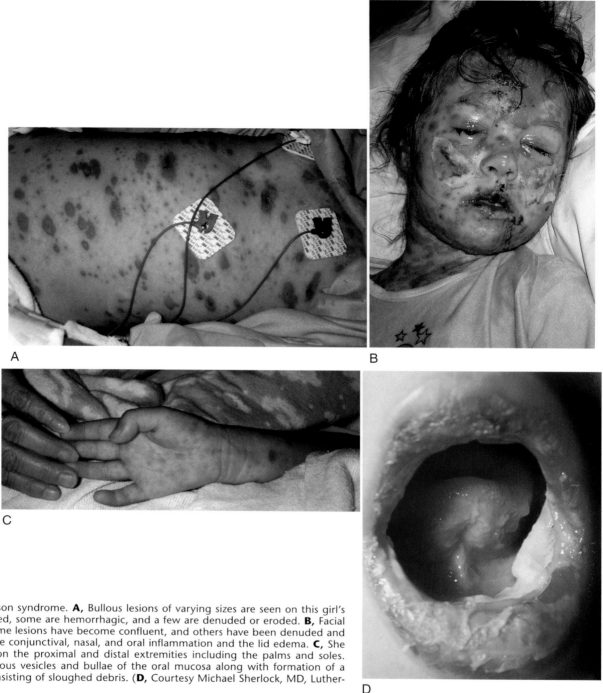

Figure 8-52. Stevens-Johnson syndrome. **A,** Bullous lesions of varying sizes are seen on this girl's trunk. Many are target shaped, some are hemorrhagic, and a few are denuded or eroded. **B,** Facial involvement is extensive. Some lesions have become confluent, and others have been denuded and then crusted. Note the severe conjunctival, nasal, and oral inflammation and the lid edema. **C,** She also had numerous lesions on the proximal and distal extremities including the palms and soles. **D,** Another child has numerous vesicles and bullae of the oral mucosa along with formation of a shaggy white membrane consisting of sloughed debris. (**D,** Courtesy Michael Sherlock, MD, Lutherville, Md.)

Stevens-Johnson Syndrome and Toxic Epidermal Necrolysis

SJS and TEN are rare, potentially life-threatening disorders characterized by widespread epidermal and mucous membrane necrosis and sloughing. In both SJS and TEN the plane of cleavage of bullae is beneath the basement membrane zone, resulting in full-thickness sloughing. Operationally, they can be distinguished by virtue of the fact that SJS tends to involve from 10% to 30% of body surface area, whereas in TEN anywhere from a third to 100% is affected, although there is some overlap. While the etiology is often unclear, hypersensitivity reactions to medications, antecedent viral infections, connective tissue disorders, and malignancy have all been implicated.

Clinically, a prodrome of fever, malaise, and sore throat usually precedes the appearance of diffuse erythroderma, which is then superseded in 24 to 48 hours by necrosis and cleavage, resulting in formation of thick-walled vesicles and bullae that often are hemorrhagic (Fig. 8-52A-C and Fig. 8-53). The Nikolsky sign is evident soon thereafter, and as bullae and vesicles slough, they leave deep bloody erosions, which then crust over. Mucous membrane involvement, particularly of the oral, conjunctival, and urethral mucous membranes, is routine and often severe. It consists of formation of fragile, thin-walled bullae that rupture early, leaving ulcerations of variable depth that are rapidly covered by a gray, yellow, or white membrane (Fig. 8-52D). On healing, mucosal adhesions and scarring may be noted. Conjunctival involvement can progress to involve the cornea, resulting in corneal scarring, and necessitates early and aggressive ophthalmologic treatment for possible prevention. Lid scarring may result in ectropion. Constitutional symptoms are prominent in

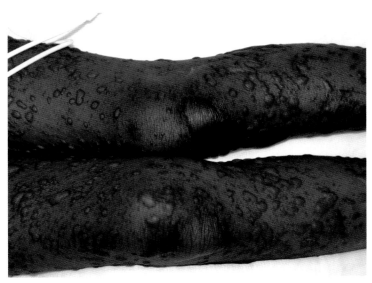

Figure 8-53. Toxic epidermal necrolysis. Three weeks after starting phenytoin for new-onset seizures, this 10-year-old experienced sudden onset of fever and malaise in association with diffuse erythroderma, conjunctivitis, and oral mucositis. Soon thereafter, thick-walled bullae formed, then rapidly sloughed, leaving deep bloody erosions. Note the extensive amount of surface area involved. (Courtesy http://www.dermatlas.org.)

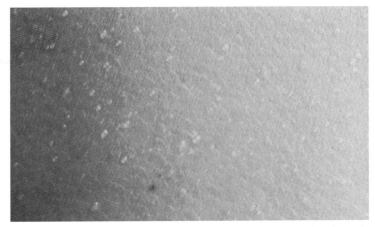

Figure 8-54. Miliaria crystallina. Found primarily over the head, neck, and upper trunk, these tiny thin-walled sweat-retention vesicles rupture readily, then quickly desquamate.

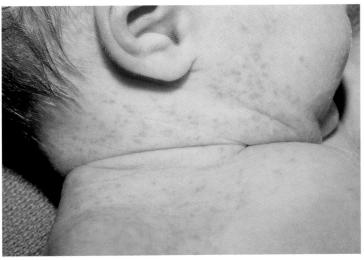

Figure 8-55. Miliaria rubra. Numerous tiny papulopustular lesions dot the skin of this infant's face, neck, and upper trunk.

both disorders and include high fever, cough, sore throat, vomiting, diarrhea, chest pain, and arthralgias. Fluid and electrolyte imbalances, caused by losses from ruptured bullae, and secondary infection are major risks and are proportionately greater in cases of TEN, given its more extensive body surface area involvement. Intensive supportive care is required to prevent complications from these fluid losses and from secondary bacterial infection, which is an ever-present danger. Recovery may take a month or more.

Although large, well-controlled trials are lacking, administration of IVIG early in the course of disease has been found to mitigate progression in some cases. Systemic steroids, on the other hand, are usually contraindicated, as they have been associated with an increased risk of morbidity from secondary infection.

Differential diagnostic considerations include staphylococcal scalded skin syndrome (SSSS) and erythema multiforme. In SSSS the plane of cleavage is high in the epidermis. Hence bullae are thin walled (see Fig. 12-18), and while mucous membranes are erythematous, they do not slough. Furthermore, Gram stain and culture of exudates from the nose and conjunctivae are positive for *S. aureus*. In EM initial lesions appear as dusky-red macules or erythematous wheals, which then evolve into bullous, target-shaped lesions, which do not tend to slough, and mucous membrane involvement, if present at all, is mild.

Miliaria

Miliaria Crystallina

Miliaria crystallina is a condition in which obstruction of the eccrine sweat ducts located high in the outer layer of the epidermis results in the formation of multiple 2- to 3-mm sweat retention vesicles. Being thin walled, these vesicles are readily ruptured (Fig. 8-54). In infants, lesions form over the head, neck, and upper trunk. In older children, they more commonly occur in areas of desquamating sunburn.

Miliaria Rubra

Sweat duct obstruction deeper in the epidermal or dermal layers produces an erythematous papulopustular eruption known as *miliaria rubra*, or prickly heat (Fig. 8-55). This rash is common in infants and children, especially over the face, upper trunk, and intertriginous area of the neck, as a result of tight-fitting clothing or use of occlusive lubricants, particularly during hot, humid weather. Wearing lightweight, loose-fitting clothing, eliminating greasy topical agents, and using corn starch assists clearing of the rash.

Infantile Acropustulosis

This remitting and exacerbating disorder of unknown etiology occurs primarily in African American boys younger than 2 to 3 years of age. Lesions begin as pinpoint erythematous papules, which evolve to form papulopustules or vesiculopustules (Fig. 8-56) that are highly pruritic. They appear in crops over the hands and feet, at times extending onto the wrists and ankles. After 10 to 21 days they resolve, only to recur within a few weeks. Ultimately, the disorder resolves by 2 to 3 years of age. Differential diagnostic considerations include scabies, dyshidrosis, erythema toxicum, and transient neonatal pus-

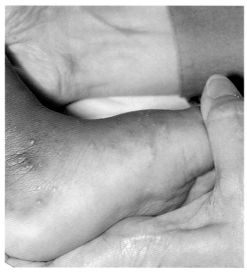

Figure 8-56. Infantile acropustulosis. Intensely pruritic papulopustular lesions are seen over the foot and ankle of this infant. He had had multiple episodes and had been treated repeatedly for scabies. (Courtesy Sylvia Suarez, MD, Centerville, Va.)

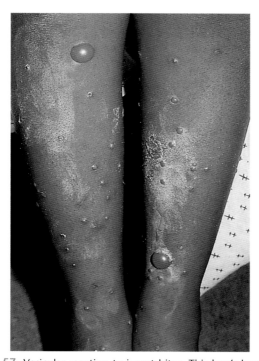

Figure 8-57. Vesicular reaction to insect bites. This boy's lower legs are studded with numerous thick-walled vesicles and bullae that have formed in response to mite bites.

tular melanosis. High-potency topical steroids applied sparingly up to twice a day and high doses of antihistamine may help relieve itching.

Vesiculation Following Insect Bites

Inflammatory reactions to insect bites, though often beginning as edematous papules, may evolve into pruritic vesicles and bullae on erythematous bases (Fig. 8-57). This is particularly true of the bites of grass and sand mites and fleas in sensitized individuals who react intensely. The eruption is frequently misdiagnosed as chickenpox or bullous impetigo. Severe pruritus, the lack of systemic complaints, localization to exposed areas (especially the

lower legs), and seasonal occurrence point to the correct diagnosis. Furthermore, the vesicles have thicker walls than those of bullous impetigo, and they do not rapidly umbilicate and crust as is true of varicella lesions. Tzanck tests and Gram stains are also negative in bullous insect bite reactions (see "Bites and Stings," later).

Reactive Erythemas

The term *reactive erythema* refers to a group of disorders characterized by erythematous patches, plaques, and nodules that vary in size, shape, and distribution. Unlike other specific dermatoses, they represent cutaneous reaction patterns triggered by a variety of endogenous and environmental agents. In children, the most common reactive erythemas include erythema nodosum, urticaria, vasculitis, and drug eruptions.

Erythema Nodosum

Erythema nodosum is characterized by symmetrical, red, tender nodules, 1 to 5 cm in diameter, which are usually located over the pretibial surfaces (Fig. 8-58A and B). Most likely, it represents a hypersensitivity reaction to streptococcal infection, sarcoidosis, tuberculosis, or other bacterial or fungal infections. Noninfectious disorders such as ulcerative colitis and regional ileitis have also been implicated. In adolescent girls, oral contraceptives are the most common cause, and a number of other medications may trigger this reaction.

Erythema nodosum is most often seen in children older than 10 years. The lesions begin as red, tender, slightly elevated nodules. These enlarge to form indurated subcutaneous plaques, and the overlying skin takes on a brownish-red or purplish-red hue within a few days. The disorder usually lasts between 2 and 6 weeks, although recurrences are common. Although any site may be involved, the shins are most commonly affected.

Differential diagnosis includes cellulitis, insect bites, thrombophlebitis, ecchymoses, and vasculitis. The fact that lesions are symmetrical, recurrent, and persistent helps exclude cellulitis and ecchymoses. Their usual pretibial and extensor location helps differentiate the lesions from thrombophlebitis. Insect bite reactions typically are pruritic, and other exposed sites such as the arms, head, and neck may be involved. The deep-seated nature of the nodules in erythema nodosum should allow differentiation from the smaller, more superficial palpable lesions of cutaneous small vessel vasculitis. However, they can mimic the cutaneous lesions seen in polyarteritis nodosum, a medium vessel vasculitis.

Treatment is directed toward the underlying cause. Nonsteroidal anti-inflammatory agents may be effective in reducing pain, and bed rest is beneficial.

Urticaria

Urticaria, commonly known as *hives,* is characterized by the sudden appearance of transient, well-demarcated wheals that are usually intensely pruritic, especially when arising as part of an acute IgE-mediated hypersensitivity reaction (Fig. 8-59A). Individual lesions usually last 1 to 2 hours but may persist for up to 24 hours. They may have an edematous white center and macular red halo (Fig.

Figure 8-58. Erythema nodosum. **A,** Note the typical red, raised, tender nodules overlying the pretibial surfaces of the legs. **B,** This 18-month-old boy developed tender, indurated, erythematous patches over his chest and abdomen after an upper respiratory infection. (**B,** Courtesy Cohen BA: Pediatric Dermatology, 2nd ed. London, Mosby, 1999.)

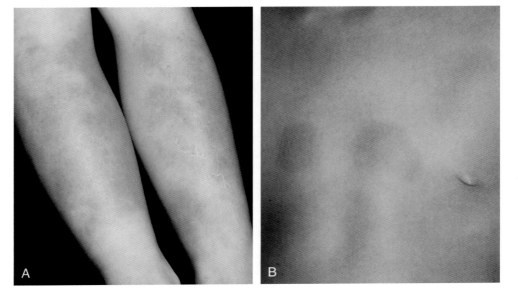

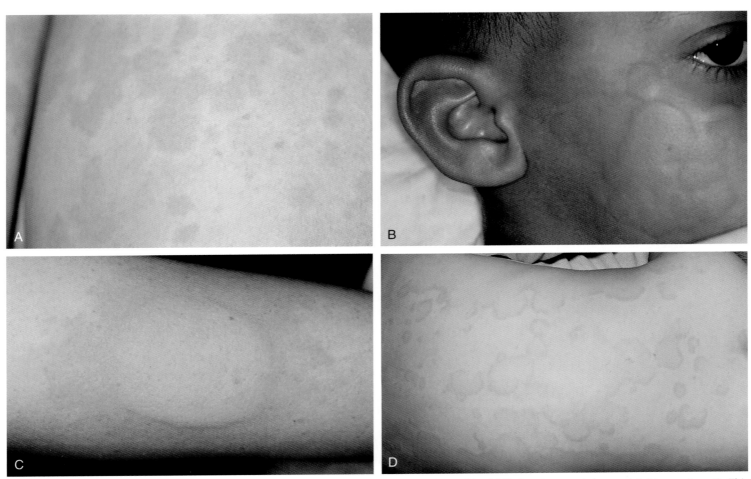

Figure 8-59. Urticaria. **A,** Typical erythematous raised wheals are seen. **B,** The wheals on this child's face have red rims and lighter centers. **C,** This patient with cold-induced urticaria has a giant whitish wheal with an erythematous halo. **D,** Gyrate urticarial plaques have evolved from individual plaques that became confluent. (**A** and **C,** Courtesy Douglas W. Kress, MD, University of Pittsburgh Medical Center.)

8-59B) or the reverse—a red center with an edematous white halo. Size can vary from a few millimeters to giant lesions greater than 20 cm in diameter (Fig. 8-59C). Central clearing with peripheral extension may lead to the formation of annular, polycyclic, and arcuate plaques, simulating erythema multiforme and erythema marginatum (see Fig. 8-59D). The reaction may involve the mucous membranes and can spread to the subcutaneous tissue, producing woody edema known as *angioedema.*

Urticaria can be caused by a variety of immunologic mechanisms including IgE antibody response, complement activation, and abnormal levels of or sensitivity to vasoactive amines. Most commonly, acute urticaria (lasting less than 6 weeks) is caused by a hypersensitivity reaction to food, drugs, insect bites, contact allergens, inhaled substances, or acute infections (especially β-streptococci infections and viral infections including mononucleosis). Chronic urticaria (lasting more than 6

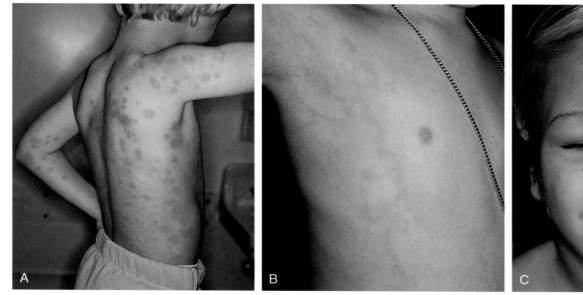
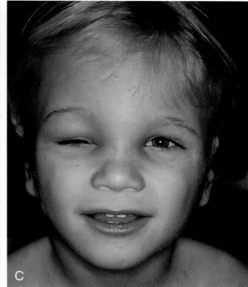

Figure 8-60. Serum sickness–like reaction to cefaclor. **A** and **B,** Extensive urticarial, target, and gyrate lesions are seen over the back, arms, and trunk. **C,** Facial edema involving the forehead was prominent in this child.

weeks) can be a sign of an underlying disorder such as occult infection (of the urinary tract, sinuses, or dentition); hepatitis B; or connective tissue disease (see Chapters 4 and 7). Urticarial lesions that remain fixed in the same location for more than 24 hours and/or heal with prolonged bruising are particularly likely to be manifestations of urticarial vasculitis.

In otherwise healthy patients who have no evidence on thorough history and physical examination to suggest occult infection or an underlying disorder and whose laboratory studies are normal, extensive testing is not warranted. Empiric treatment with oral antihistamines provides symptomatic relief and may help break the itch-scratch cycle.

Serum Sickness–Like Reaction

One relatively common acute clinical picture involves a constellation of urticarial lesions, periarticular swelling, and extremity angioedema in conjunction with acute upper respiratory infection or following use of medications such as sulfonamides, cefaclor, minocycline or the "-cillins." The urticaria is typically either nonpruritic or only mildly pruritic, and lesions evolve into target shapes or gyrate plaques simulating erythema multiforme, although they do not vesiculate (Fig. 8-60A and B). With this eruption, painful migratory periarticular swelling is seen, especially involving wrists and ankles, and often associated with bluish discoloration of overlying skin. Migratory stocking-glove angioedema, which is also painful, is common; occasionally, facial edema is seen as well (Fig. 8-60C). Following resolution of the respiratory infection or discontinuation of the offending agent, symptoms wax and wane over 1 to 3 weeks. This appears to be a T-lymphocyte–mediated reaction, and classic changes of vasculitis are not seen.

Drug Eruptions

Morbilliform Drug Eruption
Many different types of drug eruptions are seen in children. Morbilliform rashes or exanthems account for 75%

to 80% of all cutaneous drug reactions. The rash is reminiscent of measles or other viral exanthems (see Chapter 12). Erythematous macules and papules, which may range from fine to blotchy, usually begin to erupt on the face and trunk within 5 to 14 days after starting a medication. They then spread to the extremities over 1 to several days (Fig. 8-61A-C). The rash, which may be pruritic, is occasionally restricted to the extremities, or it may appear acrally (distally) at first and then spread centrally. Lesions may become confluent and generally resolve over 1 to 2 weeks with the development of mild purpura, fine desquamation, and residual postinflammatory erythema.

Fixed Drug Eruption
Fixed drug eruptions occur repeatedly at the same cutaneous site after reexposure to an offending drug. Postinflammatory hyperpigmentation is usually marked and may be the only manifestation of the rash during remissions. Morphologically and histologically, the target and bullous lesions of fixed drug reactions may be indistinguishable from erythema multiforme and may represent a localized form of EM (Fig. 8-62).

Henoch-Schönlein Purpura

Henoch-Schönlein purpura (HSP) is an inflammatory disorder with multiple predisposing conditions. It is characterized by a diffuse vasculitis involving the small postcapillary venules in the skin; gastrointestinal tract; kidneys; joints; and, rarely, the lungs and central nervous system (CNS). Although the exact etiology is unclear, the common history of antecedent upper respiratory or gastrointestinal infection suggests a hypersensitivity phenomenon resulting in a localized or widespread vascular insult. Other factors, including drugs, food, immunizations, and chemical toxins, have been implicated as well. Histologically, immune complex deposition in capillaries and postcapillary venules is associated with a leukocytoclastic vasculitis in the skin and other involved organs.

After a prodrome of headache, anorexia, and, occasionally, low-grade fever lasting 1 to a few days, patients may develop one or more of the following in any order: rash,

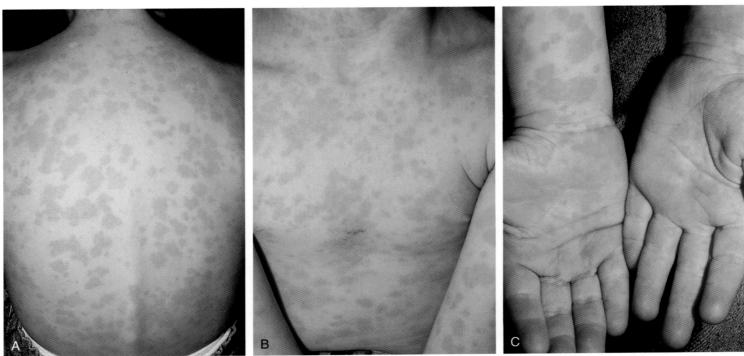

Figure 8-61. Morbilliform drug eruption. **A** and **B,** This diffuse exanthem developed on the seventh day of treatment with amoxicillin for streptococcal pharyngitis. **C,** The palms and soles were also affected.

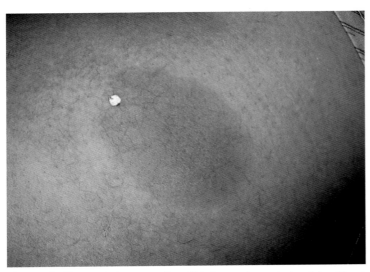

Figure 8-62. Fixed drug eruption. This hyperpigmented patch with an erythematous border developed on the flank of an adolescent taking tetracycline.

abdominal pain, arthritis, and occasionally hematochezia. Cutaneous lesions consist of erythematous macules, urticarial papules, and purpuric papules and plaques that tend to appear in crops (Fig. 8-63A to C), each resolving over 5 to 7 days, although the total duration of this waxing and waning eruption may last anywhere from 1 to 8 weeks (average, 2 to 3). Of affected children, 15% to 40% have one or more recurrences, usually within 6 weeks of resolution of the first episode.

Although in most children the initial crop consists of purpuric lesions distributed symmetrically below the waist (over the buttocks, lower abdomen, and lower extremities), in some this may be preceded by an acral or generalized urticarial eruption that is minimally pruritic and waxes and wanes over 1 to several days before the appearance of purpura. Subsequent crops of purpura usually involve the extensor surfaces of the arms, cheeks (Fig. 8-63D), and tips of the ears. The rash may also involve the trunk and genitalia. In unusually severe cases, skin necrosis may occur, heralded by the appearance of bullae.

Joint involvement consists of painful, tender periarticular swelling, especially involving the wrists, ankles, and knees. The overlying skin tends to appear ecchymotic. Stocking-glove edema of the hands and feet is also common (Fig. 8-63E and see Chapter 7). In young children, nonpruritic angioedema of the face, scalp, sacral, and/or genital areas (Fig. 8-63F) may be prominent. These phenomena wax and wane, as does the exanthem.

Gastrointestinal symptoms can precede, coincide with, or follow the appearance of cutaneous lesions. Segmental edema of the intestinal tract can cause crampy to colicky abdominal pain and may even serve as the lead point for an intussusception. Mucosal hemorrhage can be the source of gastrointestinal bleeding that can range from occult loss to massive hematochezia or hematemesis (see Chapter 17).

Up to 25% of patients develop nephritis between 1 and 8 weeks after onset of symptoms (peak, 1 to 3 weeks). This is more common in older children, and it is usually mild and self-limited. It is first detected by finding evidence of hematuria and proteinuria on urinalysis. Occasionally, nephritis is severe and progressive (see Chapter 13). CNS involvement is extremely rare, and its presence is usually heralded by severe headache, altered level of consciousness, and/or seizures following meningeal hemorrhage.

Treatment of HSP is generally supportive, although gastrointestinal, renal, and CNS vasculitis may respond to systemic corticosteroids.

The cutaneous lesions of HSP must be differentiated from acute bacterial, viral, and rickettsial infections (see Chapter 12). Negative blood cultures and classic findings on cutaneous examination and skin biopsy define HSP. Purpuric rashes associated with thrombocytopenia are more likely to be associated with petechiae and can be

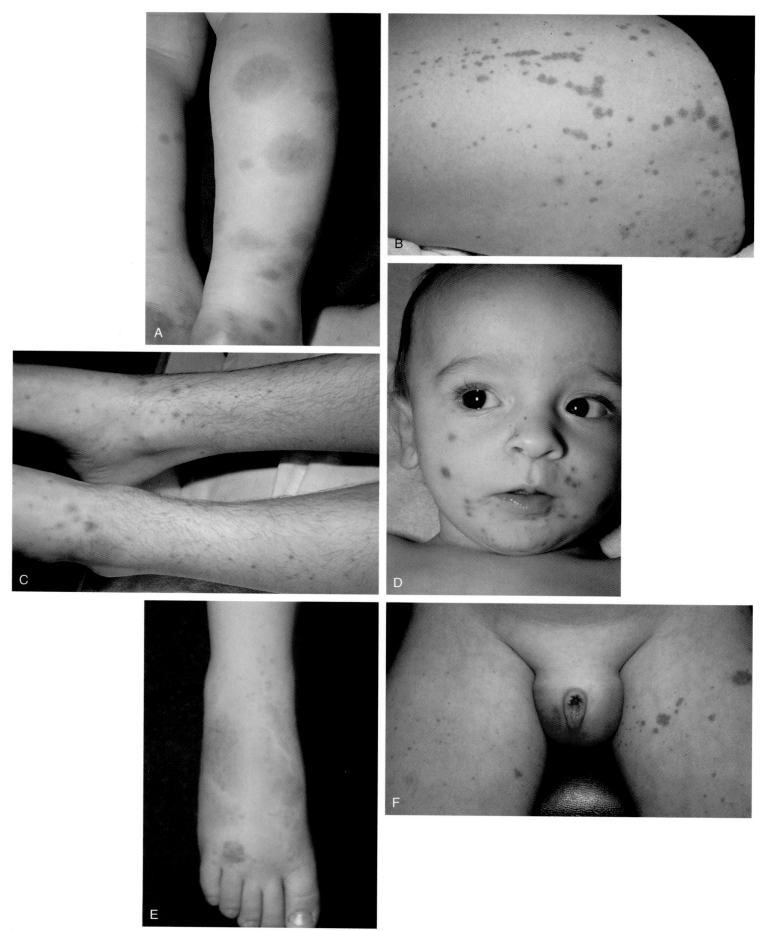

Figure 8-63. Henoch-Schönlein purpura. **A,** Palpable purpuric macules, papules, and plaques are seen over the legs and ankles of this toddler. **B** and **C,** These smaller purpuric papules are more typical and are seen initially over the buttocks, thighs, and ankles. **D,** Later crops may involve the extensor surfaces of the upper extremities, trunk, and face. **E** and **F,** Edema of the extremities, genitals, face, and scalp may be impressive.

ruled out by a normal platelet count. Finally, vasculitic rashes may also be seen in collagen vascular disorders such as lupus erythematosus, mixed connective tissue disease, and dermatomyositis (see Chapter 7). These disorders can usually be excluded by the absence of other findings.

Bites and Stings

Insect and spider bites may be associated with a number of cutaneous and systemic reactions. Lesions are found on exposed areas of skin, particularly the lower legs, arms, head, and neck. During the warm summer months they may also appear on the trunk. Protected areas (including the buttocks, groin, and axillae) are invariably spared. When bites involve the face, they can cause marked pruritic swelling that, although erythematous, is nontender and minimally indurated, if at all; rather, it tends to be soft or mushy on palpation (Fig. 8-64).

Insect Bites

Insect bites, most commonly caused by mosquitoes, fleas, mites, and flies, tend to produce mild acute local reactions including erythema, edema, and urticarial papules that are typically pruritic (Fig. 8-65A). A tiny central crust or hemorrhagic punctum may be apparent on close inspection. Occasionally, patients develop more intense hemorrhagic reactions (see Fig. 8-65B).

While mosquito and mite bites occur only during the warm months of spring, summer, and fall, flea bites can occur year round, typically in households with pets or in apartments or homes recently vacated by previous tenants or owners whose pets had fleas. Young children who only

visit on occasion with friends or relatives who have pets are also susceptible. Bites are usually found on the lower legs above the sock line but can be more diffusely distributed on crawling infants and toddlers. Like those of bed bugs, flea bites often appear in clusters of three (a clinical finding termed "breakfast, lunch, and dinner"). This stems from the fact that although fleas can jump, they cannot fly. Hence they tend to produce a localized series of bites in the same vicinity before jumping on to a new area. Excoriation caused by scratching makes them prone to secondary impetiginization. It should also be noted that not all members of a household may be sensitive to flea bites, and thereby some may "appear" to be spared. This can be a source of confusion to people who assume that if fleas are the source, everyone should be affected.

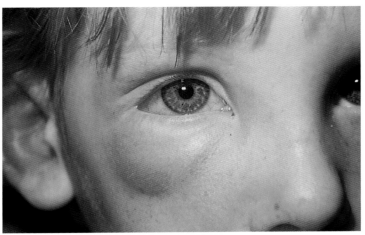

Figure 8-64. Facial swelling caused by a mosquito bite. The area was pruritic, nontender, and nonindurated. (Courtesy Michael Sherlock, MD, Lutherville, Md.)

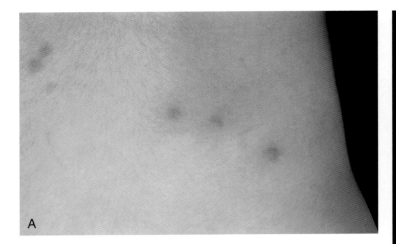

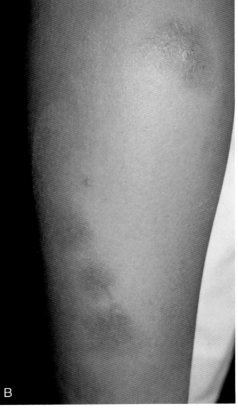

Figure 8-65. Insect bites. **A,** Multiple erythematous papules with central puncta were thought to be the result of either flea or bed bug bites. **B,** Another child had an intense hemorrhagic reaction to flea bites. (**A,** Courtesy Sylvia Suarez, MD, Centerville, Va.)

On occasion, the bites of grass or sand mites can produce frank blistering because the venom they inject contains a blistering agent that affects sensitive individuals (see Fig. 8-57).

Biting flies include sandflies, blackflies, horseflies, and gnats. The bite itself causes immediate pain and is usually followed by the development of a painful papule that sometimes vesiculates centrally.

Spider Bites

Spider bites tend to provoke more intense inflammatory reactions than those of most insects. Commonly, this consists of an area of erythema and induration that frequently becomes ecchymotic and is simultaneously painful and pruritic (Fig. 8-66). Less often, the lesions may vesiculate or even progress to develop central necrosis with eschar formation. The latter is particularly typical of the bite of the brown recluse spider.

Hymenoptera Stings

Bee, wasp, hornet, and yellow jacket stings typically produce a mild local reaction consisting of pain, erythema, and edema appearing within 2 hours after the sting (Fig. 8-67A). The honey bee leaves its stinger behind, embedded in the skin. Because this may continue to release venom for up to an hour, it should be removed as soon as possible using a horizontal scraping motion with a knife or fingernail. Grasping the stinger between forceps or two fingernails can inject more venom. Evidence indicates that topical application of a paste of papain (meat tenderizer) mixed with water may reduce the severity of local reactions, if applied within minutes of the sting.

Hymenoptera stings commonly produce a late-onset increase in swelling that is more diffuse than the initial reaction and tends to peak in 48 to 72 hours. This is the result of a delayed hypersensitivity reaction, and it is described by patients as being both pruritic and painful (Fig. 8-67B). Treatment is symptomatic.

In approximately 0.5% to 0.8% of the population (including many patients with underlying mastocytosis [see Fig. 8-83]), hymenoptera stings cause severe, acute, anaphylactic reactions within 15 minutes of the sting (see Chapter 4). This necessitates education regarding avoidance of the offending insects and immediate availability of an insect sting kit (EpiPen).

Papular Urticaria

Papular urticaria, a phenomenon seen primarily in young children, is characterized by symmetric chronic/

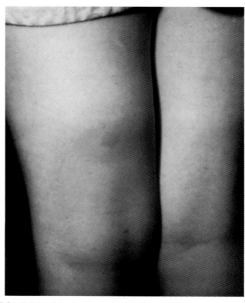

Figure 8-66. Spider bites. A marked inflammatory response consisting of a central wheal with a wide erythematous halo is seen in this child, who complained of both pain and pruritus.

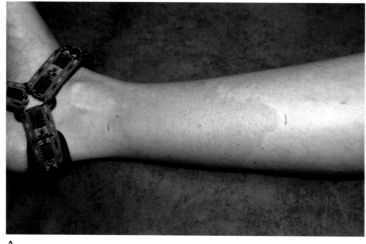

A

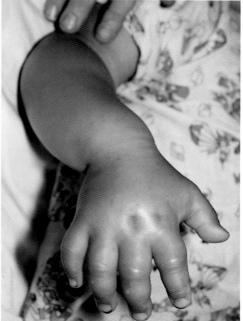

B

Figure 8-67. Hymenoptera stings. **A,** This child had an acute reaction with pain, redness, and mild swelling that developed within 2 hours of the sting. **B,** In this example of a delayed hypersensitivity response to a bee sting, marked swelling of the hand and fingers developed over 24 hours after a sting between the fingers.

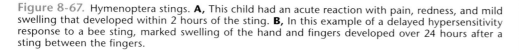

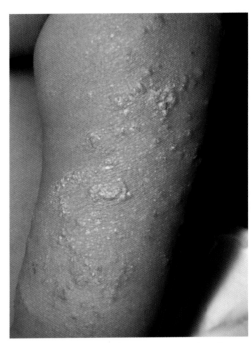

Figure 8-68. Papular urticaria. This severe, excoriated, papular reaction developed in response to recurrent flea bites. (Courtesy Michael Sherlock, MD, Lutherville, Md.)

recurrent eruptions of highly pruritic papules and wheals that tend to vesiculate centrally. Acute lesions are round, about 3 to 10 mm in diameter, and often have a central punctum. They tend to be arranged in linear or triangular clusters on exposed body surfaces such as the arms; legs; back; face; and in toddlers, the scalp. As itching is intense, the child scratches to the point of excoriation, incurring risk of secondary infection and scarring. During resolution, lesions tend to form a central crust with a surrounding collarette of scale, and ultimately (after 4 to 6 weeks) the child is left with target-shaped macules that are hyperpigmented peripherally and hypopigmented centrally. Often lesions in varying stages of evolution and healing are seen within a small geographic area (Fig. 8-68).

The disorder is the result of a hypersensitivity response induced by bites of blood-sucking insects, especially dog and cat fleas and bed bugs, and sometimes mosquitoes. Flea bites can be acquired by living in a home with pets who have fleas, in a house or apartment recently vacated by pet owners, or by visiting the home of a relative, family friend, or babysitter with pets at regular intervals. Bed bugs may be brought into the home in luggage by a family member on return from travel involving a stay in a hotel room that was infested, or after a stay at a half-way house, shelter, or hostel. Because fleas that are indoors and bed bugs bite year round, there is no seasonal predilection when they are the source.

Typically only one family member, usually the youngest child, is affected. This is because some individuals never develop hypersensitivity to the bites; others have varying thresholds of sensitization; and older individuals, sensitized in the past, have become tolerant.

Because a full-scale reaction tends to require a fairly long period of sensitization, during which the child has repeated exposure to the offending insect, few children become sensitized before their first birthday. During this period of induction of sensitization, the child reacts minimally when bitten. Once sensitized, children go through a period of variable duration (months to years) in which they experience both immediate and delayed hypersensitivity reactions to bites. Ultimately, they develop tolerance (i.e., become desensitized) and no longer react. During peak sensitivity, many experience a phenomenon known as *reactivation* in which new bites incite a delayed hypersensitivity reaction at old sites.

Identification of the offending vector and elimination of its presence can shorten the cycling. Other treatment measures include use of moisturizers, high-potency topical steroids, and oral antihistamines for acute (urticate) lesions. Good hand and nail hygiene reduce risk of secondary infection. Wearing protective clothing, avoiding going outdoors after dusk, and judicious use of insect repellent are helpful when mosquitoes are causative.

Treatment Principles for Insect Bites

General principles of therapy for insect bites consist of insect control, use of insect repellents, and application of topical corticosteroids supplemented by oral antihistamines for symptomatic relief. Parenteral administration of epinephrine, antihistamines, and corticosteroids combined with intensive supportive care may be lifesaving in anaphylactic reactions.

Infestations

Scabies

Scabies is a highly contagious infestation caused by the itch mite *Acarus scabiei*, which burrows under the skin. It is contracted by direct contact with other infested humans or fomites. The characteristic eruption appears 4 to 6 weeks after initial contact, and it is thought to represent a hypersensitivity reaction to the mites. Intensely pruritic papules, vesicles, pustules, and linear burrows appear in the finger and toe webs (Fig. 8-69A), the axillae, over the flexor surfaces of the wrists and elbows, around the nipples and waist, and over the groin and buttocks. The burrow, which is produced by the female mite, is the pathognomonic sign of scabies. It consists of a small, scaly, linear papule with pinpoint vesicles at the ends (Fig. 8-69B). In infants and toddlers the distribution differs, with the head; neck; trunk; palms; soles, dorsa, and lateral and instep portions of the feet; and lateral aspect of the wrists being more prominently involved (Fig. 8-70A-E). This age group is also more prone to developing an intense and persistent nodular reaction to the mite (see Fig. 8-70F).

In many patients, excoriation, secondary infection, or even development of a widespread secondary eczematous eruption (as a result of intense scratching) alters the appearance of or masks the primary lesions, making diagnosis more difficult. Therefore scabies must be considered in any individual who has no history of atopic dermatitis but has severe pruritus and recent onset of an eczematous rash. The distribution of scabies in intertriginous areas and over the palms and dorsa and soles of the feet helps to differentiate it from other insect bite reactions.

Although scabies can often be diagnosed clinically, an unequivocal diagnosis can be made with a skin scraping that shows a mite, mite eggs, or feces. The most important factor in obtaining a successful scraping is choice of site. Burrows and papules are most likely to be identified on the wrists, finger webs, feet, or elbows. A fresh burrow can be identified as a 5- to 10-mm raised mound with a small dark spot resembling a fleck of pepper at one end. This

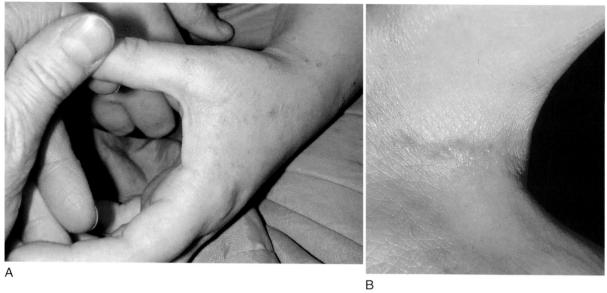

A

B

Figure 8-69. Scabies. **A,** Multiple pruritic papules, some excoriated and a few with central black dots, are seen on the wrist and dorsum of the hand. **B,** A pathognomonic scabies burrow is present in the finger web space of another child.

spot is the mite, and it can be lifted out of the burrow with a needle or the point of a scalpel blade. If a scalpel is used to scrape the burrow, it is worthwhile to place a drop of mineral oil onto the skin to ensure adherence of the scrapings to the blade. The scrapings are placed on a slide, another drop of mineral oil is added, and a coverslip is applied.

Scabies mites are eight-legged arachnids easily visible under the scanning power of the microscope (Fig. 8-71A). Care must be taken to focus through thick areas of skin scrapings so as not to miss camouflaged mites. The presence of eggs (smooth ovals, approximately one quarter to one half the size of an adult mite) or feces (reddish-brown or black pellets, often seen in clusters) is also diagnostic (Fig. 8-71B).

Eradication of scabies necessitates topical application of 5% permethrin (Elimite) cream to the patient, all household members, and close contacts (even if asymptomatic). In addition, thorough cleansing of all dirty clothing, towels, bedding, and car seat covers is essential. Two courses of treatment, a week apart, are necessary—the first to kill live mites, and the second to eliminate mites that had not hatched at the time of first application. Symptomatic therapy with oral antipruritic agents and topical steroids may be required long after the mites have been killed (i.e., until the secondary reaction has subsided). Although not yet approved in the United States for scabies, a single dose of oral ivermectin may be effective in recalcitrant cases.

Lice

Three varieties of lice produce clinical disease in humans, and all can involve the scalp hair in children. Crab lice *(Phthirus pubis)* are transmitted primarily by sexual contact. They are short and broad, with claws spaced far apart to grasp the sparse hairs on the trunk, pubic area, and eyelashes (Fig. 8-72A). They are typically found inhabiting the pubic hair and occasionally axillary hair and other body hair in adolescents and adults. Their bites produce bluish, pruritic papules that are distributed over the lower abdomen and upper thighs. Pruritus is intense, and a secondary eczematous rash may develop,

particularly in the pubic area, as a result of scratching. Young children lacking pubic and axillary hair may develop scalp or eyelash infestations after close contact with infested adults. Body lice *(Pediculus humanus corporis)* generally live in bedding or clothing, and their eggs may be found in the seams of trousers or underwear. Bites produce urticarial papules, seen primarily over the waist, neck, shoulders, and axillae, which are usually obliterated by excoriations and secondary bacterial infection.

Head lice *(Pediculus humanus capitis)* represent the most common cause of infestation in children. The lice are acquired by close physical contact; by sharing hats, combs, brushes, or scarves with an infested person; or by rubbing against upholstered furniture recently used by such a person. Head lice are long and thin, with claws spaced close together to grasp the more densely distributed scalp hairs (see Fig. 8-72B). Pruritus is the principal symptom, and the resultant scratching produces excoriations of the scalp and nape of the neck that are vulnerable to secondary infection. Occipital adenopathy is common.

Nits are seen as oval, white, 0.5-mm dots glued onto the hair shafts about 1 to 3 cm from the scalp (Fig. 8-73A), particularly above and behind the ears. These are firmly attached to the hair and do not move along the hair shafts, as do the hair casts for which they are frequently mistaken. Although nits may be seen along the entire length of the hair, they are deposited by the lice only near the scalp. Those far from the root indicate a span of perhaps months between infestation and examination. Nits are difficult to remove and may adhere as nonviable shells. Patients adequately treated for lice still have nonviable shells attached to the hair. Removal is assisted by use of a weak vinegar rinse (which is left on under a shower cap or towel for 15 to 20 minutes), followed by combing with a fine-toothed comb. Alternatively, the hair can be cut close to the scalp. This is important because the persistence of dead nits is a common cause of misunderstanding by school health care workers, who insist on retreating the children or sending them home from school. Active disease is present only if a viable organism or new nits attached close to the scalp are identified.

Diagnosis of pediculosis must be considered in patients with unexplained scalp pruritus. A careful search for the

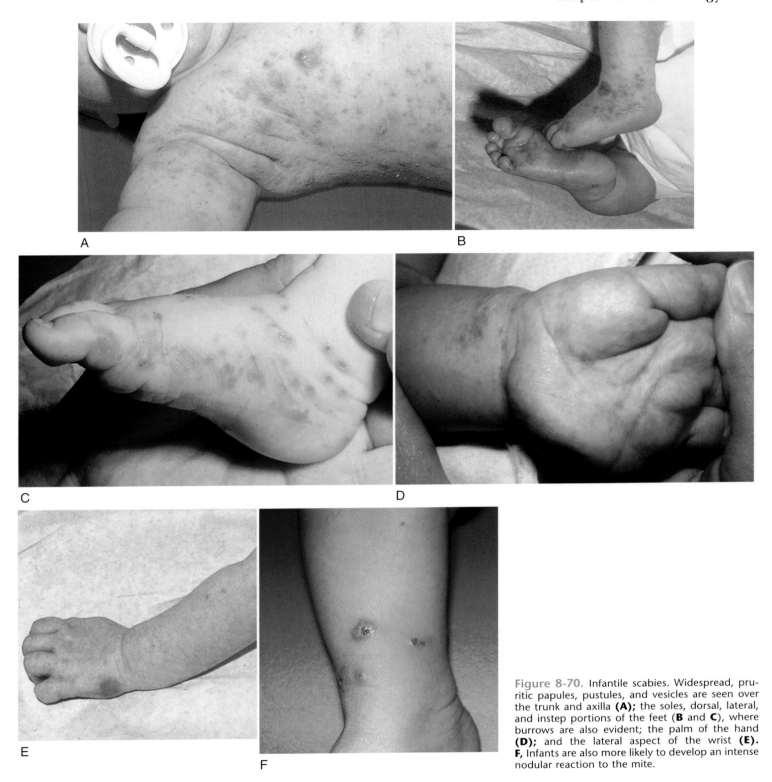

Figure 8-70. Infantile scabies. Widespread, pruritic papules, pustules, and vesicles are seen over the trunk and axilla **(A);** the soles, dorsal, lateral, and instep portions of the feet **(B** and **C)**, where burrows are also evident; the palm of the hand **(D);** and the lateral aspect of the wrist **(E).** **F,** Infants are also more likely to develop an intense nodular reaction to the mite.

organism may permit a specific diagnosis. Lice are six-legged insects visible to the unaided eye; they are commonly found on the scalp, eyelashes, and pubic areas. They are best identified close to the skin or scalp, where they can be seen moving around and where their eggs are more numerous and more obvious. Diagnosis can be made either by identifying a louse or by plucking hairs and confirming the presence of nits by microscopic examination (Fig. 8-73B).

Eradication of lice requires application of a pediculicide to infested hair-bearing areas of all household members and cleaning measures similar to those specified for ridding the house of scabies. Special attention should also be given to hats, scarves, and coat collars. Resistance to available pediculicides has been documented worldwide, and some cases may require multiple treatments or use of new agents. Permethrin 1% to 5% cream rinse is an appropriate first-line treatment, but if cure is not achieved and resistance is suspected, malathion lotion is a highly effective second-line option. However, it is important to instruct patients to avoid smoking near the patient because malathion is flammable. Lindane, an agent used in the past, is contraindicated for use in infants and children secondary to its potential for systemic absorption and neurotoxicity.

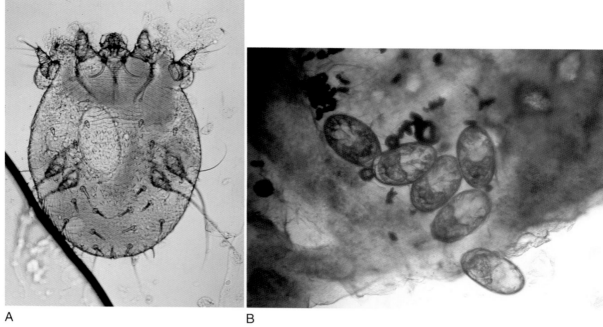

Figure 8-71. A, Microscopic appearance of an adult scabies mite obtained by scraping off the black dot at the end of a burrow. Note the small oval egg within the body. **B,** In a second specimen, no mite is seen but multiple eggs and mite feces are evident.

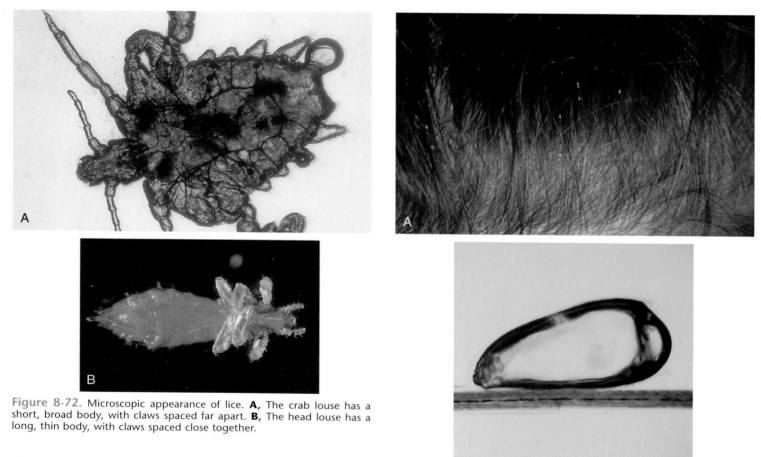

Figure 8-72. Microscopic appearance of lice. **A,** The crab louse has a short, broad body, with claws spaced far apart. **B,** The head louse has a long, thin body, with claws spaced close together.

Figure 8-73. Head lice. **A,** Nits appear as tiny white dots that adhere to the hair shafts. They are typically found 1 to 3 cm from the scalp above and behind the ears. **B,** Microscopic appearance of the nit of a head louse attached to a scalp hair. Microscopic examination distinguishes nits from hair casts and other artifacts. (**A,** Courtesy Michael Sherlock, MD, Lutherville, Md.)

Acne

Acne vulgaris, a disorder of the pilosebaceous apparatus, is the most common skin problem of adolescence. Lesions may appear on the face as early as age 8, although they usually begin to develop in the second decade of life during the onset of puberty. Other areas with prominent sebaceous follicles including the upper chest and back may be involved as well.

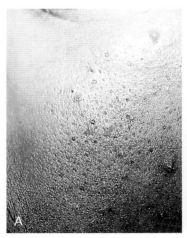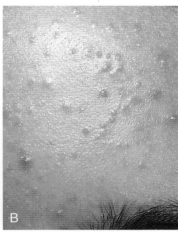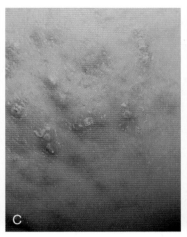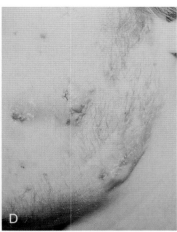

Figure 8-74. **A,** Comedonal acne with open comedones, or blackheads, seen over the cheek. **B,** Comedonal acne with closed comedones, or whiteheads, on the forehead, accentuated by side lighting. **C,** Papulopustular acne with inflamed papules and pustules over the cheeks, which responded well to antibiotics. **D,** Cystic acne shows deep cysts with marked erythema that can cause severe scarring.

The exact pathogenesis of acne is unknown. However, abnormalities in follicular keratinization are thought to produce the earliest acne lesion, the microcomedone. In time, microcomedones may grow into clinically apparent open comedones (blackheads) (Fig. 8-74A) and closed comedones (whiteheads) (see Fig. 8-74B). The entire process is driven by androgens, which stimulate sebaceous gland differentiation and growth and the production of sebum. The proliferation of *Propionibacterium acnes* in noninflammatory comedones and the rupture of comedone contents into the surrounding dermis may trigger the development of inflammatory papules, pustules, and cysts (Fig. 8-74C). Cystic acne is typified by nodules and cysts scattered over the face, chest, and back (see Fig. 8-74D). This form frequently leads to scarring.

Although therapy must be individualized, patients with mild to moderate comedonal and/or inflammatory acne respond well to a combination of topical retinoic acid, benzoyl peroxide, and antibiotics. Moderate to severe papulopustular acne warrants the use of oral antibiotics in combination with topical agents. Oral 13-*cis*-retinoic acid, or isotretinoin, should be reserved for patients with severe, scarring cystic acne recalcitrant to conservative measures.

Tumors and Infiltrations

Persistent lumps and bumps in the skin often raise fears of skin cancer. Fortunately, primary skin cancer is extremely rare in childhood, and most tumors and infiltrated lesions are benign. Hemangiomas and nevi, which can be regarded as tumors, are discussed in subsequent sections of this chapter.

Warts

Warts are benign tumors produced by human papillomavirus (HPV) infection of the skin and mucous membranes. In children they occur most commonly on the fingers, hands, and feet. The incubation period for warts varies from 1 to 6 months, and the majority of lesions disappear spontaneously over a period of 5 years. Local trauma promotes inoculation of the papillomavirus. Thus periungual lesions are common in children who bite their nails or pick at hangnails.

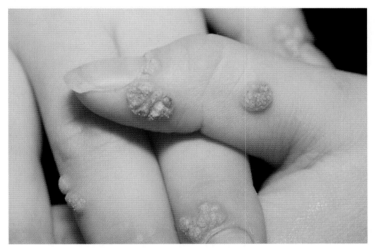

Figure 8-75. Verruca vulgaris. Dry, rough, and crusty, these common warts usually involve the hands. The periungual distribution in this girl was due in part to her habit of picking at her cuticles.

Investigators have identified more than 80 HPVs capable of producing warts, and many of these organisms produce characteristic lesions in specific locations. For instance, the discrete, round, skin-colored papillomatous (roughened) papules typical of **verruca vulgaris** (common warts) are produced by HPV types 2 and 4 (Fig. 8-75). The subtle, minimally hyperpigmented, flat warts *(verruca plana)* caused by HPV type 3 are frequently spread by picking and scratching and thus may become widespread on the face, arms, and legs (Fig. 8-76).

Plantar warts (Fig. 8-77) are associated with HPV type 1. Although not proven, the spread of these warts probably occurs through contact with contaminated, desquamated skin on shower floors, pool decks, and bathroom floors. Being much larger below the skin surface than is apparent from their external appearance, they occasionally cause pain when the patient walks. Although lesions can be confused with corns, calluses, or scars, they can be distinguished by their interruption of the normal skin lines (dermatoglyphics). Characteristic black dots in the warts are thrombosed superficial capillaries.

Warts can also be found on the trunk, oral and nasal mucosae, and conjunctivae. Anogenital lesions *(condylomata acuminata)* are usually associated with HPV types 6 and 11, and the possibility of sexual abuse must be con-

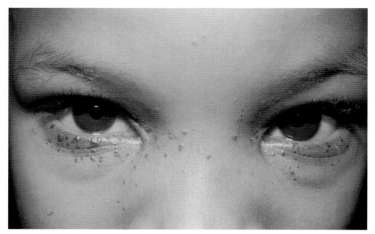

Figure 8-76. Flat warts, or verruca plana. These tiny, light brown warts are spread by scratching.

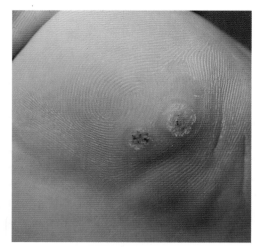

Figure 8-77. Plantar warts. Two painful lesions are seen over the ball of the foot. Note how they interrupt the normal skin lines.

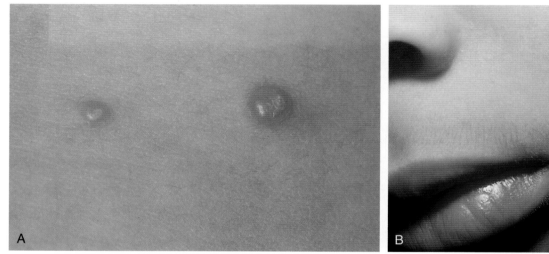

Figure 8-78. Molluscum contagiosum. **A,** In this case centrally umbilicated dome-shaped lesions are seen. **B,** Lesions have spread on the face of this boy as a result of scratching. Note that some of these lesions have protruding white centers.

sidered in children older than 3 years (with no known exposure to warts) who present with lesions at this site (see Chapter 6).

Although warts are self-limited in most children, presence of persistent and/or widespread lesions suggests the possibility of congenital or acquired immunodeficiency. Warts can become a serious management problem in immunosuppressed oncology and transplant patients, as well as those with HIV/AIDS.

Molluscum Contagiosum

Molluscum is a contagious disease caused by a pox virus, which is characterized by sharply circumscribed dome-shaped papules with waxy surfaces. Lesions can occur singly or multiply and can be pruritic. Although usually umbilicated centrally, some have protruding white centers (Fig. 8-78A and B). Lesions initially appear as pinpoint papules, then rapidly enlarge to up to 5 mm. They are found most commonly on the trunk and face, and in the axillae and genital area. Spread occurs as a result of scratching, and thus molluscum are often arranged in a linear configuration (Fig. 8-78B). Frequently, a curdlike core can be expressed from the center; microscopic examination of this material reveals typical molluscum bodies. Because

most lesions are asymptomatic and many undergo spontaneous remission within 2 to 3 years, treatment may not be necessary. However, in patients with symptomatic lesions who desire removal or in those with coexisting skin disease such as poorly controlled eczema in whom molluscum can quickly become widespread, curetting after application of topical anesthetic is curative for individual lesions and carries minimal risk of scarring. Painful destructive measures such as freezing with liquid nitrogen, electrocautery, and CO_2 laser are associated with a significant risk of scarring and recurrence and should therefore be avoided in young children. Studies looking at the efficacy of a topical immune response modifier imiquimod cream for the treatment of molluscum are ongoing.

Milia

Milia are tiny (1- to 2-mm), whitish-yellow papules that develop spontaneously on the face in neonates (Fig. 8-79). They are firm and, unlike pustules, are not easily denuded by pressure. Milia consist of small epithelial-lined cysts arising from hair follicles. They are persistent, although they may resolve spontaneously after months to years. In newborns, they usually arise without any apparent cause,

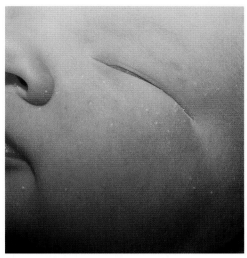

Figure 8-79. Milia. These small, whitish-yellow papules are found close to the skin surface and are particularly common around the eyes and midface.

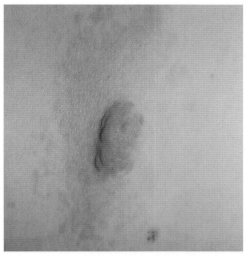

Figure 8-81. Neurofibromatosis. A soft pink neurofibroma is seen arising within a café-au-lait spot. Usually neurofibromas arise at sites that are normally pigmented.

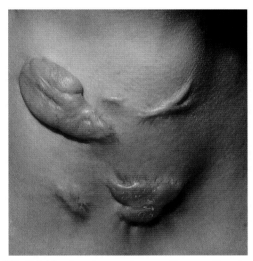

Figure 8-80. Keloids. An abnormal reparative reaction to skin injury, keloids are characterized by proliferation of fibroblasts and collagen that extends beyond the margins of the original wound.

although in older infants and children they are often seen after skin injury, such as that caused by blistering eruptions or abrasions. They are a characteristic feature of the dystrophic or dermolytic form of epidermolysis bullosa (see Fig. 8-96).

Keloids

Keloids are firm, rubbery nodules or plaques that result from the proliferation of fibroblasts and deposition of collagen following injury to the skin (Fig. 8-80). They can be pruritic or tender, especially during the active growing phase, and they may extend well beyond the margins of the original wound. This latter trait distinguishes keloids from hypertrophic scars, which remain confined to the wound margins and flatten partially within 6 months of the injury. In predisposed individuals, keloids often follow minimal injury such as abrasions, minor lacerations, acne papules, insect bites, and ear piercing. They are most commonly seen in African Americans and are more likely to develop on the ear lobes, upper trunk, and deltoid areas. Fortunately, they are not seen on the midface. Keloids may soften or regress with intralesional steroid injections alone

or in combination with surgical excision. However, recurrences are common.

Neurofibromas

Neurofibromas are solitary or multiple growths of neural tissue, presenting as soft, skin-colored or pink dermal and/or subcutaneous nodules (Fig. 8-81). The central portion of an early lesion is particularly soft, and fingertip pressure creates the illusion of pressing in a buttonhole. Neurofibromatosis 1 or von Recklinghausen disease is a syndrome characterized by the presence of multiple neurofibromas, café-au-lait spots, axillary and inguinal freckling, Lisch nodules, and various systemic findings. When considering this diagnosis, the clinician must remember that the neurofibromas usually appear after puberty, whereas in prepubertal children, café-au-lait spots are the most important cutaneous marker of von Recklinghausen disease (see Fig. 8-131A and B and see Chapter 15). Solitary neurofibromas without other stigmata of neurofibromatosis occasionally develop in normal individuals.

Mastocytosis

Cutaneous mastocytosis refers to a group of disorders characterized by dermal infiltrations of mast cells.

Mastocytoma

Isolated mastocytomas may be seen in infants. They usually appear as skin-colored or light reddish-brown, slightly indurated plaques, 1 to 2 cm in size (Fig. 8-82A). Development of a wheal-and-flare reaction after firm stroking of the lesion, known as a *positive Darier sign*, confirms the diagnosis (Fig. 8-82B). This is a response to the vascular effects of histamine released from infiltrating mast cells. Occasionally, enough histamine may be released from a large mastocytoma to cause localized blistering or systemic symptoms of flushing, wheezing, or diarrhea. Mastocytomas can be located anywhere on the body and usually resolve spontaneously by puberty.

Urticaria Pigmentosa

Urticaria pigmentosa is another form of cutaneous mastocytosis that presents with numerous small, reddish-

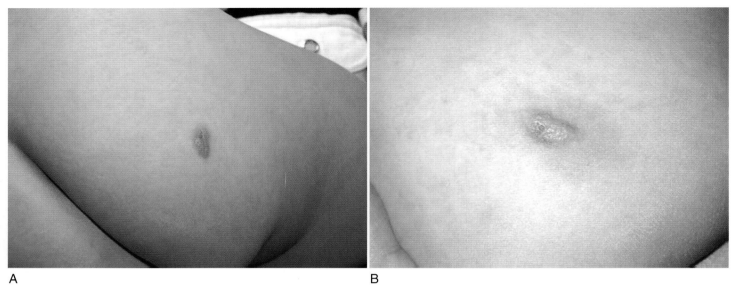

A   B

Figure 8-82. Mastocytoma. **A,** This solitary reddish-brown plaque on an infant's buttock contained numerous mast cells on histopathologic examination. **B,** Positive Darier sign. After firm stroking with a tongue blade, a wheal-and-flare appeared with an overlying bulla as a result of histamine release. This is diagnostic for mastocytoma.

brown papules or plaques, most commonly on the trunk (Fig. 8-83A-C). These may be present at birth or may appear later in childhood. They are often mistaken for café-au-lait spots but, unlike them, typically react to stroking with a wheal-and-flare reaction (Fig. 8-83B and C). Urticaria pigmentosa in children is usually limited to the skin and often resolves by adolescence. However, the bone marrow, gastrointestinal tract, and other organs may be involved. Rare systemic findings in children with urticaria pigmentosa include chronic diarrhea, gastric ulcers, flushing reactions, headaches, and failure to thrive. In infancy there is a tendency for lesions to blister, and widespread erosions may rarely result in dehydration and sepsis.

Patients with isolated mastocytomas and urticaria pigmentosa should be counseled to avoid certain medications and iodinated contrast media, which are known to cause sudden mast cell release of histamine, as these can be life threatening. Affected children should carry an EpiPen Junior because they can have a severe, even anaphylactic reaction to bee stings.

Juvenile Xanthogranuloma

Infiltration of the skin by other types of cells can also occur. An example is juvenile xanthogranuloma (JXG), in which local infiltration and proliferation of histiocytes form an isolated plaque or nodule or groups of small nodules (Fig. 8-84A and B). These asymptomatic red or yellowish-brown lesions grow rapidly in infants and young children but resolve spontaneously later in childhood. They are not associated with abnormalities of circulating lipids. In cases with multiple lesions (Fig. 8-84C) there may be associated ocular involvement. This disorder is the most common cause of nontraumatic hyphema in children. Hence ophthalmologic evaluation is important in patients with multiple or diffuse micronodular xanthogranulomas.

Langerhans Cell Histiocytosis

Langerhans cell histiocytosis (formerly known as *Letterer-Siwe disease, Hand-Schüller-Christian disease,* and

eosinophilic granuloma) is a potentially more serious disorder of proliferating histiocytes in the skin that may be associated with systemic disease. Lesions may be localized to the skin or may become more widespread with visceral involvement. Marrow failure, pulmonary disease, hepatic infiltration, and gastrointestinal lesions may result in life-threatening complications. Cutaneous lesions may be subtle and few in number or diffuse with widespread scaly papules, nodules, or infiltrative plaques (Fig. 8-85A and B). These lesions can be distinguished from seborrheic dermatitis, which they can resemble, by the presence of petechiae, bloody crusting, and firmly indurated nodules. Diagnosis is suggested by associated systemic manifestations such as hepatosplenomegaly, lymphadenopathy, and chronically draining ears (see Chapter 11). It is confirmed by skin biopsy, which shows characteristic Langerhans granules within the cytoplasm of infiltrating mononuclear cells.

Granuloma Annulare

When fully evolved, granuloma annulare is an annular eruption histologically characterized by dermal infiltration of lymphocytes around altered collagen. The lesion begins as a nodule or papule that gradually extends peripherally to form a ring. The initial papule and subsequent ring are raised and indurated, and in some cases the ring is broken into segments. The overlying epidermis is usually intact and the same color as the adjacent skin (Fig. 8-86A-C). However, it may be slightly erythematous or even hyperpigmented. Most lesions are asymptomatic, although a few are mildly pruritic. In the latter instance, superficial excoriation caused by scratching may be noted. Lesions are most commonly found on the extensor surfaces of the lower legs, feet, fingers, and hands (often overlying a joint), but other areas may be involved. They resolve spontaneously within a few months to several years, and no treatment is required. Their origin is unclear.

Granuloma annulare is most commonly confused with tinea corporis, or ringworm (see Fig. 8-35). However, the thickened indurated character of the ring and the lack of dermatitic changes such as scales, crusts, vesicles, or pustules enable clinical distinction.

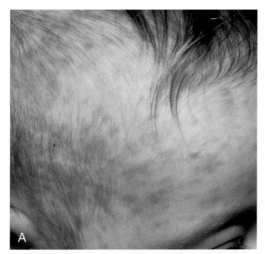

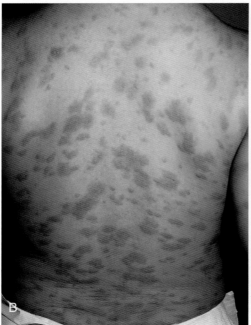

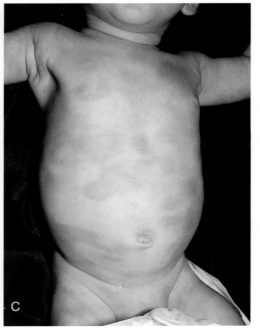

Figure 8-83. Urticaria pigmentosa. **A,** Numerous reddish-brown lesions are seen on the scalp and forehead of this toddler. **B,** Marked hyperpigmentation developed in the truncal lesions of this child. Note the wheal and flare over the right inferior scapula. **C,** Another infant also has a wheal-and-flare reaction over the left upper abdomen after accidental rubbing.

Neonatal Dermatology

The skin of a newborn differs from that of an adult in several ways: it is thinner, less hairy, has fewer sweat and sebaceous gland secretions, and has weaker intercellular attachments. During the neonatal period, common rashes or skin abnormalities may develop, and they need to be differentiated from more serious cutaneous disorders. Transient phenomena include erythema toxicum neonatorum and transient neonatal pustular melanosis. More serious diseases to be considered include systemic Langerhans cell histiocytosis and staphylococcal scalded skin syndrome.

Mongolian Spots

Mongolian spots are flat, slate-gray to bluish-black, poorly circumscribed macules. They are located most commonly over the lumbosacral area and buttocks (Fig. 8-87), although they can appear anywhere on the body. The spots range in size from 1 to 10 cm and may be single or multiple (see Fig. 6-65). Ninety percent of African American infants, up to 80% of Asian infants and those from other darkly pigmented ethnic groups, and about 10% of Caucasian newborns have these macules, which contain accumulations of melanocytes deep within the dermis. No risk of malignancy is known, and Mongolian spots usually fade without therapy by age 7.

Erythema Toxicum Neonatorum

Erythema toxicum neonatorum is a benign, self-limited, asymptomatic disorder of unknown etiology. It occurs in up to 50% of full-term infants and has no racial or sexual predisposition. Lesions usually begin 24 to 48 hours after birth but may appear up to the 10th day of life. The disorder has been described as "fleabite" dermatosis of the newborn, owing to the intense erythema with a central papule or pustule that resembles a flea bite (Fig. 8-88). The central papule or pustule is typically 2 to 3 mm in diameter and is surrounded by a much larger area of erythema. There may be a few to several hundred lesions on the back, face, chest, and extremities. The palms and soles are usually spared. A smear of material from a central pustule reveals numerous eosinophils, and concomitant circulating eosinophilia is present in up to 20% of patients. The eruption fades spontaneously within 5 to 7 days. No treatment is necessary.

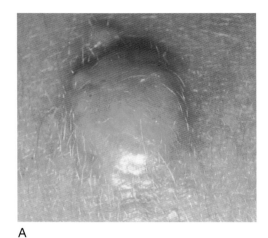

A

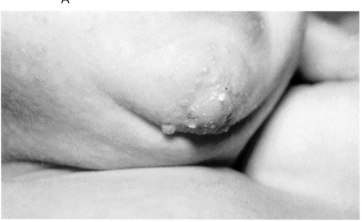

B

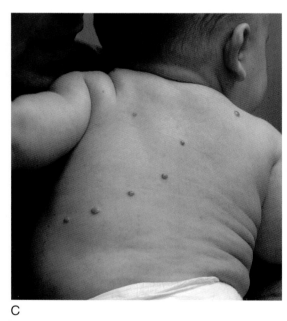

C

Figure 8-84. Juvenile xanthogranuloma. **A,** This 1-cm, yellowish nodule located on the back of a 3-month-old infant is the result of infiltration and proliferation of histiocytes. **B,** Numerous satellite papules developed around the primary lesion that appeared abruptly on the chin of this 3-month-old. **C,** Another infant has multiple micronodular juvenile xanthogranulomas, a finding that should prompt ophthalmologic referral to rule out an associated hyphema. (**B,** From Cohen BA: Pediatric Dermatology, 2nd ed. London, Mosby, 1999.)

Differential diagnosis includes transient neonatal pustular melanosis, staphylococcal folliculitis, milia neonatorum, miliaria rubra, and herpes simplex (see also Chapter 12). Infections often can be excluded clinically or with a Gram stain, Tzanck smear, and cultures, when necessary.

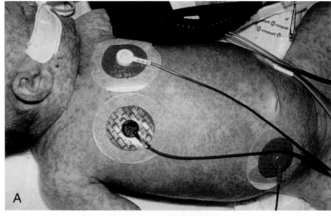

A

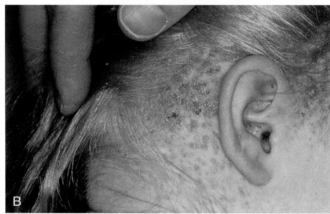

B

Figure 8-85. Langerhans cell histiocytosis. **A,** The exanthem in this 3-week-old infant began in the diaper area and rapidly generalized. Lesions were erythematous and scaly with interspersed petechiae. Associated findings included hepatosplenomegaly, diffuse adenopathy, and diarrhea with poor weight gain. **B,** In this closeup of an older child, raised infiltrative lesions with scaly surfaces, some of which have become petechial, can be seen over the neck and scalp. Chronic draining otitis is another associated finding seen in some cases. (From Cohen BA: Pediatric Dermatology, 2nd ed. London, Mosby, 1999.)

Transient Neonatal Pustular Melanosis

Transient neonatal pustular melanosis (TNPM) is a self-limited dermatosis of unknown etiology that presents at birth with 1- to 2-mm vesiculopustules or ruptured pustules that disappear in 24 to 48 hours, leaving pigmented macules with a collarette of scale (Fig. 8-89A and B). Lesions may appear anywhere on the body but are most often seen on the neck, forehead, lower back, and legs. Wright stain of a pustular smear shows numerous neutrophils; Gram stain and culture are negative for bacteria. The hyperpigmentation fades in 3 weeks to 3 months. TNPM is a benign disorder and requires no therapy. Differential diagnosis is similar to that of erythema toxicum neonatorum.

Sebaceous Gland Hyperplasia and Neonatal Cephalic Pustulosis (Formerly Neonatal Acne)

Neonatal sebaceous gland hyperplasia is a common entity consisting of multiple 1- to 2-cm yellowish-white papules usually located over the nose and cheeks of full-term infants (Fig. 8-90) and represents a normal physiologic response to maternal androgenic stimulation of sebaceous gland growth. Lesions resolve spontaneously by 4 to 6 months.

Neonates can also develop findings that resemble acne within the first few weeks of life. On close examination,

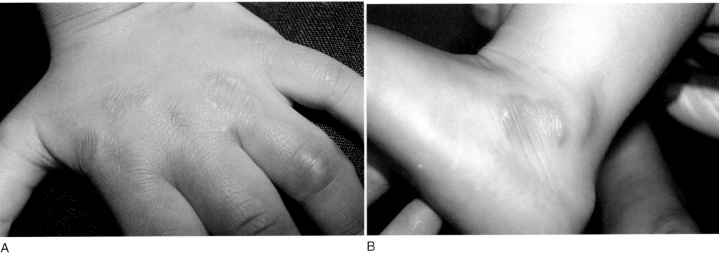

A
B

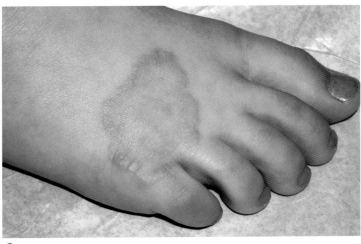

C

Figure 8-86. Granuloma annulare. **A,** Three raised, indurated rings with intact overlying skin and an early papular lesion on the ring finger are seen on a child's hand. **B,** In this infant an incomplete ring of dermal nodules overlies the lateral malleolus. **C,** In an older child this lesion on the dorsum of the foot is less raised.

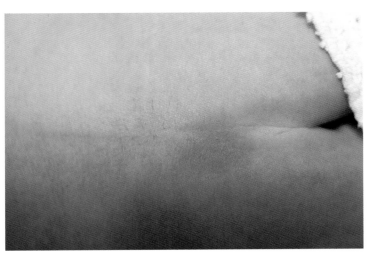

Figure 8-87. Mongolian spot. A typical slate-gray lesion is located over the lumbosacral area of this African American infant.

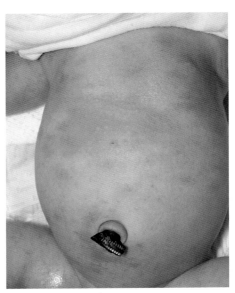

Figure 8-88. Erythema toxicum neonatorum. Numerous yellow papules and pustules are surrounded by large intensely erythematous rings on the trunk of this infant.

however, instead of true comedones, lesions are seen to consist of papules and papulopustules over the face, neck, and trunk (Fig. 8-91). It, too, is thought to be a result of hormonal stimulation of sebaceous glands, which creates a hospitable environment for overgrowth of yeast *(Malassezia sp.)*. Formerly called neonatal acne, it is now termed **neonatal cephalic pustulosis.** The condition is benign and self-limited and is best treated with topical antifungal agents.

Cutis Marmorata

Cutis marmorata is characterized by a transient, netlike, reddish-blue mottling of the skin caused by variable vascular constriction and dilatation (Fig. 8-92). It is a normal response to chilling, and on rewarming, normal skin color

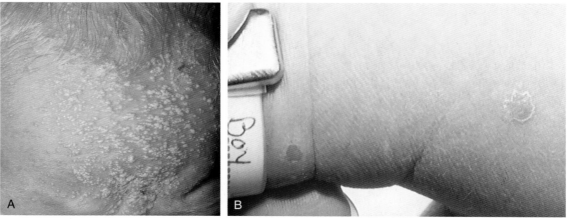

Figure 8-89. Transient neonatal pustular melanosis. **A,** A myriad of tiny pustules dot the forehead and scalp of this neonate. **B,** When the pustules rupture, a pigmented macule surrounded by a collarette of scale remains.

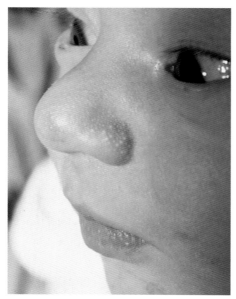

Figure 8-90. Sebaceous gland hyperplasia. Note the yellowish-white papules on the nose of this infant.

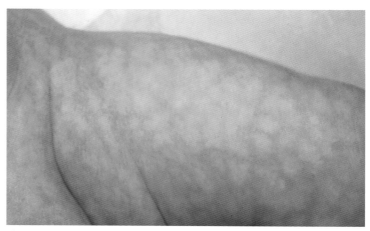

Figure 8-92. Cutis marmorata. Note the reticulated bluish-purple mottling of the skin of this infant's thigh.

returns. The discoloration occurs symmetrically over the trunk and extremities in infants. In neonates the condition usually abates by 6 months, but it may persist longer in fair-skinned individuals.

Collodion Baby

In several variants of ichthyosis, particularly lamellar ichthyosis, the infant is born encased in a thick, parchment-like scale known as a ***collodion membrane*** (Fig. 8-93). This dries and is shed in large sheets within 7 to 14 days. Significant secondary fluid, electrolyte, and heat losses can occur. Although scaling may resolve completely in some infants, most go on to develop cutaneous findings typical for the underlying ichthyosis (see Figs. 8-8 and 8-9).

Epidermolysis Bullosa

Epidermolysis bullosa (EB) is a group of inherited mechanobullous disorders characterized by the development of blisters after the skin is subjected to mild friction or trauma. The three general types are EB simplex, junctional EB, and dystrophic EB (formerly known as *epidermolytic, junctional,* and *dermolytic* forms). These types are classified according to the level at which blister formation occurs. Modes of inheritance vary with subtypes in each

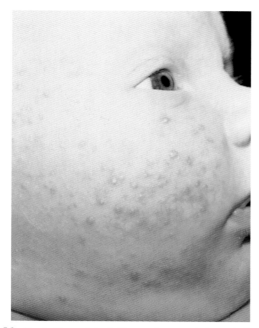

Figure 8-91. Cephalic pustulosis (formerly neonatal acne). Erythematous papules and pustules are present over the nose and cheeks.

group, and blistering, with few exceptions, occurs in the newborn period.

Epidermolysis Bullosa Simplex (Epidermolytic Epidermolysis Bullosa)

In this variant, which is usually transmitted as an autosomal dominant trait, blister formation takes place super-

ficially within or just above the basal cell layer of the epidermis. On presentation, blistering can be mild or severe and widespread (Fig. 8-94). The most common form presents in later infancy, childhood, or adolescence with blisters confined to pressure bearing areas, especially on the hands and feet, and particularly after intense physical activity. Although there is no scarring, secondary infection can occur, and atrophy may develop in some cases.

Junctional Epidermolysis Bullosa

Junctional EB, inherited as an autosomal recessive trait, usually presents at birth with bullae and erosions in a generalized distribution. Blisters form at the junction of the epidermis and dermis (Fig. 8-95). The most severe form is usually fatal during the first year of life, due to malnutrition, fluid losses, recurrent cutaneous infection, and sepsis. A milder variant resembles generalized epidermolytic EB. An uncommon subtype of this form of EB is associated with pyloric atresia and has a high mortality in the neonatal period.

Dystrophic Epidermolysis Bullosa (Formerly Dermolytic Epidermolysis Bullosa)

The dermolytic forms of EB are divided into dominant and recessive types. The plane of cleavage is deep within

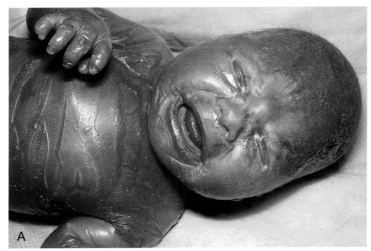

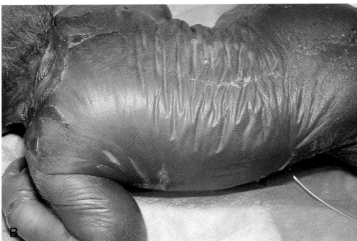

Figure 8-93. Collodion baby. **A** and **B,** A shiny transparent membrane covered this baby at birth; she later developed lamellar ichthyosis. Note the ectropion and eclabium (eversion and fissuring of the eyelid margins and lips). (From Cohen BA: Pediatric Dermatology, 2nd ed. London, Mosby, 1999.).

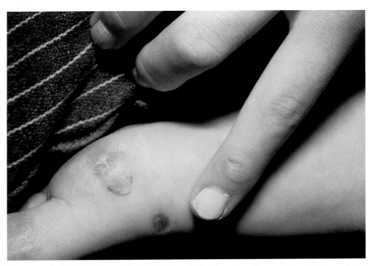

Figure 8-94. Epidermolysis bullosa (EB) simplex (formerly epidermolytic EB). Blisters form easily in pressure-bearing areas, particularly the hands and feet. Scarring does not occur.

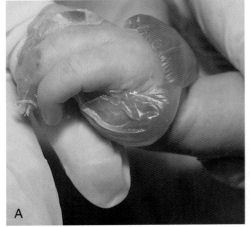

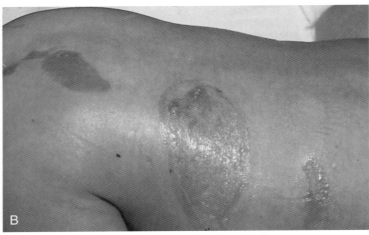

Figure 8-95. Junctional epidermolysis bullosa. Widespread involvement was seen in this infant at birth. **A,** Note the erosions and the large, intact blister over the thumb and dorsum of the hand. **B,** Large, denuded areas are evident over the back and flank.

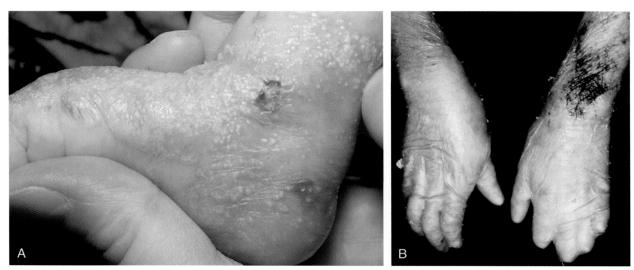

Figure 8-96. Dystrophic (formerly dermolytic) epidermolysis bullosa (EB). **A,** Blisters, erosions, and hundreds of milia are seen on the foot and ankle of this newborn. **B,** In another child with the recessive form of dystrophic EB, severe scarring encased the fingers, resulting in syndactyly.

the upper portion of the dermis. In both, scarring occurs as the blisters heal and milia are common (Fig. 8-96A). The dominant form usually results in more localized lesions (e.g., feet only) than the recessive form; patients with the latter show retardation in growth and development, severe oral blisters, loss of nails, and sometimes syndactyly (Fig. 8-96B).

Skin biopsies are helpful in distinguishing among the three general types of EB in neonates, and they are also helpful in determining prognosis. Treatment is symptomatic and supportive. Prenatal diagnosis is now possible for a number of variants for which gene markers are available. Genetic counseling is advisable.

Incontinentia Pigmenti

Incontinentia pigmenti (IP) is an X-linked, dominant disorder that affects the skin and may also involve the CNS, eyes, and skeletal system. It is seen predominantly in females and thus is thought to be fatal to males in utero. The exception is a male with genetic mosaicism for IP or an XXY male. Clinically, the disorder may present in any of three general phases, with some overlap. In the first phase, inflammatory vesicles or bullae appear on the trunk and extremities, usually within the first 2 weeks of life (Fig. 8-97A). New blisters then develop over the ensuing 3 months. At this stage a skin biopsy shows characteristic inflammation with intraepidermal eosinophils and necrotic keratinocytes. Before the blistering phase ends, the second phase, marked by development of irregular, warty papules, supervenes (Fig. 8-97B and C). These lesions resolve spontaneously within several months. A characteristic swirling or streaking pattern (referred to as a Blaschkoid distribution) of brown to bluish-gray pigmentation on the trunk or extremities marks the third phase (Fig. 8-97D and E). Interestingly, these pigmented whorls are sometimes located at different sites from those involved in the first two phases. The pigmentation, which likely represents a form of pigmentary mosaicism (see "Disorders of Pigmentation," later, and Chapter 1), lasts for many years and then gradually fades, leaving subtle, streaky, hypopigmented scars that may be the only residual cutaneous findings seen in affected mothers (Fig. 8-97F), who should be carefully examined for these markers of IP.

A number of other systemic manifestations affecting various body systems are seen in patients with IP. Up to 30% have CNS abnormalities such as seizures, mental retardation, and spasticity. Ophthalmic complications including strabismus, cataracts, blindness, and microphthalmia are seen in 35%. Pegged teeth and delayed dentition are seen in 65%. Cardiac and skeletal malformations have also been reported.

Differential diagnosis of IP in the blistering stage includes herpes simplex, bullous impetigo, and EB. Warts or epidermal nevi may mimic the warty phase. The swirled pigmentation of the third phase is quite characteristic and not likely to be confused with most hyperpigmentation disorders. It can and should be distinguished from other forms of pigmentary mosaicism given the history of antecedent vesicular and papular stages. No specific therapy is required for IP, but genetic counseling is advisable.

Hemangiomas and Vascular Malformations

Hemangiomas are benign vascular tumors or neoplasms that are dynamic, having the capacity for rapid growth as a result of endothelial cell proliferation. There are several subtypes including infantile hemangiomas, rapidly involuting congenital hemangiomas (RICH lesions), noninvoluting congenital hemangiomas (NICH lesions), kaposiform hemangioendotheliomas, tufted angiomas, and pyogenic granulomas. In contrast, vascular malformations (discussed later) are static lesions that grow only with the child.

Infantile Hemangiomas

Infantile hemangiomas constitute the most common vascular tumors of infancy and are seen in approximately 10% of infants by 1 year of age. They are seen more commonly in Caucasians, females, premature infants, and babies born to mothers with placental abnormalities. This latter phenomenon, combined with the fact that hemangiomas and the placenta express similar tissue markers (such as the glucose transporter GLUT-1), has raised the

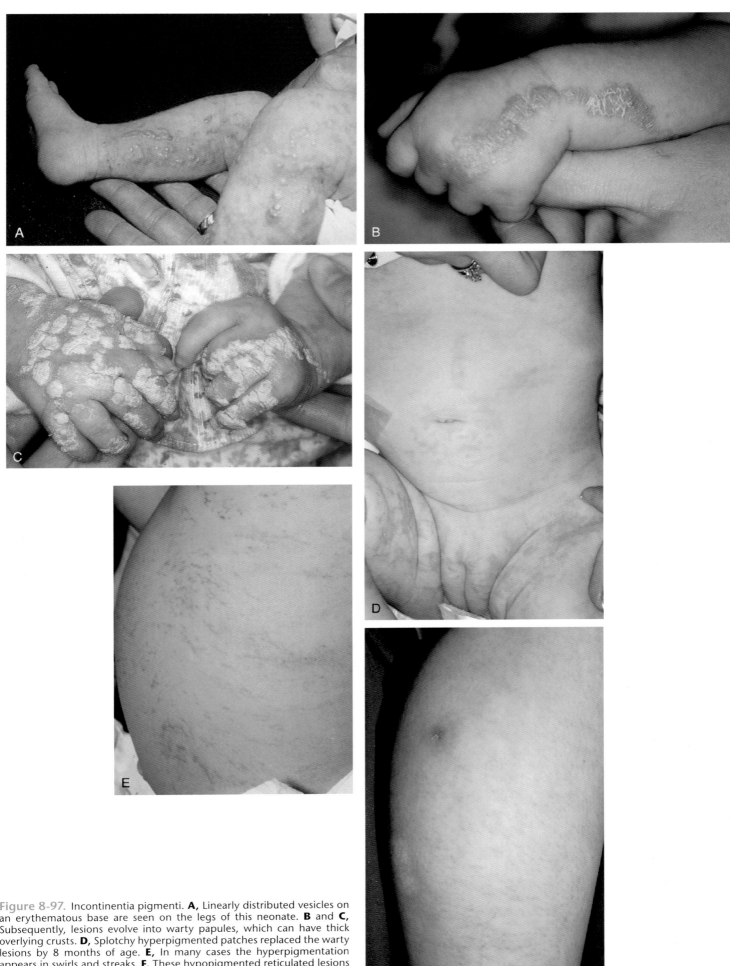

Figure 8-97. Incontinentia pigmenti. **A,** Linearly distributed vesicles on an erythematous base are seen on the legs of this neonate. **B** and **C,** Subsequently, lesions evolve into warty papules, which can have thick overlying crusts. **D,** Splotchy hyperpigmented patches replaced the warty lesions by 8 months of age. **E,** In many cases the hyperpigmentation appears in swirls and streaks. **F,** These hypopigmented reticulated lesions on the leg of an affected child's mother represent old scars in areas of prior hyperpigmentation. (**A** and **C,** From Cohen BA: Pediatric Dermatology, 2nd ed. London, Mosby, 1999.)

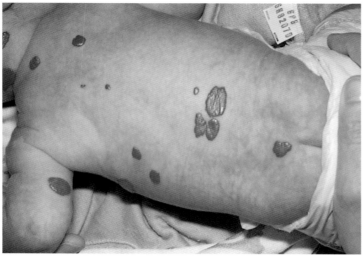

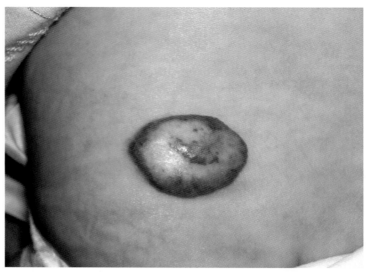

Figure 8-98. Superficial or strawberry hemangiomas. Multiple soft, red, raised lesions dot the back and arms of this otherwise healthy 1-month-old with benign hemangiomatosis. Note that a number of the lesions exceed 2 cm in diameter and are plaquelike.

Figure 8-99. Involuting hemangioma. The onset of involution is signaled by a "graying out" of the surface of the lesion.

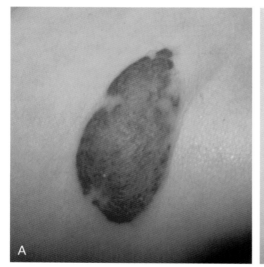
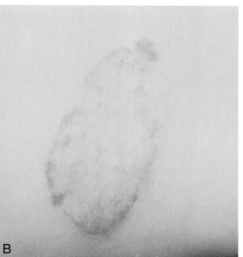
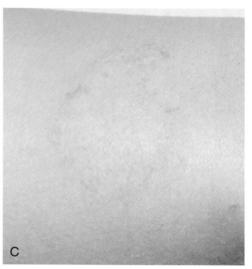

Figure 8-100. Natural history of a hemangioma. After growing for approximately 6 months, hemangiomas tend to plateau in size and then gradually involute. Note the appearance at 5 months **(A)**, at 2 years **(B)**, and almost total resolution at 5 years **(C)**.

question of whether hemangiomas may have their origin in embolized placental tissue.

While not usually present at birth, infantile hemangiomas tend to appear within several days to weeks after delivery. The initial manifestation may be slight reddening or bluish discoloration of the overlying skin. Thereafter, in the majority of cases, rapid vascular overgrowth occurs, resulting in formation of a bright red nodule or plaque with definite elevation above the surrounding skin surface (Fig. 8-98). These lesions can then grow for up to 15 months, although most peak in size by 6 to 9 months. Thereafter, they stabilize or plateau and then gradually involute at a rate of approximately 10% a year. Hence their chances of resolution are: 30% by 3 years, 50% by 5, and 70% by age 7. The onset of involution is signaled by a "graying out" of the surface (Fig. 8-99). The natural history of involution of a lesion is shown in Figure 8-100.

Although hemangiomas do involute, and families can be reassured that they will ultimately regress considerably, it is important to inform them that residual skin changes are likely. This is due to the fact that in 40% of cases the skin overlying a resolved lesion shows mild redundancy

with telangiectasias, and depending on location and maximum size, some lesions leave behind a cosmetically noticeable residue of fibro-fatty tissue (Fig. 8-101).

Clinically, hemangiomas have been described or categorized as superficial, deep, or mixed lesions, depending on the level of greatest bulk (epidermal, dermal, or subcutaneous). Superficial lesions, sometimes referred to as strawberry hemangiomas, form bright red rounded tumors and/or plaques that are well demarcated and clearly elevated above the surrounding skin surface. They are soft, compressible, and usually range in size from a few millimeters to 5 cm, although some can be much larger. In deep hemangiomas whose bulk is located deeper in the dermis or in subcutaneous fat, the overlying skin tends to have a subtle bluish hue. Further, their borders are indistinct, and they have a doughy consistency on palpation (Fig. 8-102). When placed in a dependent position, deep hemangiomas enlarge as they fill with an increased amount of blood—a finding that helps differentiate them from lymphangiomas. Most hemangiomas, however, are mixed, having both superficial and deeper components (Fig. 8-103). More than half of all hemangiomas are

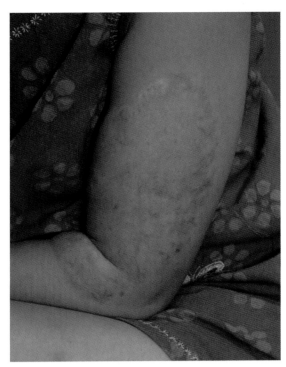

Figure 8-101. Following involution of some large hemangiomas, the patient is left with a fibrofatty residue at the site.

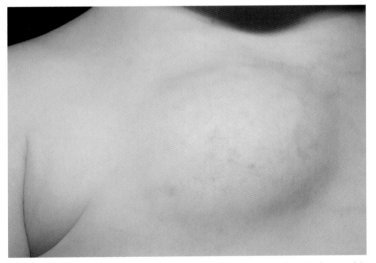

Figure 8-102. Deep hemangioma. Most of the vessels that make up this large, partially compressible lesion lie deep beneath the skin surface but still impart a bluish hue to the overlying skin. Note the indistinctness of the margins.

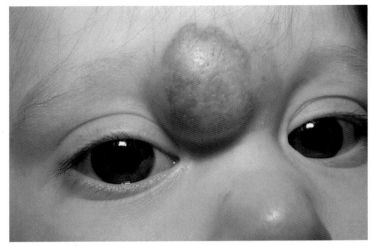

Figure 8-103. Mixed hemangioma. The hemangioma on this child's nasal bridge has both superficial and deep components.

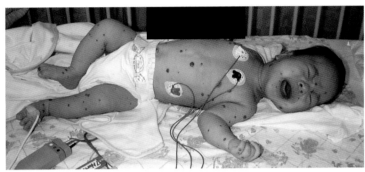

Figure 8-104. Hemangiomatosis. This infant presented with signs of congestive heart failure due to arteriovenous shunting within a large hepatic hemangioma. Note the large number of lesions and that all are less than 2 cm in diameter, rounded, and widely dispersed.

found on the head and neck, about 25% on the trunk, and the rest on the extremities.

While most infants have only a single lesion, a small proportion have multiple hemangiomas, ranging from a few to several, to a hundred or more. Those with numerous lesions are said to have hemangiomatosis. When these are limited to the skin, the condition is termed *benign* (see Fig. 8-98). In some, however, cutaneous lesions are associated with internal or visceral lesions. This appears most common in infants with numerous small (<2 cm), widely dispersed cutaneous hemangiomas (Fig. 8-104). Internal lesions can involve the liver, gastrointestinal tract, CNS and lungs, as well as other organs. Large hepatic hemangiomas often have arteriovenous shunts that precipitate high-output congestive heart failure and affected infants tend to present between 6 and 12 weeks of age with tachy-

pnea, dyspnea, and sweating with feedings and hepatomegaly. Gastrointestinal (GI) lesions are often manifest by gastrointestinal bleeding and CNS neoplasms by mass effects. Thus in young infants presenting with a large number of small, widely dispersed hemangiomas, a screening hepatic ultrasound examination and close observation for GI and CNS signs and symptoms may be advisable. It must be noted, however, that on occasion a patient with only a few or even no cutaneous hemangiomas may present with signs of an internal lesion as well (see later).

In addition to the increased risk of visceral involvement in infants with hemangiomatosis, certain sites and patterns of cutaneous hemangiomas may serve as signals for underlying lesions. The presence of hemangiomas over the lower face (lower lip, chin, preauricular area, and neck) in the "beard" distribution has a significant association with airway involvement (Fig. 8-105), and midline lumbosacral hemangiomas may be markers of underlying spinal dysraphism (see Chapter 15). Along these lines, an important syndrome newly described by Frieden and colleagues is **PHACES syndrome**. PHACES is an acronym for **p**osterior fossa malformations, **h**emangiomas (usually a plaque-like segmental hemangioma of the face), **a**rterial anomalies (including abnormal carotid arteries), **c**ardiac defects, **e**ye anomalies and **s**ternal clefting. The segmental hemangioma associated with PHACES syndrome may be present at birth and may initially mimic a port-wine stain. However, unlike port-wine stains, they are often ulcerated at the time of presentation and begin to proliferate rapidly, becoming raised and plaque-like (Fig. 8-106).

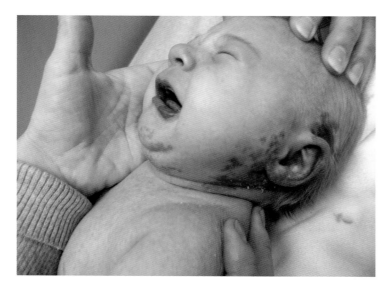

Figure 8-105. Hemangiomas involving the "beard" distribution of the lower face signal the possibility of underlying airway hemangiomas.

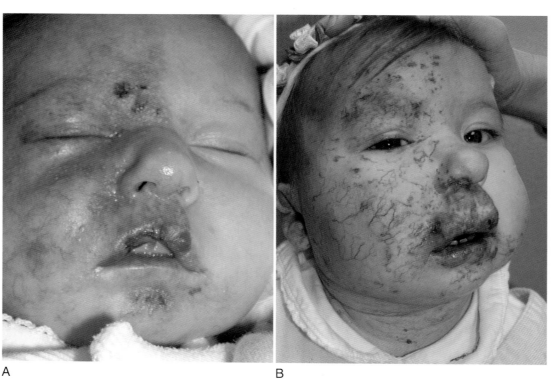

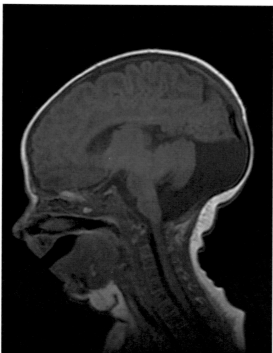

Figure 8-106. PHACES syndrome. At birth these lesions are plaquelike and may mimic a port-wine stain. However, they ulcerate early on **(A)** and then proliferate rapidly, becoming raised, as seen in the same infant at one year **(B)**. **C,** This MRI reveals a Dandy-Walker malformation in an infant with PHACES.

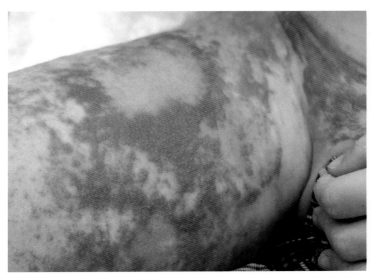

Figure 8-107. Tufted angioma. This lesion involving the right leg first appeared as a bruiselike plaque, which continued to grow well beyond infancy.

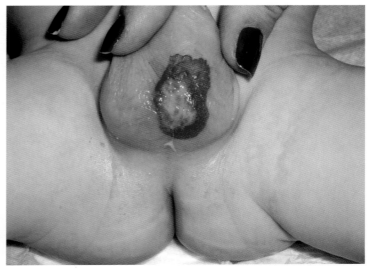

Figure 8-108. Ulcerated hemangioma. Hemangiomas located in friction- or maceration-prone areas are at risk for ulceration. When ulcerated, they cause significant pain, are vulnerable to infection, and ultimately, scarring, unless treated aggressively.

In the past it was believed that large hemangiomas, whether cutaneous or visceral, could sequester platelets, resulting in coagulopathy, a phenomenon termed *Kasabach-Merritt syndrome*, characterized by sudden enlargement of a vascular tumor accompanied by thrombocytopenia. It is now clear, however, that this potentially life-threatening condition occurs exclusively with one of two rare vascular tumors: the kaposiform hemangioendothelioma and the tufted angioma (Fig. 8-107), two distinct pathologic entities that express more lymphatic markers than hemangiomas. Both of these lesions appear more purpuric than infantile hemangiomas and need to be treated in conjunction with an oncologist because their behavior can be aggressive.

There are certain complications seen in infants with cutaneous hemangiomas that are site specific and require close monitoring because they can be associated with significant morbidity if left untreated. Periorbital and lid lesions can cause significant narrowing of the palpebral aperture, thereby occluding the visual axis. They can also compress the cornea. This constitutes an ophthalmologic emergency because, without prompt and aggressive therapy, permanent visual axis deprivation, amblyopia, strabismus, and astigmatism can result. As noted earlier, it is important to recognize that infants with hemangiomas distributed over the lower face may have similar lesions of the airway. With growth, these can cause narrowing, resulting in stridor and respiratory distress within the first few months, at times necessitating tracheotomy. Hemangiomas involving the lips, nose, or ears have a high potential for permanent disfigurement. Steroids, interferon, or surgical intervention may be indicated for lesions involving the airway or the eye.

Lesions located in areas that are prone to friction and/or maceration, such as the diaper area, intertriginous folds, and perioral region, are especially at risk of developing painful ulcerations (Fig. 8-108). This can result in bleeding, secondary infection, and ultimately scarring. Hence close attention should be paid to skin care to prevent breakdown. If ulceration does occur, treatment with wet compresses and antibacterial ointment often suffices, with pulsed-dye laser serving as an effective second-line treatment.

Considering that the majority of infantile hemangiomas cause no discomfort and, with the exceptions described earlier, pose no undue risk, and given their natural history

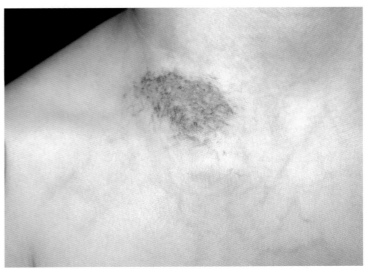

Figure 8-109. NICH lesion (noninvoluting congenital hemangioma). These lesions are present at birth and have a telangiectatic surface surrounded by a rim of pallor. (Courtesy http://www.dermatlas.org.)

of involution, conservative management (e.g., watchful waiting) is generally the best approach to management.

Recently, two new types of hemangiomas, distinguished by their presence at the time of birth and therefore termed *congenital*, have been described. The noninvoluting congenital hemangioma (NICH) is at peak size at the time of delivery but does not recede. It has a telangiectatic surface with a rim of pallor (Fig. 8-109). The rapidly involuting congenital hemangioma (RICH) also peaks in size at the time of birth, but this subtype recedes briskly, often before 1 year of life, leaving behind a characteristic atrophied plaque (Fig. 8-110). Both NICH and RICH lesions demonstrate tissue markers different from those of infantile hemangiomas and seem to have higher vascular flow, which may explain their differing clinical courses.

Pyogenic Granuloma

Pyogenic granulomas are common benign vascular tumors that resemble small hemangiomas. They are

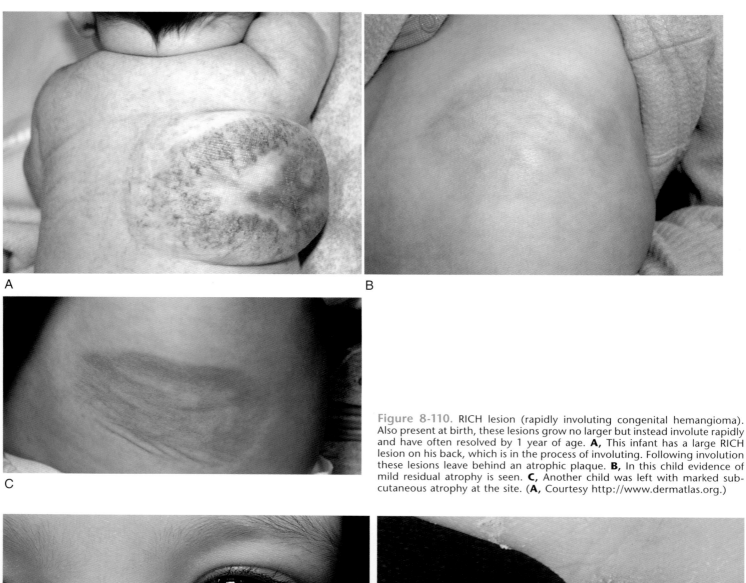

A

B

C

Figure 8-110. RICH lesion (rapidly involuting congenital hemangioma). Also present at birth, these lesions grow no larger but instead involute rapidly and have often resolved by 1 year of age. **A,** This infant has a large RICH lesion on his back, which is in the process of involuting. Following involution these lesions leave behind an atrophic plaque. **B,** In this child evidence of mild residual atrophy is seen. **C,** Another child was left with marked sub-cutaneous atrophy at the site. (**A,** Courtesy http://www.dermatlas.org.)

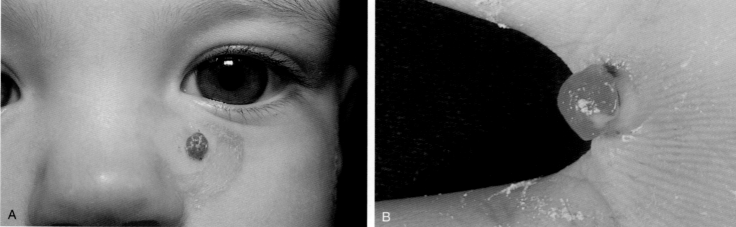

A

B

Figure 8-111. Pyogenic granuloma. **A,** A bright red, raised, hemorrhagic papule developed on an infant's cheek. **B,** Another rapidly growing friable lesion is present between this child's fingers.

thought to stem from vascular overgrowth of granulation tissue following minor trauma, or in reaction to a foreign body such as a thorn, splinter, or piece of glass. They are seen in children and young adults, and lesions are usually located on the face or an extremity, although on occasion, the trunk and mucous membranes may be involved. They consist of solitary bright red, soft nodules that are often pedunculated and average 5 to 6 mm in diameter. Their surface is friable and bleeds easily (Fig. 8-111A and B). Pyogenic granulomas are commonly confused with hemangiomas, but their onset well after the newborn period and their morphology, distribution, and course allow for

distinction between these two types of benign vascular tumors. Treatment consists of excision followed by electrodesiccation of the "feeder" blood vessels at the base. They occasionally recur, in which case repeat surgery is recommended.

Vascular Malformations

Vascular malformations are not neoplasms, but rather develop as a result of errors in morphogenesis of capillaries, veins, arteries, or lymphatic vessels (or any combination thereof). Capillary and lymphatic lesions are present at birth and, in contrast to hemangiomas, which grow rapidly and then involve, vascular malformations are static lesions that grow only in proportion to the child, and do not recede over time. Arterial, venous, and arteriovenous malformations may be present at birth but more commonly appear later in childhood or adolescence. Capillary and venous malformations are macular and easily compressible. Because they are not proliferative, they are not prone to ulceration. In this section we focus mainly on capillary and capillary/venous malformations because they are the most common vascular malformations seen in infancy. They include *salmon patches,* present in more than 70% of newborns, and *port-wine stains.*

Nevus Simplex (Salmon Patch or "Stork Bite")
The nevus simplex, which is commonly referred to as a *salmon patch* or *"stork bite,"* is a capillary malformation that is seen in the majority of infants and hence is considered a normal variant. Some experts believe that these may represent persistent fetal vessels as opposed to a true malformation, which may partly explain why they tend to fade slightly over time. Lesions are located at the nape of the neck and on the glabella, forehead, upper eyelids, and/or lower back (Fig. 8-112). They become more apparent clinically when the baby cries or strains and tend to fade or become less noticeable over the first year of life.

Nevus Flammeus (Port-Wine Stain)
The nevus flammeus, better known as a *port-wine stain* for its purple-red color, is a congenital capillary/venous malformation, consisting of dilated vessels throughout the dermis and often within subcutaneous tissues. Unlike infantile hemangiomas, these neither enlarge nor involute over time. Left untreated, however, they can develop angiomatous blebs by adolescence or adulthood. Most commonly they are located unilaterally on the face (Fig. 8-113) and, when present in the distribution of the ophthalmic branch of the trigeminal nerve, can be associated with *Sturge-Weber syndrome,* a constellation of port-wine stain, vascular malformations of the ipsilateral leptomeninges and cerebral cortex, and glaucoma. Seizures, mental retardation, and hemiplegia are possible complications (see Chapter 15 and Figs. 15-19 through 15-22). An important differential diagnostic consideration is PHACES syndrome, in which the initial lesion may resemble a facial port-wine stain before entering its phase of rapid growth (see Fig. 8-106).

A port-wine stain located over the midline occipital scalp, especially when accompanied by a hair tuft or whorl, may overlie a CNS malformation (see Fig. 15-34), just as a midline lumbosacral port-wine stain may be associated with an underlying spinal anomaly (see Chapter 15 and Fig. 15-33). An extensive port-wine stain located over an extremity may, by virtue of having an abnormally rich blood supply, result in soft tissue and bony overgrowth and hemihypertrophy, a condition known as *Klippel-Trenaunay syndrome* (see Fig. 15-23).

Nevi

Nevomelanocytic nevus is a term used to describe a group of congenital and acquired pigmented lesions located in the dermis which contain nevus cells derived from the neural crest. These cells, like melanocytes in the epidermis, have the ability to synthesize melanin. The term *nevus* also refers to a group of congenital skin lesions composed of mature or nearly mature cutaneous elements organized in an abnormal fashion. Also known as *hamartomas,* the latter may be composed of almost any epidermal or dermal structures.

Nevomelanocytic Nevi

Congenital Nevomelanocytic Nevi
Congenital forms of nevomelanocytic nevi (CNN) consist of pigmented plaques often associated with dense hair growth. At birth, lesions may be tan or light pink, with only soft vellus hairs (Fig. 8-114A). During infancy and childhood, the nevus darkens, the hair becomes more prominent, and small dark macules or nodules may appear in a pebbly array within the larger plaque (Fig. 8-114B). CNN are classified by size, specifically their greatest diameter: small being less than 1.5 cm, medium 1.5 to 20 cm, and large greater than 20 cm. A large CNN present in a segmental distribution is termed a 'giant CNN' (Fig. 8-115).

All CNN have the potential for malignant transformation, which may be heralded by development of new, darker and/or bleeding nodules within the original lesion or by sudden rapid growth of the nevus. The likelihood

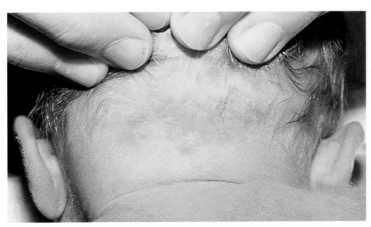

Figure 8-112. Stork bite, or salmon patch. A typical light red splotchy area is seen at the nape of the neck.

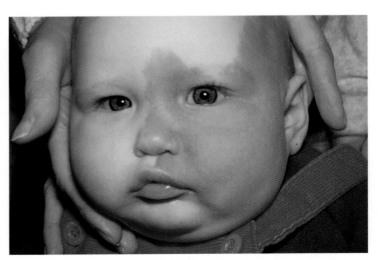

Figure 8-113. Port-wine stain. This infant has a characteristic purplish-red lesion covering nearly half of his face.

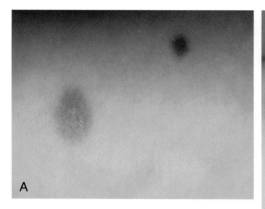
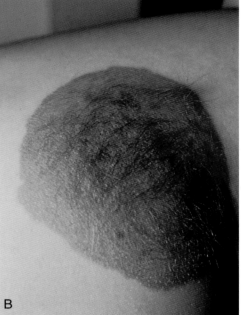

Figure 8-114. Congenital nevomelanocytic nevi. **A,** Two small nevi with differing degrees of hyperpigmentation are seen on the thigh of an infant. **B,** During adolescence this nevus developed prominent hair and dark pigmented macules and papules within its borders.

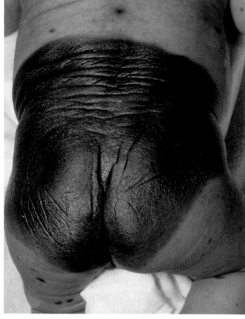

Figure 8-115. Giant nevomelanocytic nevus. This lesion covers the lower back and buttocks, is uniformly pigmented, and has smaller satellite nevi.

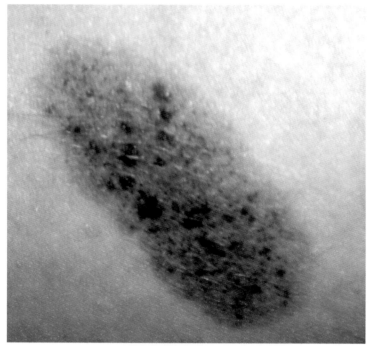

Figure 8-116. Nevus spilus. These lesions consist of light brown macules, with darker brown speckles scattered uniformly over their surfaces.

of malignant transformation is relatively low (1% to 4%) for small- to medium-sized CNN, in contrast to the much higher risk seen with giant CNN, which carry a 10% to 30% lifetime risk of progression to melanoma and which can undergo malignant change before puberty.

Although no uniformly accepted guidelines exist for management of small- to medium-size nevi, a reasonable approach is to have yearly follow-up with a dermatologist or physician skilled at monitoring patients with pigmented lesions. Excision is recommended if they begin to appear atypical or if they are located in areas that are difficult to monitor such as the scalp, groin, or interdigital spaces. Because of their higher risk, early full-thickness excision (in infancy, if possible), followed by grafting, is advisable for patients with giant CNN. However, some exceptionally large nevi may not be amenable to surgical management. In these cases impeccably close observation (facilitated by comparative photographs) is recommended, usually at

6-month intervals. Careful palpation of the entire lesion is necessary at each visit, as melanomas may arise deep within a large CNN and often are first detectable as a new palpable nodule, well before any surface change occurs.

CNN must be differentiated from other congenital pigmented spots such as urticaria pigmentosa, lentigines, café-au-lait spots, and Mongolian spots, none of which carry any significant risk of malignancy. The *nevus spilus*, which consists of a light brown macule with darker brown freckling throughout, is considered to be a variant of congenital nevus with an extremely low risk of progression to melanoma (Fig. 8-116).

Acquired Nevomelanocytic Nevi

Acquired nevomelanocytic nevi begin to develop in early childhood as small, pigmented macules 1 to 2 mm

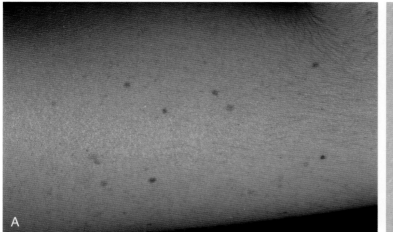
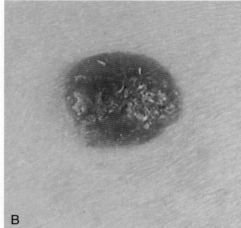

Figure 8-117. Acquired nevomelanocytic nevi. **A,** Junctional nevi. These brown macules are flat on palpation. **B,** This typical compound nevus is raised, with a regular border and uniform pigmentation.

in diameter, which are flat on palpation. At this stage the nevus cells are limited to the epidermal-dermal junction and are called *junctional nevi* (Fig. 8-117A). They then enlarge slowly and become papular or even pedunculated. In such elevated nevi, the nevus cells have proliferated into the dermis to become either intradermal or *compound nevi* (Fig. 8-117B). During puberty, these lesions may darken noticeably and increase in size. However, normal nevomelanocytic nevi rarely exceed 1 cm in diameter. They tend to be located on sun-exposed areas and are seen less frequently on the soles, palms, legs, genitalia, and mucous membranes. Generally, these nevi change slowly over months to years and warrant only observation.

Sudden enlargement of a nevus with redness and tenderness may occur because of infection of a hair follicle within the nevus or due to rupture of a follicular cyst with a secondary foreign body reaction. This may alarm the patient, prompting dermatologic evaluation. Another slower change causing concern in patients is the appearance of a hypopigmented or depigmented ring associated with mild local pruritus around a benign nevus. This is called a *halo nevus* (Fig. 8-118), and the phenomenon is caused by a cytotoxic T-lymphocyte reaction against both the nevus cells and their innocent melanocytic bystanders. As a result, the nevus tends to disappear partially or completely, and the halo eventually repigments.

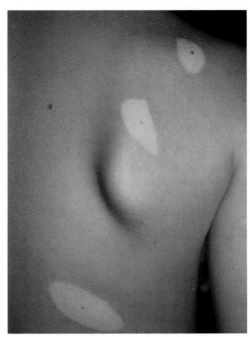

Figure 8-118. Halo nevi. Large hypopigmented halos surround three relatively small nevi on the back of this boy.

Nevi and Melanomas

Melanomas in childhood may occur de novo or develop within a giant congenital nevus. More rarely, a different type of nevus may undergo malignant transformation. Another cause of melanoma in the pediatric age group is transplacental transfer of maternal melanoma. Thus neonates born to mothers with a history of melanoma should be examined and followed carefully. Conversely, mothers of infants born with melanoma should be examined thoroughly for signs of the malignancy, and all first-degree relatives should be checked yearly for signs of melanoma.

As long as the clinical appearance of a nevus is typical, excision is unnecessary. However, a number of changes in pigmented lesions may portend the development of melanoma (Fig. 8-119). These include the following:
1. A change in size, shape, or outline, with scalloped, irregular borders
2. A change in the surface characteristics such as development of a small, dark, elevated papule or nodule within

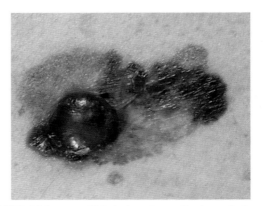

Figure 8-119. Melanoma. This lesion shows the irregularity of outline, color, and thickness typical of a melanoma.

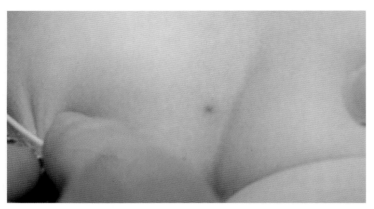

Figure 8-120. Blue nevus. This blue nodule was made up of deep nevus cells; it was firm on palpation.

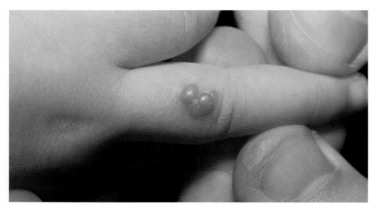

Figure 8-121. Spitz nevus. This raised red nevus grows rapidly.

an otherwise flat plaque; or flaking, scaling, ulceration, or bleeding
3. A change in color to a different shade of black or brown or to a mixture of red, white, or blue
4. Development of burning, itching, or tenderness, which may be an indication of the body's immune reaction to malignancy

Fortunately, melanomas are still rare in children. However, their incidence is increasing (at about 3% annually), and curative treatment is contingent on early diagnosis and prompt excision. Hence it is important for clinicians to have a keen awareness of diagnostic features and of worrisome changes in benign nevi that should prompt referral for possible excision. Excised specimens should be analyzed by a pathologist specialized in dermatologic pathology and in melanomas because many of the changes of dysplasia are subtle and require experience to recognize the grade.

The differential diagnosis of childhood melanoma includes congenital and acquired nevocytic nevi; the **blue nevus,** a small, firm, blue papule consisting of deep nevus cells (Fig. 8-120); traumatic hemorrhage, especially under the nails or in mucous membranes; vascular lesions such as pyogenic granuloma or angiokeratoma; and the **Spitz nevus,** a red and rapidly growing nevocytic nevus composed of spindle and epithelial cells that can be confused clinically and histologically with melanoma (Fig. 8-121).

Hamartomatous Nevi

Hamartomatous nevi are derived from embryonic ectoderm and can be composed of epidermal structures, hair

follicles *(nevus pilosis),* apocrine and eccrine glands *(apocrine* and *eccrine nevi),* fibroblasts *(connective tissue nevi),* blood vessels (salmon patch [see Fig. 8-112]), and multiple components *(nevus sebaceous).*

Epidermal nevi are quite common in pediatric patients. They are composed of epidermal structures only and must be distinguished from nevus sebaceous (see later). The lesion may be present at birth or may develop during childhood and appears as a slightly hyperpigmented papillomatous or verrucous growth (Fig. 8-122A-C). Development of and increases in verrucous changes are particularly common at puberty. Lesions may be small and localized, linear, dermatomal, or generalized. The number of differing clinical presentations is reflected in the variety of descriptive synonyms: *nevus verrucosus* for localized disease, *nevus unius lateralis* for linear or unilateral involvement, and *ichthyosis hystrix* for bilateral involvement with irregular geometric patterns. Important associations with extensive epidermal nevi are seizures, mental retardation, and ocular and skeletal defects (see Chapter 15 and Fig. 15-26). Extensive lesions have also been associated with hypophosphatemic vitamin D–resistant rickets.

Nevus sebaceous of Jadassohn is characterized by a hairless, well-circumscribed, skin-colored or yellowish waxy plaque located most commonly on the scalp, face, or neck (Fig. 8-123 and see Fig. 15-25). The lesion is usually solitary and may be linear or round. It is present at birth, although at puberty the plaque may become more verrucous, raised, and nodular (see Fig. 15-25). Histologically, epidermal proliferation is seen along with abortive hair follicles, sebaceous glands, and apocrine structures. Although it has been taught in the past that 10% to 15% of these nevi develop into secondary malignant neoplasms, recent studies suggest that this is extremely rare in children and uncommon even in adults. Many neoplasms arising from nevus sebaceous lesions, previously thought to be basal cell carcinomas, were actually benign follicular growths known as trichoblastomas. As a consequence, routine excision of nevus sebaceous in childhood is not medically necessary and can be deferred to adolescence or adulthood.

Disorders of Pigmentation

Childhood disorders of pigmentation are usually of cosmetic importance only, although some pigmented lesions are markers of multisystem disease.

Postinflammatory Pigmentary Changes

Postinflammatory hyperpigmentation (Fig. 8-124A and B) and hypopigmentation (Fig. 8-125) are the most common forms of disordered pigmentation. The phenomenon develops following inflammatory disorders of the skin such as dermatitis, acne, infection, or injury and usually resolves spontaneously over a few months. Histologically, melanocytes appear normal, but the dispersion of pigment to other cells is disturbed. Postinflammatory hypopigmentation also must be distinguished from vitiligo (see Fig. 8-127), in which there is usually a complete absence of pigment without associated scaling or history of inflammation. Tinea versicolor may present with hypopigmented patches in sun-exposed areas (or hyperpigmented lesions in clothing-covered sites), which are covered with a fine scale. KOH examination confirms the

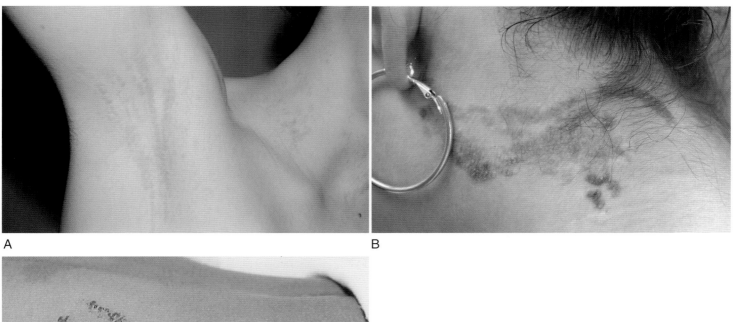

A

B

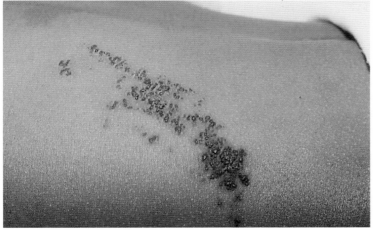

C

Figure 8-122. Epidermal nevi. **A-C,** These raised lesions vary in color depending on the child's skin tone, ranging from lightly pigmented to markedly hyperpigmented. Note the characteristic whorled array of verrucous papules best seen in **B.** All three of these children had localized lesions and were otherwise healthy. More extensive nevi may be associated with systemic abnormalities (epidermal nevus syndrome [see Chapter 15]).

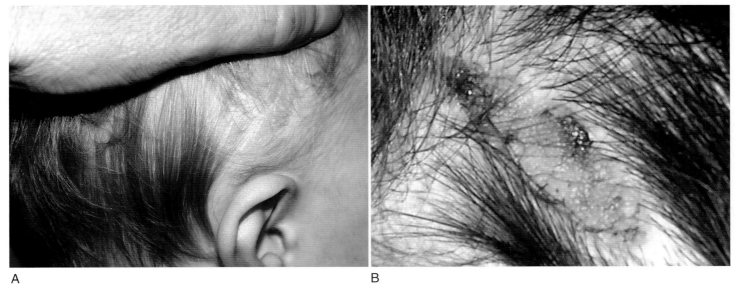

A

B

Figure 8-123. Nevus sebaceous of Jadassohn. **A,** This yellowish, hairless plaque was present on the temporal scalp at birth. **B,** In an adolescent boy the lesion has developed secondary warty growths, stimulated by pubertal androgens. (**A,** Courtesy http://www.dermatlas.org.)

correct diagnosis by demonstrating typical "spaghetti and meatballs" organisms (see Figs. 8-39 and 8-40).

Pigmentary Mosaicism

The term pigmentary mosaicism refers to a group of conditions in which affected children have genetic mosa-icism (e.g., they are born with at least two genetically different cell lines, resulting in the existence of keratinocytes of two different pigment tones). When these different populations of skin cells migrate during development, they create a whorled, fountain-like pattern of alternating hypo- and hyperpigmentation (Fig. 8-126A-C). This pattern is referred to as a Blaschkoid distribution because it occurs along the "lines of Blaschko," which are lines of embryo-

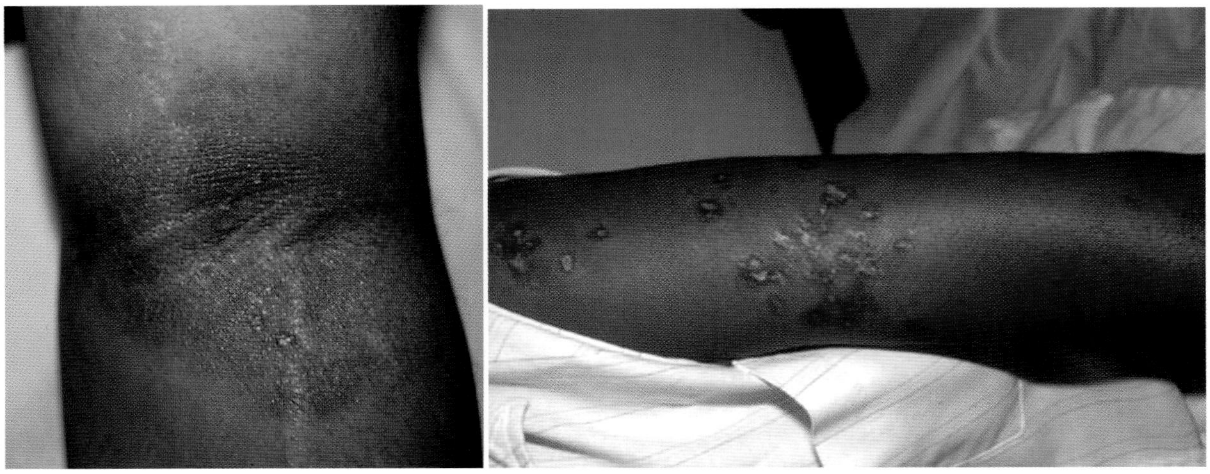

Figure 8-124. Postinflammatory hyperpigmentation **(A)** arose in a child with chronic atopic dermatitis, which provoked persistent scratching. **B,** This patient with discoid lupus provides another example of the phenomenon.

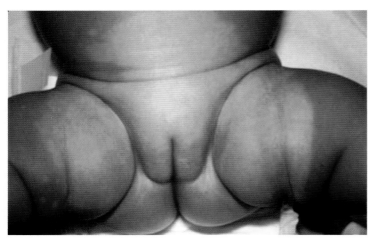

Figure 8-125. Postinflammatory hypopigmentation is evident in this infant following treatment with topical agents for seborrheic diaper dermatitis.

logic ectodermal development. They may be evident at birth and, if not, appear in infancy or early childhood. The bands are macular and are found most commonly over the trunk and respect the midline, but they can also be seen on the extremities, where they tend to be more linear. In contrast to the hyperpigmented macules of incontinentia pigmenti, those of pure pigmentary mosaicism have no antecedent vesicular or verrucous lesions.

Pigmentary mosaicism can stem from a post-zygotic mutation, an error in cell division early on in the course of embryogenesis, or as a result of random X-chromosome inactivation in X-linked conditions. The phenomenon has been reported in association with a number of different types of chromosomal mosaicism including trisomies 13, 18, and 20, among others. At least 15% of those affected have associated abnormalities of the CNS, the musculoskeletal system, and/or the eye. The more extensive the cutaneous features of whorled dyspigmentation, the more likely it is for the child to have associated extracutaneous comorbidities.

Vitiligo

In vitiligo, an acquired condition, there is partial to complete loss of pigmentation. Lesions consist of well-demarcated hypopigmented and depigmented macules and patches that are usually seen in a characteristic distribution around the eyes, mouth, genitals, elbows, hands, and feet (Fig. 8-127), although they may appear elsewhere, as in a koebnerized distribution in areas of prior friction or trauma. They enhance dramatically under a Wood's lamp. Spontaneous but slow repigmentation may occur from the edges of a lesion and around hair follicles (which retain melanocytes), resulting in a speckled appearance. Histologically, melanocytes are absent in areas of vitiligo, and evidence suggests that they have been destroyed by an autoimmune mechanism.

Ash-Leaf Spots

Congenital, well demarcated, hypopigmented macules, termed *ash-leaf spots* because of their usual lancinate shape, are often a valuable early marker of tuberous sclerosis. They appear at birth or shortly thereafter as 1- to 3-cm macular lesions on the trunk. Because they are hypopigmented, rather than totally depigmented, they are not as easily appreciated or as ivory white as the lesions of vitiligo, and their usual truncal distribution is different (see Fig. 15-13).

The identification of ash-leaf macules may be enhanced (although not as dramatically as is seen in vitiligo) by the use of a Wood's light, and this method of examination should be part of the assessment of any child, particularly one with a fair complexion, who develops idiopathic seizures in infancy. The visible purple light emitted is absorbed by normal melanin in the skin. Thus in a darkened room, areas of hypopigmentation or depigmentation appear brighter violet, whereas normally melanized skin reflects little visible light and appears dull purple or black. In addition to tuberous sclerosis, Wood's light examination may also be helpful in delineating the full extent of pigmentary changes in vitiligo and in postinflammatory hypopigmentation.

Important to recognize is that up to 0.5% of otherwise normal newborns will have an isolated hypopigmented macule, which, in the absence of other signs of tuberous sclerosis, is termed a ***nevus depigmentosus*** and represents a localized form of pigmentary mosaicism (Fig. 8-128).

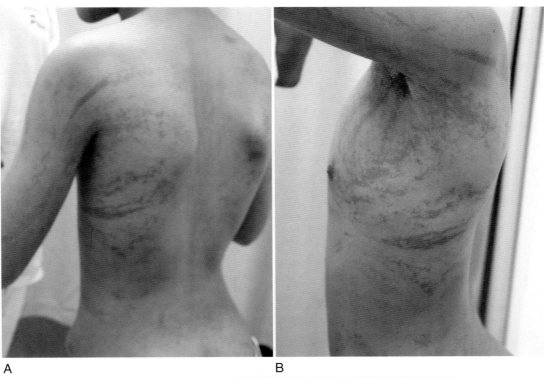

Figure 8-126. Pigmentary mosaicism. **A** and **B,** Swirling bands of alternating lighter and darker hues are seen on this adolescent's trunk, demonstrating a widespread Blaschkoid distribution. Note that they vary in width, stop at the midline, and that the streaks on the upper arm are more linear and parallel to its long axis. The patient also had a seizure disorder and significant cognitive deficits. **C,** More extensive involvement is seen over the back of another child. (**C,** Courtesy http://www.dermatlas.org.)

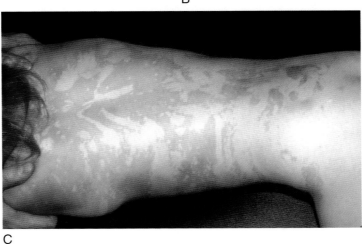

A   B

C

Albinism

The term *albinism* refers to a heterogeneous group of inherited disorders characterized by congenital hypopigmentation of the skin, eyes, and hair. It occurs in an X-linked ocular form (in which the skin appears clinically normal) and an autosomal recessive oculocutaneous form. In oculocutaneous albinism (OCA), both sexes and all races are affected equally. This form of the disorder is subdivided into a number of variants on the basis of clinical findings and biochemical markers. In the past, tyrosinase-negative and tyrosinase-positive subtypes were identified on the basis of the ability of plucked hairs to produce pigment when incubated in tyrosine. Now, DNA markers allow for identification of specific mutations. In classic tyrosinase-negative OCA, children are born without any trace of pigment. Affected individuals have snow-white hair, pinkish-white skin, and translucent or blue irises. Nystagmus is common, as is moderate to severe strabismus and poor visual acuity (see Chapter 19). Although children with tyrosinase-positive OCA may be clinically indistinguishable from their tyrosinase-negative counterparts at birth, they usually develop variable

amounts of pigment with increasing age. Eye color may vary from gray to light brown, and hair may change to blond or light brown. Most African American patients acquire as much pigment as light-skinned whites.

Because they lack the protection of melanin, patients with OCA are at high risk for early development of basal cell and squamous cell skin cancers. Hence they should be instructed in the use of sunscreens and avoidance of excessive sun exposure.

Piebaldism

Piebaldism (partial albinism) is a rare autosomal dominant disorder characterized by a white forelock and a circumscribed congenital leukoderma. The typical lesions include a triangular patch of depigmentation and white hair on the frontal scalp. The apex of this patch points toward the nasal bridge (Fig. 8-129A). Patients may also have hypopigmented or depigmented macules on the face, neck, ventral trunk, flanks, or extremities (Fig. 8-129B). Within areas of decreased pigmentation, scattered patches of normal pigmentation or hyperpigmentation may appear. The lesions are stable throughout life, although some variability in pigmentation may occur with sun exposure. Special variants of piebaldism include Waardenburg syndrome, in which leukoderma is associated with lateral displacement of the inner canthi and inferior lacrimal ducts, a flattened nasal bridge, and sensorineural deafness, and Wolf syndrome, an autosomal recessive disorder associated with neurologic deficits.

Acanthosis Nigricans

Acanthosis nigricans is characterized by hyperpigmentation and hyperkeratosis in intertriginous areas and over bony prominences. Skin lines are accentuated, and the skin surface of involved areas may have a velvety, leathery, or warty appearance (Fig. 8-130A-C). Four main forms of the disorder exist. The benign/idiopathic form is the most common and is obesity related. Onset is usually at puberty but can occur in childhood in concert with development of obesity. Interestingly, the prominence of lesions tends to lessen when the patients lose weight. An inherited form, transmitted as an autosomal dominant trait, usually presents in infancy or early childhood but becomes more prominent during adolescence. This form is also unassociated with other underlying disorders. In endocrine-associated acanthosis nigricans, the condition may antedate or appear in association with insulin resistance with or without polycystic ovary disease. More rarely, it is seen in patients with pituitary tumors. Malignancy-related acanthosis nigricans is extremely rare in childhood.

Other Pigmentary Disorders

Café-au-lait spots are tan macules that usually occur in otherwise healthy individuals but which can be an indication of neurofibromatosis 1 (von Recklinghausen disease; see Chapter 15) or McCune-Albright syndrome. In the latter, they are associated with polyostotic fibrous dysplasia of the long bones and endocrinopathy (see Chapter 9). Café-au-lait macules that are small and have smooth borders are more likely to be associated with neurofibro-

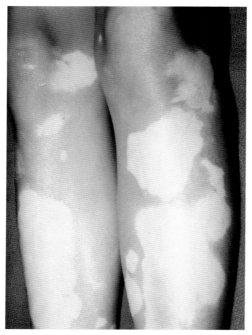

Figure 8-127. Vitiligo. Completely depigmented patches are seen on the legs. Occasionally, macules of repigmentation arise from epidermal appendages within the white patches. A characteristic distribution helps to distinguish vitiligo from other causes of hypopigmentation.

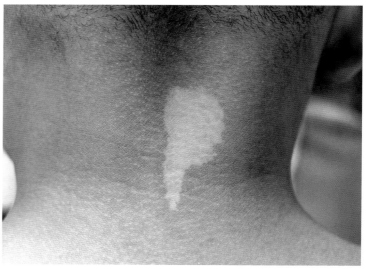

Figure 8-128. Nevus depigmentosus is a localized form of pigmentary mosaicism, seen here on the nape of the neck of an otherwise healthy child.

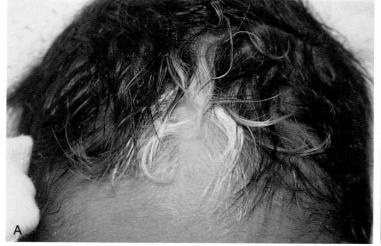
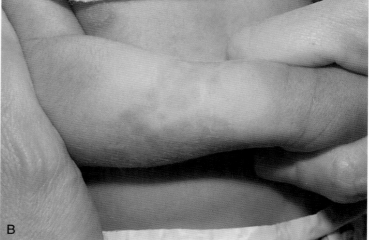

Figure 8-129. Piebaldism. **A,** A white forelock overlies a depigmented patch of scalp and forehead. **B,** The infant also has a hypopigmented patch on his arm in which smaller areas of hyperpigmentation are seen.

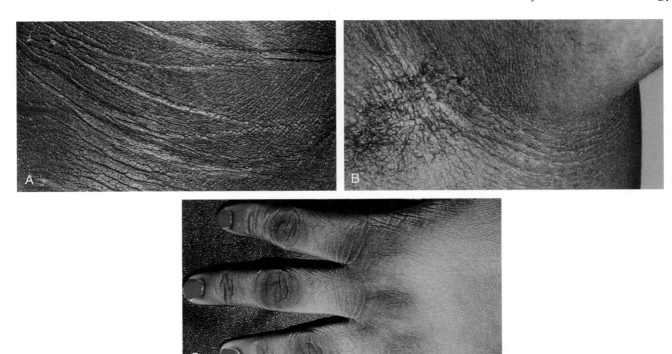

Figure 8-130. Acanthosis nigricans. **A** and **B,** Hyperpigmentation and leathery thickening of the skin are seen on the neck and in the axilla of an obese adolescent with the benign/idiopathic form of the disorder. **C,** She also had velvety hyperpigmentation and prominence of skin lines over the knuckles of her hands and other bony prominences. (From Cohen BA: Pediatric Dermatology, 2nd ed. London, Mosby, 1999.)

matosis 1 (Fig. 8-131A-C), whereas those that are large and segmental with jagged borders are more likely to be seen in association with McCune-Albright syndrome (Fig. 8-131D). Children who have café-au-lait spots in the absence of a syndrome usually have fewer than four lesions that are relatively small in size.

Swirled hyperpigmentation may be a marker of the later stages of incontinentia pigmenti (see Fig. 8-97D and E) or of pigmentary mosaicism (see Fig. 8-126). Diffuse hyperpigmentation may be seen in Addison disease and in hemochromatosis. Peutz-Jeghers syndrome is manifest by lentigo-like pigmentation of the lips (see Fig. 17-66), oral mucosa, hands, and fingers in association with benign small intestinal polyps in children (see Chapter 10 and Fig. 17-67).

Disorders of the Hair and Nails

Diseases that involve the hair and nails make up an integral part of pediatric dermatology. Hair and nails are composed of keratin produced by epidermal hair follicles and the nail matrix, respectively. Some diseases are specific to these structures, whereas others affect the skin as well. In many cases, important diagnostic clues to skin diseases and systemic disorders can be found in related abnormalities of the hair and nails.

The Alopecias

The most common diseases of the hair result in some degree of hair loss, or alopecia. Evaluation begins by determining whether scarring is present. Nonscarring alopecia can be due to growth defects causing the hair to be lost by the roots (effluvium) or by defects of the hair shaft that result in breakage.

Alopecia Caused by Systemic Insult: Telogen and Anagen Effluvium

Normal hair cycles through a growth phase lasting 3 years or more (anagen phase) and a resting phase of 3 months (telogen phase), after which the hair is shed, and the cycle then begins again. Telogen effluvium is one form of partial, temporary alopecia, which may occur 3 months after an emotional or physical stress such as a severe illness, major surgery, or high fever. It rarely causes more than 50% hair loss. In these patients the initial systemic insult induces more than the usual 20% of hairs to enter the telogen phase, and 3 months later these hairs are shed simultaneously, producing marked thinning of scalp hair until new anagen hairs regrow (Fig. 8-132). Anagen effluvium is the sudden loss of growing hairs (80% of normal scalp hairs) caused by abnormal interruption of the anagen phase. In these cases the hair shafts taper and lose adhesion to the follicle. This type of hair loss is most common after systemic chemotherapy.

Alopecia Areata

Alopecia areata is a form of localized anagen effluvium usually presenting with round or oval patches of alopecia that may be located anywhere on the scalp, eyebrows, lashes, or body. Occasionally, hair loss is diffuse or generalized. The injury causing cessation of growth is thought to be of immunologic origin. Clues to diagnosis include absence of inflammation and scaling in the involved areas of scalp and the presence of short (3 to 6 mm), easily epilated hairs at the margins of the patch (Fig. 8-133A and B). Under magnification these hair stubs resemble exclamation points because the hair shaft narrows just before its point of entry into the follicle. Another finding in many patients with alopecia areata is Scotch-plaid pitting of the nails, consisting of rows of pits crossing in a transverse and longitudinal fashion (see Fig. 8-147). The clinical course of alopecia areata is difficult to predict. The

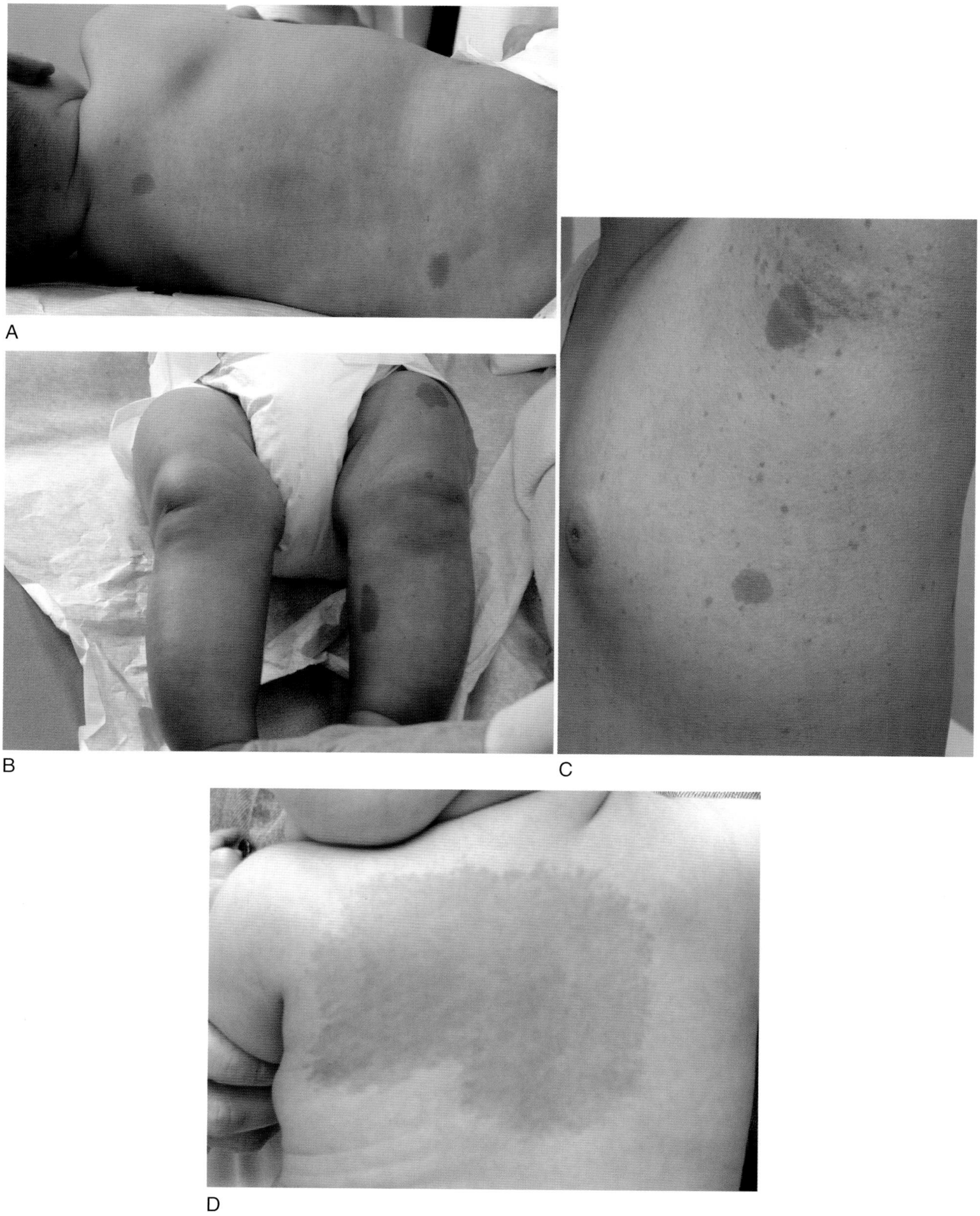

Figure 8-131. Café-au-lait macules. **A** and **B**, Small café-au-lait spots are seen in two infants with neurofibromatosis I, one fairly pigmented and one with darker pigmentation to demonstrate the differences in color of lesions with differing skin tones. Note that the lesions have smooth borders, which are typical of this disorder. The infant in **B** also has pseudoarthrosis of the tibia and fibula, with foreshortening of the left lower leg (see Chapter 15). **C,** This older boy has both café-au-lait spots and axillary freckling (Crowe's sign). The presence of six or more café-au-lait macules and axillary freckling is diagnostic for NF1. **D,** Another infant with McCune-Albright syndrome has a large café-au-lait macule located in a segmental distribution over his back. Note the jagged margins of the lesion. The child also had precocious puberty. (**C,** Courtesy http://www.dermatlas.org.)

disorder may resolve spontaneously; it may persist, with the appearance of new patches while the old patches regrow; or it may progress to total scalp (*alopecia totalis*) or even generalized whole-body alopecia (*alopecia universalis*), either of which can be permanent (Fig. 8-133C). In

severe cases it is helpful to perform a thorough search to exclude coexistent autoimmune disease such as autoimmune thyroiditis because systemically treating the comorbid condition can improve the response of alopecia to topical treatment.

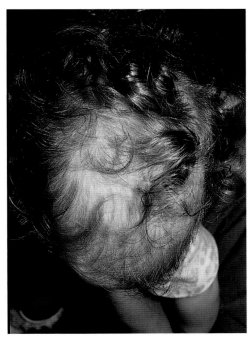

Figure 8-132. Telogen effluvium. This toddler experienced sudden partial hair loss approximately 3 months after being hospitalized for pneumococcal sepsis. (Courtesy Alejandro Hoberman, MD, Children's Hospital of Pittsburgh.)

Trichorrhexis Nodosa

Alopecia caused by hair shaft breakage is due to a structural defect of the hair, and it is easily diagnosed by microscopic examination. The most common structural defect is acquired trichorrhexis nodosa. This defect presents at any age as brittle, short hairs that are perceived by the patient as nongrowing. On gentle pulling, many hairs are easily broken. Microscopically, the distal ends of the hairs are frayed, resembling a broom (Fig. 8-134). Other hairs may have nodules, resembling two brooms stuck together. The fragility is the result of damage to the outer cortex of the hair shaft, resulting in a loss of structural support. Without this support, the weaker fibrous medulla frays like an electrical cord with broken insulation. This disorder is most common in African Americans, often arising from the trauma of combing tightly curled hairs. It is also seen after repeated or severe chemical damage to the cortex from hair straighteners, bleaches, and permanents. Because hair growth is normal, the disorder is self-limited and normal hairs regrow when the source of the damage is identified and eliminated.

Other common causes of hair loss associated with shaft abnormalities include friction alopecia, traction alopecia, and trichotillomania. All are caused by external trauma and breakage of an otherwise normal hair shaft.

Friction Alopecia

Friction alopecia (Fig. 8-135) is common on the posterior scalp of infants, where the head rubs on the pillow or bed clothes. Although worrisome to parents, this disorder

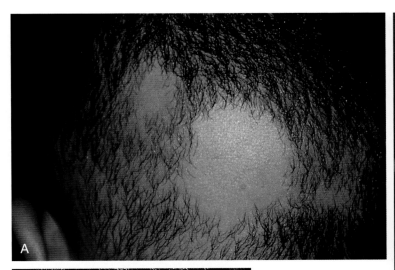

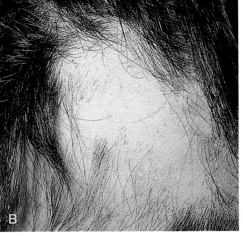

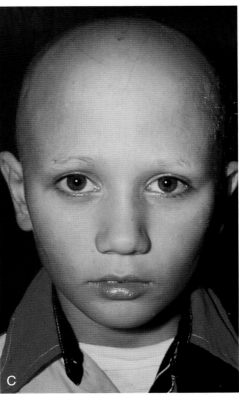

Figure 8-133. Alopecia areata. **A,** Patches of complete hair loss with otherwise normal scalp are typical of this disorder. **B,** In this closeup, small broken hairs that pull out easily are seen at the margins. **C,** In this boy the process has progressed to alopecia totalis. Note that even his eyebrows are involved. (**C,** Courtesy Michael Sherlock, MD, Lutherville, Md.)

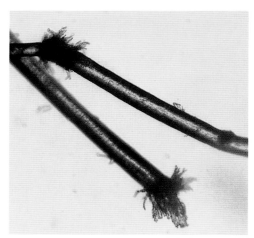

Figure 8-134. Trichorrhexis nodosa consists of a brittle hair shaft defect usually caused by overmanipulation of the hair or application of harsh chemicals. The frayed brown appearance is typical.

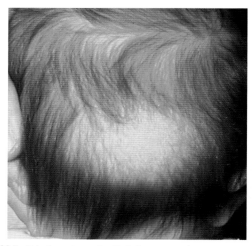

Figure 8-135. Friction alopecia. Hair loss over the occiput resulted from rubbing of the head on sheets and pillows while lying supine.

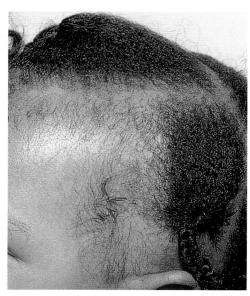

Figure 8-136. Traction alopecia. The hair thinning and loss are due to excessive traction on the hairs as a result of tight braiding.

is self-limited. It has become considerably more common since implementation of the "back-to-sleep" campaign to prevent SIDS. It can be prevented or its severity reduced by ensuring that an infant spends plenty of time on his or her tummy when awake and able to be supervised. When unusually severe or long-standing, it should raise the question of neglect, suggesting that the infant is being left to lie in his or her crib for extended periods of time.

Traction Alopecia

Traction alopecia (Fig. 8-136) is common in young girls whose hairstyles, such as ponytails, pigtails, braids, or cornrows, maintain a tight pull on the hair shafts. This traction causes shaft fractures and follicular damage. If prolonged, permanent scarring alopecia can result. On rare occasions, excess traction applied in the process of braiding can result in subgaleal bleeding and hematoma formation. This phenomenon can also be seen in child abuse victims who have been subjected to forceful hair pulling (see Fig. 6-4).

Trichotillosis (Trichotillomania)

Trichotillosis, also known as *trichotillomania,* is a fairly common disorder seen in school-age children and adolescents that mimics many other types of alopecia. It presents with bizarre patterns of hair loss, often in broad,

linear bands on the vertex or sides of the scalp where the hair is easily twisted and pulled out (Fig. 8-137). Trichotillosis is seen more commonly on the side opposite the child's dominant hand as the other hand is free to manipulate the hair while the child is engaged in other tasks. Rarely, the entire scalp, eyebrows, and eyelashes are involved. The most important clue to the correct diagnosis is the finding of short, broken-off hairs along the scalp, with stubs of different lengths in adjacent areas. This is the result of repetitive pulling and/or twisting of the hair, which fractures the longer shafts. Once broken, the hairs are too short to be rebroken until they grow longer. The scalp appears otherwise normal.

Trichotillomania is sometimes confused with alopecia areata because there are patches of hair loss with short hairs, and there may be involvement of the eyebrows and eyelashes. However, in trichotillomania, patches of hair loss are never completely bald, and the hair shafts are normal anagen hairs that are usually difficult to remove from the scalp. In addition, there are no associated nail abnormalities.

Parents and children usually vigorously deny that the alopecia could be caused by the child, and thus diagnosis rests on a high index of suspicion and recognition of the clinical findings. Although trichotillomania may occur in children with severe psychiatric disease, most cases are associated with situational stress (e.g., school phobia, marital or social problems). Trichotillomania should be distinguished from *habitual hair pulling,* twisting, or twirling seen in preschool children. This typically occurs at bedtime and naptime. Most of these young children shed the habit by the early school years.

Scarring Alopecia

Scarring alopecia in children is considerably less common than nonscarring alopecia and may be caused by a number of disorders, both congenital and acquired. Morphea (localized scleroderma) may involve the scalp with indurated, hairless plaques. Scarring alopecia may also result from severe infection (e.g., inflammatory tinea capitis) or trauma such as oil burns from hot-comb straightening of the hair. A scalp biopsy is often helpful in determining the cause of scarring alopecia.

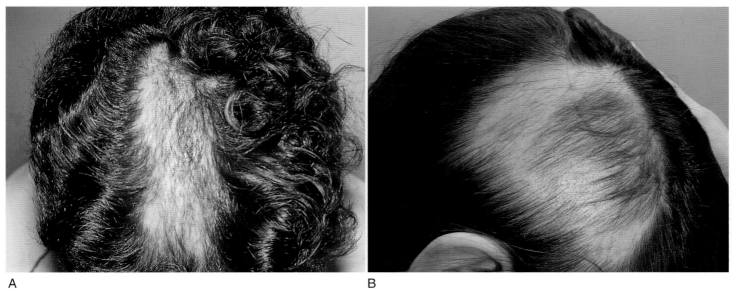

A   B

Figure 8-137. Trichotillosis, or trichotillomania. **A,** This linear patch of short broken hairs along the midline is typical of hair pulling. **B,** Another child has a unilateral geometric patch of hair loss, again with short broken hairs. Note that the scalp is normal in both cases.

Aplasia Cutis Congenita

Aplasia cutis congenita is a congenital condition characterized by absence of or failure of formation of a localized area of scalp or skin, often inherited as an autosomal dominant trait. In most cases there is a single lesion located over the vertex of the scalp. More rarely, lesions may be multiple or may involve the trunk or extremities. They may be associated with limb defects and other congenital and genetic anomalies. In the majority only the dermis and epidermis are absent; however, some lesions extend to involve subcutaneous tissue, and, in rare cases, a calvarial defect may underlie a scalp lesion.

At birth, the lesion may consist of a sharply circumscribed open and weeping ulceration, or it may be covered by a thin, often hemorrhagic membrane or crust (Fig. 8-138A and see Fig. 1-17E). Evaluation should include radiologic studies to assess depth of the lesion and a search for associated anomalies. When a hair collar sign is present surrounding the lesion (see Fig. 138D), one should rule out an underlying neural tube defect. Conservative treatment designed to protect the area from infection and injury includes application of saline compresses, topical antibiotics, and sterile dressings. Depending on the size of the lesion, healing takes place over several weeks to months, leaving a smooth atrophic and hairless scar (Fig. 8-138B and C). The disorder is easily distinguished from ulcerations due to perinatal monitor electrode insertion or blood sampling, by virtue of history. The differential diagnosis includes congenital nevus sebaceous lesions, which are raised and have an uneven, yellow, waxy surface (see Fig. 8-123), and epidermal nevi, which are typically hyperpigmented and have a raised warty surface.

Tinea Capitis (Fungal Infections of the Hair and Scalp)

Fungal infection of the hair weakens the shaft, causing breakage. This typically results in the development of multiple patches of partial alopecia, commonly referred to as *ringworm. Trichophyton tonsurans* is the organism responsible for more than 95% of cases in the United

States, and for unknown reasons, infection with this strain is endemic among African American school children, although there is some evidence of spread by inadequately disinfected barber tools. *Microsporum canis* (the dog and cat ringworm) accounts for a small percentage of cases.

Clinical presentations of tinea capitis vary. In some patients mild erythema and scaling of the scalp occur in association with partial alopecia (Fig. 8-139A). In other cases there is widespread breakage at the scalp, creating a "salt-and-pepper" appearance, with the short residual hairs appearing as black dots on the surface of the scalp (Fig. 8-139B). Occasionally, scalp lesions are annular, simulating tinea corporis. In yet other children, sensitization to the infecting organism results in more erythema, edema, and pustule formation. As the latter rupture, the area weeps and golden crusts form, simulating impetigo (Fig. 8-139C). Some cases are characterized by patches of heaped-up scale in association with small pustules (Fig. 8-139D). Less commonly, intense inflammation causes formation of raised, tender, boggy plaques or masses studded with pustules that simulate abscesses, termed *kerions* (Fig. 8-139E). Unless treated promptly and aggressively with oral antifungal agents and, in cases characterized by severe inflammation, steroids, the latter may produce scarring and permanent hair loss. Incision and drainage of kerions is not indicated because loculations are small and septae thick. Importantly, when pustules or weeping and crusting lesions involve the scalp or hair line, the infection is far more likely to be of fungal than bacterial origin. Patients with tinea capitis often have associated occipital, postauricular, and posterior cervical adenopathy (see Fig. 12-46).

Fungal infection of the scalp is readily confirmed by a KOH examination of infected hairs (Fig. 8-140). Residual broken hairs or black dots at the surface of the scalp should be scraped for KOH preparation and/or fungal culture. In the past when *Microsporum audouinii* was the most common causative organism and was easily identified by its fluorescence, the Wood's light was a useful adjunct in diagnosis. Today, however, *T. tonsurans,* the most common causative organism in the United States, does not fluoresce. Only *M. canis,* which causes 5% of cases, fluoresces bright bluish-green, still justifying its use.

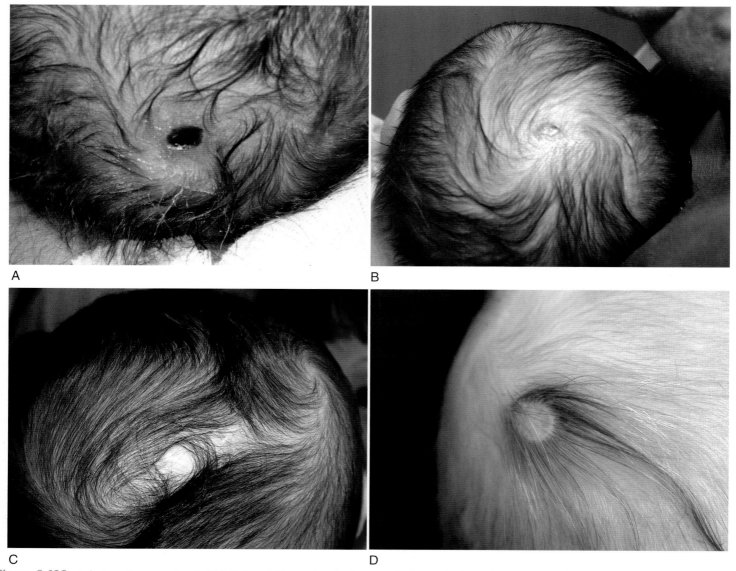

Figure 8-138. Aplasia cutis congenita. **A,** This 2-day-old has a sharply circumscribed, punched out ulceration over the vertex with a hemorrhagic crust. **B,** After 3 weeks of topical mupirocin therapy, the lesion has nearly healed. **C,** The typical atrophic hairless scar of a healed lesion is seen. **D,** Healed aplasia cutis congenita with the "hair collar sign."

Because topical antifungal agents do not penetrate deeply enough to be effective in treatment of tinea capitis, oral antifungal agents are necessary and must be administered for at least 6 weeks to 4 months to eradicate the infection. Unfortunately, risk of recurrence is high. Although griseofulvin and ketoconazole are the only oral agents currently approved in the United States for treatment of tinea capitis, recent studies show that terbinafine, itraconazole, and fluconazole are also effective and require shorter courses of therapy. However, reports of severe adverse side effects of ketoconazole have sharply curtailed its use, and studies of this agent have also raised concerns about its efficacy. Concurrent use of selenium sulfide shampoo (2.5%) during a course of oral therapy reduces spore formation and shedding and thus may help minimize the risk of spread to family members, playmates, and classmates until oral treatment is complete. Other measures useful in reducing passage of organisms to others include no communal use of brushes, combs, or hair grease jars; no sharing of hats, coats, scarves, towels, or linens; and careful washing or cleaning of combs and brushes and of potentially contaminated linen, clothing, and upholstery.

Congenital and Genetic Disorders

Some structural defects of the hair shaft are congenital in origin or associated with heritable syndromes.

Monilethrix and Pili Torti

Monilethrix is a developmental hair defect that produces brittle, beaded hair. The condition is autosomal dominant, and clinical manifestations usually appear after 2 to 3 months of age, when fetal or neonatal vellus hairs are replaced by abnormal beaded hairs (Fig. 8-141A). The scalp is most severely affected, although hair on any part of the body can be involved. The disease is permanent, although the clinical appearance of the hair may improve as the child grows older. Microscopically, regular, periodic narrowing of the hair shafts is seen (Fig. 8-141B). Breakage occurs in constricted areas close to the scalp. Care must be taken not to confuse monilethrix with *pili torti,* another structural defect in which the hair shaft is twisted on its own axis. Pili torti may be localized or generalized and also appears with the first terminal hair growth of infancy. It may be associated with Menkes

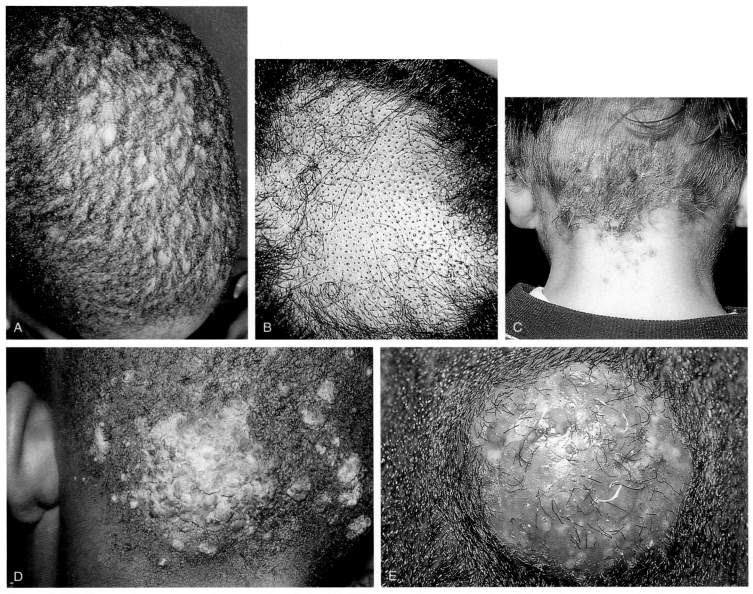

Figure 8-139. Tinea capitis can present in many guises. **A,** In this child, mild erythema and scaling of the scalp are associated with spotty alopecia. **B,** Infiltration of hair shafts by endothrix has resulted in widespread breakage at the scalp, producing a "salt-and-pepper" appearance. **C,** Superficial papules and pustules have ruptured, producing weeping and crusting lesions simulating impetigo. **D,** This variant of tinea is characterized by thick, heaped-up scale. **E,** Kerion. A boggy mass has formed as a result of an intense inflammatory response. This child, seen relatively late in the course, had near total alopecia over the involved area. Note that the lesion is studded with pustules.

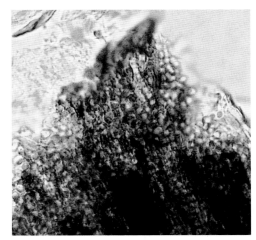

Figure 8-140. Microscopic appearance of hair shafts infected with fungi. Note the tight packing of fungal arthrospores that cause hair shaft fragility and breakage (KOH mount for endothrix).

kinky hair syndrome (Fig. 8-142), an inherited defect of copper absorption, which also affects the central nervous, cardiovascular, and skeletal systems.

Disorders Affecting the Nails

Patients may seek the advice of a physician for nail disorders because of pain or cosmetic concerns. For the physician, knowledge of nail disorders can also be helpful in detecting clues to systemic disease.

Paronychia

Paronychia is a common childhood disorder. It presents as a red, swollen, tender nail fold, usually on the side or at the base of the nail. The acute form, with sudden swelling and marked tenderness, is caused by bacterial invasion by staphylococci or streptococci after trauma to the cuticle (often from chewing), or it can develop in a child with a dermatitis that has damaged the stratum corneum barrier

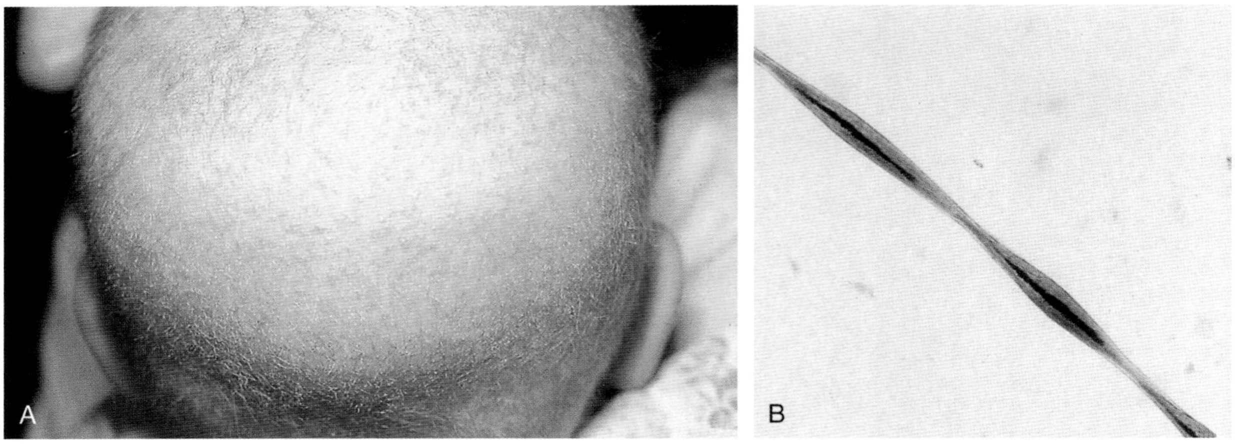

Figure 8-141. Monilethrix. **A,** Short, broken hairs give the appearance of diffuse alopecia. **B,** Microscopically, periodic narrowing of this hair shaft is evident. Hairs are brittle and break off at constricted points near the scalp.

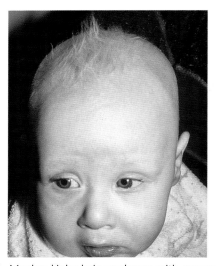

Figure 8-142. Menkes kinky hair syndrome with generalized pili torti. This infant demonstrates the characteristic features of the disorder: fair skin; blue eyes; and the fair, sparse brittle hair of diffuse pili torti. He experienced developmental regression and had a seizure disorder. (From Cohen BA: Pediatric Dermatology, 2nd ed. London, Mosby, 1999.)

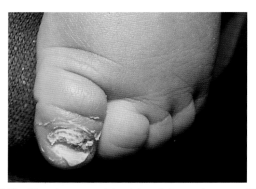

Figure 8-143. Chronic paronychia with nail dystrophy caused by candidal infection.

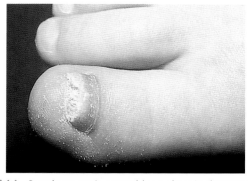

Figure 8-144. Onychomycosis caused by a chronic dermatophyte infection of the nail plate in a 4-year-old boy. This is relatively rare in prepubertal children.

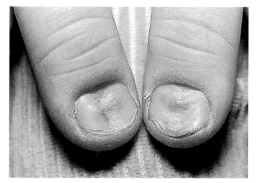

Figure 8-145. Traumatic nail dystrophy. This teenager developed median nail dystrophy as a result of chronically picking at his nails.

(see Fig. 12-32). Chronic paronychia may involve one or several nails. An associated history of chronic dermatitis or frequent exposure to water usually is present. In contrast to the acute form, tenderness is mild, although sometimes a small amount of pus can be extruded. Some degree of associated nail dystrophy often exists (Fig. 8-143). The causative organisms are *Candida* species, usually *C. albicans*. This form resolves with the use of topical antimycotics and avoidance of water.

Onychomycosis and Nail Dystrophy

Onychomycosis, or fungal infection of the nail plate (Fig. 8-144), is not as common in children before puberty as it is in adults. Thus nail dystrophy should not be treated as a fungal infection unless proven by microscopic examination or fungal culture. Dystrophic nails are seen frequently as a complication of trauma (Fig. 8-145) or of an underlying dermatosis such as psoriasis, atopic dermatitis, or lichen planus.

Trauma

Acute trauma to the nail bed may cause subungual hemorrhage, resulting in a brownish-black discoloration. This is particularly likely following crush injuries. Usually the diagnosis is simple, unless trauma is subtle. When a

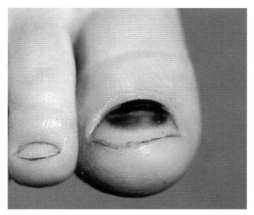

Figure 8-146. Traumatic subungual hemorrhage. Discoloration because of traumatic hemorrhage under the toenail is common in children and athletic adults. When seen at the base of a toenail, it is commonly a result of jamming the toe into the end of the shoe while running or stopping (turf toe).

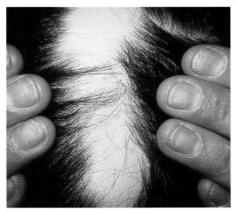

Figure 8-147. Broad, shallow, Scotch-plaid pitting of the nails associated with alopecia areata.

large, painful hematoma is produced, this should be evacuated using electrocautery to relieve pain and reduce risk of infection. Bluish-black pigmentation at the base of the great toenail, caused by jamming the toe into the end of the shoe at a sudden stop, is called *turf toe* and results in mild subungual hemorrhage (Fig. 8-146). This must be distinguished from melanoma. Concern for melanoma should heighten if pigmentation of the cuticle or proximal nail fold accompany hyperpigmentation of the nail, *Hutchinson sign*. When present, this should prompt immediate referral for a biopsy of the nail matrix to exclude melanoma. Hemorrhage, on the other hand, can be identified by the presence of purplish-brown pigment in the distal nail and normal proximal outgrowth of the nail. Chronic repetitive trauma due to development of a habit of picking at one nail with another and to long-standing rubbing of ill-fitting shoes are common sources of nail dystrophy (see Fig. 8-145).

Nail Findings in Other Dermatologic Disorders

As noted earlier, nail disorders may provide clues to other dermatologic or pediatric syndromes. For example, alopecia areata is associated with a characteristic Scotch-plaid pitting of the nails (Fig. 8-147). Similarly, psoriasis affects the nails in a number of ways that may help to distinguish it from other scaling disorders. Involvement of the nail matrix results in formation of scattered pits that are larger, deeper, and less numerous than those found in alopecia areata. Psoriasis of the nail bed, especially under the distal nail, causes separation of the nail

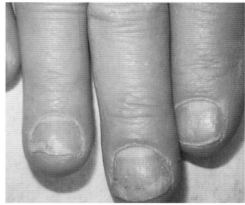

Figure 8-148. Psoriatic nails. Psoriasis affecting the nails results in onycholysis and pitting.

from the underlying skin (onycholysis) and oil-drop discoloration with heaped-up scaling (Fig. 8-148). Onycholysis alone, without pits or discoloration, may be caused by trauma, infection, nail polish hardeners, or phototoxic reactions to drugs such as tetracycline or doxycycline.

Complications of Topical Skin Therapy

An important rule in medicine is "do no harm." To follow that rule, the physician must recognize the potential for adverse side effects of the therapies prescribed.

Topical Steroids

The most commonly used topical medications are steroids. These may be classified as high, medium, or low potency, according to their biologic activity. Generally, fluorinated steroids are more potent than nonfluorinated steroids, and those in ointment bases are more active than those in cream or lotion bases. High-potency steroids should be used only for short periods of time to avoid major side effects. These side effects include skin atrophy (Fig. 8-149), telangiectases, and increased skin fragility; acneiform eruptions; permanent skin striae (Fig. 8-150); and masking or delayed recognition of infections and infestations such as tinea corporis and scabies.

Use of fluorinated steroids should be avoided on the face, eyelids, genitals, or intertriginous areas because absorption is greater and side effects are more common in these areas. Good general rules of safety are to use the weakest agent that is likely to clear the dermatitis and to avoid using topical steroids stronger than a class 5 (the most potent) in high-risk locations. If topical medication is applied to large areas, if the treated area is occluded, or if therapy is continued for a long period, adrenal suppression may result. Accidental injection of steroids into fat on attempted intramuscular injection may cause permanent subcutaneous atrophy (Fig. 8-151).

Secondary local bacterial infections and some viral infections may progress with unusual rapidity in children on topical corticosteroids. Hence patients should be instructed to look for early signs of secondary bacterial infection and return promptly if they develop. The risk of systemic viral and bacterial infections is similarly increased in patients on widespread topical or high-dose as a pro-

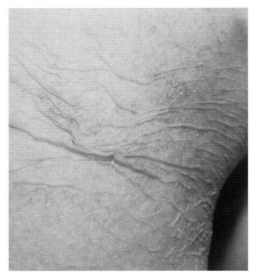

Figure 8-149. Steroid-induced skin atrophy. Topical steroids may cause marked atrophy and fragility of the skin, especially if used under occlusion regularly for more than 1 month.

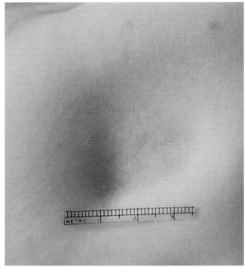

Figure 8-151. Steroid-induced subcutaneous atrophy. Injection of steroids into fat instead of muscle often produces subcutaneous atrophy. Whereas in some cases this may resolve in 6 to 12 months, in others it can be permanent.

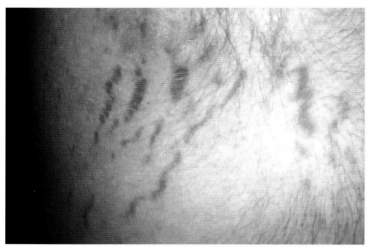

Figure 8-150. Steroid-induced striae distensae. Prolonged use of potent fluorinated steroids may cause permanent striae distensae.

longed regimen of oral steroids. All patients placed on high-dose steroids who have no past history of varicella should be alerted to return immediately for zoster immune globulin if they discover that they have been exposed to chickenpox.

Other Agents

Other complications from topical medications, such as contact dermatitis, can be easily prevented. Allergic contact dermatitis is frequently seen as a reaction to both prescribed and over-the-counter drugs. The most common allergens are neomycin, "-caine" topical anesthetics or antipruritics, and ethylenediamine (a preservative in many topical preparations). When possible, products containing these agents should be avoided. Anaphylaxis can occur even in response to topical medications, especially if applied to broken skin. Hence obtaining a history of drug allergies is important before prescribing topical agents.

Fortunately, most complications of therapy can be avoided if the physician has clear knowledge of the disease, its treatment, and the pharmacologic agents being prescribed.

Bibliography

Cohen BA: Atlas of Pediatric Dermatology. London, Mosby-Wolfe, 1993.
Cohen BA: Pediatric Dermatology, 2nd ed. London, Mosby, 1999.
Cohen BA, Lehman CU (eds): Johns Hopkins University Dermatlas. Available at http://www. dermatlas.com
Frieden IJ, Haggstrom AN, Drolet BA, et al: Infantile hemangiomas: Current knowledge, future directions. Proceedings of a research workshop on infantile hemangiomas. Pediatric Dermatology 22:383-406, 2005.
Harper J, Oranje A, Prose N: Textbook of Pediatric Dermatology. London, Blackwell Science, 2000.
Hernandez RG, Cohen BA: Insect bites—Induced hypersensitivity and the SCRATCH principles: A new approach to papular urticaria. Pediatrics 118:e189-e196, 2006.
Paller AS, Mancini AJ (eds): Hurwitz Clinical Pediatric Dermatology: A Textbook of Skin Disorders of Childhood and Adolescence, 3rd ed. Philadelphia, Elsevier Saunders, 2006.
Ruiz-Maldonado R, Parish LC, Beare JM: Textbook of Pediatric Dermatology. Philadelphia, Grune and Stratton, 1989.
Schachner LA, Hansen RC: Pediatric Dermatology, 3rd ed. New York, Churchill Livingstone, 2003.
Weinberg S, Leider M, Shapiro L: Color Atlas of Pediatric Dermatology, 2nd ed. London, McGraw-Hill, 1990.
Weston WL: Practical Pediatric Dermatology, 2nd ed. Boston, Little Brown, 1985.

CHAPTER 9

Endocrinology

Kecha A. LynShue and Selma F. Witchel

Introduction

Clinical presentations of endocrine disease can vary widely. Alterations in hormone balance result in distinct phenotypes affecting stature, timing of puberty, and body composition. The steady discovery of new genes, novel mutations, and alterations in gene expression has helped to explain at the molecular level the clinical presentation of insufficient or excessive hormone secretion, as well as altered hormone receptor activity. Despite the explosion of new information, the clinical presentations of children with endocrine disorders remain constant. The recognition of physical signs associated with these states assists in the diagnosis and treatment of imbalances of the neuroendocrine axis. The following text highlights the physical signs associated with normal endocrine function, as well as those due to hyposecretion and hypersecretion.

Normal Growth

Growth is influenced by many factors including overall health, heredity, gender, and environmental factors such as nutrition. Linear growth is rapid during the first year of life and slows between 1 and 2 years of age (Table 9-1). After 2 years of age, linear growth continues at a slower but steady rate of approximately 2 inches (5 cm) per year until adolescence. The "pubertal growth spurt" occurs during puberty. Sexual dimorphism exists in the onset of puberty between girls and boys; puberty begins at a younger chronologic age in girls. Girls experience their growth spurt during the early stages of puberty, whereas boys experience their growth spurt during midpuberty.

Because stature varies among healthy children, incremental growth rate is one of the most important elements used to assess health in a child. Subnormal growth velocity can indicate endocrine and nonendocrine disorders. The most critical tool to evaluate normal and pathologic growth is the growth chart. The Centers for Disease Control and Prevention (CDC) released updated growth charts on the basis of a broad population sample combining many different growth studies in May 2000 (Fig. 9-1A-D). These charts are readily available at http://www.cdc.gov/growthcharts. The charts not only define the 3rd and 97th percentiles for height and weight but also characterize standards for head circumferences and body mass index (BMI) defined as weight (kg)/height² (meters). In contrast to adults, for whom specific BMI values are used to define overweight and obesity, age- and gender-specific BMI values are used to classify children as overweight or underweight. Health care professionals can use the following established percentile cutoff points to identify underweight and overweight children (Table 9-2):

Although it can be normal for a child to change percentiles between birth and 18 months of age, after this age, children usually follow their growth curves fairly closely. When a child crosses percentiles in a relatively short period of time, he or she should be carefully evaluated through a detailed investigation regarding the etiology of the abnormal growth pattern. Between 4 years and adolescence, a growth rate below 4 to 5 cm per year for girls and boys is abnormal and should be assessed. Adolescence is the only time during which the rapid growth of the infant is recapitulated. For girls, a sharp increase in growth velocity is the harbinger of puberty.

Short stature with normal body proportions and decreased growth velocity can be due to endocrine, as well as nonendocrine, disorders. Exogenous pharmacologic steroid therapy often leads to growth deceleration. Non-endocrine causes include chronic illness, familial short stature, genetic disorders, and undernutrition. One common cause of short stature in children is familial or genetic short stature. The genetic growth potential of a child is heavily determined by the growth achieved by both parents and their relatives. The heritability of height has been estimated to be 0.7 to 0.8, rising to as much as 0.9 between identical twins. Common endocrine and non-endocrine causes of short stature are listed in Tables 9-3 and 9-4.

Calculation of the target height provides an estimate of a child's genetic potential. For boys, this can be calculated by adding 2.5 inches or 6.5 cm to the mean of the parents' height, and for girls, target height is calculated by subtracting 2.5 inches or 6.5 cm from the mean of the parents' heights. This information should be obtained during the initial evaluation, especially for children with concerns of tall or short stature.

Radiographic determination of epiphyseal maturation, or bone age, is often helpful in evaluating children with short stature. By convention, a radiograph of the left hand is compared with standards to determine bone age or skeletal age. Before 24 months of life, epiphyseal development is better estimated using a radiographic examination of the hemiskeleton. Children who have familial or genetically determined short stature generally have a bone age equivalent to their chronological age. The term "constitutional delay of growth" refers to children who have later onset of puberty. Typically, the bone age in children with constitutional delay is delayed, being more consistent with the children's height age rather than chronological age.

Children with constitutional delay typically have a period of decreased linear growth within the first 3 years of life. In this variant of normal growth and pubertal development, the rate of linear growth velocity and weight gain slow, often resulting in downward crossing of growth percentiles. By 2 or 3 years of age, linear growth resumes at a normal rate. Subsequently, children may grow either along the lower growth percentiles or beneath the curve but parallel to it for the remainder of the prepubertal years (Fig. 9-2). A family history of "late bloomers" or delayed puberty is common.

Genetic syndromes (such as Turner, Noonan, and Down syndromes) are examples of chromosomal abnormalities associated with short stature. Congenital disorders of bone mineralization and bone growth, such as the chondrodystrophies, represent an important cause of disproportionate short stature. When evaluating a child with a suspected chondrodystrophy, it is important to measure body proportions. A simple method of determining proportions consists of measuring the lower segment (symphysis pubis to floor) and subtracting this from the total height to determine the upper segment and then calculating the upper segment–to–lower segment ratio. This ratio, along with the arm span–to–height ratio, is used to document

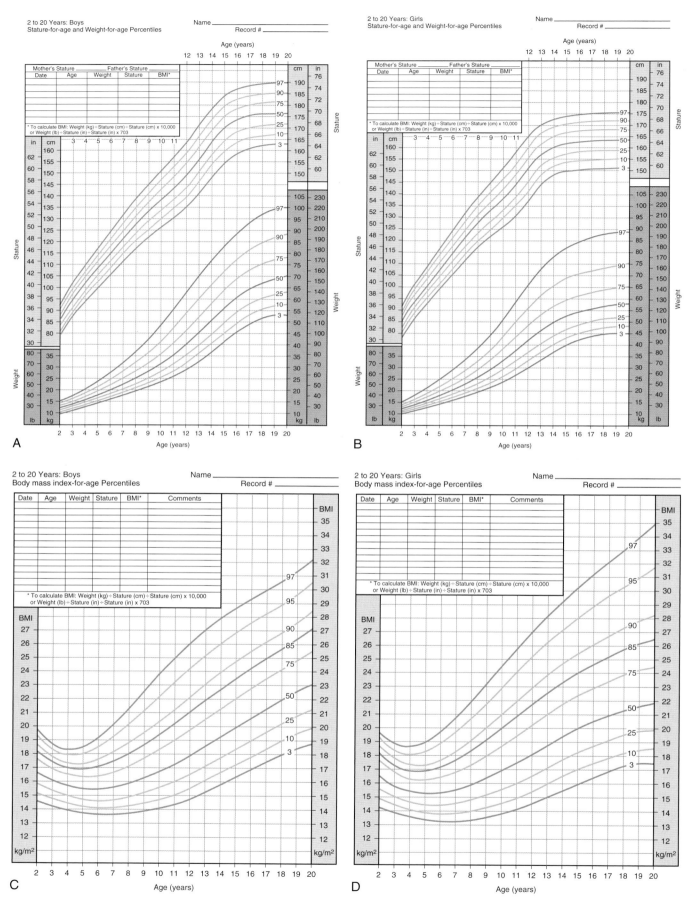

Figure 9-1. Growth charts from the Centers for Disease Control. **A,** Stature-for-age and weight-for-age for boys 2 to 20 years of age from the 3rd to 97th percentiles. **B,** Stature-for-age and weight-for-age for girls 2 to 20 years of age. **C,** Body mass index-for-age for boys 2 to 20 years old. **D,** Body mass index-for-age percentiles for girls 2 to 20 years of age. (Developed by the National Center for Health Statistics in collaboration with the National Center for Chronic Disease Prevention and Health Promotion [2000]. Available online at http://www.cdc.gov/growthcharts.)

Table 9-1 Normal Growth Rates in Children

| AGE | GROWTH RATE (PER YEAR) | |
	Inches	*Centimeters*
Birth to 1 year	7 to 10	18 to 25
1 to 2 years	4 to 5	10 to 13
2 years to puberty	2 to 2.5	5 to 6
Pubertal growth spurt—girls	2.5 to 4.5	6 to 11
Pubertal growth spurt—boys	3 to 5	7 to 13

Table 9-2 Body Mass Index Cutoff Points

Underweight	BMI-for-age <5th percentile
Normal	BMI-for-age 5th percentile to <85th percentile
At risk for overweight	BMI-for-age 85th percentile to <90th percentile
Overweight	BMI-for-age ≥95th percentile

Table 9-3 Selected Causes of Short Stature

Familial short stature (genetic)
Constitutional delay of sexual development
Malnutrition and psychosocial factors
Systemic disease
  Pulmonary
    Cystic fibrosis
    Asthma
  Cardiac and circulatory
    Congenital heart disease (cyanotic and acyanotic)
    Acquired heart disease
  Renal
    Renal insufficiency
    Pyelonephritis (chronic)
    Renal tubular acidosis
  Gastrointestinal and hepatic
    Malabsorption
    Inflammatory bowel disease
    Hepatic insufficiency
  Neurologic
    Mental retardation with growth delay
  Musculoskeletal and connective tissue
    Chondrodystrophies
    Storage diseases
    Rickets
    Skeletal dysplasias
  Immunologic
    Immune deficiencies
Syndromes associated with short stature
  Chromosomal abnormalities
    Trisomies 13, 18, 21
    Turner syndrome
    Noonan
    Progeria
    Russell-Silver
    Cockayne
    Seckel
    18q deletion
  Other syndromes
    Pseudohypoparathyroidism
    Achondroplasia
    Hypochondroplasia

Table 9-4 Endocrine Causes of Short Stature

Thyroid hormone deficiency or resistance
Cortisol hypersecretion (Cushing syndrome)
Inborn errors of steroidogenesis—adrenal hyperplasias (untreated)
Prolonged pharmacologic treatment with glucocorticoids
Disorders of the neuroendocrine GH axis
  Physical destruction of the pituitary and/or hypothalamus
  PIT-1 (transcription factors) mutations
  Somatostatin or GH-releasing hormone abnormalities
  GH gene mutations
  Laron syndrome types I and II (GH receptor or postreceptor defects)

GH, growth hormone.

subnormal growth velocity is comprehensive, with consideration of endocrine and nonendocrine disorders.

Pubertal Development

Puberty is the process through which reproductive competence is achieved and is initiated with reactivation of the hypothalamic-pituitary-gonadal axis. In humans and several nonhuman primates, adrenal pubertal maturation, indicated by increased adrenal DHEAS secretion, occurs in close temporal proximity to gonadarche. Clinical studies have demonstrated that gonadarche and adrenarche are regulated through different molecular mechanisms.

The pattern of timing of pubertal events for boys and girls is generally predictable (Fig. 9-3). For both boys and girls, mean ages for the onset of puberty vary among different ethnic groups. For white girls in the United States, mean age of onset of breast development and pubic hair growth occurs at approximately $10\frac{1}{2}$ years of age with menarche occurring at approximately $12\frac{1}{2}$ years of age. In boys, puberty usually begins between 9 and 14 years of age. This timing may be earlier for some ethnic groups, and considerable variation exists for any individual patient.

Tanner Staging

To describe the onset and progression of pubertal changes (Fig. 9-4), boys and girls are rated on 5-point scales. Boys are rated for both genital development and pubic hair growth, and girls are rated for breast development and pubic hair growth.

The stages for male *genital* development follow (see Fig. 9-4A):
Stage I (Preadolescent)—The testes, scrotal sac, and penis have a size and proportion similar to those seen in early childhood.
Stage II—There is enlargement of the scrotum and testes and a change in the texture of the scrotal skin. The scrotal skin may also be reddened.
Stage III—Further growth of the penis has occurred, initially in length with some increase in circumference. There is also increased growth of the testes and scrotum.
Stage IV—The penis is significantly enlarged in length and circumference, with further development of the glans penis. The testes and scrotum continue to enlarge, and there is distinct darkening of the scrotal skin.
Stage V—The genitalia are adult in size and shape.

whether the spine or limbs are more severely shortened. Arm span is usually equal to standing height. However, in children with achondroplasia, the long bones are disproportionately shortened. Sitting height is generally normal while the standing height is short. During adolescence, hypogonadism is often associated with increased limb length. The evaluation of a child with short stature and

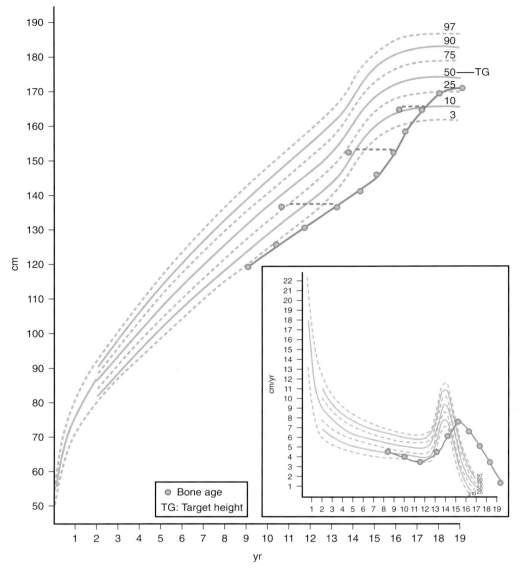

Figure 9-2. Growth curve of a child with constitutional growth delay. Note the typical pattern of growth deceleration followed by a normal growth rate.

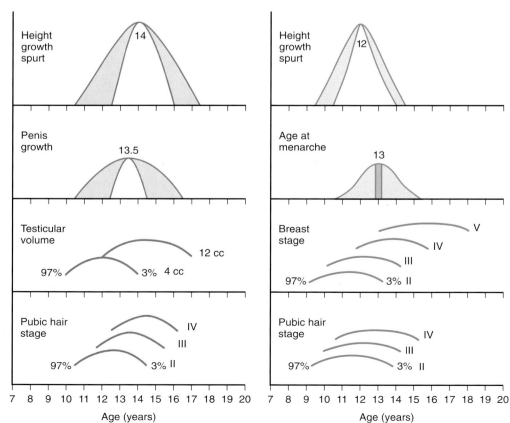

MALE PUBERTAL DEVELOPMENT

FEMALE PUBERTAL DEVELOPMENT

Figure 9-3. Schematic representation of the onset of male and female puberty. (Modified from Johnson TR, Moore WM, Jeffries JE: Children Are Different: Development Physiology, ed 2, Columbus, Ohio, 1978, Ross Laboratories, Division of Abbott Laboratories, pp 26-29. Used with permission of Ross Products Division, Abbott Laboratories, Inc., Columbus, Ohio 43215.)

The stages in male *pubic hair* development follow (see Fig. 9-4B):

Stage I (Preadolescent)—Vellous hair appears over the pubes with a degree of development similar to that over the abdominal wall. No androgen-sensitive pubic hair exists.

Stage II—Sparse development of long pigmented downy hair, which is only slightly curled or straight, occurs. The hair is seen chiefly at the base of the penis.

Stage III—The pubic hair is considerably darker, coarser, and curlier. The distribution of hair has now spread over the junction of the pubes.

Stage IV—The hair distribution is now adult in type but still considerably less than that seen in adults. There is no spread to the medial surface of the thighs.

Stage V—Hair distribution is adult in quantity and type and is described as an inverse triangle. There can be spread to the medial surface of the thighs.

The stages in female *breast* development follow (see Fig. 9-4C):

Stage I (Preadolescent)—Only the papilla is elevated above the level of the chest wall.

Stage II (Breast Budding)—Elevation of the breasts and papillae may occur as small mounds along with some increased diameter of the areolae.

Stage III—The breasts and areolae continue to enlarge, although they show no separation of contour.

Stage IV—The areolae and papillae elevate above the level of the breasts and form secondary mounds with further development of the overall breast tissue.

Stage V—Mature female breasts have developed. The papillae may extend slightly above the contour of the breast as the result of recession of the areolae.

The stages of *pubic hair* growth in females follow (see Fig. 9-4B):

Stage I (Preadolescent)—Vellous hair develops over the pubes. No sexual hair exists.

Stage II—Sparse, long, pigmented, downy hair, which is straight or only slightly curled, appears. These hairs are seen mainly along the labia.

Stage III—Considerably darker, coarser, and curlier sexual hair appears. The hair has now spread sparsely over the junction of the pubes.

Stage IV—The hair distribution is adult in type but decreased in total quantity. There is no spread to the medial surface of the thighs.

Stage V—Hair is adult in quantity, and type appears in an inverse triangle of the classically feminine type. There is spread to the medial surface of the thighs, but not above the base of the inverse triangle.

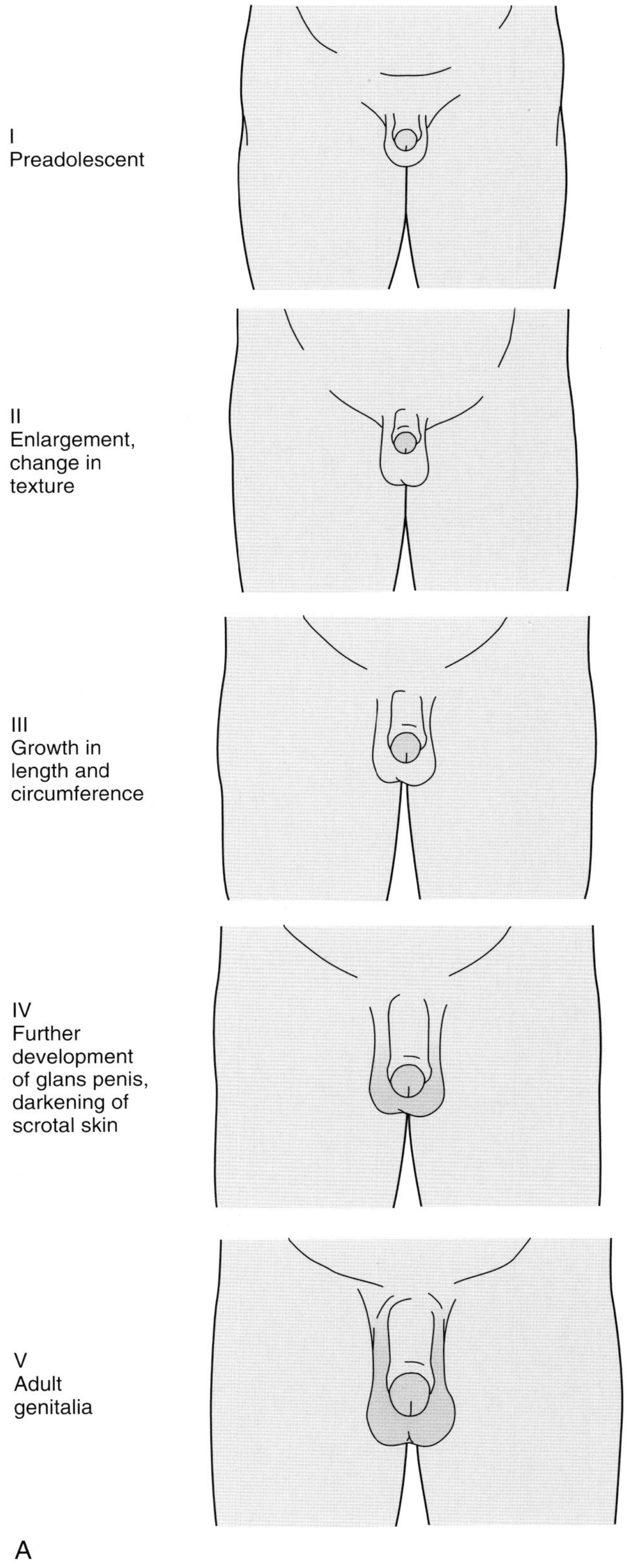

The Hypothalamus and the Pituitary Gland

The hypothalamus is derived from neuroectodermal tissue of the diencephalon and surrounds the inferior aspect of the third ventricle. Its basilar portion consists of the median eminence and pituitary stalk, which provide the common route for hypothalamic factors to reach the pituitary gland. Various regions in the hypothalamus secrete small peptide hormones that use this pathway to regulate pituitary hormone secretion. The neurohypophysis, consisting of unmyelinated axons and axon terminals, extends from the median eminence to the posterior pituitary gland.

I
Preadolescent

II
Enlargement, change in texture

III
Growth in length and circumference

IV
Further development of glans penis, darkening of scrotal skin

V
Adult genitalia

A

Figure 9-4. Schematic drawings of male and female Tanner stages show: **A,** male genital development. (*See next page for parts B and C.*)

The pituitary gland develops as a fusion of cells with different embryonic origins. There is an upgrowth of ectodermal cells from the roof of the primitive pharynx (known as *Rathke pouch*), and a downgrowth of neural tissue cells from the hypothalamus. These two distinct areas form the anterior (the adenohypophysis) and posterior (the neurohypophysis) lobes, respectively.

Both congenital and acquired abnormalities of pituitary function occur. Structural abnormalities of the central

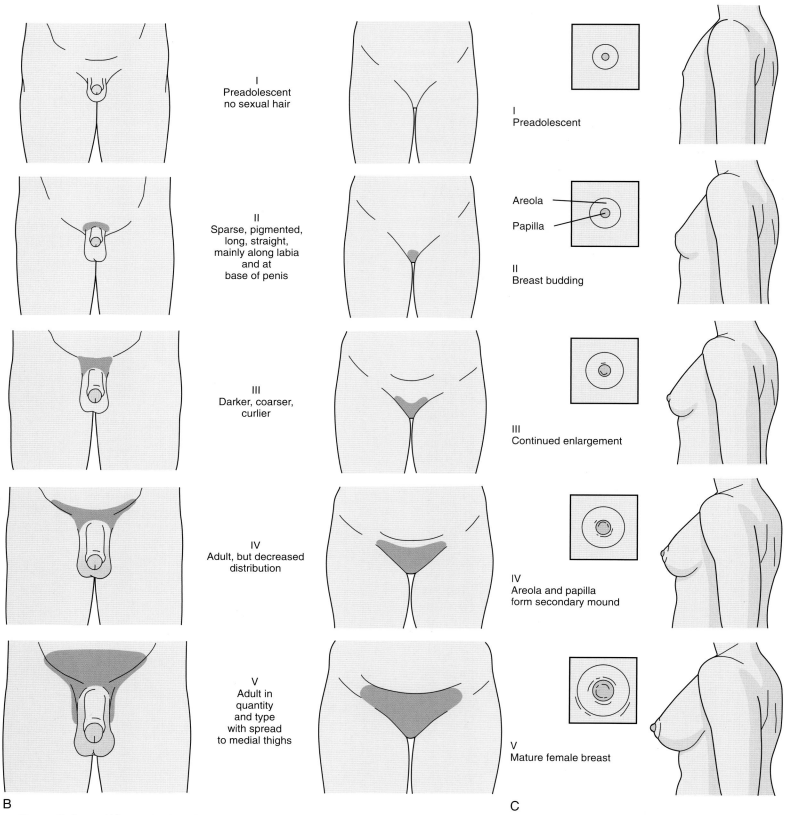

I
Preadolescent
no sexual hair

II
Sparse, pigmented,
long, straight,
mainly along labia
and at
base of penis

III
Darker, coarser,
curlier

IV
Adult, but decreased
distribution

V
Adult in
quantity
and type
with spread
to medial thighs

I
Preadolescent

Areola
Papilla

II
Breast budding

III
Continued enlargement

IV
Areola and papilla
form secondary mound

V
Mature female breast

B

C

Figure 9-4. cont'd B, pubic hair development; and **C,** breast development. (Modified from Johnson TR, Moore WM, Jeffries JE: Children Are Different: Development Physiology, ed 2, Columbus, Ohio, 1978, Ross Laboratories, Division of Abbot Laboratories, pp 26-29. Used with permission of Ross Products Division, Abbott Laboratories, Inc., Columbus, Ohio 43215.)

nervous system (CNS) such as septo-optic dysplasia (Fig. 9-5A and B) and holoprosencephaly (Fig. 9-5C) interfere with pituitary function. Craniopharyngiomas and CNS tumors can be associated with acquired hypopituitarism (Fig. 9-6). Radiation therapy for CNS tumors and traumatic interruption of the pituitary stalk are examples of additional etiologies for acquired hypopituitarism.

Anterior Pituitary

The anterior pituitary, with its diverse cell types and hormonal secretory patterns, controls many important biologic processes. It contains cells that secrete three types of hormones: corticotropin-related peptide hormones, glycoprotein hormones, and somatomammotropins. These

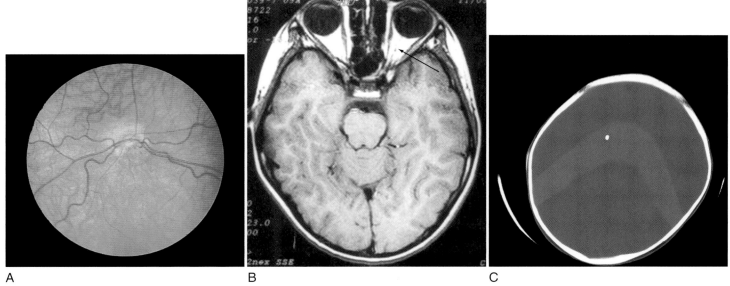

A   B   C

Figure 9-5. Congenital abnormalities of the central nervous system commonly associated with hypothalamic-pituitary dysfunction. **A,** Pale optic discs suggesting septo-optic dysplasia. This finding suggests pituitary endocrine deficiencies ranging from isolated growth hormone deficiency to panhypopituitarism. **B,** Septo-optic dysplasia as seen on MRI. **C,** Holoprosencephaly. Semilobar holoprosencephaly with a large monoventricle in a child with diabetes insipidus. (**B,** Courtesy Dr. D. Hiles, Pittsburgh, Pa.; **C,** courtesy Lynda Flom, MD, Pittsburgh, Pa.).

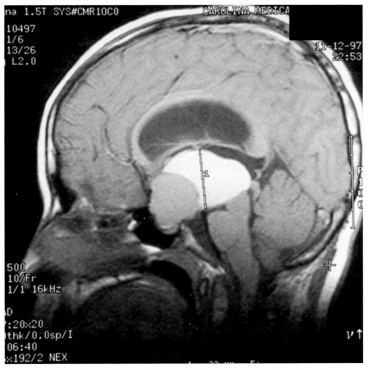

Figure 9-6. Craniopharyngioma. Heterogeneous densely enhancing suprasellar mass extending from the pituitary fossa into the hypothalamus and third ventricle.

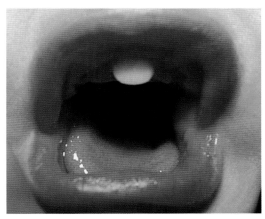

Figure 9-7. Central maxillary incisor. The presence of a single central maxillary incisor should alert the clinician to investigate the possibility of growth hormone deficiency. (Courtesy P. Lee, MD, Hershey, Pa.)

compounds have great biologic potency with tight regulation of hormone secretion using positive and negative feedback signals. Anterior pituitary hormone deficiencies cause subsequent hypofunction in the output of secondary endocrine glands with substantial consequences for growth and development. Children with a variety of midline defects have a higher incidence of hypopituitarism when compared with normal children. The child seen in Figure 9-7 has a single central incisor—an example of a midline abnormality associated with growth hormone (GH) deficiency. Thus specific alterations in physical appearance should alert physicians to an abnormality in the anterior pituitary and to subsequent secondary deficiencies (e.g., in the thyroid or adrenals).

Growth Hormone

GH modulates several complex metabolic processes. GH secretion is regulated by the relative balance between the levels of GH-releasing factor (GHRF) and somatostatin (Fig. 9-8). Both GHRH and somatostatin are secreted by the hypothalamus. The GH receptor is a single transmembrane protein. Following the binding of GH to its receptor, a second GH receptor dimerizes with the first receptor to initiate the signal transduction process. GH generates direct effects via the GH receptor signal transduction pathway and secondary effects by promoting an increase in insulin-like growth factor I (IGF-I) and insulin-like growth factor binding protein (IGF-BP3).

In children with hypopituitarism, GH treatment markedly improves growth velocity. GH stimulates an increase in lean body mass, as well as a marked increase in the size of the heart, pancreas, liver, and kidneys. It has positive effects on carbohydrate, fat, and protein metabolism and causes a decrease in body fat. GH inhibits carbohydrate uptake by muscle. This diabetogenic effect of GH action

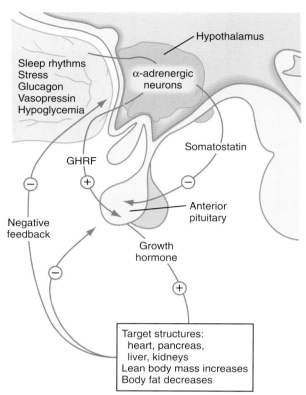

Figure 9-8. Feedback regulation of growth hormone at the level of the hypothalamus, pituitary, and target organs. GHRF, growth hormone-releasing factor.

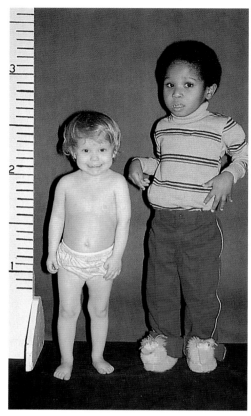

Figure 9-9. The normal 3½-year old boy (*right*) is in the 50th percentile for height. The short 3-year-old girl (*left*) has growth hormone deficiency.

is a known complication of GH hypersecretion. Typically, children with GH deficiency have normal birth weights and normal growth patterns during the first year of life, after which time their growth velocities decelerate. As seen in Figure 9-9, GH-deficient children have a characteristic "kewpie" doll appearance. They are often described as being "cherubic" because of their short stature, excess subcutaneous fat, retarded body proportion changes, and high-pitched voices. Children with hypopituitarism may present in the neonatal period with hypoglycemia. On physical examination, male infants with hypopituitarism may have small penises due to concomitant luteinizing hormone (LH) deficiency. The pulsatile nature of GH secretion necessitates provocative stimulation tests to diagnose GH deficiency.

Excessive GH secretion is uncommon in children. If GH excess begins during childhood, gigantism with increased growth velocity ensues. After closure of the epiphyses, soft tissue growth of the hands and feet and coarsening of facial features are typically the first clinical manifestations of acromegaly. Random GH, IGF-1, and IGFBP3 concentrations are usually elevated in gigantism/acromegaly.

Adrenocorticotropic Hormone

The corticotropin-related peptide hormones consist of adrenocorticotropic hormone (ACTH), α-melanocyte-stimulating hormone (α-MSH), and γ- and β-lipotropins (γ-LPH, β-LPH). These hormones are derived from a common precursor molecule, pro-opiomelanocortin. Within the subunit structure of β-LPH are the important neuroendocrine molecules, α-, β-, and γ-endorphin and enkephalin. Following posttranslational processing from this large precursor molecule, the secretion of ACTH is regulated by the level of corticotropin-releasing hormone (CRH) which is secreted by the hypothalamus. Cortisol

secreted from the adrenal gland also influences ACTH secretion by negative feedback (Fig. 9-10). Prolonged pharmacologic glucocorticoid therapy suppresses the hypothalamic-pituitary-adrenal axis with the potential for adrenal insufficiency, as well as a significant impact on growth and development.

Gonadotropins

The glycoprotein hormones include follicle-stimulating hormone (FSH) and LH. Each of these hormones is composed of two dissimilar peptide subunits. The α chain is identical for both hormones. However, the β chain is unique and confers specificity to each hormone. These hormones also contain significant amounts of carbohydrate and sialic acid residues along with their basic amino acid structures.

Secretion of LH and FSH is regulated by the pulsatile GnRH secretion. Neurons in the hypothalamus secrete GnRH in pulses that vary in amplitude and frequency during childhood and puberty. Following active secretion in late gestation and in the early neonatal period, the GnRH pulse generator becomes quiescent until the onset of puberty, which is characterized by increased GnRH secretion. Increased nocturnal LH secretion marks the reactivation of the GnRH pulse generator and onset of puberty. In primary gonadal failure, the deficiency of sex steroids interferes with negative feedback inhibition, resulting in elevated gonadotropin secretion during infancy, puberty, and adulthood.

The primary actions of FSH and LH affect gonadal function. LH binds to the LH receptor on Leydig cells to stimulate testosterone synthesis and secretion. LH stimulates ovarian theca cells to synthesize androstenedione, which serves as the precursor for estradiol synthesis. In the ovary,

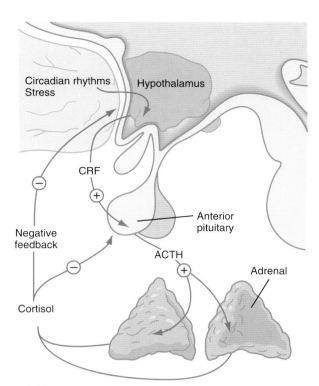

Figure 9-10. Feedback regulation of adrenocorticotropic hormone at the level of the hypothalamus, pituitary, and adrenal glands. ACTH, adrenocorticotropic hormone; CRF, corticotropin-releasing factor.

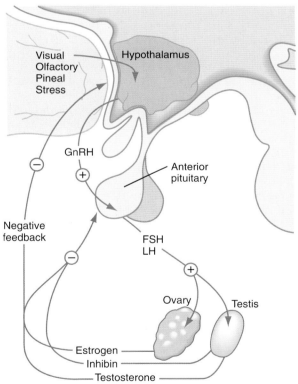

Figure 9-11. Feedback regulation of luteinizing hormone (LH) and follicle-stimulating hormone (FSH) at the level of the hypothalamus, pituitary, and gonads. GnRH, gonadotropin-releasing hormone.

FSH increases expression of aromatase, the enzyme that converts androgens to estrogens. In the testes, FSH supports Sertoli cell development and spermatogenesis (Fig. 9-11). The negative feedback effect on sex steroids on LH and FSH production is dramatically emphasized in post-menopausal women and in individuals with gonadal failure in whom marked elevations of these hormones

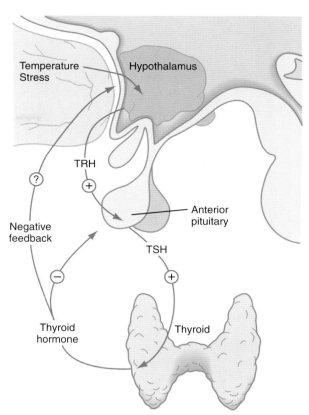

Figure 9-12. Feedback regulation of thyroid-stimulating hormone (TSH) at the level of the hypothalamus, pituitary, and thyroid gland. TRH, thyrotropin-releasing hormone.

occur. Inhibin is produced by the gonads and inhibits FSH release.

Thyroid-Stimulating Hormone

Thyroid-stimulating hormone (TSH) is a third glycoprotein hormone; its α-subunit is identical to the α-subunits of LH and FSH. Its specificity lies in its β-subunit. TSH stimulates many aspects of thyroid function. Its major role is to promote the synthesis and secretion of thyroid hormone. Mediated by the TSH receptor, TSH increases the size of the thyroid cells, vascularity of the gland, iodide uptake, thyroglobulin synthesis, and thyroid hormone secretion. The rate of TSH secretion appears to be determined by the level of circulating thyroid hormone and by the hypothalamic hormone, thyrotropin-releasing hormone (TRH), as seen in Figure 9-12. Negative feedback of TSH secretion by circulating thyroid hormone occurs mainly at the pituitary level.

Prolactin

PRL acts directly on its target organs and does not require an intermediary secondary endocrine gland. PRL's major known function in humans is the initiation and maintenance of lactation. In contrast to other anterior pituitary hormones, PRL is regulated by tonic inhibition by dopamine secreted by the hypothalamus. Congenital or acquired interruption of the hypothalamic-pituitary stalk may be accompanied by elevated prolactin concentrations reflecting decreased inhibition due to impaired hypothalamic-pituitary communication. Galactorrhea may be a clinical manifestation of hyperprolactinemia. Hyperprolactinemia can be observed with pituitary adenomas or secondary to medications such as neuroleptics, antipsychotics, estrogens, and antihypertensive medications.

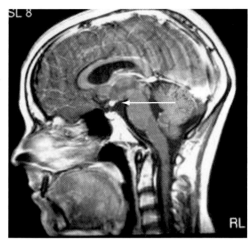

Figure 9-13. Ectopic pituitary. Note the absent normal posterior pituitary bright spot *(arrow)* within the sella on MRI. Instead, the bright spot is located in the median eminence.

Posterior Pituitary

Vasopressin and oxytocin are two evolutionarily related peptides composed of nine amino acids. These hormones are synthesized in the hypothalamus and stored in the posterior pituitary gland. Expression of vasopressin and oxytocin genes occurs in the hypothalamic paraventricular and supraoptic nuclei. On MR T1-weighted images, the posterior pituitary has a characteristic high-signal intensity. The presence of this high signal intensity adjacent to the median eminence with absence of the normal pituitary bright spot within the sella on T1-weighted images is evidence for an ectopic pituitary which is often associated with anterior pituitary hormone deficiencies (Fig. 9-13).

Vasopressin, also known as arginine vasopressin (AVP) or antidiuretic hormone (ADH), is a hormone important in water balance. It is synthesized and carried via axonal transport to the posterior pituitary, its primary site of storage. It is then released into the systemic circulation. AVP acts primarily on the kidneys at V2 receptors to aid in the reabsorption of water by affecting water permeability in the collecting duct of the kidney. At high concentrations, it also causes constriction of the arterioles through its action at V1 receptors, thereby leading to an increase in blood pressure. V3 receptors in the pituitary contribute to ACTH release by potentiating the action of CRH. Osmoreceptors in the hypothalamus detect an increase in osmotic pressure in the blood leading to increased AVP secretion and increased thirst. The combination of increased AVP secretion leading to increased renal reabsorption of free water and increased oral fluid intake will decrease osmolality. Other factors that increase AVP secretion include pain, trauma, nausea and vomiting.

Head trauma, brain tumors, encephalitis, pneumonia, and some drugs are associated with an overproduction of AVP. This can lead to inappropriate water retention and hyponatremia, known as the syndrome of inappropriate ADH secretion (siADH). The symptoms of siADH include headache, apathy, nausea, vomiting, and impaired consciousness. Underproduction of AVP results in central diabetes insipidus (DI). DI can result from pituitary tumors, head trauma, infiltrative disease processes such as Langerhans cell histiocytosis, sarcoidosis, and hemochromatosis, autoimmune hypophysitis, or from any surgery that damages the pituitary gland and hypothalamus. Familial central DI, inherited in both recessive and dominant pat-

terns, is rare and has its onset in infancy. Wolfram syndrome is an autosomal dominant form of central DI often associated with diabetes mellitus, optic atrophy, and deafness (DIDMOAD).

Nephrogenic DI is characterized by failure of the kidney tubules to respond to ADH. Genetic causes of nephrogenic DI include X-linked forms due to mutations in the V2 receptor gene and autosomal forms due to mutations in the aquaporin-2 gene. Acquired nephrogenic DI can be caused by drugs such as lithium. Psychogenic water drinking, hypercalcemia, hypokalemia, sickle cell anemia, and polycystic kidney disease can also impair renal concentrating ability.

Oxytocin secretion occurs in response to nervous stimulation of the hypothalamus. This hormone causes contraction of the smooth muscle of the uterus and also of the myoepithelial cells lining the duct of the mammary gland. Although some oxytocin is found in males, its function is unclear.

Thyroid Gland

The thyroid gland is situated in the neck or, in rare cases, at the base of the tongue or in the mediastinum. The gland originates near the base of the tongue and descends along the thyroglossal duct to its final position anterior to the trachea. The thyroid gland synthesizes thyroxine (T4) and tri-iodothyronine (T3); this process depends on the availability of iodine. Much of the circulating T4 and T3 are transported by thyroid binding globulin (TBG), albumin, and transthyretin. The free hormone is the active moiety. Inherited disorders affecting TBG concentration or acquired alterations in availability of binding sites may confound interpretation of thyroid hormone function studies.

Both overactivity and underactivity of the thyroid gland may be associated with a goiter. However, the signs of hyperthyroidism and hypothyroidism are dramatically different. The medical history and examination of the thyroid gland provide important information when evaluating a suspected abnormality in thyroid function.

As seen in Figure 9-14, the thyroid gland is usually best palpated with the examiner behind the patient. After identification of the cricothyroid cartilage, the second and third fingers are moved laterally along the trachea just medial to the sternocleidomastoid muscles. Two distinct lobes are palpable; the right lobe is usually greater in size than the left lobe. When a goiter is present, these lobes may be quite easily identified (Fig. 9-15). The texture of the gland varies with hyperthyroidism and hypothyroidism, the former usually being soft and fleshy, and the latter usually firm or bosselated. Nodules can also be palpated and may be indicative of an adenoma or carcinoma. Because the thyroid is directly supported by the trachea, having the patient swallow will elevate and depress a palpable gland along with the trachea during the swallowing motion.

Thyroid nodules are uncommon in children. A solitary thyroid nodule should raise concerns of thyroid neoplasia. Although 70% to 80% of solitary thyroid nodules prove to be benign or cystic lesions, thyroid cancer accounts for 1% to 1.5% of all childhood cancers. Clinical features suggestive of malignancy include neck irradiation, family history of medullary carcinoma, rapid growth of the nodule, fixation to adjacent structures, and enlarged lymph nodes.

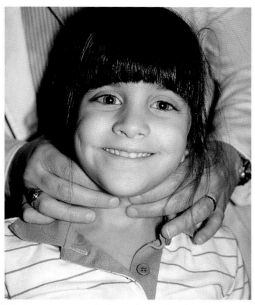

Figure 9-14. Examination of thyroid gland. The thyroid gland is best palpated with the examiner behind the patient.

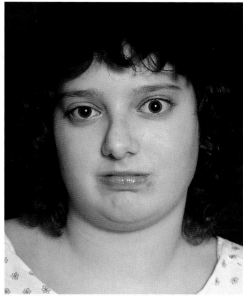

Figure 9-16. Graves disease. Mild thyromegaly and proptosis or exophthalmos are characteristic findings in patients with Graves disease.

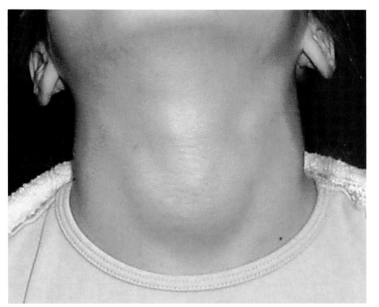

Figure 9-15. Goiter. Note an enlarged thyroid gland in a patient with Hashimoto thyroiditis easily visualized with neck extension. (Courtesy M. Parker, MD, Charlotte, N.C.).

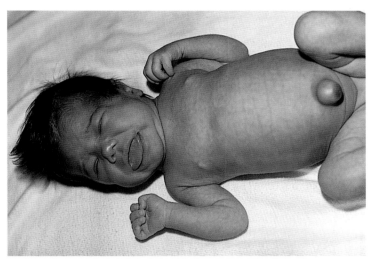

Figure 9-17. A child with cretinism. Note the broad nasal bridge, thick lips, and umbilical hernia. (Courtesy T. P. Foley, Jr., MD, Pittsburgh, Pa.)

Hyperthyroidism

Hyperthyroidism refers to excessive thyroid hormone secretion by the thyroid gland. Features of hyperthyroidism include accelerated basal metabolism, tachycardia, weight loss, increased frequency of bowel movements, heat intolerance, nervousness, widened pulse pressure, and tremor. The skin is warm and moist; hair is fine and friable. Separation of the distal margin of the nail bed, Plummer nails, may be noted. Restlessness, inability to sit still, emotional lability, short attention span, excessive sweating, and fatigue may be found. Hyperthyroidism can be due to a stimulating antibody directed against the TSH receptor (thyroid receptor antibody, TRAB, or TSII) as seen in Graves disease, adenomas or toxic multinodular goiters, activating mutations of the TSH receptor, or selective pituitary T3 resistance. Exophthalmos, a characteristic finding

of Graves disease, is usually less dramatic in children than adults, but proptosis and lid lag can be appreciated (Fig. 9-16). The hyperthyroid gland can become quite large, as much as 3 to 4 times its normal size, and is warm when palpated. A bruit may be heard over the gland. Thyroxine and triiodothyronine concentrations are elevated, and TSH concentrations are suppressed.

Hypothyroidism

Hypothyroidism, often associated with a goiter, can be congenital or acquired. Hypothyroidism can be classified as primary thyroid disease, secondary to hypothalamic-pituitary dysfunction, or due to iodine deficiency. The incidence of congenital hypothyroidism is 1 in 4000. Children with untreated congenital hypothyroidism (cretinism) develop a broad nasal bridge, coarse facial features, mental retardation, short stature, a characteristic puffy appearance of their hands, protuberant tongue, and delayed skeletal maturation (Fig. 9-17). Because treatment

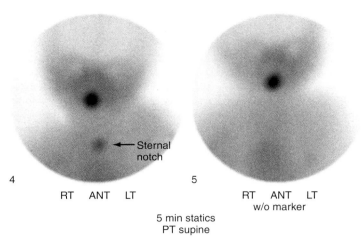

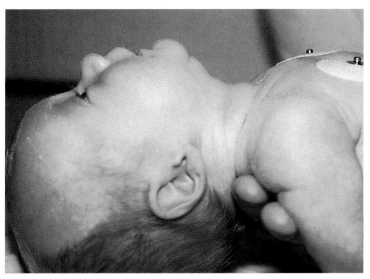

Figure 9-18. Ectopic thyroid gland. Technetium (Tc-99m) scan of an 8-day-old infant with congenital hypothyroidism. A lingual thyroid gland is identified with no functioning thyroid tissue within the anatomic thyroid bed. (Courtesy S. F. Witchel, MD, Pittsburgh, Pa.)

Figure 9-19. Examination of the neonatal thyroid gland. Examination performed by elevating the infant's trunk while allowing the head to fall back gently as shown.

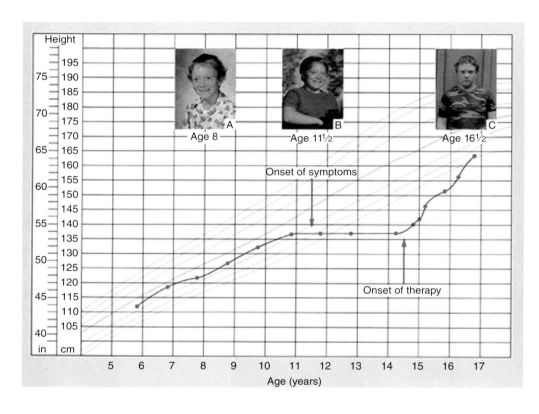

Figure 9-20. Growth curve of a child with acquired hypothyroidism. Note the sharp deceleration in growth before the onset of symptoms. Following thyroid hormone replacement, significant catch-up growth occurs. **A,** The child before onset of acquired hypothyroidism. **B,** The change in body habitus associated with acquired hypothyroidism. **C,** Resolution following thyroid replacement at indicated times.

by 3 to 4 weeks of age ameliorates these features, newborn screening programs have been implemented to identify hypothyroid infants. Despite the success of screening, thyroid function tests should still be obtained if signs and/or symptoms of congenital hypothyroidism are detected, even in the face of normal screening results. Radionuclide scanning using either technetium or iodine-123 (^{123}I) can be useful in identifying an ectopic thyroid gland (Fig. 9-18) or thyroid agenesis. Absence of radioisotope uptake is consistent with thyroid agenesis.

A goiter in an infant with congenital hypothyroidism (CH) suggests an enzymatic defect in thyroid hormone biosynthesis. To demonstrate a goiter in a newborn, the examiner's hand is best placed gently under the back and shoulder blades of the infant, and the infant's trunk is raised from the bed (Fig. 9-19). As the head falls back-

ward, the neck is elevated, and a goiter, if present, will be evident.

Acquired hypothyroidism, most frequently due to Hashimoto/chronic lymphocytic thyroiditis, may present in childhood. Typical features include dry skin, constipation, hair loss, fatigue, cold intolerance, apathy, depressed or delayed relaxation phase of deep tendon reflexes, and weakness. A sharp deceleration in growth may also be seen in children with acquired hypothyroidism, as seen in the growth curve shown in (Fig. 9-20). Family history is often positive for thyroid disease. The diagnosis is confirmed by measurement of a high TSH level and low thyroxine level. Antithyroid antibodies (thyroperoxidase and thyroglobulin) are often detected. Following institution of thyroid hormone therapy, growth velocity returns to normal. Acquired hypothalamic or pituitary disorders can cause hypothyroidism due to TRH and/or TSH deficiencies.

Thyroid hormone resistance is a rare cause of either congenital or acquired hypothyroidism. This occurs when there is resistance to either thyroid hormone or thyroid-stimulating hormone (TSH). Resistance to thyroid hormone is due to mutations in the thyroid hormone receptor β 1 (TRb1) gene and can be generalized (affecting all target tissue) or limited to the pituitary. Patients with TSH resistance have been found to have inactivating mutations of the TSH receptor (TSHR) gene. Clinical manifestations such as mental retardation and delayed bone maturation have been seen in individuals with generalized thyroid hormone resistance. Patients with partial TSH resistance are usually clinically euthyroid because they can compensate by increasing thyroid hormone levels. Those with complete TSH resistance may have profound hypothyroidism detectable on neonatal screening for CH.

Parathyroid Glands

Four parathyroid glands are located adjacent to the thyroid gland in the neck. They are responsible for the synthesis and secretion of parathyroid hormone (PTH), a hormone important in regulating extracellular calcium concentration through its effects on three principal target sites: bone, intestinal mucosa, and kidney. An increase in extracellular calcium inhibits secretion of PTH, whereas a decrease in extracellular calcium stimulates its release. In addition to calcium, there are other regulators of PTH secretion. Hypermagnesemia inhibits PTH secretion. Conversely, in states of hypomagnesemia, PTH is stimulated.

To sense the concentration of extracellular calcium and, thereby, regulate the secretion of PTH, the parathyroid cell relies on a G protein–coupled receptor, a calcium-sensing receptor (CASR). Mutations in the CASR gene have been implicated in disorders of calcium homeostasis. Activating mutations in the CASR gene have been found in families with autosomal dominant hypocalcemia, whereas loss-of-function mutations are associated with familial hypocalciuric hypercalcemia and neonatal severe hyperparathyroidism.

In the intestine, PTH does not appear to have a significant direct effect on calcium or phosphate absorption but acts indirectly by promoting the synthesis of the hormonally active form of vitamin D, 1,25-hydroxyvitamin D in the kidney, the action of which is to enhance intestinal calcium absorption. In the kidney, PTH has direct effects on the reabsorption of calcium, phosphate, and bicarbonate predominantly in the distal convoluted tubule. PTH also inhibits reabsorption of phosphate in the renal proximal tubule.

Causes of Hypercalcemia

Hyperparathyroidism

Hypercalcemia due to hyperparathyroidism is a common manifestation of the multiple endocrine neoplasia (MEN) syndrome type I. Other features of MEN 1 include islet cell tumors, Zollinger-Ellison syndrome, and pituitary tumors. Although typically a disease of adults, affected children can be identified through biochemical screening approximately 10 years before the onset of clinical symptoms. Inherited as an autosomal dominant trait, MEN 1 is associated with mutations in the menin (MEN1) gene.

Causes of Hypocalcemia

Hypoparathyroidism

Hypoparathyroidism may be congenital, surgical, autoimmune, familial, or idiopathic. Regardless of the etiology, the hallmarks of hypoparathyroidism are the same—hypocalcemia, hyperphosphatemia (phosphaturic effect of PTH is lost), and an inappropriately low or undetectable PTH level. DiGeorge syndrome (dysmorphic features, cardiac defects, immune deficiency, thymic aplasia/hypoplasia, and hypoparathyroidism) is due to a microdeletion on chromosome 22q11.2 (see Chapter 4). Approximately 10% to 20% of infants who have hypocalcemia and DiGeorge syndrome present with hypocalcemia between 0 and 3 months of age. Up to 10% of infants will present with seizures secondary to hypocalcemia.

Acquired hypoparathyroidism can be due to autoimmune disease, infiltration, or trauma. Hypoparathyroidism may be the initial feature of the autosomal recessive polyendocrinopathy-candidiasis-ectodermal dysplasia syndrome (APECED); this disorder has been associated with mutations in the autoimmune regulator (AIRE) gene located at chromosome 21q22.3.

Pseudohypoparathyroidism

Patients with Albright hereditary osteodystrophy (AHO), also known as *pseudohypoparathyroidism type Ia*, have a distinct phenotype with a round facies, short stature, obesity, skin hyperpigmentation, subcutaneous calcification, and a short thick neck (Fig. 9-21A). Shortening of the metacarpals and metatarsals is common, especially for the fourth digit (Fig. 9-21B and C). AHO results from loss of function mutations in the G_s-alpha subunit (GNAS1) gene. AHO should be suspected in a short child with hypocalcemia and a history of similarly affected family members. Affected patients have hypocalcemia, hyperphosphatemia, and extremely elevated PTH values. Because GNAS1 is an imprinted gene, the phenotype depends on the parental origin of the affected allele. When the maternal allele carries the mutation, the child typically has the phenotype of AHO and hypoparathyroidism. When the paternal allele carries the mutation, the child usually manifests only AHO. Resistance to other hormones using GNAS1, such as TSH and ADH, may be observed.

Vitamin D–Deficient Rickets

Vitamin D deficiency may result from inadequate sunlight exposure, inadequate nutrition, and/or malabsorption. Drugs that activate the catabolism of vitamin D, such as phenytoin and phenobarbital, can also worsen vitamin D deficiency in individuals with baseline marginal vitamin D stores. Vitamin D deficiency should be suspected in children with poor linear growth, delayed walking secondary to muscle weakness and bone pain, hypotonia, and anorexia. Clinical manifestations of rickets in ambulatory infants and children include genu varum or valgum (bowed legs, "knock knees") and metaphyseal flaring

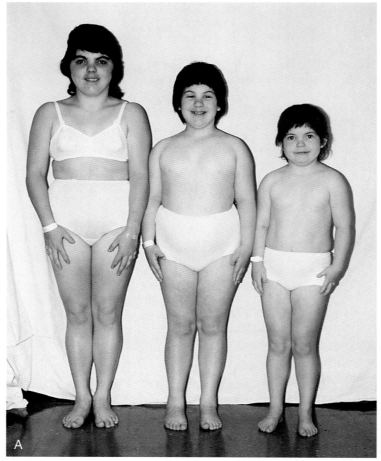
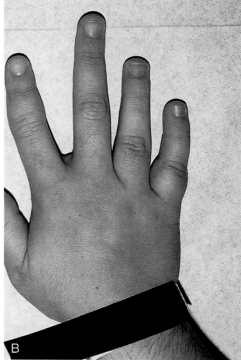
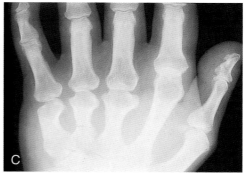

Figure 9-21. A, Albright hereditary osteodystrophy (AHO), also known as *pseudohypoparathyroidism,* is characterized by a round facies, short stature, and obesity, as seen in these three sisters. **B,** A short fourth metacarpal may be easily appreciated in this photograph. **C,** Radiograph of the hand illustrates the short fourth metacarpal seen in AHO. (**A** and **B,** Courtesy J. Parks, MD, Atlanta; **C,** courtesy J. Medina, Pittsburgh, Pa.)

(widening) (Fig. 9-22A); prominence of the costochondral junctions (rachitic rosary) (Fig. 9-22B); indentation of the lower anterior thoracic wall (Harrison's groove); frontal bossing; and, occasionally, craniotabes. Darkly pigmented and exclusively breastfed infants and children who have limited exposure to sunlight are particularly prone to developing vitamin D deficiency.

Vitamin D deficiency may also be the consequence of intestinal malabsorptive disorders such as celiac disease, biliary obstruction, gastric resection or pancreatic insufficiency. In the majority of infants and children with rickets, total calcium levels are usually borderline-normal or low, phosphate levels are low, and alkaline phosphatase activity and PTH concentrations are increased.

Causes of Hypophosphatemia

The vitamin D–resistant rickets are defined by resistance to the amounts of vitamin D generally used to treat vitamin D deficiency. Typical findings are often observed in the first months of life: radiological signs of defective mineralization on cartilage growth plates (rickets) and alterations of phosphorus homeostasis.

Pseudovitamin D–deficiency rickets (PDDR) has also been referred to as 1α-hydroxylase deficiency and vitamin D–dependent rickets type I. The clinical manifestations of this autosomal recessive condition include bone deformities, growth retardation, and weakness in early infancy. In this disorder, calcidiol concentrations may be normal while calcitriol concentrations are low due to loss of function mutations in the 1α-hydroxylase (CYP1α) gene. Vitamin D-dependent rickets type II is attributed to mutations in the vitamin D receptor gene. Additional features include growth retardation, alopecia, and extremely elevated calcitriol and PTH concentrations. Laboratory data seen in rickets are listed in Table 9-5.

Hypophosphatemic rickets is characterized by severe hypophosphatemia, postnatal growth retardation with short stature, genu varum, and dental anomalies. Muscle, bone, and joint pain and stiffness may occur. This form of rickets is associated with genetic variants in the phosphate-regulating gene with homologies to endopeptidases on the X-chromosome (PHEX) or fibroblast growth factor 23 (FGF23) genes.

Hypophosphatasia is an autosomal recessive disorder of varying severity due to loss of function mutations in the TNSALP gene. Decreased TNSALP activity leads to defective mineralization of skeletal osteoid. In addition to the radiographic findings of rickets, affected subjects have low alkaline phosphatase activity and increased urinary phosphoethanolamine excretion.

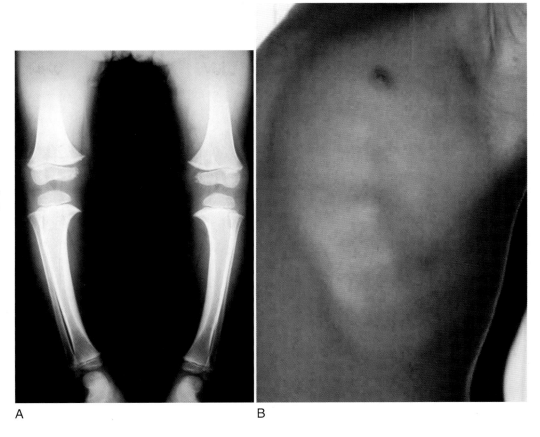

Figure 9-22. Clinical manifestations of rickets. **A,** Genu varum ("bowed legs") and metaphyseal flaring. **B,** Rachitic rosary. (Courtesy T. Thacher, MD).

A   B

Table 9-5   Laboratory Findings in Rickets

TYPE	CALCIUM	PHOSPHATE	ALKALINE PHOSPHATASE	25-HYDROXY Vit D_3	1,25-HYDROXY Vit D	PTH
Vitamin D–deficiency rickets	N, ↓	N, ↓	↑	↓	N	N
Mild	N, ↓	↓	↑↑	↓	↓, N, ↑	↑
Moderate	↓	↓	↑↑	↓↓	↓	↑↑
Severe						
X-linked hypophosphatemic rickets	N	↓↓	↑	N	N, ↓	N
Pseudovitamin D–deficiency rickets	↓↓	↓↓	↑↑↑	N	↓↓↓	↑↑↑

PTH, parathyroid hormone. From Sperling MA (ed): Pediatric Endocrinology, 2nd ed. Philadelphia, WB Saunders, 2002.

Adrenal Glands

The adrenal gland is composed of the inner adrenal medulla and the outer adrenal cortex. During fetal life, the adrenal cortex consists of the fetal adrenal cortical zone, which involutes during the first year of life and the definitive zone. The fetal zone synthesizes substrates for placental estrogen biosynthesis. At birth, the fetal adrenal is roughly twice the size of adult adrenals. Postnatally, the definitive adrenal cortex develops into the adult adrenal cortex, which synthesizes glucocorticoids, mineralocorticoids, and the so-called adrenal androgens. The adrenal medulla is responsible for the production of epinephrine and norepinephrine.

Adrenal Cortex

Cushing Syndrome

Cushing syndrome, the phenotype resulting from excessive glucocorticoids, can be due to either endogenous or exogenous steroid exposure. Rounded facies, plethora, central obesity, impaired linear growth, fatigue, and hypertension are characteristic features of Cushing syndrome (Fig. 9-23). Children with Cushing syndrome are frequently irritable. A buffalo hump as demonstrated by Figure 9-23D has been described frequently. Muscle weakness and muscle wasting occur, resulting in comparatively thin extremities (see Fig. 9-23B). Their skin is often thin and easily bruised. Loss of bone mineral density and osteopenia/osteoporosis occur with chronic glucocorticoid exposure. Delayed bone maturation may be noted.

Endogenous Cushing syndrome may be caused by adrenal tumors, pituitary adenomas (Cushing disease), or ectopic ACTH production. The differential findings in the specific etiology of Cushing syndrome are listed in Figure 9-24.

Elevated 24-hour urine free cortisol excretion or salivary cortisol measurements are two tests used to diagnosis Cushing syndrome. The high- and low-dose dexamethasone suppression tests have been used to confirm the diagnosis and assist in discerning the cause. Individuals

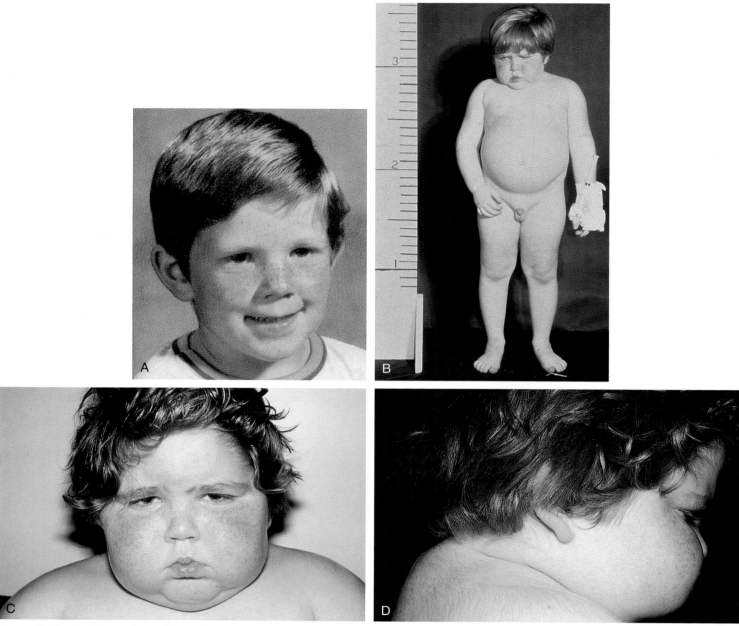

Figure 9-23. Cushing syndrome. These photographs show how dramatic the changes associated with Cushing syndrome are and how rapidly they occur. **A,** Patient before the onset of Cushing syndrome. **B,** Patient 4 months after **A** was taken. Note the centripetal obesity of the trunk compared with the extremities after the onset of Cushing syndrome. **C,** Moon facies is clearly demonstrated and should raise the diagnostic index of Cushing syndrome. **D,** Buffalo hump. Excessive adipose tissue over the lower cervical and upper thoracic spine is characteristic of Cushing syndrome.

with Cushing syndrome have a loss of normal cortisol diurnal variation. With improved imaging techniques, both head and body scans may be successful in localizing a tumor.

Adrenal Insufficiency

Patients with primary adrenal insufficiency (Addison disease) typically present with weight loss, wasting of subcutaneous tissue, and hyperpigmentation (Fig. 9-25A). Primary adrenal insufficiency is characterized by glucocorticoid and mineralocorticoid deficiencies. Little change is seen in overall growth rate. Frequently, the hyperpigmentation is striking and appears as bronzing of the skin, more obvious in flexor creases, in scars, and over the areolae of the nipples (Fig. 9-25B-D). This is due to cosecretion of ACTH and MSH (melanocyte-stimulating hormone). Vitiligo may occur as well. Frequently, patients may be confused and weak. If left untreated, patients with Addison disease weaken and vascular collapse ensues. The

decreased circulating plasma volume is reflected by the thinned narrow heart shadow seen on a chest radiograph (Fig. 9-25E). Hyponatremia and hyperkalemia are usually associated findings. Hypoglycemia and eosinophilia may occur. Autoimmune destruction of the adrenal gland has now replaced tuberculosis as the most common cause of the disease. Two autoimmune polyendocrine syndromes have also been characterized. The type I form is characterized by chronic mucocutaneous candidiasis, hypoparathyroidism, and adrenal insufficiency; it is associated with mutations in the AIRE gene. The type II form (Schmidt syndrome) is characterized by diabetes, hypothyroidism, and adrenal insufficiency.

Other causes of primary adrenal insufficiency include adrenoleukodystrophy, Wolman disease, hereditary unresponsiveness to ACTH, Allgrove syndrome, and congenital adrenal hypoplasia. Acute adrenal insufficiency due to massive adrenal hemorrhage can occur with meningitis or traumatic births.

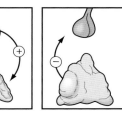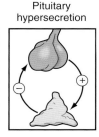

	Normal	Adrenal tumor	Pituitary hypersecretion
Plasma cortisol diurnal rhythm	10–25 µg% rhythmic	High; no rhythm	High; no rhythm
Plasma ACTH	Normal	Low	HIgh
Plasma ACTH after adrenalectomy, on normal cortisol replacement	Normal	Low	High
Plasma glucocorticoid response to ACTH	3–5 fold rise	+, 0	+
Urinary glucocorticoid response to metyrapone	2–4 fold rise	0	+
Plasma glucocorticoid response to dexamethasone	Suppressed	No fall	Partial fall

Figure 9-24. The differential diagnosis of Cushing syndrome as interpreted from the dexamethasone suppression test. (Modified from Williams RH: Textbook of Endocrinology, 6th ed. Philadelphia, WB Saunders, 1981.)

The clinical manifestations of secondary adrenal insufficiency are less fully expressed in individuals who have either isolated ACTH deficiencies or hypothalamic alterations in CRF kinetics. This is because aldosterone secretion is preserved because it is primarily regulated by the renin-angiotensin system rather than ACTH. This is well demonstrated in the girl with isolated ACTH deficiency seen before and after treatment (Fig. 9-26A and B). Although she has the clinical wasting associated with Addison disease, her skin is pale as opposed to bronze.

Congenital Adrenal Hyperplasia

The congenital adrenal hyperplasias (CAHs) are a group of autosomal recessive disorders characterized by decreased glucocorticoid biosynthesis. The specific symptoms and laboratory findings reflect the specific defect in steroidogenesis.

The most common form of CAH is 21-hydroxylase deficiency due to loss of function mutations in the 21-hydroxylase (CYP21) gene (Fig. 9-27). In this disorder, decreased glucocorticoid biosynthesis results in increased ACTH and adrenal androgen biosynthesis. The phenotype varies depending on the severity of the genetic mutation. Classic salt-wasting CAH occurs in 1 of 16,000 births and is characterized by very elevated 17-hydroxyprogesterone levels. In the most severe forms, mineralocorticoid biosynthesis is also inadequate, leading to chronic salt loss. Excessive prenatal androgen biosynthesis is associated with masculinization of the external genitalia of affected female infants. Although affected females typically have ambiguous symmetrical external genitalia with nonpalpable gonads at birth, male infants have normal male external genitalia. Typically, ovarian and uterine development are normal in virilized female infants. Hyperkalemia, hyponatremia, failure to thrive, and hypoglycemia ultimately culminating in shock ensue within 10 to 14 days of birth in the untreated infant as consequences of the severe mineralocorticoid and glucocorticoid deficiencies.

Those with simple virilizing 21-hydroxylase deficiency do not produce adequate amounts of cortisol but are able to make sufficient amounts of aldosterone to maintain normal electrolytes. Similar to classic CAH, females may have ambiguous genitalia, whereas affected males usually present later when signs of androgen excess may develop prematurely. Patients with nonclassic 21-hydroxylase deficiency produce normal amounts of cortisol and aldosterone at the expense of elevated androgen production. Younger children may present with premature pubarche, rapid growth, and advanced skeletal maturation. Affected adolescent girls may present with hirsutism, oligomenorrhea, and acne.

Less common forms of virilizing congenital adrenal hyperplasia are due to mutations in the 3β-hydroxysteroid dehydrogenase type 2 (HSD3B2) and 11β-hydroxylase (CYP11B1) genes. Loss of function mutations in the 17α-hydroxylase/17,20-lyase (CYP17) gene prevents synthesis of glucocorticoids and sex steroids. Affected females show normal female external genital development and delayed puberty, whereas affected males are undervirilized at birth; elevated mineralocorticoid concentrations can be associated with hypertension.

Adrenal Medulla

Pheochromocytoma

Pheochromocytoma is a rare catecholamine-secreting tumor derived from chromaffin cells. Clinical manifestations result from excessive catecholamine secretion from the tumor. These catecholamines include norepinephrine, epinephrine, and rarely dopamine. Symptoms may include headache, diaphoresis, palpitations, tremor, nausea, weakness, anxiety, and weight loss. Patients may present with hypertension, which may be episodic; altered mental status; or cardiac arrhythmias.

Pheochromocytoma may occur in certain familial syndromes including multiple endocrine neoplasia (MEN) 2A and 2B, neurofibromatosis, and von Hippel-Lindau (VHL) syndrome. Multiple endocrine neoplasia 2A, also known as Sipple syndrome, and 2B show autosomal dominant

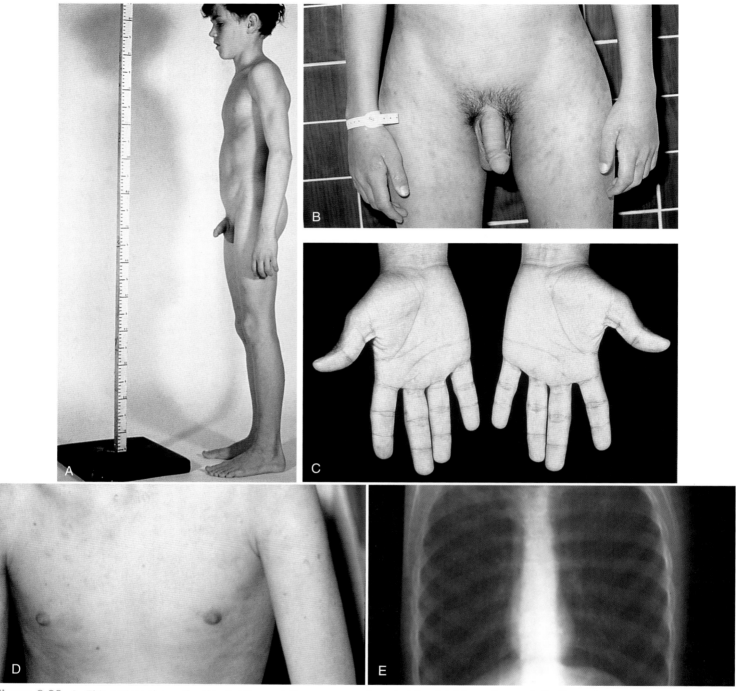

Figure 9-25. **A,** This patient shows the thin habitus and ill appearance characteristic of Addison disease. **B-D,** Hyperpigmentation may be marked. **E,** Microcardia is characteristically seen on chest radiograph. (**A-D,** Courtesy M. New, MD; **E,** courtesy J. Medina, Pittsburgh, Pa.)

inheritance and occur secondary to mutations in the RET proto-oncogene. Because medullary carcinoma of the thyroid is common in MEN 2, genetic screening to iden-tify high-risk individuals is beneficial.

In those suspected of having a pheochromocytoma, plasma metanephrines or a 24-hour urinary collection for catecholamines and metanephrine can be measured.

Sexual Differentiation

The process of sexual differentiation begins early in gestation and depends on the regulated expression of spe-cific genes and interactions of specific gene products. In the usual situation the undifferentiated gonad and related structures develop into internal and external genitalia

according to chromosomal sex (Fig. 9-28). The SRY gene, located on the short arm of the Y chromosome, plays a major role in testicular differentiation by promoting dif-ferentiation of Sertoli cells. As anticipated, mutations in the SRY gene are associated with male-to-female sex rever-sal. Through investigation of patients with aberrant sexual differentiation, other genes involved in this process have been identified. Camptomelic dwarfism and 46,XY sex reversal are usually indicative of SOX9 gene mutations. Denys-Drash syndrome, due to mutations in the WT1 gene, is characterized by Wilms tumor, nephropathy, and 46,XY sex reversal.

The child with ambiguous genitalia must be evaluated promptly. In speaking with the parents, the child should be referred to as "the baby" and not he, she, or it. An interdisciplinary approach including a pediatric endo-

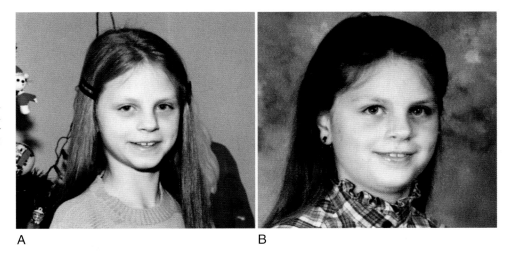

Figure 9-26. Isolated adrenocorticotropic hormone deficiency (ACTH). **A,** Young girl with isolated ACTH deficiency shows wasting and pallor rather than excessive bronzing. **B,** The same girl after therapy.

A   B

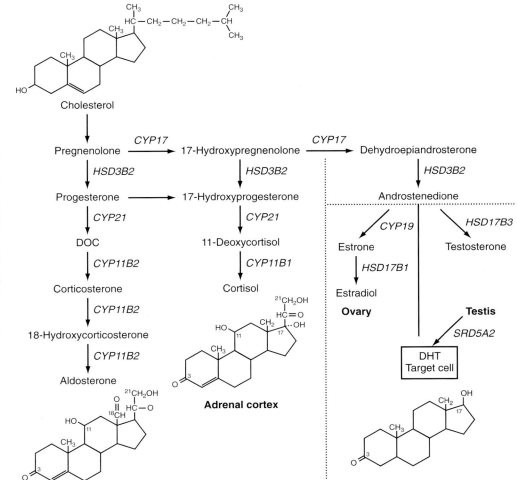

Figure 9-27. Steroid biosynthesis pathway. Pathways for the synthesis of mineralocorticoids (aldosterone), glucocorticoids (cortisol), and androgens (testosterone) are shown. Deficiency in 21-hydroxylase activity (CYP21) prevents the conversion of 17-hydroxyprogesterone to 11-deoxycortisol, resulting in an elevation of 17-hydroxyprogesterone and shunting of precursors into the pathway for androgen biosynthesis. Androstenedione is secreted by the adrenal cortex and converted to testosterone or estradiol in the periphery. Testosterone may be converted by 5α-reductase (SRD5A2) to dihydrotestosterone (DHT). Structures of cholesterol, aldosterone cortisol, and dihydrotestosterone are shown. (Courtesy K. LynShue, MD, and S. F. Witchel MD, Pittsburgh, Pa.)

crinologist, pediatric urologist, and psychologist/social worker with expertise in this area can be helpful.

The physical examination of the child directs the choice of the appropriate laboratory studies to confirm a specific diagnosis. The external genitalia should be carefully examined to determine if gonads are palpable. The magnitude of virilization and position of the urethral meatus should be noted. Asymmetrical external genitalia are typically due to gonadal dysgenesis (Fig. 9-29). Symmetrical external genitalia with nonpalpable gonads suggest a virilized XX fetus with CAH (see CAH section); the diagnosis is confirmed by an elevated 17-hydroxyprogesterone measurement.

Symmetrical genital development with palpable gonads suggests incomplete male sexual differentiation. Diagnostic entities include Leydig cell hypoplasia due to LH receptor mutations, inborn errors of testosterone biosynthesis due to mutations in steroidogenic enzyme genes, or androgen insensitivity. Determination of LH, FSH, testosterone, and dihydrotestosterone in the neonatal period is helpful because the hypothalamic-pituitary-gonadal axis is active. In complete androgen insensitivity due to loss of function mutations in the androgen receptor gene, external genital development appears to be female. Labial or inguinal gonads may be palpable, and uterine structures are absent.

Sexual appearance of fetus at second to third month of pregnancy

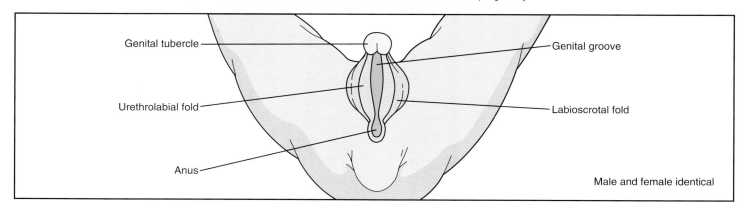

Sexual appearance of fetus at third to fourth month of pregnancy

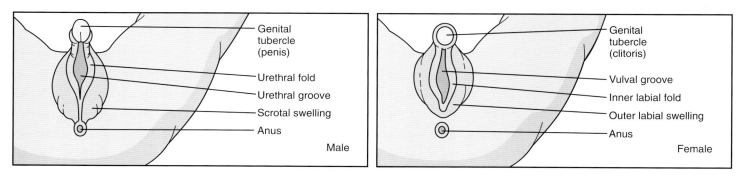

Sexual appearance of fetus at time of birth

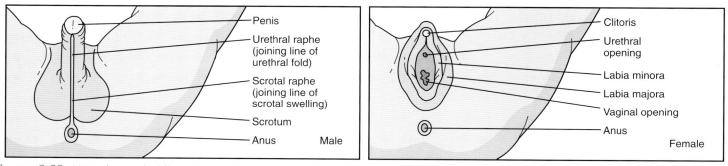

Figure 9-28. Normal sexual differentiation. Schematic drawings demonstrating differentiation of normal male and female genitalia during embryogenesis.

Persistent mullerian duct syndrome is characterized by persistence of mullerian structures in an otherwise normal 46,XY male infant. Affected infants may present with cryptorchidism or transverse testicular ectopia. This disorder can be due to mutations in the antimullerian hormone (AMH) gene or the gene for its receptor (AMHRII).

Some children born with anatomic variants, such as agenesis of the phallus (Fig. 9-30), may have neither a detectable chromosomal nor biochemical defect but rather a developmental anomaly.

Cryptorchidism

During embryogenesis, the testes migrate from their original location near the kidney through the abdomen and descend into the scrotum. Cryptorchidism, or failure of the testes to descend into the scrotum, occurs in approximately 3% of infant males. Treatment of cryptorchidism is usually delayed until 6 to 12 months of age to allow the

testicle to descend spontaneously. If there is failure of descent, an orchiopexy is performed. A cryptorchid testicle is 20 to 48 times more likely to undergo malignant transformation. Although surgical intervention may not completely alter the risk of malignancy, placing the testicle in its proper location allows for earlier detection of a suspicious mass.

Precocious Puberty

A diagnosis of precocious or early development may be made if sexual maturation begins before age 8 years for girls and before age 9 years for boys. The medical history should focus on the temporal sequence of the pubertal changes. Clinical features of androgen and estrogen effects should be noted during the physical examination. Gonadotropin-dependent precocious puberty, also known as central precocious puberty, is marked by a premature activation of the hypothalamic-pituitary-gonadal

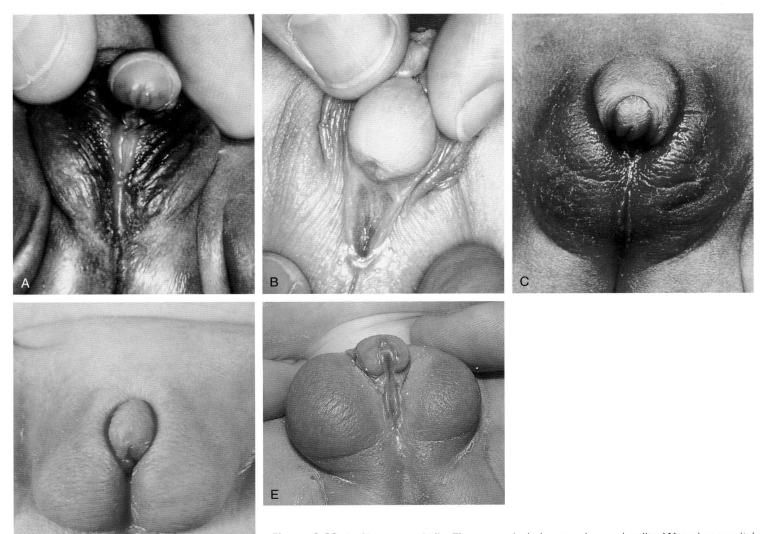

Figure 9-29. Ambiguous genitalia. These cases include a true hermaphrodite **(A)** and congenital virilizing adrenal hyperplasia **(B-E).** Note the symmetrical appearance of the genitalia. **(B-D,** Courtesy Dr. D. Becker, Pittsburgh, Pa.)

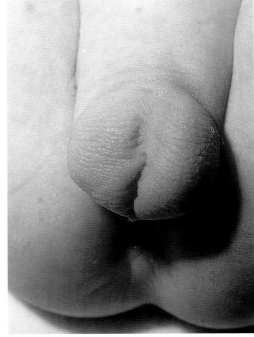

Figure 9-30. Agenesis of the phallus. Rare developmental anomaly with a normal male karyotype. (Courtesy D. Becker, MD, Pittsburgh, Pa.)

(HPG) axis. In girls, the causes of isosexual precocity (development along lines of the same sex) are related to alterations in gonadal or CNS function. Gonadotropin-dependent precocious puberty follows an early onset of pulsatile LH and FSH secretion and the subsequent response of the ovary. Hypothalamic hamartomas are composed of structurally abnormal nervous system tissue and may be associated with GnRH-dependent precocious puberty. Gelastic seizures can be associated with hypothalamic hamartomas and precocious puberty. Intracranial neoplasms are more commonly associated with precocious puberty in boys as compared with girls.

In GnRH-independent forms of precocious puberty, there is an increased production of gonadal steroids. This leads to physical changes of puberty, in the absence of activation of the HPG axis. McCune-Albright syndrome, characterized by irregular café-au-lait spots (Fig. 9-31A), polyostotic fibrous dysplasia (Fig. 9-31B), and sexual precocity, is one example of a GnRH-independent cause of precocious puberty. McCune-Albright syndrome is due to a somatic cell activating mutation of the α subunit of G protein receptor gene.

Gonadal or adrenal neoplasms secreting sex steroids, androgens, or estrogens are rare causes of precocious puberty. In boys, human chorionic gonadotropin (hCG)-secreting tumors can also cause isosexual precocity. Famil-

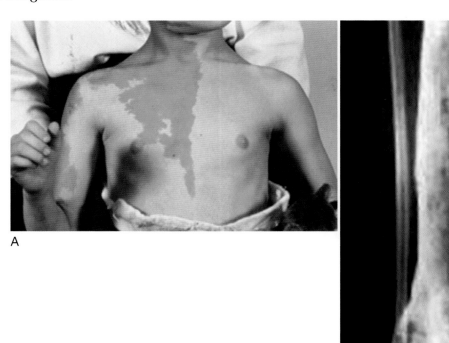

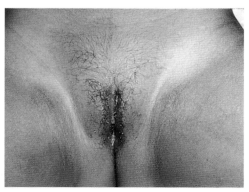

Figure 9-31. **A,** McCune-Albright syndrome. Irregular café-au-lait pigmentation over right anterior chest, shoulder, and right arm. **B,** Polyostotic fibrous dysplasia. Multiple areas of fibrous dysplasia, most commonly found in long bones and pelvis. (**A,** Courtesy National Institutes of Health, Bethesda, Md.)

ial male-limited precocious puberty or testotoxicosis is characterized by premature testicular testosterone production, testicular enlargement, and precocious puberty. It is due to constitutively active mutations of the LH receptor gene. Long-standing primary hypothyroidism in girls may be associated with isosexual precocity and inappropriate secretion of gonadotropins. Galactorrhea may occur in association with elevated prolactin levels.

Premature Thelarche

This condition occurs before expected pubertal development. The breast tissue may appear unilaterally or bilaterally and may regress or persist (Fig. 9-32). Premature thelarche is a diagnosis of exclusion and cannot be made in the presence or progression of other pubertal signs. The ingestion of exogenous estrogens, such as oral contraceptives, should always be suspected in cases of breast enlargement. Typically, premature thelarche develops during the first or second year of life without any other signs of puberty. There is no pubertal progression of this self-limited disorder. However, premature thelarche must be differentiated from other forms of progressive precocious puberty. Breast enlargement secondary to maternal hormones may occur in either sex in the immediate neonatal period.

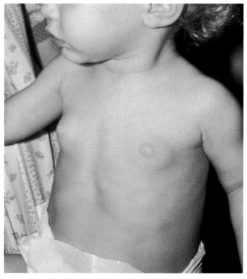

Figure 9-32. Premature thelarche. Isolated bilateral breast enlargement in a toddler with premature thelarche.

Premature Pubarche

The development of pubic hair before 8 years of age in girls and 9.5 years of age in boys is considered to be premature (Fig. 9-33). Associated findings may include axillary hair, adult-type body odor, and acne. Diagnostic considerations include premature adrenarche due to premature adrenal pubertal maturation or late-onset CAH (congenital adrenal hyperplasia). Androgen-secreting adrenal or gonadal tumors are extremely rare. Although

Figure 9-33. Premature adrenarche. Pubic hair development in a prepubertal girl with premature adrenarche.

advanced skeletal maturation is more common in CAH, ACTH stimulation tests may be necessary to distinguish late-onset CAH from premature adrenarche. To diagnose late-onset CAH, the stimulated 17-hydroxyprogesterone value should be greater than 1500 ng/dL. In children with premature adrenarche, adrenal steroid hormone concentrations may be elevated for chronological age but are normal for the degree of pubic hair development. For some girls, premature adrenarche heralds subsequent development of polycystic ovary syndrome in adolescence. Polycystic ovary syndrome is characterized by oligo/amenorrhea and hyperandrogenism.

Delayed Puberty

A common cause of delayed puberty is constitutional delay, which refers to a normal variant of the timing of puberty. Disorders of puberty can be classified as central (hypothalamic or pituitary) or gonadal in origin. Kallmann syndrome refers to hypothalamic hypogonadism. Acquired gonadotropin deficiency can be due to trauma, neoplasms, infiltrative disorders, hyperprolactinemia, or chronic illness. Anorexia nervosa, cystic fibrosis, and sickle cell anemia may be associated with delayed puberty. Turner and Klinefelter syndromes are chromosomal disorders associated with gonadal failure. Trauma, chemotherapy, and radiation therapy are additional causes of gonadal failure.

Androgen insensitivity occurs secondary to mutations in the androgen receptor gene. Androgen action is essential for retention of wolffian duct derivatives, development of the prostate, and differentiation of male external genitalia. Common clinical presenting features of complete androgen insensitivity include inguinal or labial masses in an otherwise normal-appearing female infant or primary amenorrhea in an adolescent girl. In all instances, the karyotype is 46,XY.

Patients with 17-hydroxylase deficiency have alterations in the CYP17 gene that encodes the P450C17 enzyme. This enzyme is essential for the production of cortisol and sex steroids (see Fig. 9-27). In classic 17-hydroxylase deficiency, patients with both XX and XY karyotypes are phenotypic females and both present with lack of secondary sexual development.

Mutations in various genes can lead to a variety of syndromes of dysgenesis involving the mullerian or wolffian ducts, gonads, kidneys, and adrenal glands. The Wilms tumor-suppressor gene (WT1) is essential for both gonadal and renal formation. The SF-1 (steroidogenic factor 1) and DAX1 (the duplicated in adrenal hypoplasia congenita on the X chromosome) proteins are essential for gonadal and adrenal differentiation. SOX9 and SRY are two genes important in testicular differentiation. Individuals with partial or mixed gonadal dysgenesis usually present with asymmetric genital ambiguity. Older children often present with infantile sexual characteristics and primary amenorrhea.

Turner Syndrome

Turner syndrome, due to structural or numerical aberrations of the X chromosomes, should be suspected in any short female. Typically, girls with Turner syndrome have short stature and delayed puberty due to gonadal failure. Some clinical presentations of Turner syndrome are shown in the pictures of young women reported in the original article by Turner (Fig. 9-34A and B). The wide carrying angle (cubitus valgus), shieldlike chest, and webbed neck may be easily appreciated. A more comprehensive list of physical findings in patients with Turner syndrome is listed in Table 9-6 and at the Turner Syndrome Society Web site (available on line at http://www.turner-syndrome-us.org). Evaluating for cardiac and renal anomalies in girls with Turner syndrome is important. Girls with mosaic forms of Turner syndrome may not exhibit all of these phenotypic findings. Karyotyping is diagnostic in a clinical picture suggestive of Turner syndrome. Recent studies suggest that GH treatment may significantly augment ultimate adult growth in Turner syndrome. A growth chart for untreated girls with this syndrome is shown in Figure 9-35.

Klinefelter Syndrome

Boys with Klinefelter syndrome have a 47,XXY karyotype. With puberty, the testes are noted to be small and firm. Gynecomastia and neurobehavioral difficulties are common.

For a list of other syndromes associated with endocrine dysfunction, see Table 9-7.

Diabetes Mellitus

Diabetes mellitus represents one of the most common of the chronic diseases seen by the endocrinologist. Forms of diabetes include type I diabetes (insulin-dependent dia-

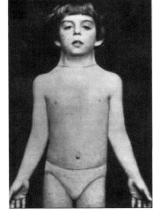
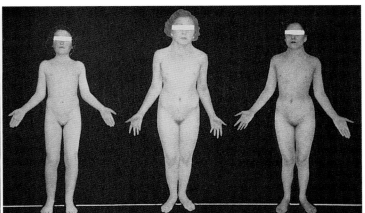

Figure 9-34. Turner syndrome. **A,** Turner used this photograph in 1938 to describe the syndrome that bears his name. This girl exhibits characteristic features of Turner syndrome including a webbed neck, broad chest, marked cubitus valgus, and low-set ears. **B,** Note the clinical heterogeneity within the syndrome.

A   B

betes mellitus, IDDM); type II diabetes (non–insulin-dependent diabetes mellitus, NIDDM); cystic fibrosis–related diabetes, drug-induced diabetes (secondary to steroids, immunosuppressive agents); and monogenic forms of diabetes (maturity-onset diabetes of the young, MODY).

Before the institution of aggressive insulin therapy, children with diabetes mellitus and short stature were seen frequently in endocrine clinics and represented instances of the Mauriac syndrome. This syndrome is characterized by poorly controlled diabetes, short stature, hepatomegaly, and sexual infantilism. Fortunately, it is rare to see a child with Mauriac syndrome. In the child with well-controlled type I, or insulin-dependent, diabetes mellitus, the growth rate should be indistinguishable from that of a normal child. However, one physical finding seen in diabetic patients is that of limited joint mobility. Figure 9-36 shows

Table 9-6	Common Clinical Findings in Turner Syndrome

Skeletal Growth Disturbances
Short stature
Short neck
Abnormal upper-to-lower-segment ratio
Cubitus valgus
Short metacarpals
Madelung deformity
Scoliosis
Genu valgum
Characteristic facies—micrognathia, high-arched palate

Lymphatic Obstruction
Webbed neck
Low posterior hairline
Rotated ears
Edema of hands, feet
Nail dysplasia
Characteristic dermatographics

Ovarian Function
Delayed puberty
Gonadal failure
Infertility

Miscellaneous Defects
Strabismus
Ptosis
Multiple pigmented nevi
Cardiovascular anomalies
Hypertension
Renal and renovascular anomalies
Hearing abnormalities

Associated Disorders
Hashimoto thyroiditis
Hypothyroidism
Alopecia
Vitiligo
Gastrointestinal disorders
Carbohydrate intolerance

Modified from Lippe BM: Primary ovarian failure. In Kaplan SA (ed): Clinical Pediatric and Adolescent Endocrinology. Philadelphia, WB Saunders, 1982.

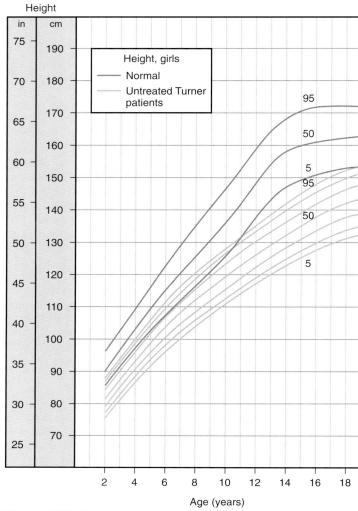

Figure 9-35. Growth curve for Turner syndrome. Superimposed is the growth curve for normal girls.

Table 9-7	Syndromes and Associated Endocrine Dysfunction

Turner syndrome	Hypothyroidism/hyperthyroidism, diabetes, ovarian failure, delayed puberty, short stature
Prader-Willi syndrome	Hypogonadotropic hypogonadism, diabetes, short stature
Klinefelter syndrome	Testicular failure
Down syndrome	Hypoparathyroidism/hyperthyroidism, short stature
Beckwith-Wiedemann syndrome	Hypoglycemia, precocious puberty
McCune-Albright syndrome	Precocious puberty, hyperthyroidism, Cushing syndrome, acromegaly
DiGeorge syndrome	Hypocalcemia
Williams syndrome	Hypercalcemia
Kallmann syndrome	Hypogonadotropic hypogonadism
Russell-Silver syndrome	Short stature
MEN 1 syndrome	Hyperparathyroidism, hypoglycemia (insulinoma), acromegaly (GH excess), Cushing syndrome, hyperthyroidism, catecholamine excess (pheochromocytoma)
MEN 2A syndrome	Catecholamine excess (pheochromocytoma), hyperparathyroidism
MEN 2B syndrome	Catecholamine excess (pheochromocytoma)
APS-1	Hypoparathyroidism, primary adrenal insufficiency
APS-2	Adrenal insufficiency, autoimmune thyroid disease or IDDM
Denys-Drash	Intersex disorders

APS-1, autoimmune polyglandular syndrome type 1—autoimmune polyendocrinopathy, candidiasis, and ectodermal dystrophy; APS-2, autoimmune polyglandular syndrome type 2—adrenal insufficiency, thyroid disease, and diabetes mellitus; IDDM, insulin-dependent diabetes mellitus; MEN, multiple endocrine neoplasia.

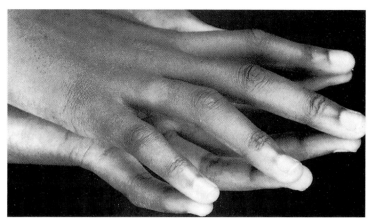

Figure 9-36. Diabetic sclerodactyly. This patient shows an inability to flatten the palms and fingers as he presses both hands together. (Courtesy A. Rosenbloom, MD, Gainesville, Fla.)

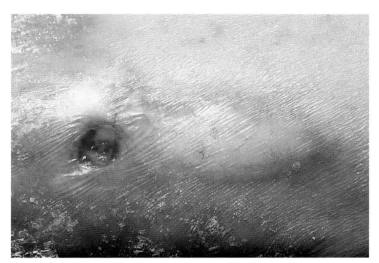

Figure 9-37. Necrobiosis lipoidica diabeticorum is characterized by the presence of yellow waxy skin lesions that exhibit reddened components. Small areas of ulceration may also be seen. (Courtesy B. Cohen, MD, Pittsburgh, Pa.)

Hypoglycemia

Signs and symptoms of hypoglycemia reflect activation of the autonomic nervous system and epinephrine release and CNS glucopenia. The differential diagnosis of hypoglycemia is broad. A useful classification divides hypoglycemia into those in which ketones are absent and those in which ketones are present (Fig. 9-38). Hypoglycemia may occur during a period of fasting or catabolic stress (Tables 9-8 and 9-9) or may be iatrogenic or drug-induced (Table 9-10).

Hyperinsulinemia and some defects in fatty acid oxidation are nonketotic or hypoketotic forms of hypoglycemia. Hyperinsulinism is a significant cause of hypoglycemia in infants and children and is the most common cause of

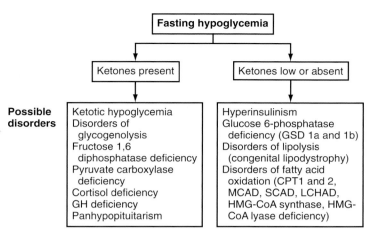

Figure 9-38. Fasting hypoglycemia. Diagnostic evaluation for fasting hypoglycemia in the presence or absence of ketosis. CPT, carnitine palmitoyltransferase; GH, growth hormone; GSD, glycogen storage disease; HMG-CoA, 3-hydroxy-3-methylglutaryl-coenzyme A; LCHAD, long-chain 3-hydroxyacyl-coenzyme A dehydrogenase; MCAD, medium-chain acyl-coenzyme A dehydrogenase; SCAD, short-chain acyl-coenzyme A dehydrogenase.

Table 9-8	Postprandial Hypoglycemia

Postgastric surgery
Diabetes mellitus
Galactosemia
Hereditary fructose intolerance
Reactive or functional hypoglycemia

Table 9-9	Fasting Hypoglycemia

Increased Substrate Utilization
Hyperinsulinism—Endogenous
Insulinoma
Mutations in SUR, KIR, GLUD, GCK
Autoimmune hypoglycemia
Infants of diabetic mothers
Beckwith-Wiedemann syndrome
Leprechaunism

Decreased Substrate Production
Inborn Errors of Carbohydrate Metabolism
Defects of gluconeogenesis
Glycogen storage diseases
Inborn Errors of Protein Metabolism
Maple syrup urine disease
Methylmalonic aciduria
Inborn Errors of Fat Metabolism
Systemic carnitine deficiency
Carnitine acetyltransferase deficiency
Hydroxymethylglutaryl CoA lyase deficiency
Acyl CoA dehydrogenase deficiency
Counterregulatory Hormone Deficiency
Cortisol
Thyroid
Glucagon
Growth hormone
Catecholamines
Ketotic Hypoglycemia
Hepatic and Renal Disease
Extrapancreatic Neoplasms
Reye Syndrome

GCK, glucokinase; GLUD, glutamate dehydrogenase; KIR, potassium inwardly-rectifying channel; SUR, sulfonylurea receptor.

the inability of a diabetic child to flatten the palms because of waxy thickened skin in the areas of the proximal and distal interphalangeal joints. Such skin has been associated with poor diabetic control. The development of specific skin lesions, such as necrobiosis lipoidica diabeticorum, may also be associated with diabetes. Figure 9-37 shows such a lipid-filled skin lesion, which may occasionally be seen in a child with type I diabetes.

hypoglycemia in the neonatal period. Hyperinsulinism may be caused by activating mutations of enzymes, such as glucokinase and glutamate dehydrogenase, by inactivating mutations of the K_{ATP} channel regulating insulin secretion, by exogenous administration of glucose lowering medications such as insulin or sulfonylureas, or by an

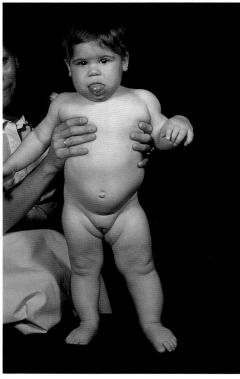

Figure 9-39. Beckwith-Wiedemann syndrome. Note hemihypertrophy on the left side, along with prominence of the tongue. (Courtesy Dr. D. Becker, Pittsburgh, Pa.)

Table 9-10	Drug-Induced Hypoglycemia

Insulin
Oral hypoglycemic agents
Ethanol
Salicylates
Propranolol
Miscellaneous other drugs
Akee fruit

Table 9-11	Causes of Secondary Obesity

Leptin Deficiency
Leptin Receptor Mutation
Endocrine Disorders
Cushing syndrome
Hypothyroidism
Pseudohypoparathyroidism
Type II diabetes mellitus
Genetic Syndromes
Prader-Willi syndrome
Bardet-Biedel syndrome
Cohen syndrome
Central Nervous System Disorders
Hypothalamic tumor
Trauma
Inflammation
Miscellaneous
Drug-induced (e.g., risperidone, tricyclic antidepressants, steroids)
Binge Eating Disorder
Bulimia Nervosa

Modified from Schneider M, Brill SR: Obesity in children and adolescents. Pediatr Rev 26:155-162, 2005.

Table 9-12	Complications of Obesity

Respiratory	**Cardiovascular**
Sleep apnea	Dyslipidemias
Snoring	Hypertension
Pickwickian syndrome	**Endocrinologic**
Asthma	Insulin resistance
Musculoskeletal	Impaired glucose tolerance
Blount disease	Type II diabetes mellitus
Slipped capital femoral	Polycystic ovarian syndrome
epiphysis	Menstrual irregularity
Gastrointestinal	**Psychological**
Gallbladder disease	Depression
Steatohepatitis	Eating disorders
	Social isolation

Modified from Schneider M, Brill SR: Obesity in children and adolescents. Pediatr Rev 26:155-162, 2005.

insulin-secreting adenoma. Syndromes such as Beckwith-Wiedemann syndrome (Fig. 9-39) may also be associated with hypoglycemia in addition to macrosomia, macroglossia, omphaloceles, hemihypertrophy and embryonal tumors. In these cases, hypoglycemia has been attributed to hyperinsulinism.

Ketotic hypoglycemia is a common cause of childhood hypoglycemia that usually presents between the ages of 18 months and 5 years with resolution of symptoms by age 8 to 9 years. Hypopituitarism, glycogen storage diseases, and disorders of gluconeogenesis are additional causes of ketotic hypoglycemia. Hepatomegaly is found in glycogen storage diseases.

Obesity and Associated Endocrinopathies

As the prevalence of obesity is increasing, clinicians are faced with the challenge presented by identifying children "at risk" for becoming overweight (see Table 9-2). Although the majority of overweight children and adolescents have exogenous obesity, genetic syndromes, hypothalamic tumors, or endocrinopathies may also present with overweight or weight gain as the initial symptom. Causes of secondary obesity are listed in Table 9-11.

Patients who are obese are at risk for developing systemic complications as listed in Table 9-12. The combination of obesity, insulin resistance, dyslipidemia, and hypertension has been termed the "metabolic syndrome" or "syndrome X." Individuals with this syndrome are at increased risk for developing type II diabetes and cardiovascular disease. Adolescent girls with hyperandrogenism, irregular menses, and chronic anovulation may also have the metabolic syndrome and polycystic ovary syndrome. An early sign of insulin resistance is acanthosis nigricans (Fig. 9-40A and B), a skin finding characterized by hyperpigmented, velvety plaques most commonly seen around the neck, in the axillae, or over joints.

Summary

As seen in the illustrations in this chapter, endocrine dysfunction results in dramatic alterations in a child's phenotype. These alterations should be readily recognized and thus direct the diagnostic approach. Careful attention to the appearance of children requiring evaluation by a physician should allow early diagnosis of endocrine disorders, resulting in prompt therapeutic intervention and restoration of the child's appearance and overall state of well-being.

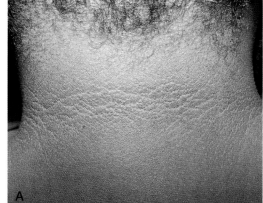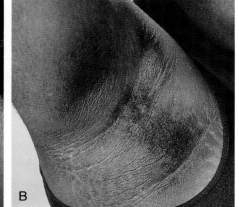

Figure 9-40. Acanthosis nigricans. Note the thickened skin and velvety appearance around the neck **(A)** and in the axilla **(B)** in this patient with polycystic ovary syndrome and insulin resistance.

Bibliography

DeGroot LJ (ed): Endocrinology, 3rd ed. Philadelphia, WB Saunders, 1995.

Kappy MS, Allen DB, Geffner ME (eds): Wilkins CJ: Principles and Practice of Pediatric Endocrinology. Springfield, Ill, Charles C Thomas, 2005.

Lifshitz F (ed): Pediatric Endocrinology: A Clinical Guide, 4th ed. New York, Marcel Dekker, 2003.

MacLaughlin DT, Donahoe PK: Sex determination and differentiation. N Engl J Med 350:367-378, 2004.

Pescovitz OH, Eugster EA: Pediatric Endocrinology. Mechanisms, Manifestations, and Management. Philadelphia, Lippincott Williams & Wilkins, 2004.

Schneider M: Obesity in children and adolescents. Pediatr Rev 26:155-162, 2005.

Scriver CR, Beaudet AL, Sly WS, Valle D (eds): The Metabolic and Molecular Bases of Inherited Disease, 8th ed. New York, McGraw-Hill, 1995.

Speiser PW, White PC: Congenital adrenal hyperplasia. N Engl J Med 349:776-788, 2003.

Partsch CJ, Heger S, Sippell WG: Management and outcome of central precocious puberty. Clin Endocrinol (Oxf) 56:129-148, 2002.

Sperling MA (ed): Pediatric Endocrinology, 2nd ed. Philadelphia, WB Saunders, 2002.

Wilson JD, Foster DW (eds): Williams Textbook of Endocrinology, 8th ed. Philadelphia, WB Saunders, 1992.

CHAPTER 10

Nutrition and Gastroenterology

CHERYL BLANK AND J. CARLTON GARTNER, JR.

Nutrition and gastrointestinal disorders are encountered daily by most pediatricians. As a world health problem, the cycle of diarrhea, poor nutrition, and consequent absorptive disorders causes untold harm. This chapter is divided into two sections, first addressing nutrition and malnutrition in children and then gastrointestinal and hepatic disorders. In this chapter we focus on entities that are commonly seen by pediatric primary care physicians.

Nutrition

Normal Infant Nutrition

Any discussion of nutrition in infancy must begin with the normal requirements (Table 10-1). Fortunately, breast milk exists worldwide. Breast milk has advantages beyond the issue of maternal-infant bonding (Table 10-2). The only supplements required are fluoride and vitamin D. In the latter part of the first year, babies fed exclusively breast milk may require additional iron. As a general rule, content and absorption of nutrients from breast milk are ideal for all infants, with the possible exception of the very low birth weight infant, who may have higher electrolyte, calcium, phosphorus, and vitamin requirements. Table 10-3 compares the major components of cow's milk–based formula, cow's milk, and breast milk.

Normal Childhood Nutrition

Given the importance of growth and development in children, awareness of nutritional status is mandatory for children's health care workers. Each pediatric visit should include a basic nutritional assessment. This process may include dietary, clinical, and detailed laboratory data. In a healthy child a brief dietary history and a plot of height, weight, body mass index, and head circumference on standard curves are sufficient. The chronically ill child may require more careful assessment to clarify acute or chronic malnutrition and plan effective therapy.

Clinical Observations of Malnutrition

Malnutrition results from an imbalance between the intake and absorption of nutrients and the rate at which the nutrients are used. This imbalance can lead to both undernutrition and overnutrition. Obesity is the result of overnutrition and has grown to epidemic proportions in the United States and other developed nations. Obesity is further discussed in Chapter 9. Undernutrition, or protein energy malnutrition, results from inadequate intake, abnormal loss of nutrients, or increased metabolic needs.

Diagnosing malnutrition is challenging. The patient's diet and food intake should be thoroughly explored. For infants, information regarding the patient's formula and how it is diluted must be obtained. For older children, quantity of food intake, food preferences, and foods avoided should be noted. Careful plotting of height, weight, and body mass index on standard growth charts over time will aid in the diagnosis of malnutrition. The Waterlow criteria assess malnutrition by plotting weight for height, indicating current nutritional status and height for age, which reflects the chronicity of malnutrition.

A traditional classification of extreme malnutrition includes marasmus, kwashiorkor, and marasmic-kwashiorkor. Marasmus, a predominantly caloric/energy deficiency with wasting of tissue, is characterized by a marked weight-for-height reduction with emaciation, loss of subcutaneous fat, lusterless and sparse hair, and poor nail growth (Fig. 10-1). Marasmus is usually seen within the first year of life and is a consequence of poor caloric, protein, vitamin, and mineral intake. Secondary effects of marasmus, such as hypothermia and bradycardia, occur late in the clinical course. Classic kwashiorkor results from a diet rich in calories but lacks protein. The initial "moon face" of kwashiorkor is often mistaken for proper nutrition. The child is often edematous, which becomes strikingly apparent after nutritional repletion (Fig. 10-2). Hepatomegaly and mental status changes are common. Skin changes in kwashiorkor patients include hyperpigmentation and hypopigmentation with a scaly, weeping dermatitis that may ulcerate and desquamate (Fig. 10-3). The rash is often more prominent in areas that are chronically irritated (e.g., the infant's groin and areas of peripheral edema) (Fig. 10-4). It resembles pellagra but is seen in areas that are not exposed to sunlight. Marasmic-kwashiorkor occurs when both patterns of malnutrition develop together, resulting in a combination of clinical features. In general, these descriptions of profound malnutrition are embraced within the term *protein-energy malnutrition*.

Failure to Thrive

The term *failure to thrive* is commonly defined as inadequate physical growth over time. It is important to remember that failure to thrive is a symptom complex and not a disease or diagnosis. The etiology for failure to thrive is vast, and the differential has often been classified into organic versus nonorganic causes. An additional classification system based on pathophysiology is frequently more appropriate. A majority of disorders that result in failure to thrive can be broken down into the following categories: inadequate caloric intake, inadequate absorption, excessive caloric/metabolic demand, or defective nutrient utilization. Table 10-4 lists possible etiologies of failure to thrive.

A detailed history, asking specific questions regarding oral intake, stooling patterns and consistency, and the presence or absence of vomiting, can often help narrow the differential diagnosis. Determining not only the volume of formula taken but how the formula was made provides information of caloric intake, as well as incorrect mixing of formula. A 3-day diet recall is most helpful because it allows the physician to review the diet over time. History of chronic illnesses and previous surgeries, especially abdominal surgery, is important to elicit. Systematic plotting of weight and height/length on standard growth curves that are specific for the child's country of origin or underlying disorder are helpful and can often prevent overinvestigation of children with normal varia-

Table 10-1	Nutritional Requirements	
AGE	CALORIES (kcal/kg/day)	PROTEIN (g/kg/day)
0-12 mo	100	2.5-3.0
1-7 yr	75-90	1.5-2.5
7-12 yr	60-75	1.5-2.5
12+ yr	30-60	1.0-1.5

Table 10-2	Advantages of Breastfeeding

Convenience
No sterilization required
Maternal-infant bonding
Less frequent hospitalizations
Passive immunity
Possible increase in IQ
Optimal absorption of nutrients, vitamins, and trace elements
Possible protection from allergen exposure
Less obesity

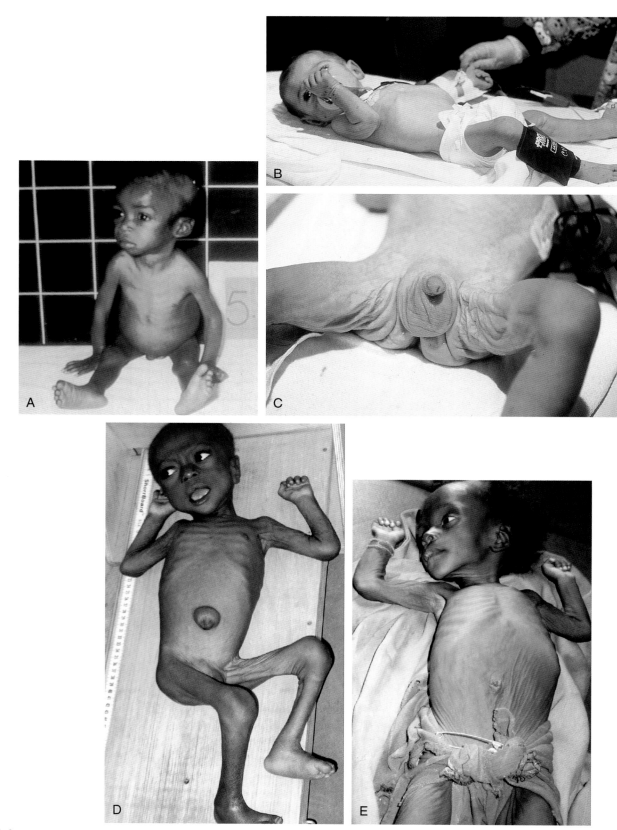

Figure 10-1. Marasmus. **A,** Note the profound wasting and sparse hair. **B** and **C,** Note the wasting of subcutaneous tissue over the thorax with prominent ribs and loose skinfolds in the groin. **D** and **E,** Note the loss of subcutaneous fat, profound wasting, loose skin folds, and sparse hair. (Courtesy Dr. Jonathan Spector, Boston.)

Table 10-3	Comparison of Milks—Selected Components		
COMPONENT	**BREAST MILK**	**FORMULA (COW'S MILK BASED)**	**WHOLE COW'S MILK**
Protein (g/dL)	1.2	1.5	3.3
Source	Human	Skim milk	Whey/casein
% calories	7	9	20
Fat (g/dL)	4	3.8	3.7
Source	Human	Soy/coconut	Butterfat
% calories	54	50	50
Carbohydrate (g/dL)	6.8	6.9	4.9
Source	Lactose	Lactose	Lactose
% calories	40	41	30
Osmolality (mEq/L)	300	290	288
Renal solute load (mEq/L)	87	90	226
Na^+ (mEq/L)	7	9	24
K^+ (mEq/L)	13	18	35
Ca^{2+} (mg/L)	340	440	1150
P (mg/L)	140	300	920
Ca/P ratio	2.2	1.5	1.3
Iron (mg/L)	0.5	0 or 12	1
Vitamin D (IU)	22	420	444
Fluoride (mg/L)	0.01	0*	0.02

*Unless water is added to concentrate.

Table 10-4	Etiologies of Failure to Thrive	
INADEQUATE CALORIC INTAKE	**INADEQUATE ABSORPTION**	**DEFECTIVE NUTRIENT UTILIZATION**
Decreased intake	Carbohydrate malabsorption (lactase deficiency)	Increased caloric need (chronic illness, such as BPD, IBD, cancer, cystic fibrosis)
Anorexia	Fat malabsorption (cystic fibrosis, chronic pancreatitis)	
Vomiting	Protein malabsorption (cystic fibrosis, intestinal lymphangiectasia, severe IBD)	
Inability to suck or swallow	Celiac disease	
Gastroesophageal reflux disease	Post–viral enteropathy	

BPD, bronchopulmonary dysplasia; IBD, inflammatory bowel disease.

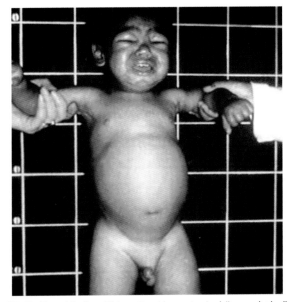

Figure 10-2. Kwashiorkor. This patient has a typical "sugar baby" appearance with generalized edema. Note the periorbital and limb edema.

tions in growth (Fig. 10-5). Crossing of growth isopleths over time should be investigated thoroughly. A careful social and behavioral history may reveal problems with parenting or the environment that are contributing to the child's failure to thrive.

Laboratory Tests and Anthropometric Measurements

Diagnostic testing, in conjunction with a detailed history and physical examination, is often helpful in determining the etiology of failure to thrive. A complete blood count and serum electrolytes are obtained routinely. Stool studies for ova and parasites, culture, *Clostridium difficile* toxin, reducing substances, or fecal elastase can suggest a possible diagnosis of infection or malabsorption. Protein malabsorption is diagnosed by determining serum protein and albumin levels, fecal alpha-1-antitrypsin level and a urinalysis. Fat malabsorption may result in altered fat soluble vitamin levels and increased 72-hour fecal fat levels. A sweat chloride test or DNA analysis will diagnose cystic fibrosis (see Chapter 16).

Laboratory testing can also be helpful in identifying some malnourished children. Although these tests are not frequently obtained, they are worth noting. Not only is the degree of malnutrition confirmed, but certain specific deficiencies may be uncovered. Unfortunately, an inexpensive laboratory test for early malnutrition is not yet available. Amino acid nomograms may aid early diagnosis but are expensive and require a sophisticated laboratory. Decreases in body proteins are helpful but reflect normal body catabolism. Consequently, retinol binding protein ($t_{1/2}$ 12 hours) and transferrin ($t_{1/2}$ 9 days) indicate more current nutritional status than the standard albumin ($t_{1/2}$ 20 to 24 days). An additional aid in assessing lean body mass is a comparison of 24-hour creatinine excretion with standard norms for height (creatinine height index).

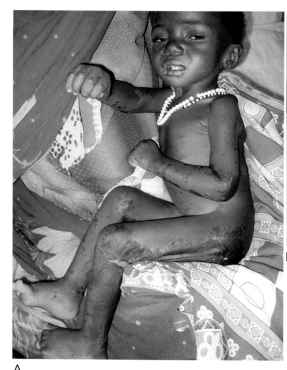

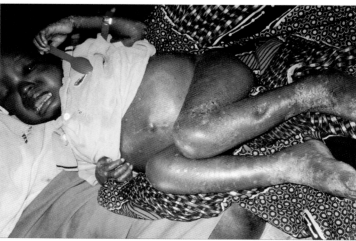

Figure 10-3. Kwashiorkor. **A** and **B,** These patients demonstrate kwashiorkor with "flaky paint" dermatosis, pigmentation changes, and pitting edema. (Courtesy Dr. Jonathan Spector, Boston.)

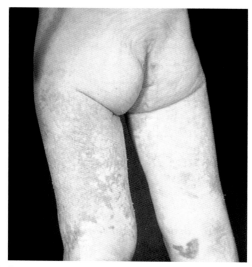

Figure 10-4. Kwashiorkor. The rash of kwashiorkor is scaly and erythematous and may weep, especially in edematous areas.

Because infection is a major cause of morbidity and mortality in the malnourished patient, a basic immunologic assessment may be indicated. Total lymphocyte counts and skin tests are adequate baseline exams since the major effects are in the T-lymphocyte system.

After the initial clinical examination of the patient with failure to thrive, anthropometric measurements could be made. These enable large groups of children to be followed sequentially, distinguishing between acute and chronic malnutrition and assessing the effects of protein or total calories. Using standard curves, such as the 2000 National Center for Health Statistics charts, height-for-age deficit (actual height ÷ expected height-for-age [50th percentile] × 100) and weight-for-height deficit (actual weight ÷ expected weight-for-height [50th percentile] × 100) may be calculated. Diminished height for age most commonly reflects chronic undernutrition, whereas low weight for

height may indicate a more acute process. Nutritional status is graded using these two parameters (Table 10-5). In addition, measurements of triceps skinfold thickness and midarm muscle circumference further delineate protein and calorie deficits (Table 10-6). The measurements must be done carefully (Figs. 10-6 and 10-7). When completed, the measurements are compared with standards and the predominant deficiencies can be defined.

Therapy

The treatment of failure to thrive and malnutrition is twofold. All attempts should be made to treat the underlying cause of the symptoms. Nutritional rehabilitation is crucial and is the major contributing factor to the treatment of these conditions. Patients with hypoproteinemia and significant changes in weight for height will need more vigorous therapy. The following formula can be used to determine both caloric and protein needs required for catch-up growth.

$$\text{Catch-up growth requirement (Kcal or g/kg/day)} = \frac{\textit{Calories or protein required for weight age}}{\text{(Kcal or g/kg/day)} \times \text{Ideal weight for age (kg)}}{\text{Actual weight (kg)}}$$

Parenteral nutrition should be considered for patients with profound injury to the gastrointestinal tract (Fig. 10-8). This advance in nutritional therapy continues to be perfected by better mixtures, less cumbersome catheters, and home total parenteral nutrition (TPN) using advanced programmable pumps. Recovery from intestinal injury is enhanced by intraluminal nutrition, which should be initiated as soon as possible. Fortunately, industrialized countries have many modified and elemental formulas for children with acute or chronic digestive disturbances. Because some causes of malnutrition may have a profound effect on intestinal absorption, several of these formulas

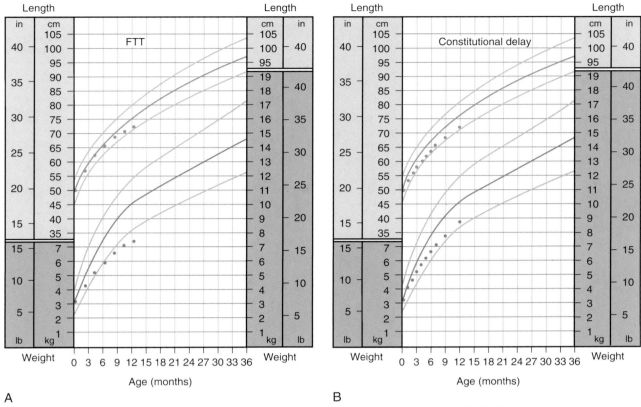

Figure 10-5. Examples of growth curves. **A,** Typical failure to thrive (FTT) with deceleration of weight gain. **B,** Slow growth but at a normal rate consistent with constitutional delay.

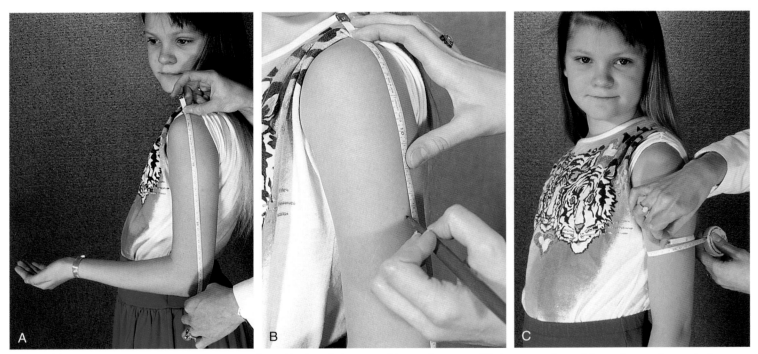

Figure 10-6. Midarm circumference. **A,** Locate the midpoint of the arm with arm bent at a 90-degree angle, and tape at acromion and olecranon processes. **B,** Mark at midpoint. **C,** Make measurement at midpoint with arm hanging loosely.

Table 10-5	Grading of Nutritional Status	
GRADE	**HEIGHT FOR AGE**	**WEIGHT FOR HEIGHT**
I	<95%	<90%
II	<90%	<80%
III	<85%	<70%

Table 10-6	Anthropometric Assessment of Nutritional Status	
MEASUREMENT	**DEFICIENCY**	**INDICATED DEFICIENCY**
Weight for age	<90% of standard	Protein-calorie
Height for age	<95%	Protein-calorie
Weight for height	<90%	Protein-calorie
Triceps skinfold	<5%	Calorie
Midarm muscle	<5%	Protein

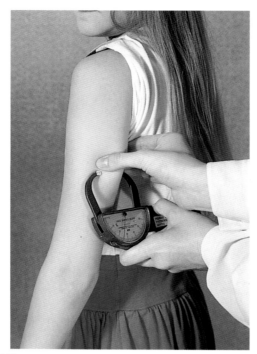

Figure 10-7. Triceps skinfold. Grasp a vertical pinch of skin and subcutaneous fat. The caliper jaw is placed over the skinfold at the midpoint mark while maintaining grasp of skinfold. Make reading to nearest 1 mm without excessive pressure. Average three readings for the final result.

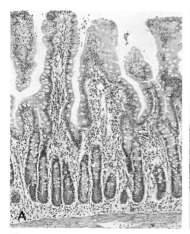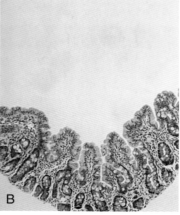

Figure 10-8. Gastrointestinal tract injury. **A,** Normal jejunal mucosa with tall villi and deep crypts. **B,** Blunted villi lead to chronic diarrhea and malnutrition.

| Table 10-7 | Nutritional Deficiencies with Characteristic Physical Signs |

VITAMIN/MINERAL	SIGN/SYMPTOM
Calcium, phosphorus, vitamin D	Rickets/osteomalacia
Vitamin A	Night blindness, xerophthalmia, Bitot spots, follicular hyperkeratosis
Vitamin C	Scurvy: bone lesions, bleeding
Vitamin E	Hemolytic anemia, peripheral neuropathy
Vitamin K	Petechiae, ecchymoses
Thiamine (vitamin B_1)	Beriberi: heart failure, increased intracranial pressure
Niacin	Pellagra: dermatitis (sun-exposed areas)
Riboflavin (vitamin B_2)	Angular stomatitis, cheilosis
Vitamin B_6	Anemia, dermatitis, neuropathy
Vitamin B_{12}	Anemia, neuropathy
Folate	Anemia
Iron	Anemia, koilonychia
Biotin	Rash, hair loss
Essential fatty acids	Rash, coagulopathy
Zinc	Rash (acrodermatitis), growth failure, delayed sexual development, ageusia
Copper	Bone changes, hypopigmentation, anemia, neutropenia
Selenium	Heart failure

may be invaluable. Knowing the specific content of each product is important. High-osmolar formulas are often not tolerated, especially by the compromised small-bowel mucosa, and may lead to worsening diarrhea.

Refeeding syndrome is a potential complication of both oral and parenteral nutritional therapy in severely undernourished patients. Profoundly malnourished individuals undergo metabolic and physiologic changes in order to survive. The reintroduction of proper nutrition may result in severe alterations in electrolyte and fluid balance. It is extremely important to monitor these parameters closely, especially for hypophosphatemia, hypokalemia, hypomagnesemia, hypocalcemia, and glucose intolerance to avoid the potentially significant morbidity and mortality associated with refeeding syndrome.

Before initiating nutritional therapy or after a period of TPN, it helps to look for specific vitamin, mineral, and trace element deficiencies. The more common and previously well-described deficiencies are listed in Table 10-7. Assigning individual findings, such as angular stomatitis, to specific deficiencies in a child with chronic, severe malnutrition is often difficult. Several deficiencies, often seen in a hospital population, are discussed subsequently.

Vitamin D deficiency results in decreased serum calcium levels, which in turn triggers parathyroid hormone to liberate calcium and phosphorus from bone in order to maintain normal serum calcium levels. Serum levels of 25-OH vitamin D are the best initial test to evaluate for vitamin D deficiency. Rickets is a consequence of vitamin D deficiency and is defined as inadequate mineralization of growing bone, or osteomalacia. Vitamin D deficiency can present in patients with liver or kidney disorders or in infants who are breast-fed without supplementation, especially dark-skinned infants with decreased sun exposure. Poor bile flow and consequent malabsorption are the primary cause in hepatobiliary disorders. Additionally, end-stage renal disease with failure of renal hydroxylation of vitamin D_3 or renal tubular wasting of phosphorus may cause poor bone matrix formation.

Children with vitamin D deficiency that results in rickets usually present at weight-bearing age with similar symptoms regardless of the cause. Poor growth, curvature of weight-bearing bones (Fig. 10-9), widening of epiphyses, and costochondral beading (Fig. 10-10) are commonly seen. Softening of the skull (craniotabes) is seen in infants. With appropriate vitamin and mineral supplementation, radiographic healing occurs, followed by bony remodeling (Fig. 10-11). In 2003 the Committee on Nutrition for the American Academy of Pediatrics recommended 200 IU/day of vitamin D for all infants and children not taking enough vitamin D–fortified foods, such as dairy products, cereals, and juices.

Deficiencies of vitamin A, E, and K, which are fat-soluble vitamins, along with vitamin D, may occur as well. Fat-soluble vitamin deficiencies are frequently associated with disorders resulting in steatorrhea. The most common disorder linked with fat malabsorption is cystic fibrosis. Vitamin A deficiency causes follicular hyperkeratosis, xerophthalmia, night blindness, and unusual shiny gray,

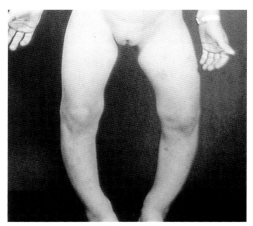

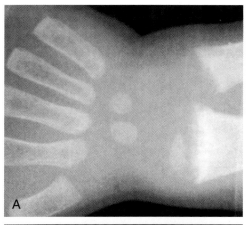

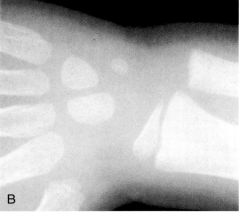

Figure 10-9. Rickets. Hypophosphatemic rickets marked by the obvious bowing of the legs.

Figure 10-11. Rickets. Radiograph of the wrist in a patient with rickets. **A,** Irregularity and widening of the epiphyses in the distal radius and ulna. **B,** With appropriate therapy, remineralization and healing occur.

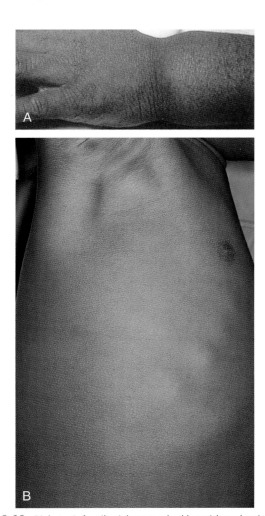

Figure 10-10. Rickets. Infantile rickets marked by widened wrists **(A)** and enlargement of the costochondral junction ("beading") **(B).** The latter occurred as the result of a rapid growth spurt after liver transplantation.

triangular lesions on the conjunctivae called Bitot spots. Clinically, vitamin E deficiency can progress from absence of peripheral deep tendon reflexes to marked ataxia. There have also been reports that retinopathy of prematurity and hemolysis are related to vitamin E deficiency. Vitamin K deficiency, seen in patients with long-standing steatorrhea or liver disease, causes prolongation of the prothrombin time and can be associated clinically with easy bleeding and bruising. Supplementation with fat-soluble vitamins is given in prophylactic doses to children at risk

of developing deficiencies and in treatment doses to children who demonstrate clinical symptoms associated with deficiencies.

Parenteral nutrition is indicated in patients who cannot tolerate nutrition via the gastrointestinal tract for greater than 3 to 5 days. Parenteral nutrition is given preferably through a central vein, allowing for more nutritionally concentrated TPN as opposed to parenteral nutrition given through a peripheral vein. The ingredients of parenteral nutrition include protein, carbohydrates, fat, electrolytes, vitamins, minerals, and trace elements.

Although parenteral nutrition has been lifesaving, especially for neonates with major intestinal disorders, numerous nutritional deficiencies have been historically discovered. Examples of this include fatty acid deficiency with the typical scaly dermatitis and zinc deficiency with alopecia, diarrhea, and acrodermatitis. With improved knowledge of parenteral nutrition, these conditions are now rare. Many unusual problems were uncovered before the reformulation of hyperalimentation mixtures. One report involved a child on hyperalimentation for 6 months who developed irritability, bone pain, and decreased hair pigmentation. Anemia and progressive neutropenia ensued, and a skeletal survey, copper, and ceruloplasmin determinations confirmed copper deficiency. Bone changes included osteoporosis, metaphyseal spurs, and periosteal new bone formation. Hematologic and bone changes reversed with copper administration (Fig. 10-12). Report of another patient requiring long-term TPN who developed a peculiar weeping dermatitis in the perioral, perianal, and lid areas along with lethargy and malaise has been documented. Changes reversed in only 4 days when intravenous biotin was added (Fig. 10-13).

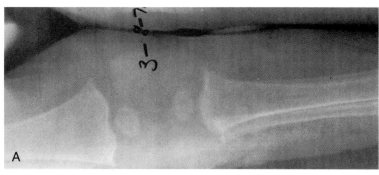
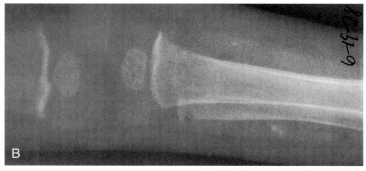

Figure 10-12. Copper deficiency. **A,** Radiograph of a child with copper deficiency reveals irregular epiphyses with spur formation, cloaking of metaphyses, periosteal new bone formation, and osteoporosis. **B,** After 3 months of intravenous copper, the child demonstrates healing of the metaphyses.

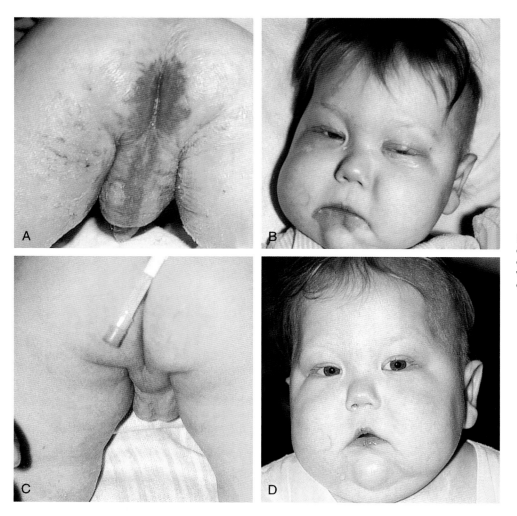

Figure 10-13. Biotin deficiency. **A** and **B,** This child on chronic hyperalimentation developed dermatitis in perianal, perioral, and lid areas along with some thinning of hair. **C** and **D,** The rash has cleared dramatically after 4 days of biotin.

Gastroenterology

Disturbances of gastrointestinal (GI) function are common in pediatric practice, perhaps second only to respiratory symptoms as a reason for office visits. This section emphasizes the major symptoms that bring patients with GI disorders to medical attention and defines entities that may be diagnosed by examination. Inflammatory bowel disease, the gastrointestinal complication of cystic fibrosis, and liver disorders are discussed later.

Abdominal Pain

Abdominal pain may be the most common abdominal complaint of children visiting the pediatrician and the pediatric gastroenterologist. The differential diagnosis of abdominal pain is vast and includes both organic and nonorganic causes. An overlap of the two also exists, making diagnosis even more difficult for the physician and more frustrating for the patient and family. The history and physical examination findings that warrant further investigation are listed in Table 10-8.

The term *functional gastrointestinal disorders* is used to define several chronic and recurrent gastrointestinal symptoms that do not have an identified organic etiology. The Rome II criteria for pediatric functional gastrointestinal disorders is a symptom-based classification system used to differentiate several subgroups of functional gastrointestinal disorders. Recurrent abdominal pain, irritable bowel syndrome, and functional dyspepsia are a few

Table 10-8	Clues to Organic Disease in Recurrent Abdominal Pain

Weight loss
Nocturnal pain
Recurrent emesis
Heme-positive stools
Abnormal physical examination findings—clubbing, perianal skin tags, abdominal mass, localized abdominal pain
Abnormal screening laboratory test results—decreased albumin, increased ESR/CRP, anemia, increased lipase/amylase

CRP, C-reactive protein; ESR, erythrocyte sedimentation rate.

examples of functional gastrointestinal disorders that cause abdominal pain.

Recurrent abdominal pain, often vague and nonspecific, affects between 10% and 20% of all school-aged children. Typically the pain is episodic, unrelated to meals, and periumbilical in location. In 1958 Apley defined recurrent abdominal pain as three or more episodes of abdominal pain over at least a 3-month time period that interferes with the child's activities of daily living. Multiple studies have demonstrated that less than 5% of these children have an organic disorder. The diagnostic criteria of irritable bowel syndrome (IBS) include abdominal pain or discomfort for at least 12 weeks in the past year along with two of the following three criteria: abdominal pain relieved by defecation, pain associated with change in stool frequency, and pain associated with change in stool form. Other symptoms that support the diagnosis of IBS include bloating, urgency, and the feeling of incomplete evacuation. Functional dyspepsia is defined as chronic or recurrent pain or discomfort located in the upper abdomen. The discomfort is often described as abdominal fullness, early satiety, bloating, belching, or nausea. The symptoms of functional dyspepsia are often aggravated with the consumption of a meal.

Peptic ulcer disease, gastritis, pancreatitis, and inflammatory bowel disease (IBD) are examples of organic causes of abdominal pain. IBD is discussed in detail later in this chapter. Appendicitis and intussusception are causes of acute abdominal pain and warrant an evaluation by a surgeon.

Peptic ulcer disease and gastritis should be considered in patients with chronic abdominal pain. In children, clues may be recurrent epigastric abdominal pain, nocturnal pain, postprandial pain, and vomiting. The use of upper endoscopy (Fig. 10-14) allows for more accurate diagnosis of both peptic ulcer disease and gastritis. The association of peptic ulcer disease, chronic active gastritis, and duodenal ulcers with *Helicobacter pylori* infections has been well documented. Endoscopic findings consistent with *H. pylori* include antral gastritis, nodularity of the antrum, and duodenal ulcers (Fig. 10-15). Treatment of *H. pylori* consists of a combination of amoxicillin, clarithromycin, and a proton pump inhibitor; or amoxicillin, metronidazole, and a proton pump inhibitor; or clarithromycin, metronidazole, and a proton pump inhibitor. The antibiotics are commonly given for 2 weeks and the proton pump inhibitor for 4 weeks. These "triple" combination regimens have been found to eradicate *H. pylori* and lead to resolution of symptoms. Although peptic ulcer disease is not yet fully established as a purely infectious disease, the theories about the etiology of peptic ulcer disease have undergone a radical shift in the past decade toward an infectious disorder. Secondary ulcer disease may also be seen as related to conditions such as systemic illness, col-

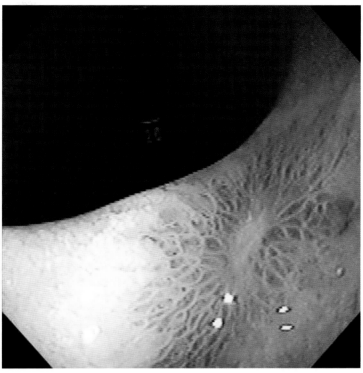

Figure 10-14. Peptic ulcer. Gastric ulcer located in the lower curvature of the stomach. Note the grayish white base of the ulcer crater and the boggy erythematous tissue surrounding the margin of the ulcer. (Courtesy Drs. Feras Alissa and Cary Sauer, Pittsburgh.)

lagen vascular disease, and drug therapy, especially nonsteroidal anti-inflammatory agents.

Pancreatitis may also be seen in children, both as an acute condition or chronic, relapsing disorder. Although gallstones (Fig. 10-16) are the most common cause of pancreatitis in adults, trauma and systemic diseases such as hemolytic uremic syndrome are the most common causes in children. Other causes of childhood pancreatitis in order of frequency are biliary tract disease; congenital anomalies (Fig. 10-17); drugs; organ transplantation; idiopathic, infectious diseases; metabolic disorders; postoperatively, malignancy; "miscellaneous" disorders; and hereditary pancreatitis. The common presenting symptoms are abdominal pain, usually in the midepigastric area, nausea, and emesis associated with elevation of pancreatic enzymes (amylase, lipase). Chronic recurrent pancreatitis may be more subtle and at times may mimic recurrent abdominal pain. Anatomic, hereditary, and idiopathic causes are much more common in chronic pancreatitis. Ultrasound and CT have aided the diagnosis of pancreatitis and the treatment of complications, such as pseudocyst formation (Fig. 10-18).

Surgical issues and the "acute abdomen" also cause abdominal pain in children. Appendicitis may not have the classic sequence or symptoms in pediatric patients, and suspicion must be high in any acute illness. Because the symptoms of appendicitis are vague and it is frequently difficult to examine pediatric patients, perforation rate for appendicitis is more common in children than in adults. An appendiceal fecalith seen on a plain abdominal x-ray or CT scan may be a good though infrequent clue (Fig. 10-19).

The classic triad of colicky abdominal pain, currant jelly stools, and vomiting are only seen in 20% to 40% of children with intussusception. Intussusception is most commonly seen in children between the ages of 3 months

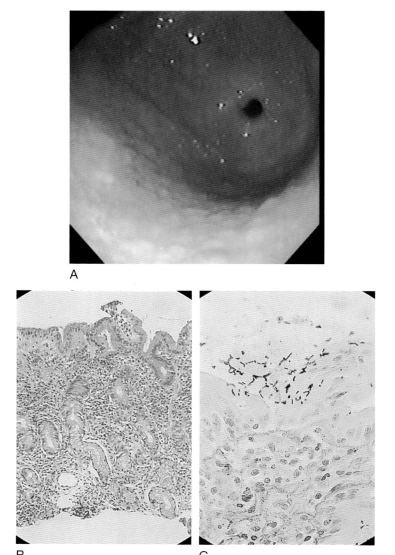

A

B

C

Figure 10-15. *Helicobacter pylori* gastritis. **A,** Nodular appearing gastric antrum consistent with *H. pylori* (Courtesy Dr. Feras Alissa, Pittsburgh.) **B,** Gastric biopsy with inflammatory infiltrate of plasma cells, neutrophils, and occasional eosinophils characteristic of *H. pylori* gastritis. **C,** Steiner silver stain (×400) demonstrates rod-shaped, spiral *H. pylori* bacteria attached to the mucosa.

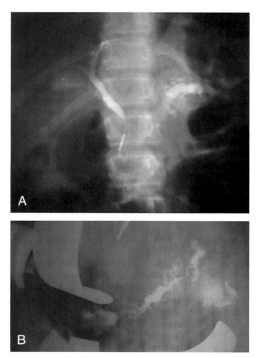

A

B

Figure 10-17. Congenital pancreatic anomaly. This 12-year-old boy had recurrent abdominal pain for 10 years. A retrograde cholangiogram demonstrated an ectatic pancreatic duct. **A,** An operative cholangiogram defined a narrow duct just before entry into the duodenum. **B,** Division of the duct and anastomosis to the jejunum led to complete resolution of symptoms.

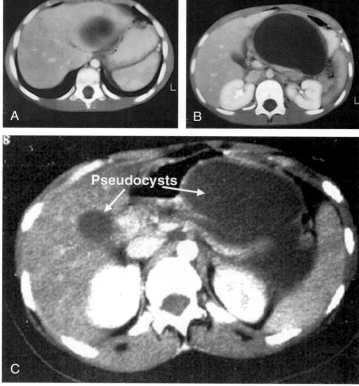

A

B

Pseudocysts

C

Figure 10-18. Pancreatic pseudocyst. Abdominal pain and emesis led to CT scan in this patient who had a bicycle handlebar injury 2 weeks earlier. **A,** Septation of the cavity. **B,** Compression of stomach and pancreas by the pancreatic pseudocyst. **C,** Two large pancreatic pseudocysts. (Courtesy Dr. Mark Lowe, Pittsburgh.)

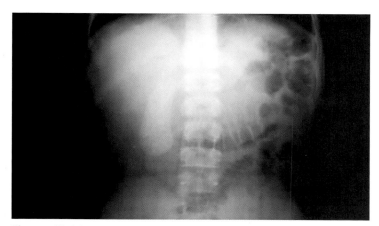

Figure 10-16. Gallstones. Plain abdominal film demonstrates gallstones in this patient with sickle cell disease and abdominal pain.

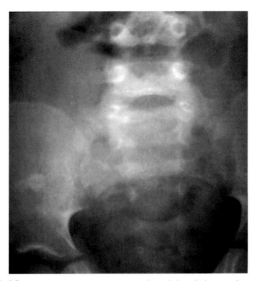

Figure 10-19. Appendicitis. An appendiceal fecalith can be seen in the right lower quadrant in this child with surgically proven acute appendicitis.

and 5 years. Older children usually have a "lead point" such as a juvenile polyp, Meckel's diverticulum, or thickened bowel associated with Henoch-Schönlein purpura as the etiology of the intussusception and require further investigation (Fig. 10-20). Neurologic symptoms, such as lethargy or seizure, are additional clues to the diagnosis. Reduction by barium enema or air enema is both diagnostic and therapeutic and simplifies management of this disorder in most instances, although surgery is occasionally necessary. Recurrence of intussusception following reduction is seen in approximately 10% of patients.

Constipation

Constipation is defined as a delay or difficulty passing a bowel movement for 2 weeks or more that results in pain and discomfort to the patient. In most children constipation is functional and without an organic cause. Painful defecation during toilet training, illness, or a stressful event often leads to stool withholding behavior and avoidance of defecation. Overflow incontinence or encopresis is the result of a chronic, distal fecal impaction leading to stretching of the rectal wall and relaxation of the internal anal sphincter. Liquid stool from the proximal colon leaks around the fecal mass, resulting in encopresis. Occasionally, major psychopathology is uncovered, especially in the older child, and appropriate intervention is necessary. Bladder dysfunction with recurrent urinary tract infections and urinary incontinence may be associated with long-standing constipation.

Examination of the child with constipation usually reveals palpable stool in the descending colon and left lower quadrant. A digital rectal examination is necessary to evaluate stool consistency, the amount of stool present in the rectum, the size of the rectum, and anal tone. A plain film of the abdomen is usually not necessary and adds little to the physical examination but can be quite revealing at times (Fig. 10-21). If the history dates to early infancy and severe constipation resulting from intestinal obstruction or obstipation is present as well, one should consider Hirschsprung disease. An unprepped barium enema radiographic study is usually diagnostic of Hirschsprung disease (Fig. 10-22), although rectal biopsy

for ganglion cells and acetylcholinesterase stain is necessary for confirmation. In older children, rectal manometric studies may help separate organic from functional disorders.

Vomiting

Recurrent vomiting is a frequent symptom in childhood. Vomiting is often associated with a viral illness but can be secondary to other entities such as pyloric stenosis, reflux, or an intestinal malrotation and volvulus.

Pyloric Stenosis

Hypertrophic pyloric stenosis is due to a narrowing of the pyloric channel secondary to hypertrophy of the pyloric musculature. The etiology of pyloric stenosis is unknown, although there is a significant associated risk of pyloric stenosis in neonates who have been given erythromycin. Pyloric stenosis usually presents in infants between 3 and 5 weeks of age. Symptoms include forceful, projectile, nonbilious emesis; persistent hunger; associated constipation; dehydration; and perhaps an unconjugated hyperbilirubinemia. Giant gastric peristaltic waves and the typical firm pyloric olive may be noted on examination (Fig. 10-23). Hypokalemic, hypochloremic metabolic alkalosis can be observed on routine laboratory tests. Diagnosis of pyloric stenosis is confirmed by an ultrasound examination that measures the thickness of the pyloric wall and the length of the pyloric channel (Fig. 10-24). Studies have demonstrated that ultrasound has a sensitivity and specificity of nearly 100% in diagnosing pyloric stenosis. In questionable cases, an upper GI barium study may confirm the diagnosis by demonstrating a narrow pyloric channel called a "string sign" (Fig. 10-25).

Reflux

Gastroesophageal reflux (GER) is defined as the passage of gastric contents into the esophagus, whereas gastroesophageal reflux disease (GERD) is the symptoms and complications of GER. Symptoms of reflux can include vomiting, poor weight gain, substernal chest pain, abdominal pain, dysphagia, esophagitis, and respiratory disorders (Table 10-9). GER is a common and usually self-limited condition beginning in early infancy. Many of these children have emesis even in the newborn nursery. Frequent episodes of nonbilious emesis beginning immediately after feeding and continuing for several hours are characteristic of reflux. GER is common during infancy and usually gradually disappears by 1 to 2 years of age. Complicated reflux (GERD) with symptoms of growth failure, aspiration, esophagitis, hemorrhage, and apnea is rare. Sandifer syndrome is described as abnormal posturing in response to reflux and is an uncommon manifestation of GERD. Additionally, psychophysiologic factors may predominate in the rumination syndrome, which may be difficult to distinguish from reflux. In late stages these children regurgitate constantly and swallow in a self-stimulating fashion, similar to a tic.

The diagnosis of GER is usually based on clinical symptoms. An upper GI series is performed to eliminate anatomic abnormalities such as pyloric stenosis, esophageal stricture, duodenal web or malrotation, but it does not diagnose reflux. Twenty-four hour esophageal pH-probe measurements confirm the presence of abnormal acid in the esophagus and can correlate symptoms with actual

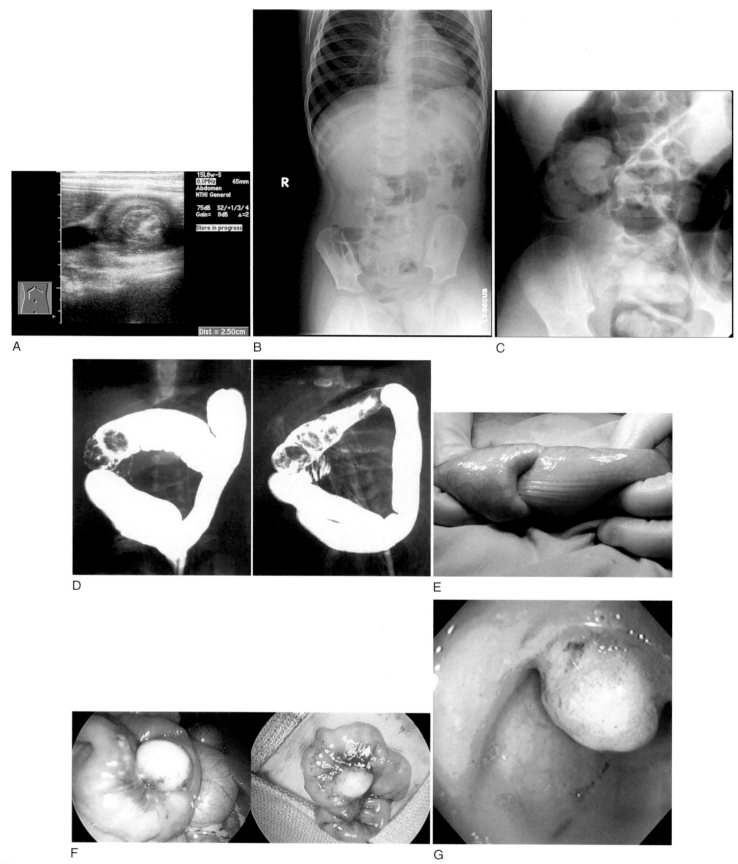

Figure 10-20. Intussusception. **A,** A "target lesion" can be seen on this ultrasound demonstrating intussusception. **B,** Occasionally, an intussusception can be seen on a plain abdominal radiograph. Note the absence of air beyond the intussusception. **C,** Air enemas are used to both diagnose and reduce an intussusception. **D,** Barium outlines the intussuscepted segment before and after it is reduced. **E,** This is an example of an intussusception seen at laparotomy, necessary when reduction is not successful during a barium or air enema. **F,** A Meckel diverticulum can be a lead point for intussusception. **G,** An intestinal polyp can act as a lead point for intussusception. (Courtesy Drs. Stefano Bartoletti and Mark Lowe, Pittsburgh.)

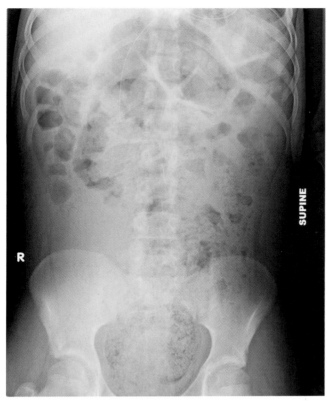

Figure 10-21. Constipation. This plain film of the abdomen demonstrates a significant amount of stool throughout the colon. Note the dilation of the rectum and colon in this child with chronic, functional constipation. (Courtesy Dr. Ann Furr, Pittsburgh.)

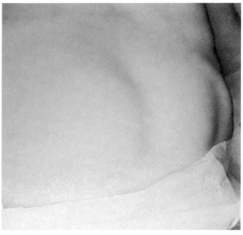

Figure 10-23. Pyloric stenosis. The giant gastric waves are best seen just after a feeding.

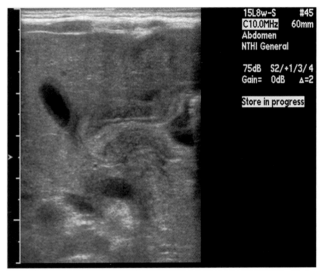

Figure 10-24. Pyloric stenosis. This ultrasound demonstrates thickening of the pyloric wall and elongated pyloric channel in an infant with pyloric stenosis.

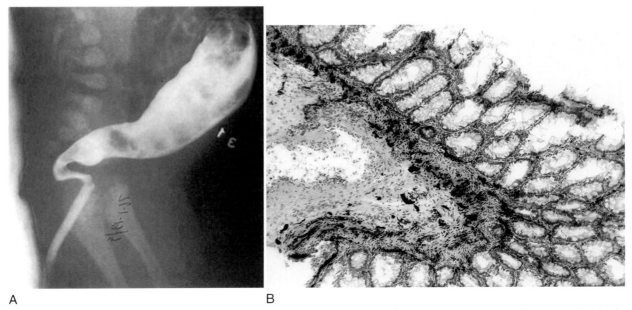

A   B

Figure 10-22. Hirschsprung disease. **A,** This barium enema demonstrates a tapered transition zone to a normal-caliber colon that is characteristic of Hirschsprung disease. **B,** This slide is specially stained with acetylcholinesterase. The increased number and size of cholinergic nerves in the lamina propria and muscularis mucosae (stains black) is diagnostic of Hirschsprung disease. (Courtesy Dr. Sarangarajan Ranganathan, Pittsburgh.)

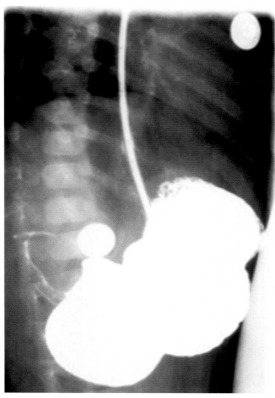

Figure 10-25. Pyloric stenosis. This typical barium study in a patient with pyloric stenosis demonstrates a "stringlike" pyloric channel.

Table 10-9	Presentations of Gastroesophageal Reflux

Regurgitation "Spitting," rumination Emesis Failure to thrive	**Respiratory** Wheezing, asthma Recurrent pneumonia Aspiration Laryngospasm Apnea
Esophagitis Irritability Colic Hiccups Anemia Hematemesis Stricture Protein-losing enteropathy Melena, occult blood loss	**Neurologic** Seizure-like episodes **Other** Clubbing of digits Sudden infant death syndrome or apparent life-threatening event
Behavioral Dystonic posturing Sandifer syndrome	

episodes of reflux. Esophagoscopy with biopsy is rarely necessary but can assess esophageal injury and can eliminate other causes of vomiting. Nuclear scintigraphy and esophageal manometric studies are rarely used to evaluate reflux.

Therapy in mild cases includes frequent small feedings and maintenance of an upright position in infants. This is usually accomplished by elevating the head of the crib. Studies have demonstrated fewer reflux events while infants are in the prone position. Because of the known increased risk of sudden infant death syndrome associated with prone positioning, supine positioning is recommended for all infants despite symptoms of reflux. The "infant seat" may worsen reflux by increasing intraabdominal pressure. Thickening feedings with rice or oat cereal (1 tablespoon/ounce) has been shown to decrease the number of vomiting episodes while not affecting the reflux index in infants. Acid suppression with

histamine-2-receptor antagonists and proton pump inhibitors has proved both safe and effective in treating reflux in infants and children. The use of prokinetic agents in the management of reflux is controversial, and studies have not demonstrated their usefulness. The exception is cisapride, which is no longer available in the United States because of its known cardiac arrhythmic side effects. Persistent, complicated reflux may require surgical intervention, most commonly with a Nissen type of fundoplication.

Intestinal Malrotation and Volvulus

Intestinal malrotation is the result of an incomplete rotation of the intestine during embryonic life. Intestinal malrotation causes the intestines not to be properly "fixed" at the mesentery. The resulting "stalklike" mesentery may serve as a focal point for twisting or volvulus of the intestine. Volvulus presents with the sudden onset of bilious emesis and abdominal pain. Bilious emesis is a surgical emergency until proven otherwise. Plain abdominal films may demonstrate paucity of air in the abdomen except for an air bubble in the stomach and one in the duodenum. An upper gastrointestinal series is the gold standard for diagnosing a malrotation and volvulus. Classically, the small intestine is rotated to the right side of the abdomen and a narrowing at the site of obstruction has a corkscrew appearance (Fig. 10-26). Under normal circumstances, the c loop of the duodenum should extend up under the antrum of the stomach and cross the midline. The c loop of the duodenum not crossing the midline is another radiologic clue of malrotation. Malrotation with an associated volvulus is a surgical emergency and must be treated as such.

Diarrhea

Diarrhea in the pediatric patient is usually acute and infectious in etiology. Chronic persistent diarrhea (>2 weeks) is a more difficult problem. Early onset, poor growth, and malnutrition suggest a congenital or more serious disorder, such as chronic protracted diarrhea. Fortunately, most older infants and children have a postinfectious or even dietary cause. A carefully performed history and examination, especially related to growth, diet, and caloric intake, may prevent excessive investigation.

Clues to the etiology of diarrhea can be found when the stool is carefully examined. Small bowel disorders result in diarrhea that is watery and free of mucus. Unabsorbed sugar is easily detected by checking the stool for reducing substances. Stool pH also may be low (<5) in the presence of carbohydrate maldigestion and malabsorption. Excessive neutral fat (triglyceride) or split fat (fatty acid) supports the diagnosis of malabsorption and can easily be detected. Neutral fat can be seen if several drops of water are added to the specimen. If 2 drops of 95% alcohol and 2 drops of stain (oil red-Sudan III) are added, smaller and more definite globules may be seen. Heating with acetic acid may be necessary to see split fat clearly under the microscope.

Infectious or inflammatory causes of diarrhea often produce stools with blood or mucus. Fecal leukocytes, another possible clue, can be seen more easily when 2 drops of water and 1 drop of methylene blue are added

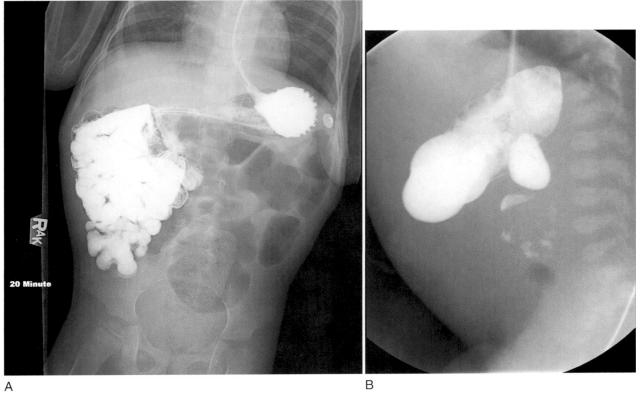

Figure 10-26. Malrotation. **A,** An upper gastrointestinal series demonstrating malrotation with the entire small bowel on the right, never crossing the midline, and the colon on the left. **B,** The corkscrew appearance of the duodenum is seen in this patient with malrotation and midgut volvulus. (Courtesy Dr. Stefano Bartoletti, Pittsburgh.)

Figure 10-27. Celiac disease. **A,** This child had a potbelly, vomiting, and weight loss as her major symptoms. Once celiac disease was confirmed, the child was placed on a gluten-free diet. Note the protruding abdomen and wasted buttocks. **B,** After 10 weeks on the diet the improvement is obvious.

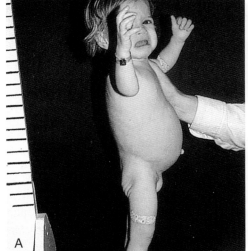
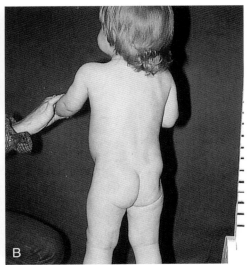

to a fresh stool smear before microscopic examination (Sondheimer). Stool culture and examination for ova and parasites can reveal fecal pathogens contributing to the patients' diarrhea. *Giardia lamblia* is occasionally the cause of diarrhea in children who are not thriving.

Whereas chronic diarrhea may be caused by malabsorption, chronic nonspecific or toddler's diarrhea is common and self-limited unless severe dietary restrictions are initiated. Stools are loose and often contain undigested fibers but no carbohydrate or fat. Occasionally, these children do better when placed on a diet containing unrestricted fat and elimination of nonmilk fluids such as juice and soda. The health beliefs of some parents, such as the benefits of low-fat, low-cholesterol foods, may contribute to the problem.

Malabsorption

Malabsorption syndromes in pediatrics range from single sugars like lactase deficiency to more complex multinutrient problems, such as those associated with short-gut syndrome. The physical signs usually are those of malnutrition. Celiac disease, or gluten sensitive enteropathy, is a chronic intolerance to dietary gluten that results in malabsorption. The incidence of celiac disease is 1 in 133 individuals in the United States. Clinical symptoms of celiac disease classically include chronic diarrhea, abdominal distention, and weight loss/failure to thrive. The classic appearance of celiac disease includes a potbelly and wasted extremities and buttocks (Fig. 10-27). However, this is probably a rare presentation of this

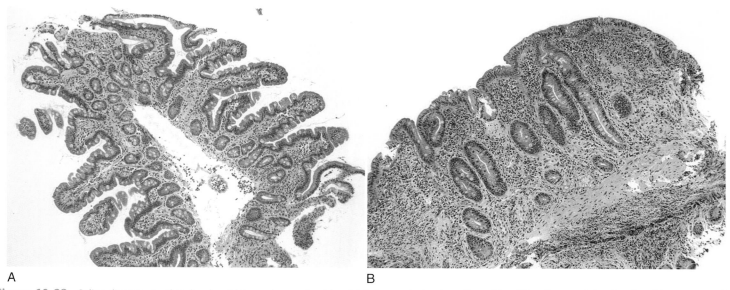

A
B

Figure 10-28. Celiac disease. **A,** This duodenal biopsy from a healthy child demonstrates long fingerlike villi and normal duodenal architecture. **B,** This is a duodenal biopsy from a child with celiac disease. Note the flattened villi, villous atrophy and the elongated crypts which are characteristic in patients with celiac disease. (Courtesy Dr. Sarangarajan Ranganathan, Pittsburgh.)

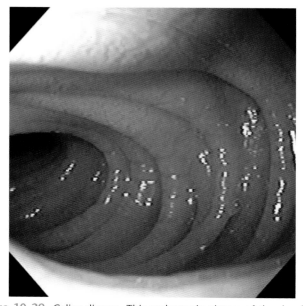

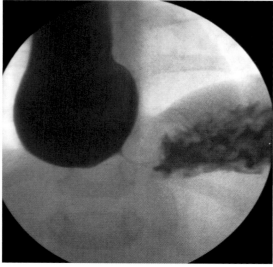

Figure 10-30. Achalasia. This barium esophagram clearly demonstrates the classic findings of esophageal dilation proximal to the lower esophageal sphincter (LES) and the "bird's beak" appearance of the narrowed LES. (Courtesy Drs. Manisha Harpavat Dave and Ryan Fischer, Pittsburgh.)

Figure 10-29. Celiac disease. This endoscopic picture of the duodenum demonstrates a smooth appearance and scalloping secondary to absent villi in a patient with biopsy-proven celiac disease. (Courtesy Drs. Mark Lowe and Cary Sauer, Pittsburgh.)

common condition. Other clinical manifestations of celiac disease include short stature, abdominal pain, constipation, arthritis, delayed puberty, anemia, and osteoporosis. Serologic testing supports the diagnosis of celiac disease, but the gold standard for diagnosis continues to be small bowel biopsies showing villous atrophy, crypt hyperplasia, and an abnormal surface epithelium (Fig. 10-28). Flattening of duodenal villi and "scalloping" can occasionally be noted during upper endoscopy (Fig. 10-29). Treatment is the complete removal of gluten (wheat, rye, barley, and oats) from the diet. Serologic testing is also used to monitor adherence to a gluten-free diet.

Dysphagia

Dysphagia is not a diagnosis, but a symptom used to describe a variety of feeding and swallowing disorders.

Other symptoms associated with dysphagia are painful swallowing, a globus sensation, and vomiting. Disorders associated with dysphagia include achalasia, eosinophilic esophagitis, and esophageal strictures secondary to caustic ingestions.

Achalasia is an uncommon disorder in children diagnosed by an esophagram (Fig. 10-30) and esophageal motility studies. Incomplete relaxation of the lower esophageal sphincter during swallowing, as well as uncoordinated peristalsis of the esophageal smooth muscles, are the dysfunctions associated with achalasia. Treatment options include esophageal dilation and injection of botulinum toxin into the lower esophageal sphincter. These procedures usually need to be repeated when symptoms return. A surgical procedure known as a Heller myotomy is a more permanent treatment of achalasia. Accidental caustic ingestions in children can result in severe esophageal injury, which heals with fibrosis and often results in strictures (Fig. 10-31). The most common

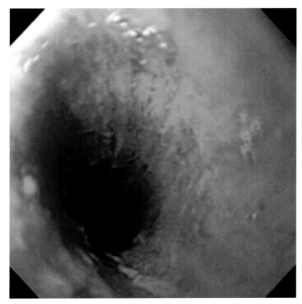

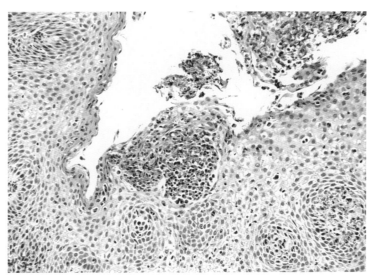

Figure 10-32. Eosinophilic esophagitis. This histologic specimen from the esophagus demonstrates numerous eosinophils.

Figure 10-31. Caustic ingestion. This endoscopic picture of the esophagus is the result of an accidental alkaline ingestion. Dysphagia and esophageal strictures requiring dilatation are common sequelae of caustic ingestions. (Courtesy Dr. Feras Alissa.)

Figure 10-33. Eosinophilic esophagitis. These endoscopic pictures of the esophagus demonstrate classic findings of eosinophilic esophagitis including linear furrowing of the esophagus **(A)** and a ringed appearance or trachealization of the esophagus **(B).** (Courtesy Dr. Feras Alissa.)

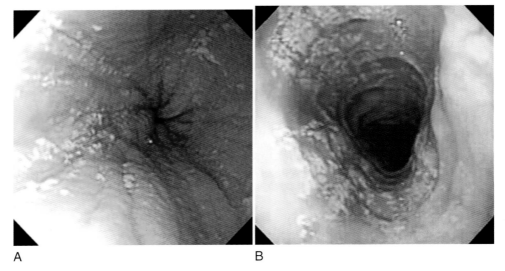

A

B

long-term symptom of an esophageal stricture is dysphagia. Repeated esophageal dilation is the treatment of choice.

Eosinophilic esophagitis is an inflammatory disorder of the esophagus that is increasingly being recognized in children. Eosinophilic esophagitis is characterized by isolated intense eosinophilic infiltration of the esophagus. Signs and symptoms of eosinophilic esophagitis are often mistaken for gastroesophageal reflux disease. They include dysphagia, vomiting, feeding refusal, heartburn, chest pain, and abdominal pain. Solid food impactions and esophageal strictures can also be presenting symptoms of eosinophilic esophagitis. Unlike reflux, eosinophilic esophagitis does not completely respond to adequate acid suppression with a proton pump inhibitor. A definitive diagnosis of eosinophilic esophagitis is made after biopsy specimens from the esophagus obtained during an upper endoscopy are examined (Fig. 10-32). The classic appearance of eosinophilic esophagitis on upper endoscopy includes linear furrowing of the esophagus, esophageal ring formation, and granularity (Fig. 10-33). The treatment of eosinophilic esophagitis has been through diet modification and corticosteroids.

Trauma

No discussion of pediatric differential diagnosis is complete without a mention of trauma or child abuse. The GI tract may figure in subtle forms of abuse, such as chronic diarrhea from laxative abuse, and feigned bleeding episodes are reported in Munchausen syndrome by proxy. Likewise, vomiting may be induced by occult trauma or abuse. Blunt injury to the abdomen, such as that from a bicycle handlebar, may produce an intramural duodenal hematoma with partial or complete obstruction and a fullness or mass on radiographic abdominal examination (Fig. 10-34). Resolution usually takes place slowly, and parenteral nutrition may be required for a period of time. As with other suspicious injuries, a skeletal survey and detailed family evaluation are mandatory if the trauma is not explained by an obvious accident.

Gastrointestinal Bleeding

Visible blood in emesis or stool is always alarming to children and their parents. Occasionally a GI bleed is not

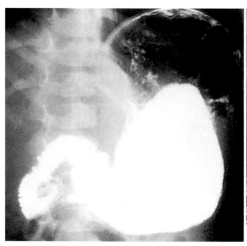
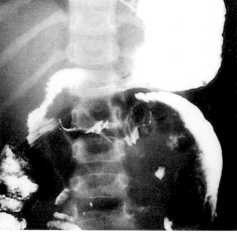

A   B

Figure 10-34. Gastrointestinal trauma. Upper gastrointestinal series demonstrates poor flow through the duodenum **(A)** and mass effect of the hematoma displacing other loops of bowel **(B)**.

Table 10-10	Causes of Gastrointestinal (GI) Hemorrhage in Children Older Than 1 Year	
UPPER GI TRACT		**LOWER GI TRACT**
Esophageal varices		Colonic polyps
Pill esophagitis		Anal fissure
Gastric ulcers		Intussusception
Gastritis		Meckel diverticulum
Helicobacter pylori		Inflammatory bowel disease
Duodenal ulcer		Infectious colitis
Inflammatory bowel disease		Hemorrhoids

detected until a patient develops iron deficiency anemia or stools are found to be guaiac positive on examination. Generally, melanotic stools, coffee ground emesis, or frank hematemesis indicate upper GI bleeding, bleeding proximal to the ligament of Treitz. Bright blood per rectum indicates loss from the lower GI tract. To determine the etiology of GI bleeding, an endoscopic examination may be required, which can be both diagnostic and therapeutic. In younger infants, particularly neonates, the diagnosis may remain unclear. The common disorders causing GI bleeding are listed in Table 10-10 (see Chapter 17) and examples seen in Figure 10-35.

Inflammatory Bowel Disease

IBD is a term used to describe both Crohn disease and ulcerative colitis. Symptoms include abdominal pain, weight loss, chronic diarrhea, rectal bleeding, and fever. Children frequently present with growth failure or delayed pubertal development as their sole presenting sign of IBD (Fig. 10-36). Whereas clinical distinctions are at times blurred, severe perianal disease with fistulas and fissures, perianal skin tags, and abscesses are diagnostic of Crohn disease (Fig. 10-37). Rectal disease is characteristic of ulcerative colitis. Histologically, Crohn disease is characterized by transmural inflammation with granuloma formation and skip areas. This deep inflammatory process accounts for the tendency to form fistulas and abscesses. Crypt abscesses are often seen in ulcerative colitis and help to distinguish this disorder from many other causes of acute colitis (Fig. 10-38). Crohn disease may affect anywhere in the GI tract and can be demonstrated on an upper GI series with small bowel follow-through with segmental narrowing, skip areas, ulcerations, and fistula formation (Fig. 10-39). Ulcerative colitis is a mucosal inflammation confined to the large bowel (Fig. 10-40). A

lead pipe appearance of the colon can occasionally be seen on a plain abdominal film (Fig. 10-41). Endoscopic findings are delineated in Figures 10-42 and 10-43. The PillCam capsule endoscopy (Given Imaging, Yoqneam, Israel) allows for direct visualization of the small intestine via a pill camera that takes two pictures a second, allowing for easier diagnosis of isolated small bowel Crohn disease not visualized on barium studies.

Extraintestinal manifestation of IBD may occur at any time or be the presenting symptom of the disease. Osteoarthropathy, or clubbing in its mildest form, may be observed in children with IBD. The earliest signs of osteoarthropathy are softening and loss of a normal angle at the base of the nail (Fig. 10-44). Many rashes accompany IBD including erythema nodosum, erythema multiforme, papulonecrotic lesions, and ulcerative erythematous plaques. Perhaps the most characteristic rash is pyoderma gangrenosum. Initial lesions are papular, then become bullous, and finally are deeply ulcerated and necrotic. The most frequent locations are the cheeks, thighs, feet, hands, legs, and inguinal regions (Fig. 10-45). Other extraintestinal manifestations of IBD include arthritis, ankylosing spondylitis, sacroiliitis, aphthous ulcers, uveitis, iritis, and sclerosing cholangitis.

Cystic Fibrosis

Cystic fibrosis is the most common inherited lethal disorder in whites, with predominantly pulmonary (see Chapter 16) and GI manifestations. All neonates diagnosed with a meconium ileus should be evaluated for cystic fibrosis (Fig. 10-46). Edema in an infant who is breast-fed or on soy formulas and consuming adequate calories should strongly suggest cystic fibrosis. These infants often appear well fed but quite thin after fluid diuresis.

The most common GI abnormality in patients with cystic fibrosis involves the pancreas (Fig. 10-47). Patients are either described as pancreatic sufficient or insufficient. Pancreatic sufficient individuals have normal fat absorption, although they may have abnormal pancreatic synthetic abilities. Recurrent pancreatitis may occur in these individuals. Pancreatic insufficiency is more common and results in steatorrhea, eventually leading to calorie and protein malnutrition, as well as failure to thrive.

Rectal prolapse occurs in approximately 20% of children with cystic fibrosis (Fig. 10-48). A sweat test should

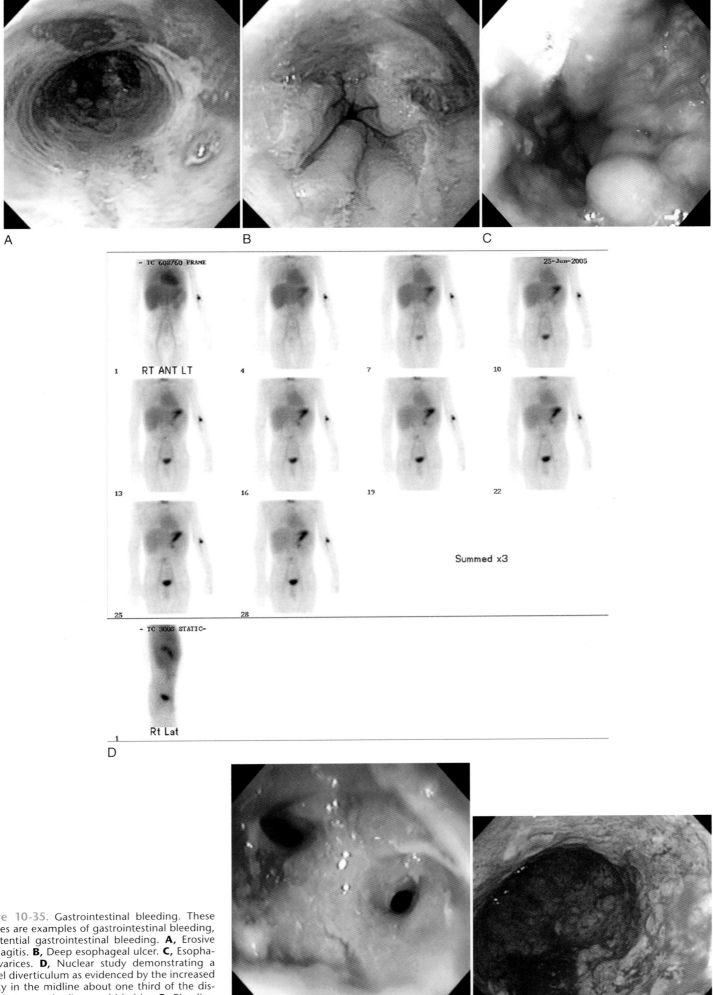

Figure 10-35. Gastrointestinal bleeding. These pictures are examples of gastrointestinal bleeding, or potential gastrointestinal bleeding. **A,** Erosive esophagitis. **B,** Deep esophageal ulcer. **C,** Esophageal varices. **D,** Nuclear study demonstrating a Meckel diverticulum as evidenced by the increased activity in the midline about one third of the distance between the liver and bladder. **E,** Bleeding terminal ileum in Crohn disease. **F,** Bleeding colon in a patient with ulcerative colitis.

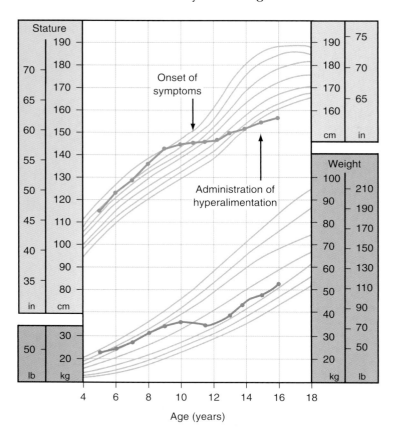

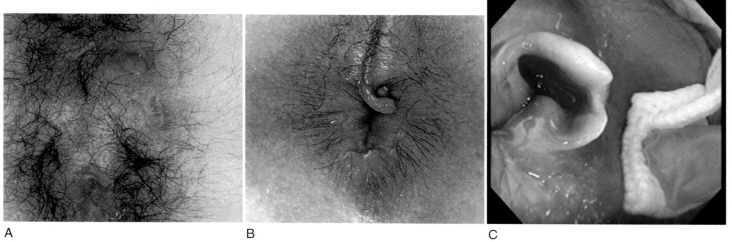

Figure 10-36. Crohn disease. This growth curve demonstrates a falloff before onset of disease symptoms and continued poor growth through many exacerbations requiring steroid therapy. Home hyperalimentation has maintained weight gain.

A   B   C

Figure 10-37. Crohn disease. **A,** The slight raised and erythematous lesion represents a perianal abscess that eventually drained. Note a scar from a previous incision and drainage procedure. **B,** Perianal skin tags are common in Crohn disease and a good clue to diagnosis. **C,** Example of a draining perianal fistula found in a child with Crohn disease. (Courtesy Dr. Feras Alissa.)

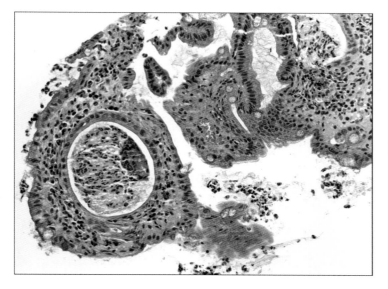

Figure 10-38. Ulcerative colitis. Pathologic image of a colonic crypt abscess in a patient with ulcerative colitis.

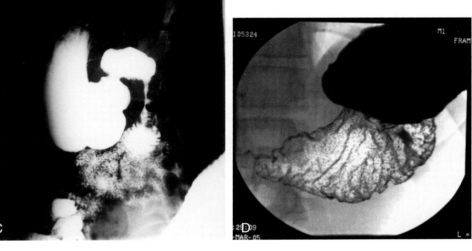

Figure 10-39. Crohn disease. **A,** Segmental narrowing of the left colon. **B,** A narrow and irregular terminal ileum. **C,** Stricturing of the duodenum. **D,** Diffuse aphthous ulcers in the stomach in a patient with Crohn disease. (Courtesy Dr. Stefano Bartoletti, Pittsburgh.)

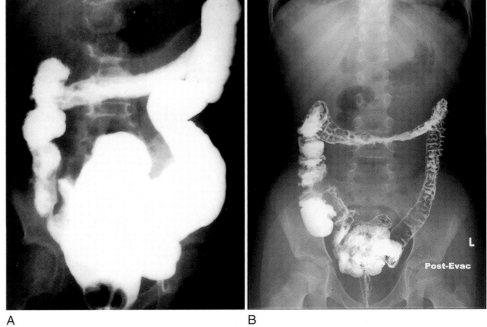

Figure 10-40. Ulcerative colitis. **A,** A narrowing and loss of haustral markings occurs, especially in the transverse colon. Mucosal irregularities are prominent in the right colon. **B,** Postevacuation barium enema in a patient with ulcerative colitis demonstrates narrowing and irregular borders indicating colon inflammation.

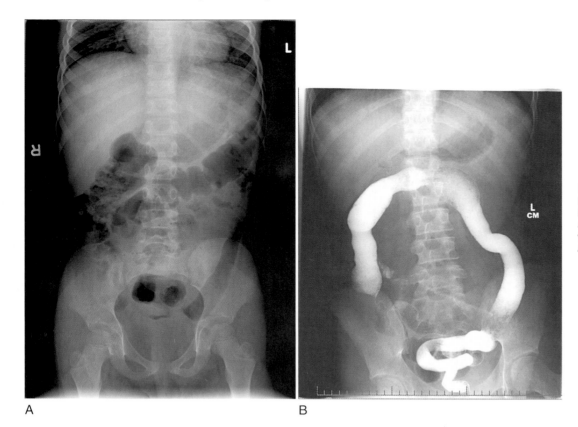

Figure 10-41. Ulcerative colitis. A lead pipe appearance to the colon can be seen on a plain abdominal film **(A)** and a barium enema **(B)** in a patient with ulcerative colitis. (Courtesy of Dr. Ann Furr, Pittsburgh.)

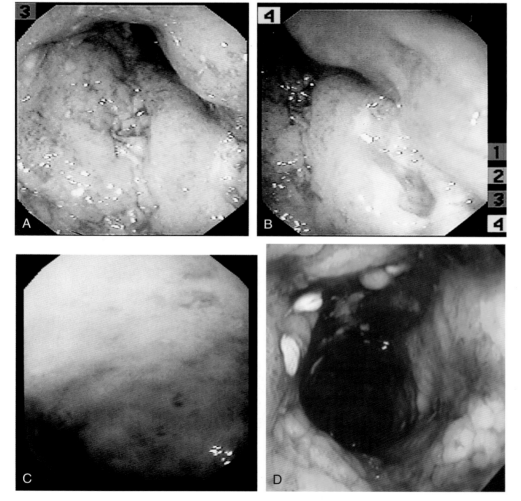

Figure 10-42. Crohn disease. Endoscopic images of a patient with Crohn disease. **A** and **B**, Note the deep, linear, ulcerated fissure. **C**, Demonstrates numerous colonic aphthous ulcers. **D**, Demonstrates a cobblestone appearance to the colonic mucosa.

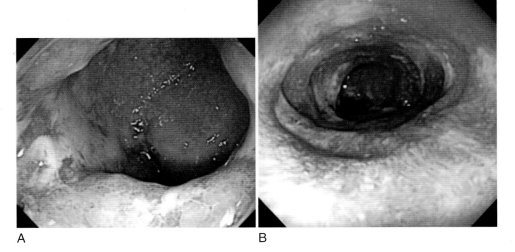

Figure 10-43. Ulcerative colitis. **A** and **B,** The entire colonic mucosa is inflamed and friable with obvious pus and bleeding.

A   B

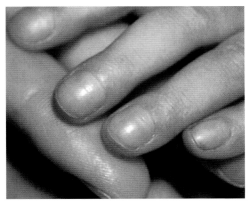

Figure 10-44. Osteoarthropathy (clubbing). Note thickening and loss of the angle at the nail bed in a child with inflammatory bowel disease.

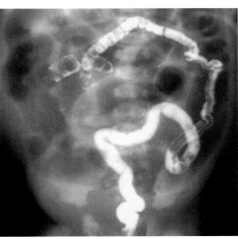

Figure 10-46. Meconium ileus. Barium enema demonstrating a microcolon secondary to meconium ileus in a neonate. (Courtesy Dr. Mark Lowe, Pittsburgh.)

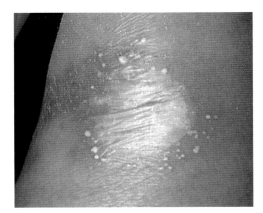

Figure 10-45. Pyoderma gangrenosum. This is a classic rash associated with inflammatory bowel disease. Initial papulopustules coalesce to form a deep necrotic lesion.

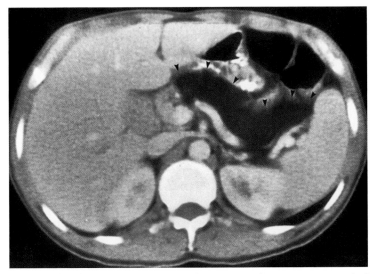

Figure 10-47. Cystic fibrosis (CF). This CT scan demonstrates a typical CF-appearing pancreas. The pancreas has been replaced by fat and appears absent. (Courtesy Dr. Mark Lowe, Pittsburgh.)

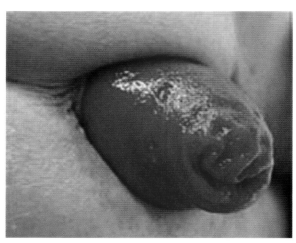

Figure 10-48. Rectal prolapse. Rectal prolapse is a relatively common finding in children with cystic fibrosis. (Courtesy Dr. Mark Lowe, Pittsburgh.)

Table 10-11	Major Causes of Neonatal Conjugated Hyperbilirubinemia

Extrahepatic	**Hepatitis**
Biliary atresia	TORCH infection
Choledochal cyst	Cytomegalovirus
Spontaneous perforation of bile duct	Hepatitis C
Choledochocele	Hepatitis B
	Human immunodeficiency virus
Intrahepatic	**Metabolic**
Idiopathic	Galactosemia
Idiopathic neonatal hepatitis	Tyrosinemia
Alagille syndrome	Niemann-Pick disease (type C)
Byler disease	α-1-antitrypsin deficiency
Anatomic	Cystic fibrosis
Congenital hepatic fibrosis with polycystic kidney and liver disease	***Chromosomal abnormalities***
	Trisomy 17, 18, or 21
	Turner syndrome

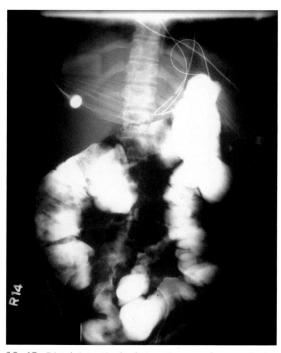

Figure 10-49. Distal intestinal obstruction syndrome. Barium enema reveals the cecal obstruction in a child with cystic fibrosis. (Courtesy Dr. Mark Lowe, Pittsburgh.)

be performed in any child with rectal prolapse because rectal prolapse often precedes the diagnosis of cystic fibrosis. *Distal intestinal obstruction syndrome* is the term used to describe a fecal impaction in the terminal ileum and cecum in patients with cystic fibrosis (Fig. 10-49). Patients present with recurrent abdominal pain, a palpable mass in the right lower quadrant, and signs of a bowel obstruction such as bilious emesis.

A wide spectrum of liver diseases occurs in patients with cystic fibrosis as well. The most common liver finding is an asymptomatic elevation of liver transaminases. Hepatic steatosis is associated with poor nutrition. Inspissated bile leads to periportal inflammation and eventually to hepatic fibrosis. Cirrhosis is rare in children. Focal biliary cirrhosis is a disorder unique to cystic fibrosis and can lead to portal hypertension, splenomegaly, and esophageal varices (see Fig. 10-35C).

Jaundice

The term *jaundice* or *icterus* refers to a yellow discoloration of the skin and sclerae caused by deposition of bilirubin. Jaundice is a clinical sign that serum bilirubin is above normal. Determining whether the hyperbilirubinemia is secondary to an elevation in conjugated or unconjugated bilirubin is crucial. Elevated conjugated bilirubin greater than or equal to 2 mg/dL or greater than or equal to 20% of the total bilirubin involves a pathologic condition, and further studies are necessary to determine its origin.

Infancy

A majority of neonatal jaundice is due to an elevation in unconjugated bilirubin. This so-called "physiologic" jaundice is due to increased bilirubin production, inadequate bilirubin excretion, or a combination of the two. The most common causes of neonatal unconjugated hyperbilirubinemia are fetal-maternal blood group incompatibility (ABO or Rh), breastfeeding, breast milk, hemolysis (glucose 6-phosphate dehydrogenase deficiency, hereditary spherocytosis), extravascular increased bilirubin due to a cephalohematoma or excessive bruising, sepsis, or congenital hypothyroidism, to name a few. Phototherapy is usually the treatment of choice for infants with an unconjugated hyperbilirubinemia.

Conjugated hyperbilirubinemia indicates a pathologic condition. The physician must determine the cause of the disorder in a timely manner because commencing medical or surgical treatment may affect outcome. The differential diagnosis for neonatal conjugated hyperbilirubinemia is immense and is usually broken down into intrahepatic and extrahepatic etiologies (Table 10-11). Clues gained during a careful and specific history and physical examination may allow the clinician to narrow the differential diagnosis.

Although not specific, a history of acholic stools may be a sign of complete biliary obstruction and will lead the physician to explore the diagnosis of extrahepatic biliary atresia. Extrahepatic biliary atresia, with an incidence of 1 in 8000 to 1 in 15,000 live births, is the most common indication for liver transplant in children. Approximately 350 children are born with this condition in the United States every year. A timely diagnosis and surgical intervention (Kasai procedure) may prevent hepatic cirrhosis, portal hypertension, and eventual liver transplantation. Extrahepatic biliary atresia may be associated with abnormalities of other organ systems, situs inversus viscerum, and polysplenia with or without congenital heart disease. Additionally, GI tract anomalies, such as malrotation (see Fig. 10-26A) and vascular anomalies (Fig. 10-50), may rarely complicate initial surgery and later liver transplantation.

Metabolic or storage diseases such as glycogen storage disease, Gaucher disease, galactosemia, and tyrosinemia may present with organomegaly along with jaundice. A choledochal cyst is a surgically correctable cause of jaundice and may be palpable (Fig. 10-51). A febrile illness in the mother during pregnancy may indicate a congenital infection in the infant resulting in a conjugated hyperbilirubinemia.

Characteristic cholestatic facies of deeply set eyes and a narrow chin along with persistent posterior embryotoxon, pulmonary artery abnormalities, and butterfly vertebrae are characteristic of Alagille syndrome or arteriohepatic dysplasia (Figs. 10-52 and 10-53). Paucity of interlobular bile ducts is the main pathologic finding found on liver biopsy. This condition has been localized to chromosome 20. Many individuals have only a few features of the disorder; prognosis is variable. These patients often suffer from xanthoma formation and severe pruritus, which occasionally are features of other chronic liver diseases (Fig. 10-54).

Childhood

Unconjugated hyperbilirubinemia occurs in older children, usually as a result of a hereditary hyperbilirubinemia syndrome. Gilbert syndrome is characterized by a mild unconjugated hyperbilirubinemia with normal liver transaminases and function. The elevated bilirubin is usually transient and occurs during times of illness, stress, or fasting. Dubin-Johnson syndrome and Rotor syndrome are autosomal recessive disorders that present with a mildly elevated unconjugated and conjugated bilirubin along with normal liver transaminases and function.

Jaundice due to conjugated hyperbilirubinemia is uncommon in older children (Table 10-12). Viral etiologies, such as hepatitis A, B, and C, are the most likely cause. Various medications, such as acetaminophen or anticonvulsants, taken in excess can result in an elevation of conjugated bilirubin.

Children with chronic liver disease and cirrhosis often have an elevated conjugated bilirubin and have many clinical features in common. The liver is usually firm and is often irregular and enlarged, although in late stages it may decrease in size. Splenomegaly follows portal hypertension. Portosystemic venous anastomoses lead to the

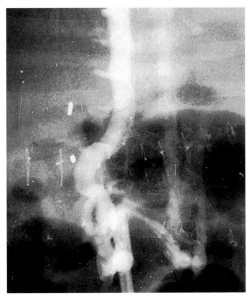

Figure 10-50. Vascular anomaly. The inferior vena cava is interrupted and continues as an azygos vein in this child with biliary atresia.

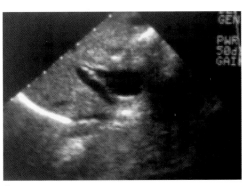

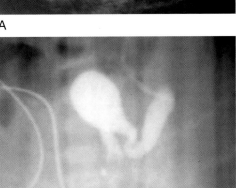

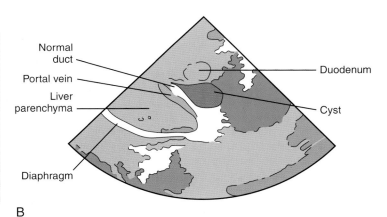

Figure 10-51. Choledochal cyst. **A** and **B,** Ultrasound and diagram of infant with obstructive jaundice demonstrates cystic structure below the liver. **C,** Intraoperative cholangiogram in same patient defines cyst and gallbladder along with hepatic and cystic ducts.

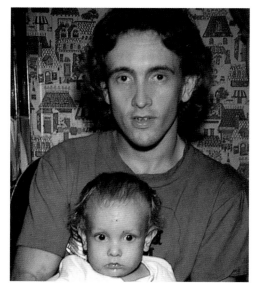

Figure 10-52. Alagille syndrome. The child has intrahepatic biliary hypoplasia, butterfly vertebrae, and mild pulmonic stenosis. The father does not have liver disease, but he does have moderate pulmonic stenosis and poor growth. Note the narrow, thin face and pointed chin of both father and child.

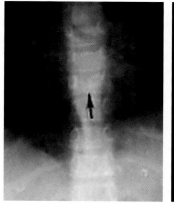 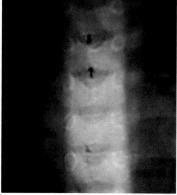

Figure 10-53. Alagille syndrome. These radiographs illustrate defects in the vertebral arches that lead to the butterfly appearance.

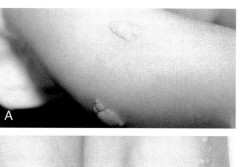

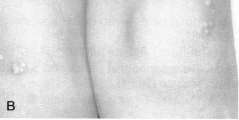

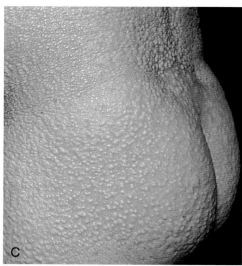

Figure 10-54. Xanthomas in chronic liver disease. Characteristic areas in the early stages of disease are pressure points such as elbows **(A)** and knees **(B)**; later, xanthomas may become generalized **(C)**.

development of dilated vessels in the abdominal wall (caput medusae) and GI tract (varices, hemorrhoids) (Fig. 10-55). Ascitic fluid may form, and, if present in sufficient quantity, produces flank dullness and a fluid wave. Ultrasonography may detect even smaller amounts of free fluid. Spider nevi, dilated vascular channels that disappear with pressure, are seen in normal adolescents but should suggest chronic liver disease if other historical or examination clues are present (Fig. 10-56).

Wilson disease is one of the chronic liver disorders that can be reversed with therapy. Presentations include hepatitis, neuropsychiatric disturbances, hemolytic anemia, and cirrhosis (Fig. 10-57). The clinician must establish a diagnosis in any child older than 4 years of age with persistent liver transaminase elevation. Serum ceruloplasmin is usually reduced, and 24-hour copper excretion elevated. However, quantitative measurement of hepatic copper may be necessary in some patients. Kayser-Fleischer rings occasionally are visible without the use of a slit lamp (Fig. 10-58). Therapy with copper-chelating agents, such as penicillamine, must be initiated before irreversible cirrhosis develops. Both the chronic liver failure and the neurologic disorder may be effectively treated by transplantation.

Table 10-12	Causes of Conjugated Hyperbilirubinemia in Older Children

Viral Hepatitis	**Metabolic**
Hepatitis A, B, C, D (acute or chronic)	α-1-antitrypsin deficiency
	Cystic fibrosis
Cytomegalovirus	Wilson disease
Epstein-Barr virus	
	Drugs
Autoimmune Hepatitis	Acetaminophen
	Anticonvulsants
Biliary Tract Disorders	Chemotherapy
Choledochal cyst	
Sclerosing cholangitis	
Cholecystitis	

Autoimmune hepatitis is defined as chronic inflammation of the liver associated with autoantibodies and hypergammaglobulinemia. Autoimmune hepatitis can present at any age but more frequently occurs during adolescence, especially in adolescent females. Patients can present with an incidental finding of hepatitis, asymptomatic jaundice or fulminant hepatitis, and liver failure. Different subclassifications of the disease have been defined on the basis of serologic autoantibodies. Treatment consists of immunosuppressive therapy with a combination of corticosteroids and azathioprine. Unresponsive patients may eventually proceed to liver transplantation.

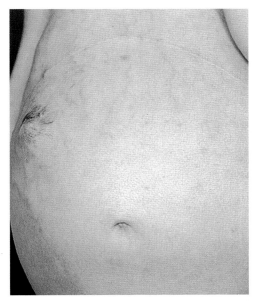

Figure 10-55. Chronic liver disease/portal hypertension. This child had biliary atresia with good bile flow after a portoenterostomy procedure. Cirrhosis developed late, with physical signs of prominent abdominal veins and ascites.

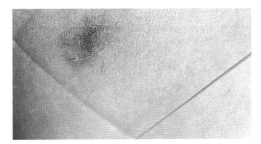

Figure 10-56. Spider nevus. The vascular lesion blanches with compression by a glass slide, but it reappears when pressure is released and is a sign of chronic liver disease.

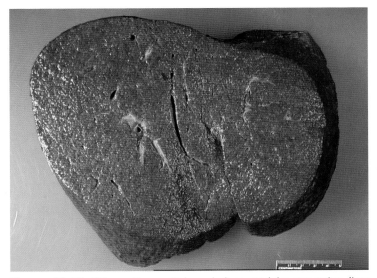

Figure 10-57. Wilson disease. Enlarged, firm, nodular appearing liver from a patient with Wilson disease who underwent liver transplant.

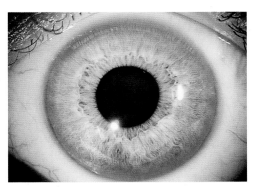

Figure 10-58. Kayser-Fleischer ring. Kayser-Fleischer ring appears as brownish discoloration in the posterior part of the cornea, as defined by slit lamp examination. Early Kayser-Fleischer rings may be seen only by slit lamp and begin at the superior and inferior poles.

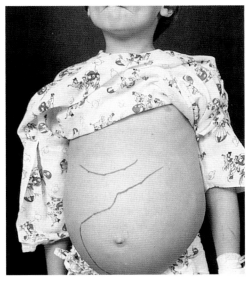

Figure 10-59. Congenital hepatic fibrosis. This clinically well child had hematemesis and hypersplenism with normal liver function studies. Note massive splenic size and large left lobe of liver. Portosystemic shunting was effective therapy.

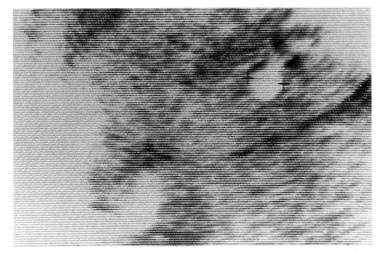

Figure 10-60. Congenital hepatic fibrosis. Ultrasound of the kidney in a patient with congenital hepatic fibrosis reveals a cystic structure.

Finally, there is one chronic hepatic disorder that usually can be recognized by examination alone. The healthy-appearing child with massive splenomegaly and a large, firm left lobe of the liver with no stigmata of chronic liver disease except GI hemorrhage almost certainly has congenital hepatic fibrosis (Fig. 10-59). These children may suffer from part of the spectrum of polycystic kidney disease in childhood, and renal function studies are warranted (Fig. 10-60). Therapy for this condition may include shunting procedures for portal hypertension because liver function may remain normal indefinitely.

Bibliography

Afzal NA, Addai S, Fagbemi A, et al: Refeeding syndrome with enteral nutrition in children: A case report, literature review and clinical guidelines. Clin Nutr 21:515-520, 2002.

Ament M: Diagnosis and management of upper gastrointestinal tract bleeding in the pediatric patient. Pediatr Rev 12:107-116, 1990.

Baker S, Liptak G, Coletti R, et al: Constipation in infants and children: Evaluation and treatment. J Pediatr Gastroenterol Nutr 29:612-626, 1999.

Balistreri WF: Neonatal cholestasis. J Pediatr 106:171-184, 1985.

Bithoney WG, Dubowitz H, Egan H: Failure to thrive/growth deficiency. Pediatr Rev 13:453-459, 1992.

Chelimsky G, Czinn S: Peptic ulcer disease in children. Pediatr Rev 22:349-355, 2001.

Corazziari E: The Rome criteria for functional gastrointestinal disorders: A critical reappraisal. J Pediatr Gastroenterol Nutr 39:S754-755, 2004.

Czaja AJ: Autoimmune liver disease. Curr Opin Gastroenterol 21:293-299, 2005.

El-Matary W, Spray C, Sandhu B: Irritable bowel syndrome: The commonest cause of recurrent abdominal pain in children. Eur J Pediatr 163:584-588, 2004.

Escher JC, Taminiau JAJM, Nieuwenhuis EES, et al: Treatment of inflammatory bowel disease in childhood: Best available evidence. Inflamm Bowel Dis 9:34-58, 2003.

Fitzgerald JF: Constipation in children. Pediatr Rev 8:299-302, 1987.

Gartner JC: Recurrent abdominal pain—who needs a workup? Contemp Pediatr 6:62-82, 1989.

Greer FR: Issues in establishing vitamin D recommendations for infants and children. Am J Clin Nutr 80:S1759-1762, 2004.

Gryboski J: The child with chronic diarrhea. Contemp Pediatr 10:71-97, 1993.

Hussain SZ, Thomas R, Tolia V: A review of achalasia in 33 children. Dig Dis Sci 47:2538-2543, 2002.

Krugman SD, Dubowitz H: Failure to thrive. Am Fam Physician 68:879-884, 2003.

Ladhani S, Srinivasan L, Buchanan C, et al: Presentation of vitamin D deficiency. Arch Dis Child 89:781-784, 2004.

Lake A: Recognition and management of inflammatory bowel disease in children and adolescents. Curr Probl Pediatr 18:379-437, 1988.

Liacouras CA, Ruchelli E: Eosinophilic esophagitis. Curr Opin Pediatr 16:560-566, 2004.

Macarthur C, Saunders N, Feldman W: *Helicobacter pylori,* gastroduodenal disease, and recurrent abdominal pain in children. JAMA 273:729-734, 1995.

McCollough M, Sharieff GQ: Abdominal surgical emergencies in infants and young children. Emerg Med Clin N Am 21:909-935, 2003.

Mews C, Sinatra F: Chronic liver disease in children. Pediatr Rev 14:436-443, 1993.

NIH Consensus Development Panel on *Helicobacter pylori* in peptic ulcer disease. JAMA 272:65-69, 1994.

Orenstein S: Gastroesophageal reflux. Pediatr Rev 13:174-182, 1992.

Orenstein S, Orenstein D: Gastroesophageal reflux and respiratory disease in children. J Pediatr 112:847-858, 1988.

Rudolph CD, Mazur LJ, Liptak GS, et al: Guidelines for evaluation and treatment of gastroesophageal reflux in infants and children: Recommendations of the North American Society for Pediatric Gastroenterology and Nutrition 32:S1-32, 2001.

Shah MD: Failure to thrive in children. J Clin Gastroenterol 35:371-374, 2002.

Shulman RJ, Phillips S: Parenteral nutrition in infants and children. J Pediatr Gastroenterol Nutr 36:587-607, 2003.

Silber G: Lower gastrointestinal bleeding. Pediatr Rev 12:85-92, 1990.

Sokol RJ: The chronic disease of childhood obesity: The sleeping giant has awakened [editorial]. J Pediatr 136:711-713, 2000.

Sondheimer JM: Office stool examination: A practical guide. Contemp Pediatr 7:63-82, 1990.

Steinberg W, Tenner S: Acute pancreatitis. N Engl J Med 330:1198-1210, 1994.

Suskind RM (ed): Textbook of Pediatric Nutrition. New York, Raven Press, 1981.

Suskind RM, Varma RN: Assessment of nutritional status of children. Pediatr Rev 5:195-202, 1984.

Tack J, Lee KJ: Pathophysiology and treatment of functional dyspepsia. J Clin Gastroenterol 39:S211-216, 2005.

Walker LS, Lipani TA, Greene JW, et al: Recurrent abdominal pain: Symptom subtypes based on the Rome II criteria for pediatric functional gastrointestinal disorders. J Pediatr Gastroenterol Nutr 38:187-191, 2004.

Walker WA, Hendricks KM: Manual of Pediatric Nutrition. Philadelphia, WB Saunders, 1985.

Weisberg P, Scanlon KS, Li R, et al: Nutritional rickets among children in the United States: Review of cases reported between 1986 and 2003. Am J Clin Nutr 80:S1697-1705, 2004.

Werlin SL, Kugathasan S, Frautschy BC: Pancreatitis in children. J Pediatr Gastroenterol Nutr 37:591-595, 2003.

Weydert JA, Ball TM, Davis MF: Systematic review of treatments for recurrent abdominal pain. Pediatrics 111:e1-11, 2003.

Wyllie R: Gastrointestinal manifestations of cystic fibrosis. Clin Pediatr 38:735-738, 1999.

CHAPTER 11

Hematology and Oncology

JEAN M. TERSAK, J. JEFFREY MALATACK, AND
A. KIM RITCHEY

Hematology

Hematologic conditions of the infant and child encompass a wide spectrum of disorders. The core of hematologic diagnosis resides in a thorough medical history and physical examination, complete blood count with reticulocyte count, and review of the peripheral blood smear. In some cases, bone marrow examination is a critical part of the diagnostic evaluation.

This chapter first highlights common hematologic conditions and selected rarer entities. In this context, peripheral blood smear and basic diagnostic tests are used to evaluate nonmalignant hematologic disease. Inherited and acquired abnormalities of the white blood cells; hemoglobin and platelets; and signs, symptoms, and evaluation of bleeding and clotting abnormalities are reviewed. Attention is then given to clinical and laboratory findings in leukemia and solid tumors.

Peripheral Blood Smear

The peripheral blood smear has two major functions. First, it provides confirmation of the values given on the standard Coulter counter printout, which may falsely report values if abnormal cells are present. For example, a falsely elevated white blood cell (WBC) count may be reported by the Coulter counter if nucleated red blood cells (RBCs) are present in the peripheral blood. The presence of RBC fragments may result in falsely elevated platelet counts. Manual review of the peripheral smear allows the diagnostician to perform the differential WBC count at the same time as examination of RBC, WBC, and platelet morphology.

A systematic approach to the evaluation of the smear can maximize the amount of information extracted. First, the slide is scanned under low power, and an area is chosen in which the RBCs are just barely touching (Fig. 11-1). Areas in which the RBCs are too dense or too sparse are fraught with artifact. Under low power, mononuclear and polymorphonuclear cells are visible. By using the high-dry or oil lens, the examiner can observe normal RBC morphology, as well as further morphologic definition of the WBC series and platelets. The normal RBC appears as a biconcave disk with an area of central pallor surrounded by an otherwise homogeneous red circle (Fig. 11-2). During childhood and adolescence, the normal RBC is about the size of the nucleus of a small lymphocyte. RBC morphology in the newborn and infant vary from this general rule. The neonatal RBC demonstrates a larger size, while the RBC of the infant and toddler is found to be smaller than that observed in later years.

After an evaluation of RBC morphology, a WBC differential count can be performed and the morphology of the cells assessed. A blood smear made from anticoagulated blood may have artifacts such as vacuolization of the WBCs. Finally, the platelets should be evaluated for number and size. Each platelet profile found on an oil immersion ($\times$970) field represents approximately 10,000 to 15,000 platelets per mm^3. The presence of large platelets suggests an active marrow with destruction of platelets rather than diminished production.

Red Blood Cell

The RBC is the most ubiquitous of the blood's cellular components. Its primary function is to mediate the exchange of respiratory gases (oxygen and carbon dioxide) between the lungs and body tissues. This is accomplished by the critical biochemical features of its oxygen-carrying intracellular component, hemoglobin (Hgb). Hemoglobin's oxygen-binding sites are completely saturated by passage of the RBC through the lungs. As the cells circulate through the systemic capillaries, the hemoglobin releases 25% of its bound oxygen to the tissues. However, the amount of oxygen released in the tissue may be significantly increased under certain conditions (fever, acidosis, level of 2,3-diphosphoglycerate), allowing some compensation for a decrease in hemoglobin. Nonetheless, a progressive decrease in the hemoglobin level eventually leads to tissue hypoxia, which triggers a release of erythropoietin. This induces an increase in RBC production, which brings the critical RBC mass back toward normal values.

Red Cell Production

RBC production usually occurs in the bone marrow, but under conditions of disease, it can also occur in extramedullary locations such as the spleen. For the first 48 hours after it has joined the peripheral circulation, a newly formed RBC, or reticulocyte, can be stained by a supravital dye for easy identification. Generally, the reticulocyte count is a reflection of the replacement of senescent RBCs. Because the RBC's life span is approximately 120 days, 0.83% of the RBC's mass must be replaced every day. Because reticulocytes maintain their staining characteristics for approximately 48 hours, the normal reticulocyte count (percentage of peripheral RBCs that is reticulocytes) is approximately 1.66%, ranging from 0.83% to 2.49%. This figure is 1% to 2% higher in menstruating women. Increased reticulocyte counts are also a reflection of increased RBC loss through hemolysis or hemorrhage. Decreased reticulocyte counts indicate decreased RBC production (Fig. 11-3).

Anemia

Increased RBC loss or decreased RBC production can result in an overall decrease in RBC mass below a critical level, leading to anemia. This is the most common abnormality of RBCs, and it is identified as a decreased hemoglobin level and decreased hematocrit. Recognition that a child's hemoglobin level is abnormal requires knowledge of age, gender, and race-related normal values. At any given age, anemia is a value greater than two standard deviations below the mean (Table 11-1). For children 6 months of age until puberty, a hemoglobin level of less than 11 g/dL is a useful definition of anemia and an indication for evaluation. Alternatively, an inappropriate drop in the hemoglobin level may also be significant: The 5-year-old child who has a hemoglobin level of 11.5 g/dL but who had a level of 13 g/dL 1 month earlier may require evaluation.

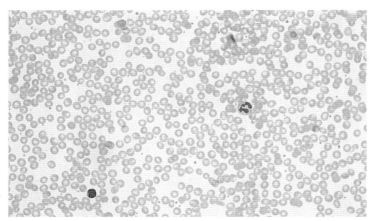

Figure 11-1. Peripheral blood smear: the appearance of a normal peripheral blood smear when viewed under low magnification (×100).

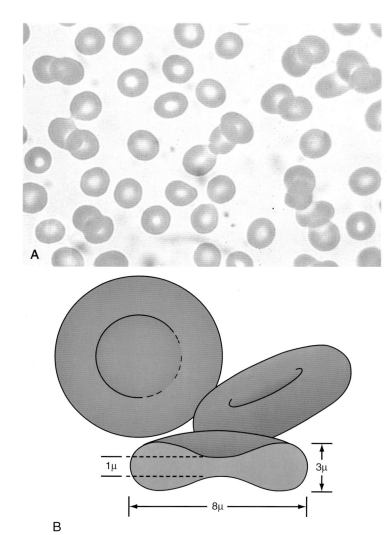

A

B

Figure 11-2. Peripheral blood smear: the appearance of a normal peripheral blood smear when viewed under high power (×400). **A,** Biconcave structure of the red blood cell (RBC). **B,** Schematic drawing of an RBC in two views demonstrating the features of the normal biconcave disk.

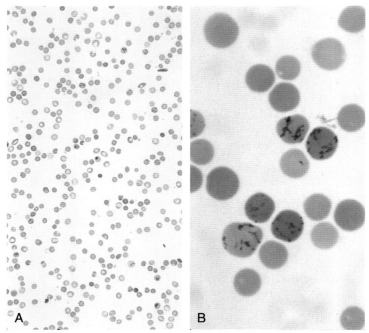

A

B

Figure 11-3. **A,** The reticulocyte: A reticulin-stained peripheral blood smear in a patient with a high (18%) reticulocyte count. The darkly stained cells are the reticulocytes seen in the peripheral blood of a patient with hemolytic anemia. **B,** High magnification of reticulocytes.

Table 11-1	Hemoglobin and Mean Corpuscular Volume (MCV) Values at Various Ages			
	HEMOGLOBIN (g/dL)		**MCV (fL)**	
AGE	*Mean*	*−2 SD*	*Mean*	*−2 SD*
Birth (cord blood)	16.5	13.5	108	98
1-3 days (capillary)	18.5	14.5	108	95
1 week	17.5	13.5	107	88
2 weeks	16.5	12.5	105	86
1 month	14.0	10.0	104	85
2 months	11.5	9.0	96	77
3-6 months	11.5	9.5	91	74
0.5-2 years	12.0	10.5	78	70
2-6 years	12.5	11.5	81	75
6-12 years	13.5	11.5	86	77
12-18 years				
Female	14.0	12.0	90	78
Male	14.5	13.0	88	78
18-49 years				
Female	14.0	12.0	90	80
Male	15.5	13.5	90	80

Modified from: Lanzkowsky P: Manual of Pediatric Hematology and Oncology, 2nd ed. Philadelphia, Churchill Livingstone, 1995.

Severe anemia from any cause may elicit symptoms of fatigue; decreased appetite; headache; and, in extreme cases, shock, congestive heart failure, or even stroke. Physical examination of the anemic child may reveal pallor, although in the fair-skinned or dark-skinned child this may be easily missed, even given an extremely low level of hemoglobin, unless palmar creases or conjunctivae are also examined for pallor (Fig. 11-4). Vital signs may be normal, but with severe anemia, tachycardia may be present.

Before embarking on a workup in a child with a low hemoglobin level, it is worth considering whether the reported blood value is accurate. Reasons for inaccuracy include poor quality control in the use of the Coulter counter; dilution of blood drawn from venous lines; and falsely elevated values, particularly in neonates when the CBC is obtained by heel or finger stick. Anemia, when it does occur, may be an isolated finding, or it may be part of the spectrum of pancytopenia in which WBC and platelet levels are also decreased. Abnormalities of greater than one cell line should alert the physician to the possibility of underlying bone marrow pathology, such as

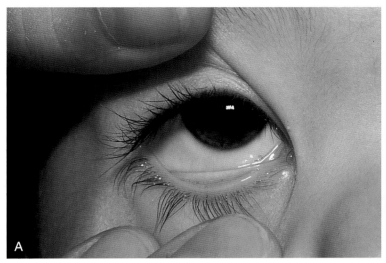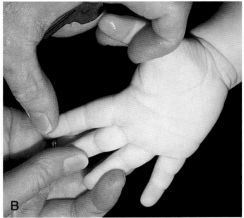

Figure 11-4. Severe anemia. **A,** Pale conjunctiva may be seen in the patient with severe anemia. **B,** Pale palmar creases are also visible in cases of severe anemia. The child in this photograph has a hemoglobin level of 4 g/dL.

marrow infiltration with malignant cells or a bone marrow failure syndrome.

Conceptually, anemia occurs as a result of one of the following:

1. Decreased bone marrow production of RBCs
2. Increased destruction of mature RBCs peripherally or of their precursors while they are still in the bone marrow (ineffective erythropoiesis)
3. Hemorrhage
4. Combinations of these factors

Anemias resulting from decreased RBC production include microcytic anemia, pure red cell aplasia, and megaloblastic anemia. Hemolytic anemias, characterized by increased RBC destruction without evidence of blood loss or ineffective erythropoiesis, include RBC membrane defects, intracellular RBC defects, and extra-RBC factors causing hemolysis.

Anemias Resulting from Decreased Red Cell Production. RBC morphology generally categorizes the type of anemia present and may suggest certain pathogenic mechanisms.

Hypochromic Microcytic Anemia

Hypochromic microcytic anemia represents the most common type of isolated failure of RBC production. Microcytosis exists when the mean corpuscular volume (hematocrit × 10 ÷ RBC number [in millions per mm³]) is low or when the RBCs themselves are smaller than the nuclei of the small lymphocytes. Hypochromia, a decrease in the concentration of intracellular hemoglobin content, is recognized when the mean corpuscular hemoglobin concentration (hemoglobin [in g/dL] × 10 ÷ hematocrit) is decreased or when the hemoglobinized rim of the RBC is less than two-thirds the diameter of the entire cell. Normally, the ratio of RBC volume to the intracellular RBC content is homeostatically maintained. As the concentration of intracellular content decreases for any reason, the volume of the cell also decreases.

The differential diagnosis of hypochromic microcytic anemia includes iron deficiency, lead poisoning, thalassemia minor (α and β types), thalassemia major (Cooley anemia), chronic infection, chronic inflammatory states, and sideroblastic anemia.

Iron Deficiency Anemia. Iron deficiency anemia is the most common pediatric hypochromic microcytic anemia. Iron deficiency is only a laboratory finding, not a diagnosis. The causes of iron deficiency must be elucidated

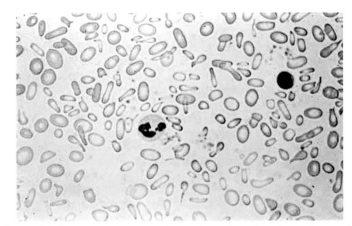

Figure 11-5. Iron deficiency results in a hypochromic, microcytic anemia. This 16-month-old patient had a history of excessive milk intake. Note the marked central pallor of the red blood cell (RBC) with a small rim of hemoglobin, as well as its small size in comparison with that of the adjacent small lymphocyte nucleus. Frequent "cigar cells" can be seen in addition to the hypochromic microcytic RBCs.

through a careful history and physical examination. Although poor nutrition is the most common cause, other causes such as hemorrhage or malabsorption must also be considered. Iron deficiency anemia occurs in infants whose rapidly increasing RBC mass outstrips the dietary iron intake. This lack of iron leads to failure of hemoglobin production and the formation of hypochromic microcytic cells. Because the normal full-term infant has adequate iron reserve to accommodate the increasing RBC mass through the first 5 months of life, iron deficiency is usually not seen until the second half of the first year of life. It is detected most often in the 10- to 18-month-old child. A second peak of iron deficiency anemia is seen during adolescence in girls.

The typical clinical history is that of an infant fed non–iron-containing whole cow milk who, from early infancy, takes large volumes of milk and little else. These children are often large, but their pallor belies their apparent robust size. Whole cow milk is not only deficient in dietary iron but often leads to an enteropathic condition with occult gastrointestinal blood loss, exacerbating the child's iron-deficient status.

Figure 11-5 shows the peripheral blood smear of a 16-month-old child who had been fed large amounts of whole milk from 3 months of age. The RBCs are microcytic and hypochromic. The number of platelets is characteristically increased (particularly when the enteropathic condition is present), although it may be normal or even decreased. In severe iron deficiency anemia, anisocytosis (varied size of RBCs) and poikilocytosis (varied RBC shape) may be prominent. Nonspecific abnormalities of RBC morphology, such as the presence of microvalocytes (cigar cells) (see Fig. 11-5) or basophilic stippling (see Fig. 11-9), may also occur. Bizarre RBC shapes are due to a three-dimensional change in structure when viewed in a two-dimensional plane of the light microscope. The microvalocyte of iron deficiency appears oval because opposite ends of the severely dehemoglobinized RBCs tend to curl up (Fig. 11-6). When viewed in two dimensions, the cell appears ovoid.

The child with iron deficiency may be asymptomatic despite a significant degree of anemia. However, when symptoms are present, irritability may be a prominent finding in the young child. Clinical consequences of severe iron deficiency anemia may have long-term implications on development as indicated by decreases in Bayley IQ scores. Affected children may manifest a peculiar physical finding termed *koilonychia*, or "spooning" of fingernails and toenails (Fig. 11-7). Glossitis may be observed in iron deficiency and other nutritional deficiencies.

Iron deficiency must be differentiated from thalassemia and lead poisoning. Although the patient history generally suggests the appropriate diagnosis, the distinction can be made, for the most part, on the basis of a few laboratory tests. Review of the peripheral smear (see Fig. 11-5) should first confirm the presence of microcytosis or hypochromia, which, like the measurements of hemoglobin, are susceptible to technical errors. In thalassemia minor, the hemoglobin is generally not less than 9 g/dL; moreover, for a given degree of anemia, the mean corpuscular volume

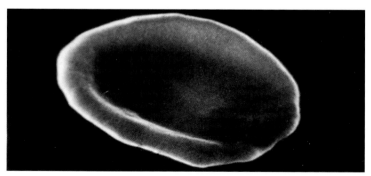

Figure 11-6. Scanning electron microscopic image of an iron-deficient RBC. Note the three-dimensional shape and curled edges.

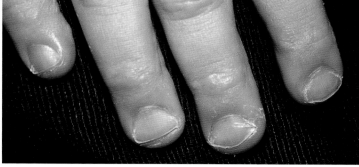

Figure 11-7. Spooning of the fingernails occurs in children with severe iron deficiency anemia.

(MCV) tends to be lower in the child with thalassemia than in the child with iron deficiency. These trends may be reflected in the Mentzer index, which mathematically relates the mean corpuscular volume to the RBC number (Mentzer index = mean corpuscular volume ÷ number of RBCs ÷ 10^6). Mentzer indices greater than 13.5 suggest iron deficiency, whereas values less than 11.5 indicate thalassemia minor. In practice the index is not always helpful because many children with mild anemias may have intermediate index values. Other helpful clues to the diagnosis can come directly from the RBC number because children with iron deficiency usually have a low RBC number, whereas thalassemia tends to result in RBC numbers greater than $5 \times 10^6/mm^3$. The RBC distribution width, or RDW, is a reflection of the degree of anisocytosis (RDW = the standard deviation of the RBC volume ÷ the MCV × 100). This value is extremely helpful in the evaluation of the patient with microcytic anemia. The RDW is large in iron deficiency and tends to be normal in thalassemia trait.

The history and physical examination, blood count, and review of the peripheral blood smear may be sufficient for diagnosis in many instances of hypochromic microcytic anemia. If the evaluation before obtaining a more specific test strongly suggests iron deficiency, a therapeutic trial of iron may be a reasonable approach. However, additional laboratory studies are often indicated. The coexistence of iron deficiency and lead intoxication is well documented, and partial response to iron therapy may indicate concurrent lead intoxication. Securing long-term follow-up of the patient is also imperative. Supplementation with oral iron must continue for approximately 2 months after return of the hemoglobin value to normal to allow for the repletion of body iron stores. The etiology of the iron deficiency anemia must be addressed to prevent recurrence.

Choosing between specific studies such as serum iron levels and total iron-binding capacity (TIBC) (used together to calculate iron saturation) or ferritin and free erythrocyte protoporphyrin (FEP) is often a matter of personal preference. In addition, when the degree of anemia is mild, the results of any combination of tests may be equivocal. FEP has the advantage of screening for lead poisoning or porphyria. FEP is not subject to significant diurnal variations. It is also unaffected by oral iron intake at the time of testing. Ferritin is an acute-phase reactant and may be elevated into the low normal range in a child with a concurrent inflammatory process. However, if ferritin is low, it is diagnostic of iron deficiency. A serum ferritin concentration of less than 12 ng/mL is suggestive of iron deficiency. Importantly, iron studies including ferritin, serum iron, TIBC, and transferrin saturation demonstrate age-related normal values. Low transferrin saturation and elevated FEP are also observed in the setting of iron deficiency.

Lead Poisoning. Lead intoxication leads to microcytic anemia. However, nonhematologic manifestations of lead intoxication, particularly neurologic complications, often dominate the picture. The spectrum of clinical presentations of lead intoxication ranges from vague symptoms of abdominal pain, vomiting, malaise, and behavioral changes to acute encephalopathic conditions, with rapid progression to coma and death. Late physical findings may include papilledema. Significant radiographic changes are also seen in lead intoxication (Fig. 11-8).

Lead intoxication occurs as a result of excessive environmental lead intake. Aerosolized and oral lead-containing environmental contaminants are major sources

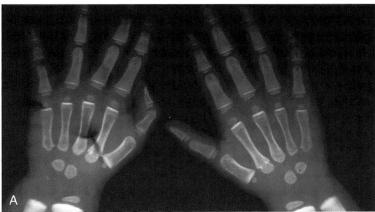

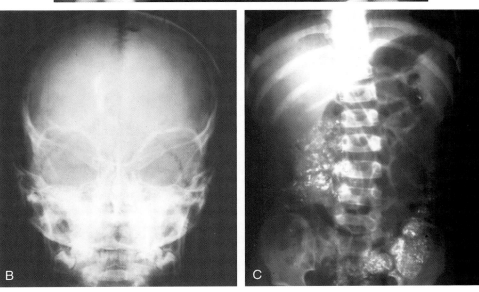

Figure 11-8. X-ray findings in lead intoxication. **A,** This hand radiograph of a child with lead intoxication reveals marked linear increases in the density of the metaphyses. These should not be confused with the growth arrest lines that may be seen after a variety of illnesses. **B,** A skull film is shown from a patient with lead intoxication and encephalopathy. Note the split of sutures indicative of increased intracranial pressure. **C,** An abdominal radiograph performed on a child with a history of pica and lead intoxication reveals radiodense, lead-containing paint chips scattered throughout the colon.

of lead intoxication. Although clearly a common mechanism in lead poisoning, pica, which is associated with the intake of flaking lead paint, represents neither the only nor the prevailing cause of lead intoxication. The finger-sucking behavior of children in homes where lead paint has become a part of house dust is perhaps a more important factor. A contaminated water supply resulting from old plumbing and deteriorating lead-containing soldered joints can cause lead intoxication in the infant (earlier than the usual "at-risk" age).

Hematologic abnormalities of lead intoxication are a direct result of the effect of lead on several cellular enzymes involved in heme production. Lead inhibits these enzyme systems, impairing iron use and globin synthesis. Thus despite normal intracellular levels, iron is unable to be incorporated into heme and hemoglobin production fails. Reduced hemoglobin production leads directly to hypochromic microcytic anemia. Basophilic stippling (Fig. 11-9) is a secondary and inconsistent hematologic manifestation of lead intoxication that occurs as a result of inhibition of yet another RBC enzyme, 5-pyrimidine nucleotidase. Although basophilic stippling is more prominent in lead intoxication, it is also present in thalassemia and treated iron deficiency. Its presence on the peripheral smear is nonspecific.

Differentiating lead intoxication from iron deficiency can, at times, be difficult. Also, lead intoxication and iron deficiency may coexist, further confusing the diagnosis. Lead poisoning and iron deficiency cause FEP to accumulate in the blood due to the inability to complete the heme biosynthetic pathway through the incorporation of iron

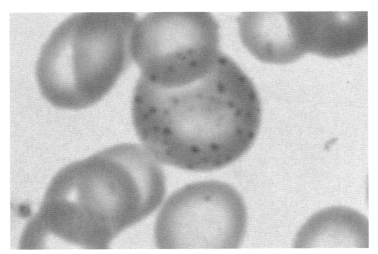

Figure 11-9. Lead intoxication leads to a hypochromic, microcytic anemia. Prominent basophilic stippling is often seen in cases of severe lead intoxication. However, this finding is not specific for lead toxicity and may also be seen in thalassemia and treated iron deficiency.

into heme. The FEP is elevated in both conditions, although extremely high levels are more common in lead intoxication. Further testing, such as determination of blood lead level, is necessary to determine the cause of elevated FEP levels. Recent information incriminating even low-level lead intoxication as a cause of disturbed cognitive function underscores the necessity for clinicians to consider this diagnosis. Silent lead intoxication with blood levels of 15 µg/dL remains a significant pediatric health problem and may not be associated with the signs of chronic high-level lead poisoning previously described.

Thalassemia. *Thalassemia* is a term applied to a group of genetic disturbances decreasing hemoglobin production and leading to anemia and/or altered levels of the various hemoglobins in the blood.

Thalassemia trait is also responsible for hypochromic microcytic anemia. In patients with β-thalassemia trait, hemoglobin electrophoresis usually reveals an increase in Hgb A$_2$ and Hgb F, whereas in patients with α-thalassemia trait the findings may be normal. This costly test is probably overused in the evaluation of hypochromic microcytic anemia. Hemograms on parents may be helpful if they show a microcytosis in at least one parent, further suggesting a diagnosis of thalassemia trait. If a diagnosis of thalassemia is suggested by any of the studies already discussed, both parents should have hemograms performed. If the child suffers from thalassemia trait, it is conceivable that both parents may also have thalassemia trait, and a subsequent child may be born with thalassemia major, a disease with serious implications regarding morbidity and mortality. Appropriate genetic counseling is indicated in this case.

Thalassemia major (Cooley anemia) causes hypochromic microcytic anemia that results from ineffective erythropoiesis caused by an imbalance between α- and β-hemoglobin chain synthesis. The peripheral blood smear shows hypochromia; microcytosis; target cells; basophilic stippling; and, often, a large number of nucleated RBCs (Fig. 11-10). β-thalassemia major is associated with increased marrow activity, which is ineffectively attempting to correct the degree of anemia. The increased marrow activity expands the marrow cavity, producing a characteristic bony hyperplasia evidenced by physical and radiographic findings (Fig. 11-11). Untreated patients with thalassemia major have chronic and severe anemia, marked hepatosplenomegaly, scleral icterus, and listlessness and may have high-output cardiac failure secondary to severe anemia. In addition, malocclusion may occur because of malar hypertrophy. This picture is not usually confused with thalassemia trait, iron deficiency, or lead poisoning. Thalassemia major generally presents after the first 6 months of life at a time when β-chain synthesis increases. Hydrops fetalis may result from α-thalassemia major. Ethnicity may be an important clue in the history: β-thalassemia trait tends to occur in patients of African or Mediterranean descent, whereas α-thalassemia trait tends to occur in patients of African or Asian origin.

β⁻-thalassemia major is largely restricted to people of Mediterranean or Middle Eastern heritage.

Chronic Inflammatory States. Chronic inflammatory states, such as chronic infection or collagen vascular diseases (particularly juvenile rheumatoid arthritis), may lead to hypochromic microcytic anemia. Although the symptoms of the child's primary illness usually clarify the diagnosis, there are occasionally cases in which a chronic subclinical infection (particularly of the urinary tract) may go undiagnosed. Differentiating a chronic inflammatory state from other causes of hypochromic microcytic anemia is usually more easily done on clinical than laboratory grounds. One laboratory study that may be of value is the serum ferritin determination. The ferritin is de-

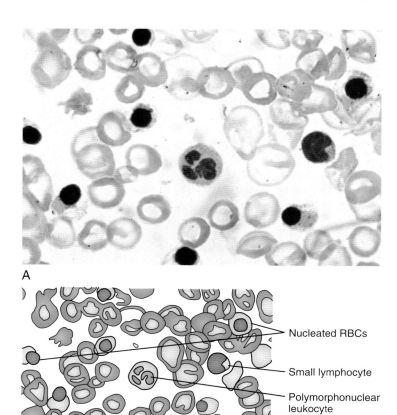

A

B

Nucleated RBCs

Small lymphocyte

Polymorphonuclear leukocyte

Figure 11-10. Thalassemia major. **A,** This peripheral blood smear in a child with thalassemia major shows a hypochromic, microcytic anemia with prominent nucleated red blood cells surrounding the polymorphonuclear cells and lymphocytes. **B,** Labeled schematic of peripheral blood smear.

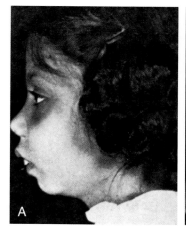

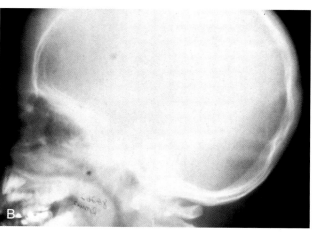

A

B

Figure 11-11. A, Maxillary hyperplasia resulting from an increased marrow space in a child with thalassemia major. **B,** Skull radiograph of the same patient demonstrates an increased marrow cavity of the skull and facial bones.

creased in iron deficiency, whereas in chronic inflammatory states it is usually elevated. Also, while serum iron is low in both iron deficiency and anemia of chronic disease, the TIBC is increased in iron deficiency and decreased in anemia of chronic disease.

Sideroblastic and Other Anemias. The sideroblastic anemias are characterized by the presence of a population of hypochromic microcytic cells in the peripheral blood, as well as sideroblasts in the bone marrow (Fig. 11-12). The sideroblastic anemias, rare in pediatrics, can be hereditary or acquired. The hereditary anemia is caused by a deficiency of an enzyme or enzyme activity required for hemoglobin production. The acquired form may arise secondary to drugs or toxins (lead being the most important of those in childhood), malignancy, inflammatory disorders, or endocrine disease. Alternatively, this disorder may be idiopathic.

Copper deficiency and chronic disease, although generally resulting in normocytic anemia, may occasionally cause a microcytic condition.

Macrocytosis

Patients with macrocytic RBC indices may have hemorrhage or hemolysis and a brisk reticulocytosis, which accounts for the large RBCs on peripheral blood smear. Such causes of macrocytosis are usually easily recognized and differentiated from macrocytic anemia on the basis of bone marrow failure syndromes, such as Diamond-Blackfan anemia, aplastic anemia, congenital dyserythropoietic anemia, and preleukemic conditions. Macrocytic anemia refers to anemia in the setting of RBCs with a mean corpuscular volume of greater than 100 fL on the Coulter indices. The differential diagnosis of macrocytosis includes reticulocytosis, Down syndrome, Diamond-Blackfan anemia, hypothyroidism, liver disease, and megaloblastic anemia.

Macrocytic Anemia with Megaloblastic Bone Marrow. These anemias constitute another group of conditions characterized by failure of adequate RBC production. Although the etiology of the megaloblastic anemias may vary, common morphologic abnormalities of the erythropoietic cells exist. The hallmark is the megaloblast, a nucleated marrow RBC with a lacy chromatin pattern and a dyssynchrony of maturation between cytoplasm and nucleus. The morphologic alterations are a direct result of decreased nucleoprotein DNA synthesis compared with cytoplasmic protein synthesis, which stems from a relative decrease in the factors needed in DNA replication, namely folate or cobalamin (vitamin B_{12}). From a morphologic standpoint, RBCs are the primary cells affected by megaloblastic changes.

On the peripheral blood smear, the RBCs are large in size (macrocytes) and display a great deal of variation in their shapes (Fig. 11-13). These macrocytic cells are generally normochromic.

Although RBCs are primarily affected in megaloblastic anemia, all of the actively dividing marrow cells fail to have normal duplication of DNA and become involved in the pathologic process. Neutrophils are the second most likely cells to display morphologic abnormalities. These cells, like the RBCs, are large, and hypersegmentation of the nucleus is a pathognomonic finding (Fig. 11-14). Neutropenia is common. The more severe and prolonged megaloblastic anemias may ultimately lead to moderate thrombocytopenia, with large bizarre platelets on the peripheral blood smear. Megaloblastic changes in each cell line are shown in Figure 11-15.

Laboratory diagnosis requires the measurement of folate and vitamin B_{12} levels in the serum and RBCs. Because a typical Western diet is unlikely to lead to folate or vitamin B_{12} deficiency, a low level of either should raise questions of altered bioavailability or peculiar diet. Goat milk is folate deficient (though in recent years many canned goat milk products are folate supplemented), and an infant on a goat milk diet may become folate depleted over time. Fad diets are often not structured thoughtfully and may lead to folate deficiency. Various drugs that decrease folate absorption (phenytoin) or interfere with folate metabolism (methotrexate) may also lead to megaloblastic changes. A pathologic condition of the gastrointestinal tract may be the primary disease causing malabsorption of folate or vitamin B_{12} and secondary megaloblastic changes. This condition may be iatrogenic if a portion of the intestines is removed for medical reasons. Pernicious anemia is a specific cause of failure of vitamin B_{12} absorp-

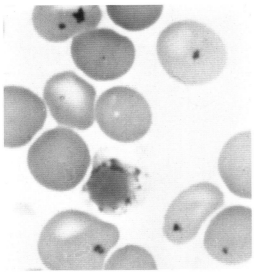

Figure 11-12. This bone marrow slide demonstrates the presence of the ringed sideroblast (iron-containing normoblast) on iron stain of the bone marrow in a patient with sideroblastic anemia.

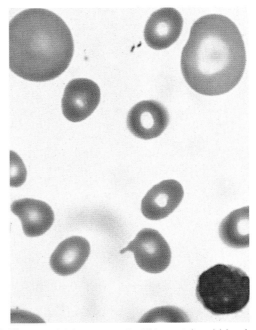

Figure 11-13. Megaloblastic anemia. This peripheral blood smear demonstrates an enlarged red blood cell (RBC, macrocyte) at the upper left of the photograph. The RBC is much larger than the normal small lymphocyte in the same field in this patient with megaloblastic anemia.

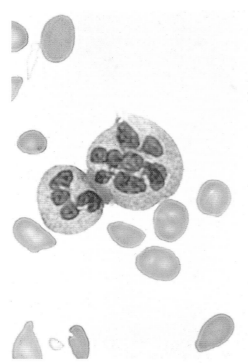

Figure 11-14. This peripheral blood smear demonstrates the presence of a hypersegmented polymorphonuclear leukocyte in a patient with phenytoin-induced folate deficiency.

	DISEASE	
Table 11-2	Features Differentiating Pure Red Cell Anemia from Transient Erythroblastopenia of Childhood (TEC)	

RBC CHARACTERISTIC	*Pure Red Cell Anemia*	TEC
Hemoglobin	Increased fetal	Normal fetal
Cellular antigen	i	I
Mean corpuscular volume	Increased	Normal
RBC enzyme activity	Normal or high	Low

RBC, red blood cell.

tion because of the absence or deficiency of the intrinsic factor required for vitamin B_{12} absorption. Glossitis (Fig. 11-16) or angular stomatitis seen in vitamin B_{12} deficiency can be a helpful physical finding in the differential diagnoses.

Macrocytic Anemia without Megaloblastic Bone Marrow. Macrocytic anemia in the absence of megaloblastic changes in the bone marrow is more suggestive of a bone marrow failure syndrome such as Diamond-Blackfan anemia. This disorder is also termed *congenital hypoplastic anemia* or *congenital aregenerative anemia*. It is characterized by the onset of anemia by 6 months of age with a low absolute reticulocyte count. Approximately 25% of patients with congenital pure red cell aplasia also have minor congenital abnormalities including thumb anomalies and/or a Turner phenotype (see Chapters 1 and 9). Some of the patients go into spontaneous remission. In others, remission may occur years after the onset of signs of the disease. In those who require treatment, the majority respond to corticosteroid therapy. The final subgroup of patients are steroid unresponsive and do not undergo remission. These patients remain transfusion dependent for the rest of their lives. Congenital pure red cell aplasia must be distinguished from an acquired disorder called transient erythroblastopenia of childhood (TEC), which is discussed in the section describing the normocytic, normochromic anemias. General differences between these two disorders are summarized in Table 11-2.

Normocytic, Normochromic Anemia
The third morphologic subgroup of anemia includes those with normochromic and normocytic RBCs. These anemias are easily analyzed on the basis of an algorithm beginning with a reticulocyte count. These normocytic and normochromic anemias with low reticulocyte counts develop because of failed RBC production. The differential diagnosis of this group includes TEC, dyserythropoietic anemia, renal disease, infection, and drug-induced aplasia.

When low-reticulocyte normocytic, normochromic anemia occurs in the presence of a decrease in WBCs and platelets, the diagnosis is more ominous and includes leukemia and tumor infiltration of the marrow.

Pure Red Cell Aplasia. Pure red cell aplasia may also be an acquired condition termed *TEC,* as mentioned previously. TEC occurs in 1- to 4-year-old children and appears 2 weeks to 2 months after a respiratory or gastrointestinal illness. Differentiating TEC from congenital pure red cell anemia is important because TEC is transient and self-limited, whereas the congenital form of red cell aplasia may be chronic. Fortunately, it has been noted that the RBCs in pure red cell aplasia have fetal characteristics, whereas the RBCs of TEC have age-appropriate characteristics (see Table 11-2). The cause of TEC remains obscure. Human parvovirus B19, known to depress erythropoiesis especially in the fetus or patients with hemolytic anemia, has been implicated as the etiologic agent in TEC in only a minority of patients. TEC may occur after many different viral infections and most likely represents altered immunity from the infection that affects erythropoiesis.

Non–TEC-acquired pure red cell aplasia is rare in pediatrics. In adults, pure red cell aplasia is sometimes suspected on an autoimmune basis and is frequently associated with thymoma. Three types of non–TEC-acquired pure red cell aplasia have been recognized. Type I has a serum IgG inhibitor of erythropoiesis and high erythropoietin levels. Type II has a low erythropoietin activity level and an erythropoietin IgG antibody. Type III has no antierythropoiesis or antierythropoietin serum antibodies. Rather, the defect appears intrinsic to the stem cell. Some of these children are preleukemic. Thymoma-associated pure red cell aplasia is extremely rare in children. Drugs, particularly chloramphenicol, have been responsible for a significant percentage of pure red cell aplasias.

The peripheral blood smear from a patient with pure red cell aplasia is often nonspecific (although it may show atypical lymphocytes as vestiges of a residual viral infection), and the bone marrow aspirate may rarely be more specific. It may demonstrate the vacuolated erythroblasts of the chloramphenicol effect or the multinucleated giant cells indicative of the rare congenital dyserythropoietic anemia (Fig. 11-17). Low reticulocyte normocytic, normochromic anemia with depressed WBCs and platelets is discussed in the section on pancytopenia.

Anemia Resulting from Increased Red Cell Destruction
Hemolytic Anemias
A normocytic, normochromic anemia with increased reticulocyte count, without evidence of blood loss, most likely results from hemolytic processes. However, the reticulocyte count may not be elevated if it is measured within a few days of the onset of hemolysis. Patients with hemolytic anemia can suffer from any of the symptoms

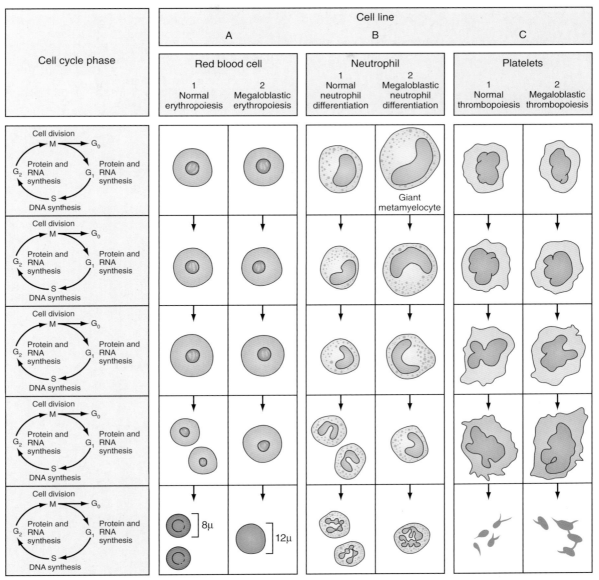

Figure 11-15. Schematic comparison of normal cellular maturation and megaloblastic differentiation of three cell lines. The cell cycle phase is identified to the left of the figure. Note that the megaloblastic cells fail to undergo replication of DNA and cellular division at the S and M phases, respectively, leading to large red blood cells; hypersegmented polymorphonuclear leukocytes; and large, bizarrely shaped platelets.

common to all anemias; in addition, they develop an indirect hyperbilirubinemia with or without clinical icterus. Other laboratory evidence of hemolysis is present including increased levels of carboxyhemoglobin, lactate dehydrogenase, and serum aspartate transaminase and decreased levels of haptoglobin.

The differential diagnosis of hemolytic anemia rests largely in the recognition of specific morphologic abnormalities on the peripheral blood smear (Table 11-3) followed by appropriate specific laboratory tests.

Normocytic, Normochromic Anemia with Elevated Reticulocyte Count. Coombs-Positive Hemolytic Anemia: Direct and indirect Coombs tests, which evaluate the patient's blood for the presence of anti-RBC antibody and complement on RBCs or in the serum, respectively, identify immunohemolytic anemia. The antibody- and complement-mediated RBC destruction produces spherocytes on the peripheral blood smear (Fig. 11-18). Coombs-positive hemolytic anemia in the newborn most often represents an isoimmune hemolytic anemia. This is caused by a maternal antibody that has crossed the placenta into the neonate, hemolyzing the newborn RBCs. Maternal antibodies form to fetal RBC antigens when fetal blood

gains entry into maternal circulation via a break in placental integrity. Maternal antibodies then cross the placenta and cause fetal RBC hemolysis. In the majority of cases of isoimmune hemolytic anemia, the maternal antibody is directed at ABO or Rh RBC antigens. When Rh antigen is the antibody target, the blood smear does not show spherocytes.

Hereditary Spherocytosis: Coombs-negative hemolytic anemia with spherocytes often represents hereditary spherocytosis (HS), which is the most common cause of genetically determined hemolytic anemia in the white population. Hereditary spherocytosis is transmitted frequently as an autosomal dominant trait, and it is named for the peculiar appearance of the RBCs on the peripheral blood smear. The RBC membrane defect, which appears to result from inherent cytoskeleton membrane instability most commonly due to spectrin deficiency, leads to loss of membrane. Membrane repair occurs, which decreases the normal RBC surface-to-volume ratio, causing the normal, bioconcave disk configuration to assume a more geometrically efficient spherical shape (Fig. 11-19). The direct consequence of this new morphology is a less pliable cell. The inability of this new cell to deform during transit

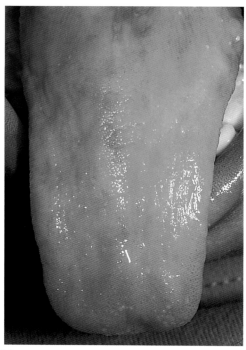

Figure 11-16. A smooth, beefy red tongue may be observed in the physical examination of a patient with vitamin B_{12} deficiency. This patient depended on total parenteral nutrition for several years without vitamin B_{12} supplementation.

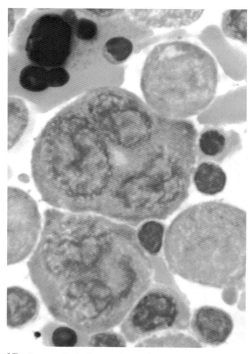

Figure 11-17. Congenital dyserythropoietic anemia type III. Note the centrally located gigantoblast present in this condition.

Table 11-3	Common RBC Hemolytic Disorders by Predominant Morphology*

Spherocytes
Hereditary spherocytosis
ABO incompatibility in neonates[†]
Immunohemolytic anemias with IgG- or C3-coated RBCs
Hemolytic transfusion reactions[†]
Severe burns or other RBC thermal injuries

Bizarre Poikilocytes
RBC fragmentation syndromes (microangiopathic and macroangiopathic hemolytic anemias)
Hereditary elliptocytosis in neonates

Elliptocytes
Hereditary elliptocytosis
Thalassemia
(Other hypochromic microcytic anemia)
(Megaloblastic anemia)

Spiculated or Crenated RBCs
Acute hepatic necrosis (spur-cell anemia)
Uremia
Abetalipoproteinemia

Prominent Basophilic Stippling
Thalassemia
Unstable hemoglobin levels
Lead poisoning[‡]

Irreversibly Sickled Cells
Sickle cell anemia
Symptomatic sickle syndromes

Intraerythrocytic Parasites
Malaria
Babesiosis
Bartonellosis

Target Cells
Hgb S, C, D, and E
Hereditary xerocytosis
Thalassemia
(Other hypochromic microcytic anemia)
(Obstructive liver disease)
(Postsplenectomy)

Nonspecific or Normal Morphology
Embden-Meyerhof pathway defects
HMP shunt defects
Adenosine deaminase hyperactivity with low RBC ATP
Unstable hemoglobin levels
Paroxysmal nocturnal hemoglobinuria
Dyserythropoietic anemia
Copper toxicity (Wilson disease)
Erythropoietic porphyria
Vitamin E deficiency
Hypersplenism

*Nonhemolytic disorders of similar morphology are enclosed in parentheses for reference. [†]Usually associated with a positive Coombs test. [‡]Disease sometimes associated with this morphology.
ATP, adenosine triphosphate; HMP, hexose-monophosphate shunt; RBC, red blood cell.
Modified from Nathan DG, Oski FA (eds): Hematology of Infancy and Childhood, 2nd ed. Philadelphia, WB Saunders, 1981.

through the splenic microcirculation leads to RBC destruction (Fig. 11-20). Most cases of HS are due to a mutation in the cytoskeletal protein spectrin. Less common defects have been described in ankyrin, a binding site for spectrin, and deficiencies of band 3 and protein 4.2 (pallidin). The characteristic smear may show increased numbers of spherocytes after splenectomy, when spherocytes are less likely to be removed from the circulation (Fig. 11-21). Osmotic fragility testing (Fig. 11-22), used commonly in patients with suspected hereditary spherocytosis, is an excellent confirmatory test but is not pathognomonic for the diagnosis.

Elliptocytosis: Hereditary elliptocytosis (Fig. 11-23) is another membrane defect morphologically distinct from hereditary spherocytosis. However, the pathophysiology of RBC destruction is similar to that in hereditary spherocytosis. Also, like hereditary spherocytosis, hereditary elliptocytosis appears to be transmitted as an autosomal dominant trait. In most instances, hereditary elliptocytosis is a mild, well-compensated hemolytic anemia that is clinically insignificant unless splenic hypertrophy develops resulting from another disease process. The elliptocyte form bears only a superficial similarity to that of the "cigar cell" of iron deficiency anemia (see Fig. 11-5). Unlike the cigar cells, the elliptocytes of hereditary elliptocytosis have normal size, have a normal mean corpuscular value,

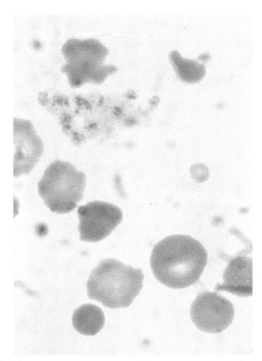

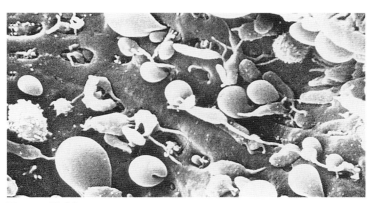

Figure 11-20. Electron micrograph of red blood cells (RBCs) traversing the splenic sinusoids. Note that the RBCs become deformed as they traverse the microcirculation of the splenic sinusoids.

Figure 11-18. Coombs-positive hemolytic anemia. Note the spherocytes and a large red blood cell with polychromasia, indicating the presence of regenerative anemia.

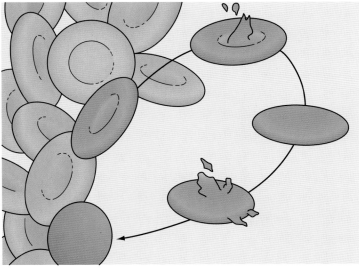

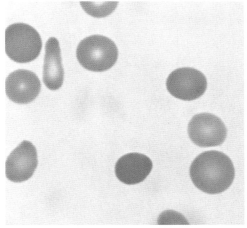

Figure 11-21. Peripheral blood smear of a patient with hereditary spherocytosis. Note the presence of small, perfectly round cells without an area of central pallor. The mean corpuscular hemoglobin concentration (MCHC) is often increased in this condition but may be normal in some cases. Reticulocyte count is also often elevated due to the shortened life span of the RBC and need for increased RBC production relative to individuals without hereditary spherocytosis.

Figure 11-19. A developing spherocyte resulting from the process of repeated membrane fragmentation, loss, and repair.

and are true elliptocytes. Elliptocytes may also be found in the peripheral blood smear of thalassemia or in megaloblastic anemia.

Acanthocytic and Echinocytic Anemia: A number of hemolytic anemias are characterized by spiculated RBCs referred to as *acanthocytes* or *echinocytes* (Fig. 11-24). Abetalipoproteinemia, which generally presents as a neurologic disorder with progressive ataxia, is also characterized by retinitis pigmentosa, fat malabsorption, and the absence of chylomicrons and very-low-density and low-density lipoproteins. Roughly 50% to 90% of the RBCs on peripheral smear are acanthocytes, which develop as a direct result of the alterations of the serum lipids. Altered membrane lipid composition changes the fluidity of the RBC, which leads to the acanthocytic form. Malabsorption of fat-soluble vitamins in abetalipoproteinemia results in vitamin E deficiency, leaving the RBCs subject to oxidative

injury. However, despite altered membrane fluidity and vitamin E deficiency, hemolysis in abetalipoproteinemia is mild.

Spur cell anemia is another disorder characterized by acanthocytes. The hemolysis in this disorder, in contrast to abetalipoproteinemia, is brisk. Spur cell anemia develops in the setting of sudden and massive liver injury arising from any cause (e.g., hepatitis with acute yellow atrophy, shock liver, hepatic infarction). The hepatic decompensation leads to increased serum lipid and cholesterol levels, which lead, in turn, to increased RBC membrane cholesterol content, thus altering RBC membrane fluidity. Spiculated cells in lesser numbers can also be seen in uremia and anorexia nervosa, as well as severe malnutrition. Probably the most frequent cause of spiculated RBCs on the peripheral blood smear is inadequate slide preparation. Thus when confronted with such a slide, review of repeated peripheral blood smears is prudent.

Target Cells: Target cells draw their name from their target-like appearance on the peripheral blood smear. They are often seen as a secondary response to a process that increases the RBC membrane or decreases the RBC content, leading to an increase in the surface-to-volume ratio of the RBCs (Fig. 11-25A). In a dried smear, the excess surface accumulates and bulges outward in the area that is normally the RBC's central pallor, producing the char-

OSMOTIC FRAGILITY

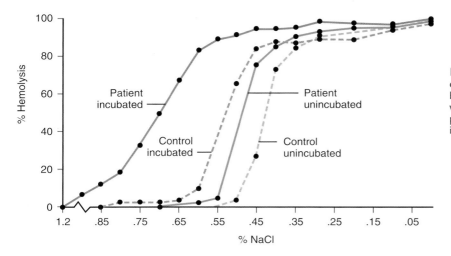

Figure 11-22. Osmotic fragility testing. The graphs show osmotic fragility pattern of unincubated and incubated red blood cells (RBCs) from a normal individual and from a patient with hereditary spherocytosis. The striking increase in fragility produced by the incubation of RBCs in hereditary spherocytosis is obvious.

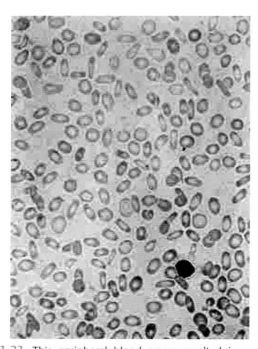

Figure 11-23. This peripheral blood smear resulted in an incidental finding of hereditary elliptocytosis in a 3-year-old child. More than 90% of the cells are elliptocytes. The child's only remarkable history was one of neonatal jaundice.

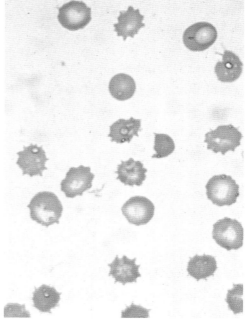

Figure 11-24. Spur cell anemia. The peripheral smear from this patient demonstrates the hematologic findings of acute hepatic necrosis. The anemia associated with the presence of these spiculated cells in the periphery can be severe.

acteristic target cell morphology. Liver diseases of any type (particularly obstructive hepatopathy), with their secondary alteration of serum lipids leading to membrane lipid loading, are well-known causes of target cell formation. Splenectomy decreases reticuloendothelial remodeling of reticulocytes, removes lipid-loaded RBC membranes, and leads to targeted RBCs. Mechanisms previously discussed which decrease RBC intracellular content, such as hypochromic microcytic anemia, also induce target formation. Finally, in a rare autosomal recessive condition, familial lecithin-cholesterol acyltransferase deficiency (characterized by anemia, corneal opacities, hyperlipidemia, proteinuria, chronic nephritis, and premature atherosclerosis), prominent target cells are seen on the peripheral blood smear.

In addition, target cells (or more accurately, pseudo-target cells) occur with various hemoglobinopathies. This happens more often in conditions associated with Hgb C, but also with Hgb S, D, and E (Figs. 11-26 and 11-27) because of aggregation of hemoglobin in the central region of the RBC (see Fig. 11-25B).

Intracellular Red Cell Defects

Hemoglobinopathies. Hemoglobinopathies often result in a characteristic and even diagnostic peripheral blood smear. They can be responsible for hemolysis resulting from unstable hemoglobin variants or altered (decreased) hemoglobin solubility.

Unstable Hemoglobin Variants: Unstable hemoglobin variants, unlike most hemolytic hemoglobinopathies, rarely have a characteristic morphology, although basophilic stippling and Heinz bodies may be noted on special staining of the peripheral blood (Fig. 11-28). The Heinz bodies represent hemoglobin aggregates that have precipitated intracellularly. RBCs in Heinz body anemia usually are normocytic but may be hypochromic as a result of RBC splenic "pitting" of precipitated hemoglobin. Because the precipitated hemoglobin may be mistaken for reticulum, reticulocyte counts may be spuriously high. Methylene blue staining of RBCs after they have incubated for a few hours can demonstrate the Heinz bodies. Hemolysis may be mild (Hgb$_{Köln}$) or brisk (Hgb$_{Bristol}$) or induced by drugs such as sulfonamides (Hgb$_{Zurich}$).

Unstable hemoglobinopathies have an autosomal dominant pattern of inheritance, and affected individuals are heterozygotes. A homozygous state would, in most cases, be incompatible with life. Congenital Heinz body hemolytic anemia is an important cause of congenital hemolytic anemia. This condition, although frequently a persistent process in the older infant, has been observed to resolve. At least some of these self-limited cases may represent the presence of unstable γ-hemoglobin, which normally disappears as the infant ages. The precipitate-

unstable hemoglobin secondarily increases membrane fragility, leading to the hemolysis seen in this disorder.

Sickle Cell Disease: Of the hemoglobinopathies that have altered hemoglobin solubility, none is as well known or as ubiquitous as sickle cell anemia. Substitution of valine for glutamic acid at position 6 in the β-chain of the hemoglobin molecule leads to the cross-linking of one β-chain to a second hemoglobin molecule's β-chain when the hemoglobin is in its deoxygenated state. This cross-linkage tips the solubility balance, leading to the sickling of the RBC (see Fig. 11-26). Although sickle cell disease is seen predominantly in black patients, it is by no means exclusive to patients of African origin, with Mediterranean and Middle Eastern peoples also being affected.

The clinical signs and symptoms of sickle cell anemia are due to decreased survival and altered rheology of the sickled RBC. As with any chronic hemolytic state, marrow cavity enlargement occurs, leading to maxillary hyperpla-

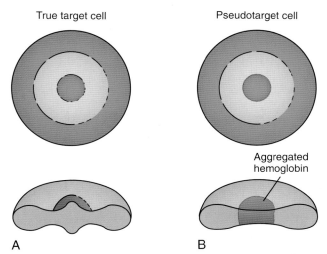

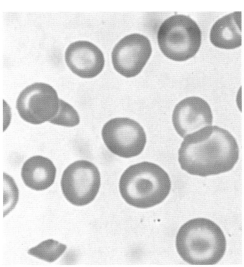

Figure 11-25. **A,** Schematic of the morphology of a target cell. **B,** Schematic of the morphology of a pseudotarget cell.

Figure 11-27. Peripheral blood smear of a child with hemoglobin SC disease. Sickle cells are seen less frequently in this disease, whereas target cells are more prominent.

Figure 11-26. **A,** Peripheral blood smear in sickle cell disease. Note the presence of sickle cells and prominent target cells. A Howell-Jolly body is also present, consistent with auto-infarction and subsequent loss of splenic function. **B,** Schematic of sickle cell and Howell-Jolly body.

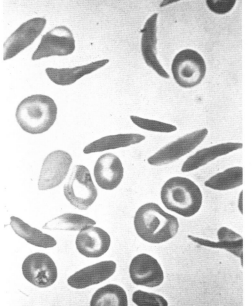

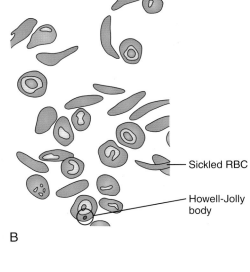

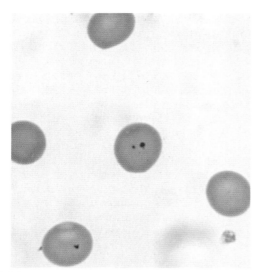

Figure 11-28. Heinz body prep. This peripheral blood smear of a 2-week-old infant with brisk hemolytic anemia demonstrates a positive Heinz body prep. The dark-staining material within two of the red blood cells shows the precipitated hemoglobin that one may see in a condition called *unstable hemoglobin.*

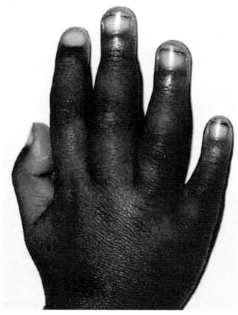

Figure 11-30. Dactylitis (hand-foot syndrome). This syndrome, in children with sickle cell disease, primarily affects toddlers. Dactylitis is seen less frequently in older children because the bone marrow of the small bones of the hands and feet loses hematopoietic activity. This loss of marrow activity is due to cortical thickening from increased use of hands and weight bearing by the feet.

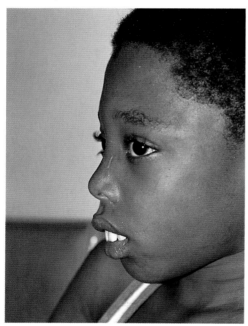

Figure 11-29. Maxillary hyperplasia. Prominent facial bones of a child with sickle cell anemia, due to enlargement of the marrow cavity in this condition of decreased red blood cell survival.

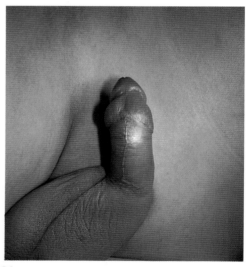

Figure 11-31. Priapism in an adolescent with sickle cell disease. Erection had persisted for 12 hours and had become extremely painful for the patient.

sia and the so-called sickle cell facies (Fig. 11-29). Sickle cells have altered rheology and lose the ability to deform in the microcirculation (see Fig. 11-20). This leads to a logjam phenomenon, causing tissue infarction and painful crises. This logjamming, also referred to as *vaso-occlusive crisis,* when occurring in certain locations, gives rise to clinical manifestations such as dactylitis (Fig. 11-30) in the toddler, priapism (Fig. 11-31), splenic sequestration, and skin ulceration.

The vaso-occlusive phenomenon may also lead to life-threatening complications of sickle cell disease: overwhelming infection with encapsulated organisms (most often *Pneumococcus*), acute chest syndrome, and stroke. The increased infectious risk in the sickle cell patient has multiple mechanisms, but by far the most important is

splenic dysfunction related to congested blood flow and then, ultimately, splenic infarction.

The peripheral smear of a patient with sickle cell disease is often diagnostic of a sickling disorder (see Fig. 11-26).

Sickle cell disease is an autosomal recessive disorder with the heterozygote having a significant but less than 50% proportion of hemoglobin of the sickle cell type. Heterozygous carriers of the sickle cell gene, although suffering a number of difficulties (e.g., poor urine-concentrating ability, occasional episodes of renal papillary necrosis with hematuria), have normal life expectancies and are virtually free of any significant consequences of their heterozygous state.

An effective screening test—the sickle cell preparation—is widely available. It identifies the child with at least 20% Hgb S. It is not useful for distinguishing sickle cell disease from the heterozygous sickle cell trait. Additionally, it may fail to detect a hemoglobinopathy related to a hemoglobin other than hemoglobin S, and it may also fail to detect a neonate who has not yet started to synthesize significant amounts of hemoglobin SS.

Hemoglobin C Disease: Though less common than sickle cell disease, disease associated with Hgb C is not rare in the African-American population. As in sickle cell disease, Hgb C disease occurs because of one amino acid change. The change, again like Hgb S, is at the sixth position of the β-chain but is a lysine rather than a valine replacement. In its homozygous form, Hgb C disease is a mild disorder characterized by hemolytic anemia and splenomegaly. The tendency of Hgb C to aggregate into precipitates is responsible for the characteristic target (actually a pseudotarget; see Fig. 11-25B) morphology of the Hgb C homozygous and Hgb C trait (heterozygous) cells on the peripheral blood smear. Vaso-occlusive phenomena are not associated with this disease, although target cells are formed on the dried peripheral blood smear. However, Hgb C, when paired in a double heterozygous state with Hgb S, results in Hgb SC disease (see Fig. 11-27) and is associated with vaso-occlusive phenomena, though less severe than Hgb SS.

Red Blood Cell Enzyme Abnormalities. Abnormalities of the RBC enzymes may also lead to hemolysis. Although almost any of the RBC enzymes involved in RBC glycolysis or free radical detoxification via the pentose shunt may be responsible for hemolysis, glucose-6-phosphate dehydrogenase (G6PD) deficiency is by far the most frequent. A second enzyme, pyruvate kinase (PK), when deficient, also leads to a hemolytic state. PK deficiency, although far less frequently seen than G6PD deficiency, is prevalent enough to deserve attention in this discussion. The blood smears of patients with RBC enzyme deficiency–induced hemolysis are often normal, although occasionally with G6PD deficiency, a suspicious morphology may be present (Fig. 11-32).

More than 370 variants of G6PD have been identified, for which enzyme activity may be normal, elevated, or severely deficient. G6PD deficiency is transmitted by a sex-linked recessive mode of inheritance. The G6PD gene is localized to the X chromosome. Heterozygous females

may rarely be affected because of inactivation of the X chromosome according to the Lyon hypothesis or because they are doubly heterozygous. Clinical syndromes may vary as well, with the degree of hemolysis paralleling inversely the level of G6PD activity. In all instances the hemolysis is due to the intracellular generation of free radicals and peroxides, which fail to be detoxified by the patient with G6PD deficiency.

Chronic hemolysis is extremely mild and subclinical in the common types. Triggered hemolysis associated with G6PD deficiency (Mediterranean type) is severe and abrupt and parallels inversely the severe enzyme deficiency. In contrast, triggered hemolysis with G6PD deficiency (A-type) may be severe but self-limited when the enzyme deficiency is mild. In addition, some agents that trigger hemolysis with G6PD deficiency (Mediterranean type) may be tolerated by patients with G6PD deficiency (A-type). A list of some drugs associated with clinically significant hemolysis in G6PD deficiency is provided (Table 11-4). Recent work has deemphasized the role of certain drug triggers. In many instances the infection being treated by certain drugs rather than the drugs themselves is responsible for the hemolysis.

Pyruvate kinase deficiency is the second most prevalent enzyme abnormality of the RBC that leads to hemolysis; however, it is a far second, indeed, with one case of PK deficiency occurring worldwide for 500,000 cases of G6PD deficiency. Autosomal recessive transmission of the enzyme defect is usually observed in PK deficiency. Like G6PD deficiency, wide clinical variability exists with PK deficiency. Mild, fully compensated hemolytic anemia, as well as severe neonatal hemolysis and hyperbilirubinemia, may occur. Hemoglobin levels range from 6 to 10 g/dL with normochromic anemia with normocytic or macrocytic indices, depending on the degree of reticulocytosis. The reticulocyte count can range from 5% to as high as 90% in the patient who has had a splenectomy. For the subgroup of patients with severe, transfusion-dependent disease, splenectomy may ameliorate or eliminate the need for transfusions. In addition to chronic hemolysis, PK deficiency may have triggered episodes (usually resulting from intercurrent infection).

Hemolysis Caused by Extra-RBC Factors

Microangiopathic Hemolysis. Hemolysis of RBCs can occur not only from intrinsic abnormalities of the RBCs but also from alterations in the RBC environment. Microangiopathic hemolytic anemia, a hematologic condition of diverse causes, is most often acquired and, rarely, congenital in origin. The hematologic picture is characterized by the presence of burr erythrocytes, schistocytes, helmet cells, and microspherocytes. In almost all cases there is concurrent thrombocytopenia. Additional laboratory studies confirm the presence of intravascular hemolysis

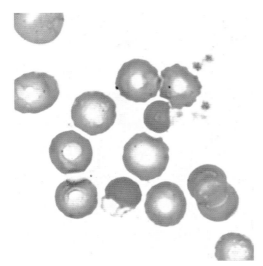

Figure 11-32. Peripheral blood smear of a patient with G6PD deficiency. This patient is experiencing a hemolytic crisis. Note the blister cells with hemoglobin condensed in the remaining (nonblistered) portion of the cell.

Table 11-4	Drugs Associated with Clinically Significant Hemolysis in G6PD Deficiency
Antimalarials	Salicylazosulfapyridine
Pamaquine	Sulfamethoxypyridazine
Pentaquine	Sulfapyridine
Primaquine	Thiazolesulfone
Quinocide	**Miscellaneous**
Antipyretics and Analgesics	Acetylphenylhydrazine
Acetanilid	Fava beans
Aminopyrine	Nalidixic acid
Antipyrine	Naphthalene
Sulfa Drugs	Phenylhydrazine
N-Acetylsulfanilamide	Toluidine blue

G6PD, glucose-6-phosphate dehydrogenase.

including elevated plasma hemoglobin levels, low to absent haptoglobin, and presence of hemosiderinuria.

Elevated serum fibrin degradation products provide evidence for disseminated intravascular coagulation (DIC). In pediatric patients, infection with shock is by far the most frequent cause of DIC. Regardless of the trigger, production of fibrin in the microcirculation and fibrin deposition in capillaries causes shearing of the RBCs as they cross the capillary beds (Fig. 11-33). In addition to RBC destruction, platelets and clotting factors are consumed. Patients may have petechiae, purpura, and persistent bleeding from venipuncture sites. Table 11-5 lists diseases known to trigger DIC.

Microangiopathic changes of the peripheral blood smear may also be seen when RBCs pass through abnormal tissues. Examples of this abnormal physiology include RBC damage in the hemolytic uremic syndrome (HUS) and thrombotic thrombocytopenic purpura (TTP). HUS is a disease of childhood that is primarily characterized by renal insufficiency. TTP is more commonly seen in adults. The patient with TTP experiences neurologic complications in addition to renal abnormalities. These disorders have in common hemolytic anemia, thrombocytopenia, and thrombotic occlusion of the microvasculature of various organs. Scientific evidence indicates that patients with familial occurrence of this syndrome may have a congenital abnormality in the processing of von Willebrand factor.

Table 11-5	Clinical Equivalent of Experimental DIC-Triggering Agents

Gram-negative septicemia
Necrotizing enterocolitis
Shock from any cause
Endothelial damage (virus, bacteria, rickettsia, heat stroke)
Trauma, burns
Ascitic fluid (LeVeen shunt)
Hypoxia-acidosis, severe hyaline membrane disease
Malignancies (acute leukemia, neuroblastoma, rhabdomyosarcoma)
Dead fetal twin
Hemolysis transfusion reaction
Small-for-gestational-age infant (placental infarct)
Purpura fulminans
Localized giant hemangioma

Modified from Corrigan JJ: Disseminated intravascular coagulopathy. Pediatr Rev 1:39-45, 1979.

Finally, a microangiopathic hemolytic anemia occurs in the Kasabach-Merritt syndrome. In this condition, blood flow within a giant hemangioma leads to a consumptive coagulopathy characterized by hypofibrinogenemia, elevated fibrin degradation products, microangiopathic fragmentation of red cells, and thrombocytopenia.

Malaria. Malaria is the most frequent cause of hemolysis on a worldwide scale. The patient who contracts the disease after being fed on by the tropical *Anopheles* mosquito is parasitized within the RBCs with organisms at the merozoite stage (Fig. 11-34). The parasitization causes a clinical picture of intermittent fever, chills, and jaundice and may lead to encephalopathy, massive hemolysis with hemoglobinuria (blackwater fever), and death. The cause of the hemolysis has been attributed to multiple mechanisms including altered RBC osmotic fragility, membrane loss of negative surface charge, direct injury by the parasite, autoimmunity, splenic pitting, and hypersplenism.

White Blood Cells

Normal values for total WBC number and differential counts are age related (Table 11-6). Black patients may have lower granulocyte counts than whites of the same age. Leukocytosis and leukopenia are common pediatric problems. Generally, these are due to increases or decreases in specific types of WBCs. Most cases of neutrophilia (Fig. 11-35), neutropenia, eosinophilia (Fig. 11-36), lymphocytosis (Fig. 11-37), lymphopenia, or monocytosis (Fig. 11-38) in the pediatric population do not represent primary hematologic disorders. The abnormalities of the blood count often represent the bone marrow response to an associated condition. The pertinent history and physical examination findings related to increases or decreases in WBC numbers are outlined throughout this atlas for various disease states.

Leukemia and Leukemoid Reactions

In some cases a leukocytosis may result from an increase in the number of immature rather than mature WBCs of any given cell line (a so-called *shift to the left*). Leukemia (Fig. 11-39) is the prototype, and Figures 11-40 to 11-43 illustrate the varied appearances of blast cells. Figure 11-44 shows a leukemoid reaction, which is characterized by a high WBC count (usually >50,000/mm^3) with an increase in the number of immature myeloid cells.

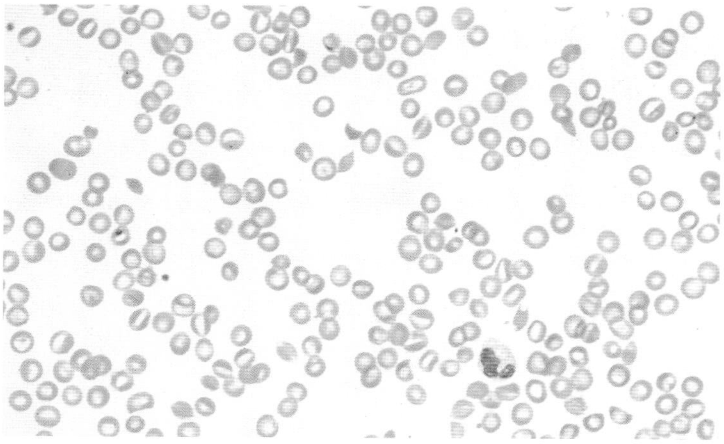

Figure 11-33. Disseminated intravascular coagulation (DIC). Peripheral blood smear of a child with meningococcemia and DIC. Note the red blood cell fragments and decreased platelet count.

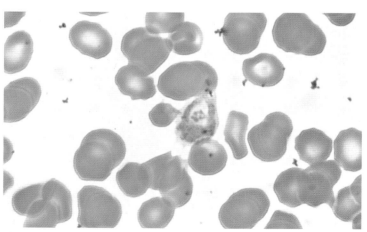

Figure 11-34. *Plasmodium vivax* malaria. This peripheral blood smear is prepared by the so-called "thick prep" method. *Plasmodium vivax* malaria is seen intracellularly in the red blood cell in the center of the smear.

Table 11-6	Normal Leukocyte and Differential Counts*			
	12 MONTHS	**4 YEARS**	**10 YEARS**	**21 YEARS**
Leukocytes, total	11.4 (6.0-17.5)	9.1 (5.5-15.5)	8.1 (4.5-13.5)	7.4 (4.5-11.0)
Neutrophils, total	3.5 (1.5-8.5) (31%)	3.8 (1.5-8.5) (42%)	4.4 (1.8-8.0) (54%)	4.4 (1.8-7.7) (59%)
Neutrophils, band forms	0.35 (3.1%)	0.27 (0-1.0) (3.0%)	0.24 (0-1.0) (3.0%)	0.22 (0-0.7) (3.0%)
Neutrophils, segmented	3.2 (28%)	3.5 (1.5-7.5) (39%)	4.2 (1.8-7.0) (51%)	4.2 (1.8-7.0) (56%)
Eosinophils	0.30 (0.05-0.70) (2.6%)	0.25 (0.02-0.65) (2.8%)	0.20 (0-0.60) (2.4%)	0.20 (0-0.45) (2.7%)
Basophils	0.05 (0-10) (0.4%)	0.05 (0-0.20) (0.6%)	0.04 (0-0.20) (0.5%)	0.04 (0-0.20) (0.5%)
Lymphocytes	7.0 (4.0-10.5) (61%)	4.5 (2.0-8.0) (50%)	3.1 (1.5-6.5) (38%)	2.5 (1.0-4.8) (34%)
Monocytes	0.55 (0.05-1.1) (4.8%)	0.45 (0-0.8) (5.0%)	0.35 (0-0.8) (4.3%)	0.30 (0-0.8) (4.0%)

*Values are expressed as cells × 10^3/μL. Mean values are given; ranges are in parentheses. Percent is for mean values.
From Altman PL, Dittmer DS (eds): Blood and Other Body Fluids. Washington, DC, Federation of American Societies for Experimental Biology, 1961.

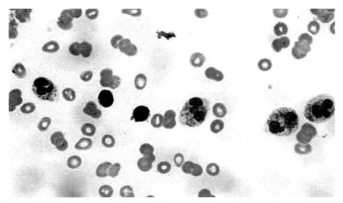

Figure 11-35. Neutrophilia and increased band forms (left shift). The pattern of a left shift of the white blood cell series is consistent with infection. The peripheral blood smear shows increased neutrophils and band forms in a child with pneumococcal sepsis.

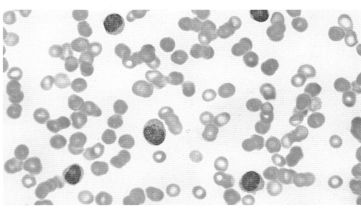

Figure 11-37. Lymphocytosis. An elevated lymphocyte count is seen in the peripheral blood smear of a child with pertussis.

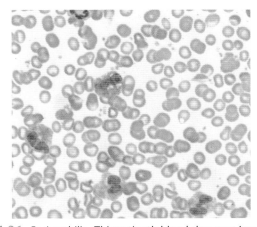

Figure 11-36. Eosinophilia. This patient's blood shows an increased WBC count and increased eosinophils due to a parasitic infection.

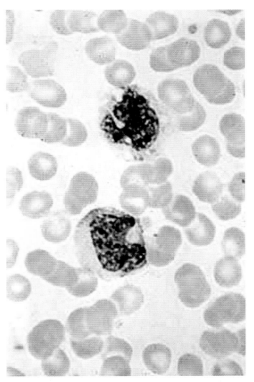

Figure 11-38. Monocytosis. The peripheral blood will often show an increased monocyte count at a time of marrow recovery after significant suppression. In this case the child is recovering from a chemotherapy-induced neutropenia.

Among the many causes of leukemoid reactions are infection and rheumatologic disorders. Leukemoid reactions must be distinguished from leukemia. Although this is definitively accomplished by a bone marrow aspirate, peripheral blood studies can assist a diagnosis. The leukocyte alkaline phosphatase level (LAP score) is increased in leukemoid reaction and decreased in chronic myelogenous leukemia. An elevated WBC count may also be associated with leukoerythroblastosis (Fig. 11-45). This term describes a finding in the peripheral blood in which increased numbers of immature granulocytes are accompanied on the smear by nucleated RBCs, RBC fragments, RBC teardrops, and large platelets. This morphologic condition has a wide differential including a spectrum of myeloproliferative disorders ranging from myelofibrosis to chronic myelogenous leukemia, polycythemia vera, and essential thrombocythemia. These conditions are rare in childhood. Patients with Down syndrome may experience a transient leukemoid reaction (transient myeloproliferative disorder) in the newborn period. Additional manifesta-

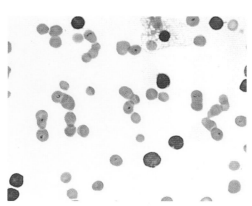

Figure 11-39. Acute lymphoblastic leukemia—peripheral blood smear. Note the presence of decreased platelets and the absence of normal white blood cells.

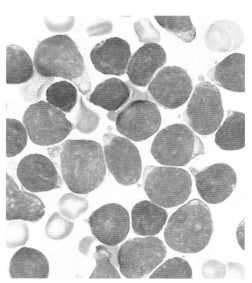

Figure 11-40. Acute lymphoblastic leukemia—bone marrow aspirate. This bone marrow aspiration is from the child whose peripheral blood is shown in Figure 11-45. Note the monotonous pattern of the lymphoblastic (L₁) cells.

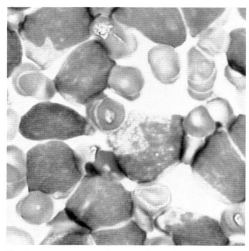

Figure 11-41. Bone marrow aspirate (L₂ lymphoblasts) in another patient with acute lymphoblastic leukemia. These lymphoblasts are larger and more heterogeneous in appearance than the L₁ lymphoblasts. Additionally, the nuclear-to-cytoplasmic ratio is lower, and nucleoli more prominent, than the L₁ lymphoblast.

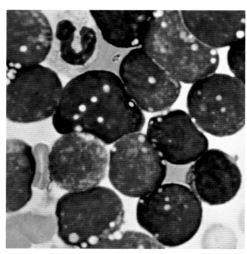

Figure 11-42. L₃ lymphoblasts. This represents the third morphologic presentation of the lymphoblast. These lymphoblasts are large, deeply staining cells that are often vacuolated. The L₃ lymphoblastic cell is characteristic of Burkitt's leukemia and lymphoma.

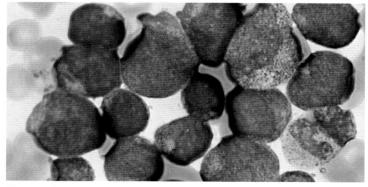

Figure 11-43. Acute myelogenous leukemia. Peripheral blood smear showing an Auer rod (red, rod-shaped figure in the cytoplasm) within a myeloblast of a patient with acute nonlymphocytic/acute myelogenous leukemia.

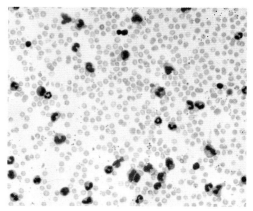

Figure 11-44. Leukemoid reaction. Elevated white blood cell (WBC) count in response to infection. The child whose blood is pictured here was documented to have pneumococcal sepsis with an appropriate WBC response.

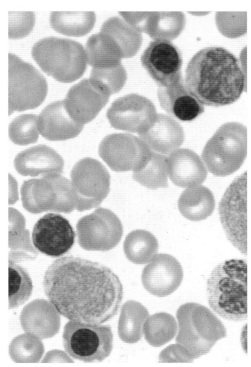

Figure 11-45. Leukoerythroblastosis. Note the presence of immature white blood cells and nucleated red blood cells, not normally found in the peripheral blood smear.

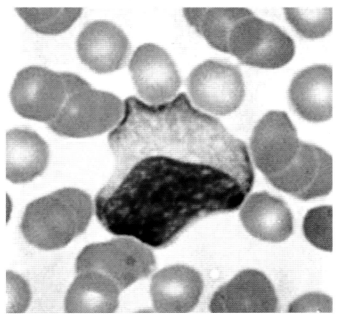

Figure 11-46. Atypical lymphocyte in the case of infectious mononucleosis. Atypical lymphocytes in the peripheral blood are often observed in patients with infectious mononucleosis. The nucleus is large, and the cytoplasm is abundant. Note that where the cytoplasm of the lymphocyte abuts the red blood cell, the lymphocyte deforms around it.

tions of this disorder include hepatosplenomegaly and circulating myeloblasts. Spontaneous remission often occurs. However, 20% to 30% of patients with Down syndrome and the transient myeloproliferative disorder develop leukemia within the first 3 years of life.

Morphologic Abnormalities

With or without an absolute increase in the numbers of specific WBC subsets, there may be morphologic abnormalities in the WBC. Increased numbers of young lymphocytes that are not lymphoblasts are often accompanied by morphologic abnormalities, the most common of which is the atypical lymphocyte (Fig. 11-46). This is a large cell with an irregular plasma membrane that often "hugs" adjacent RBCs. Its nucleus is also large, and nucleoli may be visible. The abundant cytoplasm is typically basophilic and may contain vacuoles and azurophilic granules. Morphologic subtypes of atypical lymphocytes may occur, but clinically, their recognition is of little use. Although infectious mononucleosis comes to mind when atypical lymphocytes are seen, these lymphocytes are not specific and may be present in many other situations, especially viral illnesses.

Morphologic abnormalities of the granulocytic series, although less common, may provide clues to the diagnosis. The hypersegmented neutrophil, which may be an early clue to vitamin B_{12} deficiency, has been noted previously (see Fig. 11-14). This needs to be distinguished from familial hypersegmentation by looking at the peripheral smears of family members.

Neutrophil Abnormalities

Occasionally, mature neutrophils may be abnormally large in members of a given family—the so-called hereditary giant neutrophils. The Pelger-Huët anomaly (Fig. 11-47) is usually a benign morphologic inherited anomaly, but it is sometimes acquired in adults and generally spurs a search for occult malignancy due to its known association with leukemia and lymphoma. This WBC abnormal-

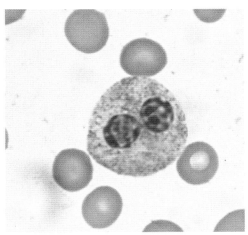

Figure 11-47. Pelger-Huët anomaly. Note the uniform bilobed nucleus of the granulocyte.

ity has also been described in association with infectious and rheumatologic disorders. Increased numbers of nuclear appendages may also be seen in the neutrophils of patients with trisomy 13 (Fig. 11-48). These, however, may be difficult to distinguish from normal neutrophil "drumsticks," which are nuclear appendages that occur in 2% to 10% of neutrophils of normal girls.

Vacuoles can occur in any WBC for a variety of reasons including artifact from anticoagulant agents, infections, or storage diseases. Certain types of inclusions, such as those seen in Gaucher disease, are limited to bone marrow histiocytes and are not detected on examination of the peripheral smear.

Toxic granulations, which are prominent azurophilic granules, are another common type of WBC inclusion. They are nonspecific but can be seen in viral and bacterial infections (Fig. 11-49). Toxic granulations must be distinguished from the hereditary dense granulation that may occasionally be present in the neutrophils of normal individuals. Döhle bodies, pale blue inclusions that usually are located peripherally in the cytoplasm of neutrophils, may coexist with toxic granulations. Together with giant platelets, Döhle bodies are seen in patients with the dominantly inherited May-Hegglin anomaly (Fig. 11-50).

Reilly bodies, or Alder-Reilly bodies, are metachromatic prominent granules when stained with toluidine blue. When present in WBCs, they are virtually pathognomonic of Hurler syndrome (Fig. 11-51). Coarse azurophilic neutrophilic granules that resemble Reilly bodies but are nonmetachromatic have been reported in Batten disease. Likewise, large greenish-brown neutrophil inclusions are characteristic of the patient with rare Chédiak-Higashi syndrome (Fig. 11-52). Such granules may appear in eosinophils and basophils as well.

WBCs may also acquire inclusions by engulfing particles from their surroundings. Erythrophagocytosis (Fig. 11-53) is a nonspecific finding that is presumably immune mediated and seen in viral infections and primary dis-

eases of the reticuloendothelial system. The LE cells of systemic lupus erythematosus are a diagnostically useful example of cellular phagocytosis, although in general, they are not seen on routine peripheral blood smears. Figure 11-54 shows a buffy-coat preparation from a patient with suspected sepsis, demonstrating intracellular bacteria. In most of these WBC anomalies, the clinical diagnosis is often suspected on the basis of presenting signs and symptoms even before the hematologic abnormality is identified. One exception to this rule is the toddler with moderate to severe neutropenia that may be chronic yet benign. The conditions of many of these children are entirely asymptomatic, and the neutropenia is an incidental finding. However, chronic benign neutropenia is a diagnosis of exclusion. The differential diagnosis is reviewed elsewhere.

Bleeding Disorders

Excessive bleeding or bruising is a common complaint during childhood. The hematologic causes (to be distinguished from child abuse, trauma, vascular anomalies) fall into two categories: disorders of platelets and coagulopathies. The child with mucocutaneous bleeding or purpura, petechiae, or ecchymoses (Fig. 11-55) is most likely to fall

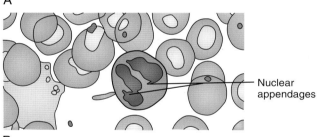
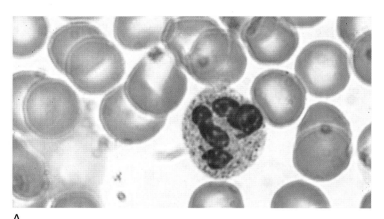

Figure 11-48. A, Nuclear appendages are normally seen in the polymorphonuclear leukocytes of girls. An increase in these appendages is seen in cases of trisomy 13. **B,** Schematic of nuclear appendages.

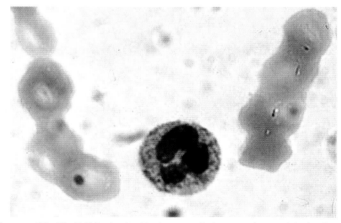

Figure 11-49. Döhle body. Toxic granulations and a Döhle body are found in the blood of this child with sepsis. The Döhle body appears as a grayish-blue staining area, which is located at the inferior border of this cell.

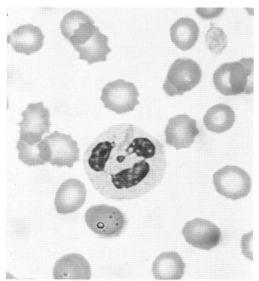
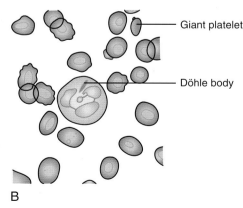

Figure 11-50. A, May-Hegglin anomaly. The peripheral blood of individuals with this condition demonstrates Döhle bodies in the white blood cells and giant platelets that may be decreased in number. **B,** Schematic of May-Hegglin anomaly.

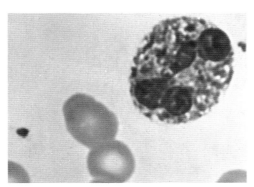

Figure 11-51. Polymorphonuclear leukocytes with prominent granules characterize Reilly bodies, as are seen in the storage disease, Hurler syndrome.

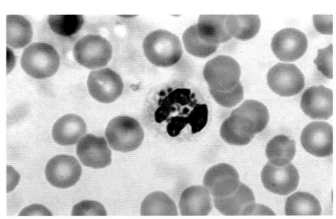

Figure 11-52. Chédiak-Higashi syndrome. Note the neutrophilic inclusion characteristic of this rare disease. (Courtesy William Zinkham, MD, Baltimore.)

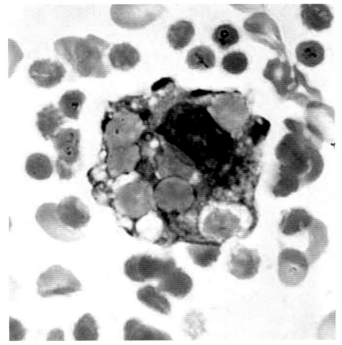

Figure 11-53. Erythrophagocytosis. Numerous red blood cells are engulfed by white blood cell cytoplasm in this peripheral blood smear of a patient with erythrophagocytosis.

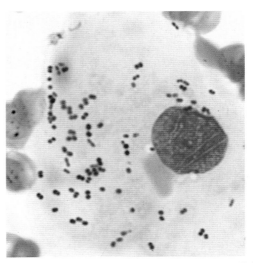

Figure 11-54. Intracellular bacteria. The presence of intracellular bacteria is detected by Wright stain of a buffy-coat smear from a neutropenic patient. Note the numerous darkly stained bacteria in the cytoplasm.

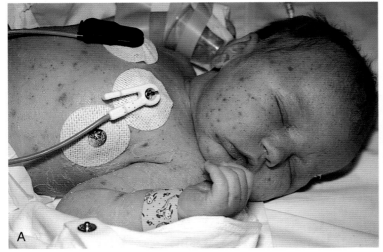

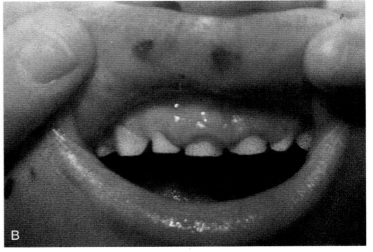

Figure 11-55. **A,** Petechiae. This infant with severe immune thrombocytopenia has visible petechiae, as well as large ecchymoses. **B,** Purpuric lesions on the oral mucosa or retina are called "wet purpura" and may suggest an increased tendency for major bleeding in the thrombocytopenic patient.

into the first; bleeding into deep tissue or joints is most likely to be a reflection of the second. Exceptions to these guidelines exist. Patients with either problem may have bleeding precipitated by trauma or surgery and may develop hematuria, guaiac-positive stools, menorrhagia, or bleeding in the central nervous system. Frequent epistaxis, although possibly related to bleeding disorders, is more likely to have a nonhematologic cause such as nose picking; dry mucous membranes; or, rarely, hypertension. Nonetheless, documentation of these problems or a positive family history usually calls for laboratory evaluation, which likely includes a complete blood count (CBC); differential count; platelet count; and a basic coagulation workup consisting of measurements of prothrombin time (PT), partial thromboplastin time (PTT), and bleeding time or closure time. The closure time is performed using a cartridge system in which the process of platelet adhesion and aggregation is simulated in vitro. This in vitro testing system provides improved reproducibility, accuracy, and reliability when compared with the standard bleeding time. Recognizing that all patients with petechiae and purpura are not thrombocytopenic is also important. These clinical manifestations may result from both quantitative and qualitative platelet defects.

Platelet Disorders

A CBC and peripheral blood smear reveal a platelet count that, if normal, is 150,000/mm^3 to 450,000/mm^3. The smear does not give information regarding the diseases of platelet function that are less often seen, but it does confirm quantitative abnormalities. Clinically, thrombocytopenia may be inapparent until counts are significantly depressed below normal and frank purpura is infrequently seen with counts greater than 20,000/mm^3. Ascertaining that the decreased platelet number is not a spurious finding by repeating the test and reviewing the blood smear is important. The child whose peripheral blood smear is shown in Figure 11-50 unfortunately underwent a splenectomy for presumed idiopathic thrombocytopenic purpura. However, the platelet count persistently was reported as less than 20,000/mm^3, whereas the manually performed platelet count number was considerably higher. The Coulter counter had ignored these large platelets and incorrectly counted them as WBCs.

Isolated thrombocytopenia may result from decreased production or from increased destruction of platelets. The etiologies for the latter are numerous and include the idiopathic or immune thrombocytopenias, hypersplenism, DIC, consumption related to intracardiac defect or bypass surgery, washout from exchange transfusion, local microangiopathic disease (hemolytic uremic syndrome), or local thrombosis (renal vein thrombosis).

DIC has already been discussed as a cause of hemolysis and occurs most often in the pediatric age range as a secondary phenomenon related to shock in bacterial or, less frequently, viral sepsis (see Fig. 11-33). DIC is also seen in Kasabach-Merritt syndrome when platelet consumption occurs within the endothelial maze of massive strawberry and cavernous hemangiomas (Fig. 11-56).

The clinical setting often helps distinguish when thrombocytopenia is due to platelet destruction as opposed to decreased production. The peripheral blood smear may reveal large or even giant platelets (Fig. 11-57). Presence of large platelets suggests an active bone marrow with peripheral destruction of platelets rather than an abnormality of production. A therapeutic trial of intravenous immunoglobulin or anti-D antibody may define the diagnosis of idiopathic or immune thrombocytopenia (ITP) in

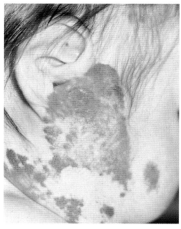
Figure 11-56. The hemangiomatous lesion in this patient resulted in Kasabach-Merritt syndrome, in which platelet consumption within the lesion leads to thrombocytopenia.

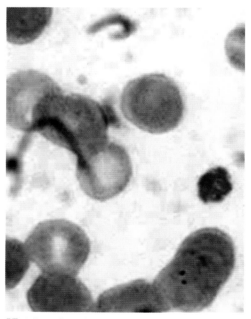
Figure 11-57. Idiopathic thrombocytopenia (ITP). Megathrombocytes (giant platelets) are often seen in the peripheral blood of patients with ITP.

the patient with isolated thrombocytopenia and large platelets. These interventions do not mask the diagnosis of a process of marrow infiltration because patients with abnormal production of platelets do not respond to this therapy. Bone marrow evaluation is necessary in the absence of response to these therapies. The bone marrow in the setting of ITP has normal to increased numbers of megakaryocytes (Fig. 11-58) and no evidence of abnormal cells. Isoimmune thrombocytopenia in the newborn occurs when fetal platelets cross the placenta into the maternal circulation and may, depending on the platelet antigens, trigger a maternal production of IgG aimed at the foreign platelet antigen. These antiplatelet antibodies can then cross the placenta and lead to infant thrombocytopenia. Isoimmune thrombocytopenia in the newborn should be suspected in the setting of a normal maternal platelet count. The neonate is at risk for hemorrhagic complications including cephalhematoma, bleeding from the umbilicus, and intracranial hemorrhage. Treatment options include washed maternal platelets and intravenous immunoglobulin.

Patients with isolated thrombocytopenia on the basis of failure of platelet production have decreased or absent megakaryocyte precursors. Differentiation of the various causes of decreased production, such as thrombocytopenia-absent radius syndrome (Fig. 11-59) and amegakaryocytic thrombocytopenia, may rest on clinical findings. Patients with this syndrome may have a number of concurrent problems such as leukemoid reactions, congenital heart disease, and failure to thrive. Their thrombocytopenia frequently resolves as they grow older. Rarely, thrombocytopenia may be caused by a combination of decreased platelet production and increased destruction. This can be seen in sepsis, collagen diseases, and Wiskott-Aldrich syndrome.

Qualitative or functional platelet defects may also lead to a bleeding diathesis. In the setting of normal platelet number and normal clotting studies, the possibility of poorly functioning platelets needs to be considered. As mentioned previously, the standard bleeding time has been replaced by the closure time at many centers. This test is more reliable and less dependent on technical factors including the person performing the test and the level of cooperation of the child. The highly specialized

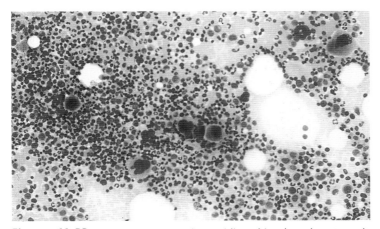

Figure 11-58. Bone marrow aspirate—idiopathic thrombocytopenia (ITP). This bone marrow aspirate shows prominent megakaryocytes consistent with the increased production and immune destruction of platelets in ITP. In children with thrombocytopenia due to decreased production, one would expect megakaryocyte numbers to be decreased.

tests necessary to confirm a diagnosis of platelet dysfunction are available in most large centers. Information in addition to that mentioned, which may point to a reason for platelet dysfunction, includes a history of drug exposure by direct ingestion by the patient or in some cases via breastfeeding (aspirin alone or as a component of another medication is the best known and affects platelet studies for the 7- to 10-day life of the platelet), history of uremia, hypothyroidism, hyperbilirubinemia, and inflammatory bowel disease. Von Willebrand disease is a heritable disorder in which platelet function abnormalities are present. Although platelet function is abnormal in this disease, it is not strictly a disorder of the platelet; rather the predisposition to bleeding and platelet dysfunction is caused by a deficiency or abnormality of von Willebrand factor. This disorder is discussed later in the review of heritable coagulation abnormalities.

Coagulopathies

Coagulopathies occur when the circulating factors necessary for normal coagulation are deficient from lack of production or from excessive consumption. Coagulopathies can occur as genetic defects, as in the decreased production of normal procoagulants (hemophilia), or as acquired conditions resulting in depressed factor production (vitamin K deficiency, liver disease) or overutilization of factors (DIC).

Whatever the cause of coagulopathy, the measurement of the PT and PTT is the first step in clarifying the diagnosis. The clotting system is shown in Figure 11-60. The PT evaluates the extrinsic and common pathways, whereas the PTT evaluates the intrinsic and common pathways. Values for these screening tests are age related so that normal newborns, especially premature infants, have prolonged PTs and PTTs compared with those of older children. These screening tests, although sensitive enough to detect the mild, moderate, or severe deficiencies of hemophilia, are normal in carriers with approximately 50% factor levels.

Heritable Bleeding Disorders
Hemophilias A and B

Although deficiencies have been reported for every procoagulant, factor VIII deficiency (hemophilia A) and factor

Figure 11-59. **A,** Child with thrombocytopenia-absent radius syndrome, also known as *TAR syndrome.* **B,** Radiograph of the same patient. Note the absence of the radius.

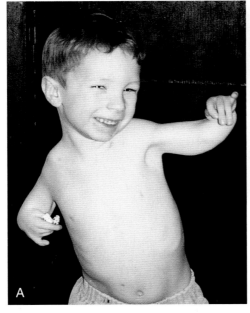

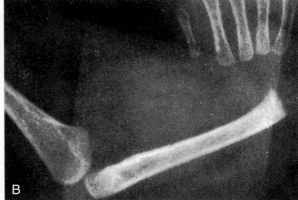

COAGULATION CASCADE

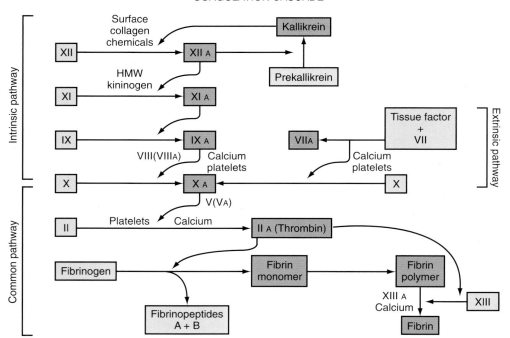

Figure 11-60. Coagulation cascade. The prothrombin time measures the extrinsic and common pathways, whereas the partial thromboplastin time measures the intrinsic and common pathways.

IX deficiency (hemophilia B) make up the majority of hemophilias. Because hemophilias A and B are transmitted in an X-linked recessive inheritance pattern, hemophilia is found nearly always in males. Hemophiliacs may have variable degrees of factor deficiency and commensurate levels of clinical disease. Patients with mild hemophilia have factor activity between 5% and 30% and, in general, suffer only from bleeding if they undergo surgery or suffer major trauma. Patients with moderate hemophilia have a factor activity of 1% to 5% and suffer localized hemorrhage in response to trauma. Finally, patients with less than 1% factor activity (the most frequent genotype) have spontaneous soft tissue hemorrhage or bleeding associated with only minor trauma.

Patients with hemophilia may present in the newborn period at the time of circumcision. Infants who escape clinical problems at that time generally do not present until 12 to 18 months of age—when they have become more mobile and minor trauma from falls precipitates bleeding. Although the clinical manifestations of hemophilia can affect any organ, the musculoskeletal, central nervous, and urinary systems predominate. The most common of the clinical manifestations include hemarthroses and soft tissue bleeding with intramuscular hematomas. Secondary hemophiliac arthropathy may also occur, with the knees, elbows, and ankles being the most commonly involved joints. Recurrent, untreated hemorrhages may lead to contractures (Fig. 11-61) and painful arthritis (Fig. 11-62). Finally, intramuscular bleeding can cause compartment syndromes with secondary peripheral nerve palsies.

Von Willebrand Disease

Von Willebrand disease is the most common, heritable bleeding disorder in which the bleeding time or closure time is generally increased with or without an increase in the PTT. The majority of cases are autosomal dominant in their inheritance pattern. The condition is frequently asymptomatic, being detected when an abnormal bleeding time, closure time, and/or PTT is noted as part of a preoperative screen. Clinical symptoms, if present, include abnormal mucosal bleeding, such as frequent epistaxis or

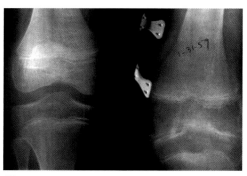

Figure 11-61. Hemophiliac arthritis. This patient with hemophilia has experienced recurrent hemarthroses. Note the widened joint space on the left knee compared with that of the normal right knee.

menorrhagia. The disease is caused by a deficiency or an abnormality of the von Willebrand factor, which is responsible for the adherence of platelets to damaged endothelium. Von Willebrand disease has multiple types, with the most common being type I. The disease may reflect a quantitative (types I and III) or qualitative (type II) defect in the von Willebrand protein. In most cases, measurement of the von Willebrand factor antigen, von Willebrand factor ristocetin cofactor activity, and factor VIII levels in plasma allow differentiation of the specific types of von Willebrand disease. Patients with a deficiency of normal von Willebrand factor may demonstrate correction of coagulation abnormalities following administration of vasopressin (DDAVP) due to its ability to cause release of von Willebrand factor stores from platelets and endothelial cells. Patients who have a qualitatively abnormal protein may require von Willebrand factor replacement through transfused donor blood products for significant bleeding or in preparation for surgical procedures. Vasopressin is not effective in qualitative defects of the protein because release of an increased amount of the abnormal protein does not result in correction of the coagulation abnormality.

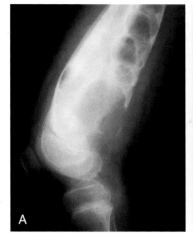 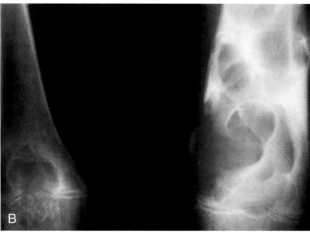

Figure 11-62. **A,** Pseudotumor of the femur. This radiographic finding has resulted from recurrent hemarthroses with subsequent bony destruction of the knee and adjacent bony structures. **B,** Note that the opposite knee also demonstrates early destructive changes in the distal femur and joint.

Acquired Coagulation Abnormalities
Acquired Disorders of Hemostasis

Decreases in clotting factor production may be acquired, as well as inherited. Hepatic synthesis of clotting factors may be depressed in vitamin K–deficient patients. Vitamin K deficiency in the newborn may be suggested by cephalhematomas, bleeding from scalp or mouth sites, or intracranial hemorrhage, particularly if there has been inadvertent omission of prophylactic vitamin K administration, breastfeeding, antibiotics, or maternal ingestion of vitamin K inhibitors in the last trimester. Prolongation of the PT and PTT is observed in disseminated intravascular coagulation. This condition is characterized by the intravascular consumption of platelets and plasma clotting factors. The abnormal accumulation of fibrin in the microcirculation leads to mechanical injury to RBCs, leading to fragmentation of RBCs and microangiopathic anemia (see Fig. 11-33). This condition is clearly associated with increased risk of bleeding.

Acquired Inhibitors of In Vitro Coagulation

The PT and PTT may be prolonged for a variety of reasons other than hemophilia or decreased factor production. The presence of an acquired inhibitor of in vitro coagulation called a lupus anticoagulant (LAC) provides one such example. The presence of an LAC may be identified by mixing the patient's plasma with normal plasma. If the PT or the PTT fails to correct when normal plasma is added, this indicates that the patient's plasma contains an inhibitor of the in vitro testing process rather than a factor deficiency. This is a critical distinction because an LAC rarely indicates an increased risk of bleeding and may even suggest a predisposition to thrombosis. Approximately 10% of patients with systemic lupus erythematosus harbor such antibodies. Patients may acquire an LAC following exposure to medications or infectious organisms. This antibody may persist for months after the exposure.

Thrombotic Disorders

Hemostasis involves a delicate balance of procoagulant and antithrombotic factors. Any condition, inherited or acquired, that disrupts this balance may lead to a bleeding tendency as described earlier or, alternatively, a predisposition to thrombosis. Risk of venous thrombosis is increased by any factor that contributes to retardation of blood flow. The most serious complication of venous thrombosis is the occurrence of embolization to the pulmonary system.

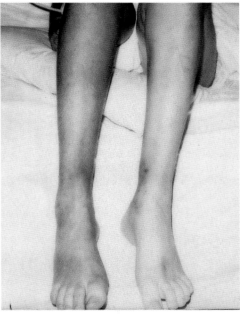

Figure 11-63. Note the swollen, discolored leg in a child with deep venous thrombosis resulting from protein C deficiency. (Courtesy R. Kellogg, MD.)

Arterial thrombosis tends to occur under conditions of rapid blood flow in which endothelial damage to the vessel wall leads to vascular occlusion. Elements of history that may suggest a hypercoagulable state include a family history of thrombosis, thrombosis at an early age (Fig. 11-63) or recurrent thrombosis, recurrent spontaneous abortions, or thrombosis during pregnancy. Predisposing conditions for venous thrombosis include indwelling catheters, severe dehydration, immobilization, and nephrotic syndrome.

Thrombotic events are rare in children relative to the occurrence of thrombosis in adults. The greatest risk periods for a thrombotic event during childhood occur during infancy and adolescence. Incidence of venous thrombosis has increased in recent years due to widespread use of central venous catheters for supportive care in the setting of many childhood diseases including the treatment of childhood malignancies.

Heritable deficiencies of anticoagulant factors including protein C, protein S, and antithrombin III (ATIII) have long been known to predispose to thrombosis. Protein C is a vitamin K–dependent glycoprotein that inhibits the procoagulant factors Va and VIIIa, thereby decreasing clot formation. Protein S is an important cofactor that is required for optimal anticoagulant activity of activated protein C. Therefore deficiency of either protein leads to an increased risk of thrombosis. ATIII is also a glycoprotein inhibitor that acts through the formation of complexes with thrombin, factor Xa, and factor IXa. This reaction accounts for the major mechanism of inhibition of thrombin, factor Xa, and factor IXa. ATIII deficiency results in loss of inhibition of these procoagulant factors, leading to a prothrombotic state. The lupus anticoagulant, discussed previously, is also associated with an increased risk of thrombosis. Finally, paroxysmal nocturnal hemoglobinuria (PNH) is a rare disorder of childhood. It is a clonal stem cell disorder in which cells demonstrate an increased sensitivity to the lytic action of complement. Clinical manifestations include abdominal and back pain, chronic intravascular hemolysis, intermittent hemoglobinuria, and diffuse venous thrombosis.

Advances in the evaluation of the hypercoagulable state include the ability to detect genetic mutations known to result in increased risk of thrombosis. These genetic conditions include factor V Leiden, the factor II prothrombin gene variant, and the methylene tetrahydrofolate reductase (MTHFR) gene mutation. The factor V Leiden mutation leads to activated protein C (APC) resistance. APC inhibits coagulation by degrading factors Va and VIIIa. Factor V Leiden is more slowly inactivated by APC, leading to increased risk of thrombosis. The prothrombin gene variant is associated with increased factor II levels in plasma and increased risk of thrombosis. The MTHFR gene mutation is a thermolabile variant associated with increased plasma homocysteine levels and increased risk of thrombosis. Genetic testing has a distinct advantage in that the results are unaffected by anticoagulant therapy if the patient has been placed on heparin or warfarin (Coumadin) before the evaluation for a hypercoagulable state. Additionally, due to the consumption of factors with large-vessel thrombus formation, interpretation of low factor levels is limited in the setting of active clotting. Results of genetic testing are unaffected by the changes in coagulation factor levels that occur during times of active thrombus formation. However, our understanding of thrombotic risk relating to these genetic mutations in children remains limited. The majority of clinical research studies to date have been in the adult population. Additional studies are necessary to further define risk of thrombosis associated for individuals in the pediatric age range.

Pancytopenia

Pancytopenia refers to a reduction in all three formed elements of the blood. In an analogous manner to anemia, pancytopenia is not a single disease entity but rather may result from a number of disease processes. Pancytopenia may occur from bone marrow failure or extramedullary cellular destruction (as seen in autoimmune disease, particularly systemic lupus erythematosus) or as a combination of depressed marrow function and increased cellular destruction. When pancytopenia is due to destruction of the formed elements of the blood, invariably there is another underlying disease. On the other hand, the pancytopenia resulting from bone marrow failure can be divided into genetically predisposed (constitutional) marrow failure syndromes, acquired marrow failure syndromes, and marrow replacement.

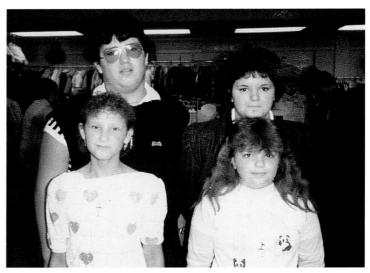

Figure 11-64. A patient with Fanconi anemia is pictured with her three siblings. This patient had a bone marrow transplant for her underlying condition. Note her diminutive size with respect to her more robust siblings.

The most frequent of the constitutional marrow failure syndromes is Fanconi anemia. Fanconi anemia is a familial disorder marked by the association of pancytopenia and marrow hypoplasia with a variable constellation of congenital anomalies of the skin, skeleton, central nervous system, and genitourinary tract (Fig. 11-64). Fragility of the chromosomes further characterizes this syndrome, and it occurs even in the absence of physical anomalies. Patients may have anemia early in life but generally develop signs of marrow failure in midchildhood. The abnormal chromosomes are the most characteristic laboratory finding, and chromosome breaks, gaps, and rearrangements are common.

Acquired marrow failure syndromes (aplastic anemia) occur as a result of an insult to the bone marrow from a variety of sources including drugs, toxins, solvents, and radiation, as well as autoimmune and postinfectious disorders. Nevertheless, 50% of aplastic anemia cases have no apparent insulting agent and are idiopathic in origin.

The clinical course of aplastic anemia from any of these causes is that of inexorable bone marrow failure with anemia, thrombocytopenia, and leukopenia, leading ultimately to death from bleeding or infection if spontaneous recovery or successful intervention fails to occur.

Although the peripheral smear reveals a paucity of platelets and WBCs with a low reticulocyte count and normochromic and normocytic anemia, a marrow aspirate and possibly biopsy generally is necessary to clarify the diagnosis in the patient with pancytopenia (Fig. 11-65).

Marrow replacement, another cause of pancytopenia, occurs with a hematopoietic malignancy such as leukemia (see Fig. 11-40) or from solid tumors invading the marrow (Fig. 11-66). A direct "crowding out" phenomenon and an alteration of the marrow "milieu" appear to contribute to marrow failure.

Acute leukemia is the most common cause of malignant replacement of marrow in childhood. The leukemic blast represents a clonal expansion of a cell at a specific stage of lymphoid or myeloid development. Clinical symptoms may include fever, fatigue, pallor, and bone pain as evidenced by limping. Acute lymphoblastic leukemia (ALL) accounts for approximately 75% of pediatric cases of acute leukemia. The peak age range is between 2 and 5 years of

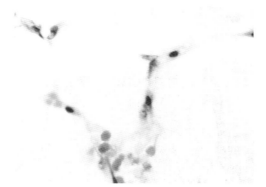

Figure 11-65. Acquired aplastic anemia—bone marrow biopsy. Note the presence of stromal marrow cells with virtually no hematopoietic elements present.

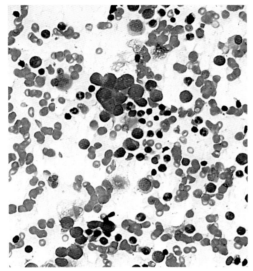

Figure 11-66. Pseudorosette formation in neuroblastoma. This pattern of tumor cells within the marrow is a characteristic of neuroblastic cells found in the bone marrow.

age. Acute myeloid leukemia (AML) is the other predominant leukemia of childhood, accounting for approximately 20% of cases. The incidence of AML is stable from birth to 10 years of age. There is a slight increase in the number of cases during the teenage years. The finding of pancytopenia, organomegaly, and lymphadenopathy in these conditions relates directly to infiltration of marrow and normal organ tissues with the expanded leukemic clone. Additional discussion of hematologic malignancy is included subsequently in the oncology section.

Pancytopenia may also be seen in hemophagocytic syndrome, also known as *hemophagocytic lymphohistiocytosis*. This term encompasses a number of disorders including conditions that are congenital or acquired. The disorder is best described as "reactive" in nature, and is due to abnormalities of the antigen-presenting and antigen processing histiocytes. This syndrome, when occurring in infants, is often of the familial or genetic type. Hemophagocytosis may also occur in association with systemic infection (viral, bacterial, fungal, or parasitic), underlying malignant disease, or as a manifestation of immune deficiency. By definition, patients must have at least two of the following hematologic abnormalities: Anemia less than 9 g/dL hemoglobin; thrombocytopenia of less than 100,000/µl; neutropenia of less than 1000 neutrophils/µl. Additional clinical findings must also be present including fever and splenomegaly. Associated laboratory

abnormalities include hypertriglyceridemia and hypofibrinogenemia. Finally, hemophagocytosis must be visualized in the bone marrow, spleen, and/or lymph nodes. These disorders are characterized by hemophagocytosis in the lymphoreticular system or central nervous system. Prognosis is dependent upon the origin as a congenital or acquired variant. The genetic form often leads to a rapid clinical deterioration with a guarded long-term prognosis. In secondary HLH, those individuals who survive their acute process, if no underlying immunodeficiency, have a more favorable prognosis.

Oncology

Pediatric malignancy is rare when compared with the incidence of cancer in the adult population. However, it remains a significant contributor to the morbidity and mortality of childhood diseases. More than 10,000 new cases of cancer are diagnosed during childhood in the United States each year. The ability to treat and cure childhood malignancies has improved dramatically over the past few decades, which is encouraging. This is due, in large part, to advances made in cooperative group clinical trials, the introduction of novel chemotherapy agents, and the improvements in supportive care for the patient receiving chemotherapy. The majority of children with cancer today will be cured. In the year 2000 an estimated 1 in 900 individuals had survived childhood cancer. Importantly, the pediatrician must be involved in monitoring the surviving children and young adults for late effects of therapy including second malignancies and organ dysfunction due to prior therapy.

The initial task of recognizing the signs and symptoms of malignancy usually falls to the pediatrician or family practitioner. The current chapter aims to review clinical presentations that should alert the primary care physician to the possibility of a malignant process. As with most pediatric conditions, the differential diagnosis varies depending on the age of the child. An immediate concern at the time of diagnosis is to prevent any tumor-related complications including neutropenia due to marrow infiltration or metabolic abnormalities due to increased cell turnover. Signs and symptoms of the most common tumors of childhood are reviewed in a manner that parallels the physical examination. This method may result in some degree of overlap, as many cancers manifest a wide spectrum of presentations that may vary in location within the body. Each tumor subtype is discussed in the context of a region in which it typically presents. For a more detailed description of specific cancers, a more comprehensive text is recommended (see Pizzo and Poplack in Bibliography).

Signs and Symptoms

Red flags that signal malignancy may be detected in the course of history taking, physical examination, or in basic laboratory testing. Table 11-7 provides a summary of signs and symptoms that should alert the physician to the possibility of a malignant process. These features may be due to the direct effect of the tumor (e.g., compression or infiltration of an organ). Alternatively, the rapid cell division may lead to metabolic abnormalities including hyperkalemia, hyperuricemia, or hypocalcemia as a manifestation of tumor lysis. True paraneoplastic syndromes are uncom-

Table 11-7	Red Flags of Malignancy

Pallor, fatigue	Headache, vomiting, lethargy
Petechiae	Lymphadenopathy
Fever without source	Hepatomegaly
Bone pain, limp	Splenomegaly
Weight loss	Abdominal mass
Anorexia	Testiculomegaly

Table 11-8	Groups at High Risk of Cancer

Hereditary cutaneous syndromes (xeroderma pigmentosum)
Neurocutaneous syndromes (neurofibromatosis)
Chromosomal abnormalities (Down syndrome, Bloom syndrome)
Hereditary or acquired immunodeficiency (ataxia-telangiectasia)
Congenital malformations or syndromes (hemihypertrophy,
   Beckwith-Wiedemann syndrome)
History of prior cancer
Intrauterine (diethylstilbestrol) or postnatal (chemotherapy) agents
Radiation
Metabolic diseases (α_1-antitrypsin deficiency)

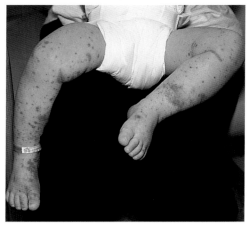

Figure 11-67. This infant has neuroblastoma and purpuric lesions relating to a tumor-related coagulopathy. Similar lesions may result from other conditions such as severe isolated thrombocytopenia and/or disseminated intravascular coagulation.

mon in the pediatric population. An example of such a paraneoplastic process occurs in a small percentage of patients with neuroblastoma. The opsoclonus-myoclonus syndrome (random eye movements and myoclonic jerking) tends to occur in patients with low-stage disease and favorable histology of the tumor. These patients therefore tend to have a favorable prognosis in terms of the cancer. Unfortunately, many are left with devastating developmental and neurocognitive deficits that relate to this rare paraneoplastic condition. Even more rare is the Kerner-Morrison syndrome, in which the patient experiences intractable secretory diarrhea, hypokalemia, and dehydration. This condition represents the secretion of vasoactive intestinal peptide and has also been described in patients with neuroblastoma. In contrast to the opsoclonus-myoclonus syndrome, the symptoms typically resolve with eradication of the tumor. The child with a new diagnosis of malignancy is sometimes asymptomatic, as may be the case in a child with a palpable abdominal mass. In other cases, nonspecific symptoms may be a prominent finding including fever, weight loss, and/or lethargy. Examples of more specific signs and symptoms in pediatric malignancy include the following: headache and morning vomiting in a patient with a brain tumor; constipation and difficulty voiding in a patient with a pelvic tumor or spinal cord compression; hypertension in a child with a renal or suprarenal tumor; bone pain and limping in a young child secondary to leukemia or, less commonly, another marrow infiltrative process.

All of these complaints are more likely to have a cause that is not malignant. However, persistence (2 weeks is a reasonable, though not absolute, guideline) or undue severity may give these signs increased significance. Similarly, in the context of a number of predisposing, underlying diseases (Table 11-8), malignancy should be considered earlier. Certainly, children with a history of one cancer, by virtue of genetics or as a "late effect" of anticancer therapy, are at greater risk of a second cancer. Cancer in a parent or sibling, although heightening anxiety about the possibility of cancer in a child, is rarely by itself a major predisposing factor. The notable exception is the infant or toddler who has an identical twin with leukemia. In this child the risk of leukemia may be as high as 25%. Retinoblastoma and Wilms tumor are also known to occur with increased frequency in offspring of individuals with these diagnoses.

The clinical findings in the child with malignancy vary greatly depending on the site of origin of the tumor. As mentioned previously, the clinical findings are presented in a regional fashion. Every attempt is made to provide a general discussion of individual pediatric cancers through a review of more characteristic physical examination findings. The discussion is not inclusive of all potential manifestations of these diseases. Its intent is to provide a fundamental understanding of the spectrum of malignant diseases of childhood along with the signs and symptoms to alert the physician to their possible presence.

Skin

Morphologic characteristics of cutaneous lesions may allow for the identification of an underlying diagnosis that suggests a predisposition to cancer, such as neurofibromatosis (see Table 11-8). Skin findings also provide a window into bone marrow function through clinical signs such as pallor, indicative of anemia, or bruising and petechiae, suggesting thrombocytopenia. Pallor may be most readily appreciated by examination of the mucous membranes including the conjunctiva and oral mucosa. If the patient is severely anemic, the palmar creases of the hand may also be demonstrably pale. Petechiae may be a normal finding on the face and upper thorax in a patient who has had forceful crying, vomiting, or coughing. Diffuse petechiae, purpura, and oral lesions are more suggestive of the presence of thrombocytopenia or platelet dysfunction (Fig. 11-67). Bruising also has a typical distribution in childhood and is often prominent on the anterior tibial surfaces of an active child. Abnormal amount of bruising or unusual sites of bruising such as buttocks or back should raise suspicion of abnormal hemostasis. If laboratory studies do not support the presence of thrombocytopenia or a coagulation disorder, the pediatrician must always be careful to consider nonaccidental trauma as the etiology.

Skin rashes may also provide clues to the specific diagnosis. In certain cases, biopsy of the skin may provide diagnostic material, thereby avoiding more invasive procedures. Nodular skin lesions may be observed in both neuroblastoma and in some cases of leukemia (Fig. 11-68). Seborrhea, which is usually a benign finding, may be one of the cutaneous manifestations of Langerhans cell histiocytosis (Fig. 11-69). This diagnosis should be considered if the rash is unusually severe or persists despite standard treatment measures. Additional physical examination findings that should increase the suspicion for this diagnosis include any erythema of gingival mucosa, organomegaly, or systemic symptoms such as irritability or failure to thrive. (Chapter 8 provides further description about this disease.) Melanoma (Fig. 11-70) is extremely rare in childhood. It most likely results from the transformation of pigmented or junctional nevi, and these pigmented lesions should be monitored for any change in size, shape, or regularity of margins. Suspicious lesions warrant biopsy. The biopsy is necessary to determine the diagnosis of a specific skin cancer. Definitive surgery depends on the histologic findings. Squamous and basal cell carcinomas (Fig. 11-71) arise most often in the setting of heritable diseases, such as xeroderma pigmentosum or basal cell nevus syndrome. These rare cases of pediatric skin cancer are also observed with greater frequency in patients who require long-term immunosuppression, such as recipients of solid organ and bone marrow transplantation.

Head and Neck

One of the most critical conditions for the clinician to recognize is the patient with increased intracranial pressure because this is a true oncologic emergency. Central nervous system tumors represent the second most common malignancy in children younger than 15 years of age. A typical history might include the occurrence of severe morning headache with associated vomiting. The physical examination may reveal the presence of papilledema or neurologic deficits, such as cranial nerve palsies. Signs and symptoms in the infant may include macrocephaly and a

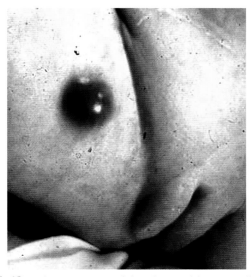

Figure 11-68. Subcutaneous nodule of neuroblastoma. Skin lesions, which are occasionally seen with leukemia or other solid tumors, may be dark ("blueberry muffin") or skin colored. (From Pearson H: Tumors of the sympathetic nervous system. In Altman AJ, Schwartz AD [eds]: Malignant Diseases of Infancy, Childhood, and Adolescence, 2nd ed. Philadelphia, WB Saunders, 1983.)

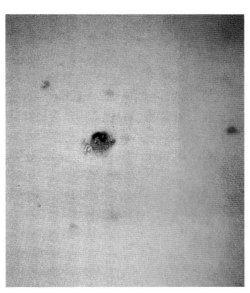

Figure 11-70. Melanoma. In addition to location (see text), suspicious signs of skin lesions include a red-brown-black color that tends to be diffuse at the periphery, crusting, bleeding, pain, or itching.

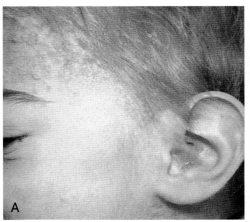
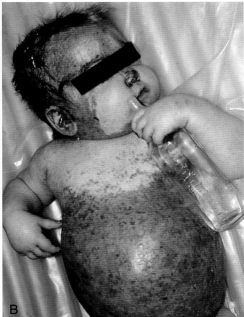
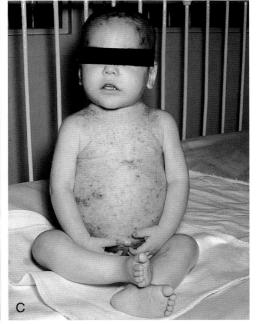

Figure 11-69. A, Langerhans cell histiocytosis (LCH). Seborrhea and chronic ear drainage may be presenting clinical features in an infant with LCH. **B** and **C,** Hemorrhagic and papular rashes are also seen in some children with this disease. (Courtesy P. Gaffney, MD, Pittsburgh.)

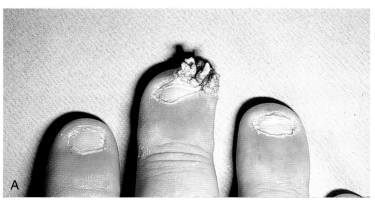

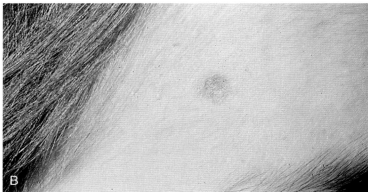

Figure 11-71. A, Squamous cell carcinoma. **B,** Basal cell carcinoma. This 7-year-old boy received prophylactic cranial radiation as part of his treatment for acute lymphoblastic leukemia 5 years before he developed a second cancer. (**A,** Courtesy J. Zitelli, MD, Pittsburgh; **B,** from Pratt CB, Douglass EC: Management of the uncommon cancer of childhood. In Pizzo PA, Poplack DG [eds]: Principles and Practices of Pediatric Oncology. Philadelphia. Lippincott Williams & Wilkins, 1988.)

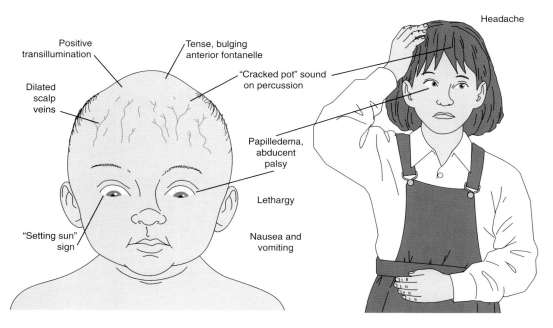

Figure 11-72. Schematic of a child with increased intracranial pressure. Macrocephaly and superficial venous distention secondary to the increased intracranial pressure are seen in this infant with a glioma of the central nervous system. The older child may instead show changes in mental status, vomiting, or focal neurologic signs. (From Stein SC: Brain tumors in children. Resident Staff Phys 26:24-28, 1980.)

bulging fontanelle due to the absence of fused sutures (Fig. 11-72). A more detailed discussion of central nervous system tumors is provided later in the section on the nervous system.

Ocular Findings

Cat's eye reflex, or leukocoria with an absent red reflex, is characteristic of retinoblastoma (see Chapter 19) and should be sought as part of the routine physical examination in the neonate and young child. This is often best appreciated from a frontal photograph of the child (Fig. 11-73) and therefore may be brought to the attention of a physician by a parent. Strabismus (see Chapter 19), particularly when first seen after infancy, may be a sign of an orbital tumor or intracranial pathologic condition and, even if intermittent, merits attention. Proptosis may be observed with several childhood tumors and may represent either a primary tumor or metastatic disease. Orbital rhabdomyosarcoma may present in this way (Fig. 11-74). Langerhans cell histiocytosis may also present with a retrobulbar mass and proptosis. The combination of exophthalmos, diabetes insipidus, and bone lesions form the classic triad that in earlier terminology had been referred to as Hand-Schüller-Christian disease, one of the histiocytosis syndromes. Finally, a child with neuroblastoma

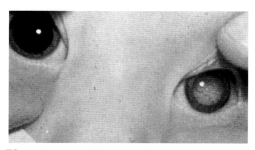

Figure 11-73. Leukocoria. Cat's eye reflex, or leukocoria, in a child with retinoblastoma. (From Abramson D: Retinoblastoma. CA Cancer J Clin 32:130-140, 1982.)

may present with metastatic disease to the orbit. The resulting condition has been referred to as *raccoon eyes* and is due to ecchymoses in the periorbital area (Fig. 11-75). Heterochromia (Fig. 11-76A), usually a benign entity, may be associated with cervicothoracic neuroblastoma (see also Chapter 19). Aniridia (Fig. 11-76B), or absence of the iris, has a known association with malignancy including the WAGR syndrome (*W*ilms tumor, *a*niridia, *g*enital abnormalities, and mental *r*etardation). Aniridia in the

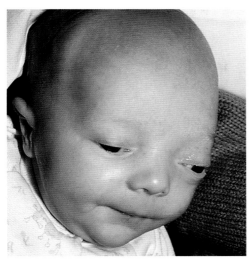

Figure 11-74. Retro-orbital rhabdomyosarcoma. This child demonstrates proptosis due to the retro-orbital tumor, as well as a large head due to the presence of increased intracranial pressure.

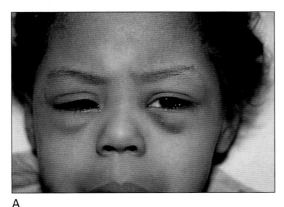

A

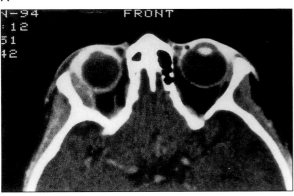

B

Figure 11-75. Raccoon eyes—neuroblastoma. This clinical finding is characteristic of retro-orbital metastatic tumor in advanced neuroblastoma. This may involve supraorbital or infraorbital areas. "Shiners" resulting from trauma or nonaccidental trauma may be a part of the initial differential diagnosis. (Courtesy H. Pearson, New Haven, Conn.)

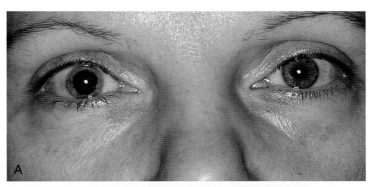

A

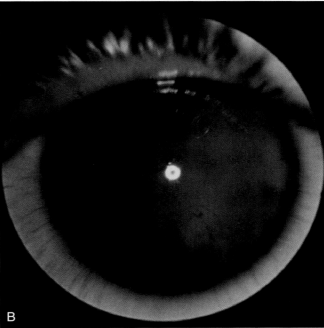

B

Figure 11-76. **A,** Heterochromia iridis in an adult. Heterochromia is associated with neuroblastoma. **B,** Aniridia. (**A,** Courtesy J. Roen, MD, New York.)

infant or toddler should prompt appropriate diagnostic studies.

Chronic draining ears are seen with Langerhans cell histiocytosis (Fig. 11-77). This diagnosis should be suspected when problems persist despite antibiotics, particularly if additional symptoms are present including skin rash, gingival abnormalities, lymphadenopathy, or organomegaly. Otorrhea may also be seen with other head and neck tumors, such as rhabdomyosarcoma. Morphologic abnormalities of the ear itself may also provide clues to a

diagnosis that may predispose a patient to malignancy. The presence of ear creases or pits may represent a manifestation of the Beckwith-Wiedemann syndrome, in which patients have a known predisposition to hepatoblastoma, Wilms tumor, and other malignancies.

A child with cancer may also present with a lesion of the orofacial region including the jaw, oral, and nasal cavities. Inappropriate loosening of the teeth may represent a clinical manifestation of Langerhans cell histiocytosis or Burkitt lymphoma. In the case of African Burkitt lymphoma, an associated jaw mass is also present (Fig. 11-78).

Orofacial Findings

Although masses such as the jaw lesion shown in Figure 11-78 are likely to be referred early to an oncologist, intraoral (Fig. 11-79) or intranasal (Fig. 11-80) masses are more likely to masquerade as nonmalignant lesions, which may forestall correct diagnosis. These may be entirely asymptomatic, or they may cause local bleeding or difficulty swallowing or breathing. Gingival hyperplasia can be seen in children with leukemia, especially the acute myelomonocytic kind (Fig. 11-81).

Although most physicians look for cervical adenopathy, it is important to remember the other lymph node groups that may be involved by focal or generalized adenopathy in leukemias, lymphomas, or solid tumors. A schematic diagram depicting the major lymph node regions is

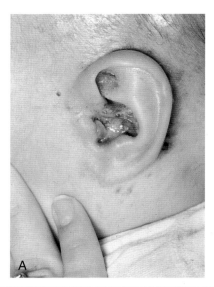

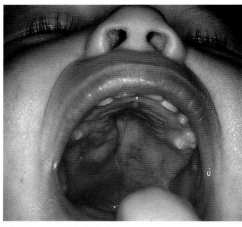

Figure 11-79. Intracranial rhabdomyosarcoma with intraoral extension. The lesion was first detected by the child's dentist and was biopsied by an ear, nose, and throat specialist who did not suspect malignancy.

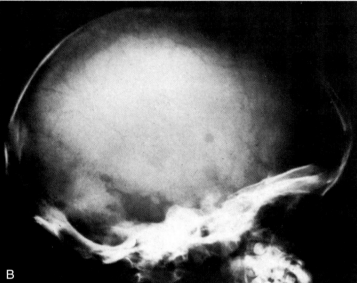

Figure 11-77. **A,** Otorrhea in a child with Langerhans cell histiocytosis. **B,** X-ray film showing destruction of the mastoid bone in the same child. (**A,** Courtesy P. Gaffney, MD, Pittsburgh.)

presented in Figure 11-82. Although large, rock-hard nodes that are fixed to the subcutaneous tissue are most convincing for malignancy, texture and size can be misleading. Because Hodgkin disease and non-Hodgkin lymphoma can occur concurrently with or after infectious mononucleosis, a positive monospot test may be a false reassurance. Therefore persistent adenopathy, even in that setting, should be followed closely. The algorithms for workup of adenopathy and indications for biopsy are reviewed in Chapter 12. Neck examination may reveal abnormalities of the thyroid. Although rare in childhood, a goiter or nodular thyroid with or without bruits may be seen in a patient with thyroid carcinoma.

Chest

External examination of the chest may disclose obvious skeletal or other chest wall masses that may be asymptomatic or associated with pain. Scoliosis has been associated with paravertebral tumors (Fig. 11-83). A discussion of tumors of muscle or bone origin is presented in the musculoskeletal section. The pediatric malignancies of this type include rhabdomyosarcoma, Ewing sarcoma, and osteosarcoma. Importantly, these tumors may present as chest wall lesions. However, subsequent discussion in this section provides a more focused review of tumors of the mediastinum. The differential diagnosis of the mediastinal mass depends to a certain extent on location. Tumors of the anterior mediastinum in children and young adults are most commonly lymphomas including both Hodgkin disease and non-Hodgkin lymphoma. Germ cell tumors and, rarely, thymomas may also be seen in this location. Masses of the middle mediastinum and/or hilar adenopathy also most commonly represent lymphoma in childhood. Disease of the lymph nodes within the chest may also indicate the presence of lymphadenopathy secondary to leukemia. Presence of a mediastinal mass in a patient with leukemia is suggestive of T-cell disease and is often associated with a high WBC count and organomegaly. Tumors of the posterior mediastinum are usually of neurogenic origin including neuroblastoma and Ewing sarcoma. In the case of neuroblastic tumors (e.g., neuroblastoma, ganglioneuroblastoma, ganglioneuroma), calcifications may be present (Fig. 11-84). Parenchymal pulmonary nodules, when tumor related, may be asymptomatic and most commonly represent metastatic solid tumor, such as a sarcoma (Fig. 11-85) or Wilms tumor. Pleural effusions may be present when malignant disease

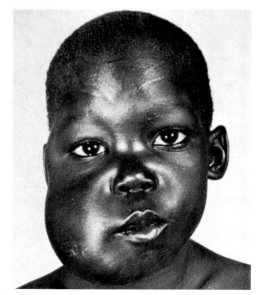

Figure 11-78. Burkitt lymphoma of the jaw in an African child. (Courtesy I. Magrath, MD, Bethesda, Md.)

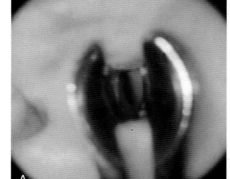

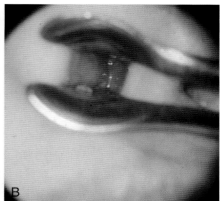

Figure 11-80. Intranasal glioma. This lesion is occluding the right nostril. The normal left nostril is also shown. (Courtesy S. Stool, MD, Pittsburgh.)

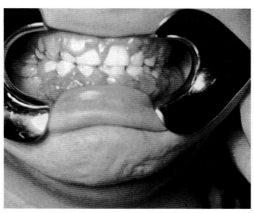

Figure 11-81. Leukemic infiltration. This photograph shows a patient with gingival hyperplasia resulting from leukemic invasion of the gums. (From Bluefarb SM: Dermatology. Kalamazoo, Mich, Upjohn, 1984).

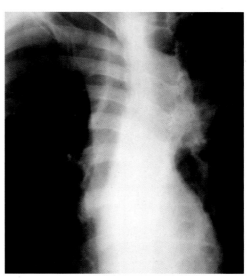

Figure 11-83. Paravertebral mass. This radiograph demonstrates the presence of a paravertebral mass with associated scoliosis.

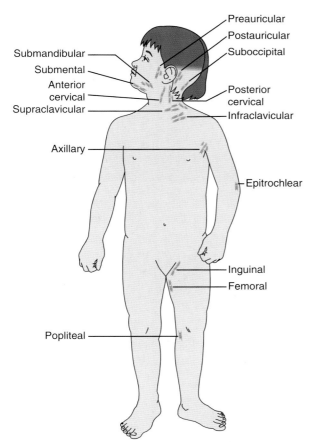

Figure 11-82. Lymph node regions. This schematic illustrates lymph node regions that are normally palpable on physical examination. Rarely, retroperitoneal nodes may become so enlarged that they are palpable.

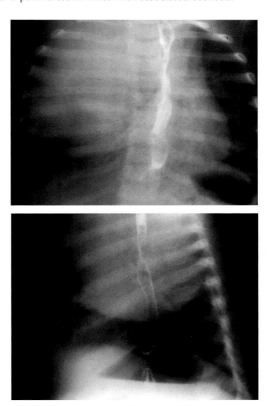

Figure 11-84. Paravertebral neuroblastoma. The posterior mediastinum is the characteristic location for an intrathoracic neuroblastoma. Calcification, not present in this x-ray film, may be seen in 50% of cases. (Courtesy J. Medina, MD, Pittsburgh.)

occurs in the chest. This is most common in the case of non-Hodgkin lymphoma (Fig. 11-86). Cytology, flow cytometry, and cytogenetics that are performed on pleural fluid may provide diagnostic material with relatively low risk in the patient with compromised respiratory status due to mediastinal disease.

Symptoms of respiratory distress may result from a primary intrathoracic process or may be due to a compromised respiratory effort from an abdominal process, such as an abdominal mass or ascites (Fig. 11-87). Pulmonary findings on physical examination and routine chest radiography allow one to rapidly distinguish an intrathoracic from an intra-abdominal process. The superior vena cava syndrome is a true oncologic emergency. It is caused by obstruction of venous return to the heart through the superior vena cava by a mass lesion. Signs and symptoms may include facial swelling and plethora, wheezing, and cough (Fig. 11-88). This syndrome may progress rapidly and lead to cardiorespiratory failure. Emergent intervention with steroid and/or radiation therapy may be required. In caring for the patient with mediastinal disease, one must also pay careful attention to electrolytes and renal function, as patients with non-Hodgkin lymphoma and T-cell leukemia are at high risk of metabolic abnormalities associated with the tumor lysis syndrome.

Abdomen

An observant parent may be the first person to detect abdominal swelling or an abdominal mass. This may

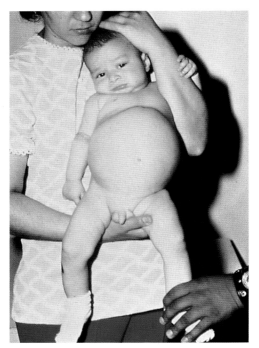

Figure 11-87. Abdominal neuroblastoma. This child has abdominal swelling with hepatosplenomegaly. Further evaluation reveals a diagnosis of neuroblastoma.

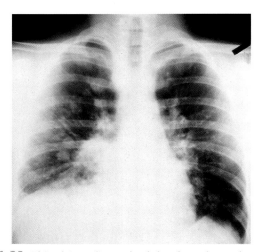

Figure 11-85. This plain radiograph of the chest shows the presence of pulmonary nodules, characteristic of metastatic sarcoma.

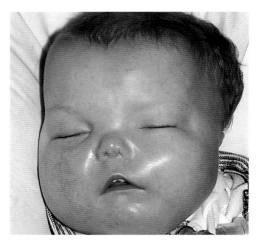

Figure 11-88. Superior vena cava syndrome. Discoloration of the face and neck with venous distention. The mediastinal masses that produce these findings often pose considerable anesthetic risk.

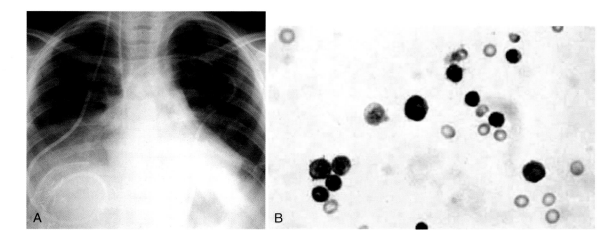

A   B

Figure 11-86. Malignant pleural effusions. **A,** The chest x-ray shows abnormal collection of pleural fluid. If malignancy is suspected, the diagnosis can sometimes be made through analysis of the pleural fluid. **B,** Cytology of the pleural fluid obtained through thoracentesis demonstrates large cells, high nuclear-to-cytoplasmic ratios, and fine nuclear chromatin, all features of malignant disease.

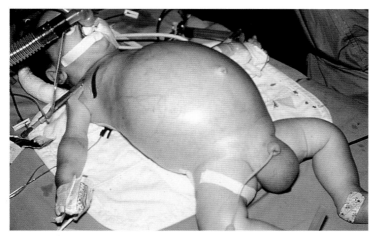

Figure 11-89. Intra-abdominal tumor. Superficial venous distention may also be seen in cases of extensive intra-abdominal tumor. (Courtesy D. Nakayama, MD, Chapel Hill, NC.)

represent hepatosplenomegaly (see Fig. 11-87) or a mass of alternative origin. A large abdominal mass may lead to the accumulation of ascites. Superficial venous distention (Fig. 11-89) may signal deep venous obstruction that also relates to the presence of intra-abdominal tumor. Patients may also demonstrate lower extremity edema and scrotal swelling in the case of male patients or labial swelling in female patients. The patient may experience respiratory difficulties due to limited chest excursion with inspiration and renal dysfunction due to external compression of renal vasculature.

The most common malignant cause of hepatosplenomegaly is leukemia or lymphoma, in which case organomegaly is due to infiltration of the involved organs with malignant cells. The abdominal mass may also reflect a primary tumor originating from an intra-abdominal organ including the kidney, adrenal gland, liver, or ovaries. Wilms tumor is the most common renal tumor of childhood. It often presents as an asymptomatic abdominal mass. Hypertension may occur due to impaired renal blood flow. Hematuria may be observed in approximately 15% of cases.

Children with neuroblastoma and other neuroblastic tumors may also present with an abdominal mass. This tumor may originate from the adrenal gland resulting in a suprarenal mass. Alternatively, a neuroblastic tumor may originate anywhere along the sympathetic neural pathway. Therefore a paraspinal mass is also a common location for neuroblastoma. Unlike Wilms tumor, many of the patients will have metastatic disease at the time of diagnosis and may appear more ill. Neuroblastoma has a wide spectrum of presenting symptomatology and prognoses. These are dependent on the patient's age at diagnosis, stage of disease, and biologic features of the tumor. In approximately 85% of cases, this neural tumor secretes excess catecholamines. The measurement of homovanillic acid and vanillylmandelic acid in the urine is an important aid to diagnosis and may be used to monitor disease status.

Non-Hodgkin lymphoma of the abdomen has a wide range of clinical presentations varying from marked retroperitoneal or mesenteric adenopathy to a clinical scenario that mimics an acute abdominal process, such as appendicitis or intussusception (Fig. 11-90).

Hepatic neoplasms are rare in childhood. The two most common hepatic tumors are hepatoblastoma and hepatocellular carcinoma. The former occurs more commonly in young children, with more than 75% of cases reported in

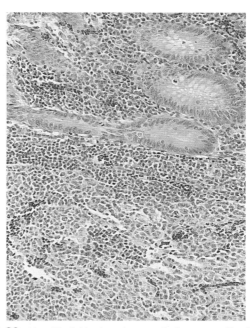

Figure 11-90. Non-Hodgkin lymphoma of the appendix. Picture of a histologic slide of the appendix, showing involvement with non-Hodgkin lymphoma. The malignant cells, predominating in the lower half of the slide, are large, with clear cytoplasm and irregularly shaped nuclei.

children younger than 3 years of age. Hepatocellular carcinoma usually occurs in older children. An elevated α-fetoprotein level may be observed in both tumors, although it is more often present in cases of hepatoblastoma. The most frequent presenting signs and symptoms for hepatic tumors include an abdominal mass with abdominal distention, anorexia, and weight loss.

A germ cell tumor of the ovary may also present as an abdominal mass. Germ cell tumors develop from the primordial germ cells of the embryo that would normally produce sperm or ova. This group of tumors is discussed further in the section on the urogenital tract.

Urogenital Tract

Involvement of the genitourinary system or sacral area by tumor in infancy or childhood often results in the presence of visible abnormalities on physical examination. However, these tumors may also occur in retroperitoneal and intra-abdominal locations. Rhabdomyosarcoma, a tumor of muscle origin, is discussed in greater detail in the subsequent section on the musculoskeletal system. However, sarcoma botryoides is a particular subtype of rhabdomyosarcoma that most often presents in the genitourinary region. This tumor has a characteristic appearance with its grapelike morphology (Fig. 11-91). Classically, it involves the vagina, but it may also involve the mucosal surfaces of other hollow organs, such as the bladder or, more rarely, the nasopharynx. Sacrococcygeal teratoma is also usually grossly apparent on physical examination (Fig. 11-92). Teratomas are embryonal neoplasms that contain tissues from all three of the germ cell layers. The sacrococcygeal location is the most common location in childhood. Other sites of origin include the pineal region, mediastinum, retroperitoneum, and ovary and testes. Although teratomas may have benign or malignant elements, nearly 20% of them exhibit malignant features. The sacrococcygeal mass must also be distinguished from a meningomyelocele and other spinal tumors. The primary discussion of Wilms tumor was in the section on abdomi-

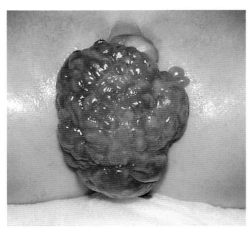

Figure 11-91. Sarcoma botryoides. A grapelike lesion present in a child with multiple congenital anomalies. The appearance of this lesion is characteristic of the sarcoma botryoides subtype of rhabdomyosarcoma.

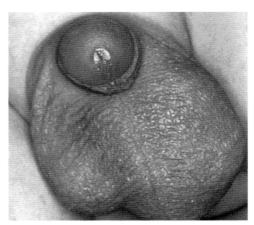

Figure 11-93. Testicular mass. This photograph demonstrates unilateral scrotal swelling in an infant with a left testicular mass.

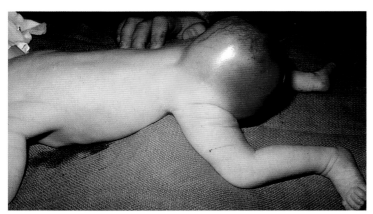

Figure 11-92. Sacrococcygeal teratoma. This teratoma has an external component and is easily visualized on physical examination. The teratoma may contain both benign and malignant elements.

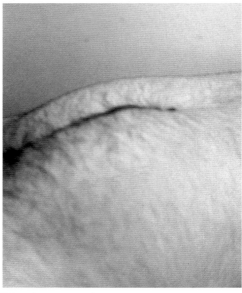

Figure 11-94. Adrenocortical carcinoma. This young girl has abdominal distention and hirsutism due to abnormal hormone production by a tumor. (Courtesy P. Lee, MD, Pittsburgh.)

nal masses. As described previously, patients with Wilms tumor may present with asymptomatic hematuria.

Testicular enlargement (Fig. 11-93) may be secondary to involvement by leukemia or lymphoma (in which case bilateral swelling may be seen) or to primary testicular tumors. Primary tumors of the testes and testicular region include germ cell tumors and paratesticular rhabdomyosarcoma. Priapism is a rare complication of chronic myelogenous leukemia resulting from sludging and mechanical obstruction due to leukemia cells and/or coagulation within the corpora cavernosa.

Abnormalities such as precocious puberty may be caused by a tumor of the central nervous system, gonads (ovaries or testes), or adrenal gland. The inappropriate endocrine-mediated physical examination findings may be the first indication of the presence of a pediatric cancer (Fig. 11-94). Early detection may have an impact on the likelihood of cure, particularly in the case of adrenal tumors.

Musculoskeletal System

Bone and joint manifestations of pediatric cancer are relatively common. Arthralgia or full-blown arthritis are well-described presentations of acute lymphoblastic leukemia. Diffuse bone pain, as discussed previously, is also common. Metaphyseal lucencies and growth arrest lines on plain radiographs are often nonspecifically associated with the diagnosis of acute lymphoblastic leukemia (Fig.

11-95). Diffuse osteopenia (Fig. 11-96) or lytic bone lesions (Fig. 11-97) may also be observed in patients with lymphoid leukemia. Similar lytic lesions and symptoms of bone pain may result from metastatic solid tumor. A rare musculoskeletal finding in the setting of pediatric malignancy is that of hypertrophic osteoarthropathy. This finding has been described in patients with hepatoma, not all of whom have advanced disease at the time of presentation (Fig. 11-98). Hemihypertrophy (Fig. 11-99) (see Chapter 9), or relative enlargement of one or more parts of one side of the body, has been associated with the subsequent development of a number of solid tumors including Wilms tumor, adrenocortical carcinoma, hepatoblastoma, and with leukemia. Although prospective studies have not been performed, the current recommendation is to perform screening abdominal ultrasound every 3 to 4 months until 6 years of age. The finding of hemihypertrophy should be distinguished from hemiatrophy, which is not a predisposing condition. A true mass involving one extremity (see Fig. 11-99C) is not usually confused with hemihypertrophy. Deep vein thrombosis may also result in asymmetry of the extremi-

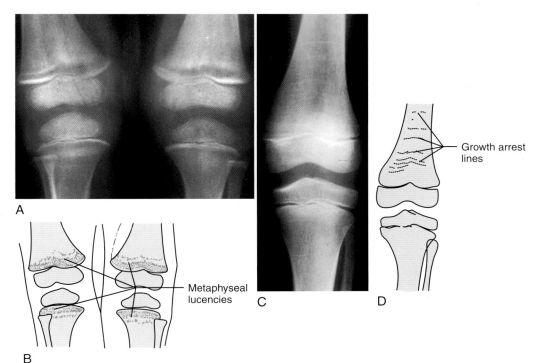

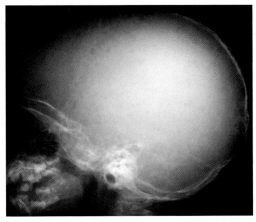

Figure 11-95. X-ray abnormalities in acute lymphoblastic leukemia (ALL). Metaphyseal (**A** and **B**) and growth arrest lines (**C** and **D**) in children with ALL. (Courtesy J. Medina, MD, Pittsburgh.)

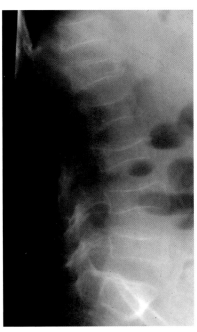

Figure 11-96. Diffuse osteopenia in acute lymphoblastic leukemia. This child was followed for many months by an orthopedist before an abnormal blood count prompted referral to a hematologist.

Figure 11-97. Lytic lesions in malignancy of childhood. This radiograph demonstrates lytic bone lesions in a child with leukemia. Similar lesions may result from metastatic solid tumors.

ties. Although this condition may relate to compression from a tumor or the presence of a paraneoplastic syndrome, thrombotic events in childhood usually represent alternative risk factors to thrombosis and are not a consequence of malignancy.

Primary bone tumors most commonly occur in the adolescent age range and should be considered when patients experience persistent pain, even in the absence of objective findings. Osteosarcoma and Ewing sarcoma are the most common bone tumors found in the child and young adult. Osteosarcoma is a primary bone tumor derived from primitive bone-forming mesenchyme (Fig. 11-100A). It is characterized by the production of osteoid. The devel-

opment of osteosarcoma appears to correlate with periods of linear bone growth, as evidenced by its peak incidence during the pubescent growth spurt and the observation that patients with osteosarcoma are taller than average for age. It is usually metaphyseal in location and involves the bones exhibiting the most rapid growth in adolescence including the femur, tibia, and humerus. Ewing sarcoma is the second most common malignant bone tumor (Fig. 11-100B). It also has its greatest incidence during the second decade of life. It is an undifferentiated tumor of bone that consists morphologically of densely packed small, round, blue cells. Unlike osteosarcoma, this tumor may also arise from soft tissue, in which case it is termed *extraosseous Ewing sarcoma*. The characteristic bone lesion is diaphyseal in location. The clinical picture may initially be mistaken as osteomyelitis due to the association of fever in approximately 30% of patients with Ewing sarcoma.

Soft tissue sarcomas represent tumors arising from muscle, connective tissue, and vascular tissue. Rhabdomyosarcoma, a tumor of striated muscle, is the most common soft tissue sarcoma of childhood. This tumor exhibits two age peaks, the first at 2 to 6 years of age and the second at 15 to 19 years of age. Rhabdomyosarcoma may originate in any site of skeletal muscle, and the most frequent presenting sign is the presence of a mass. Rhabdomyosarcoma in children in the younger age peak usually involves the head, neck, or genitourinary locations. Adolescents more commonly develop extremity, truncal, or paratesticular lesions.

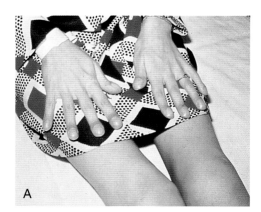

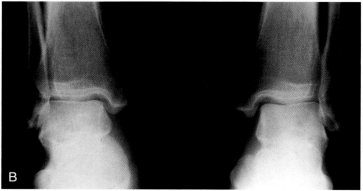

Figure 11-98. Hypertrophic osteoarthropathy. **A,** Clubbing and **B,** bone lesions in a child with hypertrophic osteoarthropathy secondary to hepatocellular carcinoma not involving the lung. (Courtesy K. S. Oh, MD, Pittsburgh.)

Nervous System

Neurologic symptoms of pediatric cancer include headache, mental status change, vomiting, seizure, and focal neurologic abnormalities. Clinical symptoms of increased intracranial pressure have been discussed in greater detail in the section on the head and neck region. Primary or metastatic intracranial tumors may also manifest as seizures, changes in mental status, or focal neurologic deficits such as cranial nerve palsy (see Fig. 11-72). Malignant and benign tumors of the central nervous system may cause these symptoms. Most pediatric brain tumors are infratentorial in location. Because these tumors usually arise in the cerebellum, patients may also present with ataxia. Spinal tumors of children may be observed anywhere along the vertebral column. The symptoms of a tumor in this location are caused by compression of the contents of the spinal canal. Pain on percussion over the vertebral column may be an early sign of cord compression and should be actively sought in the child with suspected cancer in this region. Spinal tumors often have associated weakness, with the affected muscle group corresponding to the level of the lesion. Spinal cord tumors or tumors that press on the cord may present with bowel-bladder dysfunction, paresthesias, or changes in gait.

Medulloblastoma is a malignancy of the central nervous system in childhood that originates from poorly differentiated neuroepithelial cells. Because the tumor usually arises in the cerebellum, ataxia may be a prominent symptom. Widespread seeding of the subarachnoid space may occur. Brain tumors that arise in the thalamus or hypothalamus, such as craniopharyngioma, can present with failure to thrive with or without abnormalities of sexual development (precocity or delay). Midline supratentorial tumors may also lead to visual field disturbances due to optic pathway involvement. Astrocytoma may occur in both supratentorial and infratentorial locations. Clinical presentation is dependent on the location of the tumor. Ependymoma may also occur in the supratentorial and infratentorial location. The fourth ventricle is the most common location, and obstructive hydrocephalus is the most common presenting condition. Patients with brainstem glioma most often exhibit an insidious onset of

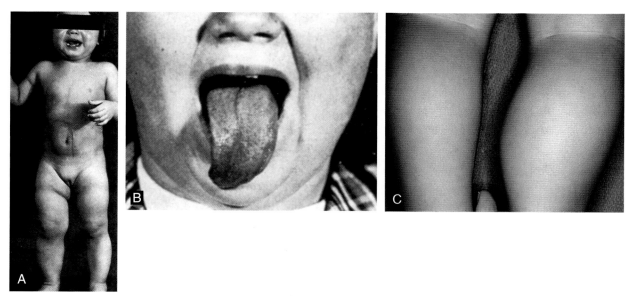

Figure 11-99. **A** and **B,** Hemihypertrophy. **C,** Asymmetry of the calf secondary to sarcoma. (**A** and **B,** Reproduced with permission from Fraumeni JF, Geiser CF, Manning MD: Wilms tumor and congenital hemihypertrophy: Report of five new cases and review of the literature. Pediatrics 40:886-899, 1967. Copyright © 1967 American Academy of Pediatrics; **C,** courtesy of D. Nakayama, MD, Chapel Hill, NC.)

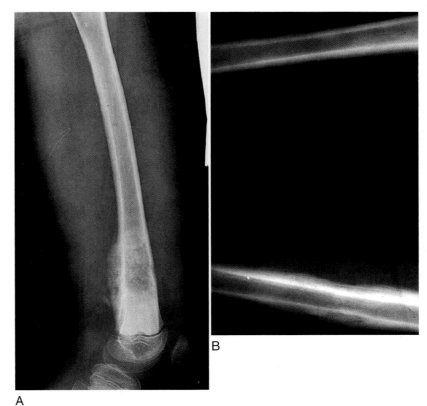

Figure 11-100. A, Osteosarcoma. X-ray film of a child with osteosarcoma showing soft tissue swelling, calcification, cortical bone destruction with increased osteodensity, and new bone formation (Codman triangle). **B,** Ewing sarcoma. X-ray film of a child with Ewing sarcoma showing cortical destruction and soft tissue swelling of the diaphysis of the femur. (Courtesy J. Medina, MD, Pittsburgh.)

symptoms with the occurrence of isolated cranial nerve deficits and long tract signs.

Post-Transplant Lymphoproliferative Disorder

Post-transplant lymphoproliferative disorder (PTLD) is a life-threatening disease that may occur following allogeneic hematopoietic stem cell transplantation or solid organ transplantation. It is not strictly a malignancy because it encompasses a heterogeneous spectrum of lymphoproliferative disorders ranging from reactive, polyclonal hyperplasias to aggressive non-Hodgkin's lymphoma. The entity of PTLD is included within this oncologic review because it may be encountered by the primary care provider caring for someone with a history of transplantation. It is most commonly an Epstein Barr virus (EBV)–driven malignancy, and symptoms and signs parallel those typically seen with primary EBV infection (e.g., fever, sweats, malaise, adenopathy). The disease occurs in those who are severely immunosuppressed and may actually resolve with the withdrawal of immunosup-

pression. However, one must balance this with the risk of graft rejection. Finally, chemotherapy or monoclonal antibody therapy may sometimes be required if resolution does not occur on withdrawal of immunosuppression.

Bibliography

Favara BE: Hemophagocytic lymphohistiocytosis: A hemophagocytic syndrome. Semin Diagn Path 9:63, 1992.

Gottschalk S, Rooney C, Heslop H: Post-transplant lymphoproliferative disorders. Ann Rev Med 56:29-44, 2005.

Hoffman R, Benz EJ, Shattil SJ, et al (eds): Hematology: Basic Principles and Practice, 3rd ed. Philadelphia, Churchill Livingstone, 2000.

Lanzkowsky P: Pediatric Hematology and Oncology. New York, Churchill Livingstone, 1995.

Miller DR, Pearson HA, Baehner RL, McMillan LW: Smith's Blood Diseases of Infancy and Childhood, 7th ed. St Louis, Mosby, 1995.

Nathan DG, Orkin S: Nathan and Oski's Hematology of Infancy and Childhood. Philadelphia, WB Saunders, 1998.

Pizzo PA, Poplack DG (eds): Principles and Practice of Pediatric Oncology, 3rd ed. Philadelphia, Lippincott-Raven Publishers, 1997.

Zucker-Franklin D, Greanes MF, Grossi CE, Marmont AM: Atlas of Blood Cells. Milan, Italy, Edi. Ermes, 1981.

CHAPTER 12

Infectious Disease

HOLLY W. DAVIS AND MARIAN G. MICHAELS

In selecting infectious diseases for presentation in an atlas format, we have chosen to emphasize common and serious disorders in which visual findings tend to be prominent. Modes of presentation, patterns of clinical evolution, and spectra of severity are stressed. The following topics are covered: infectious exanthems, mumps, bacterial skin and soft tissue infections, infectious lymphadenitis, bacterial bone and joint infections, and congenital and perinatal infections including pediatric human immunodeficiency syndrome (HIV). Because of their resurgence, we have added sections on tuberculosis and congenital syphilis. This is designed to help practitioners who have seen few, if any, cases during decades of declining incidence familiarize themselves with their modes of presentation and clinical and radiographic manifestations, thereby assisting earlier recognition and diagnosis.

Infectious Exanthems

Exanthematous disorders are numerous; commonly encountered; and, because they have many similarities, often a source of clinical confusion. In establishing a diagnosis, the clinician should attend not only to the basic character of the exanthem but also to its mode of spread, its distribution, the evolution of lesions, and the constellation of associated symptoms. In some of these illnesses the presence of a characteristic oral enanthem can be helpful in establishing the diagnosis.

Viral Exanthems

Along with mumps, three exanthems—measles or rubeola, rubella, and varicella—continue to be regarded as the "usual childhood diseases" worldwide. Although immunization has been responsible for causing a marked decrease in the incidence of measles, mumps, and rubella compared with their incidence in the prevaccine era, cases of measles (and less often mumps) still occur in children who are nonimmunized or in whom the first immunization resulted in inadequate immunity. Although varicella remains a common illness, use of varicella vaccine has decreased its frequency and has modified the skin manifestations.

Rubeola (Nine-Day or Red Measles)
Measles is a highly contagious, moderate to severe acute illness with a typical prodrome and mode of evolution. Prodromal symptoms consist of fever, malaise, dry (occasionally croupy) cough, coryza, and conjunctivitis with clear discharge and marked photophobia (Fig. 12-1A). One to two days after onset of prodromal symptoms, a pathognomonic enanthem (Koplik spots) appears on the buccal mucosa (Fig. 12-1B). The lesions consist of tiny bluish-white dots surrounded by red halos, which increase in number and then fade over a 2- to 3-day period. The exanthem is seen first on day 3 or 4, as the prodromal symptoms and fever peak in severity. It is a blotchy, erythematous, blanching, maculopapular eruption that appears at the hairline and spreads cephalocaudally over 3 days, ultimately involving the palms and soles (Fig. 12-1C-F). Once generalized, the rash becomes confluent over proximal areas but remains discrete distally. Older lesions tend to develop a rusty hue as a result of capillary leak and cease to blanch with pressure. Fading commences after 3 days, with clearing 2 to 3 days later. Fine, branny desquamation of the most severely involved areas may ensue. Generalized adenopathy may be present in moderate to severe cases.

During the acute phase of this illness, most patients are quite ill systemically. They are lethargic, have moderate to severe malaise and anorexia, and prefer to be left alone to sleep in a darkened room.

The incubation period for measles is 9 to 10 days, and patients are contagious from approximately 4 days before the appearance of rash until about 4 days after. The attack rate in exposed, susceptible people is greater than 90%. Morbidity is rather high and mortality not uncommon, especially in children of underdeveloped countries. The peak season for measles is late winter through early spring. Potential complications (resulting either from extension of the primary infection or from secondary invasion by bacterial pathogens) include otitis media, pneumonia, obstructive laryngotracheitis, and acute encephalitis. Administration of measles vaccine is highly effective in preventing this disease.

Rubella (German Measles)
Although rubella has little or no prodrome in children, adolescents, like adults, may experience 1 to 5 days of low-grade fever, mild malaise, adenopathy, headache, sore throat, and coryza. Fever, if present at all in young children, is low grade and rarely lasts more than a day. The exanthem is a discrete, pinkish red, fine maculopapular eruption, which, like measles, typically begins on the face and spreads cephalocaudally (Fig. 12-2A). The rash becomes generalized within 24 hours, then begins to fade, clearing completely by 72 hours. Forchheimer spots, an enanthem consisting of small reddish spots on the soft palate, are seen in some patients on day 1 of the rash and can be helpful in the differential diagnosis (Fig. 12-2B). Adenopathy, often generalized, is a common but not invariable feature. The occipital, posterior cervical, and postauricular nodes tend to be those most prominently enlarged. Arthritis and arthralgias are frequent in adolescent and adult female patients, beginning on day 2 or 3 and typically lasting 5 to 10 days. Large or small joints may be affected.

Many patients infected with rubella do not manifest this typical picture, however, and up to 25% of infected people are asymptomatic yet capable of transmitting the virus to others. In some, the rash may last only 1 day and may involve only the trunk; in others, the exanthem is absent and the patient appears to have pharyngitis or an upper respiratory tract infection. Because infections due to many other viruses including adenoviruses, coxsackieviruses, and echoviruses can produce a rubella-like picture, serologic testing is necessary to establish the diagnosis. Such testing is important if the patient is pregnant or has been in contact with a pregnant woman or if arthritis is a prominent feature, simulating the picture of acute rheumatic fever or rheumatoid arthritis.

The incidence of rubella peaks in late winter and early spring, and the disease is contagious in patients from a

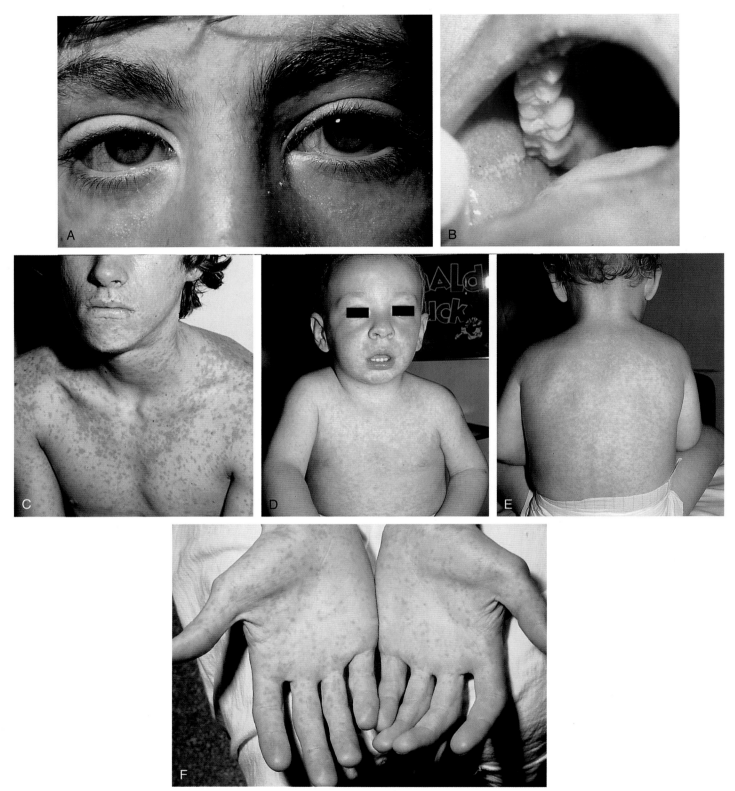

Figure 12-1. Rubeola/measles. **A,** During and after the prodromal period, the conjunctivae are injected and produce a clear discharge. This is associated with marked photophobia. **B,** Koplik spots, bluish white dots surrounded by red halos, appear on the buccal and labial mucosa a day or two before the exanthem and begin to fade with onset of the rash. **C-E,** The measles exanthem is a blotchy, erythematous, blanching maculopapular eruption that appears at the hairline and spreads cephalocaudally over 3 days, ultimately involving the palms and soles **(F).** With evolution, lesions become confluent at proximal sites. (**A, C,** and **F,** Courtesy Michael Sherlock, MD, Lutherville, Md; **B,** courtesy Robert Hickey, MD, Children's Hospital of Pittsburgh.)

few days before to a few days after appearance of the exanthem. The incubation period ranges from 14 to 21 days. Complications are rare in childhood and include arthritis, purpura with or without thrombocytopenia, and mild encephalitis. The major complication results from spread of the virus to susceptible pregnant women and

their fetuses, resulting in congenital rubella syndrome (see "Congenital and Perinatal Infections" later). When such an exposure is thought to have occurred, a specimen of blood should be obtained from the pregnant woman as soon as possible for the measurement of antibody. In addition, an aliquot of serum from this blood draw should be

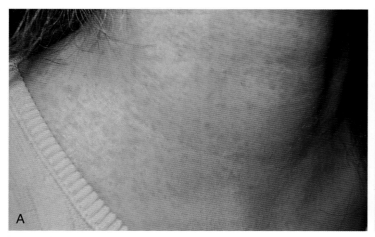 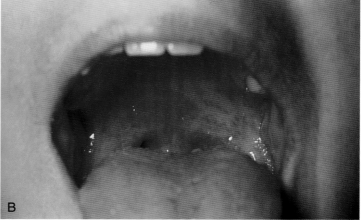

Figure 12-2. Rubella/German measles. **A,** The exanthem of rubella usually consists of a fine, pinkish red, maculopapular eruption that appears first at the hairline and rapidly spreads cephalocaudally. Lesions tend to remain discrete. **B,** The presence of red palatal lesions (Forchheimer spots), seen in some patients on day 1 of the rash, and occipital and posterior cervical adenopathy are findings suggestive of rubella. (Courtesy Michael Sherlock, MD, Lutherville, Md.)

frozen for retesting, if necessary. If the sample obtained at the time of exposure is positive for rubella-specific IgG, then the woman was likely to be immune and not at risk. If it is negative, a second sample should be obtained in 2 to 3 weeks and tested concurrently with the remaining aliquot from the initial sample. If this test is negative, a third sample should be obtained at 6 weeks. If antibody is detected in the second or third specimen, infection has occurred and the fetus is at risk.

Varicella (Chickenpox)

Varicella in the normal pediatric host is a relatively benign, albeit highly contagious, illness caused by the varicella-zoster virus. A brief prodrome of low-grade fever, upper respiratory tract symptoms, and mild malaise may occur, followed rapidly by the appearance of a pruritic exanthem. Lesions appear in crops and evolve rapidly over several hours. Most patients have three crops, although some may have only one and others may have as many as five. Initial crops involve the trunk and scalp, and subsequent crops are distributed more peripherally; thus the mode of spread is centrifugal. The presence of scalp lesions with the initial crop is often helpful in diagnosing the infection in a patient who presents early in the course of the disease. Lesions begin as tiny erythematous papules that rapidly enlarge to form thin-walled, superficial central vesicles surrounded by red halos (Fig. 12-3A). Vesicular fluid changes promptly from clear to cloudy; then drying begins, resulting in an umbilicated appearance. As the surrounding erythema fades, a central crust or scab is formed, which sloughs after several days. A hallmark of this exanthem is the finding of lesions in all stages of evolution within a relatively small geographic area of skin (Fig. 12-3B). Generally, all scabs have sloughed by 10 to 14 days. Scarring usually does not occur unless lesions become secondarily infected. It is important to recognize that in patients with preexisting dermatologic problems, the lesions of varicella, like other viral exanthems, tend to appear first and cluster most heavily at sites of prior skin irritation, such as the diaper area or sites of eczematoid dermatitis (Fig. 12-3C and D).

An enanthem is commonly seen and consists of thin-walled vesicles that rapidly rupture to form shallow ulcers (Fig. 12-3E). Other mucosal surfaces may be affected as well. Although skin lesions are pruritic, those on the oral, rectal, or vaginal mucosa and those involving the external auditory canal or tympanic membrane can be painful, necessitating analgesia. Systemic symptoms are generally mild, although low-grade to moderate fever may be present during the first few days. In most cases pruritus is the child's major complaint. In adolescents and adults the illness is more likely to be severe with prominent systemic symptoms and more extensive exanthematous involvement.

Varicella occurs year-round, with peak incidences in late autumn and late winter through early spring. The period of communicability begins 1 to 2 days before the appearance of lesions and lasts until all lesions have crusted over. The incubation period ranges from 10 to 20 days, with high secondary attack rates in susceptible people. The most common complication in normal hosts is secondary bacterial infection of excoriated skin lesions. Such infection can range from impetigo to cellulitis. Group A β-streptococcal superinfection of varicella lesions can be particularly severe, leading to myositis, sepsis, and purpura fulminans (Fig. 12-4A). Other complications, though rare, include pneumonia, hepatitis, and encephalitis. The onset of these complications is typically heralded by a secondary fever spike concurrent with an increase in general systemic symptoms. In patients with encephalitis, an altered level of consciousness along with other signs of neurologic dysfunction occurs. Reye syndrome, an encephalopathy of unclear etiology, is a well-recognized but fortunately rare complication that can occur as a child is recovering from acute varicella. Repetitive pernicious vomiting is followed by an altered level of consciousness in which periods of lethargy alternate with periods of delirium or combativeness.

In the immunocompromised host with deficient cellular immunity, varicella is a severe and often fatal disease with central nervous system (CNS), pulmonary, and generalized visceral involvement. Skin lesions are often hemorrhagic and tend to remain vesicular for a prolonged period of time (Fig. 12-4B and C). With potentially immunocompromised children who have not had varicella previously (including those on short-course, high-dose steroids), parents must be forewarned of these dangers and instructed to notify their physician immediately of any possible exposure. This enables the administration of varicella-zoster immune globulin (VZIG) within 96 hours of exposure, thus reducing the severity of illness. If VZIG is unavailable, some experts recommend prophylaxis with acyclovir starting on day 7 postexposure for high-risk patients.

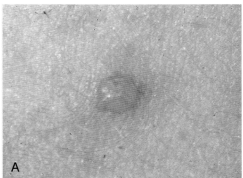

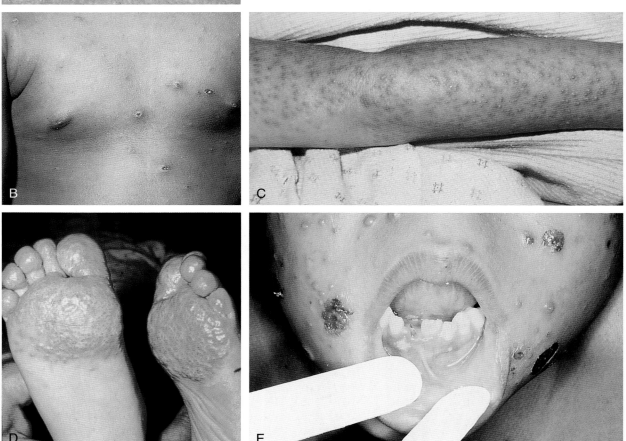

Figure 12-3. Varicella/chickenpox. **A,** The characteristic "dewdrop on a rose petal" is illustrated by this early vesicle on an erythematous base. **B,** The typical feature of lesions in all stages of evolution is seen on the trunk of this child. Note the presence of papules, vesicles, and umbilicated and scabbed lesions, all within a small area. **C** and **D,** In this child with underlying eczema, the first crop of vesicles appeared in clusters at sites previously affected by dermatitis. The flexor surface of his arm is covered with numerous discrete lesions, and vesicles are confluent over the plantar surface of his toes and on the balls of his feet. **E,** On mucosal surfaces, thin-walled vesicles may form and rapidly rupture, forming painful shallow ulcers. (**C** and **D,** Courtesy Michael Sherlock, MD, Lutherville, Md; **E,** courtesy Ellen Wald, MD, University of Wisconsin Children's Hospital.)

Adenovirus Infections

More than 40 distinct types of adenoviruses are capable of producing a variety of clinical illnesses including conjunctivitis, upper respiratory tract infections and pharyngitis, croup, bronchitis, bronchiolitis and pneumonia (occasionally fulminant), gastroenteritis, myocarditis, nephritis, cystitis, and encephalitis. An exanthem occasionally accompanies other symptoms, and a variety of rashes have been described. The eruption may consist of discrete, nonspecific, blanching, maculopapular lesions or it may be morbilliform, rubelliform, or, on occasion, petechial. Typically the rash is generalized when first noted. The most readily identifiable clinical constellation consists of conjunctivitis, rhinitis, pharyngitis with or without exudate, and a discrete, blanching, maculopapular rash (Fig. 12-5). Anterior cervical and preauricular lymphadenopathy, low-grade fever, and malaise are common associated findings. The peak season for adenovirus infections in temperate climates is late winter through early summer, and the infection is maximally contagious during the first few days of illness. The incubation period ranges from 6 to 9 days.

Coxsackie Hand-Foot-and-Mouth Disease

Of the enteroviruses, coxsackievirus group A16 produces the most distinctive exanthem, known as *hand-foot-and-mouth disease.* Patients may have a brief prodrome consisting of low-grade fever, malaise, sore mouth, and anorexia, during which lesions are absent. Within 1 to 2 days, oral lesions and soon skin lesions appear. The former usually consist of shallow, yellow ulcers surrounded by red halos. They are found on the labial and buccal mucosal surfaces, the gingivae, tongue, soft palate, uvula, and anterior tonsillar pillars (Fig. 12-6A and B). Early in the illness, small vesicles may be seen on the palate or mucosal surfaces. These enanthematous lesions usually are only mildly painful. The cutaneous lesions begin as erythematous macules on the palmar aspect of the hands and fingers, the plantar surface of the feet and toes, and the interdigital surfaces. Occasionally the buttocks may be involved as well. They evolve rapidly to form small, thick-walled, gray vesicles on an erythematous base (Fig. 12-6C to E), which may feel like slivers, be pruritic, or be asymptomatic. More than 90% of patients with disease caused by coxsackievirus A16 have oral lesions, and about two thirds have

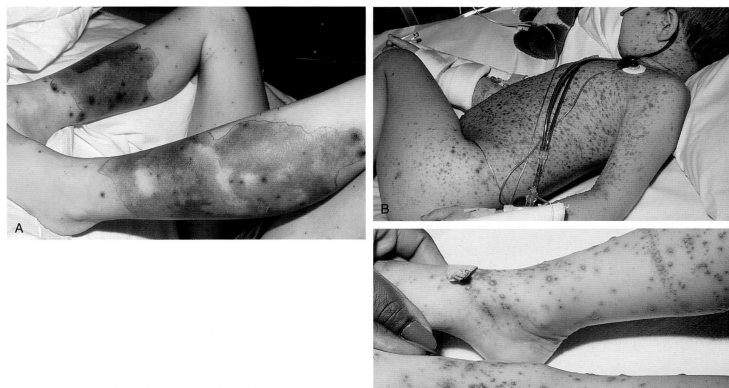

Figure 12-4. Complications of varicella. **A,** Superinfection of this child's lesions with group A β-streptococci led to purpura fulminans. **B** and **C,** Disseminated hemorrhagic varicella. **B,** In the immunocompromised child, skin lesions tend to be hemorrhagic and nearly confluent. **C,** Lesions also evolve more slowly than usual, remaining vesicular for a prolonged period.

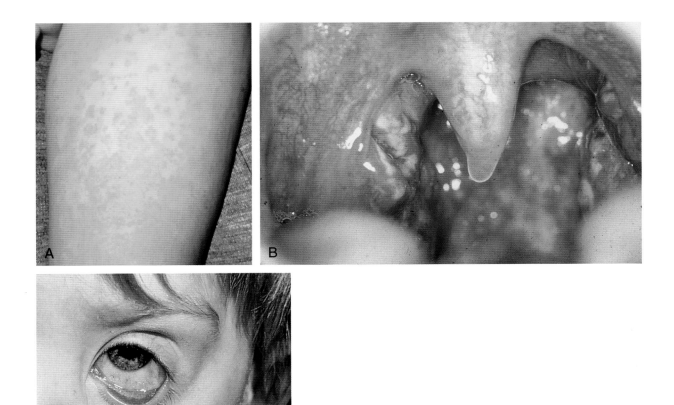

Figure 12-5. Adenovirus. **A,** This discrete, erythematous, blanching maculopapular rash was generalized when first noted and occurred in association with pharyngitis **(B)** and a nonpurulent conjunctivitis **(C).** (**A** and **C,** Courtesy Michael Sherlock, MD, Lutherville, Md.)

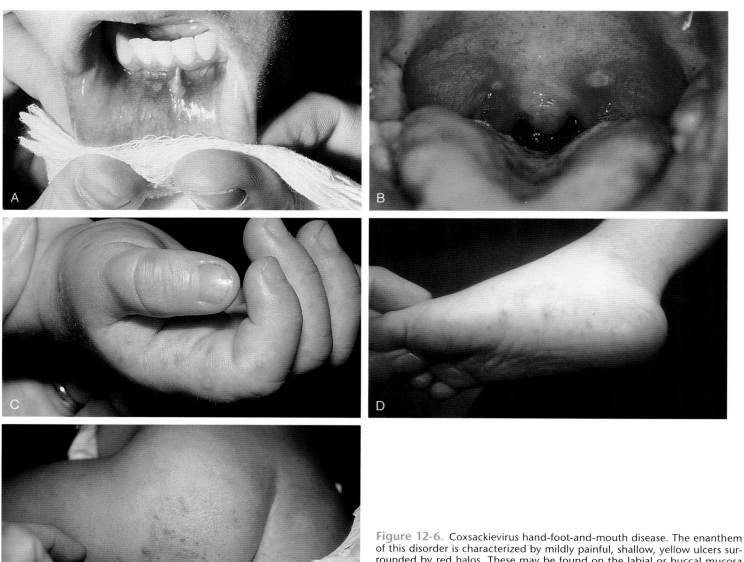

Figure 12-6. Coxsackievirus hand-foot-and-mouth disease. The enanthem of this disorder is characterized by mildly painful, shallow, yellow ulcers surrounded by red halos. These may be found on the labial or buccal mucosa **(A),** tongue, soft palate **(B),** uvula, and anterior tonsillar pillars. When oral lesions occur in the absence of the exanthem, the resulting disorder is called *herpangina.* **C** and **D,** The exanthem of coxsackievirus hand-foot-and-mouth disease involves the palmar, plantar, and interdigital surfaces of the hands and feet and sometimes the buttocks **(E).** It consists of thick-walled, gray vesicles on an erythematous base. **(D** and **E,** Courtesy Robert Hickey, MD, Children's Hospital of Pittsburgh.)

the exanthem. In those cases in which the cutaneous manifestations are absent, the process is called *herpangina* (caused by coxsackieviruses and other enteroviruses) and may resemble early herpes gingivostomatitis. However, coxsackievirus ulcers are less painful and are less often associated with the high fever and intense gingival erythema, edema, and bleeding typical of herpes (see Fig. 12-10).

Coxsackievirus hand-foot-and-mouth disease is highly contagious, with an incubation period of approximately 2 to 6 days. Symptoms last 2 days to 1 week. The peak season is summer through early fall.

Other enteroviral syndromes produced by the coxsackievirus group and by echoviruses include a mild, nonspecific febrile illness with myalgias, headache, and abdominal pain; generalized exanthems that may be maculopapular, vesicular, or urticarial; encephalitis, acute cerebellar ataxia, and myelitis; pleurodynia; myocarditis; hemorrhagic conjunctivitis; and gastroenteritis.

Erythema Infectiosum (Fifth Disease)

Erythema infectiosum is a mildly contagious illness, caused by parvovirus B19, that principally affects preschool and young school-age children. It occurs year-round, with a peak incidence in late winter and early spring. The disorder is characterized primarily by its exanthem. Fever and constitutional symptoms are unusual. Occasionally, headache, nausea, myalgias, and peripheral polyarthralgias are reported. The rash begins on the face, with large, bright red, erythematous patches appearing over both cheeks (Fig. 12-7A). These patches are warm but nontender and have circumscribed borders that are usually macular but may be slightly raised. They are easily distinguished from those of cellulitis and erysipelas (see Figs. 12-38, 12-39, and 12-41) by their symmetry and lack of tenderness, and by the absence of high fever and toxicity. The facial lesions begin to fade on the following day, and a symmetrical, macular or slightly raised, lacy, erythematous rash appears on the extensor surfaces of the extrem-

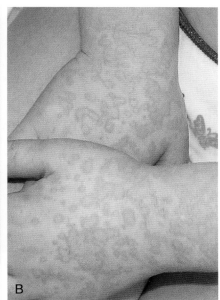

Figure 12-7. Erythema infectiosum (fifth disease). **A,** On day 1, warm, erythematous, nontender, circumscribed patches appear over the cheeks. These fade on the following day, as **(B)** an erythematous, lacy rash develops on the extensor surfaces of the extremities. (**A,** Courtesy Robert Hickey, MD, Children's Hospital of Pittsburgh; **B,** from Cohen BA, Lehman C [eds]: http://www.dermatlas.org)

Figure 12-8. Roseola infantum/exanthem subitum. **A** and **B,** The exanthem of this disorder usually appears abruptly after 3 days of high fever and irritability. It is characterized by discrete, rose-pink macules. It may be generalized at first or may start centrally and spread centrifugally. Scalp involvement is prominent.

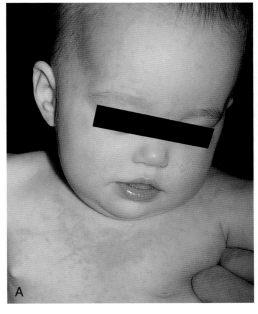

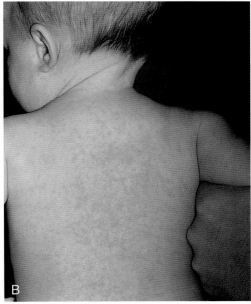

ities (Fig. 12-7B). Over the next day or so, the rash may spread to the flexor surfaces, buttocks, and trunk. Resolution occurs within 3 to 7 days of onset.

Studies have shown that the virus is transmitted primarily by respiratory secretions and that, after transmission, it replicates in red blood cell precursors in the bone marrow. It then may cause a biphasic illness, with fever and nonspecific symptoms accompanied by red blood cell suppression occurring approximately a week later, followed by the appearance of the exanthem characteristic of fifth disease 1 to 2 weeks thereafter. Viral shedding ceases before this latter phase. Although red blood cell suppression caused by parvovirus does not result in severe anemia in normal people, it can cause an aplastic crisis in patients with sickle cell disease, other hemoglobinopathies, and other forms of hemolytic anemia.

Roseola Infantum (Exanthem Subitum)

Roseola infantum is a febrile illness that primarily affects children between the ages of 6 and 36 months. The causative agent is human herpesvirus 6. The clinical course begins abruptly with rapid temperature elevation, which occasionally precipitates a febrile seizure. Anorexia and irritability are the major associated symptoms. Examination reveals no source for the fever, which is usually higher than 39° C. Administration of an antipyretic produces only a transient decrease in temperature, which then rises rapidly to its former value. Although most patients do not look toxic, many infants undergo a sepsis workup and lumbar puncture because of the combination of unexplained high fever and marked irritability. Fever and irritability persist for approximately 72 hours, whereupon the fever abruptly subsides. In most cases an erythematous, maculopapular exanthem appears simultaneously with defervescence, but in a small percentage of patients it develops 1 day before or after fever lysis. Lesions are discrete, rose-pink macules or maculopapules that begin on the trunk and then spread rapidly to the extremities, neck, face, and scalp (Fig. 12-8). They may last several hours to a day or two before resolution.

Although cases occur year-round, roseola appears to be more common in late fall and early spring. Secondary

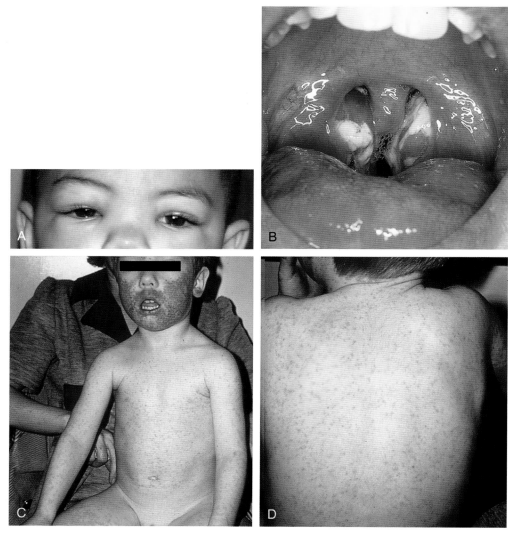

Figure 12-9. Epstein-Barr virus (EBV) mononucleosis. **A,** Eyelid edema is found in 50% of children with infectious mononucleosis. **B,** Severe pharyngotonsillitis is seen in this child, whose tonsils are markedly enlarged and covered with exudate. The uvula is erythematous and edematous. **C** and **D,** In this child with EBV mononucleosis, a diffuse, erythematous, maculopapular rash was part of the clinical picture. Lesions on his face are hemorrhagic and confluent as a result of prior irritation. (He had practiced shaving 2 days before.) Note also the swelling in the region of the tonsillar node and the fact that the child is mouth breathing as a result of adenoidal hypertrophy. (**C** and **D,** Courtesy Michael Sherlock, MD, Lutherville, Md.)

cases are uncommon, except in institutional settings. The duration of communicability is unclear, but the incubation period is thought to be 10 to 15 days.

Infectious Mononucleosis

Infectious mononucleosis is an acute, usually self-limited illness of children and young adults caused by the Epstein Barr virus (EBV). Transmission of EBV can occur by intimate oral contact (i.e., kissing), sharing eating utensils, transfusion, or transplantation. The incubation period usually ranges from 30 to 50 days, although it is shorter (14 to 20 days) in patients with transfusion-acquired infection.

In its most typical form, infectious mononucleosis is characterized by fever, fatigue, pharyngitis, lymphadenopathy, splenomegaly, atypical lymphocytosis, and a positive heterophil antibody response. Nevertheless, most young children with EBV infection do not have classic mononucleosis; instead, they tend to have either a nonspecific illness, which is clinically indistinguishable from other common viral diseases, or, less frequently, subclinical infection.

Clinical Features of Mononucleosis. The illness often begins with a prodrome, which lasts from 3 to 5 days, consisting of fatigue, malaise, and anorexia, often in association with headache, sweats, and chills. Photophobia and edema of the eyelids and periorbital tissues may be noted in some patients (Fig. 12-9A). The acute phase is usually heralded by a fever, which may show wide daily fluctuations. Pharyngitis and cervical node enlargement then become apparent. The sore throat tends to increase in severity over several days before abating and may be associated with significant dysphagia. Tonsillar and adenoidal enlargement can range from mild to marked, and the tonsillar surface may vary in appearance from one of mild erythema to one of severe exudative inflammation with palatal and uvular edema (Fig. 12-9B). Halitosis and palatal petechiae are common. Approximately one third of patients show severe pharyngeal manifestations. The anterior cervical lymph nodes are routinely enlarged, and posterior cervical adenopathy is characteristic. In classic cases the adenopathy becomes generalized toward the end of the first week. Involved nodes are firm, discrete, and mildly to moderately tender. Splenomegaly develops in approximately 50% of patients in the second to third week of illness; 10% have associated hepatic enlargement.

An exanthem is seen in 5% to 10% of patients with mononucleosis, although this percentage is greatly increased in patients treated with ampicillin or amoxicillin for pharyngeal or respiratory symptoms. Usually an erythematous maculopapular rubelliform rash, the exanthem can be morbilliform, scarlatiniform, urticarial, hemorrhagic, or even nodular (Fig. 12-9C and D).

Less common manifestations or complications of mononucleosis include pneumonitis with a pattern of a diffuse, atypical pneumonia; hematologic abnormalities, such as direct Coombs test–positive hemolytic anemia and thrombocytopenia; icteric hepatitis; neurologic disorders, such as acute cerebellar ataxia, encephalitis, aseptic meningitis, myelitis, and Guillain-Barré syndrome; and, rarely, myocarditis and pericarditis. Neurologic and hepatic involvement or widely disseminated disease occasionally can be fulminant, resulting in death. This is particularly true for immunocompromised patients. Other major complications include acute upper airway obstruction resulting from tonsillar and adenoidal hypertrophy and splenic rupture. The latter may occur spontaneously or as a result of minor trauma, repeated palpation, or the increase in intra-abdominal pressure associated with defecation. Although younger patients are somewhat less subject to the unusual manifestations and complications of mononucleosis, they are more vulnerable to acute upper airway obstruction as a result of tonsillar and adenoidal hypertrophy. This is manifested by mouth breathing, retractions with recumbency, and stertorous snoring and apnea during sleep. Moreover, children younger than 5 years of age who show significant tonsillar and adenoidal enlargement during the EBV infection are more likely to have secondary otitis media and, subsequent to resolution of the acute process, may suffer recurrent bouts of otitis media, tonsillitis, and sinusitis as a result of persistent tonsillar and adenoidal hypertrophy.

Diagnostic Methods. Several laboratory studies may be helpful in suggesting or confirming the diagnosis of infectious mononucleosis. A classic finding is a lymphocytosis with 50% or more lymphocytes and at least 10% atypical lymphocytes. These atypical lymphocytes vary in appearance, in contrast to the monotonous forms seen with leukemia. There is considerable variability, however, in the degree of lymphocytosis and in its timing. Eighty percent or more of patients have mild elevations in liver enzymes early in their disease. Most commonly the diagnosis is confirmed by the finding of heterophil antibodies in the serum toward the end of the first week or at the beginning of the second week of illness. Currently, rapid slide tests, of which the Monospot is best known, are the most prevalent method of detecting heterophil antibodies. Although the presence of heterophil antibodies is highly specific for infectious mononucleosis, the sensitivity of the test is limited, in that only about 85% of adolescents, and a much smaller percentage of younger children, with mononucleosis ever show measurable heterophil antibodies. Although EBV infection can be confirmed by measuring specific EBV antibody titers, such studies are usually reserved for patients with severe, prolonged, or atypical heterophil-negative cases of suspected EBV infection. Molecular techniques such as quantitative polymerase chain reaction (PCR) tests are also of value in cases of severe disease or in immunocompromised patients.

Differential Diagnosis of Mononucleosis. In view of the multiple modes of presentation and the wide variability in severity of illness, clinical manifestations, and clinical course, there exists a broad range of differential diagnostic possibilities. In patients presenting with fever and exudative tonsillitis, the principal diagnostic considerations include group A streptococcal pharyngitis, diphtheria, and other viral causes of pharyngitis. If lymphadenopathy and splenomegaly are the predominant features, the differential diagnosis includes cytomegalovirus infection, toxoplasmosis, malignancy, and drug-induced mononucleosis (caused by phenytoin, para-aminosalicylic acid, and diaminodiphenylsulfone). In patients with severe hepatic involvement, EBV infection can simulate other forms of viral hepatitis, as well as leptospirosis. Although the history and some aspects of the clinical picture may help in distinguishing one disease from another, specific serologic tests are often required to accomplish this.

Herpes Simplex Infections

The herpes simplex viruses produce infections that primarily involve the skin and mucous membranes, although in neonates, immunocompromised hosts, and, rarely, normal hosts, infection can result in disseminated disease and CNS involvement. Like other herpesviruses, herpes simplex virus—after producing initial (primary) infection—enters a latent or dormant stage, residing in local sensory ganglia; once latent, the virus can be reactivated at any time, causing recurrent infection. The two distinct serotypes of herpes simplex virus are types 1 and 2. Herpes simplex virus type 1 (HSV-1) is the more common pathogen and can produce a variety of clinical syndromes. In contrast, herpes simplex type 2 virus (HSV-2) is usually a genital pathogen (see Chapter 18), although occasionally it is the source of oral lesions and is the usual agent associated with neonatal herpes (see the section Congenital and Perinatal Infections).

Diagnosis of symptomatic HSV infections can often be made on clinical grounds alone, particularly in cases of primary infection. When the diagnosis is in question, a Giemsa-stained (Tzanck) smear of scrapings obtained from the base of a vesicle (see Chapter 8) usually demonstrates ballooned epithelial cells with intranuclear inclusions and multinucleated giant cells when the lesion is herpetic. Rapid antigen detection tests are more specific and sensitive than Tzanck smears. Viral cultures, obtained by unroofing a lesion and swabbing its base, yield results in 24 to 72 hours. Acute and convalescent titers are less useful and are of no help during recurrences.

Primary Herpes Simplex Infections. More than 90% of primary infections caused by HSV-1 are subclinical; nevertheless, because the virus is ubiquitous, symptomatic primary infections are common. One of the most prevalent forms of primary infection is *herpetic gingivostomatitis*. Patients with this condition typically have high fever, irritability, anorexia, and mouth pain; infants and toddlers often drool copiously. The gingivae become intensely erythematous, edematous, and friable and tend to bleed easily. Small, yellow ulcerations with red halos are seen routinely on the buccal and labial mucosa, on the gingivae and tongue, and often on the palate and tonsillar pillars (Fig. 12-10A and B). Within a short time, yellowish-white debris builds up on mucosal surfaces and halitosis becomes prominent. Thick-walled vesiculopustular lesions may also develop on the perioral skin (Fig. 12-10C). The anterior cervical and tonsillar nodes are enlarged and tender. Symptoms last from 5 to 14 days, but the virus may be shed for weeks following resolution. The illness can vary from mild to marked in severity. Young children with prolonged high fever and intense pain may become dehydrated and ketotic and should be followed closely and hydrated as needed. The diffuseness of the ulcerations and mucosal inflammation and the intense gingivitis help to distinguish this disorder from herpangina (see Fig. 12-6) and exudative tonsillitis, as well as from other forms of gingivitis.

Patients with primary herpetic infections involving the skin typically present with fever, malaise, localized lesions, and regional adenopathy. The skin lesions generally result from direct inoculation of previously traumatized skin, for example, at the site of an abrasion, burn, or small cut. Parents, siblings, and playmates with active herpetic lesions (usually cold sores) are often the source, and young

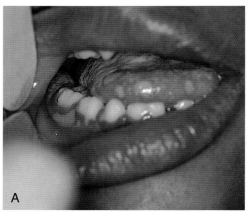
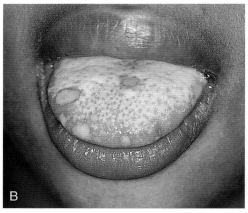
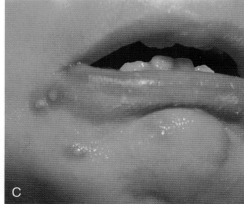

Figure 12-10. Herpes simplex infections. **A,** Herpetic gingivostomatitis is characterized by discrete mucosal ulcerations and diffuse gingival erythema, edema, and friability in association with fever, dysphagia, and cervical adenopathy. **B,** Numerous yellow ulcerations with thin red halos are seen on the patient's tongue as well. **C,** These thick-walled vesicles on an erythematous base were noted in this child, who showed early findings of intraoral involvement. (**C,** Courtesy Michael Sherlock, MD, Lutherville, Md.)

children with herpes gingivostomatitis may autoinoculate other body sites with their fingers. The lesions consist of deep, thick-walled, painful vesicles on an erythematous base; they usually are grouped but may occur singly. As they evolve over several days, the vesicles become pustular, coalesce, ulcerate, and then crust over. As a result, the lesions may simulate those of bacterial infection, but the presence of grouped vesicles and the relative sparseness of bacteria on Gram stains of vesicular fluid support the clinical diagnosis of herpes, which can be confirmed by positive findings on Giemsa stain of scrapings from the base of the lesion, rapid viral antigen detection, or viral culture.

Although the virus can infect any area of the skin, the lips and fingers or thumbs (as in *herpetic whitlow*) are the most common sites of involvement (see Figs. 12-10 and 12-11). Occasionally the eyelids and periorbital tissues are affected (Fig. 12-12); this can lead to keratoconjunctivitis, which is diagnosed on the basis of finding characteristic dendritic ulcerations on slit lamp examination (see Chapter 19). Because this complication carries a risk of causing permanent visual impairment, urgent ophthalmologic consultation is indicated whenever there is any suspicion of ocular herpetic infection.

Eczema Herpeticum (Kaposi Varicelliform Eruption). Patients with atopic eczema and other forms of chronic dermatitis are at risk for a particularly severe form of primary HSV infection and thus should avoid contact with people with active herpetic infections. Parents who have a history of recurrent herpes and a child with eczema should be instructed to be meticulous about hand washing during periods of reactivation. The illness is heralded by the onset of high fever, irritability, and discomfort. Lesions appear in crops and primarily involve areas of currently or recently affected skin. Typically they evolve to form pustules, which rupture and form crusts over the course of a few days. Occasionally these lesions become hemorrhagic (Fig. 12-13). Multiple crops can appear over 7 to 10 days, simulating varicella. However, the slower evolution of lesions, the tendency of such lesions to become hemorrhagic, their concentration in eczematoid areas, and the persistence of fever and systemic symptoms for as long as 1 week help to distinguish this disorder from varicella. Severity ranges from mild to fulminant and depends in part on the extent of the preceding dermatitis. When the area of involvement is large, fluid losses can be severe and potentially fatal. Accordingly, prompt treatment with

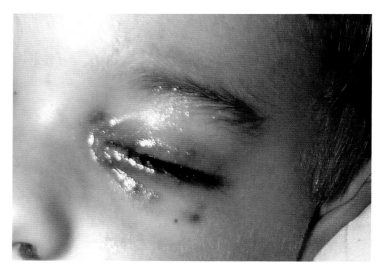

Figure 12-11. Herpetic whitlow. Grouped, thick-walled vesicles on an erythematous base that are painful and tend to coalesce, ulcerate, and then crust are the typical characteristics of a herpetic whitlow.

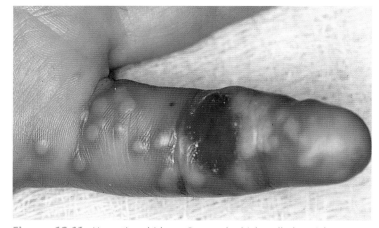

Figure 12-12. Ocular herpes may involve only the lids and periorbital skin but can spread to involve the conjunctiva, cornea, and deeper structures, with devastating results.

intravenous acyclovir is recommended. A significant risk of secondary bacterial infection also exists.

Recurrent Herpes Simplex Infection. As mentioned earlier, following primary infection, HSV becomes latent within the ganglia that lie in the region of initial involvement; reactivation of the latent virus results in localized

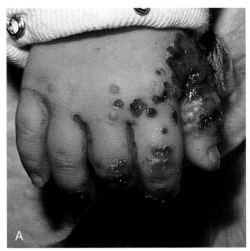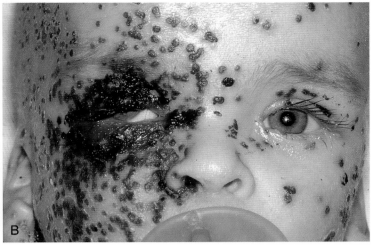

Figure 12-13. Eczema herpeticum (Kaposi varicelliform eruption). Primary herpes simplex infection in a child with underlying eczema produces crops of hemorrhagic vesiculopustular lesions limited to areas of preexisting dermatitis, which then rupture and crust. **A,** Lesions are seen on the hand of one child and on the face of another **(B).** (**A,** Courtesy Michael Sherlock, MD, Lutherville, Md.)

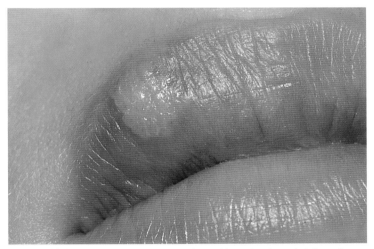

Figure 12-14. Recurrent herpes labialis (cold sore). After a brief prodrome of burning, these grouped vesicles, filled with yellow fluid, erupted on the child's upper lip.

recurrences at or near the site of previous infection. Fever, sunlight, local trauma, menses, and emotional stress are recognized triggers, and because the mouth is the major site of primary infection, labial and perioral lesions (cold sores) are seen most commonly. Many patients report a prodrome of localized burning along with stinging or itching before the eruption of grouped vesicles. These vesicles contain yellow, serous fluid and often appear smaller and less thick walled than primary lesions (Fig. 12-14). After 2 to 3 days the vesicular fluid becomes cloudy, and then crusts form. Although fever and systemic symptoms are absent, regional nodes may be enlarged and tender. The localization of the lesions to a small area helps to distinguish them from those of herpes zoster. Prodromal symptoms and discomfort help to distinguish recurrent HSV infection from impetigo and contact dermatitis.

Herpes Zoster (Shingles)

The varicella-zoster virus, like other herpesviruses, takes up permanent, albeit generally quiescent, residence in its host after initial infection (i.e., varicella). Generally the virus lies dormant in the genome of sensory nerve root cells, but it can reactivate on occasion. Mechanical and thermal trauma, infection, and debilitation all have been postulated as triggers. Immunosuppression can also pre-

dispose to reactivation. In the reactivated form, herpes zoster, lesions consist of grouped, thin-walled vesicles on an erythematous base, which are distributed along the course of a spinal or cranial sensory nerve root (Fig. 12-15). They evolve from macule to papule to vesicle and then to a crusted stage over a few days. Hyperesthesia or nerve root pain may precede, accompany, or follow the eruption and does not correlate with the severity of the rash. Pain, if present at all in pediatric patients, is rarely severe and is generally short-lived, unless a cranial nerve dermatome is involved, in which case pain can be excruciating. Fever and constitutional symptoms may or may not be part of the picture, but regional adenopathy is common.

Thoracic dermatomes are involved in most patients, followed in frequency by cervical, trigeminal, lumbar, and facial nerve regions. Cranial nerve involvement may produce a puzzling prodrome consisting of severe headache, facial pain, or auricular pain with no evident cause and lasting up to several days before appearance of the eruption. Lesions appear unilaterally on the tonsillar pillars and uvula with involvement of the maxillary branch of the trigeminal nerve; on the buccal mucosa and palate with involvement of the mandibular division; and on the face, cornea, and tip of the nose with involvement of the ophthalmic branch (Fig. 12-15D and see Fig. 20-45). When the geniculate ganglion is affected, vesicles are seen in the external auditory canal in concert with facial paralysis. Although varicella can be transmitted by patients with herpes zoster, contagion is generally less of a problem because most patients have lesions on areas that are covered by clothing and the oropharynx is not involved in most cases.

Gianotti-Crosti Syndrome

The eruption of Gianotti-Crosti syndrome, or papular acrodermatitis, though distinctive, often goes unrecognized (or is misdiagnosed). First described in association with anicteric hepatitis B, this exanthem has also been seen with infections due to other viral agents including EBV, coxsackieviruses, parainfluenza viruses, echoviruses, cytomegalovirus, and respiratory syncytial virus. Cases usually occur sporadically but occasionally occur in clusters. Most patients are between 1 and 6 years of age (range, 3 months to 15 years).

A mild prodrome consisting of low-grade fever and malaise is typical and may be associated with generalized

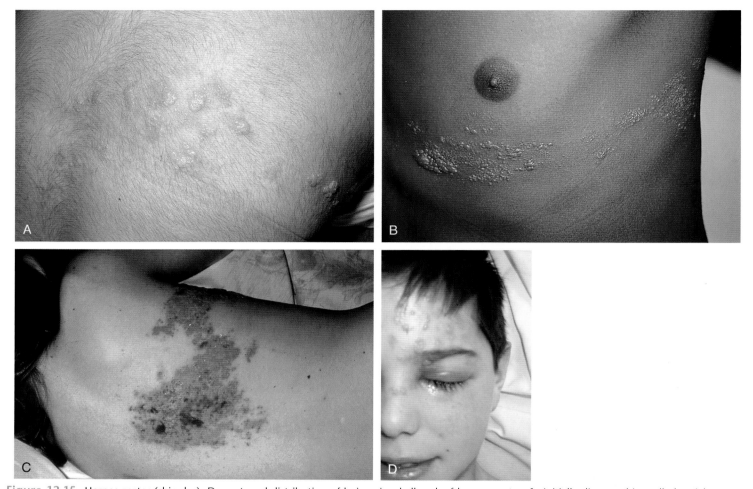

Figure 12-15. Herpes zoster (shingles). Dermatomal distribution of lesions is a hallmark of herpes zoster. **A,** Initially discrete thin-walled vesicles on an erythematous base are seen. **B,** Vesicles coalesce over a few days, and lesions then evolve to a crusted stage **(C). D,** Involvement of the ophthalmic branch of the trigeminal nerve produces lesions involving the forehead, eyelids, and nose. (**B,** Courtesy Michael Sherlock, MD, Lutherville, Md.)

adenopathy, hepatosplenomegaly (especially with hepatitis B), upper respiratory tract symptoms, and diarrhea. Within a few days the first of several crops of lesions appears abruptly. The lesions consist of discrete, firm, lichenoid papules with flat tops (Fig. 12-16A and B) and range from 1 to 10 mm in diameter, tending to be larger in infants and smaller in older children. Papules can be flesh colored, pink, red, dusky, coppery, or purpuric. They are distributed fairly symmetrically over the extremities (including the palms and soles), buttocks, and face, with relative sparing of the trunk and scalp (Fig. 12-16B), although the upper back may be involved. They tend to remain discrete but can become confluent, especially over pressure points (Fig. 12-16C), and the Koebner phenomenon may be seen. Pruritus is unusual, and there is no associated mucosal enanthem.

The exanthem often clears within 2 to 3 weeks but can persist for 8 weeks or more. Results of laboratory studies are generally nonspecific; however, liver function tests should be done, and if the results are abnormal, serologic studies for hepatitis B and EBV should be performed.

Treatment is symptomatic. Steroid creams are contraindicated because they may make the rash worse.

Bacterial Exanthems

Streptococcal Scarlet Fever

Although most commonly associated with pharyngitis and impetigo, group A β-hemolytic streptococci are frequently the cause of an illness associated with a general-

ized exanthem known as *scarlet fever*, or *scarlatina*. The exanthem is produced by an erythrogenic toxin excreted by the streptococcus. Streptococcal infections occur year-round, although pharyngitis and scarlet fever have a peak incidence in winter and spring. Transmission requires close contact to permit the direct spread of large droplets, and those with nasal infection are particularly effective sources. Anal carriers, as well as contaminated food sources, have also been responsible for outbreaks. The incubation period for scarlet fever ranges from 12 hours to approximately 7 days. The disease is contagious during the acute period, and patients may transmit the organisms during active subclinical infection as well. An average of 50% of family members living with an index case become secondarily infected, and up to half of these have subclinical disease.

Once a severe illness associated with high morbidity and mortality, scarlet fever has become a much milder illness over the past several decades. In the classic case, now seen less than 10% of the time, the patient experiences the abrupt onset of fever, chills, malaise, headache, sore throat, and vomiting; abdominal pain also may be a prominent complaint. Within 12 to 48 hours the exanthem appears and rapidly generalizes, usually beginning on the trunk and spreading peripherally, but sometimes spreading cephalocaudally. The face is flushed with perioral pallor (Fig. 12-17A). The remaining skin becomes diffusely erythematous and is covered by tiny pinhead-sized papules, giving the appearance of a sunburn with goose bumps. The texture is sandpapery on palpation, and the erythema blanches with pressure (Fig. 12-17B). The

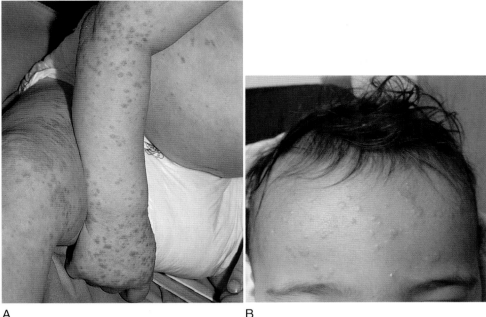

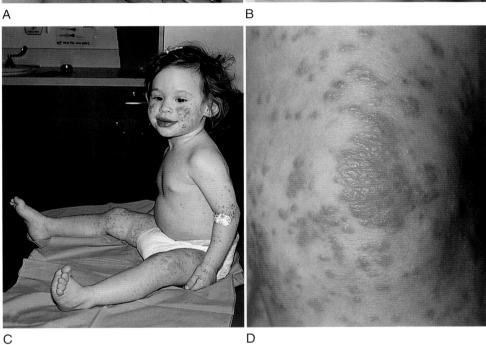

Figure 12-16. Gianotti-Crosti syndrome. **A** and **B,** Lesions consist of raised lichenoid papules with flat tops that appear in crops and tend to remain discrete. **C,** This child shows the characteristic acral distribution, with lesions involving the extremities and face but with relative sparing of the trunk. **D,** Lesions can become confluent over pressure points such as the knee.

skin may be pruritic, but it is not tender. Some patients also have urticaria and dermatographism. In severe cases, vesiculation may occur. Following generalization the rash becomes accentuated in skinfolds or creases, and 1 to 3 days after its appearance, petechiae may appear in a linear distribution along the creases, forming Pastia lines (Fig. 12-17C). Examination of the oropharynx in the "textbook" case discloses large, erythematous and edematous tonsils that are often covered by exudate, along with palatal erythema and petechiae (see Chapter 23). The uvula may be erythematous and edematous as well. The tongue also shows characteristic findings. During the first 2 days it has a white coating through which erythematous papillae project, resulting in a white strawberry tongue (Fig. 12-17D). Subsequently the white coat peels, leaving a glistening red surface with prominent papillae, a red strawberry tongue (Fig. 12-17E). Tender cervical adenopathy is noted in 30% to 60% of patients. Without treatment, the rash, fever, and pharyngitis resolve within 1 week; with treatment, improvement is relatively rapid. Desquamation occurs regardless of treatment and begins several days after onset, progressing cephalocaudally (Fig.

12-17F and G). The skin is shed in fine, thin flakes (in contrast to the thick flakes that characterize desquamation following staphylococcal exanthems [see Figs. 12-18 and 12-20]), and the extent of this process is directly proportional to the intensity of the exanthem.

Diagnosis is easy in the classic case, but the wide spectrum of disease severity and of potential manifestations can occasionally cause confusion. Fever may be absent or low grade, and malaise may be minimal. Pharyngitis may be mild (without exudate, petechiae, or marked erythema) or absent, even when the throat is the site of infection. In such cases, tongue changes may be absent as well. If streptococcal skin or wound infections are the primary site of infection, the oropharynx is normal. The appearance of the exanthem may vary as well. In some children it is patchy but continues to be most prominent near skinfolds (Fig. 12-17H). An occasional child may have diffuse petechiae. Still others may present with fever or nasopharyngitis and urticaria as their initial manifestations. In dark-skinned children, erythema and perioral pallor may be difficult to appreciate and the papules may be larger, thus producing a texture less like that of sandpaper.

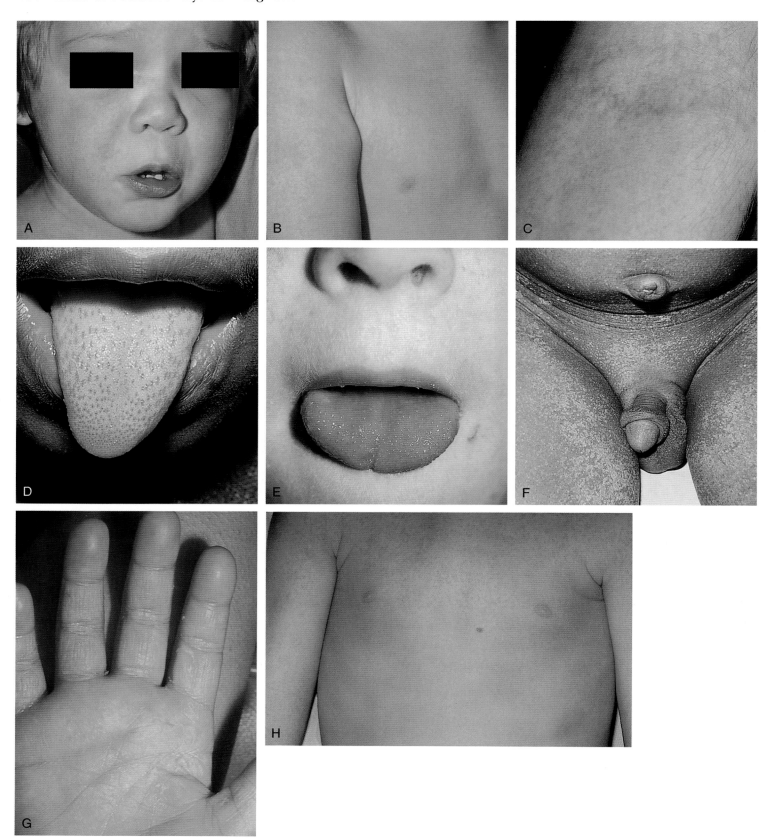

Figure 12-17. Streptococcal scarlet fever. **A** and **B,** In the classic form of this exanthem, the patient has a flushed face, perioral pallor, and a diffuse, blanching, erythematous rash that has a sandpapery consistency on palpation. **C,** Within 1 to 3 days of onset, Pastia lines may be noted. **D,** During the first 1 to 2 days the tongue has a white coating through which prominent erythematous papillae project—a white strawberry tongue. A few days later the white coat peels, leaving the characteristic red strawberry tongue with glistening surface and prominent papillae (**E**). **F** and **G,** Desquamation occurs in fine, thin flakes as the acute phase of the illness resolves and is proportional to the intensity of the exanthem. **H,** A wide spectrum of severity and manifestations exists. In this child with streptococcal scarlet fever, the rash has a patchy distribution but is accentuated in the axillae and other creases. (**A, B,** and **F,** Courtesy Michael Sherlock, MD, Lutherville, Md.)

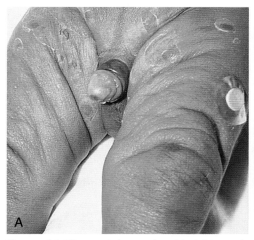
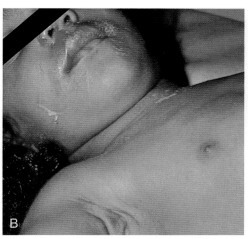
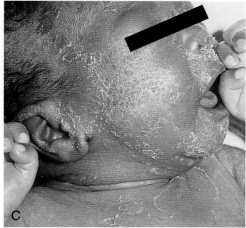

Figure 12-18. Staphylococcal scalded skin syndrome. **A,** This infant shows evidence of epidermal separation and has numerous ruptured bullae over the inguinal region and thighs. **B,** In this older child, symptoms were mild and only the skin of the face, axillae, and perineum showed signs of epidermal separation. Note the evidence of a positive Nikolsky sign on her upper lip and cheek, the result of wiping her nose. **C,** A denuded area is evident on the upper chest, and thick flakes have begun to form on the face of this infant. Culture of the purulent nasal discharge was positive for *Staphylococcus aureus*. (Courtesy Michael Sherlock, MD, Lutherville, Md.)

The recognition of scarlet fever, followed by treatment with a 10-day course of penicillin or erythromycin (in penicillin-allergic children), is important for reducing the risk of transmission and preventing rheumatic fever and pyogenic complications, the most common of which include adenitis, otitis, sinusitis, and peritonsillar and retropharyngeal abscesses. Therefore, in patients with fever or nasopharyngitis and urticaria and in children with scarlatiniform eruptions, a screening throat culture for group A streptococci should be obtained, regardless of the presence or absence of other symptoms. Poststreptococcal nephritis, however, is not prevented by antimicrobial therapy.

Staphylococcal Exanthems

Coagulase-positive staphylococci are ubiquitous organisms that are carried at any given time by approximately one third of the population. Although the hallmark of staphylococcal infection is the abscess, numerous forms of infection are seen, and at least three distinct generalized exanthematous disorders have now been identified: staphylococcal scalded skin syndrome; staphylococcal scarlet fever; and toxic shock syndrome. In each form the organisms at the primary site of infection release exotoxins, which then produce the characteristic rash. Transmission may occur by means of direct contact with persons who are infected or who are carriers. Sites of carriage include the nose, skin, axilla, perineum, hair, and nails. Spread of infection may also occur through contact with contaminated objects or food. Draining skin lesions, nasal discharge, and contaminated hands constitute particularly important sources of transmission. Traumatic or surgical wounds, burns, insect bites, areas of preexisting dermatitis, viral skin lesions, and prior viral respiratory tract infection all serve as major predisposing conditions.

Staphylococcal Scalded Skin Syndrome. A disorder seen most commonly in infants and young children, staphylococcal scalded skin syndrome is caused by phage group II coagulase-positive staphylococci. The primary infection is usually mild, with purulent nasopharyngitis, conjunctivitis, impetigo, and infections of the umbilicus and circumcision sites seen most commonly. Rarely, sepsis, pneumonia, or other severe invasive staphylococcal infections may precede the onset of the exanthem.

The infecting organisms produce an epidermolytic exotoxin, which is spread hematogenously and causes cleavage of the skin between the epidermis and the dermis. This process may begin within hours or days of the appearance of signs of the primary infection, and typically its onset is heralded by fever and irritability, often accompanied by vomiting. These symptoms are followed by the development of a diffuse erythroderma that spreads rapidly from head to toe and simulates the appearance of a sunburn. In contrast to streptococcal scarlet fever, the involved skin is tender, even to light touch. Within 1 to 3 days, thin-walled, flaccid, bullous lesions appear and rupture soon after formation (Fig. 12-18A). Simultaneously, larger portions of the epidermis begin to separate in sheets, and during this phase application of light lateral traction on the skin causes the epidermis to pull away from the dermis, leaving a raw, weeping surface; this separation of the skin in response to stroking is called the *Nikolsky sign* (Fig. 12-18B). After exfoliation the surface gradually dries, forming large, thick flakes (Fig. 12-18C).

A broad spectrum of severity exists for this syndrome. In severe cases the patient appears toxic and in considerable pain. The child may shed large portions of skin, resulting in significant fluid losses that may be accompanied by difficulties with temperature regulation. In mild cases (see Fig. 12-18B) toxicity is absent and only localized areas of skin are denuded, with the face and perineum constituting the primary sites of shedding. The causative organism can be isolated from the site of primary infection, but it is absent—at least initially—from the bullae and from sites of skin separation.

Staphylococcal Scarlet Fever. Staphylococcal infection can result in an exanthem that initially is indistinguishable in appearance from that produced by group A β-hemolytic streptococci. The illness is characterized by fever, irritability, and moderate malaise, followed by the abrupt onset of a generalized erythematous rash, often of sandpapery consistency, with accentuation in the skin creases (Fig. 12-19A). In contrast to the exanthem seen in streptococcal scarlet fever, the involved skin is usually tender, the tongue is normal, and there is no palatal enanthem. Evolution of lesions also differs, in that within 2 to 5 days the skin begins to crack, fissure, and weep, especially in the perioral and periorbital areas and in the skin creases (Fig. 12-19B). It is then shed in large, thick flakes

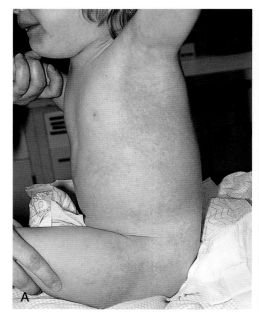

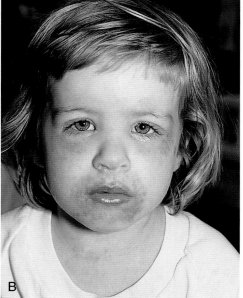

Figure 12-19. Staphylococcal scarlet fever. **A,** In this patient, nasopharyngitis and purulent conjunctivitis antedated the development of a generalized sandpaper-like rash, which was tender to the touch. **B,** The skin in the periorbital and perioral areas has begun to crack, fissure, and weep serous fluid.

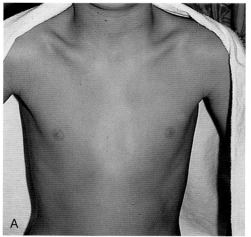

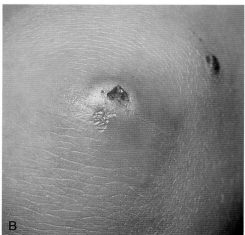

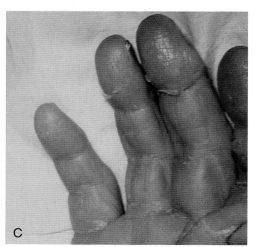

Figure 12-20. Toxic shock syndrome. **A,** This young boy presented with diffuse erythroderma, fever, chills, myalgias, headache, vomiting, and orthostatic dizziness with mild widening of his pulse pressure. **B,** Examination disclosed an infected puncture wound of the knee, which grew *Staphylococcus aureus.* Though his illness was relatively mild, the association of gastrointestinal symptoms and orthostatic changes suggested TSS, which was confirmed by laboratory studies and by subsequent desquamation **(C).** This begins periungually, and the skin is shed in thick casts. (**C,** Courtesy George Pazin, MD, University of Pittsburgh Medical Center.)

over 3 to 5 days. Local skin and wound infections are common antecedents, and their presence often enables presumptive identification of staphylococci as causative agents early in the disease. However, when nasopharyngitis is the source of primary infection, the picture can be difficult to distinguish from that of variants of streptococcal infection, in which the strawberry tongue and palatal petechiae are often absent. The same may be true if a local infection with lymphangitis is the source. In such cases the tendency for the staphylococcal rash to be tender may be the major clinical distinction, pending Gram stain or culture results. Unless the primary infection is severe enough to warrant parenteral treatment, oral antimicrobial therapy is sufficient.

Toxic Shock Syndrome. Toxic shock syndrome (TSS) is the third syndrome of staphylococcal origin characterized by a generalized exanthem. It is seen in children and adults who have localized infections caused by coagulase-positive staphylococci of phage group I or III and has been recognized in menstruating women and girls whose vaginas are colonized with these organisms. In the latter subgroup of patients (who may not have a history of prior

vaginal discharge), there is a strong correlation with tampon use, indicating that the impedance of normal menstrual flow or the presence of abrasions secondary to use of large bell-shaped tampons may contribute to the development of this syndrome. Patients with non–menstrually associated TSS often have a skin lesion, an abscess, or purulent conjunctivitis as the primary focus of infection (Fig. 12-20B).

In its full-blown form, TSS begins with a prodrome consisting of low-grade fever, malaise, myalgias, and vomiting. This is followed by an abrupt increase in fever, accompanied by chills, worsening myalgias, repetitive vomiting, abdominal pain, orthostatic dizziness, and weakness. Soon thereafter, patients show a diffuse erythroderma, mimicking a sunburn (Fig. 12-20A). Conjunctivitis with photophobia, oropharyngeal erythema, and a strawberry tongue are common features. Subsequently, severe watery diarrhea, hypotension, and oliguria may become prominent, accompanied by alterations in level of consciousness. This often necessitates massive volume replacement and vasopressor therapy. In severe cases, acute respiratory distress syndrome may develop.

Many patients have muscle tenderness and weakness, as well as diffuse abdominal tenderness without peritoneal signs. A small proportion show nonpitting edema of the face, hands, and feet. Over the ensuing days, petechiae and a secondary maculopapular rash may be noted, along with oral ulcerations. Desquamation is routine, usually beginning a week after onset of the rash. It is most prominent over the palms and soles and in the periungual areas, and the skin is shed in thick casts (Fig. 12-20C). Parenteral antimicrobial therapy directed against *Staphylococcus aureus* is designed to eradicate any focus of infection and to reduce the risk of recurrence.

Clinical and laboratory findings in severe cases point toward the existence of a process in which there is diffuse vascular leakage with third-spacing of fluids, electrolytes, and serum proteins. Secondary hypotension and hypoperfusion result in azotemia. Toxin-related hepatic changes may also be noted.

As recognition of TSS has increased, the existence of a wide spectrum of severity has become apparent. Mild cases mimic staphylococcal scarlet fever. Such patients tend to have smaller gastrointestinal losses and less difficulty with fluid shifts and attendant complications.

Meningococcal Exanthems

Neisseria meningitidis is capable of producing several clinical illnesses, two of which—acute meningococcemia and meningococcosis, or chronic meningococcemia—are characterized in part by a generalized exanthem. The organism is carried in the upper respiratory tract of humans who, though usually asymptomatic, nevertheless may transmit the organism via droplet spread of respiratory secretions to close contacts. Most people so exposed become colonized without clinical disease. Clinical illness is most common in children younger than 5 years of age, with a peak incidence between 6 and 12 months. A secondary peak of lesser magnitude is seen during adolescence and young adulthood. Susceptibility to disease appears to be related to a lack of bactericidal antibody or to a failure to produce antibody in response to infection. Antecedent viral respiratory tract infection can be a predisposing factor.

Although meningococcal infection occurs year-round, the peak season for these illnesses is late winter and early spring. Invasive disease occurs both endemically and epidemically. Persons who have intimate contact with infected patients, such as other members of the same household or persons in "closed communities" like military barracks, dormitories, or day-care centers, are at highest risk of becoming secondarily infected; and they should receive antimicrobial prophylaxis. The incubation period after exposure ranges from 1 to 10 days, with most clinical cases developing in less than 4 days. Secondary attack rates range from 0.3% to 10% and are highest during epidemic outbreaks. Any mucosal surface is subject to infection, which may remain localized or may serve as the source of invasive disease.

Meningococcal Meningitis and Acute Meningococcemia. The two major invasive forms of meningococcal disease are meningitis and septicemia, which may occur singly or in combination. Patients usually experience a prodromal period ranging from a few hours to 5 days. During this phase, symptoms of upper respiratory tract infection or nasopharyngitis in association with fever are typical. Patients may also experience lethargy, headache, myalgias, arthralgias, and vomiting. After this, an abrupt change occurs, characterized by increased fever with chills (or occasionally hypothermia), worsening malaise, and

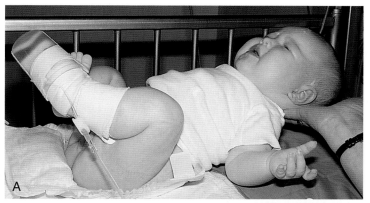
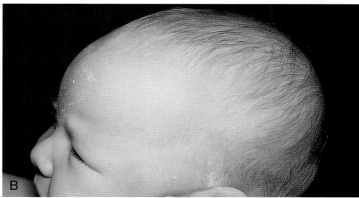

Figure 12-21. Meningitis. **A,** Nuchal rigidity and a positive Brudzinski sign are demonstrated. On attempted passive flexion of the neck, the infant grimaces with pain, neck stiffness limits flexion, and the knees and hips are flexed to reduce traction on the meninges. **B,** This infant was also found to have a bulging anterior fontanelle when sitting quietly, reflecting increased intracranial pressure.

progressive lethargy. In the 90% in whom meningitis is the primary manifestation, vomiting, irritability (often with a high-pitched cry in infants), and nuchal rigidity are prominent (Fig. 12-21A). Infants may also have a bulging fontanelle (Fig. 12-21B). Delirium, combativeness, stupor, and seizures may develop in some cases. Although some patients with meningitis also have meningococcemia, cutaneous manifestations, endotoxic shock, and disseminated intravascular coagulation (DIC) are less likely to develop in them than in those without meningeal infection and mortality is relatively low.

In contrast, approximately 10% of patients show a picture of overwhelming sepsis with little or no laboratory evidence of meningitis. In these patients the abrupt change in the clinical picture just described typically heralds the development of a rash in association with manifestations of shock including mottling, distal coolness with decreased capillary refill or cyanosis, and either widened pulse pressure or frank hypotension. Up to 85% of these patients have cutaneous lesions involving the trunk and extremities. Such lesions may consist of tender pink macules; petechiae, which may be palpably raised; and purpura, which when present is most prominent on the extremities and may progress to form areas of frank necrosis (Fig. 12-22). The combination of purpura and shock is termed the *Waterhouse-Friderichsen syndrome* and has been associated in some but not all instances with adrenal hemorrhage and secondary adrenal insufficiency. Evolution may be fulminant, resulting in prostration within a few hours, or it may be slower, occurring over a period lasting up to 24 hours. The prognosis in patients with a short prodrome, fulminant progression, and early appearance of

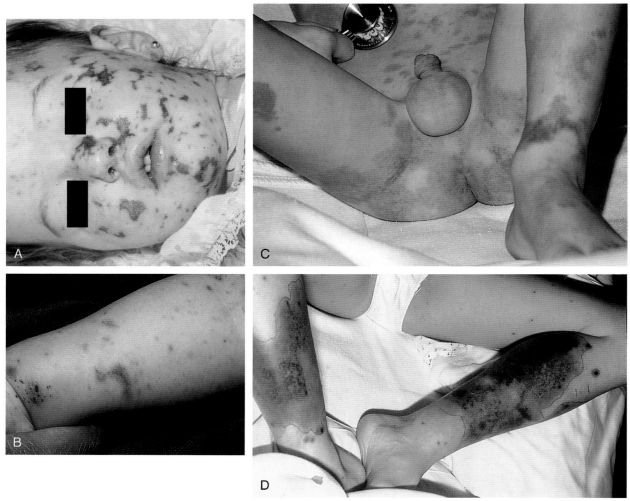

Figure 12-22. Meningococcemia. **A,** This youngster manifests the purpuric and petechial rash characteristic of acute meningococcemia. **B,** Petechiae are more apparent in this close-up of an infant. Gram stain of petechial scrapings may reveal organisms. **C** and **D,** Purpura may progress to form areas of frank cutaneous necrosis, especially in patients with DIC. (**D,** Courtesy Kenneth Schuitt, MD.)

purpuric lesions is particularly poor. More than 60% of such patients have clinical evidence of hypotension and DIC on presentation, and approximately 50% have no leukocytosis, indicating that their immune system has been overwhelmed. Only about 20% of these patients have meningitis. Mortality in such patients approaches 40%, whereas only 3% of those showing slower progression die. Most deaths occur within 24 hours of presentation and result from a combination of circulatory collapse and congestive heart failure caused by endotoxic shock and myocarditis.

In many cases the diagnosis can be suspected clinically and is confirmed by laboratory findings. Gram-stained smears of petechial lesions and buffy coat preparations often reveal gram-negative diplococci. Cultures of blood, cerebrospinal fluid (CSF), and petechial lesions should be performed unless the severity of illness precludes lumbar puncture. Because of the potential for deterioration, aggressive empirical antimicrobial therapy and vigorous supportive measures should be instituted promptly whenever meningococcemia is suspected.

Among numerous differential diagnostic possibilities are other forms of bacterial sepsis, bacterial endocarditis, Rocky Mountain spotted fever, and various other disorders characterized by thrombocytopenia. Some forms of septicemia caused by gram-negative bacilli initially may be clinically indistinguishable from meningococcal septicemia. Similarly, *Haemophilus influenzae* type B and

pneumococcal septicemia may be associated with the development of petechiae, though in these cases they are not usually palpable. The purpuric lesions of staphylococcal sepsis tend to become pustular early on, and the site of primary infection also helps distinguish infection with this organism. Adenoviral and streptococcal infections may produce petechial rashes but usually do not cause a septic picture. Other clinical characteristics help to identify patients with thrombocytopenia resulting from immune thrombocytopenic purpura, acute leukemia, and mononucleosis; the centripetal mode of spread of the petechial rash of Rocky Mountain spotted fever and the initial distribution and subsequent mode of spread of the lesions of Henoch-Schönlein purpura help to distinguish these illnesses. Differentiation can be particularly difficult in the case of a child presenting with high fever with no source other than that of an upper respiratory tract infection and a petechial rash. These findings may represent early nonfulminant meningococcemia, but they also can be part of the picture of viral illness or another bacterial process; in such cases observation or presumptive therapy may be necessary.

Meningococcosis (Chronic Meningococcemia). Meningococcosis, a disorder more indolent than acute meningococcemia, is defined as a meningococcal sepsis with a fever of greater than 1 week's duration, without meningitis. On average, symptoms are present for 6 to 8 weeks before diagnosis. In most cases symptoms are inter-

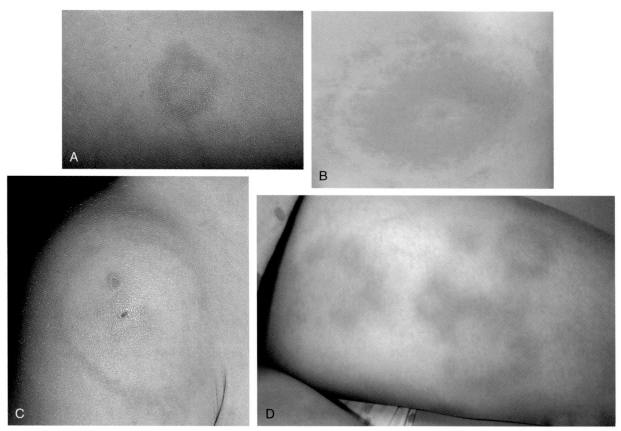

Figure 12-23. Erythema migrans/Lyme disease. **A,** This 2- to 3-cm lesion is just starting to clear centrally. **B,** This larger lesion has formed concentric circles around a central papule. **C,** Central clearing is nearly complete, and within the erythematous border the puncta of two tick bites are evident. **D,** Multiple annular lesions of differing sizes and varying degrees of central clearing are seen in this child with Lyme disease. (**A,** Courtesy Sylvia Suarez, MD, Centerville, Va. **B,** Courtesy Caroline and David Eddy. **C,** Courtesy Ellen Wald, MD, University of Wisconsin Children's Hospital. **D,** Courtesy J. Carlton Gartner Jr., MD, I. A. DuPont Hospital, Wilmington, Del.)

mittent; in all cases they consist of fever and chills (without rigor) and are associated with an exanthem in nearly 95% of cases. The rash waxes and wanes, often in association with the fever. Lesions may consist of tender erythematous, subcutaneous nodules; erythematous macules and papules; or petechiae, occurring singly or in combination. Urticarial lesions are seen occasionally. The feet, legs, upper arms, and trunk are the sites most commonly involved. Mild malaise and myalgias tend to accompany the fever and headache, and arthralgias are also common. In childhood cases swelling of hands, feet, knees, and ankles may occur intermittently, without evidence of warmth or erythema; however, when the legs are involved, the child may refuse to walk.

The diagnosis of meningococcosis can be difficult because early blood cultures are often negative (although children are more likely than adults to have positive cultures) and skin lesions are generally negative for organisms, both on smear and culture. Throat culture is usually negative as well. Leukocytosis is seen with the fever. The sedimentation rate may be normal or elevated. Thrombocytopenia is seen occasionally. Close follow-up monitoring of the clinical course, combined with repeated blood cultures, constitutes the best way to confirm the diagnosis. Of the patients whose infection goes undiagnosed and untreated, approximately one third ultimately suffer severe localized infection (after an average of 10 weeks of illness), with meningitis, carditis, nephritis, and ocular infection occurring most commonly.

Lyme Disease

Lyme disease is a multisystem, tick-borne infection caused by the spirochete *Borrelia burgdorferi*. Named for the southeastern Connecticut community where it was first discovered more than 2 decades ago, Lyme disease was originally identified as a cause of chronic arthritis. Subsequent investigation has established the multisystem nature of the illness, which primarily involves the skin, heart, nervous system, and joints.

Transmission of Lyme disease occurs when a person is bitten by an infected *Ixodes* species tick (deer tick). The *Ixodes scapularis* (formerly *Ixodes dammini*) is the most common vector and is found predominantly in the Northeast and to a lesser extent in Midwestern parts of the United States. *Ixodes pacificus* is responsible for transmission in the Western states but is not as commonly infected with *B. burgdorferi*. When not engorged, the tick is about the size of a pin head. The *Borrelia* organisms for which the tick is a vector can be harbored by any feral or domestic animal, but *I. scapularis's* preferred host and major reservoir for infection is the white-footed mouse during the tick's nymph and larval stages. Most cases occur between spring and fall when the nymph stage of deer ticks is active and people are more likely to be outdoors.

After an incubation period of 3 to 31 days, the distinctive exanthem of Lyme disease, known as *erythema migrans*, appears in approximately 50% of cases. The rash begins as a red papule or macule at the site of the tick bite and often goes unrecognized. The lesion gradually enlarges (to a median size of 15 cm), forming a large plaque, which tends to clear centrally, giving it an annular configuration (Fig. 12-23).

Occasionally, instead of clearing, the central portion develops a bluish discoloration or becomes indurated or vesicular; rarely it necroses. The exanthem may be warm to the touch, and some patients report mild pruritus, burning, or prickling sensations. Multiple secondary annular lesions or evanescent red blotches, which are smaller than the primary lesion, develop in about 25% of all patients with erythema migrans, representing early disseminated disease (Fig. 12-23D).

Although erythema migrans may be the sole manifestation of early Lyme disease, the exanthem is often accompanied by a flulike constellation of systemic symptoms that are probably the result of early hematogenous dissemination of the causative organism. These symptoms include fever (usually low grade but in some cases high spikes with chills), malaise and fatigue, headache sometimes accompanied by mild meningismus, and myalgias and arthralgias. Occasionally, nausea, vomiting, conjunctivitis, pharyngitis, a malar rash, and either regional adenopathy in association with the erythema migrans lesion or generalized adenopathy are seen.

Untreated, the erythema migrans lesion gradually resolves over 3 weeks and systemic symptoms often wax and wane over the course of several weeks. With treatment, the rash clears within several days and the systemic symptoms tend to resolve in $1\frac{1}{2}$ to 4 weeks.

Other, less common manifestations of early disseminated disease involve the nervous system and heart. Aseptic meningitis sometimes accompanied by focal neurologic signs and symptoms and unilateral or bilateral facial nerve palsy with or without CSF pleocytosis are the neurologic manifestations seen most often in pediatric patients. Optic neuritis, iritis, and keratitis are unusual. Carditis, characterized by varying degrees of atrioventricular block or myopericarditis, is rare in children.

The arthritis of Lyme disease is a late manifestation, seen in up to 50% of untreated patients. It is pauciarticular, involving large joints, especially the knee. Pain, warmth, and swelling are typical, but overlying erythema is unusual. The initial episode usually lasts about a week but can be prolonged. Thereafter, numerous recurrences may be experienced. Rarely, after a year, a chronic erosive arthritis may develop. Late neurologic manifestations include encephalitis, encephalopathy, ataxia, radiculoneuritis, and myelitis. The features of this later phase of Lyme disease are probably the result of a combination of ongoing infection and compromise of the patient's immune response.

In patients with erythema migrans, the diagnosis can be made solely on clinical and epidemiologic grounds, even in the absence of a clear history of tick bite. Results of serologic studies generally are not helpful in making a diagnosis during the early stages of the illness (although an IgM enzyme immunoassay is now available that can increase the yield). Such studies can be valuable, however, for diagnosing the disease in patients with neurologic, cardiac, or joint manifestations, especially in those with no prior history of a tick bite or erythema migrans. In patients with neurologic complications, both CSF and serum specimens should be submitted for analysis. Because commercially available test kits have been found to be unreliable, antibody studies should be done at a reference laboratory and confirmed with a Western immunoblot test to ensure maximum accuracy.

Although antimicrobial treatment can be helpful in both early and late stages of the disease, therapy should be initiated as early as possible because it not only hastens resolution of early symptoms but also prevents later complications of the disease.

Rocky Mountain Spotted Fever

Rocky Mountain spotted fever is an acute, potentially severe exanthematous disease caused by *Rickettsia rickett-*

sii. These obligate intracellular parasites are usually transmitted to humans by the bite of an infected tick, which injects organisms while it feeds on the host. Once injected, the organisms multiply in the endothelium of small blood vessels and are spread hematogenously, resulting in a widespread vasculitis characterized by focal inflammation and thrombosis with secondary vascular leakage. Because ticks are active during warm months, the peak seasons for this disorder are spring and summer. The incubation period ranges from 2 to 14 days, with an average of 4 to 8 days. Two thirds of cases occur in children younger than 15 years of age. Yearly outbreaks tend to occur in circumscribed geographic areas. Mortality is as high as 5% to 7% and often stems from failure to diagnose and treat the condition in its early phase.

Onset may be acute or gradual and is characterized by fever and headache. The headache, which may be frontal or generalized, is typically severe, unremitting, and unresponsive to analgesia. Headache may not be a major complaint in very young children, however. Other, less constant symptoms include chills, anorexia, nausea and vomiting, sore throat, abdominal pain, diarrhea, arthralgias, and myalgias. Respiratory symptoms are uncommon. The spleen is enlarged in 30% to 50% of patients, but adenopathy is not prominent. The exanthem is usually noted on or about the third day of illness, but it may appear as late as the beginning of the second week.

In most patients the characteristic appearance and mode of spread of the exanthem are the most helpful clues to clinical diagnosis. The rash begins distally on the wrists, ankles, palms, and soles, usually appearing as an erythematous, blanching, fine, macular or maculopapular eruption. It then spreads centripetally and becomes petechial (Fig. 12-24), although occasionally, lesions are petechial from the outset. In some cases the eruption is not prominent and may even be transient, making diagnosis difficult. Conjunctival injection, with photophobia and petechial hemorrhages, often develops simultaneously with the rash. Firm, nonpitting, nondependent edema, beginning in the periorbital region and then generalizing, tends to occur a few days after the onset of symptoms. In severe cases CNS symptoms develop with disease progression and range in severity from restlessness, irritability, and anxiety to confusion, delirium, and coma, with or without seizures and focal neurologic signs. Myocarditis, DIC, renal failure, and cardiovascular collapse are features of advanced disease.

White blood cell counts are normal or low in the first few days and then tend to rise. Thrombocytopenia is common. Other laboratory abnormalities include hyponatremia due to fluid shifts and renal losses; hypoproteinemia resulting from vascular and renal losses and hepatic dysfunction; abnormal liver function tests; and hyperkalemia with increasing cell death.

Because there is no diagnostic test capable of providing prompt definitive results, and because the early institution of antimicrobial treatment is crucial to a favorable outcome, the diagnosis of Rocky Mountain spotted fever must be made on clinical grounds and as early as possible. The diagnosis should be suspected in any child with fever, headache, toxicity, and a centripetally spreading petechial rash, especially when the patient's history suggests or confirms an exposure to ticks in an endemic area. Because of the potentially life-threatening nature of this infection, doxycycline is recommended as the drug of choice regardless of age (despite its usual contraindication in children younger than 8 years). Recovery is the rule if therapy is begun during the first week of illness. If treatment is

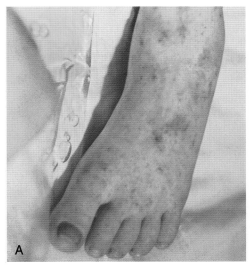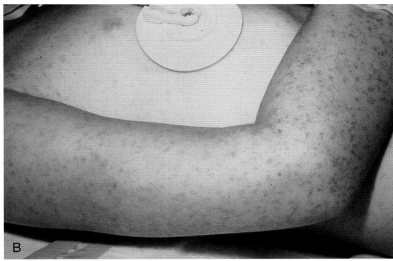

Figure 12-24. Rocky Mountain spotted fever. **A,** The exanthem characteristic of this disease first appears distally on wrists, ankles, palms, and soles. It may be petechial from the outset, or it may start as an erythematous, blanching, macular, or maculopapular eruption, which then becomes petechial as it spreads centripetally. **B,** In this child the rash has become generalized. Both petechial and blanching erythematous lesions are present. (**A,** Courtesy Ellen Wald, MD, University of Wisconsin Children's Hospital.)

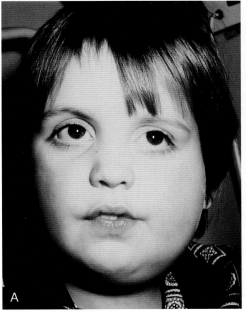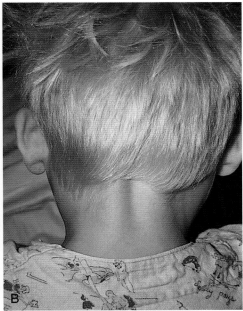

Figure 12-25. Mumps. **A,** This young boy showed unilateral parotid swelling, which was indurated and moderately tender. Visually it was appreciated best in this view, which reveals swelling anterior and inferior to his left ear. **B,** Bilateral infra- and postauricular swelling (right greater than left) can be appreciated when the patient is viewed from behind. Secondary displacement of the auricle is evident. (**A,** Courtesy G. D. W. McKendrik, MD; **B,** courtesy Michael Sherlock, MD, Lutherville, Md.)

delayed beyond the first week, however, the outcome may be unfavorable despite the institution of antimicrobial therapy and vigorous supportive measures. Subsequent serologic confirmation may be made using complement fixation tests or a variety of other assays. Immunofluorescence examination of skin biopsy specimens obtained 4 to 8 days from onset can provide earlier confirmation, but often this test is not readily available.

Mumps (Epidemic Parotitis)

Mumps is an acute viral illness that preferentially involves glandular and neural tissues. It is rarely seen in the United States since the advent of the Measles Mumps Rubella combination vaccine. Although the salivary glands, especially the parotid glands, are the most common sites of clinical involvement, the CNS and other glandular tissues may be affected as well. In up to one third of patients the infection is subclinical. Peak incidence is in late winter and spring. The incubation period is 16 to 18 days, with the disease being contagious in patients from 1 to 7 days before the onset of clinical symptoms and for 5 to 9 days thereafter. Asymptomatic children can also transmit the virus.

Prodromal symptoms consist of fever, headache, malaise, and anorexia. In the typical case these symptoms are followed within 24 hours by the onset of an earache or face pain, which older children can often localize to the region of the pinna. Pain is aggravated by chewing and by stimulation of salivation (in particular, by sour foods). Parotid swelling generally becomes noticeable within the next 24 hours, increases gradually over the ensuing few days, then abates over a similar period of time. Fever may persist for the duration of swelling but can disappear early in the course. On examination, an area of tender, indurated swelling, extending from the preauricular area through the subauricular space to the postauricular region, can be palpated (Fig. 12-25A). With pronounced enlargement the pinna is pushed up and out (Fig. 12-25B). The gland is indurated and mildly to moderately tender to palpation. The color of the overlying skin is normal. Intraoral exami-

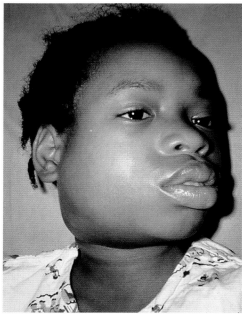

Figure 12-26. Suppurative parotitis. This patient had high fever, chills, and marked enlargement of the right parotid gland, which was severely painful and exquisitely tender. The overlying skin is erythematous, and purulent material was seen draining from the Stensen duct. (Courtesy Sylvan Stool, MD.)

nation may reveal erythema and edema of the Stensen duct. Bilateral involvement is usual, although one gland tends to enlarge before the other, and up to 25% of symptomatic patients have unilateral inflammation.

This typical picture is but one of many possible variants of clinical mumps. In some cases the parotid gland is spared and the submental or sublingual salivary glands may be the primary site of involvement. In the former instance, indurated swelling is found below the midportion of the mandible; in the latter case, bilateral submental swelling is seen externally and sublingual swelling is noted intraorally.

Preauricular swelling and induration, the Stensen duct abnormality, and the absence of prominent overlying erythema help to distinguish parotid swelling from cervical adenitis involving the tonsillar node. In confusing cases and in cases in which the submental or sublingual salivary glands are involved, closely simulating adenopathy, the patient can be given lemon juice to sip or a lemon wedge to suck. In patients with mumps, this results in a prompt enlargement of the affected gland and in pain as salivation is stimulated, whereas no such change is seen in patients with adenopathy. In cases of bacterial parotitis, the patient is likely to have high fever and show signs of toxicity. The overlying skin is erythematous, with exquisite tenderness found on palpation (Fig. 12-26). Purulent drainage from the Stensen duct can often be seen when the gland is massaged.

Although it has been estimated that up to 75% of patients with mumps may have CSF pleocytosis, symptomatic meningoencephalitis is seen only in about 10% of patients. CNS symptoms usually follow parotitis but can develop before or even in the absence of salivary gland involvement. There is a wide spectrum in the severity of these symptoms, ranging from isolated headache and malaise with fever to frank nuchal rigidity with nausea, vomiting, and severe alterations in sensorium. Fortunately, permanent sequelae are rare, although children recovering from severe mumps meningoencephalitis

may not return to normal levels of school performance for up to 6 months or a year.

Mumps orchitis is much less common in boys than in men, who have a 20% to 30% incidence. Orchitis usually follows salivary gland enlargement but may occur in its absence. Fever, chills, headache, nausea, vomiting, and lower abdominal pain are prominent and develop with the onset of painful, generally unilateral testicular swelling. Epididymitis is an invariable accompaniment. This process lasts 3 to 7 days. Oophoritis, seen in an occasional female patient, presents with a secondary temperature spike, nausea, vomiting, and severe lower abdominal pain and tenderness. Involvement may be unilateral or bilateral, and when unilateral and on the right side, it may be indistinguishable from appendicitis. Pancreatitis is an uncommon though potentially severe manifestation. Such patients tend to have sudden onset of excruciating epigastric pain in association with fever, chills, repetitive vomiting, weakness, and prostration. This, too, tends to last for 3 to 7 days. Thyroiditis, mastitis, bartholinitis, and dacryocystitis have been reported in isolated cases as well.

Bacterial Skin and Soft Tissue Infections

Superficial bacterial skin infections occur with a relatively high frequency in childhood. In most cases the causative organisms are inoculated through a small wound, such as a superficial cut, an abrasion, an insect bite, or a burn. Infection may occur at the time of the injury if the pathogen has colonized the site previously, or it may occur subsequently as the result of scratching, touching, or contamination with dirt. In some cases a preexisting dermatitis sets the stage for secondary infection by breaking down the skin barrier. The ever-present risk of infection in patients with preexisting dermatitis must be kept in mind, especially when steroids are prescribed.

Although most superficial infections are relatively minor in severity, diagnosis and proper treatment are important to reduce further spread of infection and prevent its transmission to others. Deeper skin and soft tissue infections, although less common, have the potential for causing greater morbidity and even mortality. As with superficial lesions, inoculation from an external source is the most common mode of acquisition. In many instances, however, these infections represent metastatic foci of bacteremic spread.

Group A β-hemolytic streptococci and coagulase-positive staphylococci are the organisms most commonly responsible for skin and soft tissue infections. Both organisms commonly reside in the nasopharynx, and staphylococci routinely colonize the skin, a phenomenon that is less likely, though still possible, with streptococci. Both organisms are transmitted readily by carriers or persons with active nasopharyngeal or skin infections. The fact that each pathogen produces relatively characteristic clinical features can help, to some extent, in making clinical diagnoses. Staphylococci, for example, are somewhat more likely to remain localized, stimulating suppuration and tissue necrosis, whereas streptococcal infection tends to spread along tissue planes and through lymphatics and thus is more commonly associated with secondary cellulitis, lymphangitis, and regional adenopathy. Methicillin resistant S. aureus (MRSA) has increased substantially in the community, as well as in health care settings, and cannot be clinically distinguished from methicillin-susceptible strains of S. aureus.

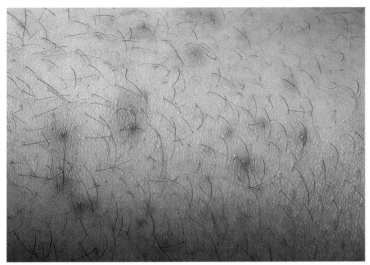

Figure 12-27. Folliculitis. The extensor surfaces of the extremities and other hair-bearing areas are the most common sites of this superficial infection of hair follicles. Lesions begin at the base of a hair shaft as erythematous nodules and then evolve to form central pustules with a thin, red rim.

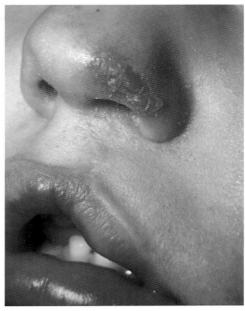

Figure 12-28. Streptococcal impetigo. This impetiginous lesion has evolved from a papule to a vesicle that ruptured, producing this characteristic honey-colored crust. (Courtesy Michael Sherlock, MD, Lutherville, Md.)

Folliculitis

Folliculitis is a superficial infection or irritation of hair follicles. The scalp, face, extensor surfaces of the extremities, and buttocks are the most common sites of involvement. Patients with dry, atopic skin and keratosis pilaris (a condition in which follicles become blocked by keratin plugs) are particularly prone to this problem (see Chapter 8). Additional predisposing factors include seborrhea, excessive sweating, poor hygiene, and topical application of or contact with oils, tars, and adhesives. In each of these situations, obstruction of follicles occurs, setting the stage for inflammation and secondary infection. After occlusion, a superficial erythematous nodule develops around the hair. The lesion then evolves into a thin-walled central pustule with a narrow, red rim (Fig. 12-27). The lesions may itch or burn and subsequently may drain and crust. Although it takes a given lesion 7 to 10 days to heal without treatment, multiple crops may occur. With scratching the infection may spread to other areas, and secondary impetiginous lesions may develop. Coagulase-positive staphylococci are the pathogens usually identified, although other skin colonizers may participate. Oral antimicrobial therapy directed at the staphylococcus and treatment or avoidance of the predisposing condition are the measures indicated to eradicate the process.

On occasion the early lesions found in some forms of tinea capitis and tinea corporis may mimic folliculitis, although itching is usually more prominent in fungal infections and the surrounding rim of erythema tends to be wider. Tinea should be suspected, especially if folliculitis is localized to the hairline of the scalp (see Fig. 8-139). Older lesions, if present, may help in distinguishing between fungal and bacterial infections. Gram stain, potassium hydroxide preparations, and cultures can be useful in evaluating questionable cases.

Impetigo

Impetigo is a superficial infection of the epidermis caused by streptococci, staphylococci, or both. Exposed portions of the body including the face, extremities, hands, and neck are the most common sites of involvement. Lesions teem with organisms and serve as a potential source of transmission to others. In temperate climates the disorder has a peak incidence in summer and early fall because of increased exposure of the body surface to insect bites, injury, and colonization by pathogenic organisms. In warm climates, impetigo is prevalent year-round. Although impetigo has traditionally been considered a streptococcal disease, recent evidence indicates that *S. aureus* has eclipsed group A streptococci as the predominant cause of impetigo. In patients without preexisting dermatitis, lesions tend to be localized, but if the child has an antecedent condition, such as eczema, the infection can spread rapidly to involve extensive areas.

In cases of impetigo caused by group A streptococci alone, the lesion begins as a papule and evolves rapidly to become a small, thin-walled vesicle with an erythematous halo. The initially serous vesicular fluid becomes cloudy and the vesicle ruptures, forming a superficial honey-colored crust (Fig. 12-28). If the crust is lifted, a shallow, smooth, weeping, erythematous base is revealed. Secondary enlargement and tenderness of the regional lymph nodes are common.

The initial macules of primary staphylococcal impetigo may evolve rapidly to form small, thin-walled pustules (Fig. 12-29A) or the larger flaccid bullae of bullous impetigo (Fig. 12-29B). The latter contain slightly cloudy fluid and are often a centimeter or more in diameter. In either instance the pustules or bullae rupture rapidly, leaving a shallow erythematous base surrounded by a superficial peeling rim (see Fig. 12-29B). In patients with more long-standing or combined infection, lesions may crust centrally and enlarge centrifugally. This may result in the formation of a superficial central scab surrounded by a bullous rim or a dried lesion with multiple concentric rings resembling an onion slice (Fig. 12-29C and D). Lesions may coalesce over time, and satellite lesions may form around larger primary lesions. Regardless of type, impetigo is frequently pruritic and the patient is stimulated to scratch, thereby spreading the infection to other sites or even inoculating the offending bacteria deeper into the skin.

The possible source of the causative organisms may be the patient's own skin or nasopharynx or those of another

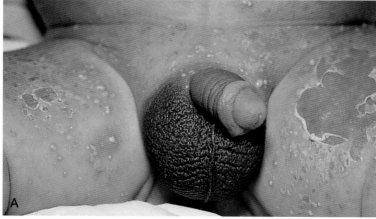

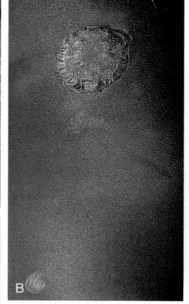

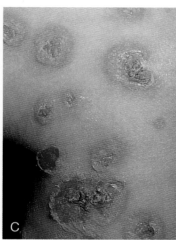

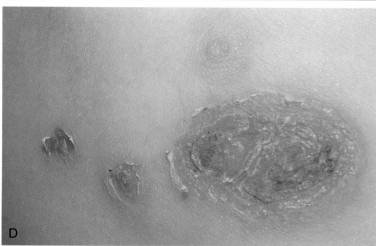

Figure 12-29. Staphylococcal impetigo. **A,** This infant with staphylococcal diaper dermatitis has multiple small, thin-walled pustules that rupture rapidly and coalesce, leaving a shallow base and a superficial peeling rim. **B,** The various stages of bullous impetigo are evident in this child. Inferiorly an unruptured flaccid bulla is seen with an older lesion above it that has spread outward and crusted peripherally; just above that, another bulla has just ruptured. **C,** In this child with staphylococcal impetigo, older lesions have central crusts with bullous rims that are spreading outward. **D,** The features of long-standing impetigo are seen in this youngster whose lesions are crusted in rings, resembling an onion slice. Note also the smaller satellites surrounding the larger primary lesion.

infected person. In patients with facial and perinasal lesions, the nose is the most likely site of origin. Oral antimicrobial therapy is preferred for eradication and is a particularly important measure if the source of infection is the nasopharynx or if the lesions are extensive, although topical antibacterial therapy with mupirocin is effective for eradicating small numbers of lesions on the extremities and may reduce the spread of infection to others. If the patient has a predisposing dermatosis, this too must be treated.

On occasion, infection with other organisms can simulate the picture of impetiginous lesions. One form of tinea capitis produces lesions identical to those of streptococcal impetigo (see Fig. 8-139C). Hence if small pustules and golden-crusted lesions are seen on the scalp or at the hairline, Gram stain and potassium hydroxide preparations are indicated to ensure the correct diagnosis. *Candida* organisms can produce tiny pustules, which rupture and have a superficial peeling rim, at times simulating staphylococcal infection in the diaper area. However, in candidal diaper dermatitis, lesions are smaller (1 to 2 mm in diameter), pustules are more evanescent, the inflammation is more diffuse, and the erythema more intense (see Fig. 8-42) than is the case in staphylococcal impetigo and staphylococcal diaper dermatitis. In confusing cases a potassium hydroxide preparation or Gram stain can be used to clarify the etiology.

Ecthyma

Ecthyma is an ulcerative skin infection that penetrates more deeply than impetigo to involve the dermis. The disorder is most prevalent in tropical climates. Poor

hygiene, insect bites, and trauma are the major predisposing factors, accounting for the fact that the lower extremities and the buttocks are the usual sites of involvement. Initially, lesions may resemble impetigo, consisting of a vesicle or a pustule on an erythematous base (Fig. 12-30A), which then ruptures and crusts over. In ecthyma, however, the lesions are painful and the crusts harder, thicker, and more adherent than they are in impetigo, and the surrounding area of erythema is indurated. The ulcerative base beneath the crust gradually deepens and enlarges. Unroofing the crust uncovers a round, deep, punched-out ulcer with raised borders (Fig. 12-30B). The size of the lesions ranges from 0.5 to 3 cm. Without treatment these lesions take weeks to heal, leaving a circumscribed scar.

In most cases ecthyma is the result of direct inoculation of organisms through the skin, with group A β-hemolytic streptococci being the usual pathogen. On occasion, staphylococci or *Pseudomonas* organisms may be the cause; when infecting a small wound, the latter pathogen is more likely to produce a central abscess that exudes a greenish or bluish purulent exudate when its crust is lifted.

Ecthyma gangrenosum is a systemic disease seen predominantly in immunocompromised patients during periods of neutropenia. It is usually caused by septicemia with *Pseudomonas aeruginosa*, during which seeding of organisms results in the appearance of metastatic skin lesions. These begin as pink macules, evolve into hemorrhagic papules, and then necrose centrally to leave a dark eschar on an erythematous base (Fig. 12-31). Subsequently, ulceration occurs, associated with deep necrosis. This metastatic form of ecthyma is distinguished easily from primary cases by virtue of the formation of multiple lesions, the presence of systemic signs of sepsis, and laboratory evidence of neutropenia.

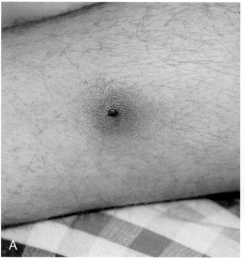
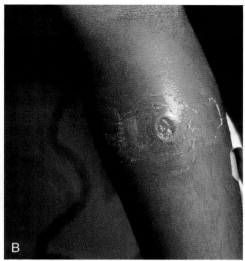

Figure 12-30. Ecthyma. **A,** In focal ecthyma resulting from the inoculation of group A streptococci, the lesion initially consists of a central vesicle or pustule (that rapidly crusts over) on a painful, indurated, erythematous base. **B,** With progression a deep, widening ulcer forms, as seen in this child after removal of the overlying crust. (Courtesy Ellen Wald, MD, University of Wisconsin Children's Hospital.)

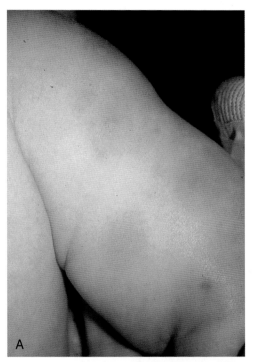

Figure 12-31. Ecthyma gangrenosum. *Pseudomonas* septicemia may result in metastatic ecthymatous lesions that begin as pink macules **(A),** become hemorrhagic **(B),** and ultimately necrose centrally to form a black eschar **(C).** (Courtesy Ellen Wald, MD, University of Wisconsin Children's Hospital.)

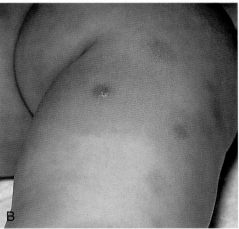
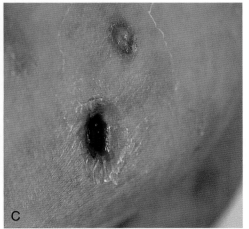

Abscesses of the Skin and Soft Tissues

Abscesses are localized collections of purulent material that are buried in a tissue, an organ, or a confined space. They result from the deep seeding of pyogenic organisms, which, in the case of abscesses involving the skin and its appendages, are usually coagulase-positive staphylococci.

As the area of inflammation expands outward, central necrosis occurs and the process tends to produce an increase in pressure, with resultant pointing toward the surface or spread along tissue planes with further local tissue destruction. Drainage is essential for healing because the abscess contents provoke a continuing inflammatory response and antimicrobials are generally unable to penetrate to the necrotic center of the lesion. Abscesses of the skin and soft tissues are categorized in part according to the site of involvement and in part according to the structure involved. The types most commonly encountered in childhood are discussed in the following sections.

Paronychia (Periungual Abscess)

A paronychia is a relatively superficial abscess that develops under the cuticle or along the nail fold of a finger or a toe. It occurs when staphylococci and occasionally streptococci gain access through a traumatized hangnail or through lesions created by clipping a cuticle or by chewing on the fingers. Occasionally an ingrown toenail is the predisposing condition; in such cases the nail, which usually was cut improperly, grows laterally into the nail fold, lacerating the soft tissue and setting the stage for infection. In typical cases, erythema, pain, and tenderness develop at the site of injury and are followed rapidly by suppuration (Fig. 12-32). The infection then advances from the portal of entry around the nail fold, and if treatment is delayed, it can burrow beneath the base of the nail, creating a subungual abscess (onychia). Occasionally, secondary lymphangitis may develop. Drainage is accomplished readily by undermining the involved portion of the cuticle and nail fold with a scalpel blade. Unless secondary complications have developed, subsequent soaking is usually sufficient to promote healing, although oral antistaphylococcal agents hasten the process.

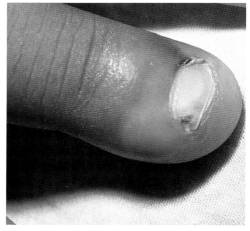

Figure 12-32. Paronychia. Chewing on a hangnail predisposed this child to the development of a paronychia. Initially, erythema developed near the hangnail and was followed rapidly by suppuration.

Abscesses of Skin Appendages

Furuncle. A furuncle, or boil, is a perifollicular dermal abscess that is usually caused by coagulase-positive staphylococci, perhaps in concert with other skin flora. It may be the result of extension of superficial folliculitis or of direct inoculation via minor trauma. Hairy areas subject to friction or maceration are particularly vulnerable. Skin contact with occlusive agents, such as oils, tars, and adhesives, is another common predisposing factor. The incidence of furuncles is much higher in older children and adolescents than it is in younger children.

The lesion begins as a small dermal nodule around a hair follicle, which initially may produce mild discomfort and itching. As it gradually enlarges, pain worsens and is aggravated by touching and motion of the involved area. With expansion, the overlying skin becomes reddened, central necrosis begins to occur, and with increased inflammation and pressure, the infection begins to seek egress. In the case of most furuncles, the abscess burrows toward the surface of the skin, which becomes thinned and shiny as the abscess becomes fluctuant (Fig. 12-33A). Application of warm compresses can hasten this process. At this point, incision and drainage are indicated. Without intervention, spontaneous drainage of bloody purulent material ultimately occurs in most cases and the patient experiences prompt relief of pain (Fig. 12-33B). In areas such as the nape of the neck or upper back, where the overlying skin is thick enough to resist external pointing, the process may take a path of lesser resistance, burrowing outward from the center through the subcutaneous tissues and along fascial planes. If this process is not interrupted by early surgical intervention, the result is a gradual formation of a *carbuncle*, which consists of an extremely painful, exquisitely tender multilocular mass of interconnected dermal and subcutaneous abscesses, with multiple points of partial drainage at the skin surface. Carbuncle formation is often accompanied by fever, chills, and increasing malaise, and there is a significant risk of secondary bacteremia. Even with treatment, sloughing and extensive scarring tend to result.

Hidradenitis Suppurativa. In hidradenitis suppurativa, an apocrine gland is the site of infection and abscess formation. Hence localization in these cases is limited to the axillae, perineum, and areolae, and the disorder affects only young people after the onset of puberty. Keratin plugging of apocrine ducts and their hair follicles appears to be a major predisposing factor, and occlusion, maceration, and poor hygiene may exacerbate the problem. The resultant obstruction fosters inflammation and provides a favorable environment for secondary invasion and multi-

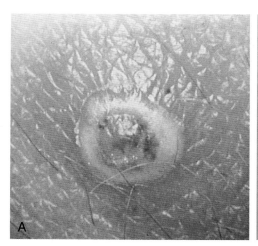
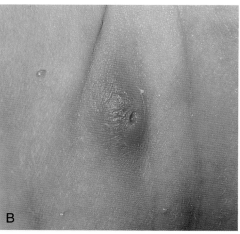

Figure 12-33. Furuncle. **A,** In this well-developed furuncle, the abscess has burrowed to the surface and the skin has thinned centrally and begun to necrose. A wide surrounding rim of erythema and induration exists. **B,** This furuncle located on the neck of a young infant had spontaneously ruptured and drained earlier in the day but was beginning to enlarge again. (**A,** Courtesy Bernard Cohen, MD, Johns Hopkins Hospital.)

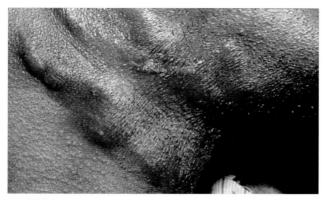

Figure 12-34. Hidradenitis suppurativa. Obstruction of apocrine ducts and hair follicles predisposes them to infection and suppuration. In this adolescent boy, the process is advanced with multiple abscesses, sinus tracts, and scarring. (From Cohen B: Atlas of Pediatric Dermatology. London, Mosby/Wolfe, 1993.)

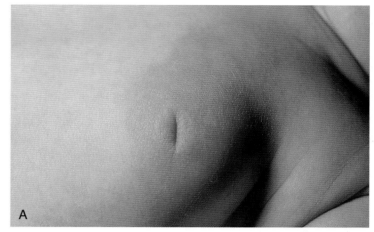

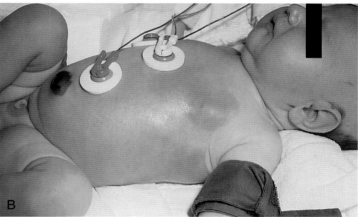

Figure 12-35. Breast abscess. **A,** The typical manifestations of a breast abscess were seen in this neonate—swelling, induration, tenderness, warmth, and erythema. With compression, pus could be expressed from the nipple. **B,** This infant was not brought to the hospital until subcutaneous rupture and extensive cellulitic spread had occurred. She was febrile, toxic, irritable, and listless on presentation.

plication of staphylococci and anaerobic bacteria. As the inflammatory process expands, the gland ultimately ruptures and an abscess forms. In contrast to the perifollicular furuncle, this infection is deeper and slower to localize and suppurate. It begins as a firm, mildly tender nodule that enlarges gradually, becoming increasingly uncomfortable and tender to the touch. With further enlargement and suppuration, the lesion(s) point to the surface and drain, although some may rupture subcutaneously. Early diagnosis, incision and drainage of fluctuant sites, institution of a prolonged course of antimicrobial therapy, wearing loose-fitting clothing, and adoption of meticulous hygienic practices may bring the problem under control. Delay in diagnosis; inadequate treatment; or, in some cases, recalcitrant disease can result in recurrence or progression with formation of multiple abscesses and sinus tracts, deep fibrosis, and scarring (Fig. 12-34) that ultimately may necessitate surgical excision.

Abscesses of Special Sites

The breasts, scalp, and perianal areas are three specific sites of abscess formation of particular importance in pediatrics. Breast and scalp abscesses are discussed in the following section. Perirectal abscesses are described in Chapter 17.

Breast Abscess. Breast abscesses occur with a small but significant frequency in pediatric patients, with incidence peaks in the neonatal and pubertal age groups. The incidence is highest in newborns of greater than 31 weeks' gestation at the time of birth, owing in part to physiologic hypertrophy of breast tissue as a result of stimulation by maternal hormones. Colonization of the skin or the nasopharynx with potentially virulent organisms (S. aureus, group B streptococci, or coliforms) during birth or in the nursery is another important predisposing factor. Up to 25% of affected infants have overt staphylococcal diaper dermatitis at the time of presentation. Minor local trauma is also thought to be a predisposing factor. Most cases occur during the second or third week after birth, but infection may occur as late as 8 weeks of age. The problem first manifests as swelling and tenderness of the affected breast. Unilateral involvement is the rule. With time, local warmth and overlying erythema become evident and it may be possible to express a purulent discharge from the nipple (Fig. 12-35A). Axillary adenopathy may be present as well. Only 25% of infants have low-grade fever, and other systemic symptoms are uncommon unless treatment is delayed. Depending on the time of presentation,

a firm, tender, nonfluctuant nodule may be found on palpation or the mass may be clearly fluctuant, indicating suppuration and necrosis. In the former instance, parenteral antibiotic therapy and close monitoring for progression are indicated. In the latter instance, prompt surgical incision and drainage are required. Broad-spectrum antimicrobial coverage should be provided pending culture results. Commonly recovered organisms include S. aureus, Escherichia coli, Salmonella species, group B streptococci, Proteus mirabilis, and mixed flora. Delay in diagnosis and institution of treatment can result in subcutaneous rupture and cellulitic spread with secondary bacteremia (Fig. 12-35B). Delay in surgical drainage of fluctuant lesions can also result in permanent loss of breast tissue, which in girls can produce a cosmetically deforming breast asymmetry that is first noted at puberty.

Breast abscesses may be seen again after puberty. Minor trauma, cutaneous infections, epidermal cysts, and duct blockages appear to be the common antecedent conditions. The clinical picture is similar to that seen in infants. S. aureus is the usual offending organism.

Scalp Abscess. As is the case with breast abscesses, pyogenic infections of the scalp are particularly common in the neonatal period. Trauma is the predominant predisposing factor, and in neonates these abscesses commonly develop at sites where scalp leads were inserted for fetal monitoring during labor. Affected infants occasionally are found to have staphylococcal diaper dermatitis as well. In most cases the infection is localized and consists of a tender nodule with overlying erythema (Fig. 12-36).

The nodule is commonly fluctuant at the time of presentation, enabling prompt incision and drainage. Staphylococci and coliforms are the major pathogens recovered. Because of the neonate's immunologic immaturity, antimicrobial therapy is also recommended and in most cases can be administered orally. On rare occasions infection is extensive and takes the form of a necrotizing fasciitis (see later discussion). In these patients and in the rare infant with a localized abscess and systemic symptoms, parenteral broad-spectrum antibiotic treatment (pending culture results) is indicated, in addition to incision, drainage, and debridement. Bacterial scalp abscesses need to be differentiated from skin manifestation of herpes neonatorum, which can present at scalp clip sites as discussed later.

When scalp abscesses are encountered in older children, care should be taken to determine the responsible pathogen. Although staphylococci may be the infecting agent, invasive fungi are more likely to be the responsible organisms. These fungi produce a thick-walled, boggy, multilocular abscess termed a *kerion* (see Fig. 8-139E). Gram stain and potassium hydroxide preparations of purulent contents and of pulled hairs are important, along with fungal culture, because, although incision and drainage (I & D) is the treatment of choice for abscesses of bacterial origin, oral antifungal and steroid therapy are indicated for the treatment of a kerion. I & D is not helpful.

Lymphangitis

Inflammation of lymphatic channels is actually a secondary manifestation of infection at a distal site. The phenomenon is the result of invasion of lymphatic vessels by pathogenic organisms, which then spread along these channels toward regional lymph nodes. Group A β-hemolytic streptococci, by virtue of elaborating fibrinolysins and hyaluronidases, are the most common source of lymphangitis, although overt lymphangitis may also develop in wounds infected by *S. aureus* and *P. aeruginosa*. Clinically, erythematous, irregular linear streaks (which may be tender) are seen extending from the primary site toward the draining regional nodes (Fig. 12-37). The primary site may be an infected wound or an area of cellulitis. Systemic symptoms consisting of fever, chills, and malaise may be present. Without appropriate antimicrobial therapy, cellulitis may develop or extend and necrosis and ulceration

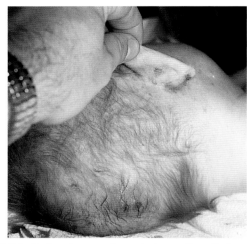

Figure 12-36. Scalp abscess. Several days after discharge from the newborn nursery this infant presented with two scalp abscesses and an impetiginous lesion behind the right ear. The surface of the larger abscess is marked by two puncture wounds, which were the site of placement of monitor leads during labor.

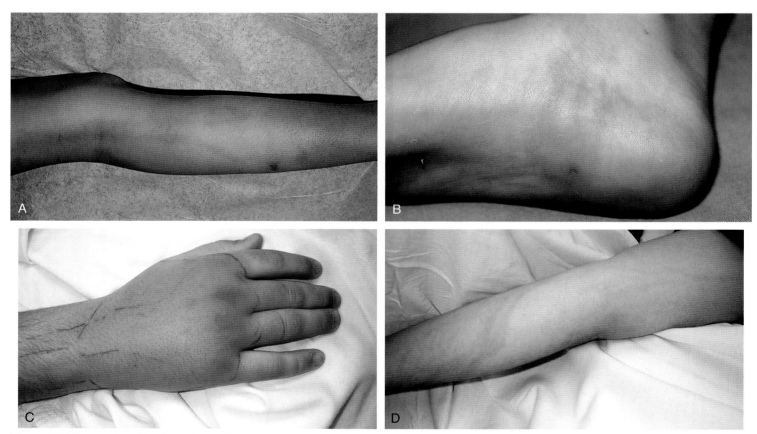

Figure 12-37. Lymphangitis. **A,** An insect bite was the source of inoculation of group A streptococci in this child, who subsequently suffered secondary cellulitis and lymphangitis. The erythematous streaks coursing up the leg were tender and slightly indurated. **B,** Three distinct lymphangitic streaks are seen coursing up the instep from an area of cellulitis surrounding a puncture wound of the foot. *Pseudomonas* was the causative organism. **C** and **D,** In this child irregular lymphatic streaks are seen coursing up the arm from a cellulitic area involving the dorsum of his hand.

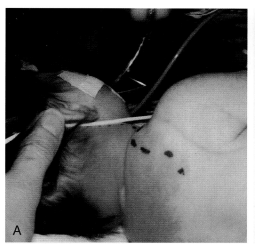
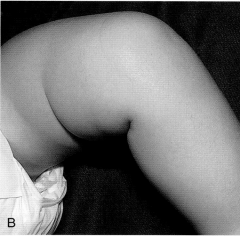
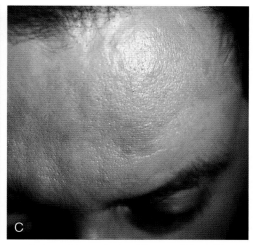

Figure 12-38. Erysipelas. **A,** This 6-week-old infant had fever, lethargy, irritability, and hypotension in association with erysipelas. The purplish-red lesion was raised, indurated, and tender. The border, though irregular, was sharply demarcated from the adjacent skin. Cultures of blood and tissue aspirate grew group A streptococci. **B,** The sharply circumscribed area of erysipelas on this toddler's leg was pink. On close inspection, one can see that the skin has a peau d'orange quality. **C,** This is seen more clearly in a close-up of an adolescent's forehead. (**C,** Courtesy James Ferante, MD.)

may occur, with the attendant risk of bacteremia. Culture and Gram stain of material from the primary site aid in the selection of antimicrobials; however, presumptive initial therapy is necessary pending culture results.

Erysipelas

Group A β-hemolytic streptococci are the source of erysipelas, an unusual and distinctive infection involving a localized area of the dermis and superficial lymphatics. The causative organisms are usually found in the upper respiratory tracts of afflicted patients and are inoculated through a break in the skin that may elude detection on presentation. Hematogenous seeding has been postulated in some cases. Systemic symptoms are prominent and precede the appearance of the characteristic skin lesion. The onset is abrupt and is heralded by fever and chills, often in association with nausea, vomiting, and headache. This prodrome is followed by the appearance of an intensely painful skin lesion that consists of a circumscribed, raised plaque that is usually deep purplish-red but which may be red or even pink (Fig. 12-38). The raised border, although irregular, is well demarcated and spreads centrifugally. Red lymphatic streaks may advance ahead of it toward the regional nodes. On close inspection the skin is seen to be edematous and may have a thickened peau d'orange character (Fig. 12-38C). On palpation it is found to be indurated, hot, and exquisitely tender. With evolution, small surface blebs containing yellow fluid may form. The face is the site most commonly involved, with the trunk, neck, and extremities being less frequent areas of localization. Patients may become bacteremic, with the development of metastatic foci of infection. Infants are at particular risk for systemic spread. The clinical picture of erysipelas is so characteristic that streptococcal infection can be presumed and parenteral antimicrobial treatment initiated. Cultures of tissue aspirate from the advancing border of the lesion and cultures of the nose and throat are typically positive for group A streptococci, as are blood cultures in septic patients.

Cellulitis

Cellulitis is an infection of bacterial origin, and subcutaneous loose connective tissue is the primary site of inflammation. With progression, the process extends centrifugally through the subcutaneous tissue and may also ascend to involve the lower dermis. Although cellulitis may develop anywhere on the body, it occurs most commonly on the extremities and face. Three major modes of origin exist:
1. Extension from a wound.
2. Hematogenous seeding.
3. Extension from a deeper infection.

Clinically, cellulitis is characterized by painful, tender, indurated subcutaneous swelling. The overlying skin is smooth, warm, often shiny, and usually erythematous (see Fig. 12-39). Occasionally it is pink or has a violaceous hue. In contrast to erysipelas, the margins or borders of both the edema and erythema are indistinct, fading imperceptibly into the surrounding tissues. Before initiation of therapy, rapid extension is the rule. Systemic symptoms are common, particularly if infection is due to hematogenous spread or to extension from deeper sites. In such cases, fever, chills, malaise, and headache are typical. Toxicity may be marked when hematogenous seeding is the source.

Wound-Related Cellulitis

Extension of infection from an external wound, such as a puncture, laceration, abrasion, or insect bite, is perhaps the most common source of cellulitis, particularly in school-age children and adolescents. Mild local erythema immediately surrounding a wound, an impetiginous lesion, or a pustule may have been noted before the abrupt onset of increased pain and the rapid evolution of subcutaneous inflammation that herald the development of cellulitis. In most cases the primary lesion is readily identifiable at the time of presentation (Fig. 12-39), but in some instances it may no longer be detectable. Occasionally, secondary infection of a preexisting dermatitis may result in a cellulitis that spreads with frightening speed (Fig. 12-40). Group A streptococci and coagulase-positive staphylococci are the organisms recovered most commonly in these circumstances. *Pseudomonas* organisms and mixed flora may be responsible for cellulitis occurring secondary to puncture wounds of the foot (see Fig. 12-37B). Although rapid peripheral spread, overt lymphangitis, and regional adenitis are regarded as highly characteristic of streptococcal infection, this same picture may be seen in patients with cellulitis caused by any of these wound-related pathogens. Fever and other systemic

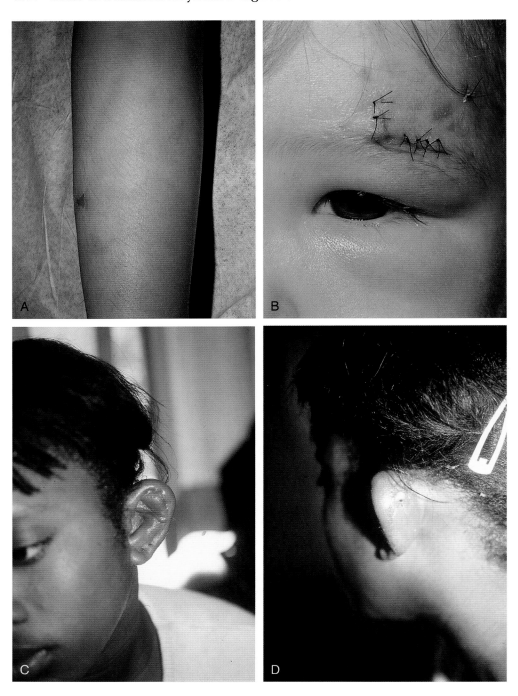

Figure 12-39. Wound-related cellulitis. **A,** The infected mosquito bite that served as the source of cellulitis in this child can be seen on the left. The area of erythema was indurated and tender. Note that the skin is smooth and the borders fade gradually into the adjacent normal skin. **B,** Mild erythema and edema are evident in the periorbital area of an infant whose laceration from a dog bite had been sutured 48 hours earlier. The edematous areas were indurated and tender. **C** and **D,** This adolescent presented with erythema, edema, and extreme tenderness caused by infection following ear-piercing. (**C** and **D,** Courtesy Robert Hickey, MD, Children's Hospital of Pittsburgh.)

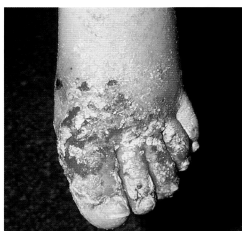

Figure 12-40. This patient with cellulitis of the foot had been on topical steroid therapy for contact dermatitis for about 48 hours when he experienced the explosive onset of swelling, redness, and pain. Impetiginous changes are apparent as well. (Courtesy Michael Sherlock, MD, Lutherville, Md.)

symptoms may be present with wound-related cellulitis but are more likely to occur with cellulitis due to hematogenous seeding or to extension of inflammation from deeper structures.

Hands, feet, and extremities are the most common sites of wound-related cellulitis. This necessitates close assessment and monitoring for further spread and for secondary neurovascular compromise. Inward spread to tendon sheaths of a hand or a foot can have disastrous consequences; hence cellulitis involving these structures must be treated aggressively, and clinical status must be monitored closely. When an extremity is encircled by cellulitis, swelling and increased pressure can result in neurovascular compromise and extensive secondary damage distally if the area is not surgically decompressed.

Gram stain and culture of material obtained from the primary wound or of tissue aspirate obtained from the point of maximal inflammation may be helpful in identifying the specific pathogen. For aspiration to be successful, a large syringe must be used to provide high-pressure suction

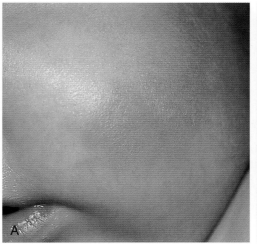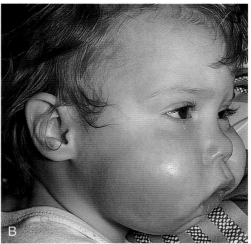

Figure 12-41. Hematogenous cellulitis. **A,** A small erythematous patch with indistinct borders appeared on this infant's cheek shortly after the onset of fever, irritability, and anorexia. On palpation it was found to be indurated and tender. Blood culture was positive for *Haemophilus influenzae* type B. **B,** In this toddler, the evolution of buccal cellulitis due to *H. influenzae* was fulminant, resulting in unusually dramatic swelling. (**B,** Courtesy Kenneth Schuitt, MD.)

and prior injection of nonbacteriostatic saline may be necessary. Blood cultures should be obtained in all patients with systemic symptoms. Prompt treatment is essential to prevent further spread and complications. Antimicrobial therapy often has to be selected empirically, pending culture results. Coverage for penicillinase-producing staphylococci is essential. Knowledge of local epidemiology of MRSA is also important for empiric coverage.

Major differential diagnostic considerations include angioedema resulting from an insect bite and delayed hypersensitivity reactions to Hymenoptera stings. The former is pruritic and nontender and often has an identifiable central punctum (see Fig. 8-64); the latter tend to be simultaneously pruritic, painful, and tender (see Fig. 8-67). Both are unassociated with systemic symptoms or with adenopathy or lymphangitis. History of trauma, presence of ecchymotic discoloration, and absence of systemic symptoms all help to distinguish swelling due to injury.

Hematogenous Cellulitis

Hematogenous seeding is another common source of cellulitis, particularly in infants and young children. Although young infants may show the sudden onset of sepsis, followed soon afterward by the appearance of cellulitis, older infants, toddlers, and preschool-age children commonly have antecedent upper respiratory tract symptoms. This prodrome is followed by the sudden development of a high fever that begins nearly simultaneously with the appearance of a nondescript area of swelling. Often this swelling is localized in the periorbital region (see Chapter 23), but at times it may be located over a cheek, the neck, or an extremity. The overlying skin rapidly becomes pink, red, or violaceous as the area of edema spreads and becomes indurated. Irritability, anorexia, and signs of toxicity become increasingly marked, in most cases prompting presentation for medical care within 24 hours. *H. influenzae* type B was once a likely source of this picture, but with widespread use of the Hib vaccine, the incidence of *H. influenzae* cellulitis has plummeted. *Streptococcus pneumoniae,* as well as group B streptococci (in infants younger than 3 months of age), are other responsible pathogens.

H. influenzae type B appears to be the sole pathogen responsible for cellulitis of the cheek, also termed *buccal cellulitis.* In this form of cellulitis, a type limited exclusively to infants, the swelling, induration, and erythema are located over the midcheek near the mandibular ramus (Fig. 12-41). Localized erythema of the underlying buccal

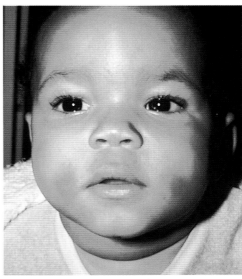

Figure 12-42. Popsicle panniculitis. This older infant, who was fond of popsicles, had bilateral areas of purplish red swelling just lateral to the corners of his mouth. He was otherwise well. On palpation, masses could be appreciated that were mildly tender, discrete, indurated, and disk shaped. These were localized areas of fat necrosis caused by cold injury. (Courtesy Michael Sherlock, MD, Lutherville, Md.)

mucosa is a common associated finding. The systemic symptomatology and exquisite tenderness help to distinguish it from "popsicle panniculitis," which results from cold injury. The latter is characterized by the formation of a mildly tender, discrete, indurated, disk-shaped, subcutaneous mass located at the angle of the mouth, with reddish purple discoloration of the overlying skin (Fig. 12-42). Systemic symptoms, induration, and tenderness also help to distinguish hematogenous cellulitis at periorbital and other sites from sympathetic swelling caused by sinusitis, which is nontender and not indurated (see Fig. 23-54), and from the pruritic nontender angioedema resulting from insect bites (see Fig. 8-64).

Because of the severity of the illness associated with buccal cellulitis and the inevitability of bacteremia with its attendant risks, expeditious evaluation and treatment are warranted. Blood cultures are positive in a high percentage of patients and may be supplemented by culture of tissue aspirates from the area of cellulitis. High-dose antimicrobial therapy should be administered parenterally, and agents selected that ensure coverage for β-lactamase–producing *Haemophilus* organisms.

Cellulitis Due to Extension of Infection from Deeper Structures

Though less common than the other forms, cellulitis resulting from extension of infection and inflammation from deeper structures may also occur. This possibility necessitates paying close attention to examination of underlying structures in evaluating any patient with evidence of cellulitis. Dental abscesses (see Fig. 20-49) and acute sinusitis (see Fig. 23-60) may underlie facial cellulitis. Osteomyelitis may produce secondary cellulitic changes in overlying soft tissues, especially after subperiosteal extension (see later discussion). Suppurative lymphadenitis and subcutaneous rupture of skin, scalp, and breast abscesses are other common sources (see Fig. 12-35B). Fever, toxicity, and other systemic symptoms are common with this form of cellulitis. Antecedent history along with the findings on careful examination usually enables identification of this type of cellulitis and recognition of the primary source.

Necrotizing Fasciitis

Variously termed *necrotizing fasciitis* or *cellulitis, synergistic cellulitis* or *gangrene, necrotizing erysipelas, streptococcal gangrene,* and more recently *flesh-eating* or *killer strep infection,* this dreaded disorder is a severe, deep, necrotizing soft tissue infection, which at a minimum involves subcutaneous tissues and fascial sheaths and often extends to underlying muscle. This process spreads relentlessly along fascial planes, producing edema, vascular thrombosis, and ever-widening necrosis, resulting in extensive soft tissue destruction. Deep surgical and traumatic wounds are major predisposing factors, although injection sites, cutaneous ulcers, abscesses, and omphalitis may serve as the initiating condition. Diabetics with vascular disease are at especially increased risk. The extremities, perineum, buttocks, trunk, and abdominal wall are the most common sites of involvement. Causative organisms include virulent strains of group A β-hemolytic streptococci, *S. aureus, P. aeruginosa, E. coli,* and mixtures of aerobes, anaerobes, and facultative gram-negative rods.

Moderate to severe systemic symptoms are prominent clinically and, along with fever, usually precede the appearance of cellulitic changes. The local area of inflammation may initially resemble ordinary cellulitis, with nonraised, indistinct margins and localized subcutaneous edema with overlying erythema. However, on careful palpation, it is often possible to appreciate that the edema and induration are deeper and far more extensive than the overlying erythema, and that the induration is unusually firm in consistency. Pain is remarkably severe early on, and the lesion is exquisitely tender. With progression, the overlying skin itself may become edematous, simulating erysipelas. Later it changes from red or purple to a patchy grayish-blue, and surface bullae, often filled with hemorrhagic fluid, may appear. At this point, numbness and decreased sensitivity to pain may be noted centrally. With further evolution, central necrosis or cutaneous gangrene supervenes (Fig. 12-43A-C). If anaerobes are involved, crepitans may become evident clinically or subcutaneous emphysema may be visible on radiographs.

As the localized process evolves, systemic symptoms increase. Signs of poor perfusion, pallor, and mottling are often accompanied by grunting respirations and alterations in level of consciousness including disorientation, obtundation, and seizures. This picture may culminate in frank prostration, often in association with generalized

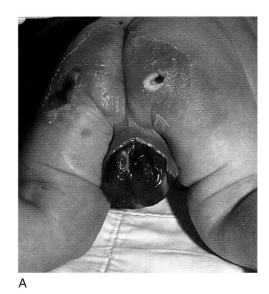
A

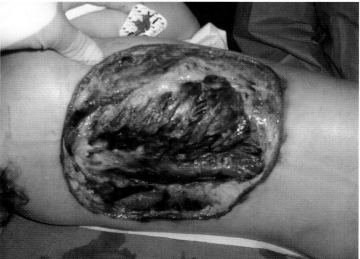
B

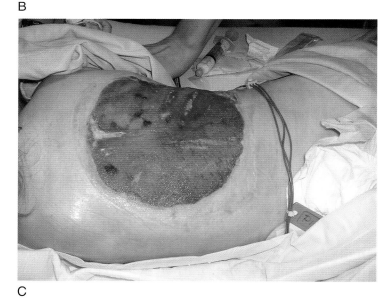
C

Figure 12-43. Necrotizing fasciitis. **A,** The extent of cellulitis and tissue necrosis is evident in this child who is recovering from necrotizing fasciitis caused by group A streptococci. On presentation he was thought to have cellulitis but was more ill systemically and appeared much more uncomfortable than would be expected. Furthermore, on presentation the area of induration extended well beyond the overlying erythema. **B,** Necrotizing fasciitis due to *Clostridium septicum* following surgical debridement in a child with presumed cyclic neutropenia. **C,** The same child 1 month later after aggressive surgical and medical management. (**A,** Courtesy Michael Sherlock, MD, Lutherville, Md.)

edema. Common laboratory findings in advanced cases include anemia resulting from hemolysis and marrow suppression, proteinuria, hypoproteinemia, hypocalcemia resulting from saponification of necrotic fat, and hyponatremia. Blood and wound cultures are routinely positive.

Mortality ranges from 8% to 70%, depending on the series reported, and morbidity and disfigurement are common in survivors. Delays in diagnosis and inadequate surgical debridement are major factors in cases with poor outcome. Hence early recognition is crucial to ensure appropriate intervention and improve prognosis. This can be particularly difficult in patients with cases resembling ordinary cellulitis that initially abate in response to antimicrobial therapy before worsening. Necrotizing fasciitis should be suspected in any patient with cellulitis (particularly around a deep wound) or omphalitis who has unusually severe pain and systemic symptoms that are out of proportion to local findings. This can enable surgical exploration before advanced skin changes and loss of sensation appear, signaling that necrosis is already extensive. If such changes are present, this process must be presumed. In early cases, findings on examination of frozen sections of biopsy material may confirm the diagnosis. Incision and passage of a probe can also be helpful. If the probe passes easily along fascial planes, the diagnosis is confirmed. Control necessitates wide excision with extensive exposure and debridement of all necrotic tissues in combination with broad-spectrum antimicrobial therapy (guided in part by Gram stain results). Aggressive supportive measures are important as well.

Infectious Lymphadenitis and Adenopathy

Lymph nodes respond to both systemic and local infections with increased cellular multiplication and activity, clinically manifested as enlargement and tenderness. Most often the enlargement is modest and, if biopsied, nonspecific hyperplasia is found histologically. This is termed *reactive adenopathy and usually resolves without a specific etiology identified*. Nodes usually are 2 cm or less in diameter, and they are discrete, slightly firm or rubbery, and mobile. Discomfort and tenderness are mild. However, in somewhat less than 25% of cases enlargement is marked, inflammation is pronounced, and a specific etiology can be identified on biopsy, a phenomenon termed *adenitis*. If the lymph node itself is infected and not just reacting to distal infection or inflammation, it can be filled with bacteria, neutrophils, and necrotic debris. Nodes usually exceed 2 to 3 cm in diameter, and overlying soft tissues may become edematous, making it difficult to distinguish exact margins. With progression, the overlying skin often becomes erythematous and may become adherent, reducing mobility. Discomfort and tenderness are moderate to marked in severity. Depending on the causative organism, suppuration may occur.

Adenopathy may be generalized or regional, but bacterial adenitis tends to be more localized. Whereas adenitis is invariably infectious in origin, adenopathy may also be a feature of collagen vascular disease or it may be of neoplastic origin. Malignant nodes are usually firm or hard in consistency but are occasionally rubbery. They may also be discrete, but, not infrequently, they are matted and often appear fixed or poorly mobile. Tenderness is unusual. Depending on the type of malignancy, the adenopathy may be isolated to one region or it may be generalized and

associated with hepatosplenomegaly and with systemic symptoms of anorexia, fatigue, weight loss, night sweats, and bone pain. Many of the infectious diseases associated with generalized or cervical adenopathy have been discussed earlier in this chapter. Some of the distinguishing features of the adenopathy characteristic of these disorders are given in Table 12-1. Neoplastic diseases are discussed in Chapter 11.

In this section we concentrate on the manifestations and causes of focal lymphadenitis. Almost any organism capable of infecting tissue can produce adenitis; hence the number of potential pathogens is large. Assessment is assisted by knowledge of the patterns of lymphatic drainage, the differential diagnostic possibilities of an inflammatory mass in a given region, and the varying clinical characteristics of adenitis produced by individual organisms.

By definition, infection of a lymph node is a secondary phenomenon occurring as a result of drainage through lymphatic vessels to a regional node. Identification of the primary source, when possible, is important in narrowing the list of potential causative organisms. In many instances, close examination of those areas in which lymphatics drain to the affected region reveals the site of inoculation. However, it is not uncommon for the primary site to have healed by the time adenitis becomes clinically manifest. In these cases, careful history taking concerning prior distal wounds or inflammation and any possible environmental exposures may disclose the identity of the probable pathogen. This can be particularly important in cases caused by organisms not readily grown on culture and in those cases in which previous administration of antibiotics has suppressed the causative organism, resulting in negative cultures.

Superficial Regional Lymph Nodes

Cervical Lymph Nodes

The cervical nodes, being numerous and draining multiple structures, are particularly common sites of acute adenitis (Fig. 12-44). In addition to the upper respiratory tract, the skin of the face, the scalp, conjunctivae, teeth, gingivae, ears, and neck all may serve as primary sites of infection. Nasal and oropharyngeal infections drain to the tonsillar and anterior cervical nodes (Fig. 12-45). Superficial facial infections and facial cellulitis may drain to the anterior cervical chain or to the preauricular or submental nodes. The occipital, posterior cervical, preauricular, and postauricular nodes receive lymphatic drainage from nearby portions of the scalp and thus may become inflamed and enlarged in connection with secondary infection of seborrhea, impetigo, wound infections, tinea capitis, or head lice infestation (Fig. 12-46). Conjunctival infections may result in adenitis of the preauricular node. The teeth, gingivae, and tongue are drained by lymphatics coursing to the submental and submandibular nodes, which can be secondarily involved in cases of dental abscess, gingivitis, and stomatitis. Infections of the external auditory canal and the auricle may drain to the preauricular or postauricular nodes, while those involving the neck may affect the anterior or posterior cervical chain.

Although the number of potential causative organisms is high, an individual pathogen can often be implicated by thorough history and physical examination. Differentiation must also be made from other masses that may be present in the cervical region, many of which are congenital and subject to secondary infection, simulating

Table 12-1	Infectious Causes of Generalized or Prominent Cervical Adenopathy			
DISORDER	**SITE(S) OF ADENOPATHY**	**CHARACTER OF NODES**	**OTHER FEATURES**	**LABORATORY FINDINGS**
EBV mononucleosis	Anterior and posterior cervical or generalized	Soft to firm, discrete, mildly to moderately tender	Pharyngitis; splenomegaly (50%); rash (15%); fever, malaise, fatigue	Atypical lymphocytosis; + Monospot (80% > 4 yr); + EBV titers; may have abnormal LFTs
CMV infection	Generalized or cervical	Soft to firm, discrete, mildly tender	Fever, malaise, fatigue; occasionally hepatosplenomegaly	Atypical lymphocytosis; abnormal LFTs; urine + for CMV on culture; + CMV titers
Toxoplasmosis	Generalized or cervical	Smooth, firm, mildly tender	Myalgias, fatigue, coryza; occasionally splenomegaly and maculopapular rash	Atypical lymphocytosis (frequent); + *Toxoplasma* titers
Brucellosis	Generalized or cervical and axillary	Discrete, may be mildly tender or nontender	History of contact with sick farm animal or ingestion of raw milk; afternoon fever and chills; sweats, malaise, headache and backache, arthralgia; splenomegaly; lasts weeks and may become chronic with metastatic abscesses	Normal or decreased WBC with lymphocytosis; + cultures and serologic tests
Rubella	Anterior and posterior cervical	Soft to mildly firm, discrete, mildly tender or nontender	Fine, discrete maculopapular rash; Forchheimer spots on palate	+ Rubella titer
Streptococcal pharyngitis	Anterior cervical	Soft to mildly firm, discrete, tender	Pharyngitis or nasopharyngitis; headache, malaise; abdominal pain; may have palatal petechiae and/or scarlatiniform rash	+ Throat culture for group A β-hemolytic streptococci
Herpes simplex	Anterior cervical and submandibular	Soft to mildly firm, discrete, mobile, tender	Gingival erythema, edema, and friability with discrete mucosal ulcers; high fever	+ Viral culture (diagnosis usually made on clinical grounds)
Coxsackievirus herpangina	Anterior cervical	Soft to mildly firm, discrete, mobile, slightly tender	Discrete ulcers on labial mucosa, gingiva, tongue, and tonsillar pillars; may have vesicles on palms and soles	+ Viral culture (diagnosis usually made on clinical grounds)
Adenovirus	Anterior cervical and preauricular	Soft to mildly firm, discrete, mobile, mildly tender	Nonspecific pharyngeal inflammation, occasionally with exudate; may have conjunctivitis	+ Viral culture

CMV, cytomegalovirus; EBV, Epstein-Barr virus; LFTs, liver function tests; WBC, white blood cell; +, positive.

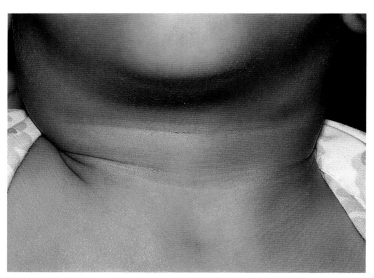

Figure 12-45. Cervical adenopathy. Bilateral enlargement of the tonsillar nodes in this child was associated with viral pharyngitis.

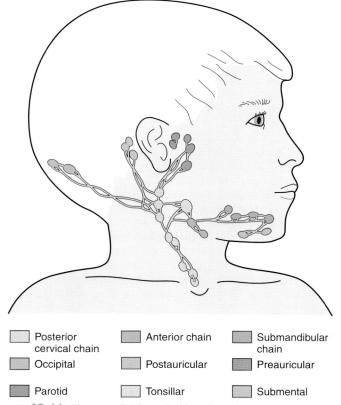

☐ Posterior cervical chain	☐ Anterior chain	☐ Submandibular chain
☐ Occipital	☐ Postauricular	☐ Preauricular
☐ Parotid	☐ Tonsillar	☐ Submental

Figure 12-44. The superficial cervical lymph nodes.

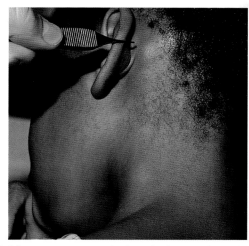

Figure 12-46. Acute postauricular lymphadenitis. This child had folliculitic and crusted scalp lesions and a tender 1.5-cm postauricular node with overlying erythema. The initial suspicion of bacterial infection was not confirmed. A potassium hydroxide preparation and fungal culture identified tinea capitis as the primary process.

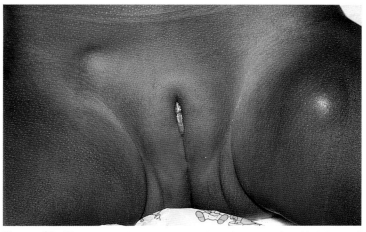

Figure 12-47. Subacute lymphadenitis of a right inguinal and left femoral node resulted in dramatic swelling in this toddler. Atypical mycobacteria were found to be causative.

adenitis. Many of these and their clinical characteristics are summarized in Table 12-2.

Axillary and Epitrochlear Lymph Nodes

More than a dozen nodes occupy the axilla. Those in the anterior pectoral portion drain the breast and chest wall, those in the lateral or midportion receive drainage from the hand and arm (see Fig. 12-51C), and those in the posterior subscapular region drain portions of the back. The epitrochlear node receives lymphatic vessels from the fingers, hand, and skin of the forearm, but it is a much less common site of adenitis than are the axillary nodes. Wound and skin infections, cellulitis, and herpes zoster are major sources of axillary adenitis in childhood.

Inguinal Lymph Nodes

The inguinal lymph nodes are divided into two groups by the Poupart ligament, with those above the ligament called *inguinal* nodes and those below it termed *femoral* nodes (Fig. 12-47, see Fig. 12-49). The inguinal group receives lymphatics from the external genitalia, anus, umbilicus, lower abdomen and back, buttocks, and upper thigh and may also drain the lower leg. Thus in addition to wound and skin infections, perianal, intra-abdominal, and genital infections may serve as sources of inguinal

adenitis. The femoral nodes primarily drain the foot and lower leg. The popliteal nodes receive drainage from the foot and lower leg, but like the epitrochlear nodes, are unusual sites of adenitis.

Having contrasted the general features of acute lymphadenitis with those of adenopathy, as well as having discussed the regions of involvement and their likely sources, we now can look at the characteristics of adenitis produced by the various causative organisms.

Acute Suppurative Lymphadenitis

Group A β-hemolytic streptococci and coagulase-positive staphylococci are responsible for causing most cases of acute lymphadenitis, regardless of anatomic region. Together they account for up to 80% of cases of cervical adenitis alone. In recent years, staphylococcal infections have surpassed streptococcal infections in frequency. Other than culture of a specimen obtained by needle aspiration, there is no way to distinguish between the two clinically, as the clinical picture for both consists of sudden, painful, and rapid enlargement, usually of a single node. The involved node is firm and exquisitely tender and may range in diameter from 2 to 6 cm (Fig. 12-48). Within 24 to 72 hours the overlying soft tissue becomes edematous and the skin erythematous. As many as 50% of patients may be febrile, and some appear toxic; bacteremia develops in a small percentage. Left untreated, suppuration occurs during the next several days and is detectable as central fluctuance. Simultaneously, thinning of the overlying skin, which also appears shiny, may be noted as the process points toward the surface (Fig. 12-49). Occasionally the abscess may point inward, rupturing into the soft tissues and dissecting along tissue planes with potentially catastrophic effects. Prompt institution of antimicrobial therapy that empirically covers *S. aureus* can significantly alter this course. When high-dose oral therapy is started before the development of overlying cellulitic changes, such changes may be prevented and enlargement halted, followed by regression. Even in patients with swelling and erythema at the start of therapy, the infection may not progress to suppuration. Patients with high fever and toxicity require parenteral treatment, as do children who fail to improve on oral medication. Suppuration necessitates incision and drainage.

Cervical nodes, especially the tonsillar and anterior cervical, are the most common sites of adenitis caused by streptococci or staphylococci. Patients are usually young children, with a peak incidence between 1 and 4 years of age. Many have an antecedent history of rhinitis, often associated with impetiginization of the anterior nares along with anterior cervical adenopathy. Cough, anorexia, vomiting, and fever can be associated findings that may persist or clear before the onset of adenitis. In older children a recent episode of pharyngitis may be reported, and in a small percentage adenitis develops in association with a peritonsillar abscess (see Fig. 23-71).

Secondarily infected dermatitis, insect bites, impetigo, and wound infections may precede the onset of adenitis in other patients, in which case the node affected depends on the primary site. These infections, as well as cellulitis, are common antecedents of axillary and inguinal adenitis caused by streptococci and staphylococci. Primary sources may be evident at the time adenitis develops, but often have already healed. Remembering that invasive forms of tinea capitis may closely mimic streptococcal and staphylococcal infection, both in the appearance of the primary

Table 12-2   Differential Diagnosis of Cervical Adenopathy/Adenitis

TYPE OF MASS	USUAL SITE(S) OF INVOLVEMENT	CHARACTER	TIME OF APPEARANCE
Lymphangioma	Preauricular, submental, submandibular, supraclavicular	Soft, compressible; transilluminates; margins often indistinct; may enlarge slightly with crying or straining; nontender unless infected	Birth to 2 years
Hemangioma	Preauricular, postauricular; may occur along or under sternocleidomastoid	Soft, compressible; margins often indistinct; enlarges with crying, straining, and dependency; nontender unless infected	Birth to 1 year; gradually enlarges during first year, then regresses
Branchial cleft cyst	Preauricular, at mandibular angle, along anterior border of sternocleidomastoid, suprasternal	Discrete; usually has overlying or nearby pore or fistula, which may retract with swallowing; nontender unless infected	Present at birth; often not noticed until infection produces enlargement, pain, and overlying erythema with or without drainage
Thyroglossal duct cyst	Midline, often at level of hyoid or just below	Discrete; usually has overlying pore or fistula; moves with tongue movement	Present at birth; often not noticed until infection produces enlargement, pain, and overlying erythema with or without drainage
Dermoid cyst	Midline, often submental or suprasternal	Discrete, smooth; doughy or rubbery; nontender; does not retract with swallowing	Infancy/childhood
Laryngocele	Just lateral to midline along anterior border of sternocleidomastoid	Soft, compressible, may gurgle on compression; enlarges with straining or crying; nontender unless infected; may have associated stridor or hoarseness; air-fluid level may be seen on radiograph	Infancy/childhood
Esophageal diverticulum	Paratracheal, usually on the left	Soft, compressible; enlarges with crying or straining; nontender; may have history of dysphagia or aspiration	Infancy/childhood
Sialadenitis	Preauricular, extending under and behind ear; submandibular, submental	Firm; mildly tender when viral; exquisitely tender when suppurative, with pus exuding from orifice; pain increased with eating, especially sour foods; elevated serum or urine amylase level	Any age
Teratoma	Midline or paramedian	Solitary; firm with irregular border; rapid increase in size; calcifications may be seen on radiograph	Infancy/childhood
Thyroid goiter	Isthmus (midline) and lobes (paratracheal)	Diffuse enlargement; usually smooth contour and soft consistency, occasionally nodular; moves with swallowing	Occasionally neonatal (with maternal ingestion of iodides); childhood in endemic areas (iodine-deficient water); childhood/adolescence in familial cases
Graves disease	Isthmus (midline) and lobes (paratracheal)	Diffuse enlargement; smooth contour and soft consistency; moves with swallowing; associated signs of thyrotoxicosis and exophthalmos	Childhood/adolescence
Hashimoto thyroiditis	Isthmus (midline) and lobes (paratracheal)	Diffuse enlargement; distinct contours; firm or rubbery; surface may be irregular; may have neck soreness and dysphagia; may have symptoms of mild hyperthyroidism	Childhood/adolescence
Thyroid carcinoma	Usually in lateral lobe or at junction of isthmus and lobe	Solitary mass; firm or hard and differs in consistency from rest of gland; may have associated adenopathy; may have past history of irradiation	Childhood/adolescence
Leukemia	Any cervical node or nodes	Firm to hard; often enlarges rapidly; may be fixed or matted; nontender; often other regions are involved; often hepatosplenomegaly; may have fever, anorexia, weight loss, bone pain, pallor, petechiae	Any age
Non-Hodgkin lymphoma	Spinal accessory, supraclavicular	Firm to hard; enlarges rapidly; may be fixed or matted; nontender; often other regions are involved; may have fever, anorexia, weight loss, bone and joint pain	5-15 years
Hodgkin disease	Anterior or posterior cervical, preauricular, supraclavicular	Firm, occasionally rubbery; slow growing; may be mobile, fixed, or matted; nontender; often otherwise asymptomatic; may have fever, malaise, weight loss, night sweats, and hepatosplenomegaly	Usually >5 years
Rhabdomyosarcoma	Nasopharyngeal, parotid, anterior or posterior cervical	When primary lesion is nasopharyngeal: symptoms of enlarged adenoids; later serosanguineous nasal discharge, weight loss, cranial nerve deficits, and secondary node enlargement When primary lesion is parotid or cervical: hard, painless, nontender mass	Any age, but more common in early childhood

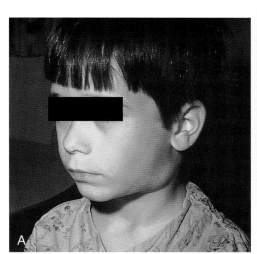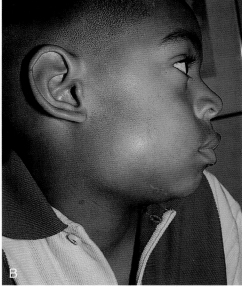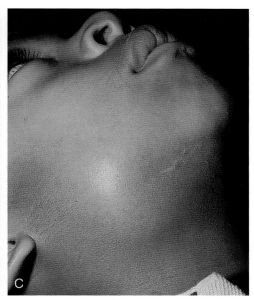

Figure 12-48. Acute suppurative lymphadenitis. **A,** This youngster was seen within 24 hours of the onset of painful enlargement of the left tonsillar node. Mild overlying edema existed, and the node was markedly tender. **B** and **C,** This boy had massive enlargement of the tonsillar node with overlying edema and mild erythema. The node was exquisitely tender, but there was no evidence of fluctuance. Group A β-hemolytic streptococci grew from his throat culture. The absence of preauricular and postauricular swelling helps to differentiate adenitis of the tonsillar node from parotitis. (**A,** Courtesy Michael Sherlock, MD, Lutherville, Md.)

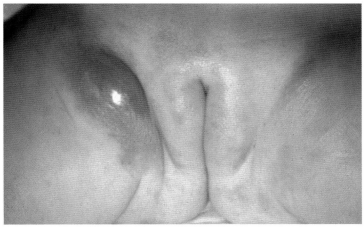

Figure 12-49. Acute suppurative lymphadenitis. Increased pain and erythema, thinning of the overlying skin, and fluctuance on palpation signal that central necrosis has occurred. (Courtesy Michael Sherlock, MD, Lutherville, Md.)

lesions and in the character of the secondary adenitis, is also important, although progression to suppuration is unusual. In these patients the occipital and/or postauricular nodes are most likely to be affected (see Figs. 12-46 and 8-139).

Although streptococci and staphylococci are the predominant pathogens causing acute lymphadenitis, occasionally anaerobic bacteria including *Actinomyces* are responsible. The vast majority of cases caused by anaerobes are secondary to dental disease including dental abscesses, gingivitis, and stomatitis; as a result, the submental or submandibular nodes are more likely to be affected. On occasion the adenitis appears simultaneously with facial cellulitis stemming from a dental abscess (see Fig. 20-49).

Actinomycotic adenitis, though unusual, has a distinctive clinical course. Enlargement of the affected node is gradual, and on palpation it is firm and lumpy, has an irregular border, and is mildly to moderately tender. Over time the center blackens and necroses, and a chronic draining sinus may form. Microscopic examination of the discharge discloses characteristic sulfur granules.

Mycobacterial Lymphadenitis

After decades of declining incidence in developed countries, the incidence of tuberculosis has begun to rise over the past several years (see the section on tuberculosis); hence *Mycobacterium tuberculosis* and nontuberculous or atypical mycobacteria (especially *Mycobacterium avium-intracellulare*) continue to be important causes of lymphadenitis. Recognition of mycobacterial lymphadenitis is important because its management is considerably different from that for lymphadenitis caused by other bacteria. Both groups of mycobacteria cause similar clinical findings. Nodal enlargement is gradual and persistent. The node is slightly to mildly tender, and initially there is little or no sign of warmth or overlying inflammation (Fig. 12-50A; see also Fig. 12-47). After a few weeks the node becomes adherent to the overlying skin, which in turn becomes thickened and tense, with overlying reddish or reddish purple discoloration (Fig. 12-50B and C). Suppuration associated with thinning of the overlying skin may occur several weeks to months after onset and may result in rupture with the formation of a chronically draining sinus. The risk of chronic drainage may be increased if aspiration is attempted. Hence this procedure is not recommended. Although the local clinical findings are similar, there are historical and other differences that can help to distinguish tuberculous lymphadenitis from atypical mycobacterial lymphadenitis.

Tuberculous Lymphadenitis

Children with tuberculosis may be of any age and frequently have a positive history of exposure to an infected adult.

Tonsillar and submandibular nodes are common sites of tuberculous lymphadenitis because of the lymphatic extension that occurs from paratracheal nodes. Supraclavicular nodes are affected as the result of drainage from apical pulmonary lesions. The posterior cervical chain is another common area. Axillary, inguinal, and femoral nodes are more likely sites of enlargement if drainage is coming from a primary skin lesion. The ipsilateral preauricular node enlarges if the conjunctiva is the site of inoc-

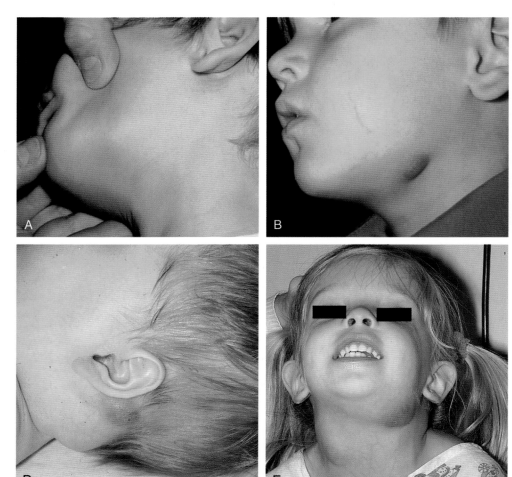

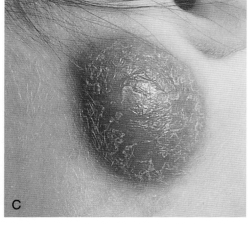

Figure 12-50. Mycobacterial adenitis. **A,** Early in the course of adenitis caused by *Mycobacterium tuberculosis* or atypical mycobacteria, enlargement of the node is gradual, tenderness is mild, and there is little or no sign of warmth or overlying inflammation. **B,** After several weeks the overlying skin becomes thickened, tense, discolored, and adherent to the node. **C,** This preauricular node was fluctuant, indicating suppuration. **D,** *M. tuberculosis* was isolated from the drainage of the postauricular node of this infant, who presented with lymphadenopathy and failure to thrive. **E,** Nontuberculous mycobacteria were isolated from the nodes of this youngster. (**A-C,** Courtesy Michael Sherlock, MD, Lutherville, Md.)

ulation. Usually a group of nodes in one region is involved if lymphatic spread is the cause. If hematogenous dissemination is the source, involvement is frequently bilateral and may be generalized; in patients with protracted hematogenous dissemination, generalized adenopathy may be present with massive nodal enlargement. The latter usually have systemic symptoms (see "Tuberculosis" later).

Initially, lymphoid hyperplasia develops as tubercles form, then necrosis and caseation supervene. Early on, nodes are firm, discrete, and nontender, but with progression they tend to become matted and adherent to the overlying skin, which often becomes discolored, thickened, and scaly (see Fig. 12-50A-C). Without treatment, spontaneous drainage ultimately occurs, leaving a draining sinus (Fig. 12-50D).

Chest radiographs reveal findings suggestive of tuberculosis in 75% of patients; the sedimentation rate exceeds 30 mm/hour in up to 80%; and the purified protein derivative (PPD) test is positive, usually with more than 10 mm of induration. Treatment of tuberculous adenitis is pharmacologic, with excision reserved for cases with chronic drainage (see "Tuberculosis" later).

Adenitis Due to Atypical Mycobacteria

Patients with atypical mycobacterial adenitis are usually younger than 4 years of age and are unlikely to have a history of exposure to tuberculosis. A submandibular, submental, preauricular, anterior cervical, inguinal, or epitrochlear node may be the site of involvement (Fig. 12-50E and see Fig. 12-47). Bilateral adenitis is unusual, generalized adenopathy does not occur, and systemic symptoms are rare. Chest radiographic findings rarely are abnormal; only one third of patients have elevated sedimentation

rates; and the PPD test is usually negative or of intermediate reactivity, with induration ranging from 5 to 10 mm. Atypical mycobacteria invariably are resistant to multiple drugs; hence excisional biopsy is generally the treatment of choice. Spontaneous regression does, however, occur over 12 to 24 months, making observation a reasonable course if suppuration or drainage has not occurred.

Adenitis Associated with Animal or Vector Contact

In many children, acute local lymphadenitis results from inoculation of a pathogen by means of an animal scratch or bite, from the bite of an insect vector transmitting a pathogen from an animal host, or from contact with a contaminated animal carcass. In some of these disorders, systemic symptoms are prominent; in others the local adenitis is the primary manifestation.

Pasteurella Multocida Adenitis

Suppurative adenitis caused by *P. multocida* may occur in patients who develop local infection at the site of a scratch or bite inflicted by a dog or cat. Soon after, the manifestations of local infection appear at the primary site (usually within 24 hours), and a regional node enlarges and becomes tender. Overlying swelling and redness are common, and suppuration may occur early. This picture is clinically indistinguishable from that of adenitis due to streptococci or staphylococci, but often *P. multocida* infection can be suspected on the basis of the history, especially the early onset of symptoms. Axillary and inguinal nodes are the most common sites of involvement.

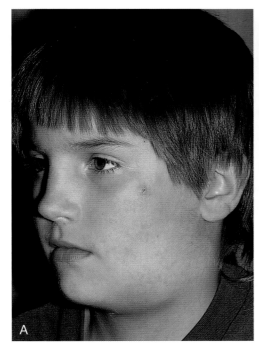
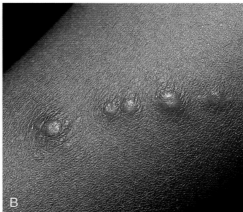
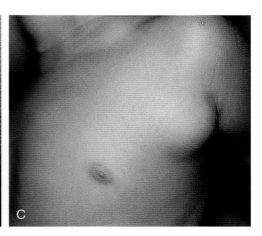

Figure 12-51. Cat-scratch disease. **A,** This boy presented with mildly painful "swollen glands." The left preauricular and tonsillar nodes were enlarged, firm, and mildly tender. An ulcerated papule, evident on his left cheek, was the site of a scratch inflicted by one of his kittens 2 weeks earlier. **B,** A line of papules is seen on the forearm of a 3-year-old at the site of a scratch inflicted by his new kitten 3 weeks before presentation. **C,** Marked enlargement of an ipsilateral axillary node had prompted his visit. The node was firm and only mildly tender. (**A,** Courtesy Kenneth Schuitt, MD.)

Cat-Scratch Disease
Although low-grade fever may occur in about 25% of affected patients, adenitis is a primary feature of cat-scratch disease, which is due to a pleomorphic bacillus that is seen on Warthin-Starry silver-stained sections of biopsied nodes. *Bartonella henselae,* a gram-negative rickettsial bacterium, is the causative agent in most cases of cat-scratch disease. Ninety percent have a history of either an antecedent cat scratch or of contact with cats, especially kittens. Although inoculation via a cat scratch is the most common means of infection, splinters, puncture wounds, and dog scratches have also been implicated. Incidence is highest in fall and winter in temperate climates, with cases occurring with equal frequency year-round in tropical areas. Most patients are in the 5- to 14-year age range, but family clusters that include younger children and adults have been reported.

Symptoms begin 3 to 30 days after inoculation, with 7 to 12 days being the most common interval. A red papule or series of papules is commonly noted at the site of inoculation (Fig. 12-51A and B). Shortly thereafter, one or more regional nodes enlarge, becoming mildly painful and tender (Fig. 12-51A and C). Involved nodes are firm, and overlying warmth and mild redness may develop within a few days of enlargement. In order of frequency, axillary, cervical, submandibular, preauricular, epitrochlear, and inguinal nodes have been reported as sites of involvement. In cases involving a preauricular node, associated conjunctivitis is common and points toward conjunctival inoculation as the source. Discomfort generally subsides in 4 to 6 weeks, but the node may remain enlarged or may fluctuate in size for months. Suppuration occurs in about one third of patients.

Diagnosis is made primarily on the basis of history, clinical picture and course, and/or findings yielded by an excisional biopsy specimen. Granulomas with microabscesses are classically seen on histopathology. Warthin Starry silver stain may reveal organisms suggestive of cat-scratch disease. Treatment is supportive. If lymph nodes are painful, suppurative aspiration can be performed and is preferable to I & D because of concerns that the latter procedure may lead to prolonged drainage and scarring. In protracted or atypical cases, excisional biopsy is suggested. The benefit of antimicrobial treatment in an immunocompetent host remains controversial.

Tularemia
Francisella tularensis may produce an illness in which adenitis is prominent, occurring in concert with systemic symptoms. Rabbits, hares, muskrats, and voles serve as endemic sources of this pathogen. Children may acquire the glandular or ulceroglandular form of the disease by handling or skinning dead animals, after an animal bite (especially that of a cat that hunts rabbits), or occasionally from the bite of an insect that serves as a vector for the pathogen. The incubation period ranges from 1 to 21 days. Onset is abrupt and characterized by fever, chills, headache, myalgias, vomiting, and possibly photophobia. Within 2 days, axillary, epitrochlear, or inguinal adenitis is noted, and soon thereafter a painful papule appears distal to the involved node at the site of inoculation. This ruptures in the ensuing day or two, forming a central ulcer with a raised edge. The involved regional node is firm and tender and may be associated with overlying erythema. Generalized adenopathy and hepatosplenomegaly may be noted in some patients, and in the second week of illness a blotchy, erythematous maculopapular rash (or occasionally a vesicular, pustular, or nodose exanthem) may appear. Without treatment, fever may persist for 2 to 3 weeks and the ulcer may take as long as a month to heal. The diagnosis is suggested by history, clinical picture, and course and is confirmed by serologic tests. Streptomycin is the treatment of choice, but intravenous gentamicin is an acceptable alternative.

Bubonic Plague
Now rare in developed countries, bubonic plague continues to sporadically afflict people who live or hunt in areas where infection is endemic in the wild rodent population. Bubonic plague is caused by *Yersinia pestis* and is usually transmitted by means of a flea bite, but on occasion inoculation occurs through a break in the skin as a result of handling an infected carcass. Thus inguinal and axillary nodes are the most common sites of bubo formation. The incubation period ranges from several hours to 10 days and ends with the abrupt onset of high fever,

chills, malaise, weakness, and headache. Pain in the area of a regional node precedes rapid nodal enlargement. The node is fixed, firm, and exquisitely tender with overlying edema. Purplish discoloration is common. The inoculation site may appear normal, or it may manifest as a skin abscess. Rapid progression of systemic symptoms occurs, with the patient appearing toxic and apprehensive and often delirious with signs of neurologic dysfunction. DIC and septic shock may supervene if treatment is not instituted promptly. If infection is suspected, the node should be aspirated to obtain material for culture, blood cultures should be performed, and broad-spectrum parenteral antibiotic therapy instituted.

General Approach to Diagnosis of Lymphadenitis

Because of the wide range of pathogens that can produce lymphadenitis, meticulous care must be taken during the clinical assessment. History taking should include questions concerning antecedent and current signs and symptoms, which may include prior wounds such as cuts, bites, punctures, splinters, or scratches distal to the inflamed node. Exposure to other ill persons or to animals, as well as recent travel, should be determined. Questions must also be asked about the presence or absence of systemic symptoms and about the rapidity of the evolution of the adenitis itself. A history of past problems and medication intake is important as well. Physical examination must include precise measurement of the size of the inflamed node, in addition to inspection of overlying soft tissue and palpation to determine contour, consistency, and degree of tenderness. The region drained by the involved node must be inspected for clues as to the probable primary source of infection. Finally, close attention should be paid to the child's general status and to other portions of the reticuloendothelial system, such as to other nodal regions, as well as to the liver and spleen.

With the preceding information, the specific pathogen may be evident on clinical grounds alone or the differential diagnostic possibilities may be considerably narrowed, permitting confirmation using a minimum of laboratory tests. Close follow-up is important for all children treated as outpatients, to monitor their clinical course and response to therapy.

Bacterial Bone and Joint Infections

Osteomyelitis

The anatomy and physiology of growing bone place children at particular risk for bacterial infection; in fact, 85% of cases of osteomyelitis occur in children younger than 16 years of age. In most series the highest incidence has been found to occur in infancy, with a secondary peak between 8 and 12 years of age. Among infants, males and females are affected with equal frequency, but among older children, males predominate in a ratio of 2:1 to 3:1. The advent of antimicrobial therapy and advances in diagnostic techniques have significantly altered the course of the disease and the outcome. Mortality has decreased from 25% in the preantibiotic era to 1% to 2%; morbidity has declined from 50% to less than 15%.

S. aureus and β-hemolytic streptococci are the most commonly identified pathogens in all age groups. Gram-negative organisms account for a small percentage of cases. *Salmonella* species are of particular importance in children with sickle hemoglobinopathies, and *Pseudomonas* organisms are often isolated in cases resulting from puncture wounds of the foot. In 15% to 30% of cases no causative organism is identified, often as a result of suppression by prior antibiotic therapy.

Once bacteria become established within bone, they stimulate an inflammatory response with the formation of exudate. As this collects, local pressure increases, promoting extension outward and causing further vascular stasis and thrombophlebitis. The resultant ischemia causes local bone necrosis. With further progression, dead bone can form a sequestrum surrounded by purulent material, which becomes inaccessible to antimicrobial penetration.

An appreciation of the anatomic and physiologic features of bone in general and of growing bone in particular is essential to an understanding of the pathophysiology of osteomyelitis in children. Nutrient vessels enter the diaphysis from the periosteum and extend to the metaphysis (or, in flat and irregular bones, to the area adjacent to the epiphysis), where terminal arterioles form loops and empty into larger sinusoidal veins. This area is one of sluggish, somewhat turbulent blood flow, which is prone to thrombosis and which serves as an ideal site for bacterial deposition in the face of bacteremia. Because they are devoid of phagocytic macrophages, the sinusoidal veins lack a major line of defense against bacteria.

In infants younger than 8 to 12 months of age, numerous additional factors assist the extension of infection once it is present. Because the epiphyseal plate has not fully formed, the nutrient arterioles penetrate into the epiphysis; hence rupture of infection into the adjacent joint is common (Fig. 12-52A). The cortex of the infant's metaphysis is thin, and the trabeculae are fewer in number, assisting penetration outward to a more loosely attached periosteum, as well as extension toward the diaphysis. Thus infants are far more likely to have extensive involvement, even with early diagnosis (Fig. 12-52B). Once the epiphyseal growth plate has formed, it serves as a relatively effective barrier to joint extension, and the frequency of secondary septic arthritis is thereby substantially reduced, although sympathetic joint effusions are not uncommon. An exception to this is hematogenous osteomyelitis involving the proximal metaphysis of the humerus or femur and of the distal fibula, where the synovium of the adjacent joint inserts so as to include the metaphysis within the joint.

Bones become infected through two major mechanisms. Hematogenous spread accounts for more than 50% of cases affecting children. Areas of rich blood supply and sluggish flow are most vulnerable to bacterial seeding; hence the metaphyseal portions of long bones and the subepiphyseal portions of flat and irregular bones are the usual sites of such involvement. Trauma may be a predisposing factor, perhaps by virtue of producing local small-vessel occlusion with secondary stasis, anoxia, and necrosis, which makes the site more vulnerable to the deposition of hematogenously spread pathogens. Children with sickle hemoglobinopathies are particularly susceptible to hematogenous osteomyelitis as a result of their vulnerability to bacteremia and sepsis and because their bones are predisposed to vascular sludging and infarction.

Spread from a contiguous focus of infection accounts for most of the remaining cases of osteomyelitis affecting children. Infections of fracture sites, surgical wounds, and puncture wounds, as well as extension of infection from

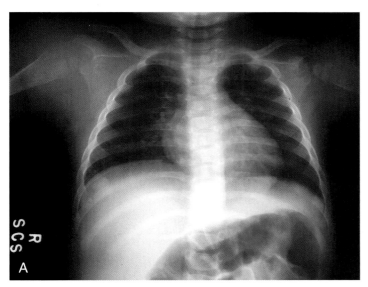

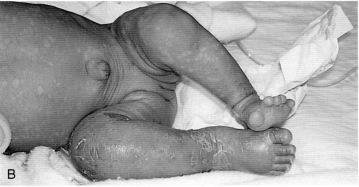

Figure 12-52. Acute hematogenous osteomyelitis in infancy. **A,** This 4-month-old who presented with a 3-day history of fever and irritability was noted to have decreased movement of the right arm and prominent swelling of the upper arm and shoulder. On x-ray examination her proximal humerus had a moth-eaten appearance, and the joint space was widened secondary to rupture of the humeral osteomyelitic lesion into her shoulder joint. **B,** Swelling of the entire leg and foot with overlying erythremia is evident in this 2½-month-old infant, who had rapid extension of osteomyelitis of the tibia.

an adjacent site of cellulitis or an abscess, serve as the predisposing conditions, with localization dependent on the original site of injury or infection.

Although important in adults, peripheral vascular disease is rarely a predisposing condition in children. If this does occur in a young person, the patient is usually an adolescent with long-standing diabetes mellitus, and the small bones of the hands or feet are the most common sites of involvement.

In addition to categorization by mode of spread or acquisition, osteomyelitis is further subdivided into acute, subacute, and chronic forms according to duration of symptoms. Of these, the acute form is by far the most common. The major clinical finding in each form is localized bone pain, which is typically constant, progressively more severe, and exacerbated by movement. Patients commonly report that the pain wakes them from sleep. The overlying soft tissues may appear normal or may be warm, mildly swollen, and occasionally erythematous, but in contrast to cellulitis, these surface findings are often subtle and induration is unusual. Spasm of overlying muscles is often intense, adding to discomfort, and the adjacent joint may be held in flexion. Beyond these common features there is a wide range of clinical expression. Appreciation of this spectrum is important to ensure early diagnosis, thus resulting in a more favorable outcome.

Acute Osteomyelitis

Acute Hematogenous Osteomyelitis. In the acute hematogenous form of osteomyelitis, the mode of presentation and the clinical findings are age dependent, although most patients present within 1 week of onset of symptoms.

Infants younger than 6 months of age often have no systemic signs of infection. However, a small percentage have low-grade fever and a few may show a frankly septic picture. Early on, irritability and anorexia are the major manifestations. Within a few days, evidence of pain on movement or of decreased use of a limb may be noted (pseudoparalysis). At this time or soon after, localized soft tissue swelling develops. This often extends rapidly to involve the entire extremity, reflecting rapid spread of infection in the underlying bone (see Fig. 12-52B). For the same reason, tenderness is also diffuse. Furthermore, multiple bones may be involved. Careful attention must be given to joint examination because of the high risk of early joint extension and secondary septic arthritis.

In children 8 months to 2 years of age, fever and signs of toxicity are common, although not universal. A history of or persistent signs of antecedent upper respiratory tract or skin infection are present in more than 50% of cases. In many patients, systemic symptoms consist primarily of fever and irritability in association with refusal to walk, a limp, or decreased use of an extremity. A small percentage present with more severe systemic symptoms including chills, lethargy, irritability, anorexia, vomiting, and dehydration. At this age children are often unable or unwilling to point to the site of discomfort, but on observation may be found to avoid moving the involved extremity or to hold a particular joint in flexion *consistently.* Soft tissue swelling and warmth may be noted overlying a metaphysis, but this is often subtle or absent in early cases and it is undetectable in cases in which the proximal femur is involved. Comparative circumferential measurements of suspected areas and painstaking care in first eliciting the child's cooperation, and then in palpating for evidence of muscle spasm or point tenderness, are well worth the effort if osteomyelitis is suspected. Even then, focal tenderness may be difficult to detect early in the course.

Children older than 2 years of age with acute osteomyelitis are usually febrile but rarely toxic. They are more likely to complain of and point to a specific site of pain, and point tenderness is generally easy to elicit unless presentation is early. Older patients describe the pain as deep, intense, and constant. Signs of adjacent joint flexion and of nearby muscle spasm are common (Fig. 12-53), but again, overlying soft tissue swelling may be subtle. Unless a sympathetic effusion has developed, the adjacent joint may be passively moved through its full range of motion, although this exacerbates the pain.

If bones other than the long bones of the extremities are the site of infection, the clinical picture can be especially confusing. Osteomyelitis of the pelvic bones can mimic numerous other conditions. Although fever and an abnormal gait are the most common presenting complaints, lower abdominal and groin pain, hip or buttock pain, sciatica, and thigh pain (with swelling) can each be prominent early complaints in individual patients. Often the initial clinical picture is more suggestive of appendicitis, pelvic abscess, or infection of the hip or femur than of pelvic osteomyelitis. To establish the diagnosis, a high level of suspicion and great care in examination are necessary. In patients presenting with abdominal complaints, the absence of rebound tenderness, lesser prominence of gastrointestinal symptoms, onset of pain in the lower

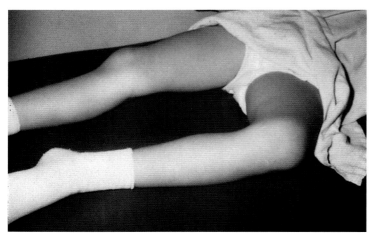

Figure 12-53. Acute osteomyelitis. Fever, hip, and thigh pain and refusal to walk were the chief complaints in this 5-year-old child with osteomyelitis of the proximal femur. On inspection she lay still, holding the left leg externally rotated and flexed at the hip and knee. This same position is also adopted by children with acute arthritis of the hip.

abdomen rather than in the periumbilical region, and normal findings on rectal examination can help to distinguish the process from that of acute appendicitis. Furthermore, although most patients have pain on hip motion in one or more planes, range of motion is either normal or only slightly limited, and with careful examination, point tenderness can usually be detected.

Acute Osteomyelitis Due to Contiguous Spread. Acute osteomyelitis resulting from the contiguous spread of infection must be suspected in patients with prior puncture wounds, deep lacerations, surgical incisions, open fractures, abscesses, or cellulitis who experience a sudden onset of increased pain at the wound site. This pain is perceived as deep, severe, and constant and is aggravated by movement. In these cases soft tissue cellulitis is a common associated finding, and fever is usual. If extension of primary soft tissue infection is the source, the patient's condition often may have worsened clinically after a period of improvement in response to antimicrobial therapy or the patient may have failed to show the expected response to therapy.

Diagnostic Methods in Acute Osteomyelitis. Standard laboratory and radiographic studies are of somewhat limited use in the diagnosis of acute osteomyelitis. The sedimentation rate is elevated in the vast majority of patients with osteomyelitis and exceeds 40 mm/hour in about 80%. This finding is helpful primarily in confirming that an inflammatory process is the source of symptoms. White blood cell counts, though sometimes elevated with a left shift in differential, may be normal in up to 50% of patients and thus are less useful.

Radiographic changes lag behind the clinical manifestations and can be subtle. The first noticeable radiographic change, usually seen about 3 days after the onset of symptoms, is the presence of deep soft tissue swelling displacing fat lines adjacent to a metaphysis (Fig. 12-54A). In the ensuing days the swelling increases, obliterating fascial planes, and then extends to involve subcutaneous tissues. These soft tissue changes can be difficult to appreciate whenever osteomyelitis involves bones of the trunk or pelvis; however, in cases of pelvic osteomyelitis, clouding of the obturator foramen, distortion of the fascial planes around the adjacent hip, or even displacement of the bladder may be detectable. If a sympathetic joint effusion is present or if rupture into the adjacent joint has resulted in secondary septic arthritis, joint space widening or bony

displacement may be evident (Fig. 12-54B; and see also Fig. 12-52A). Bone changes are not visible radiographically in untreated patients until 10 to 20 days after onset. These changes consist of periosteal elevation followed by focal evidence of bone lysis and, subsequently, by sclerosis or new bone formation at the margins of the lytic lesion (see Fig. 12-54C to E). The radiographic appearance of bone changes can be significantly delayed in patients who are being treated with an antibiotic for infection at another site, and early diagnosis of osteomyelitis and the institution of appropriate antimicrobial therapy may completely prevent development of these findings.

Technetium scanning has provided a better means of early identification and localization of sites of acute osteomyelitis. It can show abnormalities as early as 24 to 48 hours after the onset of symptoms, revealing discrete areas of increased uptake (Fig. 12-55A). The procedure has been particularly useful as a diagnostic adjunct in cases of pelvic and vertebral osteomyelitis in which the mode of presentation simulates the clinical picture of another condition (Fig. 12-55B; see Fig. 12-58C). It can also be helpful in distinguishing osteomyelitis from cellulitis, septic arthritis, and acute bony infarcts. In cellulitis, intense deep soft tissue uptake with faint diffuse uptake in underlying bone is seen; in septic arthritis the scan may be normal, or if the condition is accompanied by overlying cellulitis, the scan may show increased periarticular soft tissue uptake; in early infarcts, uptake is decreased. Technetium scans are also helpful in delineating additional areas of involvement in the small percentage of patients with multiple sites. Standard radiographs remain important in identifying fractures and malignancies, which may simulate the appearance of osteomyelitis on bone scans. Awareness that 5% to 20% of children with acute osteomyelitis can have a false-negative bone scan during the first few days is important. If suspicion remains high on clinical grounds, an MRI study can be obtained.

Vigorous attempts must be made to isolate the causative organism in order to optimize therapy on the basis of known sensitivities and a determination of bactericidal levels. Aspiration of the site of maximal tenderness or maximal uptake as revealed by bone scan or MRI can be useful in that it provides material for Gram stain and culture. In cases in which purulent material is obtained, operative drainage should be considered strongly. Even in the absence of exudate, flushing the aspirating needle with culture media often enables isolation of the causative organism. Blood cultures are positive in more than 50% of patients with acute hematogenous osteomyelitis and should be performed in all suspected cases.

Complications of osteomyelitis include secondary septic arthritis with resultant joint damage, epiphyseal injury with long-term morbidity resulting from impaired bone growth, progression to chronic osteomyelitis (now seen in less than 4% of cases), and rarely pathologic fractures. The rate of complications is highest in young infants who often have extensive bone involvement and secondary septic arthritis by the time the diagnosis is made. Care in clinical assessment and aggressive attempts to confirm the diagnosis of acute osteomyelitis as early as possible are as important in ensuring a good outcome and minimizing complications as are adequate antimicrobial therapy and recognition of the need for surgical intervention. Close collaboration between the primary care physician and the orthopedic surgeon is essential to ensure that optimal decisions are made regarding the route and duration of pharmacotherapy and the need for and timing of surgical intervention, if indicated.

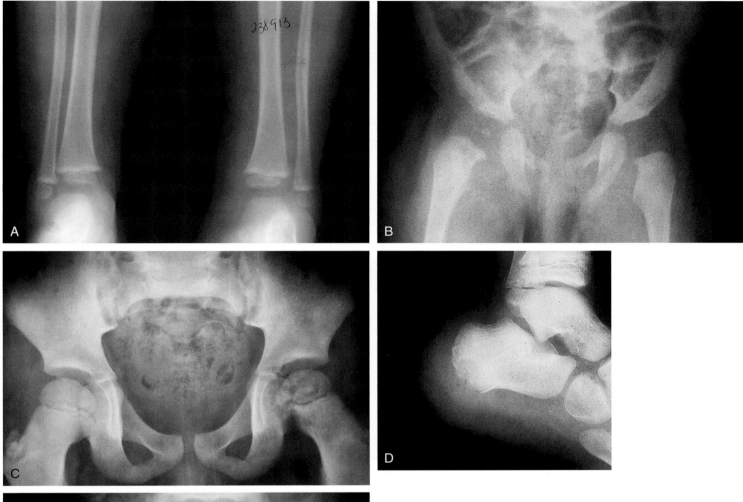

Figure 12-54. Acute osteomyelitis. Radiographic changes lag behind the clinical manifestations in osteomyelitis. **A,** The first noticeable change, occurring about 3 days after onset, is deep soft tissue swelling, seen here adjacent to the metaphysis of the distal tibia on the left. **B,** In this neonate a radiolucency is evident in the proximal metaphysis of the right femur, which is also displaced upward and laterally. On aspiration of the hip, purulent fluid was obtained, confirming the suspicion of rupture of the infection into the hip and of secondary septic arthritis. **C,** The epiphysis and proximal metaphysis of the left femur have a moth-eaten radiographic appearance in this older child. **D,** Deep and superficial soft tissue swelling overlie the radiolucent lesion of the calcaneus in this boy who acquired *Pseudomonas* osteomyelitis after a puncture wound of the heel. **E,** The late changes of a lytic lesion with sclerotic margins are seen in the right femoral metaphysis of this child who was completing his course of therapy. (**A,** Courtesy Jocelyn Ledesma-Medina, MD; **B, C,** and **E,** courtesy Roderigo Dominguez, MD, University of Texas; **D,** courtesy Ellen Wald, MD, University of Wisconsin Children's Hospital.)

Subacute Osteomyelitis

Approximately 10% of cases of hematogenous osteomyelitis have an insidious onset and a subacute course, often characterized by mild to moderate local pain in an extremity, with or without swelling. Fever is unusual, and other systemic symptoms are absent. Typically the patient has had symptoms for a few to several weeks before presentation. In some instances this subacute course appears to be related to partial suppression of the infection by antibiotics that have been administered for infection at another site (such as for otitis media, tonsillitis, or impetigo). In these patients, pain may abate during the period of antimicrobial therapy, only to worsen once they stop taking the medication. In other cases in which antibiotics have not been prescribed, reduced bacterial virulence is postulated. On examination, local tenderness is evident and overlying soft tissue swelling may be noted. By the time diagnosis is made, multiple sites are involved in up to 20% of patients. However, secondary sites may not be symptomatic.

Although white blood cell counts are usually normal, the sedimentation rate is elevated in most (but not all) patients. Blood cultures are rarely positive. Radiographs may show one of several possible findings. In children seen within a few weeks of onset who have taken antibiotics, radiographic findings may simulate the deep soft tissue swelling characteristic of early acute osteomyelitis. Other radiographic configurations include an isolated

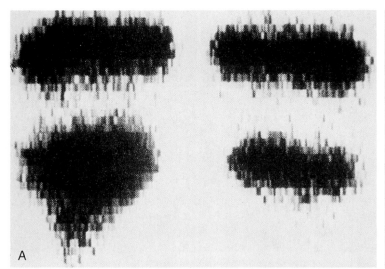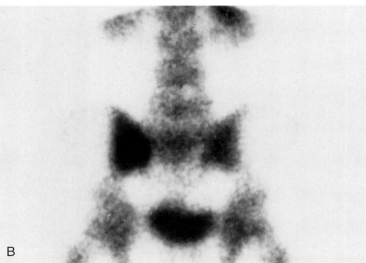

Figure 12-55. Technetium scan findings in acute osteomyelitis. **A,** In this radionuclide scan, selectively increased uptake is seen in the proximal right tibial metaphysis. The uptake in the epiphyses is normal, reflecting active bone growth. **B,** This youngster showed a puzzling picture of abdominal pain suggestive of an acute abdomen. A bone scan was obtained after other studies were unrevealing. The increased uptake in the right sacroiliac area helped to identify osteomyelitis as the source of symptoms. (Courtesy Ellen Wald, MD, University of Wisconsin Children's Hospital.)

metaphyseal radiolucency surrounded by reactive bone (Brodie abscess); a metaphyseal radiolucency with loss or disruption of cortical bone simulating a tumor; an excessive cortical reaction in the diaphysis simulating an osteoid osteoma; and multiple layers of subperiosteal new bone overlying the diaphysis, at times mimicking the appearance of Ewing sarcoma (Fig. 12-56). Although a bone scan is not of great use in distinguishing subacute osteomyelitis from a primary bone tumor, it can be helpful in revealing other sites of involvement. Because the long course, clinical picture, and radiographic findings of this infection often are indistinguishable from those of a neoplastic process, biopsy is generally required to establish the diagnosis and isolate the causative organism. In the vast majority of cases, coagulase-positive staphylococci are found. Surgical curettage, immobilization, and antimicrobials are the mainstays of treatment.

Chronic Osteomyelitis

With the advent of antimicrobial therapy and improvements in diagnostic techniques, chronic osteomyelitis has become much less common in countries where there is ready access to medical care. Delay in diagnosis, inadequate antimicrobial or surgical therapy, and unusually resistant organisms are the major factors now associated with its development. Pathophysiologically, extensive necrosis, sequestrum formation, and decompression caused by fistulization through the overlying soft tissues are characteristic findings (Fig. 12-57). Patients suffer local pain of variable severity and have chronic draining sinuses. Aggressive surgical curettage and long-term antimicrobial therapy are required to achieve resolution, but despite this, permanent functional disability and deformity are not uncommon once osteomyelitis has become chronic.

Juvenile Diskitis and Vertebral Osteomyelitis

Inflammation of an intervertebral disk space in childhood is a puzzling disorder, in terms of both its exact pathophysiology and its mode of presentation. Before the third decade of life, vascular channels penetrate through the vertebral end-plates and communicate with the intervertebral disk. Thus it is thought that hematogenously spread organisms are more likely to alight in the disk spaces of children and adolescents, whereas thereafter they may lodge in vascular arcades adjacent to the subchondral plate of the vertebra itself. This factor has been used to explain the higher frequency of diskitis in children and the relative infrequency of acute vertebral osteomyelitis before adulthood. However, differences in the clinical picture, the less frequent isolation of pathogens, and evidence that immobilization alone is effective in treating diskitis—while antimicrobial therapy is required in vertebral osteomyelitis—have led to speculation that disk space inflammation may be due to a low-grade viral or bacterial infection.

Known predisposing conditions in adults include urinary tract infections, pelvic inflammatory disease, and bowel and urinary tract surgery; in children they include upper respiratory tract infection, gastroenteritis, and genitourinary infection. The importance of antecedent trauma is unclear. Hematogenous spread may occur through the valveless veins of the Batson plexus or via the vertebral branches of the posterior spinal arteries. In both diskitis and vertebral osteomyelitis, coagulase-positive staphylococci are the organisms most commonly isolated, followed by streptococci, gram-negative enteric pathogens (including *Salmonella* and *Kingella kingae*), and corynebacteria. The lumbar spine and the lower thoracic spine are the most common sites of involvement for both entities.

The clinical picture of diskitis, which is seen predominantly in children younger than 4 years of age, is dominated by pain and progressive limp. Often, focal back pain that progressively worsens in severity is reported. In a few instances it may be perceived as primarily worse in the flank, abdomen, or hip. It is constant; may be aggravated by sitting, standing, or movement; and is typically worse at night. Children who are too young to describe their pain may initially be irritable and refuse to walk or even sit. In some cases increased irritability has been noted during diaper changes. Adoption of an abnormal posture is a frequent finding. Most commonly this posture is one of exaggerated lumbar lordosis, but in some cases the lumbar spine may be held stiff and straight. Toddlers may preferentially assume a knee-chest position. Fever is often present during the first week or two of symptoms, but it may be absent and is often low grade. Other systemic symptoms are unusual. Occasionally, abdominal disten-

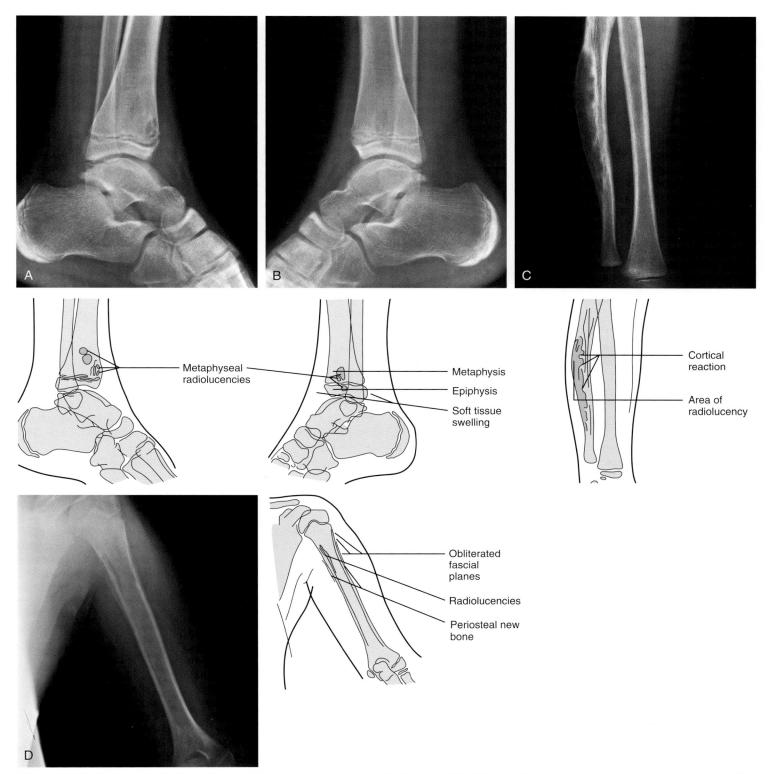

Figure 12-56. Radiographic findings characteristic of subacute osteomyelitis. **A** and **B,** This 13-year-old boy had a 7-week history of pain and swelling of both ankles. He had been treated with penicillin for presumed rheumatic fever. These radiographs show bilateral soft tissue swelling, multiple metaphyseal radiolucencies in the distal left tibia, and a radiolucency involving the metaphysis and epiphysis on the right. **C,** An extensive area of radiolucency and cortical reaction is seen in the ulnar diaphysis of this youngster. **D,** This patient complained of mild to moderate left upper arm pain for 5 weeks after an injury. Radiographic examination revealed layers of periosteal new bone, ill-defined cortical radiolucencies, and obliteration of the fascial planes. (Courtesy Department of Pediatric Radiology, Children's Hospital of Pittsburgh.)

tion is prominent, raising suspicion of intra-abdominal pathology.

Failure to remember that vertebrospinal pathology may result in a limp or refusal to walk, or in abdominal pain, and thus failure to examine carefully the backs of such patients, often results in long delays in diagnosis. Such examination may reveal paravertebral muscle spasm with

guarding and exquisite focal tenderness, although in some cases tenderness may be vague or absent. Resistance to flexion and extension of the spine are common and in the young may simulate meningeal signs. The loss of normal lumbar lordosis or the presence of local scoliosis may be noted early on. Pain on straight leg raising and hip motion may also be encountered.

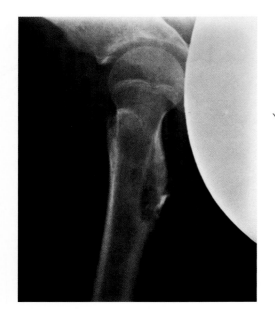

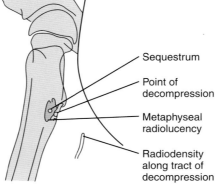

Sequestrum

Point of
decompression

Metaphyseal
radiolucency

Radiodensity
along tract of
decompression

Figure 12-57. Chronic osteomyelitis. Inadequate initial treatment resulted in progression to chronic osteomyelitis in this child. In this radiograph, taken 6 months after the onset of symptoms, a radiodense sequestrum is seen within the metaphyseal radiolucency. The process had also begun to decompress into the soft tissues of the thigh. (Courtesy Department of Pediatric Radiology, Children's Hospital of Pittsburgh.)

The sedimentation rate is elevated unless symptoms have been present for many months, but white blood cell counts are elevated only during the first few weeks. Specific radiographic changes do not appear until 2 to 6 weeks after onset, at which time disk space narrowing becomes evident. In ensuing weeks, irregularities of the adjacent vertebral end-plates become apparent. A technetium scan can reveal focal increased uptake as early as 1 week after the onset of symptoms. Culture of biopsy specimens of the disk space are commonly negative unless obtained early in the course. Most patients with diskitis improve symptomatically with immobilization alone, and the process appears to resolve after several weeks of casting.

The clinical picture of vertebral osteomyelitis, seen in older children and adolescents, usually is one of insidious onset of progressively worsening back pain that is constant, aggravated by movement, and increasingly resistant to analgesics. Usually fever is absent or low grade. Occasionally the onset is acute, with fever and generalized systemic symptoms accompanying the abrupt appearance of pain. In the rare cases encountered in young children, onset is usually acute and the clinical picture is dominated by abdominal or flank pain, with associated tenderness and often guarding. In some patients, paraspinous or spinous process tenderness, back stiffness, an exaggerated lumbar lordosis, pain on leg motion, or lower extremity weakness may be noted (Fig. 12-58). Laboratory findings in this setting are similar to those in children with diskitis, with the exception that blood cultures obtained in the acute phase are generally positive. Early radiographic findings are also similar, but frank destructive lesions of the vertebral body develop soon after the appearance of disk space narrowing is noted. Cultures of operative biopsy specimens usually yield *S. aureus*. Antimicrobial therapy is necessary to achieve clinical resolution, and surgical debridement is more likely to be required.

Septic Arthritis

Bacterial invasion of the synovial membrane with resultant septic arthritis is a condition with a high potential for long-term morbidity. Release of lysosomal enzymes by attracted leukocytes, abscess formation, the development of granulation tissue, and ischemia resulting from in-creased intra-articular pressure act in concert to damage the articular surface and promote synovial fibrosis and bony ankylosis. Early diagnosis and treatment are essential to prevent or at least minimize the extent of irreversible damage. This is hindered in many cases, however, by the fact that both the clinical picture and laboratory findings overlap with those seen in patients with viral and other forms of acute arthritis.

Septic arthritis is a disorder primarily affecting young children, with two thirds to three fourths of cases occurring in patients younger than 5 years of age. Males are affected twice as often as females. Ninety percent of cases are the result of hematogenous seeding in the course of bacteremia, and although in most cases the affected joint becomes the primary site of localization, it is not uncommon for septic arthritis to develop in a child with bacterial meningitis or pneumonia, often manifesting early in the course of treatment. Up to 40% of patients have a history or signs of an antecedent upper respiratory tract infection at the time of diagnosis. This was especially common in cases caused by *H. influenzae* type B that were frequent before the widespread use of the Hib vaccine. Streptococcal skin and soft tissue infections may antedate septic arthritis caused by this pathogen. In older children and adolescents, gonococcal urethritis, vaginitis, and cervicitis assume importance as antecedents to hematogenous seeding (see Fig. 18-37). Prior trauma may also be a predisposing factor and is reported in a significant number of cases. In approximately 10% of patients, the septic arthritis is secondary to rupture of a primary osteomyelitic lesion into the joint space. Direct penetrating injury accounts for a small percentage.

Bacterial pathogens are isolated in 65% to 75% of patients, either from synovial fluid, blood, or both. The relative frequency of pathogens varies considerably with patient age, as shown in Table 12-3. Children with sickle hemoglobinopathies occasionally suffer *Salmonella* septic arthritis. Failure to isolate an organism can be explained in some instances by suppression caused by prior antibiotic administration.

The joints affected in order of frequency are the knee, hip, ankle, and elbow. The wrist and shoulder are involved less often, with other joints being rare sites of septic arthritis. Only a single joint is affected in more than 90% of patients. *Neisseria gonorrhoeae* is the organism most

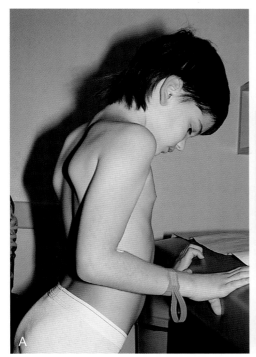
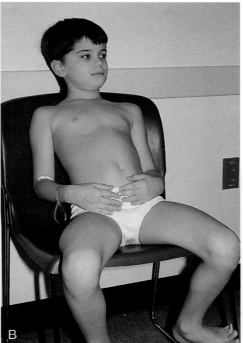
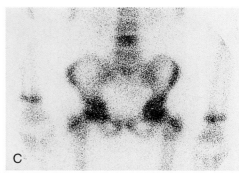
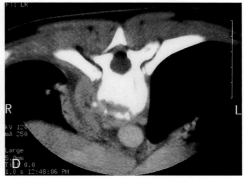

Figure 12-58. Vertebral osteomyelitis. **A-C,** This 10-year-old boy had a 2-week history of intermittent fever, malaise, and steadily worsening lower back and left hip pain, exacerbated by movement. **A** and **B,** He had an exaggerated lumbar lordosis and extreme limitation of flexion, both standing and sitting. The straight leg raising test also accentuated his pain. **C,** Bone scan revealed selectively increased uptake in the L4 vertebral body. **D,** This 13-year-old girl had an 8-week history of intermittent throbbing pain in her midback with a few days of fever. Pain was worse on arising and in the evening, with prolonged standing and with lying down. She had a markedly elevated sedimentation rate and tenderness to deep palpation in the lower thoracic region. MRI done at the time of biopsy shows fragmentation of the body of T8 with extension of infection into the paraspinous tissues on the right. The biopsy specimen showed that the paraspinous mass consisted of granulation tissue with numerous polymorphonuclear leukocytes and plasma cells and grew *Staphylococcus aureus* on culture. (**C** and **D,** Courtesy Department of Pediatric Radiology, Children's Hospital of Pittsburgh.)

Table 12-3	Relative Frequency of Pathogens in Septic Arthritis According to Age		
NEONATE	**1 MONTH-2 YEARS**	**2-5 YEARS**	**>5 YEARS**
S. aureus	Group A streptococci	*S. aureus*	*S. aureus*
Group B streptococci	*S. pneumoniae*	Group A streptococci	Group A streptococci
Gram-negative enteric pathogens	*N. meningitidis*	*N. meningitidis*	*N. gonorrhoeae*
	P. aeruginosa	*S. pneumoniae*	*P. aeruginosa*
	Salmonella species	*H. influenzae* type B	
	H. influenzae type B		

commonly associated with multiple joint involvement, but other pathogens may be responsible, particularly coagulase-positive staphylococci and *H. influenzae* type B. The hip and shoulder joints, if involved, are particularly prone to damage because clinical signs may be subtle and thus diagnosis is often delayed. Further, because the synovium inserts distal to the epiphysis of the proximal humerus and femur, compromise of the blood supply to the epiphysis is more likely to occur as a result of increased intra-articular pressure.

The typical clinical picture of hematogenous septic arthritis is one of a young child who presents with moderate to high fever and signs of toxicity, in association with severe localized joint pain, overlying swelling, and marked limitation in range of motion. The fever may be quite acute in onset, or it may have been present for a few days, but the child tends to be seen soon after the onset of joint symptoms. Variations in this picture depend in part on the age of the patient, the joint involved, the causative organism, and the duration of symptoms. Infants and toddlers cannot describe focal pain, and thus they tend to present with fever and irritability, the latter aggravated by movement. Refusal to bear weight or decreased use of an

extremity may or may not have been noted by the family. When a knee, ankle, wrist, or elbow is involved, local swelling and warmth are usually evident (Fig. 12-59). However, early on the swelling may be subtle, high fever may make any warmth difficult to distinguish, and surface erythema is often absent. Whenever a hip is involved, swelling and warmth are not evident externally and pain may be referred to the knee or thigh. Often the position adopted by the patient is the best diagnostic clue. To minimize intra-articular pressure and pain, the child prefers to lie still with the knee and hip flexed and with the hip externally rotated (see Fig. 12-53). In cases of septic arthritis of the shoulder, subtle swelling may or may not be evident, but the shoulders may not be held at the same level and the arm on the involved side is held against the chest to splint the joint.

Septic arthritis of the sacroiliac joint (see Fig. 12-55B), which accounts for about 1% of cases, can present a particularly confusing picture, often mimicking hip or intra-abdominal disease. Only one third of patients have an acute presentation, the remainder having a subacute course. Buttock pain, limp, and fever are the most common presenting complaints. Up to one third of patients

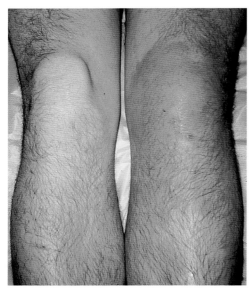

Figure 12-59. Septic arthritis. This adolescent boy awoke suddenly at 3 AM with severe left knee pain. By 8 AM he was febrile and had marked swelling with overlying erythema and extreme limitation of movement. Examination of joint fluid revealed gram-positive cocci in chains, with a white blood cell count of 24,000/mm³. Cultures were positive for group A streptococci. (Reprinted from the clinical slide collection on Rheumatic Diseases © 1991, 1995. Used by permission of the American College of Rheumatology.)

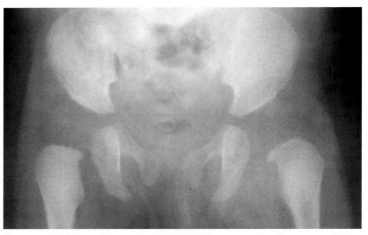

Figure 12-60. Radiographic findings characteristic of septic arthritis. Although radiographs may be normal early on, joint space widening can be detected in most cases. In this infant, who presented with fever, toxicity, and refusal to move the left leg, capsular swelling and lateral displacement of the proximal left femur are readily apparent. (Courtesy Roderigo Dominguez, MD, University of Texas.)

complain of unilateral radicular pain. Findings of lower abdominal and rectal tenderness in association with normal hip motion may fool the examiner who fails to recognize that leg and buttock pain necessitate meticulous examination of the lower back. Such an examination reveals tenderness over the involved sacroiliac joint, and pelvic compression replicates the pain, as does hyperextension of the ipsilateral hip with the patient supine and dangling his or her leg over the edge of the table.

Limitation of joint motion and evidence of pain on motion are perhaps the most valuable clinical clues to the diagnosis of septic arthritis. Limitation is usually severe unless presentation occurs early, and motion provokes marked discomfort. In young patients with fever and decreased use of an extremity but without clear-cut swelling, localization is often possible if, after careful inspection and palpation for bony tenderness, each joint of the extremity is gently moved while the examiner carefully guards the other joints, without touching them. Diagnosis can be particularly difficult in neonates and infants, who may be afebrile and often have no systemic symptoms. In such cases, decreased use of an extremity is often the earliest clue. Pain on motion is usually evident, however, even before the appearance of localized swelling.

When septic arthritis results from rupture of a focus of osteomyelitis into a joint, distinction between the two processes can be difficult to establish clinically. Focal pain is generally of longer duration, but because most cases occur in infants younger than 8 months of age, this clue is often unavailable. In older children the hip, shoulder, and ankle are the major sites of this secondary form of septic arthritis. These children usually have a history of prolonged focal pain, antedating a brief period of respite (due to decompression of the infected bone), followed by the sudden return of pain that is markedly aggravated by joint motion. In the days following a penetrating joint injury, a sudden increase in pain and swelling should prompt immediate suspicion of secondary septic arthritis.

Because of the high cost of delays in diagnosis in terms of morbidity, any child with fever, acute onset of pain, and limited motion of a joint should be presumed to have septic arthritis until proved otherwise. These findings should prompt expeditious diagnostic investigation. Plain radiographs with comparison views should be obtained without delay and inspected carefully for even subtle signs of joint space widening or capsular distention, although findings may be normal in early cases. If the hip is the suspected site of pathology, lateral and upward displacement of the femoral head may be noted along with displacement of the gluteal fat lines (Fig. 12-60). A bone scan is perhaps the best method of evaluating the child with suspected septic arthritis of the sacroiliac joint and is also useful in identifying patients with underlying osteomyelitis.

Arthrocentesis should be considered early, as examination of joint fluid is the study most likely to yield definitive results. A heparinized syringe should be used to prevent spontaneous clotting. Positive findings on Gramstained specimens are particularly helpful; cultures are positive in 60% or more of cases. Pleocytosis is common, with two thirds of patients having a white blood cell count of more than 50,000/mm³. Remembering, however, that there is considerable overlap with nonbacterial arthritis in terms of the cell counts, differential counts, and protein and glucose levels found on examination of synovial fluid is crucial.

Peripheral white blood cell counts and sedimentation rate may add suggestive evidence, but again there is overlap with viral arthritis. Up to 20% of patients have white blood cell counts under 10,000/mm³, although most have a significant leftward shift. The sedimentation rate may be markedly elevated, but it is under 40 mm/hour in up to 45% of patients. Blood cultures are positive in up to 40% of cases. As cultures of joint fluid from patients with disseminated *N. gonorrhoeae* infection are often negative, it is important to culture blood, skin lesions, throat, and cervix or urethra when this agent is suspected.

Diagnosis thus depends on assessment of the assembled data including clinical course, physical findings, and results of multiple laboratory studies. Even with negative findings on Gram stain, empirical antimicrobial therapy selected to cover the most likely pathogens (see Table 12-3) should be started, pending culture results, in patients in whom septic arthritis is deemed likely on the basis of the available findings. As is true of osteomyelitis, collaboration between pediatric and orthopedic colleagues is crucial, for drainage of infected material is essential to ensuring a good outcome.

Any disorder associated with acute arthritis must be considered as part of the differential diagnosis of septic arthritis. In some instances the clinical picture of an obvious viral or vasculitic syndrome enables differentiation. The polymigratory picture of acute rheumatic fever and the much less acute onset of juvenile rheumatoid arthritis help to distinguish these conditions. Adenopathy, visceromegaly, anemia, and radiographic changes help distinguish malignant joint infiltration.

Tuberculosis

After decades of steady decline, tuberculosis has shown a disturbing increase in incidence in the United States in recent years. This appears to be related to a combination of factors: the human immunodeficiency virus (HIV) infection epidemic (which predisposes to the reactivation of prior infection and to the development of active and rapidly progressive disease with new infection); a decline in the services of departments of public health; the rise in the homeless population and of barriers in access to health care; and an increase in the immigration of people from places where tuberculosis is prevalent. Worldwide, famine, war, and natural disasters that create large numbers of refugees; crowded living and working conditions; and sweat-shop-type labor practices involving long working hours and the employment of child laborers spawn conditions that favor the acquisition of tuberculosis and its spread. In addition, poor compliance with the lengthy treatment regimens required has led to increased transmission of ever-more-resistant organisms. Those at high risk in the United States include people from ethnic and racial minority groups, especially of low socioeconomic status living in overcrowded conditions in populous urban areas; immigrants and foreign-born adoptees from Southeast Asia, China, Latin America, Haiti, and Eastern Europe; the homeless; migrant workers; elderly persons living in nursing homes; prisoners in correctional institutions; HIV-positive or immunosuppressed people; children in close contact with adults in these groups; and health care professionals. Most are located in seven states—California, Florida, Georgia, Illinois, New York, South Carolina, and Texas (border states or states with large immigrant populations or large pockets of people living in extreme poverty).

Transmission

Tubercle bacilli are transmitted from person to person, with the usual source being aerosolization of organisms from an adult or adolescent with active pulmonary, especially cavitary, disease. Children with primary tuberculous disease rarely transmit infection because they have a relatively small number of organisms, if any, in endobronchial secretions and are rarely able to cough forcefully enough to expel them.

Infants and toddlers living with or in close contact with an infectious adult, and adolescents and young adults helping to care for infectious people are at especially high risk for infection. Thus parents, grandparents, older siblings, nannies and sitters, housekeepers, and boarders are the major sources of transmission to children. Less often, teachers, school bus drivers, coaches, and nurses have been source cases.

The portal of entry in more than 98% of instances is the lung; it is estimated that the inhalation of as few as one to three bacilli in a single aerosolized droplet can result in infection. Rarely a superficial skin or mucous membrane lesion may be the site of inoculation. Congenital infection can occur if a pregnant woman experiences lymphohematogenous spread during gestation or has tuberculous endometritis. Health care professionals are at particular risk when handling specimens of infected secretions or body fluids and contaminated syringes or instruments such as lavage tubes and bronchoscopes.

Pathogenesis

Once the organism has gained entry, there is a silent period of incubation lasting 3 to 10 weeks. The larger the inoculum, the shorter the incubation period and the more severe the signs and symptoms of the primary infection. The end of the incubation period is marked by the development of hypersensitivity to the organism, as manifested by a positive PPD skin test (Fig. 12-61), and can be accompanied by fever of 1 to 3 weeks' duration. During this time, the patient's inflammatory response intensifies in the *primary complex,* which has three components: (1) the primary focus or site at which the bacilli have lodged (usually a subpleural alveolus, which can be at any site in either lung); (2) the inflamed lymphatics that drain the area; and (3) inflamed regional lymph nodes. Macrophages migrate to the primary focus, transform into epithelioid cells, and gather into clusters, forming a tubercle. If the host's immune response is effective, the lesion is walled off and then gradually resolves and disappears. If the host response is less effective, bacilli multiply and the primary focus can caseate centrally. Thereafter, organisms in the lesion can travel along lymphatics to regional nodes, provoking more inflammation along the track and in the nodes. Infection can then spread by way of other lymphatics to more distant nodes—most commonly the paratracheal, anterior cervical, and abdominal nodes. New foci may heal, become dormant with the risk of later reactivation, or progress.

Affected nodes that enlarge and caseate can cause numerous complications. For example, hilar nodes press-

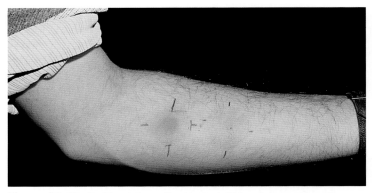

Figure 12-61. Positive tuberculin skin test. This adolescent boy became infected as a result of living with and helping to care for a grandfather whose chronic "smoker's cough" was ultimately discovered to be a manifestation of chronic cavitary tuberculosis. He had a greater than 15-mm induration. (Courtesy Kenneth Schuitt, MD.)

ing on an adjacent bronchus set up sympathetic inflammation in its wall, leading to partial obstruction as the result of a combination of compression and edema collection. Occasionally the inflammatory process damages the cartilaginous rings, resulting in secondary collapse. In other cases it progresses to perforate the bronchial wall, releasing caseous material into the lumen. This may form an obstructive plug or provoke the formation of granulation tissue. Alternatively, organisms released from the caseous material may then travel through the airways to infect other parts of the lung. Rupture of a caseous subpleural primary focus or node results in pleural effusion. Enlarged caseous subcarinal nodes may compress the esophagus, causing dysphagia, or may rupture into it, producing a bronchoesophageal fistula. Infected nodes can compress the subclavian vein, resulting in edema of the ipsilateral upper extremity, or compress the recurrent laryngeal or phrenic nerves. They may also rupture into the mediastinum, or they may erode into adjacent blood vessels, setting the stage for miliary spread.

The host's ability to mount an effective response to inhibit replication of tubercle bacilli and contain the primary infection depends on several factors. Very young and therefore immunologically immature children, malnourished children, adolescent girls, pregnant women, and immunodeficient or immunosuppressed people are at particular risk for progression of disease. Recent infection, especially pertussis or viral infections such as measles, influenza, and varicella, also increases the susceptibility to tuberculous infection and progression. Genetic selection for resistance in populations living in endemic areas and acquired resistance appear to be somewhat protective.

Clinical Forms of Tuberculosis

Infection without Disease

Patients with this latent form of tuberculosis have a positive skin test reaction (see Fig. 12-61) but no clinical signs or symptoms of disease and normal chest x-ray findings. Although many of these children never manifest signs of primary infection, if the infection goes unrecognized and untreated, there is a 10% chance of reactivation of their tuberculosis later in life; thus they serve as a major reservoir. Other patients in this category simply have been identified very early and will go on to suffer clinical disease if treatment is not instituted. Patients with underlying HIV infection have a 10% risk of reactivation each year.

Tuberculous Disease

Patients who have evidence of tuberculosis on chest x-ray or clinical signs and symptoms of pulmonary or extrapulmonary infection are said to have tuberculous disease. The risk of developing disease after infection exceeds 40% for infants, is 24% to 25% for children between 1 and 10 years of age, and is 15% for those between 11 and 15 years of age.

Primary Pulmonary Tuberculosis. The symptoms of primary pulmonary tuberculosis, which are typically insidious in onset, are often attributed to viral illness. Some children have low-grade fever with no apparent source, together with mild anorexia and decreased activity. Others may have associated rhinorrhea, nasal congestion, and pharyngeal erythema and are mistakenly thought to have a viral upper respiratory tract infection. On occasion, erythema nodosum may develop in concert with the fever. Chest examination is generally normal, even in patients with abnormal chest radiographs. Rarely children present with a more dramatic "pneumonic" mode of onset, with high fever, tachypnea, and signs of toxicity. In such cases the clinical findings are those characteristic of lobar pneumonia, with rales, rhonchi, and bronchial breath sounds heard on auscultation and dullness noted on percussion. Patients with either mode of onset tend to show improvement over a few days to a few weeks, though some may be noted to tire easily and be less active than usual. Without specific treatment, some develop low-grade afternoon fevers weeks later that may persist for as long as a few months.

Radiographic findings characteristic of primary pulmonary tuberculosis may be limited to enlarged hilar (Fig. 12-62A) or carinal nodes (seen best on lateral views); faint, cloudy infiltrates that extend to the pleura (Fig. 12-62B); or a lobar infiltrate (Fig. 12-62C) in patients exhibiting the "pneumonic" picture. Infiltrates contain the primary complex and, like it, can be located anywhere in either lung.

Endobronchial Tuberculosis. When enlarged nodes cause bronchial obstruction (usually 3 to 6 months after infection, and most commonly in children younger than 2 years of age), focal hyperaeration or fan-shaped, segmental parenchymal *collapse-consolidation infiltrates* are seen (Fig. 12-63). The latter consist of the primary focus and secondary inflammation and atelectasis. Sometimes narrowing of a bronchial lumen is noted. Infants affected by this endobronchial process often have a harsh, paroxysmal cough that mimics that of pertussis, along with wheezing and rhonchi noted on auscultation. The cough is often worse when the infant is lying supine than when prone. Respiratory distress may be noted during the course of an intercurrent infection. Older children generally have no cough but can manifest the auscultatory findings. With or without treatment, consolidation-collapse lesions can reexpand and resolve; clear with residual calcification of the primary complex and regional node (Ghon complex); or go on to scarring, with progressive contraction of the involved pulmonary segment in association with bronchiectatic changes. Calcification may persist or start resorbing within a few years. Occasionally, it progresses to ossification and formation of true bone.

Pleural Effusion. Rupture of a caseous subpleural, primary focus or lymph node can also occur 3 to 6 months after initial infection. This usually occurs in school-age children. The caseous material provokes an intense pleural reaction with the formation of a proteinaceous effusion. This can be localized or generalized. Pleural effusion can also result from hematogenous spread, as well as from direct extension of infection from a subpleural focus. Clinically, development of pleural effusion is heralded by the abrupt onset of fever, chest pain, and shortness of breath and is manifested by decreased chest wall movement and decreased breath sounds, dullness to percussion, and egophony on examination. When the effusion is massive, respiratory distress is evident. Pleural fluid is usually clear or slightly cloudy, greenish yellow, often blood tinged, high in protein, and usually low in glucose. Leukocytes predominate early, lymphocytes later, with counts ranging from 300 to 10,000 cells/mm^3. Bacilli are present in small numbers. Radiographs may show clouding of a lower lung field with obliteration of the diaphragm or, in the event of massive effusion, total "white-out" of the lung with mediastinal shift.

Progressive Primary Pulmonary Tuberculosis. Progressive primary pulmonary tuberculosis occurs in infants

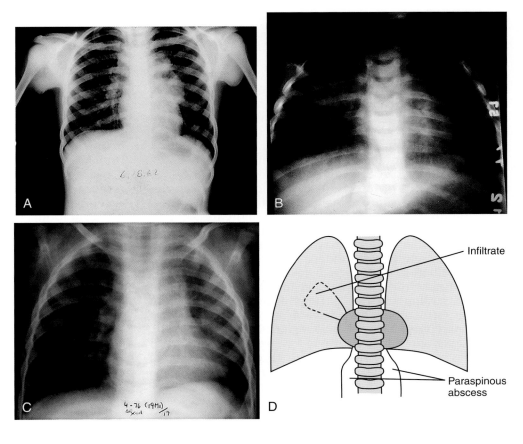

Figure 12-62. Primary pulmonary tuberculosis. **A,** Marked enlargement of hilar nodes without a pulmonary infiltrate is seen in this asymptomatic child. She was tested as part of a contact investigation, and this chest radiograph was obtained because her skin test was positive. **B,** A hazy infiltrate involving a segment of the right upper lobe is seen extending from the hilum to the pleura. This child also has tuberculous spondylitis with a paraspinous abscess, the shadow of which is seen below the diaphragm **(D). C,** In this boy who presented with a pneumonic clinical picture, a hazy infiltrate occupies the entire left upper lobe. (**A** and **B,** Courtesy Jocelyn Medina, MD; **C,** courtesy Richard Towbin, MD, Children's Hospital of Philadelphia.)

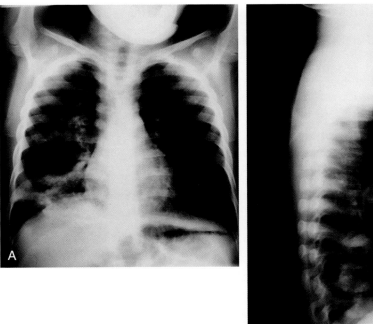

Figure 12-63. Progressive primary pulmonary tuberculosis (endobronchial). This 8-year-old girl initially had fever, cough, and mild tachypnea. She was treated with antibiotics for presumed bacterial pneumonia but showed only partial clinical improvement. Repeat radiographs obtained a month later showed progression. A purified protein derivative test was then done and was positive. **A** and **B,** She has a collapse-consolidation lesion involving the right lower lobe, with a primary cavity. (Courtesy Ellen Wald, MD, University of Wisconsin Children's Hospital.)

and young children whose primary focus steadily enlarges, caseates, liquefies, and empties its bacilli-laden contents into a bronchus. The organisms then disseminate through the airways to the rest of the lung, setting up new foci of infection. Clinically these patients have remittent fever, cough, apathy, and malaise, along with anorexia and weight loss. Over time they begin to appear listless and chronically ill. Wet rales may be heard over the site of the primary cavity. Radiographically a small cavity is seen at the site of primary focus, along with a collapse-consolidation lesion (see Fig. 12-63) and later diffuse infiltrates. On rare occasions, a large caseous, primary focus can cause a pneumothorax, bronchopleural fistula, or caseous pyothorax if it ruptures into the pleura. Alternatively, it may rupture into the mediastinum, after which caseous material may track upward to the supraclavicular fossa.

Lymphohematogenous Spread and Miliary Tuberculosis. Miliary tuberculosis occurs when bacilli are disseminated from an involved node of the primary complex by means of the bloodstream to distant sites. In some patients this is clinically occult and occurs early during the incubation period or shortly thereafter. Major sites of seeding include the pulmonary apices, spleen, and superficial nodes. In some cases, evidence of resulting metastatic lesions is seen 2 to 4 months later, when the child has a nonspecific illness characterized by low-grade fever and fatigue, splenomegaly, and generalized adenopathy, sometimes associated with papulonecrotic skin lesions. Others remain asymptomatic, and their metastatic lesions may either remain dormant or reactivate years later.

Acute miliary spread occurs in some patients (usually within 6 months of infection) when a caseous node ruptures directly into a vessel. Organisms in seeded foci may die or set up new foci that are then walled off and become dormant or may progress, expand, and cause further complications. Miliary disease may be detected incidentally in an infant or child who undergoes chest radiography as part of evaluation for low-grade fever without an apparent source. Other children experience insidious progression of symptoms following intercurrent measles, influenza, or pertussis; still others may have a more abrupt onset of fever, tachypnea, lethargy, and weakness accompanied by hepatosplenomegaly. Within a few weeks, symmetrical tubercles of uniform size are seen throughout the lung fields (Fig. 12-64) and rustling breath sounds can be heard on auscultation. Skin lesions, which may be nodular, purpuric, or papulonecrotic, may appear as well.

A subset of infected children exhibit a process known as *protracted hematogenous spread,* which involves repeated episodes of release of organisms into the bloodstream. These patients have high sustained or spiking fever; leukocytosis (with white blood cell counts up to 40,000/mm³); and marked, generalized, nontender adenopathy, and they look quite ill. Within a few weeks, mottled pulmonary lesions of varying size are seen. Polyserositis and multiple bony lesions tend to develop, along with crops of papulonecrotic skin lesions, which form after each episode of seeding.

Extrapulmonary Tuberculosis

Tuberculous Meningitis. Following lymphohematogenous or miliary spread, caseous foci may develop in the brain and meninges. Fifty percent of infants and children with miliary tuberculosis go on to develop meningitis. Extension of infection or rupture of one of these foci into the subarachnoid space results in tuberculous meningitis, which usually develops within 3 to 6 months of initial infection in children younger than 6 years of age. The

resulting exudate is thick and gelatinous. It infiltrates meningeal and cerebral vessels, causing vasculitis with secondary occlusion and infarction; it impedes CSF flow and resorption, often resulting in a communicating hydrocephalus; and it collects at the base of the brain, impinging on the optic chiasm and the third, sixth, and seventh cranial nerves.

Often preceded by a viral illness or head injury, the onset of symptoms is usually gradual, beginning with anorexia, fever, pronounced apathy, irritability, and emotional lability, often with headache. Within a week or two, drowsiness, vomiting, meningismus, a sluggish pupillary response, and cranial nerve palsies supervene, often accompanied by hyperreflexia and seizures. Confusion, disorientation, dysarthria, tremors, and athetosis are other findings that may be seen during this phase. Untreated, the condition progresses to coma, the syndrome of inappropriate antidiuretic hormone, opisthotonic or decerebrate posturing, the Cushing triad, and death. CSF pressure is usually elevated, and the fluid is clear (though often xanthochromic); cell counts range from 50 to 500 cells/mm³, with leukocytes predominating early and lymphocytes later. The protein content is elevated (often markedly), and glucose levels are usually low. Early diagnosis and the institution of antituberculous therapy can significantly reduce morbidity and mortality, but even with treatment, complications are common in survivors.

Skeletal Tuberculosis. Skeletal tuberculosis is an extrapulmonary manifestation seen in 1% to 6% of children with untreated primary infection; it becomes clinically evident within 6 months to 3 years after the initial infection. Very young children are at greatest risk because of the high rate of blood flow through their growing bones. It can start as a metaphyseal endarteritis following hematogenous seeding; it can develop by means of extension from lymphatics, especially from a paravertebral node to a vertebra; or it can arise as the result of direct local or hematogenous spread from a neighboring bone.

Formation of granulation tissue and caseation characterize the inflammatory process, which ultimately results in pressure necrosis and the formation of a cold abscess, which can then rupture into an adjacent joint or surrounding soft tissues (see Fig. 12-62B). The vertebrae; bones about the knee and hip; and, in infants, the phalanges are the most common sites involved. Other than the phalanges, involvement of non–weight-bearing bones is unusual. As is often the case with osteomyelitis, a history of antecedent trauma before the onset of symptoms is frequently obtained. Fever is absent or low grade, unless the lesions develop as part of the process of protracted hematogenous spread. Pain is often relatively mild in comparison with that associated with other forms of bacterial osteomyelitis.

Tuberculous spondylitis usually involves the vertebral bodies of two or more thoracic vertebrae but can affect lumbar vertebrae as well. Clinically, nocturnal pain, manifested by crying in the night and restless sleep; low-grade fever; and later postural change (stiff back, kyphosis) and gait disturbance (with all weight-bearing joints kept slightly flexed) are prominent. Patients with lumbar disease adopt a wide-based stance and gait. Pain may be localized to the back or referred to the chest or abdomen. When cervical vertebrae are affected, pain may be localized to the neck or referred to the occiput or arms; the child may have difficulty holding up the head, and torticollis is often present. Occasionally an opisthotonic posture is adopted. On examination, severe paraspinous muscle spasm, marked limitation of flexion, pain on percussion, and

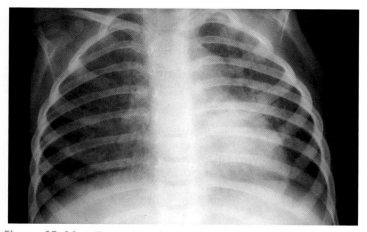

Figure 12-64. Miliary tuberculosis. Two weeks after miliary spread, this infant's lung fields are symmetrically dotted with tiny tubercles. (Courtesy Richard Towbin, MD, Children's Hospital of Philadelphia.)

hyperreflexia with clonus may be evident. When there is an associated paraspinous abscess, swelling and fluctuance may be noted adjacent to the site of maximal tenderness. Initially radiographs show slight disk space narrowing; subsequently mild wedging and partial collapse of the vertebral body occur. Later, bony destruction (Fig. 12-65) and ultimately pancake collapse of the vertebral body occur, resulting in kyphotic angulation-Pott disease. Complications include paravertebral, psoas, and retropharyngeal abscesses, as well as neurologic abnormalities secondary to associated spinal cord compression, inflammation, and vasculitis. Because the spinal canal widens caudally, compression is more likely the higher the level of the vertebrae involved.

Involvement of bones about the knee results in pain, stiffness, and limp, which can be intermittent. Limitation of motion varies depending on the extent of associated synovial inflammation. Unilateral thigh or knee pain and limp are the most common modes of presentation of acetabular or proximal femoral disease.

The dactylitis seen in infancy is characterized by painless fusiform swelling of the fingers or toes. Radiographically, affected phalanges, and sometimes metacarpals, initially show fusiform enlargement and increased density. Later, cystic changes are seen.

Tuberculous Pericarditis. Seen in less than 5% of children with progressive pulmonary tuberculosis, tuberculous pericarditis can result from direct invasion of organisms from an adjacent infected lymph node, from rupture of an adjacent primary focus into the pericardial sac, or from lymphatic spread from subcarinal nodes. A hemorrhagic exudate collects and may progress to tamponade. Patients tend to have low-grade fever, anorexia, and rarely chest pain. On examination a pericardial friction rub is usually apparent; with large effusions, heart sounds are diminished and a narrow pulse pressure is noted.

Tuberculous Adenitis. Tuberculous adenitis is discussed earlier in "Infectious Lymphadenitis" (see Fig. 12-50).

Tuberculosis in Adolescence. Adolescents may suffer a primary infection or experience reactivation of earlier disease. The latter is more likely if the primary infection occurred after 7 years of age. The period of the adolescent growth spurt, especially in girls of low socioeconomic status, is the time when the risk of the reactivation or the development of progressive primary disease is greatest. With reactivation, the new lesion develops in the same lobe as that of the old primary complex and tends to

remain localized; there is a relatively low risk of hematogenous spread or extension to regional nodes because of prior development of hypersensitization. Affected patients have cough and fever, often accompanied by chest pain, and may exhibit hemoptysis. Anorexia with weight loss and easy fatigability are common. Chest findings may be normal early on, but moist rales may be heard over the apices after cough or on end-expiration. Small round or wedge-shaped infiltrates or linear streaks with mottling may be evident on chest radiograph. This and progressive primary disease can evolve to chronic cavitary disease within a few years if appropriate treatment is not instituted.

With progression, weight loss and fatigue increase and an early-morning cough productive of increasing amounts of sputum becomes bothersome. Daily fevers and night sweats are common, and an appearance of chronic illness supervenes. Wet rales, bronchial breath sounds, wheezing, and dullness to percussion are typical physical findings. Radiographs may reveal mottling, patchy infiltrates, segmental or lobar opacification, and cavitary changes, which may be unilateral or bilateral.

Tuberculin Testing

The gold standard of skin testing for tuberculosis is the Mantoux test with 5 tuberculin units (0.1 mL) of purified protein derivative (PPD). This is injected intradermally on the volar surface of the forearm, with the needle bevel up and oriented perpendicularly to the long axis of the arm. After injection, which when done properly, raises a wheal, the 27-gauge needle should be left in place for a few seconds to prevent leakage from the injection site. The test should be read by a health care professional 48 to 72 hours later; this is done by measuring the diameter of any induration that develops at the site, again at a right angle to the long axis of the arm (see Fig. 12-61). The test is rarely negative in infected children; anergy is seen only in those who have overwhelming infection or are immunosuppressed and is occasionally seen in a child with an intercurrent viral infection. Use of multiple puncture tests as screening tools should be abandoned because they cannot be standardized. Interpretation of a positive test is based on associated risk factors (Table 12-4).

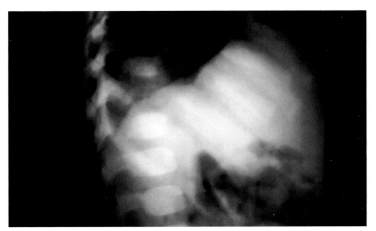

Figure 12-65. Tuberculous spondylitis. Extensive bony destruction of the T12 vertebral body along with mild collapse of T11 is seen. (Courtesy Jocelyn Medina, MD.)

Table 12-4	Interpretation/Risk Factors for Positive Purified Protein Derivative (PPD) Test
DEGREE OF INDURATION THAT REPRESENTS A POSITIVE TEST	**RISK FACTORS**
≥5 mm of induration	Known close recent contact with an infected patient Immunosuppressed HIV positive Currently on steroids Chest radiograph showing old healed lesions
≥10 mm of induration	High-risk racial or ethnic group (émigrés from an endemic area) Younger than 4 years of age Underlying medical condition that increases risk for severe disease (e.g., diabetes, malignancy, chronic renal failure, malnutrition)
≥15 mm of induration	No risk factors

Case Finding

The most efficient and cost-effective means of identifying infected children is through contact investigation of persons known to be in close contact with an adolescent or adult with pulmonary tuberculosis. Conversely, if a child is found to be positive, household members and others in close contact should be tested to find the source case.

Because of the low prevalence of tuberculosis in most parts of the United States, routine yearly skin testing is not indicated. However, children from high-risk groups should be tested routinely and all new immigrants should undergo PPD testing.

Diagnosis

Most children with tuberculosis are diagnosed by means of skin testing performed as a result of contact investigations prompted by identification of an infectious adult. Cultures remain essential, for diagnosis and identification of drug-resistant organisms. However, in young children with primary pulmonary tuberculosis, sputum is unavailable for culture, the yield from early-morning gastric aspirates is only about 40%, and the yield from specimens obtained by bronchoscopy is often not much better. Hence cultures of sputum from source-case adults (which have a much higher yield) are often the best means of obtaining organisms and testing their susceptibility to antituberculosis drugs, thereby guiding selection of a treatment regimen.

Other specimens that can be used for cultures include pleural fluid and preferably a pleural punch biopsy specimen from patients with pleural effusion; CSF from patients with meningitis; lymph node biopsy specimens or aspirates from patients with adenitis; bone marrow biopsy or liver biopsy specimens from patients with miliary disease or protracted hematogenous spread; joint fluid or synovial biopsy specimens from patients with tuberculous arthritis; and skin biopsy specimens from patients with cutaneous lesions.

Treatment Principles

Appropriate therapy with antituberculous drugs prevents the development of disease in children who are asymptomatic, halts the progression of disease, and prevents complications. Further, it dramatically reduces the risk of subsequent reactivation. In infectious adults and adolescents, therapy is aimed not only at managing the disease, but at rendering the person noninfectious as quickly as possible.

Tubercle bacilli thrive in large numbers in the well-oxygenated environment of an open pulmonary cavity but replicate much more slowly, sometimes intermittently, or become dormant in caseous lesions and within macrophages. Naturally resistant organisms are routinely found in patients with large populations of organisms. Therefore agents are selected for their ability to kill organisms in differing environments and to prevent the development of secondary drug resistance. The choice and number of drugs and duration of therapy are determined by the stage and severity of the disease at diagnosis; by epidemiologic data regarding the likelihood of drug resistance; and results of cultures and susceptibility testing, if available. The course of therapy must be lengthy (even with new shorter regimens) to ensure that slowly growing bacilli are eliminated and to give the patient's own host resistance time to kill organisms that persist, despite therapy. This necessitates close follow-up and the support of health care workers to assist compliance; in some cases, direct supervision of medication administration is necessary.

Children younger than 4 years of age have a high risk for severe disease from *M. tuberculosis*. Accordingly, they should be started on prophylaxis if they have been exposed to an infectious adult, even if their PPD is negative and until they are retested 3 months after exposure. Medication can be discontinued if the repeat test is again negative. Children who have a positive PPD without evidence of disease can take a single agent for 9 months. Children with primary pulmonary tuberculosis are treated first with a combination of three drugs for 2 months and then with two drugs to complete a 6- to 9-month course. Those with milder forms of extrapulmonary disease are treated similarly, but for 9 to 12 months. Patients with tuberculous meningitis and those suspected of having resistant organisms are treated initially with four medications, pending the results of susceptibility tests, and treatment is continued for a minimum of 12 months.

Administration of corticosteroids in concert with antituberculosis agents decreases the severity of the inflammatory response and attendant vasculitis and thereby reduces morbidity and mortality in patients with severe complications, such as meningitis, miliary disease with alveolar-capillary block, massive pericardial and pleural effusions, and marked hilar adenopathy that produces respiratory embarrassment.

Congenital and Perinatal Infections

Numerous pathogens that produce relatively mild or even subclinical disease in children and adults can cause severe disease with devastating sequelae in children who acquire such infections prenatally or perinatally. Toxoplasmosis, rubella, cytomegalovirus (CMV), herpes simplex virus (which comprise the TORCH syndromes), and syphilis are well-known sources of pathology. In addition, sepsis, meningitis, pneumonia, and other infections caused by numerous perinatally acquired bacterial pathogens, including tetanus in underdeveloped countries, cause significant neonatal morbidity and mortality, especially in infants born prematurely. Because of the breadth of this subject and space limitations, we have limited discussion to disorders that tend to have distinctive physical findings.

Congenital Toxoplasmosis

Toxoplasma gondii is an intracellular protozoan whose definitive host is the cat. Oocysts are shed in the feces and can survive in soil for years. Infection of humans is acquired primarily from the ingestion or inhalation of oocysts excreted in cat feces or consumption of raw or undercooked meat from animals who acquired infection from oocysts in the soil. Occasionally, transmission occurs by means of transfusion or organ transplantation. Although most cases of infection in children beyond the neonatal period are thought to be subclinical, a mononucleosis-like syndrome and cervical adenopathy have been identified as clinical features, and it may well be that in many cases the clinical picture simulates a viral illness and thus the true cause goes unrecognized.

Prenatally acquired infection has the potential to cause serious harm to the developing fetus. In the United States an estimated 1 to 2 per 1000 live-born infants have congenitally acquired toxoplasmosis. Maternal infection during pregnancy results in fetal infection less than 50% of the time, however. The risk of transmission to the fetus increases as gestation advances, but the severity of fetal injury is greater the earlier the infection occurs during pregnancy. Major sites of involvement are the CNS, retina, choroid, and muscles. Seventy percent of congenitally infected infants appear normal at birth, about 10% to 20% are overtly symptomatic, and approximately 10% have detectable chorioretinitis without other abnormalities (see Chapter 19). Infected infants without signs of disease and those with mild chorioretinitis alone are at risk for progressive ocular and, on occasion, CNS involvement if the infection is not diagnosed and treated. In many instances, however, the diagnosis is not suspected until evidence of visual impairment, strabismus, or developmental delay prompts careful ophthalmologic and neurologic assessment.

In symptomatic newborns the classic constellation of hydrocephalus, chorioretinitis, and intracerebral calcifications points toward the diagnosis of congenital toxoplasmosis. However, most often the clinical picture simulates that of other congenital infections, especially cytomegalovirus infection. Affected infants tend to be small for gestational age, may be microcephalic or hydrocephalic, develop early-onset jaundice, have hepatosplenomegaly and diffuse adenopathy, and can have petechial and purpuric lesions or a generalized maculopapular rash. Seizures can occur, and CSF examination may show a pleocytosis with an increased protein content and xanthochromia. Skull radiographs or a head CT scan may reveal diffuse cortical calcifications (Fig. 12-66), in contrast to the periventricular pattern seen in infants with congenital cytomegalovirus infection. Interstitial pneumonitis and myocarditis may be prominent features as well. These infants are at high risk of suffering severe neurodevelopmental sequelae, if they survive. Other infected infants may appear normal initially but may rapidly develop signs of neonatal myocarditis with minimal CNS manifestations, although they, too, may have cerebral calcifications, as do many infants with apparently isolated chorioretinitis.

Diagnosis can be confirmed by demonstration of a positive IgM or IgA assay within the first 6 months of life. Double-sandwich enzyme immunoassays or immunoabsorbent assays for *T. gondii*–specific IgM should be used in infants suspected of having congenital toxoplasmosis. Thorough ophthalmologic, auditory, and neurologic evaluations are also indicated. In addition, a head CT scan should be obtained and CSF examined. To halt further and future progression of the disease, all infected infants, whether symptomatic or not, warrant prolonged treatment (up to 1 year) with a combination of pyrimethamine (supplemented with folic acid) and sulfadiazine. This should be instituted and administered in consultation with appropriate specialists.

Congenital Rubella

Widespread use of rubella vaccination has thankfully made congenital rubella a rarity in developed countries. Although normally a benign infection, rubella can lead to severe consequences if acquired in utero. Even if asymp-

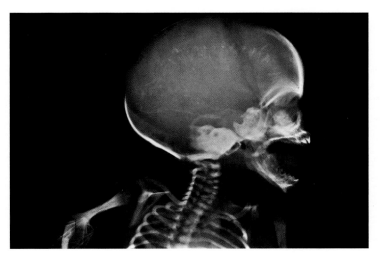

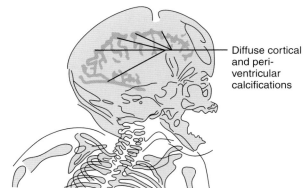

Diffuse cortical and peri-ventricular calcifications

Figure 12-66. Congenital toxoplasmosis. Microcephaly, ventricular dilatation, and cerebral calcifications were prominent findings in this infant with severe congenital toxoplasmosis. (Courtesy Department of Pediatric Radiology, Children's Hospital of Pittsburgh.)

tomatic infection occurs in the mother, rubella can be transmitted across the placenta to the developing fetus. The earlier in gestation the infection occurs, the greater the potential for injury. Close to 40% of fetuses infected during the first 8 weeks spontaneously abort or are stillborn, and 25% have gross anomalies noted at birth. Ultimately, 85% of live-born infants infected in the first trimester suffer adverse consequences, as do 35% of those infected between weeks 13 and 16. Infection after 4 months' gestation does not appear to cause disease. The most commonly encountered anomalies are central diffuse cataracts; congenital heart disease (patent ductus arteriosus, pulmonary artery stenosis, pulmonary valvular stenosis); and sensorineural deafness (usually bilateral, occasionally unilateral), seen singly or in combination.

Thus there is a wide range of clinical manifestations. Some infants at risk are normal. Some appear normal at birth but later are found to have hearing loss. Some are small for gestational age and at birth have evidence of congenital heart disease and ocular anomalies, including microphthalmia, glaucoma, cataracts that may be central or diffuse, and pigmented retinopathy (see Chapter 19). Many of these infants develop jaundice within 24 hours of birth and have hepatosplenomegaly and diffuse adenopathy as well. Although usually present at birth, ocular findings may be missed unless a careful ophthalmologic examination is performed.

Ten to twenty percent of live-born infants with congenital rubella show signs of severe disseminated infection at or shortly after birth. In addition to early-onset jaundice, hepatosplenomegaly, and adenopathy, they often have

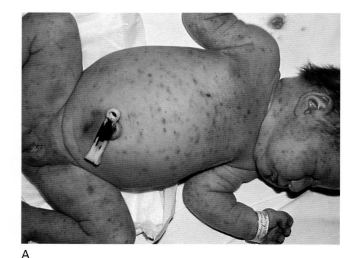

A

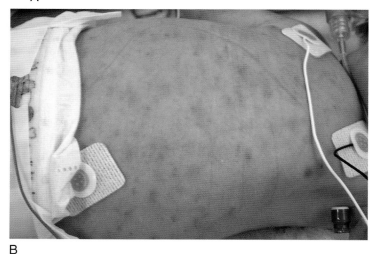

B

Figure 12-67. Congenital infections. **A** and **B,** Congenital rubella: Both of these newborns had the full-blown picture of the "expanded rubella syndrome" including a generalized blueberry muffin rash, diffuse petechiae, hepatosplenomegaly, the early onset of jaundice, and neurologic depression. The infant shown in **A** is jaundiced and has bluer lesions. **B,** This infant with congenital cytomegalovirus infection has nearly identical findings to those in the newborn with rubella in **A.** (**A,** Courtesy Michael Sherlock, MD, Lutherville, Md.)

signs of myocarditis with ischemic changes on electrocardiograms, interstitial pneumonitis, thrombocytopenia with petechiae and purpura, and CNS dysfunction that may range from lethargy and hypotonia to frank meningoencephalitis. Radiographs may reveal bony abnormalities consisting of metaphyseal lucencies and irregular epiphyseal mineralization. In some cases a rubelliform rash or a characteristic raised, bluish, papular eruption, termed a *blueberry muffin rash,* may be evident as the result of dermal erythropoiesis (Fig. 12-67A). Most of these severely affected infants are microcephalic, in addition to being small for gestational age. In countries with universal vaccination programs, infants with these findings are more likely to have congenital CMV infection (Fig. 12-67B). Survivors of this "expanded rubella syndrome" are highly likely to be deaf and have significant psychomotor retardation.

In a small percentage of infants with congenital rubella, delayed manifestations may surface. These include anemia toward the end of the first month; the insidious onset of interstitial pneumonitis; and the appearance of a chronic, generalized rubelliform exanthem at 3 to 4 months of age. Still later, immunodeficiency may be detected. Feeding

difficulties, chronic diarrhea, and failure to thrive are common.

Infants with congenital rubella are chronically and persistently infected and tend to shed live virus in urine, stools, and respiratory secretions for up to a year. Hence, they should be isolated when in the hospital and kept away from susceptible pregnant women when sent home. Diagnosis can be confirmed by viral culture and specific IgM titers.

Congenital Cytomegalovirus Infection

A ubiquitous virus of the herpesvirus family, CMV infects approximately 1% of all live-born infants while in utero. Infection of the fetus can develop from either primary infection of the mother or reactivation of virus acquired earlier. However, primary infection is believed to be associated with a higher risk for symptomatic disease in the infant. Approximately 10% of infected infants have symptoms at birth. Similar to other TORCH syndromes, findings include small size for gestational age, micro-cephaly, thrombocytopenia, hepatosplenomegaly, hepatitis, intracranial calcifications (see Fig. 15-27), chorioretinitis, and hearing abnormalities. Some affected babies can be born with a "blueberry muffin" appearance similar to that of congenital rubella (see Fig. 12-67B). Another 10% to 15% of congenitally infected infants may not manifest problems until later in infancy or childhood when they are found to have sensorineural hearing loss and/or developmental delays. Children identified with congenital CMV infection should have routine hearing assessments until 5 years of age because hearing loss can be progressive.

Neonatal Herpes Simplex Infection

Infants born vaginally to mothers with primary genital herpes simplex infection have a 50% risk of acquiring disease. In contrast, less than 5% born to mothers with recurrent lesions develop herpes neonatorum. Risk of infection increases with prolonged rupture of membranes. Typically the mother is asymptomatic and the infant appears totally normal at birth. Signs of infection may develop any time within the first 4 weeks but usually appear 4 to 8 days postpartum. Infection may be localized to the skin, eye, mouth, or CNS, or it may be systemic. In the latter instance, onset begins with fever or subnormal temperature in association with lethargy, poor feeding, vomiting, and jaundice. The liver and spleen are enlarged and often remarkably firm. Respiratory distress supervenes, followed by a picture that is indistinguishable from that of septic shock with DIC. Approximately three fourths of affected infants have typical herpetic skin or mucosal lesions (Fig. 12-68A and B). The scalp and face are the sites most commonly involved (Fig. 12-68C). Occasionally lesions are limited to the conjunctiva or to the oral mucosa. In the absence of these lesions, accurate diagnosis is extremely difficult. The prognosis is relatively good for infants with localized skin, eye, or oral involvement if they are treated promptly with intravenous acyclovir. If untreated, most of these infants will progress to CNS and/or disseminated disease. Mortality of infants with disseminated disease is high, exceeding 50%, but has been reduced by early recognition and systemic antiviral therapy. The survival rate is better in those with localized CNS disease

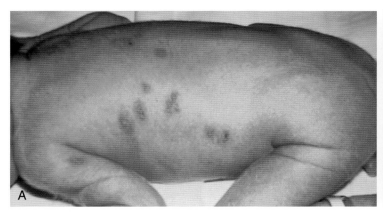

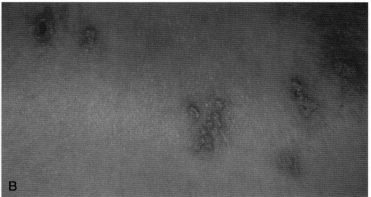

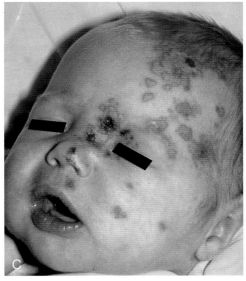

Figure 12-68. Neonatal herpes simplex type 2 infection. **A** and **B,** Although the child was normal at birth, fever, lethargy, and decreased feeding suddenly developed in this infant at 6 days of age. On examination, multiple grouped vesicular lesions were noted on the trunk and scalp. The liver and spleen were markedly enlarged and firm. He had a fulminant course resembling that of septic shock and died within 24 hours. **C,** Vesicular lesions are found most commonly on the scalp and face, as demonstrated in this infant. (**A** and **B,** Courtesy Michael Sherlock, MD, Lutherville, Md.)

than in those with systemic infection, but severe morbidity results in both.

Less frequently, infections may occur prenatally as a result of ascent from the lower genital tract through ruptured membranes or as a result of maternal viremia. In the event of prenatal acquisition, the infant may die in utero or may be born with jaundice, skin lesions, and signs of systemic infection.

Congenital Syphilis

Initial hopes of eradicating syphilis with the advent of penicillin in the mid-20th century proved to be premature, for as prevalence of disease waned, so did funding for its control programs, and dramatic resurgences occurred in the 1960s and again in the 1980s. Concomitantly, an increase in congenital infection mirrored the rise in incidence of syphilis in women of childbearing age. Fortunately, revitalized control programs once again have decreased the incidence. However, hopes for eradication have yet to be realized, and it remains important for physicians to be able to recognize the clinical manifestations of syphilis. Its congenital form is discussed here. Manifestations in adolescents are presented in Chapter 18.

Women most at risk of acquiring and transmitting syphilis to their infants are young, of low socioeconomic status, have multiple sex partners, and live in an area where syphilis has become endemic. Drug use and the practice of trading sex for drugs substantially increase risk of acquisition and complicate efforts to trace sexual contacts. Adding to the risk of fetal transmission is the fact

that women at greatest risk of acquiring the disease often fail to seek or receive inadequate prenatal care, thus delaying prenatal diagnosis and treatment.

Congenital syphilis results from hematogenous spread of *Treponema pallidum* from an infected mother through the placenta to the developing fetus, resulting in disseminated disease. It appears that risk of transmission to the fetus is greatest when the mother acquires disease during or shortly before pregnancy (i.e., when she is in the primary, secondary, or early latent phase of the disease). Infection early in gestation can result in stillbirth, hydrops fetalis, prematurity, or neonatal death. Live-born infected infants may or may not have obvious signs and symptoms at the time of delivery. Those who do not may develop clinical manifestations during the neonatal period or weeks, months, or even years later if the disease goes undiagnosed and untreated. The earlier the onset, the poorer the prognosis. Although the reasons for delay in symptom onset are not fully understood, it appears that when delivery occurs while the mother is in the incubation period, and is thus seronegative, long-delayed onset is more typical.

Infants who are symptomatic at birth tend to have evidence of intrauterine growth retardation, hepatosplenomegaly, direct and indirect hyperbilirubinemia, Coombs-negative hemolytic anemia, thrombocytopenia, generalized lymphadenopathy (including epitrochlear nodes), and mucocutaneous lesions. These lesions are often vesicular or bullous and ultimately rupture to form superficial crusted erosions or ulcerations. The rash is generalized and includes palms and soles. When skin lesions appear after the first month, they are more likely to be

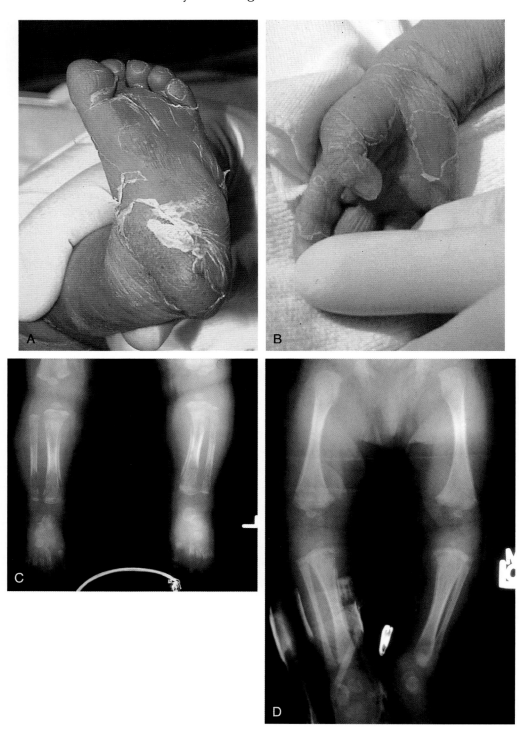

Figure 12-69. Congenital syphilis. **A** and **B,** Desquamation of the foot and hand are seen in this infant with congenital syphilis. **C,** This 3-month-old who presented with untreated congenital syphilis had diffuse periosteal reaction of the tibias and generalized demineralization. **D,** Wimberger sign, the osseous destruction of the proximal tibial metaphysis, is seen in another affected infant. (**A** and **B,** Courtesy Pablo Sanchez, MD, and Walid Salhab, MD, University of Texas Southwestern Medical Center; **D,** courtesy Manuel P. Meza, MD, Children's Hospital of Pittsburgh.)

papulosquamous or maculopapular, resembling those of secondary syphilis in older individuals (see Fig. 18-32). They tend to be oval in shape; pinkish red in color; and distributed predominantly over the back, buttocks, posterior thighs, and soles, although perioral and palmar lesions may be present. Over time these lesions tend to turn brown in color, and fine desquamation of the palms and soles may be noted (Fig. 12-69A and B). Three to four months after delivery, affected infants may develop typical condylomata lata—moist papular or warty lesions around the nose and mouth and in intertriginous areas. Mucosal lesions, termed *mucous patches,* consist of patchy white lesions seen over the palate and other mucosal surfaces. Characteristic snuffles may develop between a week and a few months of age. Affected infants have an increasingly profuse rhinorrhea, in which the nasal discharge can be

blood tinged, when there are associated ulcerations of the nasal mucosa. A hoarse cry is commonly seen with snuffles. The nasal discharge, mucosal lesions, and moist cutaneous lesions teem with organisms.

Widespread symmetrical skeletal involvement is seen radiographically in essentially all infants with congenital syphilis (see Fig. 12-69C and D), although only about 15% have symptoms of pain. Their discomfort is manifested as irritability and pseudoparalysis of Parrot, in which decreased limb movement, especially of the upper extremities, is noted. Osteochondritis, evident on x-ray examination as early as 5 weeks, is characterized by horizontal radiopaque bands often with adjacent lucent lines that are seen in the metaphases, along with irregular demineralization of the lateral aspect, which creates a mottled appearance. In the proximal tibias the medial portion of the metaphyses can be demineralized as well, a phenomenon termed the *Wimberger sign* (see Fig. 12-69D). Radiographic evidence of periostitis is generally not seen until about 3 to 4 months of age and is characterized by the formation of one or more layers of periosteal new bone extending along the length of the diaphyses of long bones (see Fig. 12-69C and D).

CNS involvement is common in infants with full-blown clinical disease but also can be found in some who are otherwise asymptomatic. Accordingly, CSF examination is recommended for all infected infants. Untreated infants can go on to develop meningitis with a clinical picture that simulates that of acute bacterial meningitis. However, CSF examination reveals a monocytosis with moderately elevated protein and a normal glucose. Chronic meningovascular inflammation may become evident later in the first year. This can progress to fibrosis, resulting in hydrocephalus and cranial nerve palsies (especially of cranial nerves VII, III, IV, and VI) along with regression in developmental milestones. In the second year, progressive cerebral endarteritis may cause focal infarctions with secondary strokelike symptoms and seizures.

All of the symptoms of "early congenital syphilis" just described are the direct result of active infection. Manifestations of "late congenital syphilis" are usually sequelae or stigmata of prior disease activity but can in some instances be due to persistent disease. They may be seen in up to 40% of cases and include the following:

1. Maldevelopment of permanent teeth
   - Hutchinson teeth—the upper central incisors are smaller than normal, barrel shaped, and notched in the center of the incisal surface
   - Mulberry molars—abnormal cusp development results in formation of multiple peripheral cusps and a central cusp
2. Interstitial keratitis—development of a ground-glass appearance of the cornea and scleral vascularization, which have their onset around puberty
3. Eighth nerve deafness
4. Skeletal stigmata due to sclerotic changes
   - Sabre shin
   - Frontal bossing
5. Cartilaginous stigmata due to gummatous breakdown and/or ulceration
   - Saddle nose deformity
   - Palatal perforation
6. Clutton joints—painless hydrarthrosis of the knees
7. Rhagades—fissuring of the skin in the perinasal and perioral areas
8. Mental retardation and, more rarely, chronic neurosyphilis with paresis, or less commonly, tabes dorsalis

Testing all pregnant women for syphilis and promptly treating those who are seropositive constitute the mainstay in preventing congenital syphilis. Infants should be further evaluated and treated if the mother did not receive treatment or may have been inadequately treated. The latter should be suspected if a nonpenicillin regimen was used, if there was less than a fourfold decrease in her serum titer following treatment, or if treatment was administered less than a month before delivery.

Neonatal Tetanus

Tetanus is an exceptionally painful acute neuromuscular disorder caused by release of a neurotoxic exotoxin by *Clostridium tetani*. The bacterium, a gram-positive anaerobic rod, forms terminal spores that are highly resistant to heat and antiseptics. Prevalent worldwide, the organism is present in the intestines of humans and animals. Accordingly, it is widespread in soil and is found in especially large numbers in the cultivated soil of rural areas fertilized by manure. It is also present in dust and dirt in urban areas. When organisms are inoculated along with dirt or soil into a wound with devitalized or necrotic tissue, they find ideal anaerobic conditions for spore germination. Once they have germinated, spores release two exotoxins; tetanolysin and tetanospasmin. Tetanolysin assists with potentiating infection, while tetanospasmin is one of the most potent neurotoxins known. The toxin diffuses locally, binding irreversibly to presynaptic terminals of lower motor neurons where it impedes neuromuscular transmission, and, acting on the motor end-plates of nearby skeletal muscle cells, it interferes with contraction-relaxation mechanisms. Additional toxin is believed to spread via the bloodstream and lymphatics to yet other peripheral nerve terminals, and some leaves the inoculum site traveling via retrograde axonal transport to lower motor neuron cell bodies in the spinal cord and brainstem. There it migrates across synapses to inhibitory interneurons and blocks release of neurotransmitters, thereby suppressing their inhibitory control. Lacking effective inhibition, patients experience persistent muscular rigidity and periodic spasmodic contractions of voluntary muscles, which are extremely painful. The toxin's action on autonomic nerves also results in disinhibition.

Neonatal tetanus is a generalized form of the disorder seen in infants born to unimmunized or inadequately immunized mothers and is usually the result of contamination of the umbilical stump. Cutting the cord with an unclean instrument, application of dirty dressing materials, and/or the cultural practice of placing mud or dung on the stump to hasten cord separation may be the source of the inoculum.

Affected neonates are still seen in significant numbers in more than 50 (mostly underdeveloped) countries worldwide, and neonatal tetanus has its highest incidence in parts of eastern and southern Asia and sub-Saharan Africa. In those areas incidence is highest among the poor who have little or no access to health care, are poorly educated regarding safe and sanitary birthing practices, and often whose cultures make them suspicious of health care providers and immunizations. Significant underreporting of the disease, especially in remote areas where births and deaths often go unrecorded, makes it impossible to know the exact incidence, but it is estimated to be somewhere in the vicinity of 500,000 cases per year. Mortality is high—95% of cases with no treatment and 25% to 90% for infants receiving treatment, depending on its quality.

The incubation period for neonatal tetanus ranges from 3 to 4 days to 2 weeks, with onset of symptoms usually occurring 6 to 7 days after delivery. Initially the baby appears restless and irritable and seems to have difficulty suckling. Within 1 to 2 days, trismus (lockjaw) due to masseter rigidity, dysphagia with drooling, and noisy respirations are noted. These are associated with neck, back, and shoulder stiffness. Subsequently there is rapid cephalocaudal progression of muscular rigidity from neck to back and abdomen, and then the extremities. Opisthotonic posturing is typical, and hands are held fisted and toes fanned out. Orbicularis oris spasm produces the appearance of a sardonic grin termed *risus sardonicus* (Fig. 12-70A and B). These manifestations are accompanied by fever and the onset of painful tonic or tetanic spasmodic contractions of voluntary muscles, which range from mild to severe, can last a few to several minutes, and can be

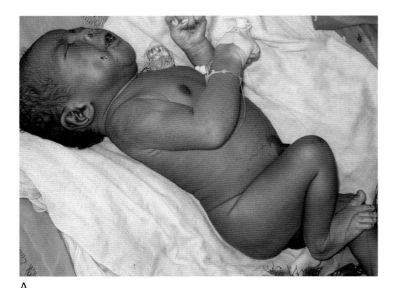

A

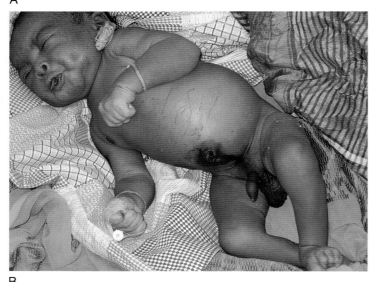

B

Figure 12-70. Neonatal tetanus. **A,** This newborn demonstrates the trismus (locked jaw) and fixed smile of risus sardonicus that are typical of tetanus. Note as well the clenched fists and fanned toes. **B,** Viewed from the side, his opisthotonic posturing is more evident. (Courtesy Jonathan Spector, MD, Boston.)

precipitated by even minimal external stimuli. Masseter, orbicularis, and pharyngeal rigidity make sucking difficult, if not impossible, and significantly impair swallowing. Spasms involving laryngeal muscles and the diaphragm can cause severe respiratory embarrassment. Symptoms of autonomic disinhibition include periods of excessive sweating, hypertension, tachycardia, and arrhythmias. Complications include aspiration, atelectasis, pneumonia, fractures of vertebrae and long bones, and respiratory arrest. In survivors, clinical improvement tends to begin about 2 weeks after onset of symptoms with a gradual decrease in fever, degree of rigidity and frequency, and intensity of spasms. Resolution then proceeds gradually over the ensuing 6 weeks. Many surviving infants show persistent signs of developmental delay, problems with balance, and some degree of muscle atrophy. Later, when old enough, these children may complain of easy muscle fatigue and cramping.

The diagnosis of tetanus must be made clinically. Laboratory studies are unhelpful.

Successful treatment regimens include the following:

- Prompt administration of tetanus immune globulin to neutralize any free or unbound toxin
- Good local wound care
- Administration of penicillin or metronidazole
- Good supportive intensive care in a dim, quiet room with minimal stimulation
- Neuromuscular blockade and sedation to reduce pain, severity of spasms, and rigidity and allay anxiety
- Intubation and ventilation as needed for respiratory compromise
- Attention to nutrition often via total parenteral nutrition
- H_2 blockers to prevent stress ulcers
- Initiation of immunization with tetanus toxoid
- After-care physical therapy

Effective prevention measures in areas where tetanus remains endemic necessitate aggressive outreach immunization campaigns (often to remote areas) aimed especially at women and girls of childbearing age, as well as unimmunized or inadequately immunized pregnant women. These efforts must be combined with carefully tailored and culturally sensitive education programs (to overcome cultural taboos) that emphasize safe and sanitary birthing practices and cord care, as well as conveying the importance and safety of immunizations.

Human Immunodeficiency Virus and Acquired Immunodeficiency Syndrome

HIV-1 is a retrovirus and is the major etiologic agent of acquired immunodeficiency syndrome (AIDS) throughout the world. A second virus, HIV-2, is endemic in West Africa and accounts for the remainder of AIDS cases. HIV is a ribonucleic acid virus that is trophic for $CD4^+$ (helper) T lymphocytes, as well as some monocytes, macrophages, and microglial cells of the central nervous system that bear $CD4^+$ surface markers. The virus becomes integrated into the host genome and hence persists in the infected individual for life.

More than 9000 children (younger than 13 years of age) in the United States have been reported to the Centers for Disease Control and Prevention (CDC) with AIDS, and more than half of these children have died. Estimates suggest that more than 2 million children worldwide have been infected with the virus. Of these children, the vast majority acquire the virus perinatally from their HIV-infected mothers. This is particularly true in technologically advanced countries as superb screening procedures are available to ensure the safety of blood supplies. Without intervention, there is a 15% to 30% risk of transmission of HIV from an HIV-infected mother to her offspring. However, in 1994 a large multicenter, randomized, double-blind study proved that maternal-to-child transmission of HIV could be reduced with the use of zidovudine given to HIV-infected women orally during the second and third trimesters, intravenously intrapartum, and to the offspring for the first 6 weeks of life. Subsequent studies using combination therapy with highly active antiretroviral agents were even more successful, preventing almost all vertical transmission of HIV in non–breast-feeding populations. However, these therapies are often unavailable to women in poorer countries of the world because of costs and logistics. Worldwide estimates suggest that 17 million women of childbearing age are currently infected with HIV. Not only can transmission occur during the time of delivery, but also postnatally through breast milk. These staggering figures, along with the problem of accessing these individuals for antenatal and postnatal therapy, tell a sobering story that sorely needs to be addressed.

Blood bank screening procedures introduced in 1985 have virtually eliminated the risk of transmission from exposure to HIV-infected blood products in countries that can afford to use them. Like adults, adolescents acquire HIV through high-risk behaviors, such as unprotected sexual activity and needle sharing. Adolescents account for less than 1% of cases of AIDS reported to the CDC. However, given that it takes an average of 10 years for acquired HIV to progress to AIDS, it is clear that much adult AIDS can be ascribed to HIV infection acquired during the teenage or young adult years. HIV is not transmitted by casual contact with an HIV-infected individual in normal living conditions and school settings. Under unusual circumstances, contact between HIV-infected blood and open skin lesions or mucous membranes of an uninfected individual can result in virus transmission.

The timing of symptom development in untreated HIV-infected children varies. Approximately one third of infants present rapidly in the first months or year of life with one or more of the characteristic AIDS-indicator conditions, suggesting intrauterine infection. The majority of other children infected with HIV present in the first few years of life with a more indolent course, and only a small percentage of children develop symptoms years later akin to what is seen with adults.

HIV-infected infants often present with failure to thrive (Fig. 12-71), developmental delay or loss of developmental milestones, hepatosplenomegaly, lymphadenopathy, candidal skin or mucosal infections (Fig. 12-72), chronic diarrhea, chronic lymphoid interstitial pneumonitis, and recurrent or particularly severe bacterial infections. The last include sepsis, pneumonia, meningitis, abscess, or recurrent episodes of cellulitis, otitis media, and sinusitis. Common pathogens are *S. pneumoniae, H. influenzae, Salmonella, S. aureus,* and gram-negative organisms.

HIV infection is often suspected because of a history of maternal high-risk behaviors or because of a child's clinical presentation. Approximately 50% present with symptoms of HIV infection by the age of 1 year and 82% by 3 years. Increasing attention to testing all women during pregnancy allows for intervention and prevention of perinatally transmitted infection.

Although, as noted earlier, bacterial infections are often seen in HIV-infected infants, opportunistic infections related to defects in cell-mediated immunity also occur. One of the most common of these is *Pneumocystis jiroveci* (formerly *P. carinii*) pneumonia (PCP) (Fig. 12-73), which occurs in more than one third of untreated symptomatic HIV-infected children. Other opportunistic infections include *Mycobacterium avium* complex, candidal esophagitis, cytomegalovirus infection, cryptosporidiosis, persistent or disseminated herpes simplex virus, cryptococcosis, and toxoplasmosis and unusually extensive cases of molluscum contagiosum (Fig. 12-74). Of particular note is *M. avium* complex, which may cause fever, weight loss, diarrhea, and abdominal pain.

An especially devastating feature of HIV infection is the encephalopathic condition that leads to developmental delay, loss of developmental milestones, and behavioral alterations. Also seen are pyramidal tract signs, paresis, ataxia, pseudobulbar palsy, and decreased tone. CT scans and MRI studies often show severe brain atrophy with increased ventricular size and calcifications in the basal ganglia and frontal lobes (Fig. 12-75). The course of HIV-related neurologic disease is variable and may be intermittent, static, or relentlessly progressive.

Table 12-5	Selected Abnormalities of the Immune System in AIDS

Lymphopenia (more common in adults)
Decreased helper T lymphocytes (T4)
Decreased helper-to-suppressor ratio (T4/T8 ratio)
Decreased T- and B-lymphocyte mitogen responses (pokeweed, phytohemagglutinin, concanavalin A)
Decreased specific antibody response to antigen
Increased immunoglobulin levels (IgG, IgD, IgA, IgM, IgG subclasses)
Deficient serum isohemagglutinin levels
Positive test for antinuclear antibodies
Positive Coombs test
Positive circulating immune complex levels

Lymphoid interstitial pneumonitis, leading to chronic interstitial pneumonitis, can be seen in children with HIV (Fig. 12-76). This form of chronic lung disease presents insidiously over the course of several years with cough; wheezing; clubbing of the fingers (Fig. 12-77); hypoxemia; radiologic features of a diffuse reticulonodular infiltrate; and, at times, hilar and mediastinal adenopathy. Children with this condition often have lymphadenopathy, hepatosplenomegaly, parotid gland enlargement, and a longer survival than children who have opportunistic infections.

As with many immunodeficiencies, malignancies also occur in children with AIDS, although at rates significantly lower than in adults. Kaposi sarcoma (Fig. 12-78) and lymphoma have been reported in affected children, particularly in countries with endemic human herpes virus 8, such as sub-Saharan Africa.

Other clinical manifestations of HIV include diarrhea, hepatitis, pancreatitis, cardiomyopathy (Fig. 12-79), eczema, nephrotic syndrome, and pancytopenia. HIV infection therefore presents with a multitude of clinical pictures. The clinical pattern of disease reflects direct HIV infection, as well as the immune system dysregulation caused by the viruses, including evidence of immunodeficiency and autoimmune disease. A variety of immunologic abnormalities occur with HIV infection (Table 12-5).

Diagnosis of HIV infection in children older than 18 months of age is reliably established by detecting serum IgG antibodies to a number of specific HIV antigens using two assays. The enzyme-linked immunosorbent assay (ELISA) is used as a highly sensitive screening test. Serum reported as positive by ELISA assay needs to be confirmed by the Western blot assay, which, to be considered positive, must indicate the presence of antibodies against a requisite number of HIV-specific antigens. In rare instances when an HIV-infected child has a B cell deficiency, detection of viral particles by polymerase chain reaction is recommended even if the child is older than 18 months of age. In contrast, definitive diagnosis in children less than 18 months of age relies on the detection of viral particles. This is because of the ubiquitous presence of passively acquired maternal antibodies (including IgG antibodies against HIV) in newborns of HIV-infected mothers. Accordingly, conventional antibody assays only establish exposure to an infected mother, not true infection of the infant.

Detection of proviral DNA using the polymerase chain reaction (PCR) amplification technique has proved to be a powerful tool in establishing the diagnosis of HIV infection in infants and is relied on early in life. Sensitivity, however, is only about 30% in the first week of life and

FAILURE TO THRIVE IN A CHILD WITH AIDS

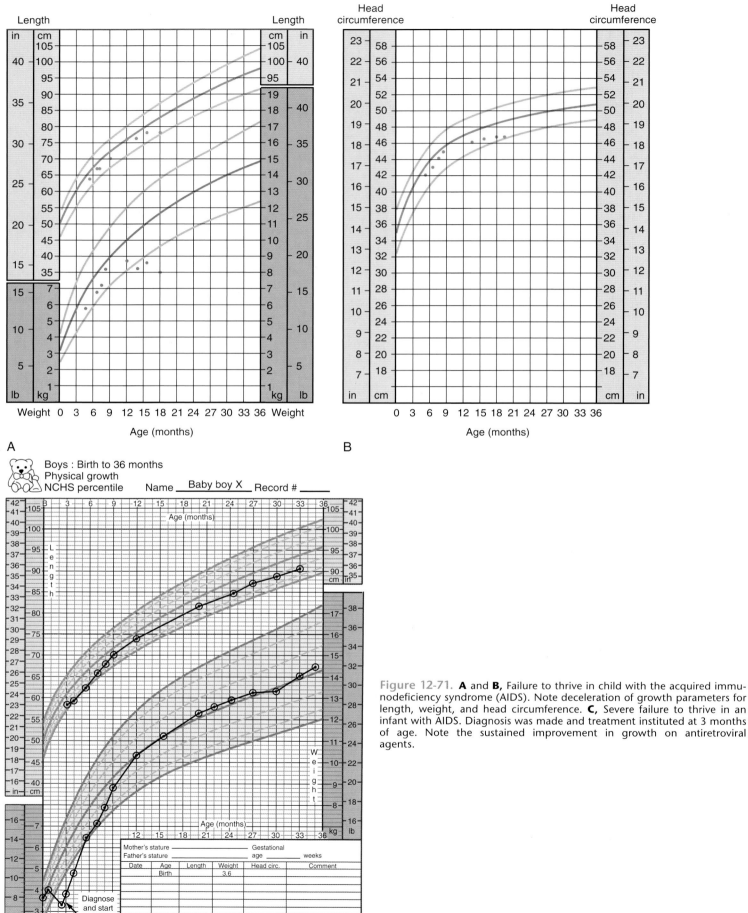

Figure 12-71. **A** and **B,** Failure to thrive in child with the acquired immunodeficiency syndrome (AIDS). Note deceleration of growth parameters for length, weight, and head circumference. **C,** Severe failure to thrive in an infant with AIDS. Diagnosis was made and treatment instituted at 3 months of age. Note the sustained improvement in growth on antiretroviral agents.

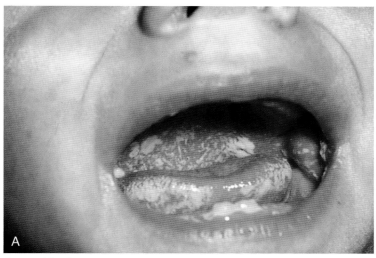

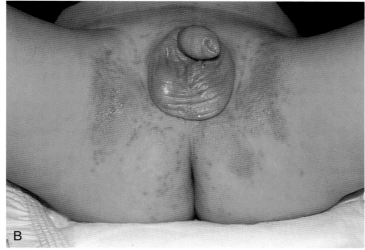

Figure 12-72. Child with AIDS. **A,** Oral thrush. **B,** Candidal diaper dermatitis. (**A,** Courtesy G. B. Scott, MD, and M. T. Mastrucci, MD, Miami.)

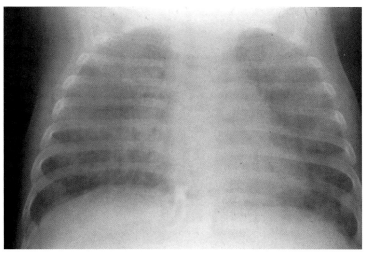

Figure 12-73. *Pneumocystis jiroveci* pneumonia in a child with AIDS. Note diffuse bilateral haziness. (Courtesy G. B. Scott, MD, and M. T. Mastrucci, MD, Miami.)

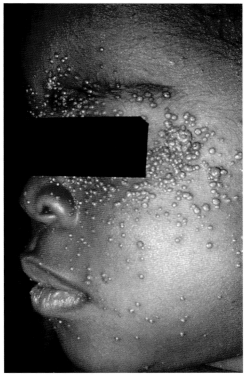

Figure 12-74. Severe molluscum contagiosum in a patient with AIDS. (Courtesy G. B. Scott, MD, and M. T. Mastrucci, MD, Miami.)

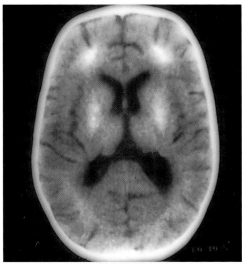

Figure 12-75. CT scan in infant with AIDS. Note the frontal lobe and basal ganglia calcification and increased ventricular size secondary to cerebral parenchymal volume loss.

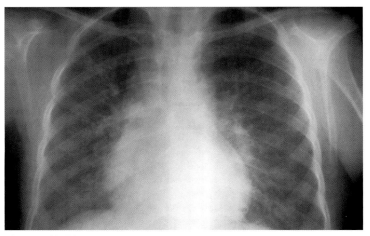

Figure 12-76. Lymphoid interstitial pneumonitis in a child with AIDS. Note the diffuse bilateral reticulonodular infiltrates.

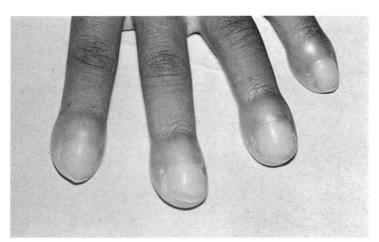

Figure 12-77. Clubbing in patient with lymphoid interstitial pneumonitis and AIDS. (Courtesy G. B. Scott, MD, and M. T. Mastrucci, MD, Miami.)

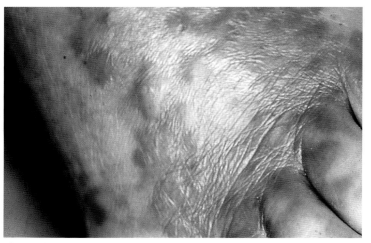

Figure 12-78. Cutaneous manifestations of Kaposi sarcoma. The purplish hyperpigmented plaques and nodules are characteristic.

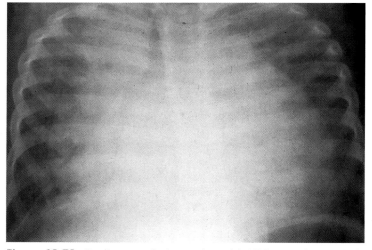

Figure 12-79. Cardiomyopathy in a patient with AIDS. Note the massively increased heart size. (Courtesy G. B. Scott, MD, and M. T. Mastrucci, MD, Miami.)

used. Conventional p24 antigen detection is not sufficiently sensitive to make it a useful technique in diagnosing HIV infection in infants. HIV culture, although useful, is time consuming and only performed in specialized research laboratories.

Therapy can be divided into that needed during the evaluation phase of infants born to mothers infected with HIV and that for children conclusively diagnosed with HIV. Zidovudine, as noted earlier, is used for the first 6 weeks of life to attempt to prevent transmission from mother to infant. Trimethoprim-sulfamethoxazole is used as prophylaxis against PCP until a child has had at least two negative HIV PCR tests obtained between 1 and 6 months of age or until the infected child is at least 12 months of age. Children infected with HIV who have CD4 counts less than 15% of total T lymphocytes should remain on PCP prophylaxis. In general, combination antiretroviral therapy is strongly recommended for all infected infants younger than 12 months old and for all symptomatic children. The exact treatment regimens are changing rapidly and are beyond the limits of this chapter.

New therapies for HIV itself and its related complications have changed the prognosis of this disease. Although not a cure, these treatments allow children infected with HIV to grow and develop into relatively healthy toddlers and children and attend school in age-appropriate classes. Accordingly, early diagnosis and aggressive management are critical. Most importantly, however, is identification and treatment of HIV-infected pregnant women to improve their health and prevent transmission to the newborn altogether.

Bibliography

American Academy of Pediatrics, Committee on Infectious Diseases: Report of the Committee on Infectious Diseases—Red Book 2003, 26th ed. Evanston, Ill, American Academy of Pediatrics, 2000.
Barton LL, Feigin RD: Childhood cervical lymphadenitis: A reappraisal. J Pediatr 84:846-852, 1974.
Barton LL, Friedman AD: Impetigo: A reassessment of etiology and therapy. Pediatr Derm 4:185-188, 1987.
Bingham PM, Galetta SL, Athreya B, Sladky J: Neurologic manifestations in children with Lyme disease. Pediatrics 96:1053-1056, 1995.
Cherry JD: Newer viral exanthems. Adv Pediatr 16:233-286, 1969.
Chesney PJ, Davis JP, Purdy WK, et al: Clinical manifestations of toxic shock syndrome. JAMA 246:741-748, 1981.
Clain A: Demonstrations of Physical Signs in Clinical Surgery, 17th ed. Bristol, England, John Wright-PSG, 1986.
Dich VQ, Nelson JD, Haltalin KC: Osteomyelitis in infants and children. Am J Dis Child 129:1273-1278, 1975.
Feigin RD, Cherry JD: Textbook of Pediatric Infectious Disease, 3rd ed. Philadelphia, WB Saunders, 1992.
Fleisher G, Ludwig S, Campos J: Cellulitis: Bacterial etiology, clinical features and laboratory findings. J Pediatr 97:591-593, 1980.
Hanshaw JB, Dudgeon JA, Marshall WC: Viral Diseases of the Fetus and Newborn, 2nd ed. Philadelphia, WB Saunders, 1985.
Hurwitz S: Clinical Pediatric Dermatology, 2nd ed. Philadelphia, WB Saunders, 1993.
Krugman S, Katz SL, Gershon AE, Wilfert CM: Infectious Diseases of Children, 9th ed. St Louis, Mosby, 1992.
Lascari AD, Bapat VR: Syndrome of infectious mononucleosis. Clin Pediatr 9:300-304, 1970.
Leibel RL, Fangman JJ, Ostrovsky MC: Chronic meningococcemia in childhood. Am J Dis Child 127:94-98, 1974.
Long SS, Pickering LK, Prober CG: Principles and Practice of Pediatric Infectious Diseases. New York, Churchill Livingstone, 2000.
Mandell GL, Douglas RG Jr, Bennet JE: Principles and Practice of Infectious Diseases, 4th ed. New York, Churchill Livingstone, 1995.
May M: Neck masses in children: Diagnosis and treatment. Pediatr Ann 5:517-535, 1976.
Morrey BF, Bianco AJ, Rhodes KH: Septic arthritis in children. Pediatr Clin North Am 6:923-934, 1975.
Nixon GW: Acute hematogenous osteomyelitis. Pediatr Ann 5:65-81, 1976.

increases to more than 90% by the end of the first month. A positive test should be confirmed on a separate blood sample. Two negative HIV DNA PCR tests (the first after 1 month of age and the second after 4 months of life) strongly support the absence of mother-to-child transmission. Quantitative HIV RNA amplification can also be

Rapkin RH, Bautista G: *Haemophilus influenzae* cellulitis. Am J Dis Child 124:540-542, 1972.

Remington JS, Klein JO: Infectious Diseases of the Fetus and Newborn Infant, 5th ed. Philadelphia, WB Saunders, 2000.

Salzar JC, Gerber MA, Goff CW: Long-term outcome of Lyme disease in children. J Pediatr 122:591-593, 1993.

Season EH, Miller PR: Primary subacute pyogenic osteomyelitis in long bones of children. J Pediatr Surg 11:347-353, 1976.

Shapiro ED: Lyme disease. In Burg FD, Ingelfinger JR, Wald ER, Polin RA (eds): Current Pediatric Therapy, 15th ed. Philadelphia, WB Saunders, 1996.

Starke JR, Jacobs RF, Jereb J: Resurgence of tuberculosis in children. J Pediatr 120:839-855, 1992.

Steere AC: Lyme disease. N Engl J Med 321:586-596, 1989.

Toews WH, Bass JW: Skin manifestations of meningococcal infection. Am J Dis Child 127:173-176, 1974.

Tofte RW, Williams DN: Toxic shock syndrome: Evidence of a broad clinical spectrum. JAMA 246:2163-2167, 1981.

Wannamaker LW, Ferrieri P: Streptococcal infections—updated. DM October:1-40, 1975.

Wilson HD, Haltalin KC: Acute necrotizing fasciitis in childhood. Am J Dis Child 125:591-595, 1973.

CHAPTER 13

Nephrology

DEMETRIUS ELLIS

The manifestations of renal and genitourinary disorders range from readily apparent gross structural abnormalities to subtle abnormalities of the urinary sediment. In this chapter, examples of physical findings, as well as characteristic urinary findings and radiographs, are used to demonstrate the broad spectrum of these disorders in the pediatric population.

Essentials of Medical History and Physical Examination

The medical history and physical examination often provide clues implicating a renal or genitourinary disorder. Congenital but often nonheritable genitourinary disorders are diagnosed with an increasing frequency by high-resolution ultrasonography during the second and third trimesters and may include obstructive disorders, such as posterior urethral valves, multicystic dysplasia, polycystic kidney disease, prune-belly syndrome, or renal agenesis. Oligohydramnios and fetal compression signs reflect reduced urine production associated with some of these disorders and may result in early postnatal death as a result of associated pulmonary underdevelopment. Unilateral and, less frequently, bilateral cystic dysplasia is the most common cause of abdominal mass in newborns. A large placenta may be a telltale sign of congenital nephrotic syndrome of the Finnish type, in which severe proteinuria precedes birth. Failure to urinate during the first 24 hours of life should prompt evaluation for obstruction of the kidneys, ureters, or bladder. Urinary tract infection (UTI) should be a consideration in all febrile infants, particularly during the first 2 weeks of life, even in the presence of documented sepsis, meningitis, or other sources of infection. Urinary tract anomalies including vesicoureteral reflux and megaureters distending the abdomen are common in infants and young children with well-documented UTI. Children with true polyuria or polydipsia, rather than urinary frequency, may have a renal concentrating defect, such as nephrogenic diabetes insipidus, or salt-losing nephropathy, such as nephronophthisis.

Failure to thrive, lethargy, or irritability and recurrent emesis are common manifestations of renal disease in infants and may be associated with metabolic acidosis and other electrolyte disturbances. Occasionally, the renal disorder is discovered because of deliberate studies obtained after discovering dysmorphic features, imperforate anus, vertebral abnormalities, fetal alcohol syndrome, or other disorders that have a renal component.

Family pedigrees may assist the diagnosis of congenital or heritable disorders such as cystinuria, cystinosis, oxaluria, and polycystic kidney disease and thereby lead to a variety of preventive measures before children become symptomatic. Hypertension in infants without aortic coarctation is most often a result of a renovascular disorder, such as renal venous thrombosis (infants of diabetic mothers, hyperviscosity syndrome, dehydration); arterial thrombosis (caused by embolism in patients with ventricular septal defect or patent ductus arteriosus or a result of umbilical artery catheterization); or renal artery stenosis. Asphyxia at birth or severe dehydration, sepsis, or shock may lead to acute tubular necrosis and oliguric renal failure.

Hypertension in the older child may cause headache, dizziness, recurrent emesis, epistaxis, or visual disturbances. In severe cases secondary congestive heart failure may occur, particularly if there is a history of oliguria, impaired renal function, or glomerulonephritis. Renal disorders account for most cases of hypertension, particularly in the preadolescent child in whom primary or essential hypertension is rare. The presence of café-au-lait spots, neurofibromas, fibrous-angiomatous lesions of the skin, thyroid enlargement, abnormal pulses, or bruits over the renal arteries or major vessels may point to a specific diagnosis.

Gross or microscopic hematuria is the most common reason children are referred to outpatient pediatric nephrology clinics. The medical history is critical to pinpointing the correct cause of hematuria because it assists the elimination of a large number of possibilities. These possibilities include complications in the neonatal period necessitating umbilical artery line placement that may result in renal or aortic occlusive disease, bronchopulmonary dysplasia managed with loop diuretics leading to hypercalciuria or nephrocalcinosis, use of medications that lead to tubulointerstitial nephritis or coagulopathies, congenital heart disease leading to subacute bacterial endocarditis with secondary immune complex renal disease or thromboembolic disease, hemophilia, thalassemia, sickle cell disease, and other thrombotic or hemolytic disorders. The social history is particularly important in newborns because it may suggest child abuse, trauma, or Munchausen syndrome by proxy as the cause of the hematuria. Fever without an apparent source and symptoms of frequency, dysuria, back pain, or nocturia may suggest a UTI. The presence of hematuria or renal failure in other family members may suggest polycystic kidney disease, whereas a similar history together with neurosensory hearing loss may indicate Alport syndrome. Menarche is at times confused with hematuria.

In children with gross hematuria with or without flank or abdominal pain and absence of urinary casts or significant proteinuria to suggest a glomerulonephritis, a family history of nephrolithiasis or a history of high dietary intake of salt, dairy products, or vitamins suggests hypercalciuria. Apart from hematuria with urinary casts, an acquired glomerulonephritis may be indicated by a history of an antecedent pharyngitis or concurrent infection, pallor, edema, rapid weight gain, arthritis, or arthralgia together with a purpuric or malar rash, which may suggest a diagnosis of Henoch-Schönlein purpura, systemic lupus erythematosus, or petechiae associated with hemolytic uremic syndrome. A history of direct or indirect trauma may explain the hematuria in the active and otherwise healthy adolescent.

Failure to grow in the absence of an obvious nutritional deficit may be a sign of a chronic renal disorder in any child. Evaluation of such a disorder should include a careful urinalysis; complete blood cell count; and measurement of blood urea nitrogen (BUN), serum creatinine, bicarbonate, alkaline phosphatase, calcium, and phosphorus levels.

Urinary Screening and Urinalysis

Urinalysis

The current American Academy of Pediatrics recommendation is to perform a urinalysis at 5 years of age and in sexually active adolescents. However, many pediatricians continue to perform screening urinalysis more frequently including in infancy, young childhood, late childhood and adolescence. Furthermore, urinalysis may be indicated on the basis of medical history and urinary symptoms or as a prerequisite for participation in organized sports. A carefully performed urinalysis may expedite the diagnosis of various disorders and prevent the performance of unnecessary, costly, and invasive studies. For instance, a child with persistent painless hematuria without microscopic presence of pyuria or bacteriuria need not undergo ultrasonography, cystoscopy, voiding cystourethrography, or dimercaptosuccinic acid (DMSA) scan. Alternatively, if such a child also has cellular casts the diagnostic studies may focus on glomerulonephritis.

A clean catch or midstream urine sample is preferred for urinalysis. Ideally this sample must be processed within 1 hour to prevent bacterial overgrowth, solute crystallization, or dissolution of cells or casts. The routine urinalysis consists of three basic steps: gross inspection, dipstick, and microscopic examination. Abnormalities commonly encountered on urinalysis are shown in Figure 13-1.

Gross Inspection

On gross inspection, the color of urine may be described as clear, yellow, dark yellow, green, brown, tea colored, pink, clear red, grossly bloody, blue, or even black. A comprehensive list of chemicals that may impart a specific color to the urine has been compiled by the U.S. Food and Drug Administration and may be accessed on the Internet at http://vm.cfsan.fda.gov/~lrd/colorfac.html.

Smoky urine is indicative of stagnated blood that has decomposed and the iron component has oxidized in the renal tubules. This commonly occurs in glomerulonephritis.

Clear red urine may suggest hemoglobinuria.

Red urine that tests negative by the dipstick may be due to numerous factors including foods, dyes, drugs, and pigments (Table 13-1). A special case is the "red diaper syndrome" in infants, which is due to urate excretion or overgrowth of *Serratia marcescens*. Yellow urine that becomes black to brown on exposure to air suggests alkaptonuria or increased excretion of homogentisic acid. Yellow-brown urine may be seen in obstructive jaundice and is due to oxidation of bilirubin to biliverdin. Blue urine, or "blue diaper syndrome," is due to Hartnup disease (neutral aminoaciduria) and is also seen in tryptophan gastrointestinal malabsorption syndrome, in which indigotonin or indigo blue are excreted in the urine.

Screening by Dipstick

The modern dipstick is a marvel of modern biochemistry. Each small square is chemically engineered to be sensitive, specific, and cost effective for the substance it detects. Despite these advantages, screening by this method has been criticized as being so sensitive that disorders may be suspected in the absence of a pathologic condition, thereby resulting in unnecessary evaluation, costly studies, and anxiety on the part of the child and his or her family. It may also miss significant renal pathology that is not associated with hematuria or proteinuria.

Glucosuria (excess sugar in urine) generally denotes diabetes mellitus. On rare occasions, however, glucosuria may represent a familial benign disorder termed *renal glucosuria*, which occurs in the absence of hyperglycemia and is caused by one of several defective proximal tubular glucose transporters. Dipsticks usually employ the glucose oxidase reaction for screening, which specifically detects glucose but may miss other reducing sugars such as galactose and fructose. For this reason, most newborn and infant urines are routinely screened for reducing sugars by methods other than glucose oxidase (e.g., the Clinitest, a modified Benedict's copper reduction test).

The hematest square contains orthotoluidine that lyses intact urinary erythrocytes, and the free hemoglobin gives a color reaction proportional to the number of erythrocytes (RBCs) present in the urine sample. The sensitivity of detecting three or more RBCs per high-power field (hpf) in centrifuged urine ranges from 91% to 100%, with a specificity of 65% to 99%. Free hemoglobin or myoglobin in patients with systemic disorders leading to high plasma concentrations of such pigments also reacts with orthotoluidine.

Protein is detected by the tetrabromophenol reagent, which relies on the principle that certain pH indicators show a different pH, or pH "error," in the presence of protein as opposed to the absence of protein. This test is particularly sensitive for albumin and less so for other proteins. Hence, significant small-molecular-weight proteinuria resulting from systemic overproduction or due to insufficient proximal tubular reabsorption in children with tubulopathies may be underestimated or missed by this test.

The nitrite test is often positive in children with UTI because of bacterial breakdown of urinary nitrates. With proven UTI this test has a sensitivity of 35% to 85% and a specificity of 92% to 100%.

The leukocyte esterase test is often positive due to release of this enzyme from intact or lysed neutrophils in individuals with UTI. This test has a sensitivity of 72% to 97% and a specificity of 64% to 82%. In adults and older children (but not in infants) the presence of both positive nitrite and leukocyte esterase tests has both positive and negative predictive values that approach 100%, whereas either test alone has a much lower predictive value for UTI.

Ketones may be detected by the combined presence of sodium nitroprusside and alkaline buffer reagent, which reacts with acetoacetate (diacetic acid), acetone and beta-hydroxybutyric acid produced by starvation or diabetes mellitus and beta-hydroxybutyric acid.

Specific gravity (SG), which is a measure of the total solute in urine and depends on both the concentration and molecular weight of solutes, may be quantitated by the N-Multistix SG, Bayer Corporation, Elkhart, Ind. Specific gravity contrasts with osmolality, which depends only on the concentration of solutes in urine. The SG square on the dipstick test consists of pretreated electrolytes with a specific association constant (pKa). Hydrogen ions are released in direct correlation to the concentration of ions in the urine. This causes the pH indicator (bromophenol blue) to turn acidic in direct proportion to the ionic strength in the urine, which in turn corresponds to specific gravity. High urinary protein concentrations give a high SG value by this method. In healthy individuals, about 0.001 unit of SG equals 40 mOsm/kg H_2O. Thus an SG of 1.010 corresponds to 400 mOsm/kg H_2O, 1.020 equals 800 mOsm/kg H_2O, and 1.030 equals 1200 mOsm/kg H_2O. Children with low fluid intake or dehydration or

Figure 13-1. **A,** *Left,* Starch granules commonly seen in urine. Notice variable size (7 to 40 μM), irregular shape with rounded corners, central indentation. *Right,* "Maltese cross" appearance can be seen with polarized light. Talc particles have similar appearance. Do not confuse these with lipid droplets seen in children with nephrotic syndrome and lipiduria, which are spherical with clear centers and usually measure less than 7 μM across. **B,** Mites (shown), pinworm ova *(Enterobius vermicularis),* or vegetable fibers and other fecal artifacts may be washed into the urine from the urethra or vaginal introitus. **C,** Tubular epithelial cells in a child with toxic tubulopathy due to amphotericin toxicity. **D,** Transitional epithelial cells arising from the renal pelvis, ureter, or bladder may appear pear shaped and can be confused with tubular epithelial cells as seen in **C.** Transitional cells are much larger in size, with smaller distinctive nuclei. These cell types may be found in very small numbers in healthy children. **E,** Yeast hyphae *(arrow)* and leukocytes in an immunosuppressed child. **F,** Wright-Giemsa staining showing eosinophiluria associated with tubulointerstitial nephritis and acute renal failure in a child with hypersensitivity to methicillin. **G,** Calcium oxalate crystals, usually seen in acid urine, with characteristic octahedral or star-shaped pattern in a child with hematuria associated with hypercalciuria. **H,** Four-sided form of uric acid crystals; other forms include amorphous, six-sided bipyramidal or whetstone crystals. **I,** Coarse granular casts composed of degenerated cellular elements in a child with chronic IgA nephritis. Notice the typical parallel borders and refractivity of casts in general.

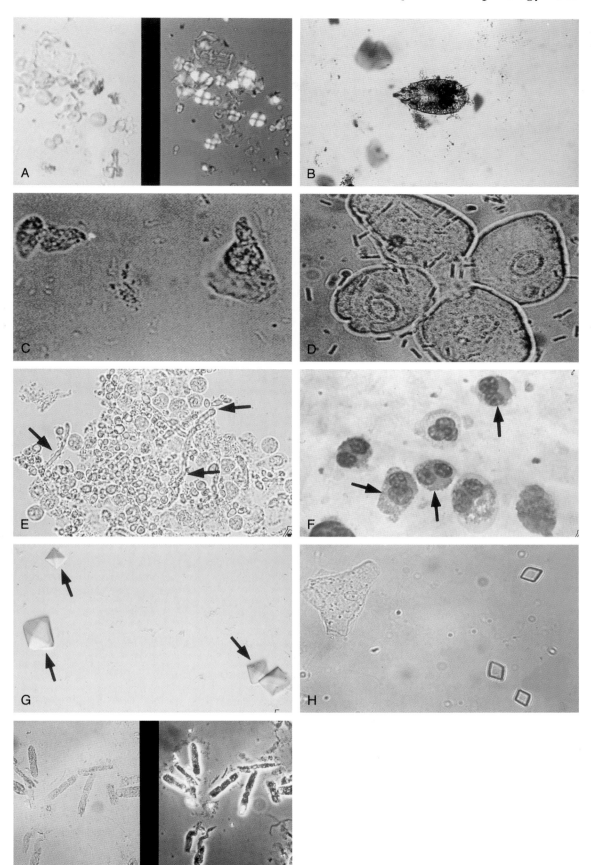

Table 13-1	Causes of Red or Discolored Urine without Hematuria

Pink, Red, Cola-Colored, Burgundy
Drug and food ingestion: Aminopyrine, chronic mercury or lead, benzene, phenolphthalein, phenytoin, carbon tetrachloride, sulfonethylmethane, dinitrophenol, anthocyanin, azo dyes, beets, blackberries, chloroquine, deferoxamine mesylate, ibuprofen, methyldopa, nitrofurantoin, phenazopyridine, rifampin, rhodamine E, sulfasalazine, *Serratia marcescens,* urates (red diaper syndrome)
Dark Brown, Black, Orange
Disease associated: Alkaptonuria, homogentisic aciduria, melanin, methemoglobinemia, tyrosinosis
Drug and food ingestion: Alanine, resorcinol, thymol, Pyridium

Reproduced with permission from Boineau FG, Lewy JE: Evaluation of hematuria in children and adolescents. Pediatr Rev 11:101-107, 1989. Copyright © 1989 American Academy of Pediatrics.

those receiving hyperosmolar radiocontrast media have high SG. Low SG may be found in healthy children with high fluid intake or in those who are unable to concentrate the urine because of tubulointerstitial disorders or because of inadequate secretion of antidiuretic hormone.

Microscopic Examination

Meticulous examination of the urine sediment begins with centrifugation of 10 mL of freshly voided urine for 5 minutes at 3000 rpm. Such standardized preparation enables semiquantitative comparison of sequential samples in individual patients and often provides invaluable information concerning the etiology of numerous renal disorders, as well as the anatomic location of hematuria or pyuria. Abnormalities commonly encountered on microscopy are shown in Figure 13-1. Dysmorphic RBCs, best seen in uncentrifuged urine with phase microscopy, are usually of glomerular origin as opposed to urologic origin. White blood cells (WBCs) coated with antibody tend to become agglutinated or clumped. Such clumped WBCs are indicative of pyelonephritis or interstitial nephritis rather than cystitis. The presence of tubular epithelial cells is abnormal.

Scanning of the entire slide may be necessary to detect small numbers of casts. Although this is time consuming, it is a rewarding practice because the presence of casts is indicative of intrinsic renal injury and may spare the child unnecessary uroradiographic studies.

Hyaline casts form on polymerization of Tamm-Horsfall glycoprotein, which is a well-characterized mucoprotein uniquely found in the ascending limb of Henle and distal convoluted tubule. Small quantities of hyaline casts may be found in healthy individuals, but larger numbers of hyaline casts occur in proteinuric disorders. In the distal convoluted tubule or in the collecting duct WBCs, RBCs, or tubular cells may become trapped in the hyaline matrix to produce casts. Muddy-brown granular or epithelial cell casts are seen in acute tubular necrosis. Granular casts form from disintegration of cellular elements. These are always pathologic and may be found in most cases of glomerulonephritis. Wide casts may derive from dilated tubules, which occur in individuals with advanced renal disease.

Crystals are best identified in fresh urine that is of near body temperature. Uric acid crystals and urates are found in urine with a pH below 6, whereas phosphates precipitate in urine with a pH above 6.5. Both urates and phosphates precipitate when the urine specimen is refrigerated. Crystals may be found in healthy individuals and in patients with urolithiasis or hyperuricemia, or in individ-

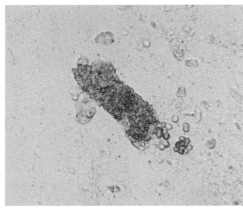

Figure 13-2. Red blood cell cast from a patient with poststreptococcal glomerulonephritis. These casts are almost always associated with glomerulonephritis or vasculitis and virtually exclude extrarenal disorders of bleeding.

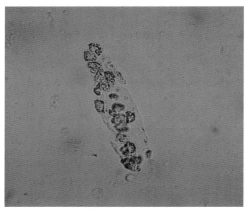

Figure 13-3. White blood cell cast from a patient with chronic glomerulonephritis.

uals with a specific drug intake or poisoning (e.g., ethylene glycol). Exceptions include flat hexagonal crystals, which are pathognomonic of cystinuria.

Glomerular Disorders

Nephritis and Nephrosis

In children suspected of having a glomerular disease, the urinary sediment can provide important clues that may expedite the diagnosis and help formulate therapeutic plans. A classic example of nephritic syndrome is that of acute poststreptococcal glomerulonephritis, in which the urinalysis reveals variable levels of proteinuria and granular red (Fig. 13-2) and, less frequently, white (Fig. 13-3) blood cell casts. On the other hand, the urine of children with classic nephrotic syndrome, such as minimal change disease, shows heavy proteinuria (>40 mg/m^2/hr), free fat droplets and oval fat bodies, and little or no hematuria or other sediment abnormalities.

Unlike patients with nephrotic syndrome, those with acute nephritic syndromes are usually hypertensive, have darkly colored urine, and have a depressed glomerular filtration rate. Several disorders exhibit features of both nephritis and nephrosis. The nephrotic syndrome in childhood is generally the result of one of five primary disorders: minimal change disease, mesangial proliferative glomerulonephritis, focal glomerulosclerosis, membranous nephropathy, and membranoproliferative glomerulonephritis. Minimal change disease is the most common, accounting for more than 70% of all cases of nephrosis in children. This disease is so named because of its virtually normal light microscopic histology, negative immunofluorescence, and fusion of epithelial cell foot processes on electron microscopy. Laboratory features include selective proteinuria, normal complement levels, decreased IgG levels, and increased IgM levels. Minimal change nephrotic syndrome is relatively benign, with more than 95% of patients maintaining adequate renal function.

Mesangial proliferative glomerulonephritis exhibits diffuse proliferative changes with negative or variable deposition of mesangial IgG, IgM, and C3. It represents about 10% of nephrosis cases in childhood. Serum complement levels are normal, but hematuria is common.

Focal glomerulosclerosis accounts for 10% to 15% of nephrotic syndrome in childhood. It demonstrates focal and segmental sclerosis, with IgM and C3 deposition within affected glomeruli. Hematuria, pyuria, poorly selective proteinuria, and normal C3 levels are characteristic of laboratory features. The majority of children with mesangial proliferation or focal glomerulosclerosis progress to renal failure about 6 years after the onset of the disease.

Membranous glomerulopathy is an uncommon cause of nephrotic syndrome in children, and it has unique histopathologic changes seen by microscopy. Capillary walls appear thickened, and the basement membrane has argyrophilic spikes on special staining. IgG deposits can be seen within the capillary walls, and electron microscopy shows subepithelial deposits. Protein excretion is variably selective, the serum C3 value is normal, and patients are prone to renal vein thrombosis. Ultimate renal function is maintained in 50% to 70% of children with this disorder.

Membranoproliferative glomerulonephritis is subdivided into two main types. Type I has lobular changes along with the mesangial proliferative changes and subendothelial deposits seen on electron microscopy. Hematuria is common, and the serum C3 level is intermittently low. More than half of patients avoid chronic dialysis. Type II disease has C3 capillary and mesangial immune deposits. Hematuria, persistently reduced serum C3 levels, and the presence of C3 nephritic factors are laboratory features of type II. The disorder is also known as *dense deposit disease* because of enhanced osmiophilic staining observed by electron microscopy. Unlike type I, almost all patients with type II disease progress to end-stage renal disease.

Acute Glomerulonephritis

The most common causes of acute glomerulonephritis in children include poststreptococcal or postpneumococcal glomerulonephritis, IgA nephritis, Henoch-Schönlein purpura, and hemolytic uremic syndrome. In some instances these disorders may have an aggressive clinical course characterized by oliguria, hypertension, and rapid reduction in glomerular filtration rate, in which case the designation of rapidly progressive glomerulonephritis (RPGN) is given. The renal biopsy in such patients often demonstrates cellular or acellular crescents and inflammatory infiltrates. Several other chronic glomerulonephritides, such as membranoproliferative glomerulonephritis and membranous glomerulopathy, may also evolve into RPGN.

In addition to the clinical symptoms, the antinuclear antibody titer, streptococcal titers, quantitative serum immunoglobulin concentrations, and C3 and C4 levels are often helpful in differentiating several of the glomerulonephritides. Serum complement levels are particularly helpful because only a few of these conditions are associated with depressed complement levels. In poststreptococcal glomerulonephritis, the complement levels are only transiently reduced and return to normal concentrations within 8 weeks after onset of the renal symptoms.

A typical situation is that of a child 3 to 10 years of age, whose symptoms during the preceding few days have included mild periorbital edema, headache, and decreasing urine output. The urine is described as being smoky or tea colored. Medical history reveals that 2 weeks earlier the patient experienced a febrile illness with painful pharyngitis for which he or she received no medical attention. Clinical examination reveals a blood pressure of 140/105 mm Hg, mild periorbital edema, and tenderness on palpation of the kidneys. A urinalysis shows the following values: 2+ protein, 3+ blood, and an SG of 1.020. Red blood cell casts (see Fig. 13-2) are seen on urinalysis. Laboratory studies are consistent with mild renal insufficiency. Also found are a protein excretion of 1.1 g/24 hr, a low plasma C3 level, and elevated streptozyme and anti-DNAase B titers, evidence that strongly implicates a streptococcal infection in the pathogenesis of the glomerulonephritis. Generally, complete and spontaneous recovery of all renal abnormalities occurs within 5 weeks with conservative management, although hematuria may persist for about 1 year or longer.

Chronic Glomerulonephritis

White blood cell casts may be seen in the urine sediment of patients with acute or chronic glomerulonephritis and vasculitis, as well as pyelonephritis and other disorders resulting in tubulointerstitial nephritis. The cast shown in Figure 13-3 occurred in a child with systemic lupus erythematosus whose only symptom was mild back pain. Urinalysis demonstrated 2+ protein, microhematuria, pyuria without bacteria, and red and white blood cell casts. Diagnosis was confirmed by immunologic findings including low serum C3 and C4 levels, a positive fluorescent antinuclear antibody titer, and antibodies against double-stranded DNA. Renal biopsy revealed diffuse proliferative lupus nephritis. Note that formation of tubular casts is aided by diminished urine flow, high urinary solute concentration, and the hyaline matrix of plasma- and tubule-derived protein in which cells become embedded. Several acute glomerular syndromes may progress to chronic glomerulonephritis. In the final stages, many such patients develop hypertension and severe renal failure (uremia). On renal ultrasonography, the kidneys appear small and fibrosed.

Henoch-Schönlein Purpura

Three weeks after a respiratory infection, a 2-year-old boy experienced symptoms of generalized malaise, abdominal pain, periorbital edema, and difficulty walking "as if his legs were hurting." One day later he developed an ecchymotic, purpuric rash, the characteristic clinical manifestation of Henoch-Schönlein purpura. The rash covered the extensor surfaces of the extremities and the buttocks but spared the trunk. Individual lesions faded over 1 week, but new lesions appeared or recurred over several weeks. Other cutaneous manifestations of the vasculitic lesions in this disorder are shown in Figures 13-4 and 13-5.

Some patients initially develop an urticarial-type eruption that subsequently becomes macular or maculopapular. Occasionally, younger patients develop an angioneurotic-like edema of the scalp, face, or dorsum of

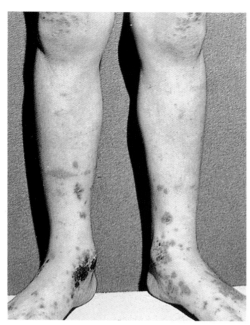

Figure 13-4. Henoch-Schönlein purpura. Vasculitis resulted in cutaneous necrosis below and anterior to the right malleolus.

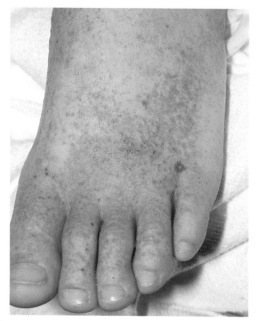

Figure 13-5. Henoch-Schönlein purpura. The typical vasculitic rash is evident in the dorsum of the foot of this 15-year-old boy. He went on to develop rapidly progressive glomerulonephritis and pulmonary hemorrhage, which were managed by pulse methylprednisolone.

the hands or feet. Of children with Henoch-Schönlein purpura, 90% have a prodrome consisting of an upper respiratory infection 1 to 3 weeks before the onset of symptoms and 80% have melena, hematemesis, and/or arthritis mostly involving the ankles and knees. About half of the patients have renal involvement ranging from simple microhematuria and a variable degree of proteinuria to oliguria and renal failure. In contrast to adults, use of multiple medications is rarely related to the onset of this condition in children.

This condition has no distinct biochemical features. Some patients have leukocytosis and an elevated serum IgA level. In the absence of severe proteinuria, hypoalbuminemia and edema are often a result of protein-losing

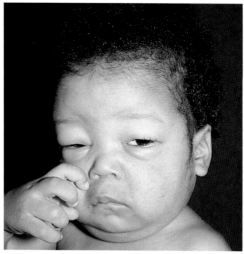

Figure 13-6. Minimal change disease in a 2-year-old boy with nephrotic syndrome. Eyelid edema in any child should prompt the performance of urinalysis, rather than the presumption of allergy.

enteropathy. Platelet counts and coagulation studies are normal. The skin rash is essential for the diagnosis of Henoch-Schönlein purpura because the renal abnormalities may otherwise closely resemble a similar disorder known as *IgA nephropathy (Berger disease).*

Nephrotic Syndrome

Children with nephrotic syndrome rarely have an underlying systemic illness or a history of drug intake and thus are designated as having primary or idiopathic nephrotic syndrome. Patients with poststreptococcal glomerulonephritis, Henoch-Schönlein purpura, IgA nephritis, or systemic lupus erythematosus, as well as rare patients treated with nonsteroidal anti-inflammatory agents, lithium, colchicine, and other drugs, may also be associated with nephrotic-range proteinuria (i.e., $\geq 40\,mg/m^2/hr$).

Minimal change disease is the single most common cause of idiopathic nephrotic syndrome in childhood. Generalized edema and rapid weight gain are characteristic features of this condition, with the former showing a predilection for the eyelids, pleural spaces, abdomen, scrotum, and lower extremities (Figs. 13-6 and 13-7). Although edema per se usually provokes few complaints from most patients, at times it may be disfiguring, and it may produce skin induration and breakdown, or interference with respiratory, genitourinary, or gastrointestinal function. Symptoms may occasionally be confused with allergic edema. However, the findings of severe proteinuria, hypoalbuminemia, and hypercholesterolemia usually lead to correct diagnostic and treatment measures.

Of special interest is nephrotic syndrome presenting in the newborn period or in the first 2 to 3 months of life. Acquired immunodeficiency syndrome has recently been added to the list of systemic diseases underlying infantile nephrotic syndrome and is increasingly recognized as a cause of this disorder in infants and young children. Focal glomerulosclerosis is the most common underlying histopathologic lesion.

Hematuria

Isolated gross or microscopic hematuria is probably the most common symptom prompting nephrologic assessment in children. Many such children have symptomless

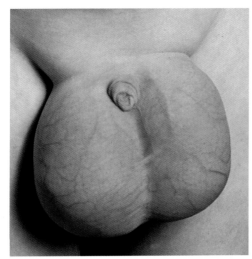

Figure 13-7. Nephrotic syndrome. Severe scrotal edema in a 6-year-old boy.

Table 13-2	Evaluation of Nephrolithiasis

Clinical History
Family history of nephrolithiasis
Immobilization or other protracted illness or stress
High dietary purine intake
Excessive salt or calcium ingestion
Large and infrequent meals
Excessive intake of vitamins or over-the-counter medications
Symptoms of UTI or history of pyelonephritis
Source and calcium content of drinking water
Polyuria or polydipsia

Physical Diagnosis
Band keratopathy and other signs of hyperparathyroidism
Elfin facies and other features of Williams syndrome

Radiologic Studies
Ultrasound—especially sensitive in identifying renal calculi and nephrocalcinosis
KUB—for the identification of ureteral stones; radiopaque stones include calcium oxalate and cystine
Spiral CT—identifies urologic abnormalities and confirms obstruction; especially helpful in detecting radiolucent calculi, such as uric acid, urates, matrix, and xanthine
^{125}I-hippurate scan—may provide differential renal function or suggest obstruction

Urinary Studies
Urinalysis—may reveal pyuria or bacteriuria; inability to lower urinary pH or to concentrate the urine; or flat, hexagonal crystals pathognomonic of cystinosis
Urine culture
Screening with cyanide-nitroprusside (cystinosis)
Timed urine collections on two or more occasions for determination of the following values: creatinine, sodium, potassium, calcium, phosphorus, magnesium, oxalate, citrate, cystine, and uric acid

Biochemical Studies
Creatinine, BUN, electrolytes, total CO_2, albumin, calcium, phosphorus, magnesium, and uric acid; plasma parathyroid hormone levels if indicated
Chemical analysis of gravel or stones

BUN, blood urea nitrogen; KUB, plain films of kidneys, ureters, and bladder; UTI, urinary tract infection.

microscopic hematuria often detected during routine office visits or physical examinations required before participation in sport activities. Because of the large number of conditions associated with persistent hematuria in children, several algorithms have been devised to aid in the systematic evaluation of this condition (Fig. 13-8).

History and clinical symptoms may point toward trauma, viral or bacterial cystitis, drug-induced hematuria, or other causes. Detection of the most common causes of hematuria including glomerulonephritis or UTI can be readily achieved by the finding of cellular casts in a carefully performed examination of the urinary sediment or by appropriate bacterial cultures. Moreover, the absence of red blood cells in a child with positive *o*-toluidine reagent color change on the dipstick may lead to the correct diagnosis of conditions associated with rhabdomyolysis or hemolysis.

Once these simple measures are undertaken, biochemical techniques are used to investigate renal function, hyperexcretion of metabolites resulting in nephrolithiasis, hemoglobinopathies, bleeding diathesis, or immunologic assessment of an underlying glomerulonephritis. Measurement of calcium and creatinine concentrations in a single voided urine sample should also be included in the minimal initial assessment of asymptomatic hematuria because hypercalciuria is found in a large proportion of such children. Identification of possible disorders by such methods may help determine the need for further assessment. Thus the finding of a nephritic sediment obviates the need for any radiologic procedures, whereas the presence of a single well-documented UTI in a child younger than 8 years of age may be an indication for imaging procedures. In the absence of any physical signs, such as an abdominal mass to suggest Wilms tumor or neuroblastoma, malignancies of the kidney or urinary tract rarely present with isolated gross or microscopic hematuria. Renal ultrasonography coupled with Doppler evaluation of the renal vessels is useful in screening for the presence of tumor, polycystic kidney disease, or renal venous thrombosis in infants. CT or nuclear magnetic resonance techniques may provide detailed anatomic resolution of such masses.

Invasive cystography or arteriography is rarely necessary in the evaluation of structural lesions underlying isolated hematuria in children. A technetium ^{99m}Tc-dimercaptosuccinic acid renal scan may disclose renal scars suggestive of chronic pyelonephritis in children with or without vesicoureteral reflux. Finally, a renal biopsy may be helpful in making a definitive diagnosis in cases of suspected renal parenchymal disease manifested by hematuria.

Pediatric Nephrolithiasis

The diagnosis of nephrolithiasis should be entertained in any child with acute onset of flank or abdominal colicky pain. In children, renal colic is poorly localized and is often described as diffuse abdominal pain. Small stones may produce no pain at all and are detected only after an episode of gross hematuria, pyuria, or UTI. Thus a strong index of suspicion is required on the part of the clinician so that appropriate diagnostic studies are undertaken. Relatively few children pass gravel or stones, and the kind of crystals found in the urine are rarely of diagnostic value. Although dietary phytate is a more common cause of endemic stones in the Far East and UTI is more common in Europe, metabolic disorders predominate in children with nephrolithiasis in the United States. The clinical history and laboratory evaluation often reveal the cause of the stones. Biochemical analysis of the calculus is therefore of little diagnostic importance. One diagnostic approach to pediatric nephrolithiasis is shown in Table 13-2.

The most common calculus found in children consists of calcium oxalate. Such calculi frequently occur in chil-

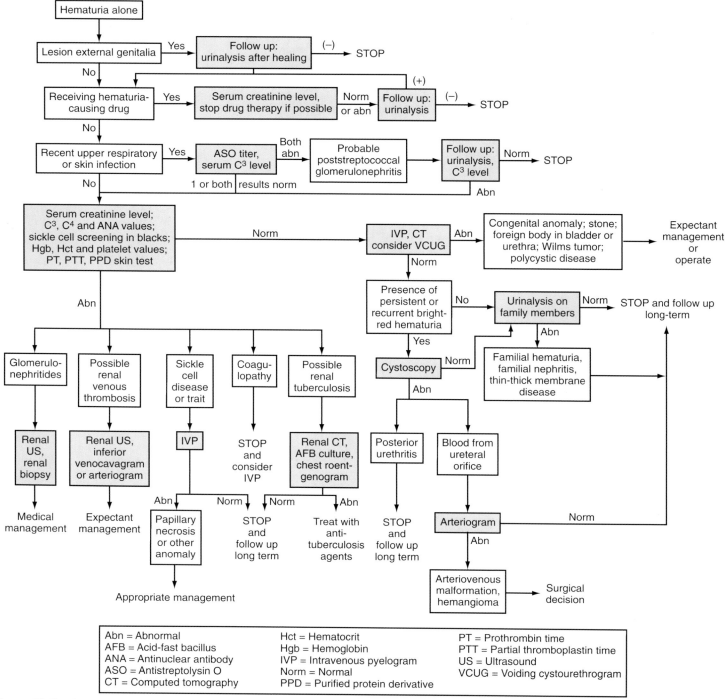

Figure 13-8. Algorithm for diagnosis of hematuria. (From Brewer ED, Benson GS: Hematuria: Algorithms for diagnosis. JAMA 246:877-880, 1981. Copyright © 1981, American Medical Association.)

dren with idiopathic hypercalciuria, which may be silent or manifested by painless microscopic or recurrent gross hematuria for many years before frank nephrolithiasis occurs. Hypercalciuria is found in 35% of all children evaluated for hematuria. Screening for hypercalciuria may be done using a single voided urine specimen; a fasting calcium-to-creatinine ratio exceeding 0.21 in a child older than 6 years is highly suggestive of this condition, which may then be confirmed by a 24-hour urine collection having a calcium content greater than or equal to 4 mg/kg body weight. The nonabsorptive form of hypercalciuria appears to have an autosomal dominant inheritance underlying a renal tubular defect and net loss of calcium

independent of the amount of dietary calcium ingested. The absorptive form may be associated with increased serum concentrations of calcitriol resulting in increased fractional absorption of calcium at the intestinal level. Premature infants who have been given high doses of furosemide to control fluid retention associated with bronchopulmonary dysplasia may develop hypercalciuria, nephrolithiasis, and nephrocalcinosis. Other disorders predisposing to nephrolithiasis include hyperparathyroidism, cystinuria (Fig. 13-9), hyperoxaluria, defects of purine metabolism and distal (type I) renal tubular acidosis (Fig. 13-10). UTIs and obstructive uropathy are also important. Laboratory studies and the radiologic location

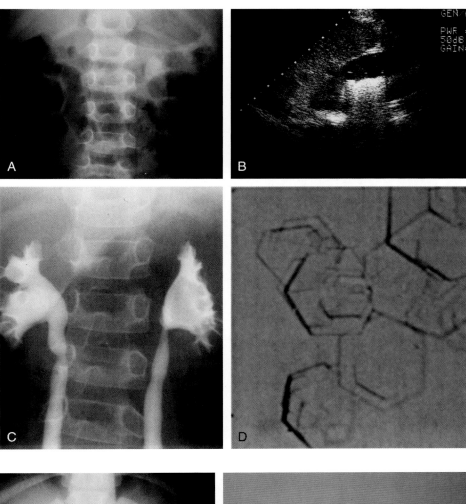

Figure 13-9. Cystinuria. A 6-year-old boy, born of a consanguineous marriage, presented with diffuse abdominal pain, oliguria, and mild renal failure. **A,** Plain film of the abdomen showed a slight opacity in the area of the left kidney. **B,** Renal ultrasound demonstrated a distinct shadow produced by the calculus. **C,** An intravenous pyelogram showed relatively radiolucent stones within the left renal pelvis. Multiple small calculi produced the dilation and partial obstruction of both ureters. **D,** Pathognomonic flat hexagonal cystine crystals were noted on urinalysis.

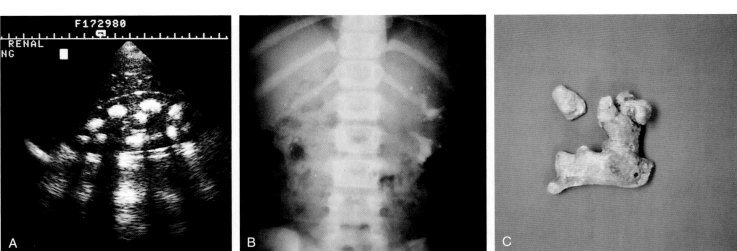

Figure 13-10. Renal tubular acidosis. **A,** Renal ultrasound demonstrates severe nephrocalcinosis in an 8-year-old girl who failed to thrive because of familial type I renal tubular acidosis. Note the multiple echogenic shadows produced by the calcium deposits within the renal parenchyma. **B,** A staghorn calculus in the left renal pelvis of another child with renal tubular acidosis. **C,** Appearance of staghorn calculus removed at operation. The shape of such calculus generally conforms to the pelvocaliceal system.

and appearance of the stone often provide clues to the cause and treatment of the nephrolithiasis.

Apart from available medical therapies and traditional surgical techniques, specific conditions may be treated by newer modalities, such as extracorporeal shock-wave lithotripsy and stone fragmentation through pulse laser energy.

Renal Venous Thrombosis

Volume depletion secondary to diarrhea or vomiting, hypotension, hypercoagulable or hyperviscosity states (hematocrit more than 65%), or indwelling catheters in the vicinity of the renal veins especially predispose infants to renal vein or intrarenal venous thrombosis (Fig. 13-11). Older children with severe nephrotic syndrome are also prone to this disorder. Among children, 75% of all cases of renal venous thrombosis occur in the first month of life, and 50% of all cases are bilateral. The typical clinical features of renal vein thrombosis are a palpable renal mass in 60% of infants and hematuria and thrombocytopenia, which occur in more than 90% of the patients. Renal function may be normal, particularly in unilateral renal vein thrombosis or in bilateral disease that does not result in oliguria. The renal ultrasound is the diagnostic procedure of choice, particularly when coupled with Doppler examination of the renal and adjacent major vessels (Fig. 13-12).

Vesicoureteral Reflux

Vesicoureteral reflux is a congenital condition in which the normal valve mechanism of the ureterovesicular junction is impaired, leading to reflux of bladder urine into

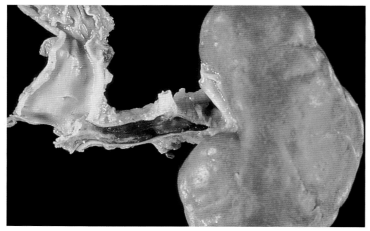

Figure 13-11. Renal vein thrombosis. A 12-year-old boy with ulcerative colitis died following a bout of severe diarrhea and dehydration. Apart from dural sinus thrombosis, the left renal vein contained this partially organized clot.

the ureter or kidneys. In a young child with UTI, such reflux of infected urine is a major risk factor for the development of pyelonephritis, renal scarring, and chronic renal damage.

The severity of vesicoureteral reflux is assessed by the findings on voiding cystourethrograms and classified according to the following international grading system (Fig. 13-13):

Grade I—reflux into the ureter only (Fig. 13-14).

Grade II—complete reflux into the ureter, pelvis, and calices without any dilation of the structures (Fig. 13-15).

Grade III—complete reflux with mild dilation or tortuosity of the ureter, and mild dilation of the renal pelvis but only slight blunting of the caliceal fornices (Fig. 13-16).

Grade IV—complete reflux with moderate dilation of the ureter, renal pelvis, and calices; complete obliteration of the sharp angle of the fornices with maintenance of the papillary impressions of the calices (Fig. 13-17).

Grade V—gross dilation and tortuosity of the ureter with gross dilation of the renal pelvis and calices; obliteration of the papillary impressions of the calices (Fig. 13-18).

Grades I through III have a high rate of spontaneous resolution, and patients with such findings may be placed on suppressive antibiotic regimens to ensure maintenance of sterile bladder urine. Grades IV and V are generally associated with significant anatomic abnormalities of the ureteral orifice, and they often require surgical correction.

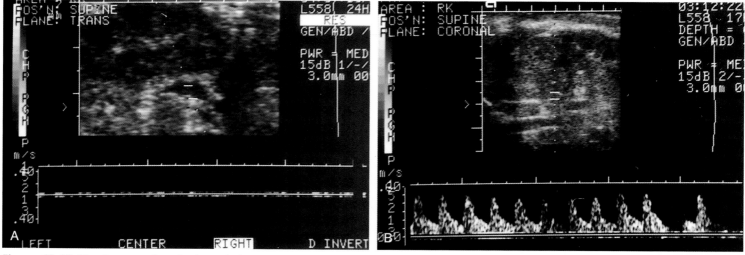

Figure 13-12. Renal venous thrombosis. A plethoric 2-day-old infant of a diabetic mother (hematocrit 75%) was found to have an abdominal mass in the right abdomen on routine physical examination. Evaluation disclosed hematuria and thrombocytopenia without elevation in BUN or serum creatinine concentrations. **A,** Notice the absence of venous pulsations in the lower panel on the Doppler study of the right renal vein while arterial pulsations remained intact. **B,** Subsequent serial renal ultrasound studies showed a progressive reduction in the size of the right kidney despite recanalization of the venous thromboses.

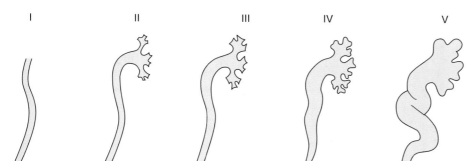

I   II   III   IV   V

Figure 13-13. Grades of vesicoureteral reflux, schematically presented.

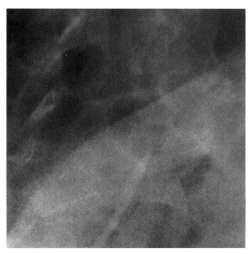

Figure 13-14. Grade I reflux: cystourethrogram shows reflux only into the ureter.

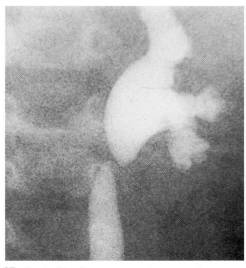

Figure 13-17. Grade IV reflux: cystourethrogram shows complete reflux with moderate dilation of the ureter, pelvis, and calices; complete obliteration of sharp angle of fornices.

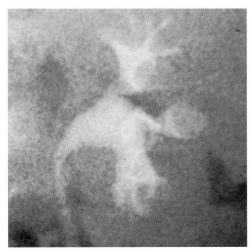

Figure 13-15. Grade II reflux: cystourethrogram shows complete reflux into the ureter, pelvis, and calices; no dilation.

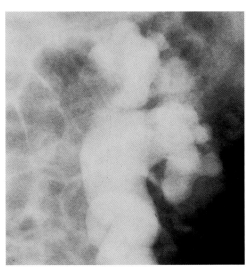

Figure 13-18. Grade V reflux: cystourethrogram shows gross dilation of the ureter, pelvis, and calices; obliteration of the papillary impressions of the calices.

Bacterial Cystitis

Young children whose symptoms include an acute onset of fever, emesis, dysuria, suprapubic pain, and a urinary sediment such as that shown in Figure 13-19 should be suspected of having bacterial cystitis. By far the most common organism cultured from patients with acute or chronic urinary tract infections is *Escherichia coli; Pseudomonas* or *Proteus* organisms are occasionally found, particularly in patients with abnormal genitourinary anatomy.

The dipstick test detects nitrite (produced by urinary pathogens by conversion of dietary nitrates) and leukocyte esterase (released by polymorphonuclear leukocytes present in urine). When both tests are positive, both the positive and negative predictive values are nearly 100% accurate in predicting UTI. Although these are good screening tests in older children with symptomatic or asymptomatic bacteriuria, they are impractical in infants because of stool contamination resulting in an increased rate of false-positive samples. Screening infants for UTI

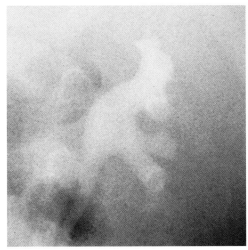

Figure 13-16. Grade III reflux: cystourethrogram shows complete reflux with mild dilation of the ureter and renal pelvis but only slight blunting of the calices.

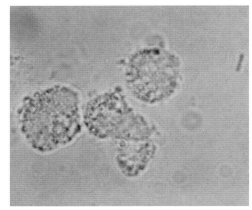

Figure 13-19. White blood cells and a rod-shaped organism seen on high-power view of unspun urine suggestive of bacterial cystitis.

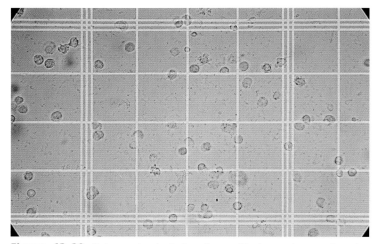

Figure 13-20. Enhanced urinalysis using a Neubauer hemocytometer (×200) showing numerous white blood cells (>10 WBC/mm³) indicative of a urinary tract infection.

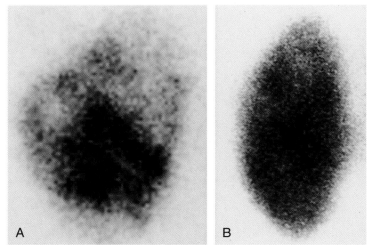

Figure 13-21. Dimercaptosuccinic acid (DMSA) scan. The image in **A** is abnormal, with numerous filling defects indicative of pyelonephritis, whereas the image in **B** is normal.

Table 13-3	Sensitivity, Specificity, and Predictive Values of Standard versus Enhanced Urinalysis					
	STANDARD			**ENHANCED**		
	Cx+*	**Cx–†**	**Total**	**Cx+**	**Cx–**	**Total**
Test+	21	5	26	27	2	29
Test+	11	661	672	5	664	669
TOTAL	32	666	698	32	666	698
Sensitivity		65.6%			84.5%	
Specificity		99.2%			99.7%	
Positive predictive value		80.8%			93.1%	
Negative predictive value		98.4%			99.3%	
Prevalence		4.6%			4.6%	

*Cx+, Culture positive, 50,000 cfu/mL.
†Cx–, Culture negative.
From Hoberman A, Wald ER, Perchansky L, et al: Enhanced urinalysis as a screening test for urinary tract infection. Pediatrics 91:1196-1199, 1993.

has markedly improved with the use of enhanced urinalysis. Unlike standard urinalysis performed in uncentrifuged urine obtained by catheterization or suprapubic aspiration in which prediction of UTI is based on greater than five white blood cells and any number of bacteria per high-power field, enhanced urinalysis consists of counting white blood cells in such a urine sample in a Neubauer hemocytometer (Fig. 13-20) and counting bacteria in a Gram-stained smear. UTI is then predicted on the basis of the finding of greater than 10 white blood cells per mm³ plus any number of bacteria present in 10 oil fields examined. On the basis of results from the Children's Hospital of Pittsburgh (Table 13-3), enhanced urinalysis is more sensitive (84.5% vs. 65.6%) and has a higher predictive value (93.1% vs. 80.8%) than standard urinalysis in predicting UTI in febrile infants.

Although the diagnosis of UTI is established by appropriate urine cultures, the site of infection may not be apparent when considering the symptoms or urinalysis findings alone. DMSA scanning (Fig. 13-21) performed during a febrile, well-documented UTI is the earliest and most sensitive test available for detecting children with pyelonephritis at risk for developing renal scarring, as well as for detecting children with previous renal scars. Renal ultrasonography and intravenous pyelography, although less reliable, may also be useful in health care centers in which DMSA scanning is unavailable. We currently recommend that children younger than 8 years of age with

abnormal DMSA scans undergo standard micturition cystourethrography under fluoroscopic monitoring to obtain the best baseline anatomic definition and to assess bladder capacity and emptying. If vesicoureteral reflux is found, future monitoring may be done by nuclear voiding cystourethrography, which limits radiation exposure. Such studies usually define structural abnormalities leading to obstructive nephropathy or vesicoureteral reflux and are essential in planning the medical and surgical management of these patients.

Developmental and Hereditary Disorders

Developmental Abnormalities

The number of congenital malformations associated with renal abnormalities is too large to discuss individually in this chapter. Renal abnormalities should be suspected in any child with one or more congenital abnormalities. In this chapter, only a selected number of syndromes are considered in which renal abnormalities are serious, relatively common, and easily diagnosed by the physical findings.

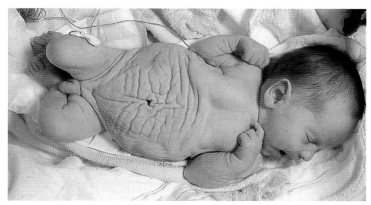

Figure 13-22. Prune-belly syndrome. This newborn shows the wrinkled and redundant skin covering the abdominal wall. On palpation, no abdominal muscular tone could be detected.

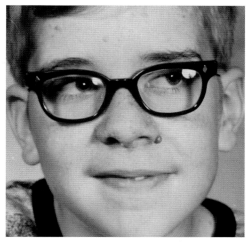

Figure 13-23. Tuberous sclerosis. Six-year-old boy with characteristic papules distributed across the bridge of the nose and the nasolabial folds. He was originally diagnosed as having polycystic kidney disease because of abdominal distention and bilateral renal enlargement before the onset of any skin lesions.

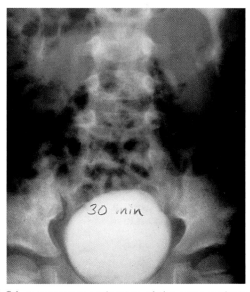

Figure 13-24. Intravenous pyelogram of the same patient as in Figure 13-23 shows enlarged kidneys with the collecting system stretched and distorted by multiple soft tissue masses representing renal angiomyolipomas.

Prune-Belly Syndrome (Eagle-Barrett Syndrome)

This syndrome usually consists of the absence of abdominal musculature, renal and urinary tract abnormalities, and cryptorchidism (Fig. 13-22). Boys are affected more severely and 20 times more frequently than girls. Although there is generally no ureteral obstruction, the ureters are dilated and tortuous, and 75% exhibit reflux. The bladder is enlarged despite low renal pelvic and intravesical pressures. Infection is common because of urinary stasis.

The major determinant of prognosis in these patients is the degree of associated cystic renal dysplasia. Intestinal malrotation is a common associated abnormality; anomalies of the limbs and heart may occur, but these are uncommon. Infertility in males is universal even when it is possible to surgically place the testes into their normal intrascrotal position. Libido and orgasm, however, remain normal. Early orchiopexy may improve the chances for fertility and prevent testicular neoplasia.

Tuberous Sclerosis

Tuberous sclerosis is a neurocutaneous syndrome inherited as an autosomal dominant trait with marked variability of expression. The full syndrome is characterized by myoclonic seizures, mental deficiency, foci of intracranial calcifications, depigmented "ash leaf" cutaneous patches, and pathognomonic skin lesions known as fibroangiomatous nevi (adenoma sebaceum). The skin lesions may be present during the first year of life but may go unnoticed until 4 to 7 years of age when they take the form of discrete yellowish papules distributed along the bridge of the nose and the nasolabial folds (Fig. 13-23). Patients with tuberous sclerosis may have hamartomas in many organs and tissues. Renal angiomyolipoma causing genitourinary symptomatology may suggest the diagnosis of polycystic kidney disease (PKD) in patients with minimal skin or central nervous system involvement (Fig. 13-24). Although small asymptomatic cysts are common in autopsy cases of tuberous sclerosis, large renal cysts may be discovered early in infancy and suggest the diagnosis of autosomal dominant PKD. Hypertension and renal insufficiency may further confuse the diagnosis. In such instances the diagnosis of tuberous sclerosis is confirmed by family history and the development of other features of the syndrome.

Imperforate Anus

Because of common embryologic origins and the anatomic proximity of the genitourinary and lower gastrointestinal tracts, children with imperforate anus have a high incidence of genitourinary and lower spinal abnormalities. A high imperforate anus (at or above the supralevator muscle) (Fig. 13-25) is associated with a 50% incidence of genitourinary anomalies, mainly unilateral renal agenesis, neurogenic bladder, or vesicoureteral reflux. In boys, one usually finds a fistulous communication between the blind end of the rectal pouch and the prostatic urethra. In girls, the rectum often communicates with the vagina or posterior fourchette. All children with imperforate anus should undergo evaluation of the genitourinary tract with renal ultrasound and voiding cystourethrography and must be monitored for UTI.

Posterior Urethral Valves

The most common obstructive lesions of the lower urinary tract in male infants are posterior urethral valves. Such folds traverse the urethra from a point just distal to the verumontanum to the proximal limit of the membranous urethra and obstruct urinary flow with consequent enlargement of the prostatic urethra, hypertrophy of the bladder neck, trabeculation of the bladder, and significant dilation of the upper urinary tract. Infants with posterior urethral valves may experience renal failure and profound electrolyte imbalance. Older children may have abdominal masses, voiding disturbances, or infection. Diagnosis is made radiologically by voiding cystourethrography (Fig. 13-26) and confirmed endoscopically. Although urinary diversion is frequently required, some patients can be treated directly with transurethral valve ablation. Surgery is usually successful in achieving urinary drainage, but in many cases associated renal dysplasia may lead to chronic renal failure during infancy or childhood.

Crossed Renal Ectopy

Children with the developmental anomaly of crossed renal ectopy generally have an abdominal mass or hematuria following minor trauma. Obstruction at the ureteropelvic junction is common. The location of the ectopic

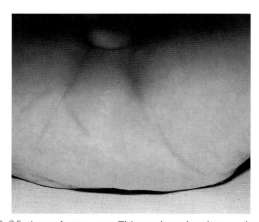

Figure 13-25. Imperforate anus. This newborn boy has an absent median raphe and anal atresia. On further study, he was found to have agenesis of the right kidney, severe dysplasia in the left kidney, and a communication of the blind-ended rectal pouch and the prostatic urethra.

kidney may be cryptic, as in the pelvic region, and can be best demonstrated by a renal radionuclide scan. Crossed renal ectopy, renal agenesis, and/or duplication of the collecting system are often found in association with Klippel-Feil syndrome (Fig. 13-27) but have also been associated with cervicothoracic vertebral anomalies and müllerian duct aplasia in girls.

Horseshoe Kidney

Horseshoe kidney results from fusion of the lower renal poles during development (Fig. 13-28). Although generally asymptomatic, patients with horseshoe kidney may have (1) hematuria after trauma to the pelvic area; (2) a midline abdominal mass; or (3) a ureteropelvic junction obstruction, a common associated finding in this condition.

Duplication of the Urinary Collecting System

Duplication of the urinary collecting system is one of the most common of all genitourinary abnormalities. It is sometimes familial and more common in girls than in boys. About 30% of the duplications are bilateral (Fig. 13-29) but with much variation in the extent of duplication. This condition occurs when the kidney is penetrated by two separate ureteral buds during nephrogenesis. When present, vesicoureteral reflux usually occurs in the ureter from the lower pole, whereas ureteral obstruction occurs almost exclusively in the ureter from the upper renal segment. Reflux into a duplicated system is unlikely to resolve spontaneously. These associated problems may predispose patients to recurrent infection or hydronephrosis necessitating surgical correction.

Hereditary and Metabolic Disorders

Identification of specific genes and gene transcripts associated with a multitude of genetic disorders involving the kidneys has vastly elucidated the diagnosis and pathophysiology of many cystic and metabolic disorders.

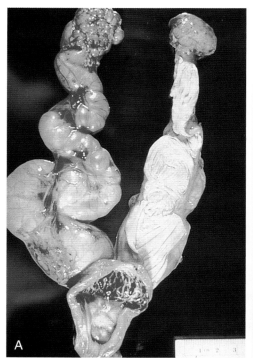

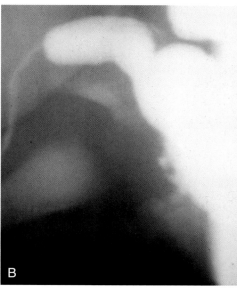

Figure 13-26. A, Posterior urethral valves. Notice the marked enlargement and tortuosity of the ureters and the small, thick-walled, muscular bladder noted on autopsy of this newborn. **B,** An antemortem voiding cystourethrogram shows a dilated proximal urethra typical of this condition.

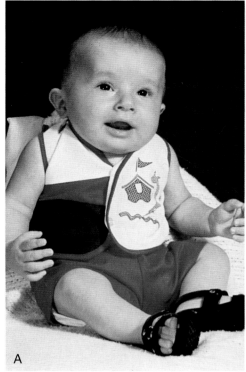
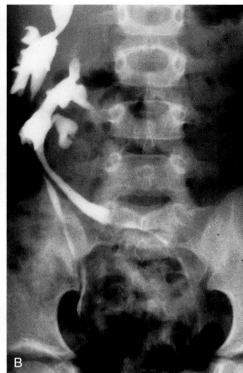

Figure 13-27. Klippel-Feil syndrome. **A,** Short neck (fused cervical vertebrae) and nonfunctioning right thumb caused by lack of tendons to this digit. Intravenous pyelogram **(B)** reveals crossed renal ectopia of the left kidney, whereas the ureter from the left kidney crosses the midline and inserts into the left side of the trigone.

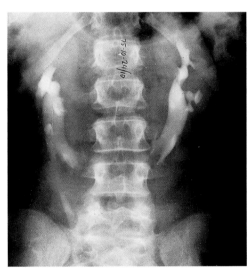

Figure 13-28. Horseshoe kidney. This excretory urogram was performed as part of the evaluation for gross hematuria following abdominal injury in the child. Notice the unusual and oblong configuration of the collecting system resulting from fusion of the lower renal poles.

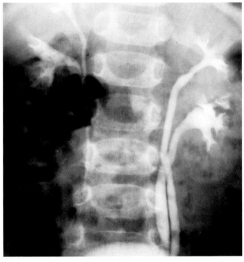

Figure 13-29. Duplication of the urinary collecting system is seen bilaterally in excretory urography of a child with recurrent pyelonephritis. This was the result of vesicoureteral reflux in the ureter from the left lower pole. Ureteral duplication is incomplete on the right side (Y-type).

Polycystic Kidney Disorders

In 1990 Kissane devised a useful classification and overview of the renal cystic disorders of childhood. Only four of the most common and most important forms of PKD are presented here. Although autosomal dominant PKD (ADPKD) and cystic renal dysplasia are far more common (1 in 1000 population), autosomal recessive PKD (ARPKD; 1 in 20,000 population) is a much more serious disorder during childhood. Cystic renal dysplasia has no defined inheritance pattern and is often associated with other syndromes. Nephronophthisis, or medullary cystic disease complex, although less common than the other three disorders, is an important cause of end-stage renal disease in childhood. Renal cystic disease may also be an important component of numerous other syndromes (Table 13-4) that are not discussed in this chapter.

Autosomal Recessive. With the exception of the most severe manifestations of ARPKD, prenatal diagnosis by renal ultrasonography is usually unreliable until the second half of pregnancy. This disorder has variable expression, so the severity of the cystic malformation often determines the age and mode of presentation. About 85% of cases begin during infancy. Oligohydramnios and associated pulmonary hypoplasia may result in life-threatening respiratory difficulties and talipes in the neonate, whereas abdominal masses and hypertension are common indications in later infancy; hepatic enlargement, portal hypertension, growth failure, and progressive renal insufficiency occur more commonly in the school-age child. Pancreatic cysts are rare and usually do not produce digestive difficulties. Hyponatremia often occurs in infancy and may relate to nonosmotic release of

Table 13-4	Syndromes Associated with Cystic Kidneys

SYNDROME	INHERITANCE
Meckel-Gruber	AR
Jeune thoracic dystrophy	AR
Short rib polydactyly	AR
Zellweger cerebrohepatorenal	AR
Tuberous sclerosis	AD
von Hippel-Lindau	AD
VATER association	NI
Renal-retinal dysplasia	AR
Ivemark	AR
Fryns	AR
Trisomy 21, 13, or 18	—
Oral-facial-digital, type I	XL
Laurence-Moon-Bardet-Biedl	AR
Kaufman-McKusick	AR
Hypothalamic hamartoma	NI?
Lissencephaly	Variable
Prune-belly	NI?
Ehlers-Danlos	Variable
Branchio-oto-renal	AD
Roberts	AR
DiGeorge	Variable
Smith-Lemli-Opitz	AR
Turner	—
Noonan	—
Joubert syndrome	AR
Bardet-Biedl syndrome	AR/Variable
Nephronopthisis	AR
Caroli disease	AR

AD, autosomal dominant; AR, autosomal recessive; NI, not inherited; XL, X-linked.

From Zerres K, Volpel MC, Weiss H: Cystic kidneys: Genetics, pathologic anatomy, clinical picture, and prenatal diagnosis. Hum Genet 68:104-135, 1984.

vasopressin, particularly in the setting of pulmonary disease, excessive renal salt wasting, extracellular volume contraction, and inadequate dietary salt replacement.

Congenital hepatic fibrosis is frequently present in this condition and may predominate over kidney involvement in some of the patients. Because of portal tract hyperplasia and fibrosis, hypersplenism and hematemesis are frequent in such patients. Liver pathology may be similar in other autosomal recessive syndromes associated with PKD (see Table 13-4).

It has become increasingly apparent that the ultrasonographic findings in ARPKD are not specific and may resemble those of ADPKD, particularly after infancy. Because of this and because the signs and symptoms can occur at various ages with either disorder, ARPKD has replaced the former designation of "infantile PKD." The abnormal gene is located on chromosome 6, but unlike ADPKD parental involvement is rare. Thus a normal renal ultrasound in both parents supports the diagnosis of ARPKD rather than ADPKD.

In children with ARPKD the cysts are initially small but can enlarge with age to produce palpable flank or abdominal masses (Fig. 13-30). The condition may be differentiated from bilateral hydronephrosis of any cause by thorough radiologic evaluation, which may include sonography, cystography, and intravenous pyelography. The intravenous pyelogram in Figure 13-31 shows a characteristic mottled nephrogram, with retention of the contrast material in dilated medullary and cortical collecting ducts producing brushlike medullary opacification with streaks radiating to the outer portion of the kidney. This correlates well with the pathologic findings in such kidneys of cystic dilation localized to the medullary and cortical collecting ducts. This localization is best demonstrated by isolated nephron microdissection (Fig. 13-32).

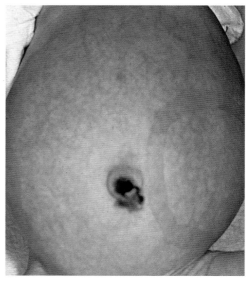

Figure 13-30. Autosomal recessive polycystic kidney disease. Note the marked abdominal distention and bilaterally enlarged kidneys, as indicated by the outlined area. Congenital hepatic fibrosis frequently accompanies this disorder.

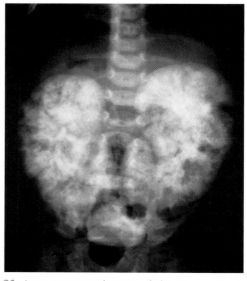

Figure 13-31. Intravenous pyelogram of the same patient as in Figure 13-30 shows the characteristic mottled nephrogram, with brushlike medullary opacification secondary to retention of contrast material in dilated cortical and medullary collecting ducts.

Autosomal Dominant. ADPKD is one of the most common inherited disorders and accounts for 10% of all patients with end-stage renal disease in the United States. Cysts may arise from all nephron segments. Two gene mutations present on the short arm of chromosome 16 account for the majority of individuals with ADPKD, with the *ADPKD1* gene comprising 90% of the cases and an even greater fraction of the more symptomatic individuals. Even within ADPKD1 families there is much variability in the phenotypic expression of the many extrarenal manifestations and in the severity of the renal disease and its clinical course. With current high-resolution renal ultrasonography, up to 90% of one half of the presumed gene carriers younger than 20 years of age have detectable cysts. The false-negative ultrasonographic diagnosis for ADPKD in this age group is 8%. Compared with children with fewer than 10 cysts at the time of diagnosis of ADPKD, those with more than 10 cysts have a similar creatinine

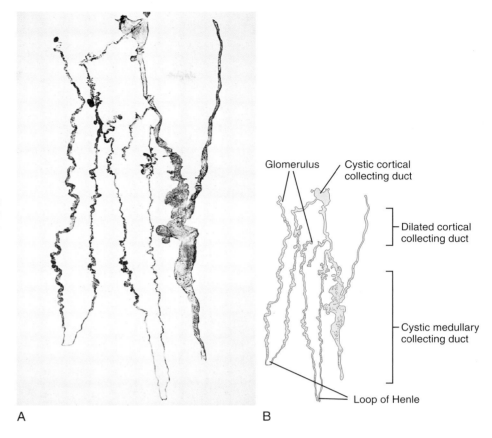

Figure 13-32. **A** and **B,** Cystic areas are apparent in the microdissected tubule and collecting duct shown in this photograph. (Courtesy G. Fetterman, MD, Pittsburgh.)

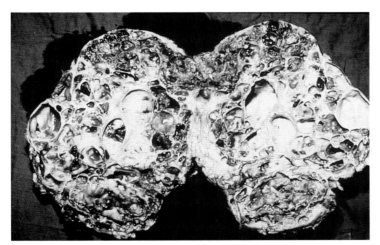

Figure 13-33. Autosomal dominant polycystic kidney disease. Note the replacement of normal renal parenchyma by large fluid-filled cysts.

clearance but are more likely to complain of flank or back pain or urinary frequency and have a greater incidence of palpable kidneys, inguinal hernias, palpitations, hypertension, and urinary concentrating defect. Pathologically the cysts become large and asymmetrical and involve all parts of the nephron (Fig. 13-33).

Because of the psychological and practical (insurability, participation in sports) implications, it is recommended that an ultrasonographic diagnosis be pursued only in children at risk of developing ADPKD who manifest hypertension or those participating in contact sports who may be at risk for recurrent gross hematuria that may adversely affect the renal prognosis. Genetic linkage analysis may be done for prenatal diagnosis and family planning purposes or may be limited to individuals with a family history of PKD who are asymptomatic, have a nondiagnostic ultrasound, and wish to donate a kidney.

Except for children with enlarged kidneys and large cysts detected in infancy, renal failure or nephrolithiasis caused by ADPKD rarely occurs in childhood. Similarly, extrarenal manifestations including rupture of intracranial aneurysm, colonic diverticula, or symptomatic mitral valve prolapse are rare. Children with acute onset of "thunder clap" headache or neurologic symptoms that suggest impending rupture or compression of an intracranial aneurysm should undergo urgent magnetic resonance angiography.

Liver cysts may occur in ADPKD but are rarely associated with liver dysfunction or portal hypertension. A liver biopsy may help to differentiate ADPKD from ARPKD because congenital hepatic fibrosis is also found in ARPKD and is present only rarely in ADPKD.

Cystic Renal Dysplasia. Pathologically, abnormal renal morphogenesis includes processes leading to both deficient parenchyma (hypoplasia) (Fig. 13-34) and abnormally differentiated parenchyma (dysplasia) (Figs. 13-35 and 13-36). These conditions often coexist and, despite the presence of cysts, the kidneys may be too small to appreciate by bimanual examination (i.e., bracing the flank and back with the fingers of one hand while gradually producing deep abdominal compression with the other hand). When bilateral, these renal disorders are frequently detected during the first few weeks of life. The infant usually demonstrates poor weight gain, pallor, emesis, and tachypnea. Many of the early symptoms are secondary to metabolic acidosis resulting from renal insufficiency. The amount of urine output bears little relationship to the degree of renal failure as reflected by the serum creatinine level and BUN concentration. Collectively these conditions constitute the most common cause of chronic renal failure in children.

Patients with renal hypoplasia often have gastrointestinal, central nervous system, cardiac, and pulmonary abnormalities, but other abnormalities of the genitouri-

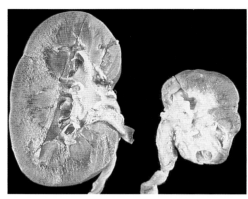

Figure 13-34. Unilateral renal hypoplasia/dysplasia. In contrast to the normal right kidney, the left kidney is markedly small. The parenchyma in the upper pole is normal, but microscopic examination of the lower pole showed several morphologic features of dysplasia.

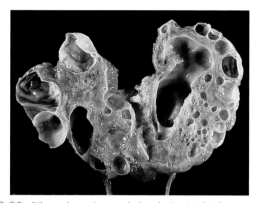

Figure 13-35. Bilateral cystic renal dysplasia. Multiple cysts of various sizes are seen throughout the cortex and medullary regions of a newborn with severe renal failure.

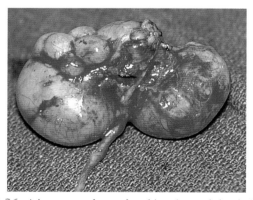

Figure 13-36. A less severe form of multicystic renal dysplasia involving mainly the midportion of the kidney.

nary tract are rarely present. Obstruction of the gastrointestinal or genitourinary tract is commonly found in patients with dysplasia. Less common anomalies may include Down syndrome, tracheoesophageal fistula, ventricular septal defect, and lumbosacral dystrophies.

Cystic dysplasia may be a major component of several syndromes with distinct additional malformations (see Table 13-4). Many of these syndromes have defined inheritance patterns. The overall risk for siblings of children with isolated forms of dysplasia or hypoplasia is usually less than 10%, but it may be higher if one of the parents has renal agenesis or a kidney that is affected by the same process. Pediatricians should be aware of several of the more common syndromes described in the paragraphs that follow.

Multicystic Dysplasia. Multicystic dysplasia is the most common cystic disorder in children and the most common cause of abdominal mass in newborns. It is usually unilateral. In typical cases there is complete loss of the renal architecture, and microscopically there are primitive ducts, fibrosis, and islands of cartilage representing the distinctive features of dysplasia. The condition may be discovered by prenatal sonography, or it is often diagnosed during the neonatal period after palpation of a "lumpy" intra-abdominal mass of variable size that often transilluminates. Because atresia of the ureter is usually present, urine output and renal function depend on the presence of bilateral involvement and the degree of associated renal dysplasia. Very large multicystic kidneys can interfere with respiration or produce mechanical intestinal compression. Radionuclide scanning, renal ultrasonography, and retrograde urography are usually sufficient to establish the diagnosis.

The unaffected contralateral kidney is usually hypertrophied and has normal corticomedullary differentiation and no evidence of obstruction. Obstructive disorders, such as posterior urethral valves, urethral atresia, or ureteroceles obstructing a duplicated ureter draining the upper pole (especially in girls with wetness between episodes of normal voiding), may be associated with morphologic features of dysplasia. Biliary dysgenesis (congenital hepatic fibrosis) has rarely been associated with renal dysplasia.

Because a large percentage of multicystic kidneys spontaneously involute and are rarely the cause of hypertension, infection, or tumor development, the prevailing opinion is that unilateral and asymptomatic multicystic kidneys do not need to be removed. However, correction of any associated ureteral abnormalities that may be present in the contralateral kidney is of vital importance.

Juvenile Nephronophthisis or Medullary Cystic Disease. Juvenile nephronophthisis and medullary cystic disease share similar morphologic features including prominent tubulointerstitial fibrosis and cysts that vary in number and size. The cysts are not prominent in most children, prompting the diagnosis of nephronophthisis, particularly if the disorder is autosomally inherited. The cysts usually enlarge with advancing renal failure. Juvenile nephronophthisis accounts for 2.4% of all children with end-stage renal disease in the United States. Polyuria and polydipsia as a result of a concentration defect and, at times, severe salt wasting are prominent clinical features. An ultrasound or abdominal CT scan may reveal normal-sized or small kidneys and loss of corticomedullary differentiation with or without medullary cysts. Hepatic fibrosis is probably the most important manifestation associated with juvenile nephronophthisis. Adults with this disorder have more prominent renal cysts and an autosomal dominant inheritance; thus it may be more aptly designated as medullary cystic disease.

Potter Sequence

Potter sequence can occur in any renal cystic or dysplastic disorder severe enough to produce oligohydramnios or anhydramnios. Oligohydramnios leads to a complex syndrome of fetal compression. Although chronic leakage of amniotic fluid may cause oligohydramnios, it most commonly occurs secondary to decreased fetal urine formation because of renal agenesis or severe underlying renal structural disorders. In the extreme example of renal

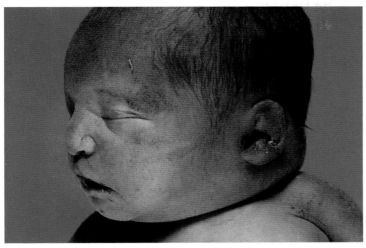

Figure 13-37. Potter facies. This infant with bilateral multicystic dysplasia died at 12 hours of age with pulmonary insufficiency. The altered facies produced by the fetal compression syndrome of oligohydramnios includes small, posteriorly rotated ears; micrognathia; a beaked nose, and wide-set eyes. (Courtesy T. Macpherson, MD, Magee-Women's Hospital, Pittsburgh.)

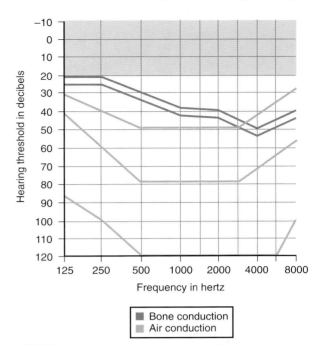

Figure 13-38. In Alport syndrome, a loss of high-frequency auditory perception may be found in 40% of patients. Because the hearing deficit may be most marked at frequencies between 2000 to 8000 Hz, it may be initially detected only by audiometric testing.

agenesis the virtual absence of amniotic fluid during fetal life leads to pulmonary hypoplasia and fetal compression, which consequently results in abnormal positioning of the hands and talipes, and altered facies characterized by abnormally small, posteriorly rotated ears; a small chin; a beaked nose; and unusual facial creases (Fig. 13-37). Such newborns have what is known as *Potter sequence,* and they usually die of respiratory insufficiency secondary to the severe associated abnormalities of pulmonary development.

Alport Syndrome

Alport syndrome, or hereditary progressive nephritis, is characterized by recurrent hematuria, progressive renal failure, and neurosensory deafness. Alport syndrome is transmitted by autosomal dominant inheritance with variable penetrance. The majority of affected individuals have an abnormal type IV collagen as a result of an abnormal X-linked gene present on chromosome 13, known as the *COL4A5* gene. However, a number of mutations have been defined that modify the clinical expression of the disease. The classic clinical presentation is persistent or recurrent hematuria that may be recognized early in childhood. Proteinuria is absent or mild in the early stages of the disease but increases as the disease progresses. The course is commonly one of slowly progressive renal failure, often accompanied by hypertension that is more severe in boys than in girls. The majority of patients with Alport syndrome have neither deafness nor ocular defects, but loss of high-frequency auditory perception occurs in up to 40% of patients and thus may be used as a clinical marker in family studies (Fig. 13-38).

Alport syndrome must be differentiated from the many benign forms of childhood hematuria including thin glomerular basement membrane disease and other progressive glomerular disorders. Diagnosis relies on careful family history, audiologic or ocular abnormalities, renal histopathologic features such as the presence of foam cells and glomerular sclerosis on light microscopy (Fig. 13-39), and ultrastructural alterations of the glomerular capillary basement membrane (Fig. 13-40). No specific treatment exists for this disorder; progressive end-stage renal disease is managed with dialysis and renal transplantation.

Hypophosphatemic Rickets

Rickets is a disturbance of growing bone in which defective mineralization of the matrix leads to an abnormal accumulation of uncalcified cartilage and osteoid. Hypophosphatemic vitamin D–resistant rickets is an X-linked inherited disorder that, unlike other forms of childhood rickets, is clinically characterized by normal muscle tone and strength, absence of tetany or convulsions, growth failure, and the predominance of rachitic changes in the lower extremities. Biochemical differentiation consists of hypophosphatemia, normal plasma calcium and bicarbonate levels, normal parathyroid hormone and 1,25-hydroxyvitamin D levels, a plasma 1,25-dihydroxyvitamin D concentration that is low for the level of hypophosphatemia, and absence of aminoaciduria. The pathogenesis of the disorder is believed to involve a renal tubular phosphate leak that is accompanied by an inappropriately low 1,25-dihydroxyvitamin D synthesis by renal tubular cells. The characteristic radiologic features of hypophosphatemic rickets, as in all forms of childhood rickets, include early widening of the spaces between the end of the metaphyses of long bones and an overall decrease in bone density (Fig. 13-41).

The objective of treatment is to promote healing of the rickets and increase growth velocity through normalization of serum phosphorus and alkaline phosphatase concentrations while avoiding hypercalcemia, hypercalciuria, hyperoxaluria, and hyperparathyroidism. These goals are best accomplished by the judicious combined use of oral phosphate and calcitriol. Because nephrocalcinosis and eventually decreased glomerular filtration rate may occur in association mainly with phosphate supplements, regular biochemical and renal ultrasonographic monitoring is essential in determining the lowest amounts of oral phosphate and calcitriol doses that achieve the treatment objectives while minimizing the complications.

Cystinosis

Cystinosis is an autosomal recessive metabolic disorder characterized by the intralysosomal accumulation of

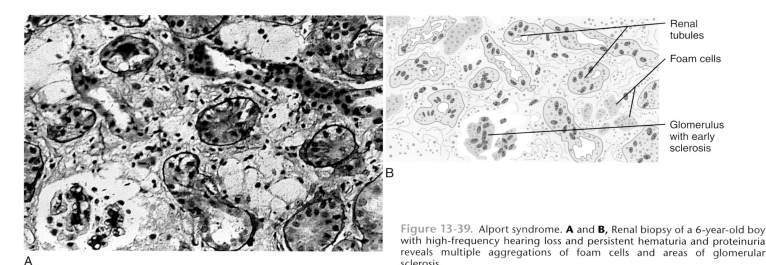

Figure 13-39. Alport syndrome. **A** and **B,** Renal biopsy of a 6-year-old boy with high-frequency hearing loss and persistent hematuria and proteinuria reveals multiple aggregations of foam cells and areas of glomerular sclerosis.

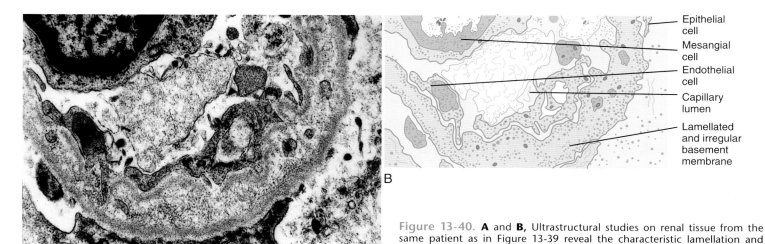

Figure 13-40. **A** and **B,** Ultrastructural studies on renal tissue from the same patient as in Figure 13-39 reveal the characteristic lamellation and irregularities of the glomerular basement membrane, diagnostic of Alport syndrome.

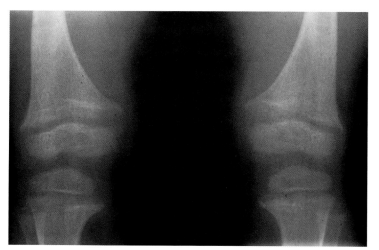

Figure 13-41. Hypophosphatemic rickets. Radiograph of the knees of a 2-year-old girl with bowlegs. Note the widened space between the metaphyses and epiphyseal ossification center, cupping and splaying of the metaphyses of the femur and tibia, and an overall decreased density of bone. (Courtesy M. Goodman, MD, Children's Hospital of Pittsburgh.)

cystine in most body tissues. After degrading intracellular protein, the cystinotic lysosomes are unable to transport cystine into the cytoplasm because of a defect in the lysosomal transporter, cystinosin. In its nephropathic form, the disease causes global proximal tubular dysfunction (Fanconi syndrome) and progressive glomerular damage.

The clinical manifestations of this renal tubular dysfunction include failure to thrive; renal tubular acidosis; and rickets, which results from persistent urinary losses of bicarbonate and phosphorus. Also associated with this disorder are low-molecular-weight proteinuria and glycosuria.

Cystinotic children show a number of clinical features not obviously related to the renal abnormalities. The majority have blond hair and a fair complexion; this, in association with growth failure and rickets, results in a strikingly similar appearance between unrelated patients. Clinical diagnosis is established by ophthalmologic examination, which detects a characteristic peripheral retinopathy, and by slit lamp examination, which detects the deposition of crystalline material in the conjunctiva and cornea. Diagnosis is confirmed by the finding of cystine crystals in the bone marrow of affected patients (Fig. 13-42) and by the presence of elevated levels of cystine in fibroblasts or peripheral leukocytes.

Treatment of nephropathic cystinosis consists of correction of the metabolic abnormalities induced by the tubular dysfunction. Patients thus receive alkali, phosphorus, potassium supplements, and often vitamin D analogues. Despite such therapy, renal function progressively deteriorates, and most patients require end-stage renal disease therapy in the first decade of life. No specific treatment is available for this metabolic disorder. Early treatment with cysteamine markedly delays but does not prevent multiorgan injury. Patients with this condition may benefit

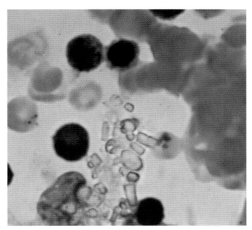

Figure 13-42. Cystinosis. The finding of cystine crystals in bone marrow aspirate from affected individuals, as seen here, may aid the diagnosis.

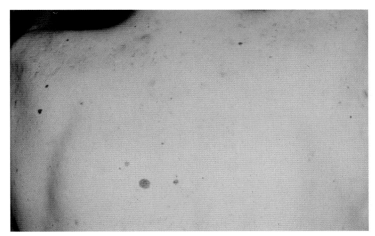

Figure 13-43. Fabry disease. The small, reddish purple papules are angiokeratomas. This young man had hematuria and minimal proteinuria but no renal insufficiency.

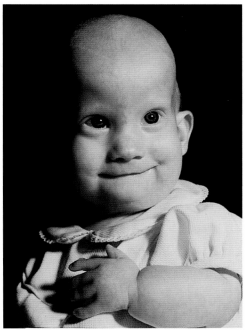

Figure 13-44. Jeune syndrome evident by brachycephaly, short stubby fingers, alopecia, and short stature in a 2-year-old girl with moderate renal failure.

from synthetic growth hormone because growth failure may persist despite successful kidney transplantation.

Angiokeratoma Corporis Diffusum (Fabry Disease)

The diagnosis of Fabry disease is usually made in childhood by recognition of its characteristic dermal telangiectasias, especially over the trunk (Fig. 13-43). This is one of the renal X-linked disorders for which prenatal diagnosis is possible through measurement of α-galactosidase (ceramide trihexodase A) in amniotic fluid cells or chorionic villi, or by gene analysis. The absence of this enzyme leads to lysosomal accumulation of an abnormal neutral glycosphingolipid in the vascular smooth muscle of the glomeruli, heart, sympathetic ganglia, and skin. Peripheral nerve involvement results in limb paresthesias and pain. Thrombosis and hemorrhage in these vessels may result in myocardial or cerebrovascular ischemia, and progressive renal failure is usually preceded by hypertension, proteinuria, and hematuria.

Jeune Syndrome

Because many of the children born with Jeune syndrome have severe and usually lethal pulmonary agenesis, the condition is also known as *asphyxiating thoracic dystrophy*. However, many children overcome the early respiratory difficulties and may exhibit a small thoracic cage, brachycephaly, short limbs, abnormal radiologic features

of the pelvic bones, and a variety of renal manifestations ranging from mild to moderate glomerular or tubular changes to microcystic renal dysplasia (Fig. 13-44). At the Children's Hospital of Pittsburgh, we have successfully transplanted four uremic children with Jeune syndrome and noticed marked improvement in their growth and bone disease, as well as excellent neurologic and intellectual development.

Denys-Drash Syndrome

Denys-Drash syndrome is characterized by Wilms tumor, male pseudohermaphroditism, and nephropathy. Although most children with this condition have an abdominal mass, there may be a history or clinical evidence of edema, reflecting the severe proteinuria. Because 70% of such children have nephrotic syndrome in the first month of life, they are often misdiagnosed as having congenital or Finnish-type nephrotic syndrome. However, instead of the typically microcystic proximal tubule, widened Bowman space, and mesangial proliferation found in the latter disorder, the characteristic lesion is that of diffuse mesangial sclerosis (Fig. 13-45). This progressive disorder leads to hypertension, hyperkalemia that is disproportionate to the reduction in glomerular filtration rate (hyporeninemic hypoaldosteronism), and progression to renal failure at 1 to 4 years of age. Despite the absence of ambiguous genitalia, the phenotypically female youngster whose biopsy is shown in Figure 13-45 had an XY karyotype and absence of testes, ovaries, fallopian tubes, and uterus on abdominal laparotomy performed at the time of renal transplantation.

Alagille Syndrome

The main components of Alagille syndrome, which is also known as *arteriohepatic dysplasia*, are absence of intrahepatic bile ducts leading to cholestatic jaundice, unusual facies, posterior embryotoxon, vertebral defects, and pulmonary artery hypoplasia. Children with this condition have high circulating concentrations of total cholesterol, phospholipids, triglycerides, pre-beta and

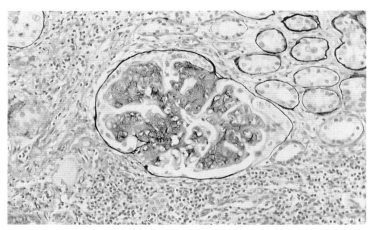

Figure 13-45. Denys-Drash syndrome. Distinctive glomerular lesion of diffuse mesangial sclerosis. Notice the spongy and "solid" appearance of the mesangium without proliferative changes and the obliteration of the capillary lumina. Interstitial inflammation and dilated tubules are also apparent.

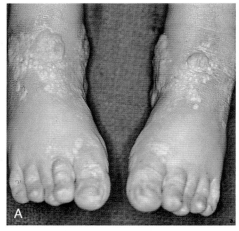

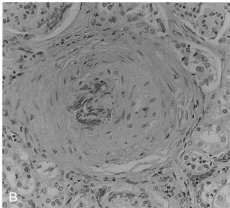

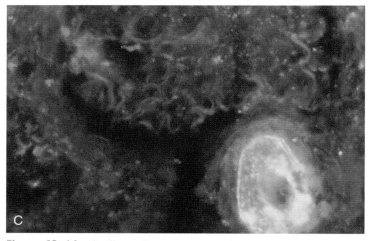

Figure 13-46. Alagille syndrome. **A,** Notice the large xanthomatous subcutaneous deposits of cholesterol in the dorsal aspect of the feet in this 5-year-old boy. **B,** Renal failure occurred secondary to diffuse renal arteriolar occlusion caused by lipid-laden endothelial cells and macrophages. **C,** Striking autofluorescence of the lipids is seen within such occluded vessels.

beta-lipoproteins, and elevated apolipoproteins. Thus large lipid accumulations in the skin and other tissues are common (Fig. 13-46A). Various renal abnormalities have been increasingly appreciated in association with Alagille syndrome. In one report, 18 of 26 such patients had glomerular lesions characterized by mesangial lipidosis. Although severe renal dysfunction is uncommon, children surviving advanced stages of liver failure may also develop severe renal failure. The latter may occur in association with liver failure ("hepatorenal syndrome") or may result from marked occlusion of renal arteries by lipid-laden or foam cells as shown in Figure 13-46B and C.

Renovascular Hypertension

Renal Artery Stenosis

Although only 5% of pediatric hypertension is caused by renal artery stenosis, detection of this abnormality is particularly important because a cure usually can be achieved. The basic pathophysiology of all renovascular hypertension involves activation of the renin-angiotensin-aldosterone system. If a lesion in the minor or major branches of the renal artery significantly decreases renal perfusion pressure, it causes an increased renin release from the affected kidney. The high plasma renin activity leads to increases in angiotensin II levels with subsequent increases in total peripheral vascular resistance. This also leads to increased adrenal aldosterone production with resultant renal sodium and water retention and expansion in extracellular fluid volume.

Renovascular hypertension should be suspected in any hypertensive child with the physical finding of high-pitched bruits heard in the flank or abdominal areas or when stigmata of syndromes associated with arterial abnormalities are present (e.g., neurofibromatosis type I, homocystinuria, Marfan syndrome, phakomatoses). Patients with renovascular hypertension may show abnormalities on intravenous urography (delayed appearance of contrast in the affected kidney, difference in renal length, ureteric notching), abnormalities on radionuclide renal scans, or elevated plasma renin activity. Renal arteriography together with selective renal vein renin sampling is

the definitive diagnostic procedure for all pediatric patients with suspected renovascular hypertension.

Intrinsic diseases of the renal artery include fibromuscular dysplasia, thrombotic and embolic lesions, aneurysms, arteritis, and arteriosclerosis. The lesions of fibromuscular dysplasia involve multiple areas of stenosis alternating with aneurysmal dilation in the distal two thirds of the main renal artery (Fig. 13-47). Although difficult to differentiate from fibromuscular dysplasia histologically, the narrowing of the renal artery associated with neurofibromatosis generally begins within 1 cm of the origin from the aorta, distinguishing it from the distal involvement of fibromuscular dysplasia (Fig. 13-48). The

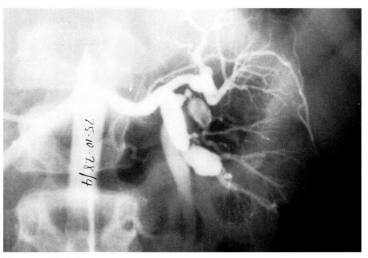

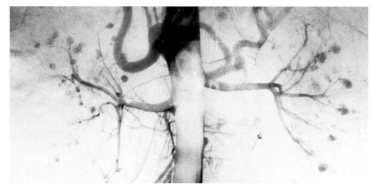

Figure 13-49. Polyarteritis nodosa. This arteriogram is from a 12-year-old girl with weight loss, fever, abdominal pain, and malignant hypertension. Note the diagnostic features of renal involvement including multiple thrombi and aneurysms.

Figure 13-47. Fibromuscular dysplasia. Arteriogram of a 12-year-old patient with malignant hypertension shows multiple areas of stenosis alternating with aneurysmal dilation in the distal segment of the renal artery.

lowed by autotransplantation of the remaining kidney at a later time.

Hirsutism

Although many endocrinologic causes of hirsutism exist, a number of drugs used in children with renal disorders can produce this condition. Marked hirsutism generally accompanies the use of minoxidil or diazoxide, which are potent antihypertensive agents causing direct relaxation of arteriolar smooth muscle. Cyclosporine, used widely to combat tissue allograft rejection after organ transplantation, has a dose-dependent effect on hair growth. Hirsutism and alteration in body image may be a major determinant of drug compliance, particularly in adolescent girls undergoing organ transplantation.

Chronic Renal Failure

Renal Osteodystrophy

Renal insufficiency leads to secondary hyperparathyroidism principally through inadequate renal synthesis of calcitriol (1,25-dihydroxyvitamin D) and by decreased renal clearance of dietary phosphate. This in turn leads to impaired mineralization of cartilage and bone, resulting in rickets and osteomalacia, and an excess of parathyroid hormone, which leads to osteitis fibrosa cystica, the classic bone disease seen in primary hyperparathyroidism. In any given patient each of these pathologic processes may occur with varying severity, giving a wide range of clinical and radiologic presentations, known as renal osteodystrophy. In children, renal osteodystrophy is clinically characterized by growth retardation, bone pain, deformity or fracture of long bones, and tissue calcification. The radiologic features in children include increased thickness and fraying of the radiolucent zone in the region of growth plates; subperiosteal erosion of the cortices of long bones and phalanges; and changes in bone density including osteoporosis, osteoclerosis, coarsening of the trabecular pattern of long bones (Fig. 13-50) or, rarely, brown tumors (Fig. 13-51).

Typically, this disorder becomes clinically evident when glomerular filtration rate falls below 50 mL/min/1.73 m^2 and is a common and often major complication among children undergoing dialysis. Management includes dietary phosphate restriction, calcium-containing dietary phosphate binders, which reduce intestinal phosphate

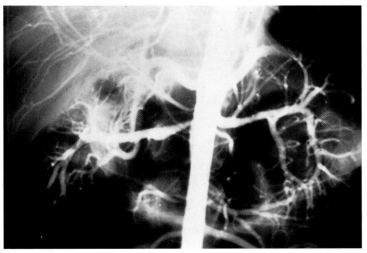

Figure 13-48. Neurofibromatosis in a 13-year-old with mild mental retardation and a blood pressure of 140/100 mm Hg. Arteriogram shows narrowing of the renal artery close to its origin from the aorta, in contrast to the distal involvement of fibromuscular dysplasia.

majority of pediatric patients with polyarteritis nodosa have renal involvement with hypertension, which leads to arterial lesions characterized by multiple thrombi and aneurysms (Fig. 13-49). Such arteriographic findings are diagnostic in the child with hypertension accompanied by weight loss, fever, and systemic manifestations of diffuse arteritis.

Correction of renovascular hypertension caused by intrinsic disease of the renal artery includes surgical revascularization of the kidneys or dilation of discrete stenoses by transluminal angioplasty. Diffuse arteritis, which may cause renovascular hypertension in children with underlying systemic diseases, is treated medically with corticosteroids, immunosuppressives, or anticoagulants depending on the nature of the primary disease process. Young children with bilateral renal artery stenosis together with coarctation of the abdominal aorta represent a most challenging management problem. The small-caliber vessels and possible scarring in the vessel walls render bypass or reconstructive surgery a most difficult task. Transluminal angioplasty is also ineffective in most cases. This problem has been successfully managed by staged bypass of the coarctation and autotransplantation of one kidney, fol-

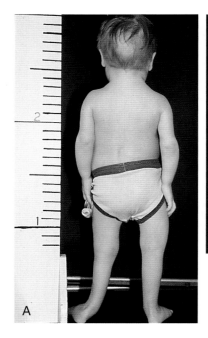

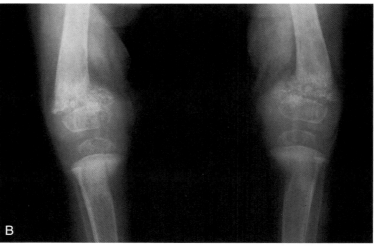

Figure 13-50. Autonomous hyperparathyroidism and severe renal osteodystrophy in a 6-year-old boy with renal failure caused by posterior urethral valves. **A,** Bossing of the occiput. **B,** Radiograph shows distal femoral and proximal tibial areas, as well as subperiosteal erosion of the cortical bone and active rickets in the epiphyseal ossification centers.

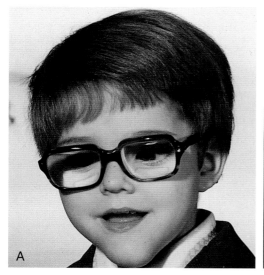

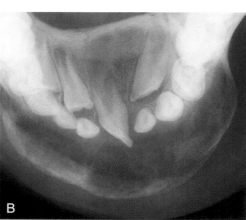

Figure 13-51. Renal osteodystrophy. **A,** This 5-year-old boy with moderate renal failure secondary to obstructive uropathy was admitted for evaluation of loose teeth and marked protrusion of the mandible. **B,** Surgical exploration of a radiolucent mandibular tumor was cancelled after biochemical evaluation was consistent with renal osteodystrophy. Biopsy revealed a brown tumor resulting from intense osteoclastic activity and bone resorption. Medical treatment resulted in regression of the tumor and the prognathia, bone remineralization, strengthening of the dental ridge, and dental preservation.

absorption, and calcitriol to aid intestinal calcium absorption and to suppress parathyroid hormone (PTH) secretion. However, such regimens often result in hyperphosphatemia and hypercalcemia with subsequent vascular and soft tissue calcification. To help reduce these complications, newer regimens advocate administration of calcium-free, metal-free phosphate-binding agents such as sevelamer, vitamin D analogues such as doxecalciferol or paricalcitol to more selectively suppress PTH, and calcimemetic agents, which act directly on the parathyroid cell calcium-sensing receptor such as cinacalciet. Optimal control of secondary renal hyperparathyroidism by such means together with control of metabolic acidosis is essential in promoting linear growth in young children.

Anemia of Renal Failure

Severe anemia in chronic renal failure is principally caused by the inability of the damaged kidneys to secrete

sufficient amounts of erythropoietin. In untreated children with end-stage renal failure, the hemoglobin levels are often lower than in adults (5 to 7 g/dL) and severely limit the tolerance to physical activity. In the past patients developed the facial features and radiographic appearance of Cooley anemia (Fig. 13-52). Currently attention to nutrition, iron status, replacement of folic acid, and other erythroactive water-soluble vitamins lost through dialysis, along with administration of recombinant erythropoietin, has resulted in a marked improvement in quality of life. This aids in preventing hemosiderosis, allergic reactions, infections, and other risks associated with frequent blood transfusions.

Growth Failure

Growth failure remains a major problem for children receiving dialysis and may persist following successful renal transplantation. Recombinant human growth

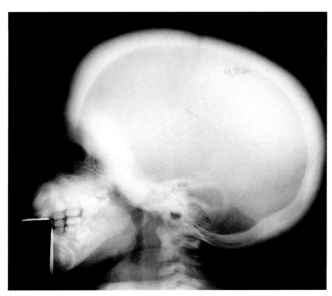

Figure 13-52. Anemia of renal failure. Note the facial and radiologic features of extramedullary erythropoiesis in the same child shown in Figure 13-51. Notice the thickened cranial table with the brushlike projections.

hormone therapy has been extremely efficacious in promoting growth of such children before renal transplantation. Precautions may be necessary if growth hormone therapy is continued after renal transplantation. This agent is effective even in children with normal concentrations of secretional endogenous growth hormone.

Bibliography

Alagille D, Estrada A, Hadchouel M, et al: Syndromic paucity of interlobular bile ducts (Alagille syndrome or arteriohepatic dysplasia): Review of 80 cases. J Pediatr 110:195-200, 1987.

American Medical Association, Board of Trustees: Clinical laboratory tests and standards. JAMA 255:373, 1986.

Bradley M, Schumann B: Examination of urine. In Henry JB (ed): Todd-Sanford-Davidsohn Clinical Diagnosis by Laboratory Methods. Philadelphia, WB Saunders, 1984, p 380.

Brewer ED, Benson GS: Hematuria: Algorithms for diagnosis. JAMA 246:877-880, 1981.

Fogazzi GB: Crystalluria: A neglected aspect of urinary sediment analysis. Nephrol Dial Transplant 11:379-387, 1996.

Frick GM, Gabow PA: Hereditary and acquired cystic disease of the kidney. Kidney Int 46:951-964, 1994.

Gilli G, Berry AC, Chantler C: Syndromes with a renal component. In Holliday MA, Barratt TM, Vernier RL (eds): Pediatric Nephrology, 2nd ed. Baltimore, Williams & Wilkins, 1987.

Goldraich NP, Goldraich IH: Update on dimercaptosuccinic acid renal scanning in children with urinary tract infection. Pediatr Nephrol 9:221-226, 1995.

Graff L: In Biello LA (ed): A Handbook of Routine Urinalysis. Philadelphia, JB Lippincott, 1983.

Grupe WE: Relapsing nephrotic syndrome in childhood. Kidney Int 16:75-85, 1979.

Guay-Woodford LM, Torres VE: Genetic diseases of the kidney. NephSAP (ASN) 4:161-238, 2005.

Habib R, Dommergues JP, Gubler MC, et al: Glomerular mesangiolipidosis in Alagille syndrome (arteriohepatic dysplasia). Pediatr Nephrol 1:455-464, 1987.

Harms E: Prenatal diagnosis of inborn errors of metabolism with renal manifestations. Pediatr Nephrol 1:540-545, 1987.

Kaplan BS, Kaplan P, Rosenberg HK, et al: Polycystic kidney disease in childhood. J Pediatr 22:867-880, 1989.

Kaplan MR: Hematuria in childhood. Pediatr Rev 5:99-105, 1983.

Kissane JM: Renal cysts in pediatric patients: A classification and overview. Pediatr Nephrol 4:69-77, 1990.

Klau G, Watson A, Edefonti A, et al: Prevention and treatment of renal osteodystrophy in children on chronic renal failure: European guidelines. Pediatr Nephrol 21:151-159, 2006.

Laufer J, Boichis H: Urolithiasis in children: Current medical management. Pediatr Nephrol 3:317-331, 1989.

McCrory WW: Glomerulonephritis. Pediatr Rev 5:19-25, 1983.

Sibley RK, Mohan J, Mauer SM, Vernier RL: A clinicopathologic study of forty-eight infants with nephrotic syndrome. Kidney Int 27:544-552, 1985.

Stapleton FB: Idiopathic hypercalciuria: Association with isolated hematuria and risk for urolithiasis in children. Kidney Int 37:807-811, 1990.

Strauss J, Abitbol C, Zilleruelo G, et al: Renal disease in children with the acquired immunodeficiency syndrome. N Engl J Med 321:625-630, 1989.

U.S. Preventive Services Task Force: Screening for asymptomatic bacteriuria, hematuria and proteinuria (AFP Publication No. 389-395). 1990.

West CD, McAdams AJ: The chronic glomerulonephritides of childhood: Parts I and II. J Pediatr 93:1-12, 167-176, 1978.

Zerres K: Genetics of cystic kidney disease. Pediatr Nephrol 1:397-404, 1987.

CHAPTER 14

Urologic Disorders

MARK F. BELLINGER

The manifestation of many congenital urological malformations, acquired disorders, and the result of common urological surgical procedures may produce visible or palpable findings on physical examination. Some clinical presentations are unique. In other cases, disorders of varying etiology may present similar signs, symptoms, and physical findings. Differential diagnosis is central to an appreciation of pediatric urologic disorders.

Physical Examination

Items of patient and family history may prove to be important in consideration of the differential diagnosis of urological disorders. A family history of urinary infection, hydronephrosis, vesicoureteric reflux, cystic kidney disease, compromised fertility, or genital malformation may indicate the presence of heritable urinary anomaly.

Examination begins with a general overview of the patient. Hemihypertrophy, congenital scoliosis, an abnormal gait, facial or external ear deformities, or the presence of multiple congenital anomalies may be associated with urologic disorders. Abdominal examination should begin with inspection for visible masses, followed by gentle palpation. Enlarged kidneys are usually palpable as upper abdominal or flank masses. An enlarged bladder or lesion of gynecologic origin may be palpable as a midline mass arising out of the pelvis. Abdominal masses should be characterized as cystic or solid; smooth, lobulated, or irregular; fixed or mobile; and tender or nontender.

The groin should be examined for inguinal gonads. Gonads palpable in the groin are frequently quite mobile and may move during examination from the inguinal canal almost into the scrotum, or lateral to the scrotum toward the perineum. They may also move from a palpable position in the groin to disappear into the abdomen during examination, so high testes may be palpable on one examination and nonpalpable on the next. The sensitivity of palpation or detection of inguinal testes and other masses may be increased by the use of soap or lubricant on the examiner's fingers. It may be difficult to palpate an inguinal testis by trying to "pinch" it between the fingers, whereas lubricated fingers gliding over the inguinal canal may easily detect a gonad as it slides beneath the fingers. The best technique is to place the fingers flat overlying the inguinal canal above the level of the internal inguinal ring and slide them slowly toward the pubis, then over the pubis toward the scrotum and down over the perineum lateral to the upper scrotum. On occasion, a vas and spermatic cord palpable in the groin (most notably where it passes over the pubic tubercle) may end in a small "nubbin" (remnant of an atrophic testis), which may be palpated in the upper scrotum. The structures of the inguinal canal should be examined in a similar fashion to detect thickening of the cord structures that may be seen in the presence of an inguinal hernia or communicating hydrocele. Masses in the inguinal canal may also represent an inguinal hernia containing bowel, omentum, or bladder (or ovary in girls, perhaps a testis in a phenotypic female with androgen insensitivity) (Fig. 14-1), communicating hydrocele or hydrocele of the cord or malignancy of the paratesticular tissues or cord structures (i.e., sarcoma). Inguinal lymphadenopathy is usually detected lateral to the inguinal canal.

Genital examination should include both inspection and palpation. The penis should be of appropriate length and diameter. Penile stretch length can be determined by using a ruler or tongue blade pressed against the pubic symphysis as the penis is gently stretched alongside it and the position of the tip of the glans marked for measurement. A concealed or buried penis may occur after circumcision or may be congenital. In most cases, hidden penises are retractile, in large part due to a thick suprapubic fat pad. Most cases of buried penis will resolve with time, whereas in severe cases the tethering may be due to dysgenetic fascial attachments and requires surgical correction. It may be difficult to determine the difference between the two in younger boys. The foreskin should be examined for adhesions to the glans, which may represent merely residual preputial fusion to the glans that will resolve spontaneously, or preputial skin bridges, which can occur after circumcision and require surgical division. The urethral meatus should be examined for size and location. The presence of chordee (ventral penile curvature) or a suggestion of its presence should be noted. The size and degree of development of the scrotum and the location and size of the testes are determined. Retractile testes should come well into the dependent portion of the scrotum when the room is warm and the patient is relaxed. If it is difficult to determine whether the testes are undescended, retractile, or normal, repeat examination may be helpful. The epididymis should be palpated and examined for tenderness or the presence of masses. The spermatic cords should be examined for the presence of abnormal findings (thickening, masses, varicocele). The cord is most easily examined as it crosses over the pubic tubercle. Male patients should be examined in both the supine position and in the standing position with and without Valsalva.

In the female patient the introitus should be inspected to confirm a normal size and location of the clitoris, the urethral meatus, the vaginal introitus, and hymenal ring.

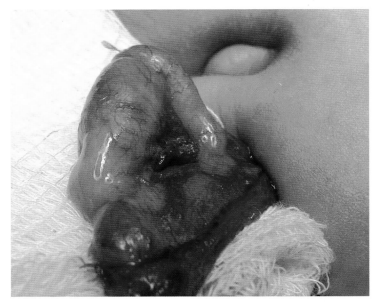

Figure 14-1. Androgen insensitivity. Left inguinal testis in an XY phenotypic female with androgen insensitivity.

Labial masses, swelling, or adhesions (fusion) may completely conceal the introitus. Lysis of labial adhesion may be necessary to allow examination of the introitus. Masses protruding from the urethral meatus or located near or originating in the vicinity of the meatus should be noted. Vaginal or urethral discharge or the presence of hymenal tags or an imperforate hymen may be seen. Posterior displacement of the vaginal introitus with a short or mucosalized perineal body is abnormal. The appearance and position of the anus should be noted. Rectal examination may be performed to assess sphincter tone or to help characterize abdominal or pelvic masses.

The lower back should be examined for hair tufts, clefts, sinus tracts, or other signs of spinal dysraphism. A general neurologic examination and testing of the anal wink, bulbocavernosus reflex, and lower extremity reflexes should be performed, especially if neurovesical dysfunction is suspected. The bulbocavernosus reflex is assessed by a brisk squeeze of the glans penis or clitoris or a tug on an indwelling Foley catheter. A positive response, which indicates an intact sacral reflex arc, is indicated by reflex contraction of the anal sphincter and bulbocavernosus muscle. Absence of the reflex strongly suggests the presence of a sacral neurologic lesion.

Antenatal Urinary Tract Dilation

Detection of urinary tract dilation (hydronephrosis, hydroureteronephrosis, pyelectasis, pyelocaliectasis) in the fetus is common, either during screening for a fetal anomaly or as a serendipitous finding (Fig. 14-2). All fetal urinary tract dilation demands postnatal evaluation. Most cases of hydronephrosis, even of a significant degree, are not detectable by physical examination of the neonate. Because only the most severe cases present as an abdominal or flank mass, a distended bladder, or generalized increase in abdominal girth and thus lead to immediate uroradiologic evaluation, most questions surround those infants with modest fetal hydronephrosis and a normal postnatal physical examination. All infants with fetal urinary dilation should have postnatal ultrasonography. In severe bilateral cases, ultrasound may be performed urgently, whereas in less severe hydronephrosis, ultrasound examination may best be performed 3 to 10 days after delivery to allow increased urine production to fill out dilated systems that may be relatively decompressed in the immediate postnatal period, especially in a relatively dehydrated infant. When postnatal ultrasound is normal (spontaneous resolution of fetal hydronephrosis occurs in up to 20% of cases) (Fig. 14-3), follow-up ultrasound should be performed at several months and at 1 year because delayed reappearance of dilation has been reported.

When postnatal hydronephrosis is documented, complete radiographic evaluation is indicated. If dilation is severe, renal function poor, or coexistent anomalies demand it, evaluation should be performed as soon as possible. Voiding cystourethrography is an integral part of the evaluation of every infant with hydronephrosis and should be the first study performed in all cases to rule out both infravesical obstruction and vesicoureteric reflux (see Fig. 14-2B). Subsequent evaluation with intravenous urography, radionuclide scan, or both may be appropriate to assess function and document whether true obstruction or mere dilation is present. If the infant is in stable condition (particularly when the lesion is unilateral or moderate in degree with good renal function), radionuclide evaluation should be delayed for 4 to 6 weeks to allow improved glomerular filtration, making studies more accurate. If nonobstructive dilation is documented, long-term follow-up may document gradual resolution of the hydronephrosis in some cases and persistent dilation in others.

Posterior Urethral Valves

Valvular obstruction of the posterior urethra is a common cause of infravesical obstruction in males. Presentation may be associated with prenatal hydronephrosis (see Fig. 14-2), urinary tract infection, incontinence, or renal failure. Although the classic presentation of infants and older children with urethral valves is a diminished urinary stream, few children are actually evaluated because of this symptom. Neonates may present with severe pulmonary hypoplasia and renal failure or with bladder distention and hydroureteronephrosis. Older boys with

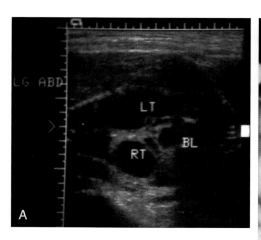

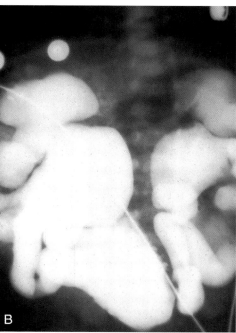

Figure 14-2. Fetal hydronephrosis. **A,** Fetal ultrasonography performed to assess gestational age reveals bilateral fetal hydronephrosis and a distended bladder. **B,** Voiding cystourethrogram reveals posterior urethral valves and severe bilateral vesicoureteric reflux. BL, bladder; LT, left kidney; RT, right kidney.

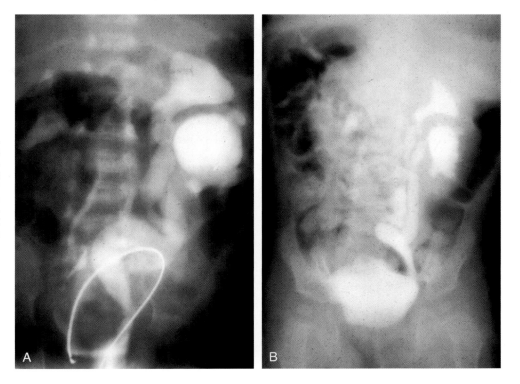

Figure 14-3. Postnatal hydronephrosis. **A,** Intravenous pyelogram at 1 month of age shows incomplete left ureteral duplication with hydroureteronephrosis of both ureters. **B,** Intravenous pyelogram at 4 months of age without surgical intervention reveals spontaneous improvement in hydroureteronephrosis. Subsequent diuresis renogram showed equal renal function and prompt washout; the hydronephrosis completely resolved by 2 years of age.

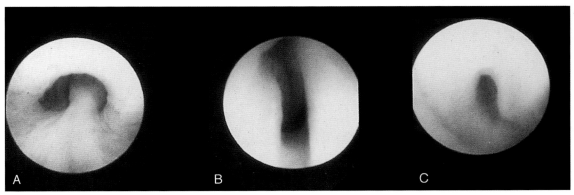

Figure 14-4. Posterior urethral valves. **A,** Endoscopic view of a normal posterior urethra and verumontanum. **B,** Type II urethral valves. The sail-like right and left leaflets are partially disrupted superiorly. **C,** Type III urethral valves. These almost complete iris-diaphragm valves cause a more significant obstruction than type II leaflets.

unrecognized urethral valves may present with symptoms ranging from incontinence to renal failure. Voiding cystourethrography is the key to the diagnosis of urethral valves. In most cases endoscopic fulguration of urethral valves is undertaken (Fig. 14-4A-C). In some cases cutaneous vesicostomy may be indicated, especially in tiny babies in whom urethral instrumentation may be problematic. Rarely is upper tract diversion (ureterostomy or pyelostomy) indicated. The ultimate prognosis for renal function depends on the state of the renal parenchyma (dysplasia) and of bladder compliance (poorly compliant bladders with diminished elasticity may fail to allow reflux or hydronephrosis to improve after valve ablation and may be associated with a worse prognosis for continence and renal function).

Cryptorchidism

Cryptorchidism occurs in approximately 33% of premature and 3% of full-term boys. Observing gradual testicular descent over several weeks in a premature infant is not unusual. Cryptorchidism is associated with many syndromes but rarely with urinary tract anomalies. The exception is congenital monorchism, which may be associated with ipsilateral renal agenesis. Renal ultrasound is indicated. Hypospadias associated with even unilateral cryptorchidism should raise the question of intersex anomalies, and karyotype should be determined in the neonate (Fig. 14-5). When bilateral nonpalpable testes are present in infancy, endocrinologic evaluation (serum FSH, LH, testosterone) may determine whether functional testicular tissue exists. The infant with cryptorchidism should be monitored closely, with hormonal or surgical treatment undertaken at about 6 months of age.

Prune-Belly (Eagle-Barrett Triad) Syndrome

Prune-belly syndrome has a fascinating constellation of physical findings and occurs almost exclusively in boys at a rate of 1 in 35,000 to 50,000 live births. The triad includes abnormal abdominal musculature (variable degrees of muscular laxity, which may be asymmetrical); abdominal cryptorchidism; and floppy dysmorphic urinary tracts, most with vesicoureteric reflux (Fig. 14-6). Plain abdominal radiography demonstrates the bell-shaped thorax and abdomen seen in this syndrome. The typical prune-belly refluxing ureter, with increasing tortuosity in the lower portion, is revealed by voiding cystourethrogram or intravenous urogram. Because of the severe risk of sepsis associated with urinary tract infec-

tion, urethral catheterization should only be undertaken with the utmost care to prevent infection and with antibiotic prophylaxis. Megalourethra may be seen. Associated with the syndrome in most patients are prostatic hypoplasia and dimples on the lateral aspects of the knees, which some experts believe are secondary to an exaggerated cross-legged position in utero. Gastrointestinal and cardiac anomalies occur in a proportion of patients, but the factor that most determines longevity is the presence and degree of renal dysplasia.

Anomalies of the Urachus

The urachus extends from the bladder dome to the umbilicus and is usually a vestigial structure during extrauterine life. Several lesions may result from persistence of the urachus: patent urachus, vesicourachal diverticulum, urachal cyst, and alternating urachal sinus. Many of these lesions go unrecognized for long periods before becoming symptomatic. Patent urachus results when the urachal lumen fails to obliterate and the bladder communicates with the umbilicus (Fig. 14-7). Umbilical drainage, inflammation, or infection may result. Voiding cystourethrography is important in the evaluation of possible urachal disorders and to exclude infravesical obstruction. The differential diagnosis includes persistent omphalomesenteric duct. Urachal cysts may become infected and present in infancy through adulthood with suprapubic or infraumbilical pain, tenderness, a palpable mass, or abdominal wall inflammation (Fig. 14-8). Urinary tract infection with irritative voiding symptoms or sepsis may result. Ultrasonography or CT may aid in diagnosis. Urachal diverticula are usually clinically inconsequential unless they are large enough to cause urinary stasis and infection. Because unrecognized urachal remnants may be the source of carcinoma in adults, many cases with a poor prognosis due to delayed detection, even asymptomatic urachal lesions, should be excised.

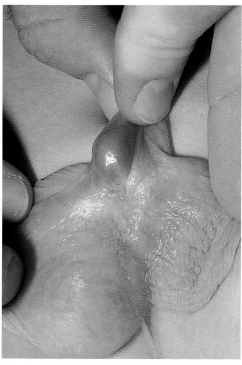

Figure 14-5. Intersex. Hypospadias and left cryptorchidism in a neonate found to have mixed gonadal dysgenesis with a mosaic karyotype.

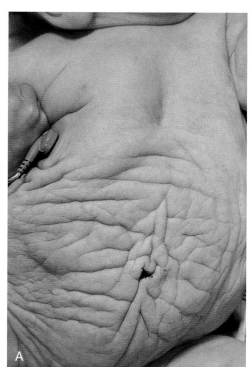

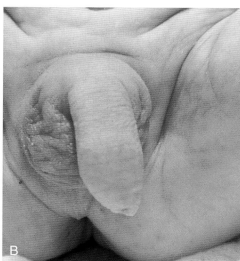

Figure 14-6. Prune-belly syndrome. **A,** Classic appearance of a wrinkled abdomen in a neonate. In older babies, the belly is less wrinkled and more floppy. **B,** Empty scrotum of the same infant.

Hydronephrosis

Ureteropelvic Junction Obstruction

Lesions of the ureteropelvic junction (UPJ) are a common cause of hydronephrosis. UPJ obstruction may present as antenatal hydronephrosis, neonatal flank mass, urinary tract infection, or recurrent abdominal pain in the older child and adolescent. In many cases of significant obstruction the kidney may not be palpably enlarged. UPJ obstruction may be documented by ultrasound or intravenous pyelography and confirmed by retrograde pyelography (Fig. 14-9A). Voiding cystourethrography is important, particularly in infants, because vesicoureteric reflux may coexist with UPJ obstruction. In some cases reflux is the primary lesion, with the UPJ kink as a secondary lesion (Fig. 14-9B), whereas in other cases, severe reflux may be the primary lesion with a secondary kink at the ureteropelvic junction, which may or may not prove to be obstructive (Fig. 14-9C). Not all hydronephrotic kidneys are truly obstructed. In borderline cases, radionuclide diuresis renography (Lasix renal scan) (Fig. 14-10) or percutaneous antegrade pressure perfusion studies (Whitaker test) may be necessary to determine whether surgical intervention is warranted. Some dilated but unobstructed infant kidneys spontaneously return to a normal or near-normal appearance with time (see previous discussion).

Megaureter

The term *megaureter* is descriptive of a large ureter, with or without intrarenal hydronephrosis (Fig. 14-11). Megaureters may be the result of massive vesicoureteric reflux or obstruction at the ureterovesical junction, or they may be nonobstructive. Experience with neonatal megaureters has shown that many of these lesions, when studied by diuresis renography or Whitaker protocols, are found to be nonobstructive. Some resolve spontaneously. The repair of true obstructive megaureters requires excision of the abnormal distal ureter and reimplantation of the tapered segment into the bladder. A nonrefluxing megaureter is thought to be due to either local neurologic or, more likely, muscular abnormalities of the distal ureter that interfere with normal peristalsis. Megaureters may be discovered on antenatal ultrasonography or present as a source of urinary tract infection. Calculi may form in them.

Multicystic Renal Dysplasia

Multicystic renal dysplasia (see Chapter 13) is the second most common cause of renal enlargement in the neonate and may be discovered by antenatal ultrasound, serendipi-

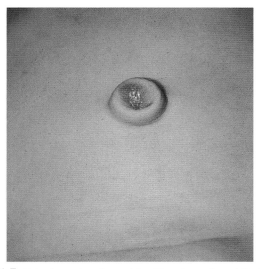

Figure 14-7. Patent urachus in a girl with recurrent umbilical drainage and inflammation.

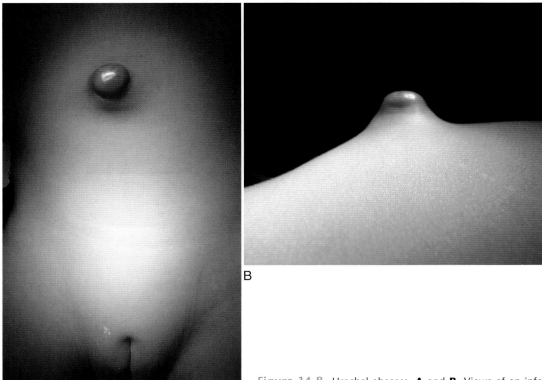

A

B

Figure 14-8. Urachal abscess. **A** and **B**, Views of an infected urachal abscess in a girl with fever and abdominal pain.

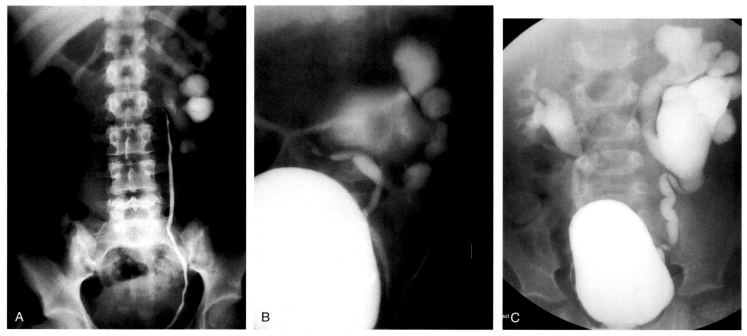

Figure 14-9. Ureteropelvic junction obstruction. **A,** Retrograde ureterogram defines obstruction at the ureteropelvic junction. **B,** The coexistence of vesicoureteric reflux and ureteropelvic junction obstruction is seen in this voiding cystourethrogram. **C,** Voiding cystourethrogram demonstrates a nonobstructive kink at the left ureteropelvic junction.

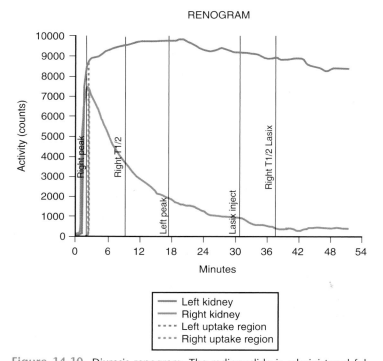

Figure 14-10. Diuresis renogram. The radionuclide is administered followed by a diuretic. The curves show a normal right kidney (prompt decrease in counts as the radionuclide is washed out of the collecting system) and an obstructed left kidney (only a small fraction of the radionuclide is slowly drained out of the collecting system).

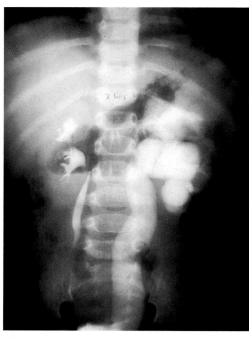

Figure 14-11. Megaureter. Intravenous pyelogram shows a left megaureter with hydroureteronephrosis and a normal right kidney and ureter.

tously, or during the evaluation of an abdominal mass. Multicystic renal dysplasia must be differentiated from hydronephrosis, and the combination of ultrasonography and radionuclide scan is usually diagnostic because, although the ultrasound appearance may be similar, multicystic kidneys rarely function on scan (Fig. 14-12). Because contralateral vesicoureteric reflux is common, voiding cystourethrography should be performed in all patients to detect reflux into the solitary functioning kidney. A percentage of multicystic kidneys (at least 15%

but perhaps much higher) spontaneously involute as determined by follow-up ultrasonography, and there is still debate about the indications for nephrectomy. The Urology Section of the American Academy of Pediatrics has instituted a registry for longitudinal follow-up of these patients. It appears that the potential for hypertension, infection, and malignancy in these kidneys is small.

Simple Renal Cysts

Simple renal cysts were thought to be rare in children until the advent of high-resolution ultrasound technology. They are now frequently detected, albeit much less

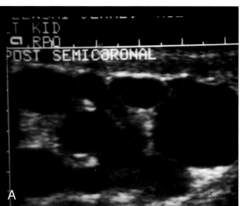 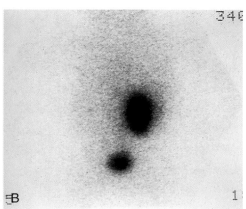

Figure 14-12. Multicystic dysplasia. **A,** Ultrasound examination of a multicystic kidney. **B,** Nuclear medicine scan of a nonfunctional left multicystic dysplastic kidney (posterior view). The top area of contrast represents the right kidney, and the lower one is the bladder.

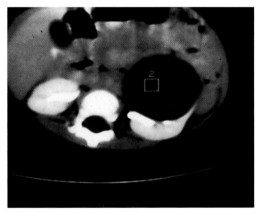

Figure 14-13. Simple renal cyst. CT of a huge left renal cyst, which presented as a left upper quadrant abdominal mass.

commonly than in adults, in whom the incidence increases with age. As a result, the traditional admonition to surgically explore all cysts in children has been replaced with the policy of radiographic evaluation similar to that in adults. Simple cysts should be treated as benign. Most renal cysts are discovered serendipitously while evaluating the urinary tract for infection-related symptoms, but large cysts occasionally present as abdominal masses. Radiologic evaluation usually includes ultrasonography, but CT (Fig. 14-13) and even cyst puncture for aspiration and contrast studies may be used to confirm the nature of the cyst. The differential diagnosis includes cystic Wilms tumor, multilocular cystic dysplasia, duplication anomaly with hydronephrosis, calyceal diverticulum, and adult polycystic disease.

Cutaneous Urinary Diversion

Although permanent urinary diversion in children is rarely performed in this age of intermittent catheterization and urinary tract reconstruction, temporary diversion still has an important role in difficult situations. Understanding the anatomic relationships of urinary stomas is an integral part of caring for children with diversions.

Cutaneous pyelostomy The renal pelvis is marsupialized to the skin (Fig. 14-14). This is an uncommon diversion except in small infants with severe hydronephrosis and compromised renal function.

End ureterostomy A single stoma is created, which usually requires using the distal ureter (Fig. 14-15).

Loop ureterostomy A double-barreled stoma is created, allowing access to both the proximal and distal ureter (Fig. 14-16).

Intestinal diversion An isolated segment of bowel is interposed between the skin and ureters. The normal continuity of the intestinal tract is restored (Fig. 14-17).

Cutaneous vesicostomy This is probably the most commonly created temporary diversion in children, usually in cases of urethral valves, neuropathic bladder, prune-belly syndrome, and occasionally severe vesicoureteric reflux. A vesicostomy is basically a vesicocutaneous fistula, and in the small infant it is simply covered with a diaper (Fig. 14-18).

Appendicovesicostomy This is a continent diversion intended to allow intermittent catheterization of the bladder when urethral access is difficult (Fig. 14-19). The stoma is frequently concealed in the umbilicus.

Nephrostomy This percutaneous or operatively placed catheter is a temporary urinary diversion or upper tract access for contrast or manometric evaluations (Fig. 14-20).

Exstrophic Anomalies

Classic Exstrophy

Bladder exstrophy occurs in approximately 1 of every 40,000 live births. It predominates in boys and is thought to result from premature rupture of the cloacal membrane. The infant is usually otherwise healthy. Examination reveals a red mucosal surface of varying size on the infraumbilical abdominal wall, which represents the entire bladder opened as a book. On the inferior bladder surface the trigone and ureteral orifices are visible, freely effluxing urine. The penis is epispadiac and lies dorsally tethered against the bladder. When the penis is retracted downward, the entire mucosal surface of the urethra is seen to be splayed open (Fig. 14-21A and B). In severe cases the penis may be bifid or rudimentary, and gender assignment may be questionable. The scrotum may be normal or bifid, and testes may be undescended. Inguinal hernias are common. The pubic symphysis is widespread. In girls a hemiclitoris and duplicate vagina are common (Fig. 14-21C and D). The delicate bladder surface should be kept moist until urologic consultation is obtained. Prompt upper tract evaluation and neonatal closure are routine. Pelvic osteotomy may be necessary to achieve successful closure.

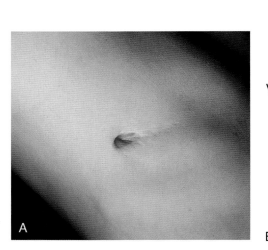
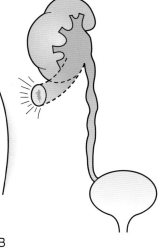

Figure 14-14. Cutaneous pyelostomy.

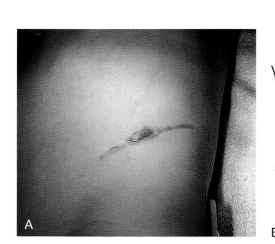
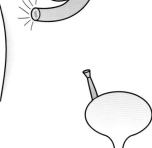

Figure 14-15. End ureterostomy.

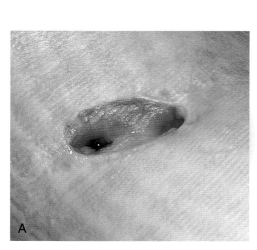
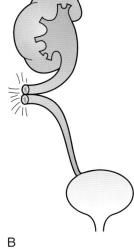

Figure 14-16. Loop ureterostomy. Note double-barreled stoma.

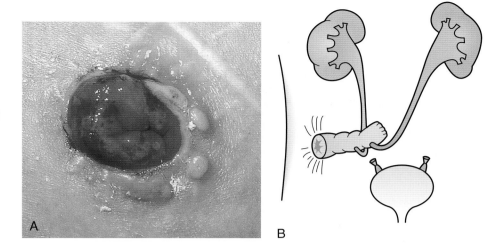

Figure 14-17. Ileal conduit stoma (intestinal diversion).

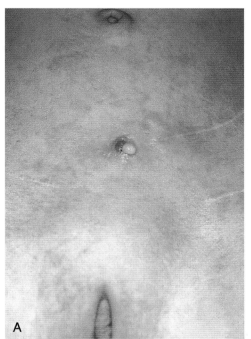

Figure 14-18. Cutaneous vesicostomy.

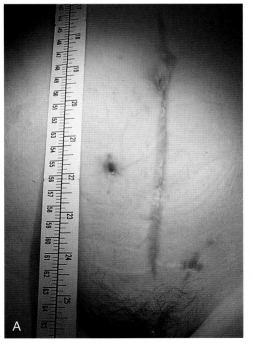

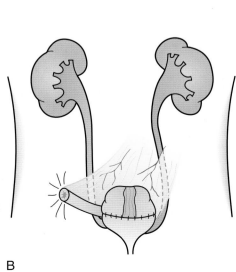

Figure 14-19. Appendicovesicostomy.

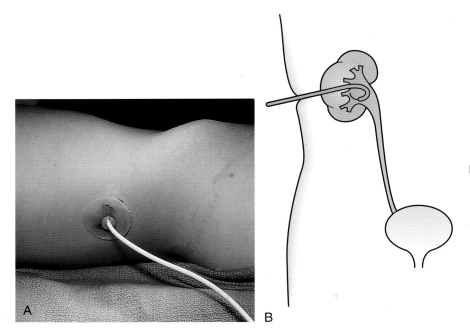

Figure 14-20. Percutaneous nephrostomy.

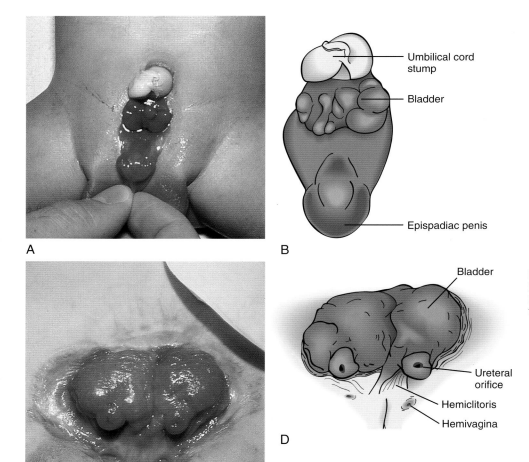

Figure 14-21. Exstrophy. **A** and **B,** Classic bladder exstrophy in a boy infant with a small bladder. **C** and **D,** Bladder exstrophy in a girl. Note the separated openings to each hemivagina.

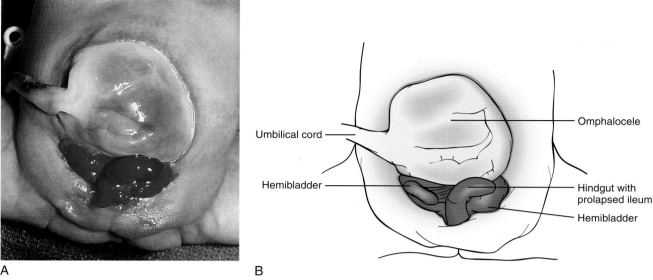

Figure 14-22. Cloacal exstrophy.

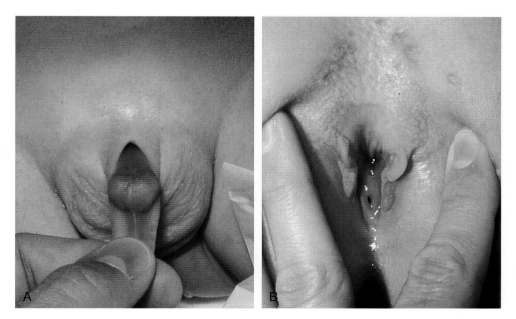

Figure 14-23. Epispadias. **A,** Penopubic epispadias with incontinence in a boy infant. **B,** Epispadias in a girl reveals a patulous urethra and widespread hemiclitoris.

Cloacal Exstrophy

Cloacal exstrophy is a rare anomaly (1 in 200,000 births). It represents an embryologic mishap similar to that resulting in classic exstrophy, except that rupture of the cloacal membrane occurs before the urorectal septum has completed its descent to separate the hindgut from the bladder. The resulting constellation of anomaly is severe, with long-term survival little better than 50% in most cases. Most children have a large omphalocele, and the majority have myelomeningocele and hydrocephalus. Examination of the exstrophic mucosa reveals that the bladder is divided into two widely separated halves, with a strip of bowel mucosa in the middle (Fig. 14-22). This strip is the ileocecal segment, usually accompanied by a long, prolapsed tubular structure, which is the terminal ileum. Separate orifices enter the appendix (or appendices) and a short, blind colon. The anus is imperforate. The genitalia are usually hypoplastic with the genital primordia widely separated at either side of the exstrophic cloaca. A female gender assignment is commonly thought to be appropriate because of the extreme difficulty that may be encountered in creation of a functional phallus in many cases, although gender assignment is now a controversial topic. A multispecialty approach should be taken to the infant with cloacal exstrophy.

Epispadias

Epispadias may represent the middle or opposite end of the spectrum of exstrophic anomalies, depending on the severity of the lesion. Approximately 55% of patients are boys with penopubic epispadias and urinary incontinence. These boys have a palpably and radiographically widened pubic symphysis and a broad spadelike penis with the urethra opened fully on its dorsal surface up to the level of the bladder neck. The penis is usually tethered dorsally, and the patient is usually incontinent (Fig. 14-23A). A smaller percentage of boys demonstrate only penile or balanitic (glanular) epispadias. These boys have normal urinary continence. In girls with epispadias (the most rare cases of epispadias), incontinence is usually accompanied by a wide urethra and a bifid clitoris (Fig. 14-23B). The

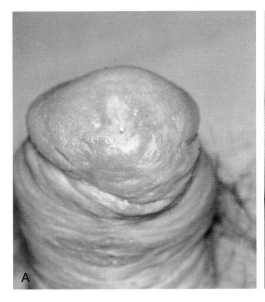
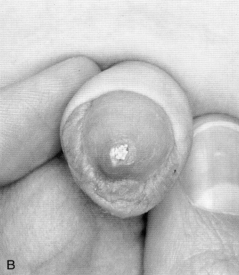

Figure 14-24. Urinary retention. **A,** Urinary retention secondary to severe chronic balanitis (balanitis xerotica obliterans). **B,** Urinary retention secondary to an impacted urethral calculus.

cosmetic appearance of the genitalia in both genders can be improved by genitoplasty, but the larger problem is incontinence, which is accentuated by small bladder capacity. Staged surgical correction is the rule. Renal ultrasonography and voiding cystourethrography should be performed in all cases.

Urinary Retention

Acute urinary retention in infants and children is usually voluntary and associated with severe acute cystitis, urethritis, meatitis (in boys), or vaginitis. In boys, urethral stricture (congenital, traumatic) and meatal stenosis with meatitis (Fig. 14-24A) should be considered. Urethral valves are more likely to cause dysuria or straining without complete retention. Retention in girls is unlikely to be caused by even severe labial adhesions, so uncommon lesions such as a prolapsed ureterocele should be considered. Bladder or urethral calculi can also cause retention, and these (Fig. 14-24B) can be diagnosed by a plain abdominal film and ultrasound examination. Pelvic masses (bladder, prostate, or genital rhabdomyosarcoma or other malignancy [Fig. 14-25]; uterine or ovarian masses; hydrocolpos; or hydrometrocolpos) secondary to imperforate hymen or vaginal atresia, sacrococcygeal tumors, or tumors of neural origin may cause retention due to neurological involvement of the sacral nerve roots or due to bladder neck or urethral compression. Severe constipation may similarly cause retention by a sheer mass effect. Acute neurologic changes associated with spinal cord injury or tumor or transverse myelitis may cause neurogenic retention. Intermittent catheterization may be extremely valuable in managing the bladder until diagnostic evaluations can be completed.

Neurovesical Dysfunction

Neurovesical dysfunction in childhood may be either congenital (meningocele, myelomeningocele, intradural lipoma, diastematomyelia, sacral agenesis) or acquired (trauma, transverse myelitis, spinal cord tumor). Independent of etiology, the evaluation and management of the

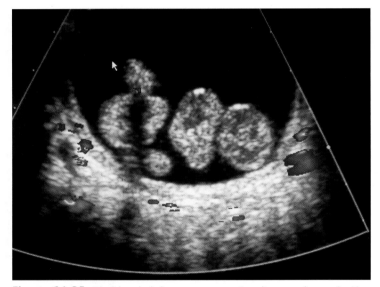

Figure 14-25. Bladder rhabdomyosarcoma. An ultrasound examination of the bladder in a boy who presented with urinary retention. The study reveals polypoid lesions of a botryoid rhabdomyosarcoma, which obstructed the bladder outlet, causing urinary retention.

child with neurovesical dysfunction are extremely important to preserve renal function, prevent renal damage from infection, and provide social continence. Physicians caring for an infant with neurovesical dysfunction should ensure that periodic evaluation of the child's urinary tract is carried out. This evaluation may include radiographic or urodynamic studies, which should be repeated several times during the first year of life or after injury and at least yearly thereafter or as indicated. Danger signs may include infection, fever, or a change in normal pattern of bladder or bowel continence (Fig. 14-26).

Uninhibited bladder contractions and discoordinated voiding may be seen in other neurologic conditions, and these may result in bladder dysfunction severe enough to cause not only incontinence or retention of urine but also upper tract deterioration. Multiple sclerosis and other demyelinating diseases are examples. Severe cerebral palsy is frequently associated with incontinence, although upper tract deterioration is uncommon.

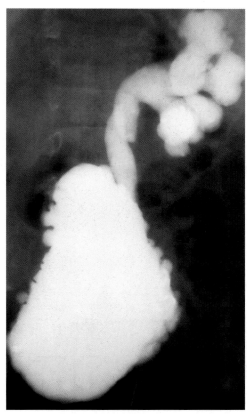

Figure 14-26. Neurovesical dysfunction. Severe bladder trabeculation and vesicoureteric reflux in a child with myelomeningocele.

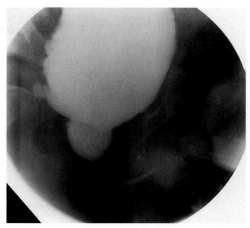

Figure 14-27. Voiding dysfunction. Voiding cystourethrogram of a boy with Hinman-Allen syndrome shows severe dilation of the prostatic urethra thought to represent urethral valves. Severe bilateral hydronephrosis resulted from vesicoureteric reflux.

Non-Neurogenic Vesical Dysfunction

The "non-neurogenic neurogenic bladder," or what is termed *Hinman-Allen syndrome*, is a little-known but important entity that may result in incontinence and renal failure. This syndrome represents a learned disorder of micturition and usually presents as day and night incontinence, fecal soiling, and urinary tract infection. Many children display behavioral problems. This syndrome seems to be at the far end of the spectrum of the frequency syndrome of childhood, and its slightly more prevalent and symptomatic cousin, dysfunctional voiding, are two symptomatic diagnoses seen with increasing frequency by both pediatricians and pediatric urologists. Most children with dysfunctional voiding have some degree of incontinence and fecal soiling. Some have urinary urgency to the point of incontinence, although overflow incontinence from a full bladder may also occur (the lazy bladder syndrome). On occasion, the child may display disordered micturition without symptoms of incontinence and may have only urinary tract infection as a symptom of the dysfunction. In severe cases in which bladder function is severely disordered and detrusor/sphincter discoordination is severe, the child's bladder may appear to have the configuration of a bladder that has suffered damage from intravesical obstruction or neurovesical dysfunction (Fig. 14-27).

The diagnosis of dysfunctional voiding is one of exclusion, made after ruling out occult neuropathy such as a tethered spinal cord (CT or MRI scan of the lumbosacral spine), and infravesical obstruction (voiding cystourethrogram and urodynamic evaluation) because the uroradiographic findings often mimic neurovesical dysfunction or obstruction. If child and family are cooperative, bladder retraining using a timed, double-voiding regimen may be effective, frequently augmented with biofeedback. In severe cases, intermittent catheterization may be necessary to reverse hydronephrosis. When renal function is in jeopardy and patient cooperation is minimal, temporary urinary diversion may be appropriate. Many children with this disorder require behavioral or psychological therapy in combination with thoughtful urologic management.

Anomalies of the Male Genitalia

Hypospadias

Hypospadias is a common anomaly that occurs in approximately 1 in 250 male births. The configuration of the urethra varies from mild glanular hypospadias to severe perineal hypospadias with chordee (ventral penile curvature). In describing the appearance of the hypospadiac penis, it is important to refrain from nonspecific terms such as *first-degree* and *minimal*. Proper definition of the anomaly should give an accurate description of the location of the meatus (glanular, coronal, subcoronal, distal shaft, midshaft, proximal shaft, penoscrotal, scrotal, perineal) and the presence or absence of chordee (Fig. 14-28). When hypospadias is associated with cryptorchidism, karyotype should be determined. Voiding cystourethrography is not indicated in hypospadias except in severe lesions or in boys with a history of urinary tract infection. Renal sonography is more likely to be abnormal in boys with proximal hypospadias. Infants with hypospadias should not be circumcised because the dorsal preputial skin may be necessary for penile reconstruction. Repair is usually undertaken at approximately 6 months of age.

Chordee

Chordee (ventral penile curvature) without hypospadias occurs much less frequently than chordee with hypospadias. Chordee may be a minor problem related to skin tethering; may be a result of abnormal development of the urethra and ventral penile structures; or may be due to a congenitally short urethra, in which case surgical correction requires division of the urethra and interposition of a skin tube. If chordee is suspected in the neonate, circumcision should be delayed until examination under

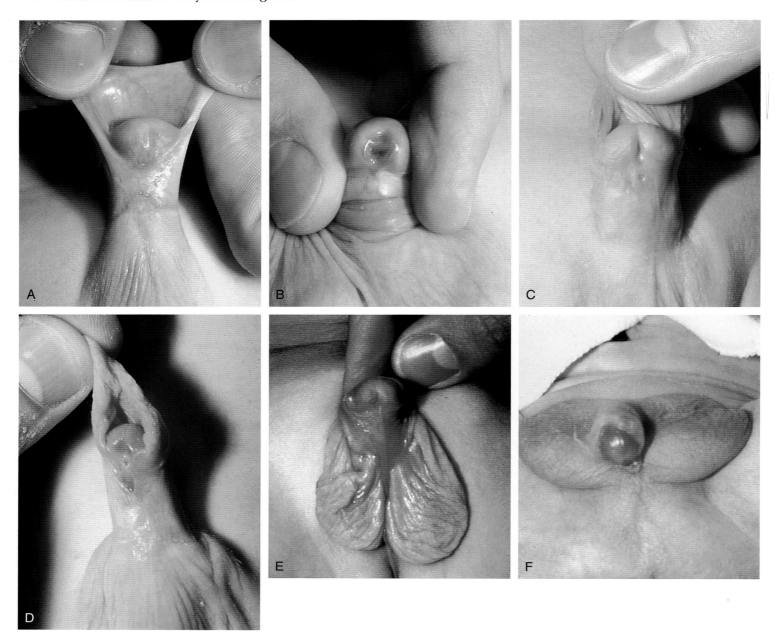

Figure 14-28. The various forms of hypospadias, revealing location of the meatus. **A,** The typical appearance of the "dorsal hood" prepuce seen in association with hypospadias. **B,** Glanular hypospadias. **C,** Subcoronal hypospadias. **D,** Midshaft hypospadias. **E,** Scrotal hypospadias with bifid scrotum but without chordee. **F,** Perineal hypospadias with chordee.

anesthesia and artificial erection can determine whether either circumcision or repair is appropriate (Fig. 14-29).

Penile Torsion

Torsion of the penis may be congenital or acquired. Congenital torsion may be severe and related to anomalous development of the corporal bodies, but, most commonly, it is mild and related to dysgenetic subcutaneous fascia (Fig. 14-30). In many cases the ventral median raphe is seen to spiral around the shaft. Most penile torsion is counterclockwise. Acquired torsion may occur after circumcision or hypospadias repair.

Webbed Penis

This minor anomaly is easily corrected with a V-Y scrotoplasty (Fig. 14-31). Webbing is caused by the transposition of scrotal skin onto the ventral penile shaft at the

penoscrotal junction. The ill effects are purely cosmetic in nature.

Buried Penis

Buried penis may occur as a primary finding in the neonate, but it is most common after circumcision (Fig. 14-32). Buried penis is usually the result of a thick suprapubic fat pad; it resolves with normal development. In severe cases, dysgenetic subcutaneous fascial bands bind the penis down. Buried penis after circumcision may be similar to congenital buried penis, and observation may be the rule. In this situation, removal of more skin might leave the penile shaft skin deficient. If caused by a severe phimosis that covers the glans completely, surgical intervention may be necessary to open the phimotic ring and remodel the shaft skin. In severe cases, which do not resolve into early adolescence, surgical reconstruction may be necessary.

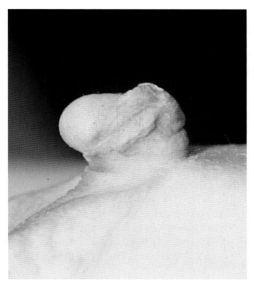

Figure 14-29. Chordee not associated with hypospadias.

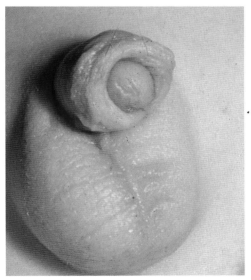

Figure 14-30. Mild counterclockwise penile torsion.

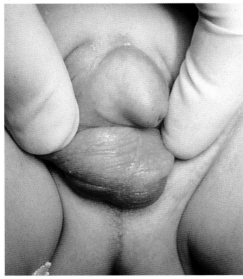

Figure 14-31. Webbed penis.

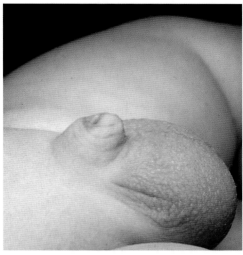

Figure 14-32. Buried penis after circumcision.

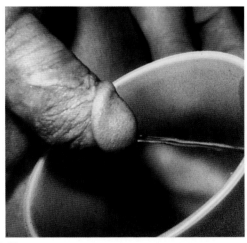

Figure 14-33. Meatal stenosis. Observation of the urinary stream in suspected meatal stenosis reveals a full stream, ruling out significant meatal stenosis.

Postcircumcision Concerns

Meatal Stenosis

Relative meatal stenosis is common after circumcision, secondary to mild recurrent meatitis. Mild to moderate stenosis is usually asymptomatic, but dysuria, strangury, or deflection of the urinary stream may bring the child to a physician's office. Mere examination of the meatus is insufficient to document stenosis, and the urinary stream should be observed for a thin or upward stream or for bulging of the meatus (Fig. 14-33). In many cases referred for evaluation, the urinary stream appears normal and no intervention is necessary. Meatotomy in the office under local anesthesia is curative.

Meatal Bridges

These unusual lesions appear to result from meatal stenosis in which the ventral aspect of the meatus recanalizes, leaving a bridge of skin across the meatus that may cause dysuria or deflection and spraying of the urinary stream (Fig. 14-34).

Preputial Adhesions and Skin Bridges

Fibrinous adhesions are a result of incomplete retraction of the prepuce during normal development or after circumcision. These adhesions resolve spontaneously with normal hygiene and development. Fibrous adhesions (preputial skin bridges) result when the free edge of the circumcising incision adheres to the glans penis and, not properly cared for, fuses to the glans. The resulting bridge of skin may cause penile torsion or trap smegma, causing recurrent inflammation or infection (Fig. 14-35). Circumferential skin bridges may be quite disfiguring, and the repair of these can be challenging. Proper instruction on care of the infant penis after circumcision should prevent most of these bridges from forming.

Microphallus

Microphallus (micropenis) is a small, normally formed penis more than two standard deviations below the mean (<1.9 cm stretch length in neonates) (Fig. 14-36). Important to obtain is an accurate penile stretch length and corporal shaft diameter by using a rigid ruler placed on the pubic symphysis and stretching the penis to extend the glans as far as possible along the ruler, while not stretching the prepuce. Microphallus is thought to result from failure of normal penile growth after 14 weeks' gestation. Two primary causes of the failure of penile growth may be hypogonadotropic hypogonadism (failure of the hypothalamus to produce GnRH) and primary testicular failure (deficient testosterone production) (hypergonadotropic hypergonadism). Karyotype should be determined. Follicle-stimulating hormone (FSH), luteinizing hormone (LH), and testosterone levels should be measured in addition to a diagnostic human chorionic gonadotropin (HCG) stimulation test to assess testicular function. Evaluation of the pituitary/hypothalamic function should be carried out by measurements of serum, glucose, sodium, potassium, cortisol, and thyroid hormone levels, and perhaps an MRI to assess the anatomy of the hypothalamus and midbrain. Although a great deal of controversy exists about the long-term outlook for penile growth at puberty and about the appropriateness of female gender reassignment in infancy, most authors suggest a diagnostic trial of testosterone for 3 months before making a final decision about gender assignment. An increasing impetus is toward the male sex of rearing.

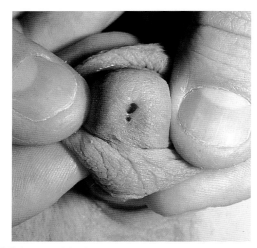

Figure 14-34. Meatal bridge.

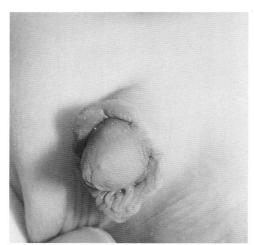

Figure 14-35. Preputial skin bridges after circumcision.

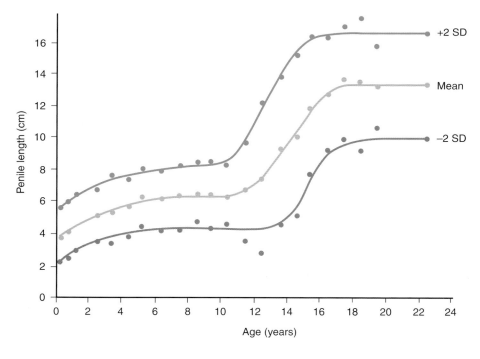

Figure 14-36. Cumulative frequency curves of penile length for age. (From Lee PA, Mazur T, Danish R, et al: Micropenis. I: Criteria, etiologies, and classification. Johns Hopkins Med J 146:156-163, 1980. © Johns Hopkins University Press. Reprinted with permission of The Johns Hopkins University Press.)

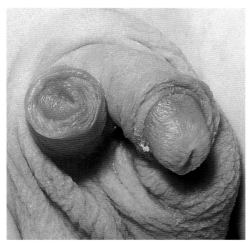

Figure 14-37. Diphallus. Both of these penises were functional. Continence was normal.

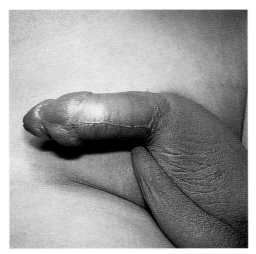

Figure 14-38. Priapism.

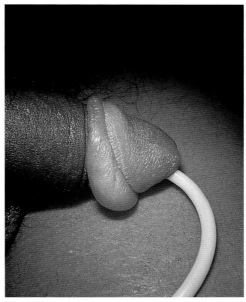

Figure 14-39. Paraphimosis. Catheterized patient with edematous prepuce proximal to the glans.

Diphallus

Diphallus is a rare entity usually associated with severe deformities of the lower urinary tract and genitalia. Complete evaluation of the upper and lower urinary tract is mandatory. In most cases of diphallus, one penis is dominant in erectile and urethral function, but in some, the bladder is septate or duplicated, and each phallus plays a significant role (Fig. 14-37).

Priapism

Priapism is a persistent, painful erection in which the corporal bodies are firmly erect but the glans is soft (Fig. 14-38). The shaft and preputial skin may become edematous, and the pain of priapism is usually severe. Priapism in children is usually related to an underlying disease state as opposed to the more common idiopathic variety seen in adults. It is most frequently associated with sickle cell disease but may be seen in relation to pelvic malignancy, leukemia, blunt perineal trauma, or secondary to acute spinal cord injury. Sickle cell–related priapism should initially be treated as any other sickle cell crisis, with oxygenation, exchange transfusion, and systemic alkalinization. Surgical therapy may be necessary to irrigate the corpora cavernosa or perform a cavernosal-spongiosal shunt or vascular bypass.

Acute Balanitis and Posthitis

These inflammatory lesions (balanitis, of the glans; posthitis, of the prepuce) are most common in uncircumcised boys with infection from the entrapped smegma beneath the foreskin. Usual treatment involves slight dilation of a snug preputial opening, warm baths, and a broad-spectrum antibiotic for a few days if the process is severe. Candidiasis or other causes should be treated appropriately. Whether balanitis or posthitis indicates the need for circumcision is determined on an individual basis once the acute inflammation has resolved.

Paraphimosis

Phimosis describes the inability to retract a tight, scarred prepuce. If a tight prepuce is retracted over the glans to the level of the corona (paraphimosis), the constricted ring of skin may act as a tourniquet applied to the distal shaft and glans, and ischemia may result (Fig. 14-39). Treatment may involve manual compression of the glans and edematous prepuce to allow reduction of the tight band. In severe cases when reduction of the paraphimosis cannot be achieved manually, a dorsal slit must be performed, surgically dividing the phimotic band. Circumcision may be appropriate after an episode of paraphimosis.

Lesions of the Scrotum and Scrotal Contents

The scrotum is composed of several fascial and muscular layers containing the spermatic cord and its contents, as well as the testes and their appendages. Any layer of the scrotal wall or any of the contents of the scrotum may produce a clinically evident lesion. Each testis is an ovoid structure lying in a vertical plane in its hemiscrotum in

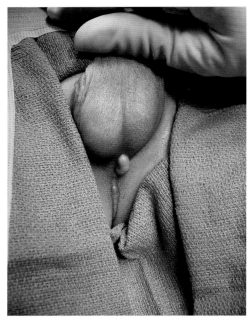

Figure 14-40. Median raphe cysts of the perineum and posterior scrotum.

which it is quite mobile, moving up and down with crem-asteric contraction and relaxation and separated from the contralateral testis and scrotal contents by the fibrous median septum. Posterior and slightly lateral to the testis lies the epididymis, which may be closely applied to the body of the testis or attached by a somewhat longer meso-epididymis. The appendix testis and appendix epididymis are small embryologic remnants attached to the upper anterior testis or head of the epididymis. These structures are not palpable in the normal state and are not constant findings in all boys.

Median Raphe Cysts

Epithelial inclusion cysts of the median raphe of the scrotum and perineum are not rare (Fig. 14-40). Although isolated cysts may be seen, a more common finding is a chain of cysts extending along the midline of the perineum and scrotum. The cysts are filled with white or yellow epithelial debris and are usually asymptomatic, although infection of the cyst contents may occur. The cystic lesions appear to represent infolding of skin during fusion of the labioscrotal folds during formation of the external genita-lia. Excision of the median raphe and cysts should be performed carefully in one elongated excision, leaving behind no area of microscopically encysted skin that might subsequently enlarge into a clinically evident cyst.

Acute Scrotum

The acute scrotum is a urologic surgical emergency until proven otherwise. It is most imperative to rule out torsion of the spermatic cord. The most important aspects of evaluating the patient with an acute scrotum are history and physical examination. The nature of the onset of pain and swelling is important, as is a history of dysuria, fever, hematuria, previous urinary tract infection, urethral instrumentation, and scrotal or perineal trauma. Exami-

nation of the scrotum starts with the normal testis, while observing the involved testis for its size, location, and anatomic orientation. The skin and wall of the scrotum are examined for edema, inflammation, and fluctuation. Mobility of the testis should be assessed, as should the presence or absence of a cremasteric reflex ipsilateral to the involved testis. Laboratory evaluation includes uri-nalysis, white blood cell count, and testicular flow scan or color Doppler examination if appropriate. The bottom line is expeditious evaluation with a liberal approach to exploration if the diagnosis is uncertain.

Torsion of the Spermatic Cord

Torsion of the spermatic cord is the most significant condition that must be excluded in cases of scrotal pain and swelling (Fig. 14-41). Because the testis deprived of its normal blood supply has at most a few hours before irre-versible injury destroys spermatogenic potential, acute swelling of the scrotum is a diagnostic and surgical emer-gency until torsion has been adequately excluded as a cause. Torsion may occur at any age.

Antenatal torsion is thought in most cases to represent extravaginal torsion or torsion of the entire scrotal con-tents including the covering tunics. It occurs during descent of the testis and usually presents at birth as a firm, nontender mass high in the scrotum or at the scrotal inlet. Frequently there is fixation to the overlying skin as a part of the inflammatory response. Although a point of current controversy, the classic teaching has been that these testes are not salvageable and that it is more important for the contralateral testis to have normal scrotal fixation and not be prone to asynchronous torsion. Although "salvage" of a testis after antenatal torsion is unlikely, acute torsion can occur during delivery and may rarely be a reversible situ-ation. Synchronous or asynchronous contralateral torsion may occur. A scrotal mass at birth should thus be consid-ered a surgical emergency until proven otherwise. Many pediatric urologists now feel that immediate exploration of both testes should be undertaken to assess viability of the involved testis and, more importantly, to ensure the safety of the solitary surviving testis. The risk of general anesthesia must be considered.

Intravaginal torsion (within the tunica vaginalis) may occur at any age. Most patients have acute, painful swell-ing of the scrotum, and many also have lower abdominal pain, nausea, and vomiting. It is not unusual for a boy to awaken with pain, but torsion can also occur after scrotal trauma or during almost any activity. On occasion, torsion has a much more insidious onset as a dull scrotal pain of subacute nature. Dysuria is usually absent, and urinalysis is normal, but leukocytosis may be noted. Examination may vary depending on the time elapsed after the acute episode. Most patients are uncomfortable. The scrotum early on may appear normal but soon becomes red and swollen, with the testis elevated because of foreshortening of the spermatic cord. The contralateral testis may have a more transverse orientation than normal. In the acute stage, a hydrocele may develop. The testis may have an abnormal orientation, with the epididymis located in an abnormal position due to torsion of the cord. The crem-asteric reflex is usually absent, and elevating the testis to the pubic symphysis increases pain (negative Prehn sign). When inflammation has progressed, the scrotum becomes a firm, homogeneous mass in which all anatomic land-marks are lost.

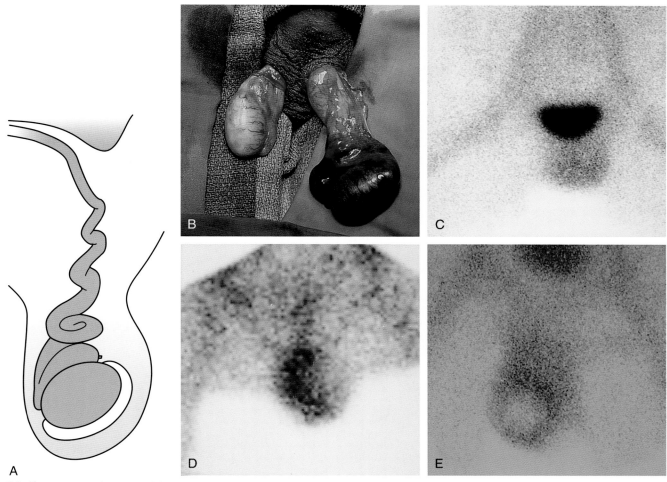

Figure 14-41. Intravaginal torsion of the spermatic cord. **A,** Torsion of the spermatic cord. **B,** Surgical exploration and detorsion of left spermatic cord. The left testis was necrotic. The right testis also shows bell-and-clapper deformity. **C,** Nuclear blood flow scan showing normal flow to both testes. The dark area above the scrotum is the bladder full of radionuclide, which is excreted in the urine. **D,** Nuclear blood flow scan showing increased flow to the right testis resulting from epididymitis. **E,** Nuclear blood flow scan showing the classic bull's-eye configuration of a missed torsion of the right testis.

If torsion is suspected, attempting to detorse the cord by gentle twisting in either direction may allow the cord to untwist, at least partially. If detorsion occurs, relief of pain is instantaneous. Nuclear blood flow scan or color Doppler ultrasound, if immediately available, may be helpful in many instances. A normal nuclear medicine scrotal scan shows identical flow to both testes (see Fig. 14-41C). When the scrotum contains an inflammatory process, blood flow is increased on the involved side (see Fig. 14-41D), whereas in the presence of an acute torsion, blood flow is diminished. A missed torsion, in which the scan is performed several hours or days after torsion occurs, appears as a central area of diminished flow surrounded by a halo of increased activity (see Fig. 14-41E). Color flow Doppler imaging has proven to be a superior alternative to nuclear medicine imaging in almost all cases of acute or chronic scrotal conditions, offering not only determination of the presence or absence of blood flow to the testis, but also anatomic information about the scrotum and its contents not available in nuclear medicine studies. When torsion of the spermatic cord is diagnosed, immediate surgical exploration is warranted (see Fig. 14-41A).

Torsion of Testicular Appendages

The appendix testis and appendix epididymis are embryologic remnants that are normally undetectable on routine examination. Torsion of an appendix, which can occur in the early pubertal age group, may be difficult to differentiate from torsion of the spermatic cord. Early after the onset of acute scrotal pain, a small tender mass may be palpable on the upper anterior surface of the testis or epididymis (Fig. 14-42A). In light-skinned children, the swollen, dark, infarcted appendage may be visible through the scrotal skin (the "blue dot" sign of Dresner) (Fig. 14-42B and C). In later presentations the entire testis and scrotum may become inflamed and indistinguishable from torsion of the spermatic cord. Color flow Doppler examination may indicate increased blood flow, and an enlarged torsed appendage may be visualized.

Epididymitis

Epididymal inflammation may be bacterial or nonbacterial in etiology. Nonbacterial inflammation may be caused by reflux of sterile urine into the ejaculatory ducts or ectopic insertion of a ureter into the seminal vesicle or vas deferens. In many cases of nonbacterial epididymitis, anatomy is normal and no obvious etiology is evident. Nonbacterial epididymitis is much more common than bacterial inflammation. The clinical presentation of epididymitis may be indolent or acute, as with torsion. Fever often accompanies bacterial epididymitis, and the urinary sediment may reflect infection. Examination of the

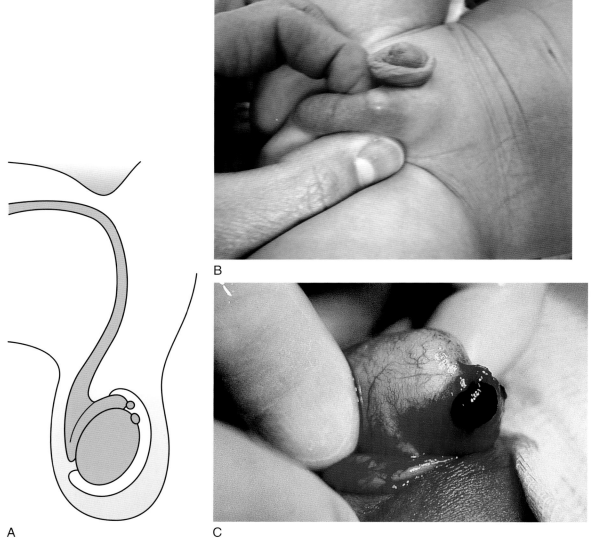

Figure 14-42. A, Torsion of appendix testis or epididymis. **B,** Examination of the left hemiscrotum in a case of torsion of the appendix testis reveals a "blue dot" sign. **C,** Operative findings after torsion of an appendix epididymis.

scrotum in early stages demonstrates a tender, slightly swollen epididymis (Fig. 14-43), but later the entire scrotal contents are replaced by an inflammatory mass. The cremasteric reflex is present, and elevation of the testis on the pubis may relieve pain (Prehn sign). A radionuclide scan or color Doppler examination demonstrates increased blood flow. Ultrasound may show an enlarged epididymis. If torsion of the spermatic cord cannot be excluded, surgical exploration must be carried out promptly. All children with bacterial epididymitis should undergo complete upper and lower urinary tract radiographic evaluation after resolution of the acute process. Scrotal abscess formation may result from bacterial epididymitis. Nonbacterial epididymitis is treated expectantly. Administration of nonsteroidal anti-inflammatory medication and limitation of activity including bedrest for 48 hours in cases with severe scrotal swelling usually results in rapid improvement of clinical symptoms.

Undescended Testes

See the earlier discussion in "Physical Examination."

Chronic Scrotal Swelling

Varicocele

A varicocele consists of dilated veins of the pampiniform plexus of the spermatic cord (Fig. 14-44). Varicoceles occur primarily on the left side and may be found before puberty. They may be bilateral. The postulated causes of varicocele vary from hormonal to hydrostatic. The postulated cause of testicular injury from varicocele varies from hormonal deficiencies to temperature effects. Most varicoceles decompress in the supine position. Those that do not decompress or those that present with acute onset on either side may lead to concern about lesions in the kidney or retroperitoneum causing obstruction to venous outflow. Most varicoceles are asymptomatic and are noted by the child incidentally or discovered on routine examination. Pain secondary to varicocele is uncommon, but a dull aching may occur in large varicoceles.

Infertility is found in approximately 33% of adults with varicoceles, and because semen analyses are not generally available in children, controversy has arisen over the proper management of adolescents. Ablating varicoceles in adolescents with testicular growth failure ipsilateral to

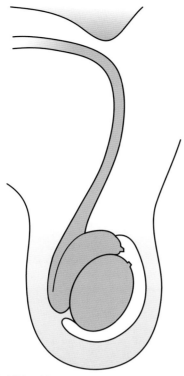

Figure 14-43. Epididymitis.

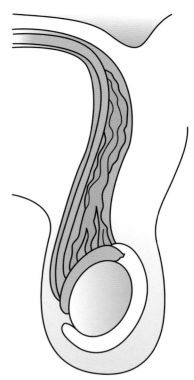

Figure 14-44. Varicocele.

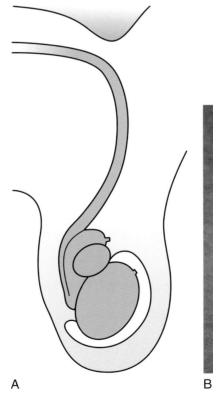

Figure 14-45. Spermatocele **(A)** and operative appearance of large spermatocele **(B).**

A

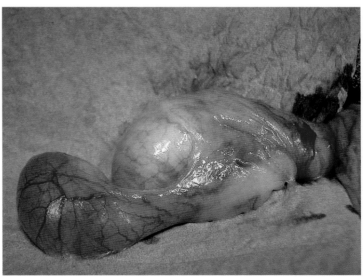

B

the varicocele, or in those with bilateral varicocele, is common practice. In patients with minimal or no testicular atrophy, observation and serial measurements of testicular volume are indicated, with the option to perform varicocele ablation if ipsilateral testicular growth failure becomes evident.

Spermatocele

Spermatoceles or epididymal cysts are common in adolescents. They are painless cystic masses located in the epididymis (commonly in the upper pole) (Fig. 14-45). They vary in size but are usually less than 1 cm in diameter. They are mobile, transilluminate, and do not vacillate in size, although gradual enlargement may occur. Ultrasound examination may be helpful if the diagnosis is in doubt. Spermatoceles contain sperm dand are essentially retention cysts of the epididymis or tubules of the rete testis. Excision is not usually recommended in routine symptomatic cases but may be appropriate for painful or enlarging cysts.

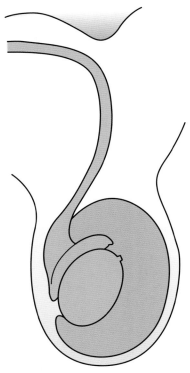

Figure 14-46. Hydrocele.

Hydrocele

Hydroceles are fluid accumulations within the tunica vaginalis or processus vaginalis (Fig. 14-46). They may be small or large, are usually painless even if they are large, and may be tense enough to obscure palpation of the testis. They transilluminate. Simple scrotal hydroceles are common in neonates and usually resolve spontaneously over several months. When examining an infant with huge hydrocele, examination of the lower abdomen should be performed to rule out the presence of an abdomino-scrotal hydrocele. The presence of an abdominoscrotal hydrocele may be noted if compression of the scrotal hydrocele causes enlargement of a lower quadrant mass. Ultrasound may confirm this finding. Large hydroceles may present in adolescence without an obvious etiology. In adolescent cases when the testis cannot be palpated, an ultrasound examination should be done to verify that the testis is normal. If the processus vaginalis remains patent, a communicating hydrocele results and may present with periodic increase and decrease in scrotal size. In these cases, thickening of the inguinal spermatic cord may be noted. If a segment of processus vaginalis fails to obliterate, trapping fluid in midcord, a hydrocele of the cord may result. These may also communicate with the peritoneum through a patent processus vaginalis and thus may vacillate in size. When the diagnosis of an inguinal mass is uncertain, imaging (ultrasound or CT) or exploration may be warranted because soft tissue sarcomas may originate from spermatic cord and paratesticular tissues.

Testis Tumors

Malignant tumors of the testis may occur at all ages, from neonate to adulthood. Most testis tumors present as a firm, painless mass within the testis. Large masses may seem to replace the testicular parenchyma. The mass may be smooth or irregular to palpation. On occasion, a sudden enlargement of a tumor or bleeding within the tumor may

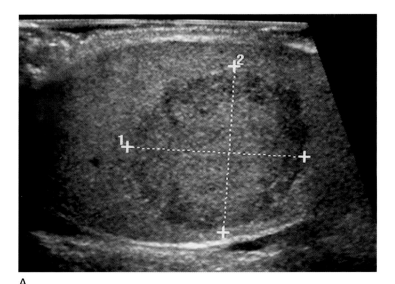

A

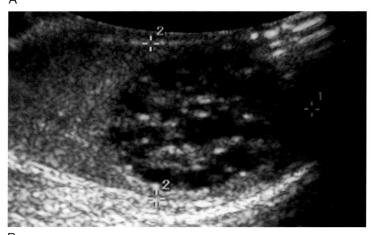

B

Figure 14-47. Testis tumor. **A** and **B**, Ultrasound examination of two patients with palpable testis tumors.

cause a painful, rapid enlargement of the involved testis. Solid masses within the substance of the testis should be considered malignant until proven otherwise. Testicular ultrasound is helpful in the evaluation of testicular masses (Fig. 14-47).

Lesions of the Female Genitalia

Labial Hypertrophy

Rarely, hypertrophy of one or both labia majora may cause unilateral or bilateral prominence of the labial structure. Herniation of an ovary into the labium should be easily ruled out by physical examination. Vascular or lymphatic malformations must be ruled out in bilateral lesions, but many unilateral cases are idiopathic (Fig. 14-48). Resection of the hypertrophic tissue may be indicated when the lesion appears to be idiopathic.

Labial Adhesion (Fusion)

Labial adhesions (fusion) are common in the prepubertal age group. They represent fusion of the labia minora, postulated to be the result of inflammation of the thin

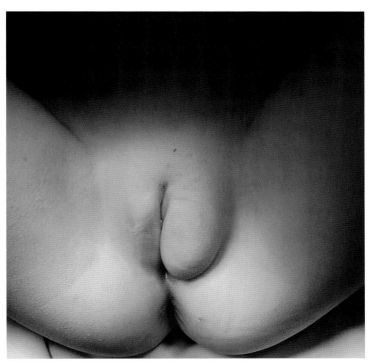

Figure 14-48. Idiopathic hypertrophy of left labium majus.

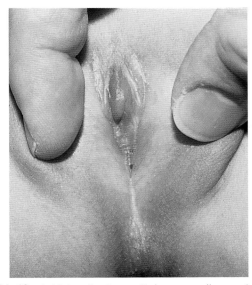

Figure 14-49. Labial adhesions. Only a small opening remains anteriorly.

labial mucosa that simply adheres in the midline. Fusion begins posteriorly and may progress until almost complete fusion results (Fig. 14-49). On inspection, the vaginal introitus may be closed with the exception of a small anterior opening. Severe fusion may be associated with dysuria, postvoid dribbling as the urine voided into the vagina drains out, or urinary tract infection. Although most adhesions lyse spontaneously as puberty approaches and the vaginal epithelium cornifies, problems of hygiene and discomfort bring many girls to the physician for evaluation and treatment.

Labial fusion must be separated mechanically. Lysis may be managed by parents at home, merely cleansing the introitus in an anterior-to-posterior motion, and applying a petroleum or other ointment to diminish mucosal irritation. Lysis can also be performed easily in the office: merely spreading the labia or mechanically separating the adhesions with an ointment-covered gloved finger will

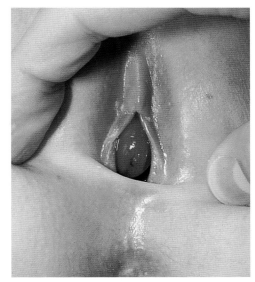

Figure 14-50. Urethral prolapse. This is a chronic case in which the initial hemorrhagic nature of the acute prolapse has resolved with observation, leaving a protuberant, edematous urethra.

usually suffice. No anesthetic should be necessary. Some practitioners feel that lysis should be followed by the application of estrogen cream to the area for several days to thicken the vaginal mucosa. Unfortunately, many physicians think that the mere application of estrogen will cure the problem. This is untrue. After lysis, simple hygiene should prevent recurrence.

Urethral Prolapse

Prolapse of the urethra occurs almost exclusively in black girls. Its cause is unknown. The presentation is usually bloody spotting, with occasional mild dysuria. Examination reveals a reddened or dark circumferential prolapse of the urethra with an otherwise normal introitus (Fig. 14-50).

Introital Polyps

Small polyps may originate from the urethral meatus or hymenal ring (Fig. 14-51). These usually are thin mucosal tags that cause no symptoms and require no specific treatment. Fleshy polyps or multiple polyps should be examined closely and biopsied to exclude malignancy such as sarcoma botryoides (see Chapter 11).

Prolapsed Ureterocele

Prolapse of a large ureterocele through the urethral orifice should be considered in the differential diagnosis of all interlabial masses in infants and children (Fig. 14-52). Ureteroceles are cystic dilations of the distal ureter, which are located in the bladder or urethra and may prolapse through the urethral meatus as reddened or even necrotic mucosal surfaces. A prolapsed ureterocele, unlike urethral prolapse, does not present a symmetrical orifice but rather presents an asymmetrical protrusion through the urethra. Catheterization alongside the prolapse may locate the lumen of the urethra. Prolapse of a ureterocele may be associated with a palpable distended bladder or flank mass (hydronephrosis). Ultrasonography of the bladder and

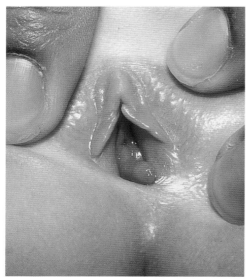

Figure 14-51. Introital polyp. A small polyp of the posterior vaginal fourchette.

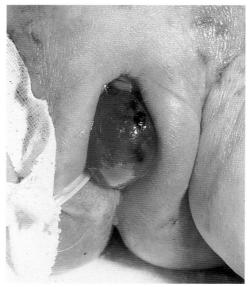

Figure 14-52. Prolapsed ureterocele. The catheter enters the urethra.

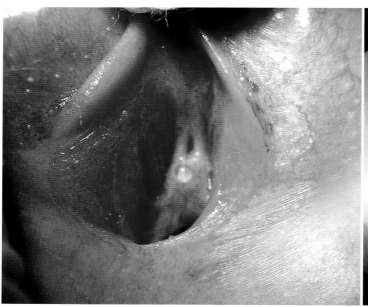

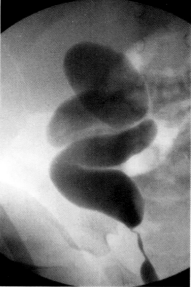

Figure 14-53. Ectopic ureter. **A,** A drop of urine exits from the orifice of an ectopic ureter located just below the urethral meatus in the urethrovaginal septum. **B,** Retrograde pyelography of the same ureter reveals a huge, tortuous ureter subtending the upper pole of a right complete ureteral duplication. Heminephrectomy cured the patient's incontinence.

A

B

kidneys demonstrates unilateral or bilateral hydronephrosis or hydronephrosis of a segment of a complete ureteral duplication, usually the upper pole of an obstructed renal unit. Voiding cystourethrography with intravenous urography or radionuclide studies and occasionally direct puncture of the ureterocele with contrast injection may be appropriate to define the anatomy of the malformation.

Ectopic Ureter

Ureteral ectopia may be associated with a single collecting system or a complete duplication of the collecting system (complete ureteral duplication). In females, an ectopic ureter may drain into the bladder neck, urethra, urethrovaginal septum, vagina, or uterus. Girls with ectopic ureter into the urethra, urethrovaginal septum, or vagina may have a normal voiding pattern but with a continuous dribbling incontinence of small amounts of urine. In some of these girls, a tiny ectopic ureter may be seen to drip urine from the introitus (Fig. 14-53).

Paraurethral Cysts

Cystic lesions of the paraurethral or vaginal mucosa may be found on routine examination and are usually asymptomatic. They rarely cause voiding symptoms and occasionally present in older girls as palpable interlabial masses. Normal mucosa overlies the cyst, which usually displaces the urethral meatus slightly from the midline. Most cysts rupture spontaneously, but aspiration or marsupialization may be necessary (Fig. 14-54).

Congenital Obstruction of the Vagina

Vaginal obstruction may occur as a result of an imperforate hymen, vaginal atresia or septa, or urogenital sinus malformation. Fusion anomalies of the müllerian structures may result in a septate vagina or bicornuate uterus with one obstructed segment. Neonates may have abdominal masses or urinary retention; girls with didelphic or bicornuate uterus may have pelvic pain or menstrual irregularities at puberty. Examination of the infant may reveal a distended vagina (hydrometrocolpos) with a bulging hymenal membrane. If a vaginal septum or atresia is the cause of the obstruction, external genital examination may be normal and a complete pelvic examination with vaginoscopy may be necessary. Ultrasonography of the pelvis may be helpful, but pelvic CT or MRI scan may give the most anatomic information (Fig. 14-55). All girls with uterine or vaginal anomalies should have imaging of the upper urinary tract given the high incidence of upper tract anomalies in this group. As a corollary, girls with proven unilateral renal agenesis should be followed through puberty for the development of müllerian anomalies, commonly uterus didelphys with an obstructed uni-

lateral uterine horn or vagina ipsilateral to the side of the absent kidney. Pelvic ultrasound examination in the peri-pubertal period is a good way to follow these girls.

Ambiguous Genitalia

Human genitalia begin as undifferentiated structures that early in gestation are identical in both sexes. The combined effects of genetic, hormonal, and local influences modify the structure and function of the genitalia to produce genital structures appropriate to the gender of the individual (see Chapter 9). When abnormal development occurs, genitalia of indeterminate nature may result. The recognition of abnormal genitalia is the first step in the evaluation of intersex. The combination of hypospadias and bilateral or unilateral cryptorchidism should be considered as representative of intersex until proven otherwise. Examination of the genitalia in suspected intersex cases should include assessment of phallic length and diameter; presence or absence of gonads and their size; assessment of labioscrotal and perineal anatomy; rectal examination; ultrasonography, MRI or CT of the pelvis; and flush genitogram (urethrogram) to delineate urethral or vaginal structures. A full genetic and endocrine evaluation should be carried out as well (Fig. 14-56).

Genital Ambiguity Associated with Imperforate Anus

The embryologic deformity that produces a high imperforate anus in girls occasionally also influences the formation of the external genitalia by presumed local factors. The end result may be genitalia that appear to be masculinized (Fig. 14-57).

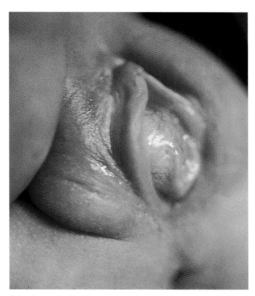

Figure 14-54. Paraurethral cyst.

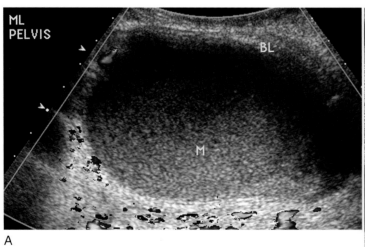

A

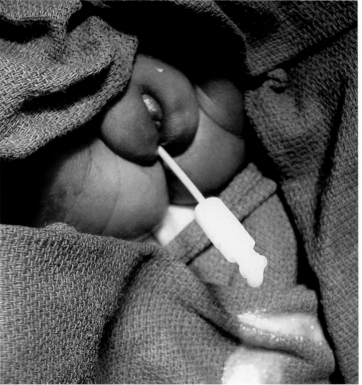

B

Figure 14-55. Hydrometrocolpos. **A,** Sagittal ultrasound of the pelvis in a neonate with a large pelvic hydrometrocolpos secondary to distal vaginal atresia. "M" delineates the mass (hydrometrocolpos), and "BL" defines the anteriorly displaced and compressed bladder. **B,** Catheter drainage of released white mucoid drainage, with disappearance of the pelvic mass.

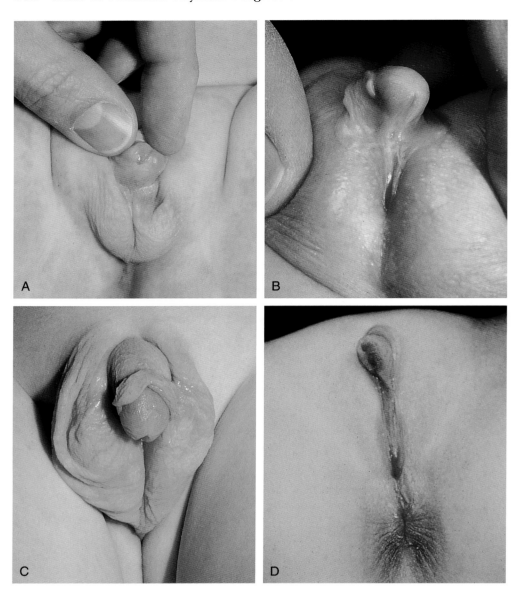

Figure 14-56. Various causes of genital ambiguity. **A,** Congenital adrenal hyperplasia. **B,** Mixed gonadal dysgenesis. **C,** True hermaphrodism. **D,** Posteriorly displaced urogenital sinus.

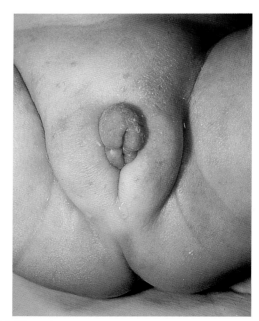

Figure 14-57. Ambiguous genitalia in a girl with a high imperforate anus.

Genital Trauma

Injury to the genitalia may be the result of minimal trauma or may be a part of multiple trauma. Although genital trauma may not be life threatening, proper management may be important to the later well-being and psychosocial development of the patient. This is particularly important in children. Trauma to the penis or scrotum should always raise the question of urethral injury (Fig. 14-58A). This is easily ruled out in the emergency department or x-ray department by injecting contrast (intravenous contrast in case of extravasation into vascular structures) through the urethral meatus, using a blunt-tipped syringe or a small catheter. Once urethral injury has been excluded, urethral catheterization can be performed safely. Scrotal trauma mandates critical evaluation of the testes. Scrotal ultrasound may be necessary to rule out testicular rupture or laceration. When injury is discovered, examination and repair should be performed in the operating room (Fig. 14-58B and C). Scrotal and testicular trauma is not uncommon in breech delivery, when the scrotum is the presenting part. Prompt urologic assessment should be sought. Ultrasound examination of the testes may be helpful if massive edema or hematoma precludes thorough examination. If injury is suspected, surgi-

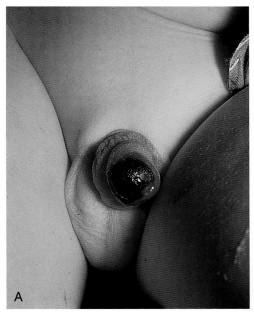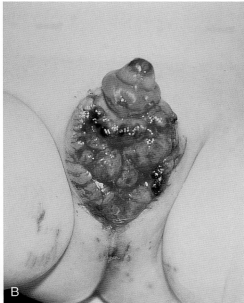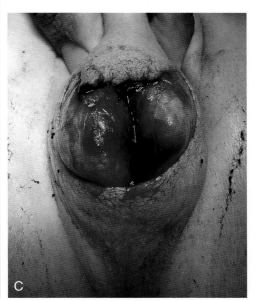

Figure 14-58. Genital trauma. **A,** Trauma to the glans penis from a falling toilet seat. A common injury that is usually best served by observation unless the urethra is disrupted. **B,** Perineal trauma. The testes were injured, but the urethra was intact. **C,** Scrotal trauma. The testicular tunics were intact, and primary skin closure produced an excellent result.

cal exploration is the most conservative approach. Trauma to the female genitalia and perineum usually requires examination under anesthesia to allow a complete evaluation of the injury, with concomitant repair when necessary.

Bibliography

Belman AB, Kaplan GW: Genitourinary Problems in Pediatrics. Philadelphia, WB Saunders, 1981.

Gillenwater JY, Grayhack JT, Howards SS, Mitchell ME (eds): Adult and Pediatric Urology. Philadelphia, Lippincott Williams & Wilkins, 2002.

Lee PA, Mazur T, Danish R, et al: Micropenis. I: Criteria, etiologies, and classification. Johns Hopkins Med J 146:156-163, 1980.

Walsh PC, Retik AB, Vaughan ED, Wein AJ (eds): Campbell's Urology. Philadelphia, WB Saunders, 2002.

Williams DI, Johnston JH (eds): Paediatric Urology. London, Butterworth, 1982.

CHAPTER 15

Neurology

RAJIV VARMA, SHELLEY D. WILLIAMS,
AND HENRY B. WESSEL

Neurologic Examination

The primary objective of the neurologic examination is to assess the functional integrity of the central nervous system (CNS) and the peripheral nervous system (PNS) and to detect and localize any sites of neurologic dysfunction. Techniques and interpretation of the pediatric neurologic examination are based largely on knowledge of normal growth and development. The examination is preceded by a thorough history of the presenting problem including timing and mode of onset; course; and a past medical history that focuses on the antenatal, perinatal, and neonatal periods for possible prior insults (e.g., bleeding, infection, hypoxia, drugs, trauma). Abnormalities of birthweight; the need for resuscitation after delivery; early neonatal problems with hypoglycemia, hypocalcemia, or severe jaundice; and abnormalities in activity or difficulty feeding shortly after birth often serve as red flags. This is followed by a detailed history of behavior; growth and development with attention to evidence of delay, slowing, cessation, or regression of developmental milestones; and any possible association with prior illness or trauma. Obtaining a family history of neurologic, neuromuscular, or developmental problems is also important.

The traditional systematic neurologic evaluation proceeds from assessment of mental status and language functions through evaluation of cranial nerves, gross motor function, muscle strength, gait and station, balance and coordination, sensory systems, and deep tendon reflexes. It is applicable to older children and adolescents without significant modification from the evaluation geared to the adult. Tools essential to the neurologist include the reflex hammer, bright penlight, ophthalmoscope, and stethoscope. For evaluation of the primary sensory modalities of light touch, pain, temperature, and vibration, wisps of cotton, sterile disposable pins, glass test tubes (to hold hot and cold water), and a tuning fork (256 Hz for children and young adults, 126 Hz for older persons) are used. A collection of small, common objects (e.g., coins, buttons, keys) to be identified by feel alone are useful for assessment of cortical sensations of stereognosis. Derangements of primary sensory function may be present with lesions at the level of the nerve roots, plexuses, or peripheral nerves. If a particular area of decreased sensation is identified in part of a limb, careful delineation of its boundaries often suggests root (dermatomal), plexus, or peripheral nerve involvement (Fig. 15-1A and B).

Neurologic examination of the younger child requires flexibility and a gentle, staged approach. The first stage consists of observation, much of which can be done while taking the history as the infant sits in the parent's lap or while the toddler or older child plays with toys. The child's level of alertness and interest in people and the environment are assessed. Facies, head shape, body habitus, spontaneous movements, position, and posture are noted, along with spontaneous vocalizations and quality and pitch of cry in infants. In the child old enough to walk, stance and gait, as well as the ability to run, stoop and recover, climb onto a stool, and rise from the floor (when developmentally appropriate) are observed. These observations provide a good general impression of the child's developmental level and abilities.

Much of the remainder of the neurologic examination also lends itself to play, and in stage 2 a more detailed assessment of mental status, language, handedness, and fine and gross motor skills is performed by engaging the child in play. A selection of rattles, keys, spinning and mechanical toys, dolls, cars, small blocks, noise makers, tennis balls, hand puppets, crayons, and picture books supplement the traditional instruments. If further observation of gait is necessary, the examiner can have the child walk to or with the parent. Children older than 4 years of age love to show what they can do when asked to walk on their heels or toes, hop, or do tandem gait along a line. Pat-a-cake games are popular for testing rapidly alternating movements with young children. Then with the child comfortable and rapport established, the hands-on examination is initiated with the child still dressed and in the parent's lap. Trying to catch the otoscope light as it is shown over various parts of the body can precede following the light with the eyes and looking at it. For infants and toddlers, following a face or spinning toy is still better for testing extraocular movements (Fig. 15-2). Having a parent jingle keys at the child's eye level and asking the child to look at the sound while looking in the child's eyes assists the ophthalmoscopic examination in older preschool and young school-age children (Fig. 15-3). Asking young children to make faces, stick out their tongues, and blow up balloons are other helpful techniques in assessing cranial nerves.

Tone is assessed by observing resistance to passive motion. Then active motion and motion against resistance are checked. Older preschoolers and school-age children love showing their muscles, and push-pull games can be used to test muscle strength, especially when the child's efforts are admired. Deep tendon reflexes can often be tested at this time with only the shoes off. These are normally brisk, or 3+, in the young infant, becoming 2+ by 6 months of age. If directly tapping on the tendon seems upsetting to the child, it may help to place a finger over the tendon to be percussed and tap that. In infants and toddlers, it is often easier to elicit the ankle jerk by placing a finger over the ball of the child's foot and gently dorsiflexing it before percussing the Achilles tendon (Fig. 15-4). Preschoolers and young children love having the examiner express surprise and pleasure when reflexes are elicited.

Finally the parent is asked to help undress the child, and the remainder of the examination proceeds with the parent providing reassurance and assistance as needed. During this stage, head circumference is measured in the infant and toddler, and the head, midline of the neck and back, and skin are carefully examined for abnormalities. Muscles are inspected for symmetry, and extremity circumference is measured a set distance from a bony landmark if asymmetry is suspected, and abnormal muscle movements are noted. The appropriate disappearance or persistence of primitive reflexes is determined in infants (see Chapter 3). The Babinski reflex is difficult to elicit and interpret during the first year because stroking the sole of the foot may simply stimulate withdrawal or plantar flexion. Using the Oppenheim technique—running the thumb down the medial surface of the tibia—gives a more interpretable response (Fig. 15-5). Evaluation of sensation

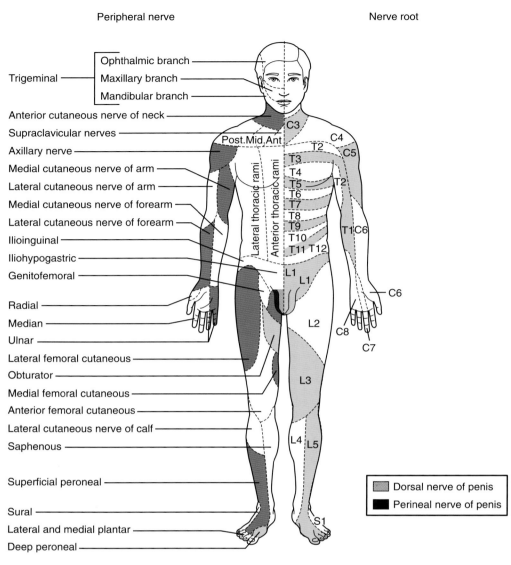

Peripheral nerve

Nerve root

Trigeminal
- Ophthalmic branch
- Maxillary branch
- Mandibular branch

Anterior cutaneous nerve of neck

Supraclavicular nerves

Axillary nerve

Medial cutaneous nerve of arm

Lateral cutaneous nerve of arm

Medial cutaneous nerve of forearm

Lateral cutaneous nerve of forearm

Ilioinguinal

Iliohypogastric

Genitofemoral

Radial

Median

Ulnar

Lateral femoral cutaneous

Obturator

Medial femoral cutaneous

Anterior femoral cutaneous

Lateral cutaneous nerve of calf

Saphenous

Superficial peroneal

Sural

Lateral and medial plantar

Deep peroneal

Post. Mid. Ant

Lateral thoracic rami

Anterior thoracic rami

C3 C4 C5 T2 T3 T4 T5 T6 T7 T8 T9 T10 T11 T12 L1 L1 L2 L3 L4 L5 C6 C7 C8 T1 C6 S1

Dorsal nerve of penis
Perineal nerve of penis

Figure 15-1. Cutaneous sensory innervation. The segmental or dermatomal (nerve root) distribution is shown on the left side of the body, and the peripheral nerve distribution on the right side of the body. **A,** Anterior view.

A

is difficult in the younger child and is generally limited to appreciation of light touch and pin prick. These may be assessed with minimal discomfort using a partially unbent paper clip.

Neurologic examination of the newborn is highly specialized. The essential components of the neonatal examination include assessment of gestational age, growth patterns, dysmorphic features, motor tone, postures, spontaneous activity, cry, respiratory patterns, brainstem reflexes, response to bright light, response to noxious stimuli, developmental reflexes, and deep tendon reflexes (see Chapter 2). Normal findings vary with gestational age. The immaturity of the newborn's CNS, with functioning largely at a subcortical reflex level, may conceal all but the most severe neurologic deficits—hence the often deceptively normal examination of the newborn with hydranencephaly.

The most prevalent neurologic disorders in childhood are related to CNS infection, ingestions, congenital malformations, perinatal insults, trauma (including abuse), progressive neurodegenerative or neuromuscular processes, and metabolic disorders. This chapter concentrates on selected neurologic disorders accompanied by physical signs that can be detected on visual inspection.

Neurocutaneous Syndromes

The neurocutaneous syndromes or phakomatoses are congenital, often inherited disorders with prominent cutaneous and neurologic manifestations. The simultaneous involvement of the skin and nervous system, both derivatives of embryonic ectoderm, suggests that these disorders may be caused by an unknown abnormality of the embryonic epiblast. Although the clinical and pathologic features of the phakomatoses are diverse, these syndromes share a propensity for malformations and hamartomatous tumors of multiple organs. Among the more frequently encountered phakomatoses are neurofibromatosis, tuberous sclerosis, Sturge-Weber syndrome, ataxia-telangiectasia, and linear sebaceous nevus.

Neurofibromatosis 1

Neurofibromatosis 1, or NF-1 (previously known as von Recklinghausen disease), is the most common of the neurocutaneous syndromes and affects about 1 in 3000 individuals. Although usually inherited as an autosomal

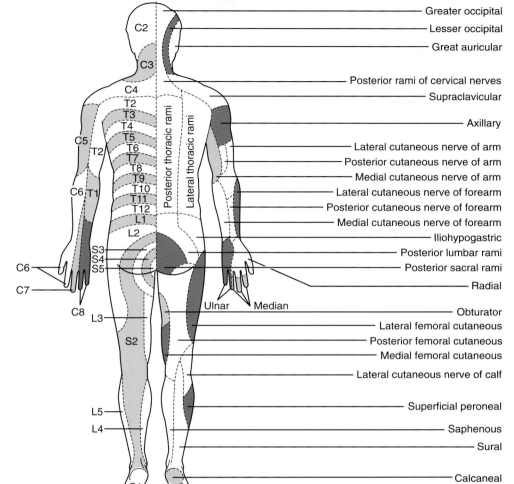

Nerve root

Peripheral nerve

Greater occipital
Lesser occipital
Great auricular
Posterior rami of cervical nerves
Supraclavicular
Axillary
Lateral cutaneous nerve of arm
Posterior cutaneous nerve of arm
Medial cutaneous nerve of arm
Lateral cutaneous nerve of forearm
Posterior cutaneous nerve of forearm
Medial cutaneous nerve of forearm
Iliohypogastric
Posterior lumbar rami
Posterior sacral rami
Radial
Obturator
Lateral femoral cutaneous
Posterior femoral cutaneous
Medial femoral cutaneous
Lateral cutaneous nerve of calf
Superficial peroneal
Saphenous
Sural
Calcaneal
Lateral plantar
Medial plantar

Ulnar   Median

Figure 15-1 cont'd. B, Posterior view. (Modified from Simon RP, Aminoff MJ, Greenberg DA: Clinical Neurology, 4th ed. Stamford, Conn., Appleton & Lange, 1999.)

B

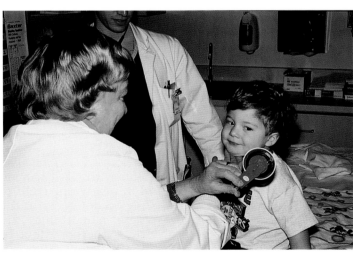

Figure 15-2. Testing extraocular motion. Older infants and toddlers tend to be captivated by spinning or sparkling toys and readily follow the objects, making it easy to test such motion.

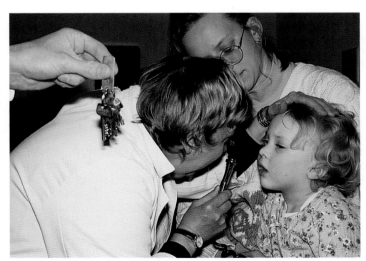

Figure 15-3. Ophthalmoscopic examination. Having a parent hold and jingle keys at the child's eye level and asking the patient to look at the sound enhances the child's ability to focus, assisting good visualization of the retina in young children.

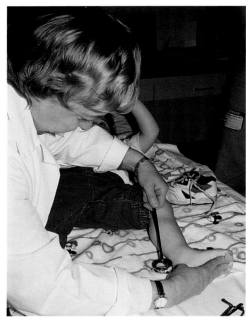

Figure 15-4. Achilles reflex. Gently dorsiflexing the foot before percussing the Achilles tendon makes it easier to elicit this reflex.

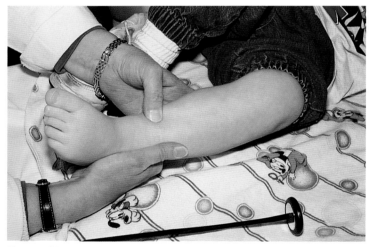

Figure 15-5. Oppenheim technique for checking the Babinski response. Running the thumb down the medial surface of the tibia produces a more interpretable response in infants and toddlers because it avoids stimulation of a plantar flexion or withdrawal response.

Table 15-1	Diagnostic Criteria for Neurofibromatosis 1 (NF-1)

Diagnostic criteria are met if two or more of the following are found:

- Six or more café-au-lait macules >5 mm in greatest diameter in prepubertal children and >15 mm in greatest diameter in postpubertal individuals
- Two or more neurofibromas of any type or one plexiform neurofibroma
- Axillary or inguinal freckling
- Optic glioma
- Two or more Lisch nodules (iris hamartomas)
- A distinctive osseous lesion such as a sphenoid dysplasia or thinning of long bone cortex with or without pseudarthrosis
- A first-degree relative (i.e., parent, sibling, or child) with NF-1, according to these criteria

dominant disorder, up to 50% of cases may be sporadic (i.e., the result of new mutations). The *NF1* gene has been localized to chromosome 17q. Neurofibromin, its gene product, acts as a tumor suppressor, and its function is altered in affected patients. Characteristic clinical manifestations include multiple hyperpigmented skin macules (café-au-lait spots), axillary or inguinal freckling, multiple skin neurofibromas, and iris hamartomas (Lisch nodules). Associated abnormalities may include optic gliomas; other CNS tumors of glial or meningeal origin; neurofibromas of spinal or peripheral nerves; pheochromocytoma, macrocephaly, cognitive impairment; and bony abnormalities. Diagnostic criteria for NF-1 are summarized in Table 15-1.

Multiple café-au-lait spots, the most frequently encountered cutaneous abnormality, are brown hyperpigmented macules with smooth margins, usually most numerous over the trunk (Fig. 15-6A and see Fig. 8-131A-C). Other abnormalities of cutaneous pigmentation may include axillary or inguinal freckling or extensive areas of hyperpigmentation (Fig. 15-6B and C). Hyperpigmented skin lesions almost always precede neurologic symptoms and often increase in size and number with advancing age. They are not necessarily present at birth and may be inconspicuous in early childhood, becoming more prominent at puberty. Ninety-seven percent of NF-1 patients have at least five café-au-lait spots by 20 years of age.

Although multiple café-au-lait spots are a clinical hallmark of NF-1, they may also occur as an autosomal dominant trait unassociated with the other features of neurofibromatosis. Genetic investigations in such families have excluded linkage to the NF-1 locus on chromosome 17, indicating a distinctly different genetic association. Multiple café-au-lait spots can be found, as well, in a variety of other conditions (Table 15-2). They are a prominent feature of McCune-Albright syndrome, the additional manifestations of which include skeletal dysplasia and endocrine abnormalities. Those seen in McCune-Albright syndrome are often large and have irregular ("coast of Maine") margins (see Fig. 8-131D), in contrast with the smooth ("coast of California") borders characteristic of the hyperpigmented lesions of NF-1. Café-au-lait spots also may be encountered in tuberous sclerosis and neurofibromatosis 2 (NF-2) but are seldom prominent. They are present in about 10% of the general population (typically four or less in number) and are not by themselves a sign of disease.

Additional cutaneous manifestations of NF-1 may include extensive plexiform neuromas at the terminal distribution of nerve fibers (Fig. 15-7 and see Fig. 8-81) or small subcutaneous nodules—neurofibromas—scattered along the course of nerve trunks (Fig. 15-8).

Pigmented hamartomas of the iris, termed *Lisch nodules,* are seen in more than 90% of patients with NF-1 who are older than age 6 and can be found in nearly one third of younger individuals (Fig. 15-9). They do not occur in the normal population. Although these hamartomas are asymptomatic and do not correlate with the extent or severity of other manifestations, they are helpful in establishing the diagnosis.

Short stature and macrocephaly are common in NF-1 patients, and skeletal abnormalities are found in 51% (Fig. 15-10). The characteristic findings include the following:

1. Severe angular scoliosis with dysplasia of the vertebral bodies (Fig. 15-10A)
2. Defects of the posterior-superior wall of the orbit

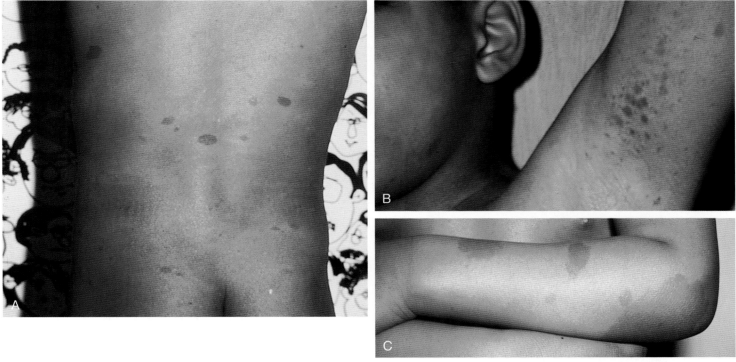

Figure 15-6. Neurofibromatosis 1 (NF-1). Clinical manifestations of cutaneous pigmentary abnormalities. **A,** Most common are multiple café-au-lait spots over the trunk. **B** and **C,** Also seen are axillary freckling and extensive areas of hyperpigmentation. (Courtesy Michael Sherlock, MD, Lutherville, Md.)

Table 15-2 Conditions Associated with Café-au-lait Lesions

DISORDER	CLINICAL FEATURES
Neurofibromatosis	Most common in NF-1, rare in NF-2 (see sections on NF-1 and NF-2 and Table 15-3)
Tuberous sclerosis	See Table 15-4
McCune-Albright syndrome	Polyostotic fibrous dysplasia, precocious puberty, endocrine dysfunction
Watson syndrome	Features of Noonan syndrome (webbed neck, hypertelorism with antimongoloid slant, low-set ears, pulmonic stenosis, low intelligence), plus meets criteria for NF-1
Epidermal nevus syndrome	Verrucous skin lesions, scoliosis, aortic coarctation, mental retardation
Bloom syndrome	Severe intrauterine and postnatal growth retardation, photosensitivity, telangiectatic erythema of cheeks/face
Ataxia-telangiectasia	Ataxia, conjunctival telangiectasia, recurrent sinopulmonary infections
Silver syndrome	Intrauterine growth retardation, hemihypertrophy, syndactyly, triangular facies, premature sexual development
Gaucher disease	Opisthotonos, splenomegaly, cranial nerve dysfunction, regression of motor milestones
Turner syndrome	Short stature, webbed neck, coarctation of aorta, delayed puberty
Fanconi anemia	Aplastic anemia, hyperpigmentation, short stature, mental retardation, congenital anomalies of bone, heart, eye, kidney
Multiple lentigines (LEOPARD) syndrome	Multiple small lentigines, hypertelorism, pulmonic stenosis, cryptorchidism, mild growth retardation, sensorineural deafness

3. Congenital bowing and thinning of the cortices of long bones and pseudarthrosis of the tibia, fibula (Fig. 15-10B and see Fig. 8-131B), femur, or clavicle (see Fig. 6-77)
4. Disorders of bone growth associated with elephantoid hypertrophy of overlying soft tissue
5. Erosive bony defects produced by contiguous neurogenic tumors
6. Scalloping of the posterior margins of the vertebral bodies corresponding to saccular areas of dilation of the spinal meninges (Fig. 15-10C)

Patients with NF-1 can be affected with various tumors of the brain, spinal cord, and peripheral nerves, although with a much lesser frequency than in patients with NF-2. Optic nerve glioma is the most common CNS tumor and affects 15% of NF-1 patients. It often presents as progressive visual loss with optic atrophy and tends to be less aggressive than in patients without NF-1. Ependymo-

mas, meningiomas, and astrocytomas also have been reported.

Magnetic resonance imaging (MRI) scans frequently show areas of increased signal intensity on T2-weighted images of the globus pallidus, brainstem, or cerebellar white matter (Fig. 15-11). Believed to represent hamartomas, these regions of abnormal signal intensity do not appear to correlate with neurologic dysfunction. However, their presence helps confirm the diagnosis of NF-1. Computed tomography (CT) seldom demonstrates corresponding abnormalities.

Learning disabilities and behavior problems are common and may affect up to 40% of NF-1 patients. Although their full-scale intelligence quotient is generally lower than the general population, severe mental retardation is rare. Approximately 10% of NF-1 patients have seizures.

A small percentage of NF-1 patients have dysplasia of the renal or carotid arteries. Renal artery stenosis can

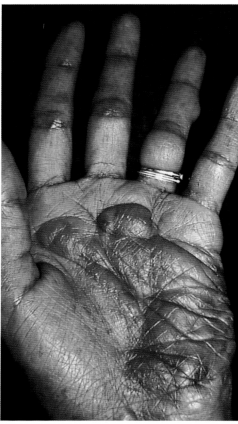

Figure 15-7. Neurofibromatosis 1 (NF-1). Extensive plexiform neurofibroma of the palm. (Courtesy Michael Sherlock, MD, Lutherville, Md.)

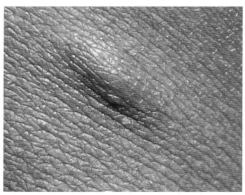

Figure 15-8. Neurofibromatosis 1 (NF-1). Subcutaneous neurofibroma along the course of a nerve trunk. (Courtesy of Michael Sherlock, MD, Lutherville, Md.)

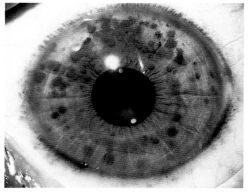

Figure 15-9. Neurofibromatosis 1 (NF-1). Pigmented hamartomas of the iris (Lisch nodules).

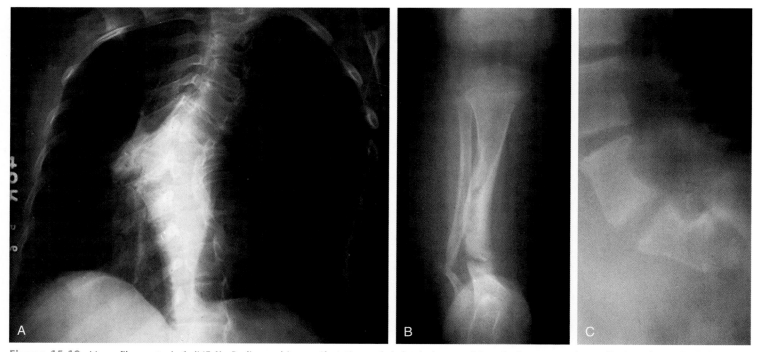

Figure 15-10. Neurofibromatosis 1 (NF-1). Radiographic manifestations of skeletal abnormalities. **A,** Severe angular scoliosis and vertebral dysplasia. **B,** Congenital bowing and pseudarthrosis of the tibia and fibula. **C,** Scalloping of the posterior margins of the vertebral bodies resulting from dural ectasia. (Courtesy Department of Radiology, Children's Hospital of Pittsburgh.)

cause systemic hypertension, and adult NF-1 patients may develop pheochromocytoma with concomitant hypertension. Cerebral artery dysplasia can include moyamoya syndrome with abnormal vessels of the circle of Willis, predisposing to cerebral infarction in children and cerebral hemorrhage in adults.

Neurofibromatosis 2

Neurofibromatosis 2, or NF-2 (also known as *bilateral acoustic neurofibromatosis*), is a distinct genetic disorder characterized by autosomal dominant inheritance of bilateral acoustic neuromas with a penetrance of more than

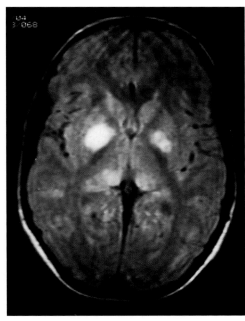

Figure 15-11. Neurofibromatosis 1 (NF-1). T2-weighted MRI demonstrates high signal-intensity areas in the region of the globus pallidus bilaterally. (Courtesy Division of Neuroradiology, University Health Center of Pittsburgh.)

Table 15-4	Diagnostic Criteria for Tuberous Sclerosis

Major Features
Facial angiofibromas or forehead plaque
Nontraumatic ungual or periungual fibroma
Hypomelanotic macules (i.e., ash-leaf spots [≥3])
Shagreen patch (connective tissue nevus)
Multiple retinal nodular hamartomas
Cortical tuber
Subependymal nodule
Subependymal giant cell astrocytoma
Cardiac rhabdomyoma, single or multiple
Lymphangiomyomatosis
Renal angiomyolipoma

Minor Features
Multiple randomly distributed pits in dental enamel
Hamartomatous rectal polyps
Bone cysts
Cerebral white matter radial migration lines
Gingival fibromas
Nonrenal hamartoma
Retinal achromatic patch
"Confetti" skin lesions
Multiple renal cysts

Definite tuberous sclerosis: Two major features or one major and two minor features
Probable tuberous sclerosis: One major plus one minor feature
Possible tuberous sclerosis: Either one major feature or two or more minor features

Modified from Roach ES, Gometz MR, Northrup H: Tuberous Sclerosis Complex Consensus Conference: Revised clinical diagnostic criteria. J Child Neurol 13:624-628, 1998.

Table 15-3	Diagnostic Criteria for Neurofibromatosis 2 (NF-2)

- Bilateral eighth nerve masses seen with appropriate imaging techniques (e.g., CT, MRI) or
- A first-degree relative with NF-2 and a unilateral eighth nerve mass, or two of the following:
- Neurofibroma
- Meningioma
- Glioma
- Schwannoma
- Juvenile posterior subcapsular lens opacity

95%. NF-2 occurs in approximately 1 in 50,000 people. It results from a mutation of the *NF2* gene on the long arm of chromosome 22. The NF-2 gene product, merlin or schwannomin, serves to suppress tumor formation, and its dysfunction leads to the common occurrence of CNS tumors in NF-2 patients. Most patients eventually develop bilateral acoustic neuromas (vestibular schwannomas).

Symptoms usually first appear in the teens or early twenties, when pressure on the vestibulocochlear or facial nerve complex results in impaired auditory discrimination, hearing loss, tinnitus, unsteadiness, or facial weakness. Presenile lens opacities, found in half the patients examined, may precede the onset of symptoms referable to acoustic neuroma. Other Schwann cell tumors of cranial nerves, spinal roots, or the spinal cord, as well as multiple CNS tumors of meningeal or glial origin, may develop. Cutaneous manifestations such as café-au-lait spots, cutaneous neurofibromas, and axillary or inguinal freckling are less common in NF-2 than in NF-1, and Lisch nodules are not typical. Diagnostic criteria for NF-2 are summarized in Table 15-3.

Tuberous Sclerosis

Tuberous sclerosis (TS) is inherited as an autosomal dominant trait. Two genes appear to cause the disorder: *TSC1* located on chromosome 9q and *TSC2* on chromosome 16q. Their gene products (hamartin for *TSC1* and tuberin for *TSC2*) have tumor suppressor activity, which is dysfunctional in affected patients. Both genes produce similar phenotypes when expressed. Although 1 in 6000 to 9000 people in the population carry a *TS* gene, expression is highly variable and full expression of disease is seen in only 1 in 150,000 members of the population. Most carriers have hypopigmented macules (ash-leaf spots) as their only manifestation. Spontaneous mutation appears to account for the majority of newly diagnosed cases, and in up to 2% of patients without a positive family history, the disorder may be the result of germline mosaicism.

The more prominent features of this neurocutaneous disorder include seizures (96%), mental retardation (60%), intracranial calcification (49%), tumors of various organs (including the brain, heart, liver, and kidneys), and cutaneous lesions. Seizures are the most frequent presenting complaint. Clinical expression can be quite variable even among affected members of the same family. Diagnostic criteria are summarized in Table 15-4.

The characteristic skin lesion of tuberous sclerosis is the angiofibroma *(adenoma sebaceum)*. These are seen as erythematous papules distributed over the nose and malar region of the face (Fig. 15-12). Approximately 40% of children with tuberous sclerosis demonstrate these lesions by 3 years of age.

Hypomelanotic macules with irregular borders, termed *ash-leaf spots,* are another common cutaneous manifestation (Fig. 15-13A and B). These generally appear earlier than adenoma sebaceum and may be present at birth. They are detectable by 2 years of age in more than half of affected children. They resemble vitiligo but differ in that they are not completely devoid of melanin. In fair-skinned infants, these nevi may be demonstrable only under Wood light.

Another valuable cutaneous marker is the *shagreen patch,* a plaque of thickened skin with a cobblestone or orange-

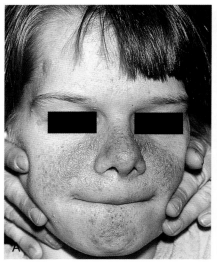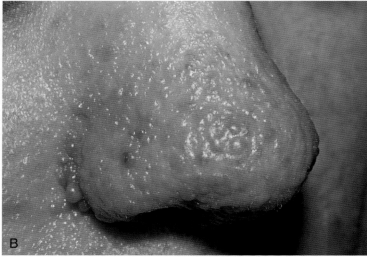

Figure 15-12. Tuberous sclerosis. **A,** This adolescent boy had adenoma sebaceum in a characteristic malar distribution and chin lesions as well. **B,** A closeup view of nasal lesions is shown.

peel texture often seen on the dorsal aspect of the trunk (Fig. 15-14). Histologically, the shagreen patch is a connective tissue nevus.

Additional dermatologic manifestations of tuberous sclerosis include periungual fibromas (Fig. 15-15) and macular areas of hyperpigmentation. Recognition of the cutaneous features can suggest an etiologic diagnosis in some patients with mental retardation or seizures. Oral examination may reveal pitting of dental enamel.

In patients with tuberous sclerosis, CT scans often demonstrate subependymal nodules seen as intracranial calcifications that appear as multiple scattered areas of increased density adjacent to the walls of the lateral and third ventricles (Fig. 15-16). CT is superior to MRI for demonstration of small calcifications. No relationship has been established between the extent of periventricular calcification and clinical severity as judged by developmental function or seizure frequency. CT may also demonstrate asymptomatic but typical intracranial calcifications in individuals who lack external manifestations of the disorder. This can help identify subclinical cases and improve the accuracy of genetic counseling in affected families.

The characteristic gross abnormality of the brain in TS is the presence of multiple gliotic nodules (hamartomas) of varying size, which constitute the tubers for which this disorder is named. These are located over the convolutions of the cerebral hemispheres and beneath the ependymal lining of the lateral and third ventricles. Heterotopic nodules of identical structure may be found in the cerebral white matter as well. Although cortical tubers are rarely apparent on CT scans, they are readily identified by MRI studies (Fig. 15-17). Severely affected patients have a greater number of cerebral cortical lesions detected by MRI scans, suggesting that MRI may be useful in predicting eventual clinical severity in young children with newly diagnosed tuberous sclerosis. Tumors may arise from cortical or subependymal tubers, complicating the course of the disease by producing increased intracranial pressure and other symptoms associated with intracranial mass lesions. Up to 80% of patients with tuberous sclerosis develop seizures of variable types that are often difficult to control. Infantile spasms are common and may be the presenting symptom leading to diagnosis. Patients with a history of infantile spasms and those who develop other types of seizures when very young tend to have more severe seizure disorders and poorer cognitive function.

Subependymal giant cell astrocytomas (Fig. 15-18) can affect 10% of tuberous sclerosis patients and are clinically manifested by symptoms of obstructive hydrocephalus. The site of obstruction is often at the level of the foramen of Monro in the lateral ventricles. Such patients may present with signs of increased intracranial pressure, behavior change, or worsening seizure control.

Visceral lesions associated with tuberous sclerosis include cardiac rhabdomyoma, renal angiomyolipomas, pulmonary lymphangiomyomatosis, and hepatic hamartoma. Cardiac rhabdomyomas occur in up to two thirds of patients and may be multiple. They tend to regress over the first few years of life and are usually asymptomatic, though occasionally an affected newborn may have obstructive congestive heart failure. About three fourths of tuberous sclerosis patients have renal angiomyolipomas, which are often bilateral and multiple. Most remain clinically silent, but tumors greater than 4 cm in size are more likely to be symptomatic and may cause hematuria or proteinuria. Renal disease is the most common cause of death in adults with the disease and may be manifest as flank pain, hematuria, or retroperitoneal hemorrhage. Renal cysts occur earlier and less often than do angiomyolipomas. Rarely, children with tuberous sclerosis can present in infancy with polycystic kidney disease. Chronic renal failure and malignant transformation of renal tumors are rare. Pulmonary lymphangiomyomatosis affects less than 2% of patients, mostly females, and is rare before the adult years. Symptoms include dyspnea, spontaneous pneumothorax, and hemoptysis. Hepatic hamartoma is clinically insignificant.

Sturge-Weber Syndrome

The cardinal manifestations of Sturge-Weber syndrome are as follows:
1. A vascular malformation or port-wine stain over the face that involves the cutaneous distribution of the ophthalmic division of the trigeminal nerve
2. Ipsilateral leptomeningeal angiomatosis with associated intracranial calcifications
3. A high incidence of mental retardation and ipsilateral ocular complications

The port-wine stain (Fig. 15-19) is usually present at birth and consists of a pink-to-purple macular cutaneous

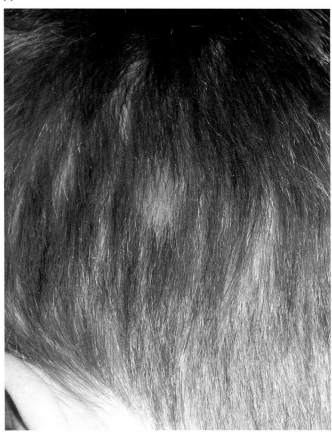

A

B

Figure 15-13. Tuberous sclerosis (TS). **A,** An ash-leaf spot is an oval depigmented nevus with irregular borders. **B,** This child with TS has numerous hypopigmented macules over his scalp, and the hair growing from these is hypopigmented as well (a phenomenon termed *poliosis*). (Courtesy Robin Gehris, MD, Children's Hospital of Pittsburgh.)

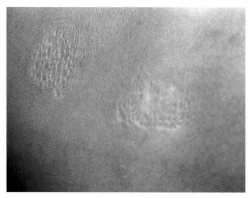

Figure 15-14. Tuberous sclerosis. Shagreen patch. This plaque of thickened skin with a cobblestone texture is distinctive but is one of the less common cutaneous manifestations. (Courtesy Michael Sherlock, MD, Lutherville, Md.)

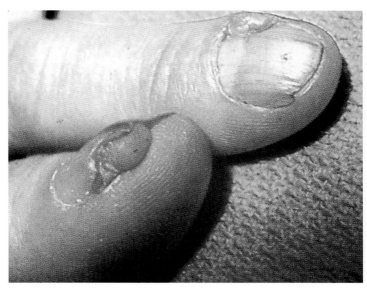

Figure 15-15. Tuberous sclerosis. Periungual fibromas. These nodular lesions can occur singly or multiply in the ungual or periungual areas. (Courtesy Michael Painter, MD, Children's Hospital of Pittsburgh.)

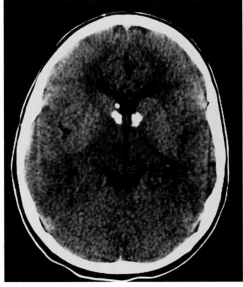

Figure 15-16. Tuberous sclerosis. This CT cut through the foramina of Monro shows the multiple periventricular calcific deposits characteristic of this disorder. (Courtesy Division of Neuroradiology, University Health Center of Pittsburgh.)

vascular malformation. Only patients with lesions involving the cutaneous distribution of the ophthalmic division of the trigeminal nerve (i.e., forehead and upper eyelid) are at risk for associated neuro-ocular complications (Fig. 15-20). Repeated ophthalmologic and CT examinations are indicated only in this high-risk group, which has a 10% to 20% incidence of associated intracranial angiomas.

The coincidence of seizures and a facial port-wine stain should suggest the diagnosis of Sturge-Weber syndrome, which can be confirmed by CT scan (Fig. 15-21). These scans may be normal at birth but subsequently show areas of gyriform contrast enhancement corresponding to the

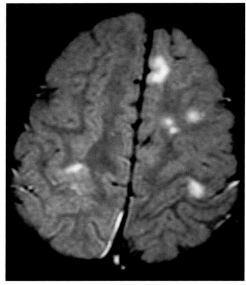

Figure 15-17. Tuberous sclerosis. MRI demonstrates multiple cortical tubers that appear as areas of increased signal intensity in this T2-weighted image. The signal abnormalities arise predominantly within the white matter subjacent to the tuber. (Courtesy Division of Neuroradiology, University Health Center of Pittsburgh.)

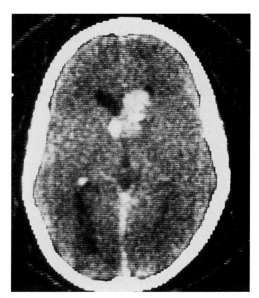

Figure 15-18. Tuberous sclerosis. CT scan demonstrates a large subependymal astrocytoma, which intermittently obstructed the ventricular system, producing episodic symptoms of increased intracranial pressure. (Courtesy Division of Neuroradiology, University Health Center of Pittsburgh.)

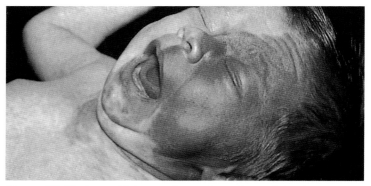

Figure 15-19. Sturge-Weber syndrome. A nonelevated purple cutaneous vascular malformation, often termed a port-wine stain, is seen in a trigeminal distribution, including the ophthalmic division.

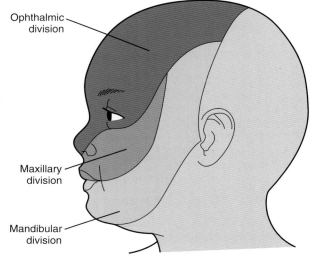

Ophthalmic division

Maxillary division

Mandibular division

Figure 15-20. Sturge-Weber syndrome. Cutaneous distribution of the division of the trigeminal nerve. Only patients with facial port-wine stains that involve the ophthalmic division are at risk for associated neuro-ocular symptoms.

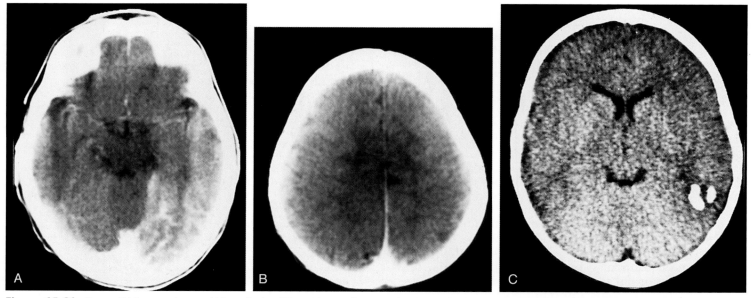

Figure 15-21. Sturge-Weber syndrome. Although the CT scan is usually normal at birth, findings such as gyriform contrast enhancement, seen here in the left occipital, temporal, and parietal lobes (A), and associated hemispheric atrophy (B) may be observed as early as 4 months of age. Serpiginous parenchymal calcifications may be found in the older child (C). (Courtesy Division of Neuroradiology, University Health Center of Pittsburgh.)

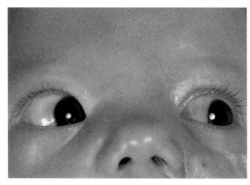

Figure 15-22. Buphthalmos. Enlargement of the cornea of the right eye is evident. This is one of the associated ocular findings in Sturge-Weber syndrome and should prompt urgent evaluation for associated glaucoma. (From Booth IW, Wozniak ER: Pediatrics. Baltimore, Williams & Wilkins, 1984.)

leptomeningeal angiomatosis. Serial examinations often demonstrate progressive ipsilateral cerebral atrophy. Additional findings may include serpiginous calcifications of brain parenchyma underlying vascular malformations of the pia. These intracranial calcifications are first seen on CT scan but become evident on plain skull films by the end of the second decade.

Associated ocular abnormalities are often encountered. Buphthalmos (corneal enlargement) or a coloboma may be present at birth, and glaucoma frequently develops in infancy or later childhood (Fig. 15-22). Dilated vessels in the sclera, conjunctiva, and retina are common, and angiomatous malformations of the choroid occasionally occur.

The estimated incidence of facial cutaneous angioma is 1 in 5000, and the estimated frequency of the complete syndrome is 1 in 30,000. Among patients with the complete syndrome, seizures occur in 90%, and contralateral hemiparesis eventually develops in one third. Early developmental milestones are often normal, but about 50% develop cognitive difficulties ranging from mild to severe. Behavioral problems are common. Patients with refractory epilepsy are more likely to be more severely delayed. Although most cases are sporadic, genetic determination has not been ruled out. No cases of direct transmission from parent to child have been reported, however.

Klippel-Trénaunay Syndrome

Patients with Klippel-Trénaunay syndrome (KTS) are born with a port-wine stain that is usually located over the lateral aspect of one leg. Less often an arm and a leg may be affected. In rare instances more extensive, even bilateral, involvement is seen. The surface lesion is associated with an underlying vascular malformation, which provides an unusually rich blood supply to soft tissue and bony structures that results in hypertrophy (usually hemihypertrophy) and lymphedema (Fig. 15-23A and B). These features are often evident in the newborn, and progressive enlargement occurs during the first few years. Most cases are sporadic. However, a few cases have been reported to be autosomal dominant.

Ataxia-Telangiectasia

Ataxia-telangiectasia is a multisystem, autosomal recessive degenerative disorder characterized by ataxia, oculocutaneous telangiectasia, immunodeficiency, and a high incidence of neoplasia. The nature of the basic underlying

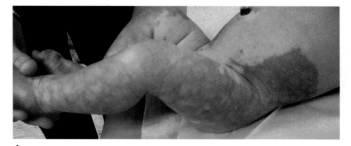

A

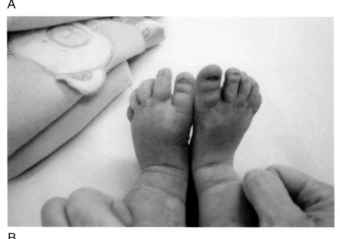

B

Figure 15-23. Klippel-Trénaunay syndrome. **A,** This infant with K-T-S is unusual in that he has vascular malformations involving both lower extremities, which extend upward over the lateral aspects of the abdominal wall. **B,** In this view of his feet, one can appreciate a greater degree of hypertrophy on the right.

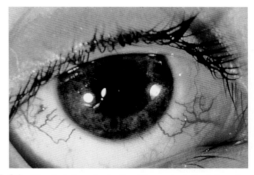

Figure 15-24. Ataxia-telangiectasia. Characteristic telangiectases in the bulbar conjunctiva usually develop between 3 months and 6 years of age.

defect is unknown. Ataxia is the usual presenting feature, and the course of the neurologic disturbance is rather stereotypic. Tremors of the head may be seen before 1 year of age, and unsteadiness of gait is evident when the child first walks. Progressive global ataxia and slurred, scanning, dysarthric speech are typical during the early school-age years. Loss of deep tendon reflexes and impairment of position and vibratory sensation are evident by the end of the first decade. Adolescence is marked by choreoathetosis, dystonic posturing, gaze apraxia, and progressive dementia.

The characteristic cutaneous manifestations of this disorder appear by 6 years of age. Telangiectases first appear on the bulbar conjunctivae (Fig. 15-24) and develop later over the malar regions, ears, antecubital fossae, neck, and upper chest.

Neuropathologic changes are widespread, with the cerebellum being the site of maximal degeneration. Loss of Purkinje and basket cells, thinning of the granular cell layer, and mild changes in the molecular layer are characteristic findings.

Systemic manifestations include major defects in cellular and humoral immunity. Deficiencies of IgA and IgM are characteristic and together with impaired cellular immunity contribute to susceptibility to the recurrent sinus and pulmonary infections that mark this disorder, as well as to the tendency to develop malignancies of the lymphoreticular system (most commonly ALL or lymphoma) during adolescence or early adulthood (see Chapter 4). Serum α-fetoprotein levels are elevated, which serves as a nonspecific marker. Adult family members of patients, especially mothers, may also be susceptible to malignancy, breast and lung cancer being the most common.

Linear Sebaceous Nevus

The nevus sebaceus of Jadassohn is usually present at birth, manifest as a yellowish-tan, waxy linear lesion (Fig. 15-25) that contains a papillomatous excess of sebaceous glands. This nevus may be found on the scalp, face, neck, trunk, or extremities. With time, the lesion becomes unsightly. This eventuality and a 15% to 20% risk of malignant degeneration have led practitioners to recommend early surgical excision. Although usually seen as an isolated abnormality in otherwise normal individuals, an association with seizures and mental retardation has been reported. The risk of neurologic abnormalities is greatest when the cutaneous lesion is located in the midfacial area.

Epidermal Nevus Syndrome

Epidermal nevus syndrome is a congenital neurocutaneous disorder in which an epidermal nevus is seen in association with neurologic dysfunction. The latter may include seizures, paresis, mental retardation, and develop-

mental delay. Unilateral hemimegalencephaly with intractable seizures is the commonest CNS abnormality. Disorders of segmentation/migration and multiple other structural CNS anomalies have been reported. Extra-CNS congenital defects may involve connective tissues, especially the skeleton, as well as ocular, cardiac, and genitourinary systems. The skin lesions are hamartomatous (derived from embryonic ectoderm) and characterized by hyperplasia of the epidermis and adnexal structures. They are usually present at birth, although some may appear later in the first year. They appear as raised, often warty hyperpigmented lesions typically in a linear pattern (Fig. 15-26). They may enlarge subsequently but tend to stabilize in size by puberty. Most cases are sporadic, although a small number are autosomal dominant.

Incontinentia Pigmenti

Incontinentia pigmenti is a rare, X-linked dominant syndrome with cutaneous, neurologic, ophthalmologic,

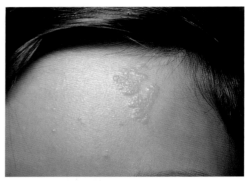

Figure 15-25. Linear nevus sebaceus of Jadassohn. This yellowish-tan, waxy-appearing lesion became elevated at puberty and was associated with seizures and mental retardation.

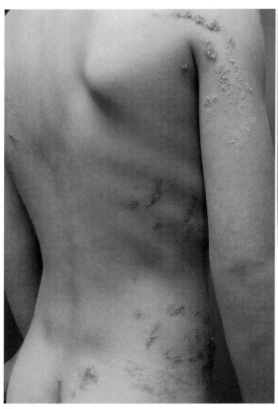

A

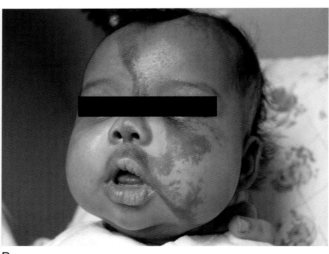

B

Figure 15-26. Epidermal nevus syndrome. **A,** Hyperpigmented verrucous papules are seen unilaterally over the upper arm, trunk, hip, and lumbosacral area of this adolescent boy. He had had a seizure in infancy and was learning disabled. **B,** In this infant, raised hyperpigmented lesions are present on the left face and both sides of the forehead and were associated with intractable seizures. (Courtesy Robin Gehris, MD, Children's Hospital of Pittsburgh.)

Table 15-5 Causes of Macrocephaly

EARLY INFANTILE (BIRTH-6 MO)	LATE INFANTILE (6 MO-2 YR)	EARLY TO LATE CHILDHOOD (AFTER 2 YR)
• Hydrocephalus (progressive or arresting) — Induction disorders (congenital malformations) • Spina bifida cystica, cranium bifidum, Chiari malformations (types I, II, and III), aqueductal stenosis, holoprosencephaly • Mass lesions — Neoplasms, A-V malformations, congenital cysts • Intrauterine infections — Toxoplasmosis, cytomegalovirus infection, syphilis, rubella — Perinatal or postnatal infections • Bacterial, granulomatous, parasitic — Peri- or postnatal hemorrhage • Hypoxia, vascular malformation, trauma • Hydranencephaly • Subdural effusion — Hemorrhagic, infectious, cystic hygroma • Normal variant (often familial)	• Hydrocephalus (progressive or arresting) — Space-occupying lesions • Tumors, cysts, abscesses — Postbacterial or granulomatous meningitis — Dysraphism • Dandy-Walker syndrome, Chiari type I malformation — Posthemorrhagic • Trauma or vascular malformation • Subdural effusion • Increased intracranial pressure syndrome — Pseudotumor cerebri • Lead, tetracycline, hypoparathyroidism, steroids, excess or deficiency of vitamin A, cyanotic congenital heart disease • Primary skeletal cranial dysplasia (thickened or enlarged skull): osteogenesis imperfecta, hyperphosphatemia, osteopetrosis, rickets • Megalencephaly (increase in brain substance) — Metabolic CNS diseases: leukodystrophies (e.g., Canavan, Alexander), lipidoses (Tay-Sachs), histiocytosis, mucopolysaccharidoses — Proliferative neurocutaneous syndromes: von Recklinghausen, tuberous sclerosis, hemangiomatosis, Sturge-Weber — Cerebral gigantism • Soto syndrome — Achondroplasia — Primary megalencephaly • May be familial and unassociated or associated with abnormalities of cellular architecture	• Hydrocephalus (arrested or progressive) — Space-occupying lesions — Preexisting induction disorder — Aqueductal stenosis — Chiari type I malformation — Postinfectious — Hemorrhagic • Megalencephaly — Proliferative neurocutaneous syndromes — Familial • Pseudotumor cerebri • Normal variant

From Gabriel RS: Malformations of the central nervous system. In Menkes JH (ed): Textbook of Child Neurology, 2nd ed. Philadelphia, Lea & Febiger, 1980.

and dental manifestations. It is caused by a mutation in the *NEMO* gene.

Neurologic and ophthalmologic problems often become manifest during early infancy and are reported to occur in about 30% of patients. They may include seizures, CVA, developmental delay, mental retardation, and microcephaly. Cutaneous features are described in Chapter 8 (see Fig. 8-97).

Central Nervous System Malformations

Malformations of the CNS are a leading cause of neurologic and developmental disability in infants and children. Although CNS malformations are not necessarily accompanied by external dysmorphic features, disturbances of cranial volume, abnormalities of head shape, and skin lesions overlying the dorsal midline should alert the physician to the possibility of associated CNS dysmorphogenesis.

Macrocephaly

Macrocephaly is defined as a head circumference greater than two standard deviations above the mean for age, gender, and gestation. This abnormality can be caused by a myriad of conditions (Table 15-5) including hydrocephalus (excessive accumulation of cerebrospinal fluid [CSF]);

intracranial mass lesions (tumors, subdural effusions); thickening or enlargement of the skull (primary skeletal dysplasias); and a true increase in brain substance (megalencephaly). The latter is seen in Soto syndrome, achondroplasia, neurocutaneous syndromes, and certain lipidoses, leukodystrophies, and mucopolysaccharidoses. Primary megalencephaly may occur as a benign familial trait.

Evaluation of the child with a head that is abnormally large or appears to be growing at an excessive rate should include the following:
1. Serial measurements of head circumference
2. Measurement of the parents' head circumferences and exploration of family history for evidence of macrocephaly or neurologic and cutaneous abnormalities
3. Developmental history
4. Careful examination for evidence of increased intracranial pressure, developmental delay, skeletal dysplasia, abnormal transillumination, cranial bruits, ocular abnormalities, or organomegaly

Plain skull radiographs may provide evidence of increased intracranial pressure (see Fig. 15-38), identify intracranial calcification (Fig. 15-27), or detect primary skeletal dysplasias (Fig. 15-28). CT or MRI scans allow assessment of ventricular size and permit detection of intracranial mass lesions and chronic subdural effusions. CT is the method of choice for demonstrating intracranial calcification and detecting fresh blood.

Hydrocephalus
Hydrocephalus is caused by an imbalance between CSF production and resorption that is of sufficient magni-

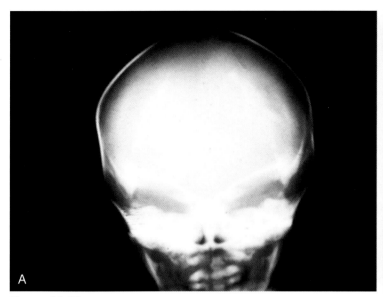

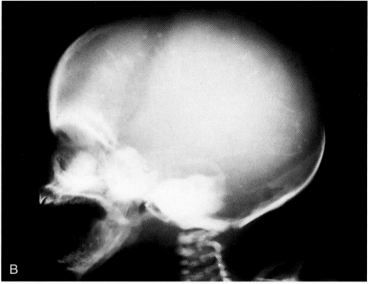

Figure 15-27. Macrocephaly. Frontal **(A)** and lateral **(B)** radiographs reveal bilaterally symmetrical, paraventricular cerebral calcifications in association with cranial enlargement in an infant with congenital cytomegalovirus infection. (Courtesy Department of Radiology, Children's Hospital of Pittsburgh.)

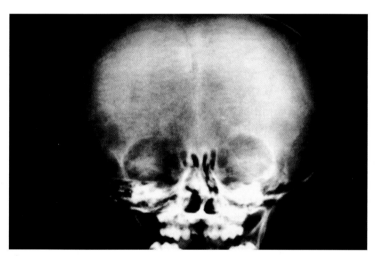

Figure 15-28. Macrocephaly. Plain skull radiographs allow detection of primary skeletal dysplasias. In this case, note the mosaic rarification of the cranial vault and multiple wormian bones characteristic of osteogenesis imperfecta. (Courtesy Department of Radiology, Children's Hospital of Pittsburgh.)

tude to result in a net accumulation of fluid within the ventricular system. Impaired CSF resorption may occur secondary to obstruction of CSF pathways within the ventricular system (noncommunicating hydrocephalus) or as a result of obstruction of the subarachnoid space (communicating hydrocephalus). Hydrocephalus secondary to CSF overproduction is rare but does occur in some cases of choroid plexus papilloma (see Fig. 15-42). Noncommunicating hydrocephalus is often due to aqueductal stenosis or congenital malformations of the fourth ventricle, and it is a common complication of tumors or vascular malformations of the posterior fossa that compress the cerebral aqueduct or obstruct outflow from the fourth ventricle. Causes of communicating hydrocephalus include intracranial hemorrhage, meningitis, cerebral venous or dural sinus thrombosis, and diffuse infiltration of the meninges by malignant cells.

The clinical manifestations of hydrocephalus in infancy are stereotypic. The head is excessively large at birth or grows at an abnormally rapid rate, becoming macroce-

phalic over the first few months. The forehead is disproportionately large, and the face appears small in relation to the calvarium. The scalp is thin and glistening, and its veins are distended, often becoming strikingly dilated when the infant cries. The anterior fontanelle is large, tense, and nonpulsatile, and the sutures are excessively wide (Fig. 15-29A). Divergent strabismus, abducens nerve paresis, and impaired upward gaze are important ocular findings. With severe hydrocephalus, there may be forced, conjugate downward deviation of the eyes so that the inferior half of the iris is hidden by the lower eyelid, producing the "sunsetting" sign (Fig. 15-29B). Neurologic abnormalities include developmental delay, persistence of early infantile automatisms, and spasticity and hyperreflexia of the lower extremities. CT or MRI scans demonstrate enlargement of the ventricular system and thinning of the cortical mantle and may provide additional anatomic information concerning the etiology (Fig. 15-29C).

Infantile hydrocephalus must be distinguished from other causes of macrocephaly in infancy such as chronic subdural hematoma, expanding porencephalic cyst, and certain degenerative disorders that may produce abnormal enlargement of the head (see Table 15-5). In premature infants with suspected hydrocephalus, the normally rapid rate of postnatal head growth must be taken into account.

Dandy-Walker Malformation
The Dandy-Walker malformation is a primary developmental abnormality characterized by progressive cystic enlargement of the fourth ventricle beginning early in fetal life. This is accompanied by enlargement of the posterior fossa and upward displacement of the tentorium, torcula, and transverse sinuses. Associated hydrocephalus is almost universal, and may be present at birth or may develop later, during infancy or childhood. Of affected individuals, 60% show signs of hydrocephalus and increased intracranial pressure by 2 years of age.

Clinical manifestations of Dandy-Walker malformation are variable and depend on the severity and rate of progression of the associated hydrocephalus. A child with a symptomatic condition often has an unusually prominent bulging occiput in addition to the usual findings of hydrocephalus. In children younger than 1 year of age, trans-

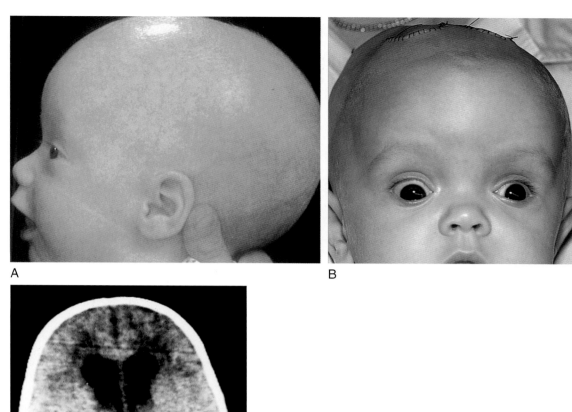

Figure 15-29. Infantile hydrocephalus. **A,** Characteristic enlarged head, thinning of the scalp, distended scalp veins, and a full fontanelle. **B,** Paresis of the upward gaze is seen in an infant with hydrocephalus resulting from aqueductal stenosis. Paresis is more apparent on the right. This phenomenon is often termed the *sunsetting sign.* **C,** CT scan demonstrates a dilated ventricular system and thinning of the cortical mantle. (**A,** From Booth IW, Wozniak ER: Pediatrics. Baltimore, Williams & Wilkins, 1984; **B,** courtesy Albert Biglan, MD, Children's Hospital of Pittsburgh. **C,** Courtesy Division of Neuroradiology, University Health Center of Pittsburgh.)

illumination of the skull effectively demonstrates the posterior fossa cyst (Fig. 15-30A). Ataxia, nystagmus, and cranial nerve deficits may also be prominent features.

Plain skull radiographs demonstrate posteroinferior enlargement of the cranial vault, thinning and ballooning of the occipital squama, and upward displacement of the torcula. CT or MRI scans confirm the presence of a large posterior fossa cyst, a small cerebellar remnant, and associated hydrocephalus (Fig. 15-30B).

Hydranencephaly

Hydranencephaly is a severe anomaly of the brain characterized by the absence of the cerebral hemispheres despite intact meninges and a normal skull. Affected children often appear deceptively normal at birth, with little to suggest the presence of a severe brain abnormality (Fig. 15-31A). Because newborns function at a subcortical reflex level, even complete absence of the cerebral hemispheres may not interfere with normal reflexes. However, within the first few weeks of life, developmental arrest, decerebration, hypertonia, and hyperreflexia become apparent in the infant with hydranencephaly. Most of these infants

do not live beyond 6 to 12 months, although survival for several years is occasionally reported. Seizures are common, and progressive enlargement of the head may complicate nursing care.

The diagnosis may be suggested if, on transillumination of the skull, the entire calvarium is lit up (Fig. 15-31B). However, severe hydrocephalus and bilateral subdural hygromas may present a similar appearance.

CT scan demonstrates a large, water-dense cavity replacing the cerebral hemispheres with islands of residual brain tissue seen at the base (Fig. 15-31C). To distinguish this disorder from massive bilateral subdural hygromas, cerebral angiography is required to confirm absence of the cerebrum.

Microcephaly

Microcephaly is defined as a head circumference more than two standard deviations below the mean for age, gender, and conceptual age. Apart from cases resulting from premature closure of the sutures (generalized craniosynostosis), microcephaly reflects an abnormally small brain and can be a symptom of any disorder that impairs

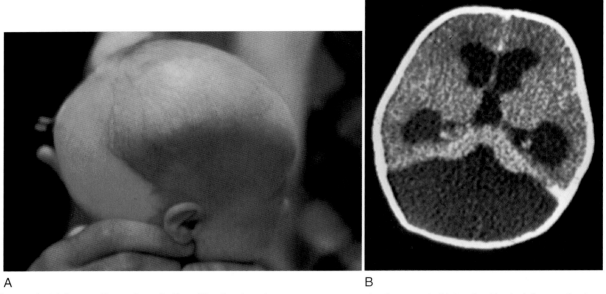

A　　　　　　　　　　　　　　　　　　　　　B

Figure 15-30. Dandy-Walker malformation. **A,** Transillumination demonstrates a posterior fossa cyst. Note also the bulging occiput, prominent scalp veins, and enlargement of the head. **B,** CT scan shows a posterior fossa cyst, a small cerebellar remnant, and associated hydrocephalus. (**A,** Courtesy Michael J. Painter, MD, Children's Hospital of Pittsburgh.)

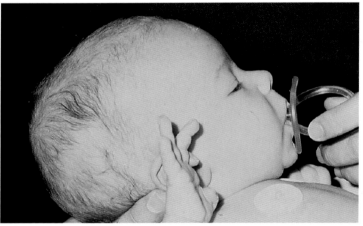

Figure 15-31. Hydranencephaly. **A,** Patient, age 3 weeks, has a deceptively normal appearance with little to suggest a severe brain abnormality. **B,** Transillumination of the skull lights up the entire calvarium, suggesting the diagnosis. **C,** CT scan demonstrates replacement of the cerebral hemispheres by a large, water-dense cavity with residual islands of brain tissue in regions of the occipital poles and right inferior temporal lobe. (**C,** Courtesy Division of Neuroradiology, University Health Center of Pittsburgh.)

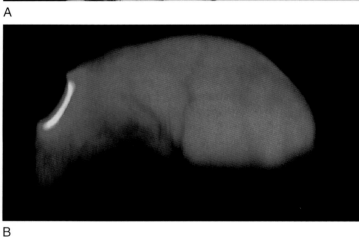

A

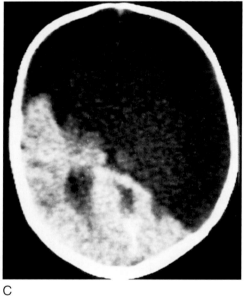

B　　　　　　　　　　　　　　　　　　　　　C

brain growth (Table 15-6). The neurologic manifestations range from minor (e.g., poor fine motor skills, mild intellectual impairment) to profound (e.g., decerebration, chronic vegetative state). Diagnostic evaluation should include a family history, prenatal history, a search for associated congenital anomalies, karyotyping, amino acid screening, and serologic studies for intrauterine infection. Plain skull radiographs can detect craniosynostosis, whereas CT scan is useful in identifying intracranial cal-

cifications. MRI is preferred for delineation of recognizable patterns of CNS dysmorphogenesis.

Midline Defects and Occult Spinal Dysraphism

Development of the human nervous system begins early in the third week of gestation with the proliferation of ectodermal cells in the dorsal midline to form the neural plate. By the end of the fourth week, the neural plate has invaginated and then fused in the midline to form the neural tube. The cerebrum, diencephalon, midbrain, and brainstem develop from the rostral portion of the neural tube. The caudal portion separates from the overlying ectoderm, forming the precursor of the spinal cord, and is surrounded by mesodermal elements destined to form the vertebral bodies and supporting soft tissue structures. Midline spinal cord and vertebral skeletal defects, termed *spinal dysraphism,* result from defective closure of the caudal portion of the neural tube. Abnormal neural tube closure beginning early in the embryologic sequence produces dysraphic states involving both neural and skeletal elements (myelomeningocele [see Fig. 1-12C]), whereas closure defects occurring later produce congenital anomalies restricted to the posterior elements of the vertebrae (spina bifida occulta).

Occult spinal dysraphism is a defect of intermediate severity in which vertebral anomalies are associated with underlying intraspinal tumors or developmental abnormalities. Its presence is often (though not always) betrayed by cutaneous and subcutaneous abnormalities centered over the midline of the back, such as a hairy patch (Fig.

15-32A), skin tag, port-wine stain, hemangioma, subcutaneous lipoma (Fig. 15-32B), cutis aplasia, or sinus tract (Fig. 15-32C). Infants with atypical dimples or clefts (>5 mm) that are located more than 2.5 cm from the anus also have an increased incidence of underlying malformations, whereas those with simple blind dimples located within the gluteal cleft or within 2.5 cm of the anus do not. Although neurologic abnormalities are commonly associated with the lesions mentioned earlier, they are by no means universal. Figure 15-33 shows a child with a large lumbosacral hemangioma who did not have any associated neurologic abnormality.

Midline defects are not limited to the caudal portion of the neural tube but can occur over the head and neck as well. Most notably, these include encephaloceles. These may be obvious in their appearance (see Fig. 1-12A), may have no external findings (see Fig. 23-37), or may be associated with an overlying scalp lesion such as a vascular malformation (Fig. 15-34).

Because early diagnosis and neurosurgical intervention can prevent the onset and/or progression of neurologic deficits, newborns with midline cutaneous or subcutaneous stigmata and those with atypical dimples or clefts should undergo radiologic screening. Ultrasonography has proved to be the best tool for this purpose before ossification of the posterior vertebral elements (at 3 months) because it not only can detect vertebral defects and spinal anomalies but also can be used to assess cord motion. If this reveals an underlying malformation or anomaly, follow-up MRI and neurosurgical referral are indicated. Common intraspinal lesions include dermoid tumors, intraspinal lipomas (Fig. 15-35), and diastematomyelia (Fig. 15-36).

Although some patients with occult spinal dysraphism may show signs of neurologic dysfunction and talipes equinovarus from birth, most develop symptoms insidiously after a symptom-free interval. Dysfunction usually begins at approximately 3 years of age, but many do not develop problems until school age or adolescence. Presenting complaints may include back or leg stiffness; clumsiness; mild weakness or numbness of

Table 15-6	Causes of Microcephaly

Genetic Defects Autosomal recessive defects Autosomal dominant defects **Disorders of Karyotype** Trisomies Deletions Translocations **Intrauterine Infections** Rubella Cytomegalovirus infection Toxoplasmosis Congenital syphilis Herpesvirus infections	**Antenatal Irradiation** **Exposure to Drugs and Chemicals during Gestation** Ethyl alcohol exposure (fetal alcohol syndrome) Phenytoin exposure Trimethadione exposure Methyl mercury exposure **Maternal Phenylketonuria** **Perinatal Insults** Traumatic Anoxic Metabolic Infectious

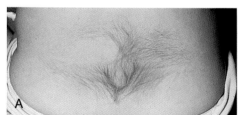

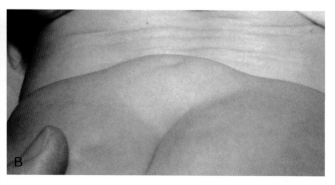

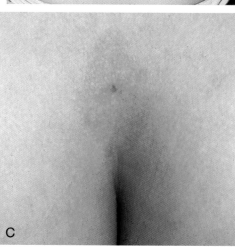

Figure 15-32. Cutaneous and subcutaneous markers of occult spinal dysraphism. **A,** Note the hairy patch over the lumbar region, here associated with diastematomyelia. **B,** The soft subcutaneous mass seen overlying the sacrum of this infant was determined to be a lipoma. **C,** Sacral sinus tract associated with intraspinal dermoid tumor. (**A** and **C,** Courtesy Michael J. Painter, MD, Children's Hospital of Pittsburgh. **B,** From Cohen BA: Atlas of Pediatric Dermatology, London, Mosby-Wolfe, 1993.)

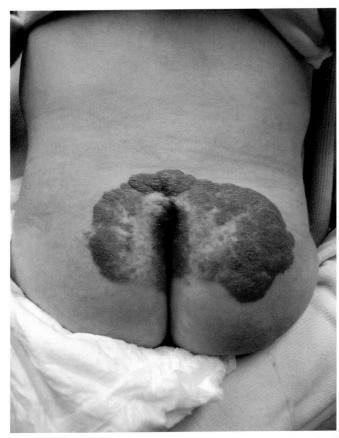

Figure 15-33. Lumbosacral hemangioma. This child has a large lumbosacral hemangioma which extended well below the surface and wrapped around the vertebral column but regressed promptly and was not associated with any abnormality of the underlying neural or bony structures. (Courtesy Robin Gehris, MD, Children's Hospital of Pittsburgh.)

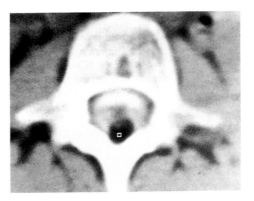

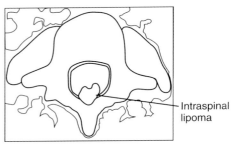

Figure 15-35. Occult spinal dysraphism. CT scan demonstrates an intraspinal lipoma in a child with a subcutaneous lipoma over the lumbar spine.

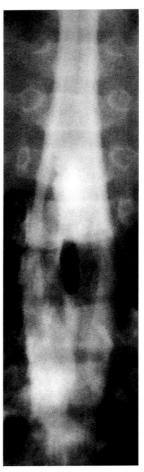

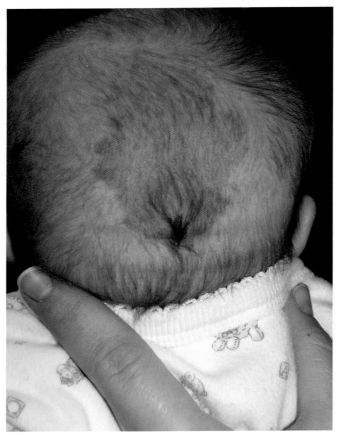

Figure 15-34. Midline vascular malformation with an underlying atretic encephalocele in an infant who had no signs of neurologic dysfunction. (Courtesy Robin Gehris, MD, Children's Hospital of Pittsburgh.)

Figure 15-36. Diastematomyelia. This 6-month-old infant had progressive inturning and plantar flexion of the left foot and a slightly deviated gluteal cleft. On myelogram, her spinal cord splits at L1, coursing around a bony spur at L2, then rejoins at L4-L5. She also had complete spinal dysraphism of L2-L4 and partial dysraphism at L1 and L5.

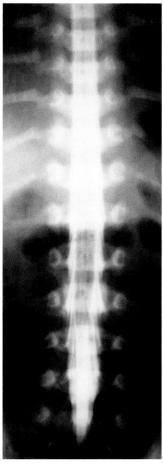

Figure 15-37. Tethered cord resulting from a tight filum terminale. On myelography, the conus medullaris is pulled down to L3-L4 by a tethered filum terminale, the upper portion of which is thickened. Presenting symptoms included weakness of plantar flexion, eversion of the feet, and bladder dysfunction. (Courtesy Charles Fitz, MD, Children's Hospital of Pittsburgh.)

the lower extremities; or problems with bowel or bladder dysfunction.

Objective findings may consist of decreased tone and decreased deep tendon reflexes in the lower extremities; patchy decreases in sensation; and foot deformities consisting of broadening and shortening, deepening of the arch, and contractures of the toes (see Fig. 21-110). Symptoms of associated tethering of the spinal cord may be present in infancy, but often their onset is delayed until the child enters a period of rapid growth and develops back, leg, or buttock pain; signs of lower limb spasticity; and, on occasion, bowel and bladder dysfunction. These symptoms presumably are due to progressive deformation of the tethered cord, which is not free to "ascend" normally within the spinal canal as the rate of linear growth of the vertebral column outpaces that of the spinal cord. Tethering of the spinal cord by an anomalous filum terminale (Fig. 15-37), producing similar signs of progressive neurologic dysfunction, can occur in the absence of associated cutaneous abnormalities, vertebral defects, or intraspinal tumors.

Increased Intracranial Pressure

The cranial cavity is occupied by the brain, blood, and CSF. An increase in the volume of any of these compartments, unless accompanied by a concomitant decrease in one or both of the other compartments, results in increased intracranial pressure. Increased intracranial pressure can result from a wide variety of disorders and is itself hazardous. Recognition of associated signs and symptoms permits early diagnosis and prompt intervention to forestall progressive brain injury or catastrophic neurologic deterioration.

Primary Signs and Symptoms

The clinical manifestations of increased intracranial pressure vary with age. In infants, examination of the anterior fontanelle allows reliable assessment of intracranial pressure. In the normal, quiet infant held in an upright or sitting posture, the anterior fontanelle is flat or slightly concave. Under these conditions, an anterior fontanelle that bulges above the contour of the calvaria and that is excessively firm on palpation is always abnormal (see Figs. 15-29A and 12-21B). Because the cranial sutures are not fused in infants and young children, increased intracranial pressure rapidly produces separation of the bony plates of the skull. In infants, this can be detected by palpation; in older children, skull radiographs may be necessary to identify widened cranial sutures (Fig. 15-38A). Prominent convolutional markings on the inner table of the skull (Fig. 15-38B) are a less useful radiographic sign because they are frequently seen on skull radiographs of normal children. However, when secondary to increased intracranial pressure, they are preceded by suture diastasis and changes in the sella turcica (Fig. 15-38C). An excessive rate of head growth is a prominent feature of chronically increased intracranial pressure in infants and children up to 3 years of age. Associated findings may include frontal prominence and distended scalp veins (see Fig. 15-29A). If the ability to compensate for increased intracranial pressure by expansion of the calvaria is exceeded, other symptoms appear. These may include listlessness, irritability, poor feeding, vomiting, failure to thrive, paresis of upward gaze (see Fig. 15-29B), increased tone, hyperactive stretch reflexes, and a high-pitched cry. Papilledema is uncommon.

In older children and adults the most consistent clinical features of increased intracranial pressure include headache, vomiting, visual disturbances, and papilledema. Headaches are of variable severity. They may be constant or intermittent and generalized or localized to frontal, temporal, or occipital regions. In some, but by no means all cases, they recur on early rising or awakening and are accompanied by vomiting. The headaches may be exacerbated by sneezing, coughing, or straining. Vomiting resulting from increased intracranial pressure is no different from vomiting from other causes. It is seldom projectile and is not necessarily accompanied by headache.

Horizontal diplopia (double vision) secondary to paralysis of one or both abducens nerves is the most common visual disturbance. Initially, double vision may occur only on lateral gaze toward the side of the paretic lateral rectus muscle. This may be intermittent and may not be accompanied by limitation of ocular motility sufficient to be seen by the examiner. With progression, diplopia becomes constant and is present even with the eyes in the primary position, and an internal strabismus results (Fig. 15-39). Selective vulnerability of the sixth cranial nerve to increased intracranial pressure may be explained by its long intracranial course and proximity to rigid structures. Other visual disturbances may include transient obscurations, visual field deficits, and impaired upward gaze.

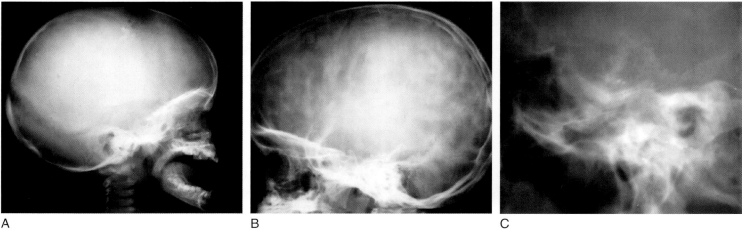

A   B   C

Figure 15-38. Findings of increased intracranial pressure that may be seen on standard skull radiographs. **A,** Widening of the cranial sutures. **B,** Prominent convolutional markings on the inner table of the skull (beaten silver skull). **C,** Erosion of the sella turcica, in this case resulting from a craniopharyngioma. (**A,** Courtesy Department of Neuroradiology, University Health Center of Pittsburgh; **B** and **C,** courtesy Jocelyn Medina, MD.)

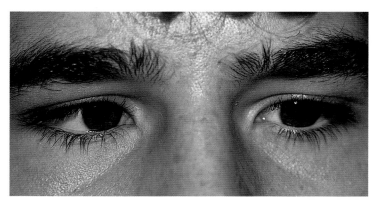

Figure 15-39. Left abducens (sixth cranial nerve) palsy. This boy presented with headaches and diplopia and was found to have papilledema and a left abducens palsy. Note that his left eye cannot move past the midline on left lateral gaze. (Courtesy Kenneth Cheng, MD, Children's Hospital of Pittsburgh.)

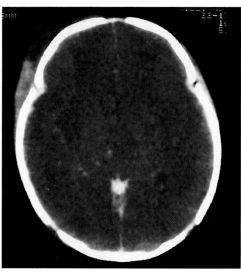

Figure 15-41. Cerebral edema. CT performed 24 hours after severe hypoxic-ischemic injury. Note the obliteration of the cerebral ventricles, the loss of gray-white matter differentiation, and the homogeneous "ground-glass" appearance. (Courtesy Department of Neuroradiology, University Health Center of Pittsburgh.)

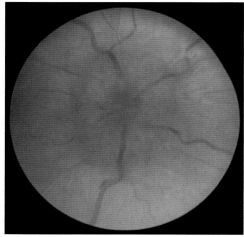

Figure 15-40. Papilledema. Fundus photograph shows blurring of the optic disk margin, elevation and hyperemia of the optic nerve head, and distention of the retinal blood vessels. (Courtesy Kenneth Cheng, MD, Children's Hospital of Pittsburgh.)

Sustained intracranial hypertension produces papilledema, a passive swelling of the optic disk (Fig. 15-40). The observation of papilledema in a child with headache, vomiting, or visual disturbances confirms the presence of increased intracranial pressure. The absence of venous pulsations or the presence of associated flame-shaped

hemorrhages can help distinguish papilledema from other causes of blurred optic disk margins.

Increased intracranial pressure may be accompanied by changes in personality and behavior, deteriorating school performance, decreased appetite and activity, and alterations in level of consciousness.

Etiologies

Causes of increased intracranial pressure include cerebral edema, mass lesions, trauma, CNS infections, pseudotumor cerebri, and hydrocephalus.

Cerebral Edema
Cerebral edema (Fig. 15-41), an expansion of brain volume resulting from an increase in brain content of water and salt, is a response of brain tissue to a variety of insults. Vasogenic cerebral edema results from the alterations in vascular permeability produced by brain tumor, trauma, abscess, and hemorrhage. Cytotoxic cerebral edema, caused by swelling of brain cells (neurons and

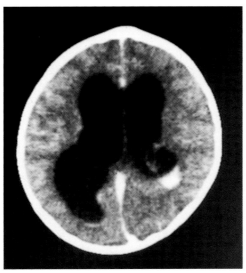

Figure 15-42. Choroid plexus papilloma. CT of an infant with excessively rapid head growth. There is an enhancing mass within the body of the left lateral ventricle and associated ventricular enlargement (hydrocephalus) secondary to excessive secretion of CSF by the tumor. (Courtesy Michael Painter, MD, Children's Hospital of Pittsburgh.)

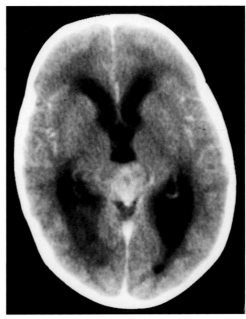

Figure 15-44. Pineal region tumor. CT scan of a patient with headache, lethargy, vomiting, and paresis of upward gaze shows an enhancing mass lesion in the pineal region and severe obstructive hydrocephalus. (Courtesy Department of Neuroradiology, University Health Center of Pittsburgh.)

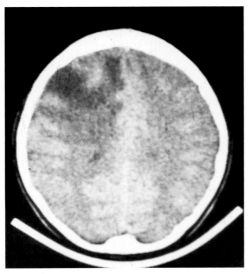

Figure 15-43. Hemispheric oligodendroglioma. CT scan of a patient with seizures demonstrates a low-density mass lesion in the right frontal lobe. (Courtesy Michael Painter, MD, Children's Hospital of Pittsburgh.)

glia), usually results from infection, hypoxia, ischemia, or toxins.

Intracranial Mass Lesions

Tumors, intracranial hemorrhages, abscesses, and vascular malformations produce increased intracranial pressure by occupying space, causing cerebral edema, obstructing CSF pathways, and altering blood flow.

Intracranial Tumors. *Choroid plexus papillomas,* by secreting an excess of CSF, cause communicating hydrocephalus (Fig. 15-42). Although astrocytomas of the cerebral hemispheres (Fig. 15-43) often manifest as seizures or contralateral motor difficulties, symptoms of increased intracranial pressure are the initial manifestations in 37% of cases and are present at the time of diagnosis in 80%. *Pineal region tumors* (Fig. 15-44) frequently obstruct the third ventricle or cerebral aqueduct, producing signs and symptoms of increased intracranial pressure accompanied by *Parinaud syndrome* (impairment of the upward gaze with preservation of the downward gaze and retraction-

convergence nystagmus with attempted upward gaze) resulting from compression of the periaqueductal gray (see Fig. 15-29B). *Hypothalamic region tumors* such as craniopharyngioma (Fig. 15-45) manifest as growth retardation or failure of sexual maturation accompanied by visual field defects resulting from compression of the optic chiasm. Hydrocephalus occurs in 25% of cases.

Headache and vomiting accompanied by disturbances of gait and coordination are frequent presenting manifestations of posterior fossa tumors such as cerebellar astrocytoma, medulloblastoma, and ependymoma. Midline tumors involving the cerebellar vermis can produce truncal ataxia (Fig. 15-46A), whereas mass lesions of the cerebellar hemispheres often cause unilateral limb ataxia and horizontal nystagmus (Fig. 15-46B). The cardinal manifestations of brainstem glioma (Fig. 15-47) are cranial nerve palsies associated with contralateral hemiplegia and ataxia. Increased intracranial pressure is not an early feature.

Brain Abscesses. Brain abscesses (Fig. 15-48) are uncommon in the absence of predisposing factors such as chronic otitis or sinusitis, chronic pulmonary infection, dental abscesses, cyanotic congenital heart disease, or immunosuppression. Unless accompanied by prodromal symptoms of fever, headache, lethargy, and malaise, brain abscesses may be impossible to distinguish from other intracranial mass lesions on clinical grounds.

Intracranial Hemorrhage. *Spontaneous intracranial hemorrhage* (Fig. 15-49) secondary to rupture of a vascular malformation or arterial aneurysm is rare in the pediatric population. Leakage of small amounts of blood into the subarachnoid space produces symptoms (e.g., fever, headache, stiff neck) that mimic those of bacterial meningitis. In such cases the correct diagnosis may first be suspected when lumbar puncture yields grossly bloody fluid. The presentation of large subarachnoid hemorrhages is catastrophic, with sudden onset of excruciating headache followed by collapse and evidence of increased intracranial pressure.

Head trauma results in increased intracranial pressure by provoking cerebral edema or causing intracranial hemorrhage. The modes of presentation of *cerebral contusion,*

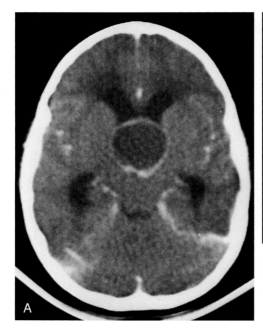

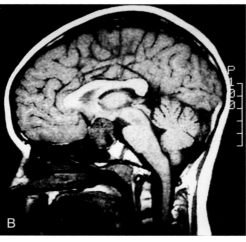

Figure 15-45. Craniopharyngioma. **A,** CT scan shows a large, spherical suprasellar mass, obliteration of the third ventricle, and associated hydrocephalus. **B,** MRI scan provides superior visualization of the anatomic relationship of this tumor with the optic chiasm and hypothalamus. (Courtesy Department of Neuroradiology, University Health Center of Pittsburgh.)

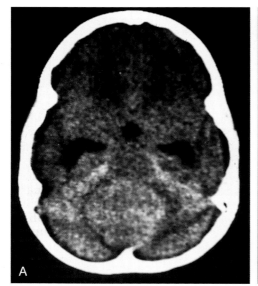

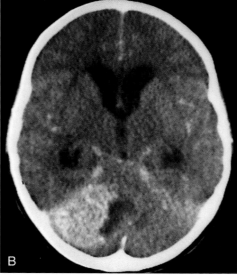

Figure 15-46. Cerebellar neoplasms. **A,** Midline ependymoma filling the fourth ventricle and invading the cerebellar vermis. **B,** Glioblastoma of the right cerebellar hemisphere. (**A,** Courtesy Michael Painter, MD, Children's Hospital of Pittsburgh; **B,** courtesy Department of Neuroradiology, University Health Center of Pittsburgh.)

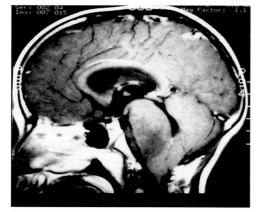

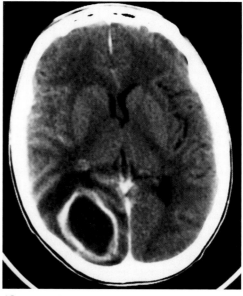

Figure 15-47. Brainstem glioma. This 6-year-old girl had a 2- to 3-month history of personality change, decreased school performance, and intermittent urinary retention and constipation; a 3-week history of ataxia and vague upper back pain; and a 6-day history of severe frontal headache with vomiting after breakfast. She had diplopia secondary to left sixth nerve palsy, nystagmus, right facial weakness, slurred speech, dysphagia with drooling, torticollis, an unbalanced gait with a tendency to list to the left, dysmetria greater on the left, and bilateral papilledema. Her MRI scan showed marked enlargement of the pons resulting from a mass lesion extending into the brainstem and compressing the fourth ventricle, causing hydrocephalus. (Courtesy Charles Fitz, MD, Children's Hospital of Pittsburgh.)

Figure 15-48. Brain abscess. CT scan demonstrates a low-density mass lesion with an enhancing rim and surrounding edema in an immunosuppressed patient with an *Aspergillus* abscess. Bacterial abscesses and neoplasms can present a similar CT appearance. (Courtesy Department of Neuroradiology, University Health Center of Pittsburgh.)

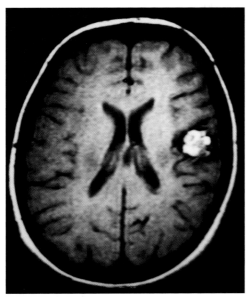

Figure 15-49. Intracranial hemorrhage. Enhanced MRI scan demonstrating a cerebral hemangioma with associated old hemorrhage. (Courtesy Michael J. Painter, MD, Children's Hospital of Pittsburgh.)

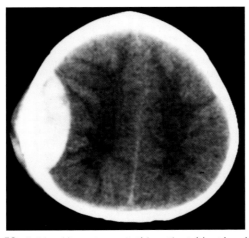

Figure 15-50. Epidural hematoma. In this patient, blunt head trauma was followed by vomiting, progressive obtundation, and decreased movement of the left arm and leg. The CT scan showed a large, lens-shaped epidural hematoma over the right hemisphere. (Courtesy Department of Neuroradiology, University Health Center of Pittsburgh.)

subdural hematoma, and posttraumatic cerebral edema are discussed in Chapter 6. The features of *epidural hematoma* (Fig. 15-50) in childhood, which differ from those encountered in adults, are emphasized here. Infants and young children with epidural hematoma frequently suffer no immediate loss of consciousness after the traumatic event. Associated linear skull fractures are less common than in adults, and the source of bleeding into the epidural space is generally ruptured epidural veins rather than lacerations of the middle meningeal artery. Hence the evolution of symptoms is slower, and the typical adult picture of immediate loss of consciousness, followed by a brief lucid interval and then collapse, is not seen until adolescence. Often, persistent lethargy and intermittent vomiting are the only initial signs. On early assessment, some affected children and adolescents demonstrate a slowed reaction time, especially when responding to questions (as if there is a processing delay). Severe headache, papilledema, and localizing signs may not emerge for several hours to days. Once neurologic signs and symptoms appear, they may progress rapidly to coma and death or evolve slowly over several days before producing brainstem compression.

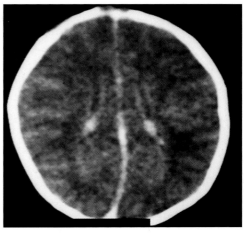

Figure 15-51. Bacterial meningitis in an infant with fever; lethargy; nuchal rigidity; and a tense, distended fontanelle. The CT scan shows contrast enhancement of the cortical gyri and ependyma of the lateral ventricles. (Courtesy Department of Neuroradiology, University Health Center of Pittsburgh.)

Meningitis
Bacterial meningitis (Fig. 15-51 and see Fig. 12-21B) produces increased intracranial pressure by causing cerebral edema and impairing reabsorption of CSF. Signs and symptoms are discussed in Chapter 12. Although cerebral edema and intracranial hypertension may complicate the course of viral encephalitis, the usual presentation is with seizures, behavioral change, and altered level of consciousness.

Other Causes
Pseudomotor Cerebri. Pseudotumor cerebri is a syndrome of increased intracranial pressure that occurs in the absence of hydrocephalus or an intracranial mass lesion. The disorder may be associated with the use of certain drugs (e.g., steroids, tetracycline, vitamin A, oral contraceptives); can occur as a complication of otitis media or sinusitis; and can be caused by a variety of endocrine and metabolic disturbances. Another risk factor is obesity. It is also more common in adolescent girls. However, in many instances pseudotumor is idiopathic. The presenting symptom is headache. Papilledema is the rule, and abducens nerve palsy is common (see Figs. 15-39 and 15-40). There may be associated nausea and vomiting, but most children do not appear acutely ill. Many patients have visual obscurations. Progressive papilledema may lead to optic atrophy, and treatment is essential to prevent loss of vision. Pseudotumor cerebri is a diagnosis of exclusion. A CT or an MRI scan must be done to rule out hydrocephalus or a mass lesion. Examination of the cerebrospinal fluid is unremarkable apart from increased opening pressure.

Neurocysticercosis. Neurocysticercosis is another disorder that can present with signs of increased intracranial pressure. It is the most common CNS parasitic infestation worldwide and is endemic in Mexico, Central and South America, parts of Asia including China, Africa, and India. Neurocysticercosis is being seen with increasing frequency in developed countries, often in immigrants from or recent visitors to endemic areas. Cerebral cysticercosis occurs when larvae of the pork tapeworm (*Taenia solium*) encyst in CNS tissues. Eating contaminated pork carrying the *T. solium* larvae leads to acquisition of the intestinal tapeworm. Cysticercosis results from fecal-oral transmission of the ova shed by the adult intestinal tapeworm and is often transmitted to affected children by family, household, or community contacts who carry the adult *T. solium* tapeworm. Following transmission, hematogenous spread to neural, ocular, or muscular tissues can occur. Seizures are

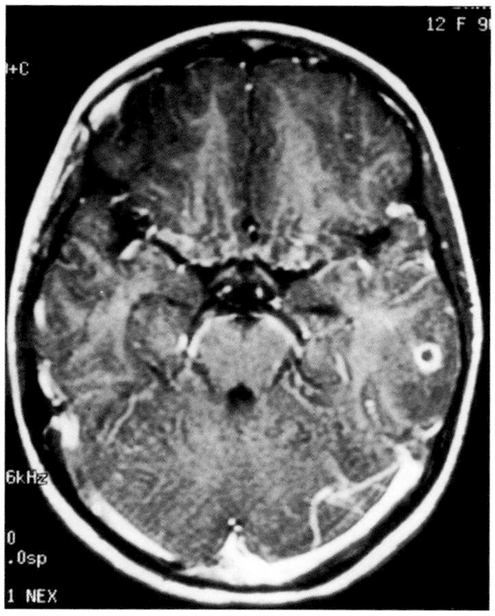

Figure 15-52. Neurocysticercosis. This 12-year-old presented with focal seizures and chronic headaches after recent travel to an endemic area. MRI revealed a small ring-enhancing cyst in the left temporal lobe with surrounding edema, felt to be consistent with neurocysticercosis. (Courtesy Patricia Crumrine, MD, Children's Hospital of Pittsburgh.)

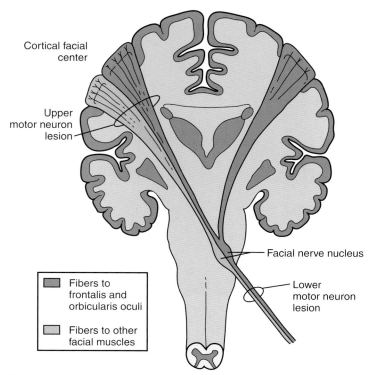

Figure 15-53. Central motor control of the facial muscles. The portion of the facial nerve nucleus that supplies the lower half of the face receives predominantly crossed fibers originating from the opposite cerebral hemisphere; the portion that innervates the upper half receives fibers from both cerebral hemispheres. (Modified from Haymaker W: Bing's Local Diagnosis in Neurological Diseases, 15th ed. St Louis, Mosby, 1969.)

the most common presenting sign of neurocysticercosis and are often accompanied by headache. Less commonly, patients can develop meningitis as a result of inflammatory reactions to ruptured cysts or they may present with signs and symptoms of increased intracranial pressure due to obstruction of CSF pathways by cysts, resulting in noncommunicating hydrocephalus. Findings on neuroimaging vary depending on the stage of development of the organism and range from nonenhancing cysts to ring-enhancing lesions to calcified nodules. Lesions may be single or multiple. Single enhancing cysts are most common in children living in North America (Fig. 15-52).

Facial Weakness

The cortical motor center controlling the muscles of facial expression is located in the lower third of the precentral gyrus (Fig. 15-53). Motor fibers arising in the cerebral cortex travel through the corona radiata, internal capsule, and cerebral peduncle into the pons, where the majority decussate to supply the facial (seventh) nerve nucleus on the opposite side. Some fibers, destined to terminate in the portion of the facial nerve nucleus that innervates muscles in the upper half of the face, do not decussate. Thus whereas the portion of the facial nerve nucleus that supplies the lower half of the face receives predominantly crossed fibers originating from the opposite cerebral hemisphere, the portion that innervates the frontalis muscle and the orbicularis oculi muscle has bilateral supranuclear control.

Peripheral Facial Weakness

A lesion of the seventh nerve nucleus or emergent facial nerve results in flaccid weakness of the entire face on the same side. On the affected side the face is smooth, with flattening of the nasolabial fold; drooping of the corner of the mouth; and inability to smile, frown, retract the corner of the mouth, wrinkle the forehead, or close the

eye (Fig. 15-54). Causes of peripheral facial weakness include infection, trauma, hypertension, a cerebellopontine angle mass, tumors of the pons, and acute idiopathic paralysis (Bell palsy).

Central Facial Weakness

With a lesion above the level of the facial nerve nucleus (i.e., an upper motor neuron lesion), there is weakness of the lower part of the face on the opposite side but relative sparing of the upper portion of the face. The ability to wrinkle the forehead (frontalis muscle) and to voluntarily close the eyes (orbicularis oculi muscle) is preserved (Fig. 15-55).

Neuromuscular Disorders

Weakness is the most common presenting symptom of neuromuscular disease. If time is taken to determine the ways in which the weakness interferes with normal activities and uncover the types of tasks that the patient finds difficult, the distribution and severity of muscle weakness can be predicted from the clinical history. Determining the mode of onset and pattern of progression of the symptoms is essential in the differential diagnosis and selection of diagnostic studies. Because many neuromuscular disorders are genetically determined, a complete family history must be obtained.

Essential components of the physical examination of patients with neuromuscular disease include inspection, palpation, percussion, evaluation of deep tendon reflexes, and assessment of muscle strength. Inspection can reveal

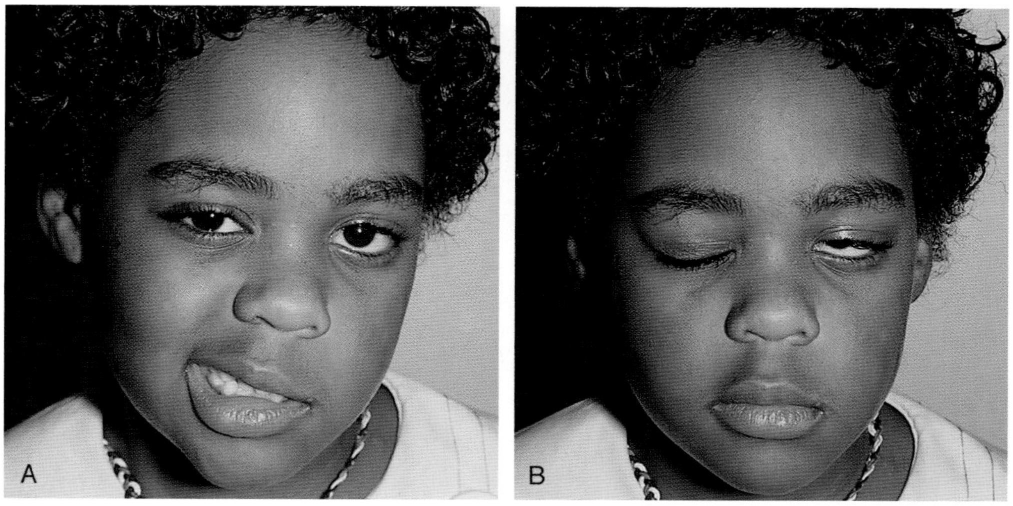

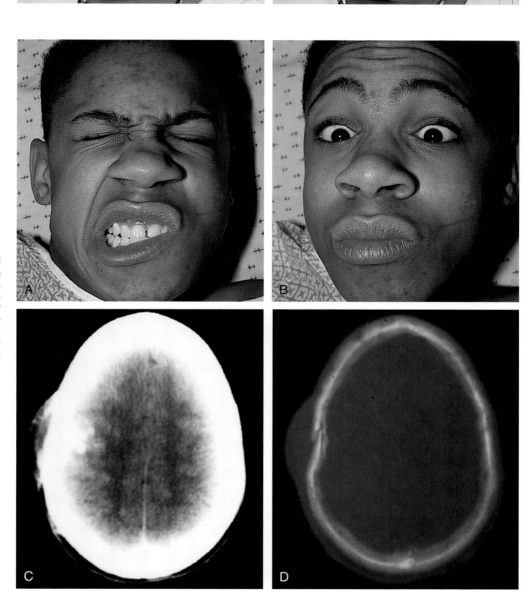

Figure 15-54. Peripheral facial weakness. Flaccid weakness of the entire left face resulting from a lesion of the left facial nerve. **A,** Flattening of the nasolabial fold and inability to retract the corner of the mouth. **B,** Inability to fully close the eye.

Figure 15-55. Central facial weakness. **A** and **B,** Weakness of the left face with relative sparing of the upper portion secondary to a lesion of the right cerebral hemisphere. There is flattening of the nasolabial fold and inability to retract the corner of the mouth, but the ability to close the eye and wrinkle the forehead is preserved. **C** and **D,** CT scans show the depressed fracture of the temporal bone that was responsible for this central facial palsy.

muscle wasting and atrophy (or conversely hypertrophy), abnormal spontaneous activity, and abnormal resting postures. Palpation permits assessment of muscle consistency, determination of muscle tone (with observation of resistance to passive motion), and detection of muscle tenderness. Percussion is useful in detecting myotonia. Assessment of muscle strength includes individual muscle testing and functional evaluation. The strength of individual muscles is recorded using a standardized system such as the following:

0 No contraction
1 Flicker or trace contraction
2 Active movement with gravity eliminated
3 Active movement against gravity

Table 15-7	Clinical Features of the Muscular Dystrophies				
	DUCHENNE	**BECKER**	**FASCIOSCAPULOHUMERAL**	**LIMB-GIRDLE**	**MYOTONIC**
Inheritance	X-linked recessive	X-linked recessive	Autosomal dominant	Autosomal recessive	Autosomal dominant
Age at onset	Early childhood	Late childhood, adolescence	Variable: childhood through early adult life	Childhood to early adulthood	Highly variable
Pattern of weakness	Pelvic girdle, shoulder girdle	Pelvic girdle, shoulder girdle	Face, shoulder girdle	Pelvic girdle, shoulder girdle	Face, distal limbs
Rate of progression	Rapid	Slow	Very slow	Variable	Variable
Associated features	Pseudohypertrophy of calves	Pseudohypertrophy of calves	None	Pseudohypertrophy rare	Myotonia
Systemic features	Mental retardation, abnormal electrocardiogram, cardiomyopathy	Occasional mental retardation	None	None	Frequent mental retardation, heart block, cataracts, premature balding, testicular tubular atrophy, diabetes

4 Active movement against gravity and resistance
5 Normal power

Functional evaluation of muscle strength is accomplished by observing the patient rising from the floor, rising from a chair, stepping onto a stool, climbing stairs, walking on the heels, hopping on the toes, and raising the arms above the head. This evaluation permits rapid detection of proximal weakness of the hips and shoulders and distal weakness of the legs.

Duchenne Muscular Dystrophy

The muscular dystrophies are genetically determined disorders characterized by progressive degeneration of skeletal muscle, usually after a latency period of seemingly normal development and function. The various clinical types of muscular dystrophy are traditionally classified on the basis of patterns of inheritance, distribution of initial weakness, age of onset of clinical manifestations, and rate of progression (Table 15-7).

Duchenne muscular dystrophy, affecting 1 in 3500 male births, is characterized by X-linked recessive inheritance; early onset; symmetrical and initially selective involvement of pelvic and pectoral girdles; pseudohypertrophy of the calves; high levels of activity of certain serum enzymes, notably creatine kinase; and relentless progression leading to wheelchair confinement by adolescence and death from cardiorespiratory insufficiency by age 20 years.

Duchenne muscular dystrophy is caused by a deletion mutation affecting the Xp21 region on the short arm of the X chromosome. Dystrophin, the large cytoskeletal protein normally encoded by this gene locus, is absent from the muscle fibers of patients with Duchenne muscular dystrophy. The precise function of dystrophin in maintaining the integrity of muscle and the mechanism by which dystrophin deficiency produces progressive muscle destruction remain to be determined. Becker muscular dystrophy, an allelic disorder affecting 1 in 30,000 male births, is distinguished clinically by later age at onset, slower rate of progression, and longer survival and biochemically by the presence of dystrophin of abnormal molecular weight. Approximately 70% of patients with Duchenne or Becker muscular dystrophy have detectable dystrophin mutations on routine DNA testing of peripheral blood. The remaining 30% are diagnosed by dystrophin analysis of muscle biopsy tissue.

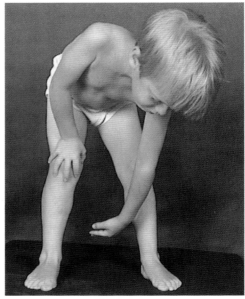

Figure 15-56. Duchenne muscular dystrophy. This child, age 5, has difficulty rising from the floor. Unilateral hand support on the knee is required to get erect.

Clinical manifestations of Duchenne muscular dystrophy do not usually appear until the second year of life or later. Early developmental milestones are normally attained, although the first attempts at walking may be delayed. Gait is often clumsy and awkward from the start, and the ability to run is never normally attained. Difficulty in climbing stairs, frequent falls, and progressive difficulty in rising from the floor are early features. To rise from the floor, the child may at first need only to push with one hand on a knee (Fig. 15-56). However, as weakness of the extensors of the hips becomes more pronounced, rising from the floor becomes increasingly difficult and requires the use of the hands to "climb up the legs" (the Gower maneuver) (Fig. 15-57).

Progressive gluteal weakness leads to the assumption of a compensatory posture characterized by a broadened base, accentuated lumbar lordosis, and forward thrusting of the abdomen (Fig. 15-58). Although weakness of the arms is not a common early symptom, proximal upper extremity weakness is easily detected on clinical examination when the child is lifted with the examiner's hands placed beneath the arms. There is marked laxity of the

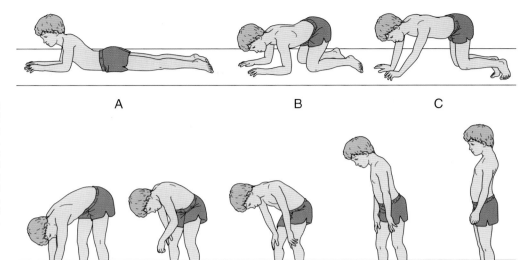

Figure 15-57. The Gower maneuver. This series of diagrams illustrates the sequence of postures used in attaining the upright position by a child with Duchenne muscular dystrophy. **A-C,** First, the legs are pulled up under the body, and the weight is shifted to rest on the hands and feet. **D,** The hips are then thrust in the air as the knees are straightened, and the hands are brought closer to the legs. **E-G,** Finally, the trunk is slowly extended by the hands walking up the thigh. **H,** The erect position is attained.

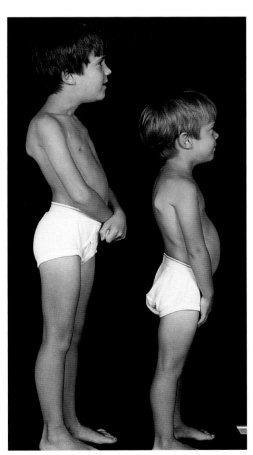

Figure 15-58. Compensatory posture in Duchenne muscular dystrophy. These brothers, ages 5 and 8, show the progression of compensatory postural adjustments with broadening of stance, accentuated lumbar lordosis, and forward thrusting of the abdomen, all more pronounced in the older boy.

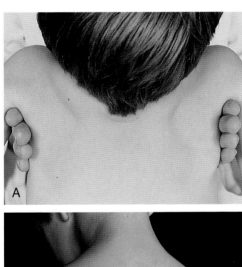

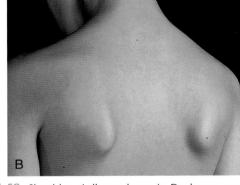

Figure 15-59. Shoulder girdle weakness in Duchenne muscular dystrophy. **A,** This child, age 5, demonstrates weakness and hypotonia of the shoulder girdle musculature. Upward displacement of the shoulders and abnormal rotation of the scapulae are seen when the child is lifted with the examiner's hands under his arms. **B,** Spontaneous winging of the scapulae can be noted in this 8-year-old.

shoulder girdle musculature associated with upward displacement of the shoulders and abnormal rotation of the scapulae (Fig. 15-59A). In addition, spontaneous winging of the scapulae may be prominent (Fig. 15-59B).

Weakness of the neck flexors, as evidenced by marked head lag when the child is pulled to sit from the supine position (Fig. 15-60), is an early finding. Enlargement of muscles, particularly in the calves (Fig. 15-61), is a common feature by 5 or 6 years of age. The abnormally enlarged muscles have an unusually firm, rubbery consistency on palpation. Early in the clinical course, this increase in muscle volume may result from true hypertrophy, with muscle strength proportional to bulk. Later, infiltration by fat and connective tissue sometimes maintains this bulk despite loss of muscle fibers. This is called *pseudohypertrophy.*

Charcot-Marie-Tooth Disease

Charcot-Marie-Tooth disease, also known as *hereditary motor-sensory neuropathy type I (HMSN-I)*, is an autosomal dominant demyelinating form of peroneal muscular atrophy. DNA studies have distinguished two genetic disorders, HMSN-IA, associated with a gene mutation of chromosome 17, and HMSN-IB, caused by a mutation on chromosome 1. Both share similar clinical features. The onset of symptoms is usually in the second decade, with presenting complaints being foot deformities and gait abnormalities. Often, pes cavus or hammer-toe deformities develop in early childhood long before more overt symptoms appear (see Fig. 21-109). The clinical picture is quite variable, and because most affected persons do not consult a physician for their neurologic problems, the majority of cases remain undiagnosed. The astute physician considers the diagnosis when a patient who presents with unrelated symptoms is found to have pes cavus or hammer-toes and symmetrical distal weakness.

Muscle weakness and atrophy begin insidiously in the foot and leg muscles. The intrinsic muscles of the foot are often affected first, followed by involvement of the peronei, anterior tibial, long toe extensor, intrinsic hand, and gastrocnemius muscles. Weakness and atrophy may even spread to the more proximal muscles of the leg and forearm. The degree of muscle wasting is often mild; however, in some cases the loss of muscle mass in the distal lower extremities is severe, giving rise to a striking "stork-leg" appearance (Fig. 15-62A). With involvement of

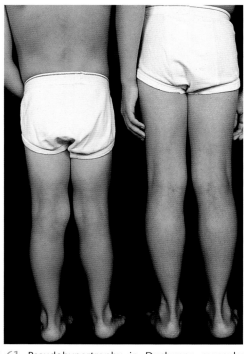

Figure 15-61. Pseudohypertrophy in Duchenne muscular dystrophy. Note the enlargement of the calves in brothers, ages 5 and 8.

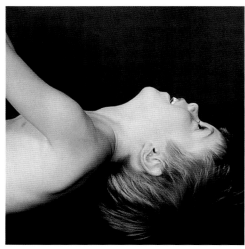

Figure 15-60. Neck muscle weakness in Duchenne muscular dystrophy. This 5-year-old boy has neck flexor weakness. Note the marked head lag when the patient is pulled to sit from the supine position.

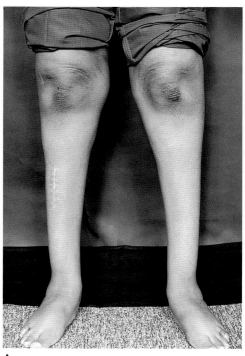

A

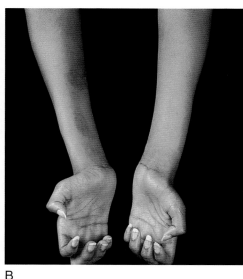

B

Figure 15-62. Charcot-Marie-Tooth disease. **A,** This patient, age 15, with distal muscular atrophy of the lower extremities demonstrates the "stork-leg" appearance. **B,** She also has atrophy of the forearm and intrinsic hand muscles resulting in a "claw-hand" deformity.

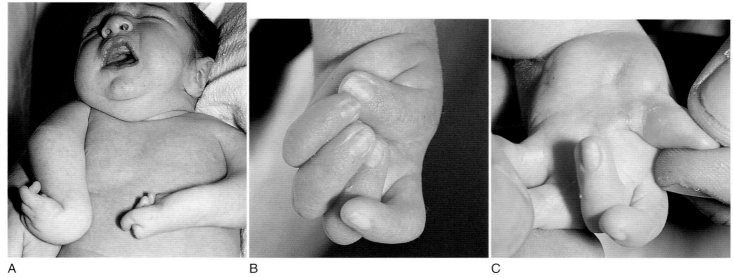

A   B   C

Figure 15-63. Congenital cervical spinal atrophy. **A,** This 2-day-old infant has flaccid paresis limited to the upper extremities and associated congenital flexion contractures. **B,** Wasting and atrophy of the intrinsic hand muscles with flexion contractures of the fingers and poorly developed transverse palmar creases **(C)** were also present.

the distal upper extremities there may be obvious wasting of the intrinsic hand muscles and development of secondary "claw deformities" (Fig. 15-62B). Deep tendon reflexes are lost first in the gastrocnemius and soleus muscles, and subsequently in the quadriceps femoris muscle and upper limbs. Sensation may be mildly impaired in the distal lower extremities.

Congenital Cervical Spinal Atrophy

Congenital cervical spinal atrophy is a rare disorder that is manifested at birth by dramatic flaccid paresis of the upper extremities (Fig. 15-63A). The presence of congenital flexion contractures suggests chronic denervation that must have occurred in utero and allows this syndrome to be distinguished from injury to the cervical spine or brachial plexuses during delivery (see Chapter 2). Abnormalities in the formation of the transverse palmar creases are present in all cases (Fig. 15-63B and C), suggesting an antenatal insult during the first trimester. The disorder is nonprogressive.

Myotonia Congenita

Myotonia congenita is an inherited disorder of skeletal muscle in which muscle stiffness is the only complaint. Autosomal dominant and autosomal recessive forms are related to different mutations of the skeletal muscle chloride channel gene on chromosome 7. The clinical symptoms are rather stereotypic. After a period of inactivity, the muscles stiffen and are difficult to maneuver; however, with continued activity, the stiffness diminishes and movement becomes almost normal. Typically, the child moves clumsily with a stiff, awkward gait and falls often. However, as activity continues, the child begins to walk freely and with adequate "warm-up" can run without difficulty.

Generalized muscular hypertrophy is a frequent finding on examination, with affected children often having an unusually well-developed, athletic appearance (Fig. 15-64).

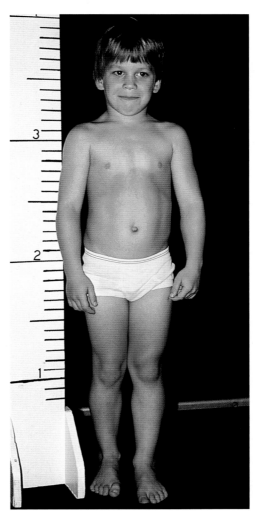

Figure 15-64. Body habitus in myotonia congenita. This 8-year-old boy demonstrates generalized muscular hypertrophy, giving him a well-developed, athletic appearance.

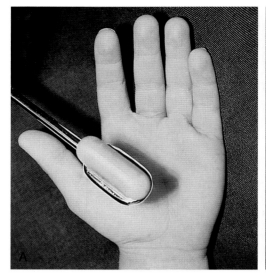
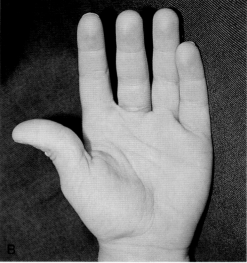

Figure 15-65. Myotonia congenita, delayed muscle relaxation. Percussion of the thenar eminence **(A)** is followed by involuntary opposition of the thumb and visible contraction of the muscles of the thenar eminence **(B),** which lasts for several seconds.

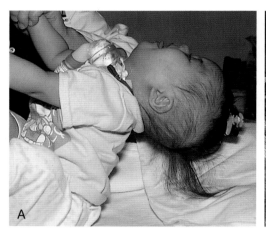
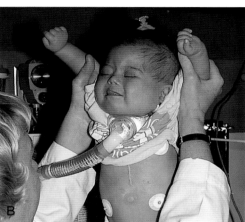

Figure 15-66. Hypotonic infant. **A,** Abnormal traction response. When the infant is pulled up from the supine position, her head falls into extreme extension and her arms fail to flex to counter the traction applied by the examiner. **B,** When held under the arms, she tends to slip through the examiner's hands.

This belies their sedentary habits and physical ineptitude resulting from muscle stiffness. Clinically, myotonia may be demonstrated by observing delayed relaxation of the muscles after sustained voluntary contraction such as clenching of the hand. Myotonia may also be elicited by percussion of the thenar eminence (Fig. 15-65).

The Hypotonic Infant

Because depression of muscle tone is clinically manifest by paucity of movement, unusual postures, diminished resistance to passive movement, and increased range of movement of joints, the hypotonic infant has been likened to a rag doll. The legs lie externally rotated and abducted, with their lateral surfaces in contact with the bed while the arms are extended at the sides or flexed so that the hands lie beside the head. When the infant is pulled up by the hands from the supine position (traction response), the head falls into extreme extension, and the limbs fail to flex to counter the traction (Fig. 15-66A). In horizontal suspension with the chest and abdomen supported by the examiner's hand, the infant with hypotonia drapes limply like an inverted U, and when held under the arms, tends to slip through the examiner's hands (Fig. 15-66B). Because maintenance of normal postural tone requires functional integrity of both the CNS and PNS, hypotonia is a common symptom of many disorders

Table 15-8	Differential Diagnosis of Hypotonia
DISORDERS OF THE CNS	**DISORDERS OF THE PNS**
Chromosome disorders	Spinal muscular atrophies
Trisomy	Congenital polyneuropathies
Prader-Willi syndrome	Transient neonatal myasthenia
Other	Congenital myasthenic syndromes
Other genetic defects	Congenital muscular dystrophy
Static encephalopathies	Myotonic dystrophy
Congenital malformation	Fukuyama type dystrophy
Perinatal acquired	Other
encephalopathy	Congenital myopathies
Postnatal acquired	Metabolic myopathies
encephalopathy	Systemic illness
Inborn errors of metabolism	Benign congenital hypotonia
Amino acid disorders	
Organic acid disorders	
Urea cycle disorders	
Peroxisomal disorders	
Lysosomal disorders	
Neonatal spinal cord injury	

affecting the brain, spinal cord, peripheral nerves, and muscles (Table 15-8). Hypotonia also occurs as a nonspecific manifestation of systemic illness. The term *benign congenital hypotonia* is reserved for infants with isolated depression of postural tone that resolves with growth and maturation, usually by 1 year of age. It is often a diagnosis of exclusion.

Childhood Epilepsy

The overall incidence of epilepsy follows a bimodal distribution, peaking in children younger than 5 years of age and in adults older than 65 years of age. A classification of epileptic seizures detailed in Table 15-9 divides them into those of focal onset (partial seizures) and those with bilateral cortical representation from the outset (generalized seizures). *Simple partial seizures* have no associated impairment of consciousness and may represent simple motor or sensory phenomena. Patients with *complex partial seizures* experience seizure spread to cortical and subcortical areas resulting in alteration in consciousness. Some partial seizures may secondarily generalize to contralateral brain areas, with loss of consciousness, often with bilateral convulsive features.

Generalized seizures may be convulsive or nonconvulsive in nature. In children, nonconvulsive generalized sei-zures often present as absence epilepsy. Other generalized seizures such as tonic, tonic-clonic, atonic, and myoclonic are defined by the type of motor activity observed.

Absence seizures are typically brief in duration (5 to 20 seconds) and are characterized by sudden staring or arrest of activity with abrupt recovery. They are often associated with facial automatisms such as eye flutter, chewing, or ocular supraversion (Fig. 15-67). The incidence of absence epilepsy peaks in children between the ages of 3 and 8 years; however, onset can be in adolescence. The disorder has a strong genetic predisposition and usually occurs in children who are otherwise neurologically and intellectually normal. It is often outgrown by late childhood or during adolescence. A typical electroencephalogram (EEG) pattern seen in affected individuals consists of generalized 3-per-second spike-and-wave discharges (Fig. 15-68),

Table 15-9	Classification of Epileptic Seizures
CURRENT TERMINOLOGY	**OTHER NAMES**
1. Partial seizures	Jacksonian, adversive, or
Simple partial (consciousness not impaired)	focal motor seizures
Motor signs	
Special sensory (visual, auditory, gustatory, vertiginous, or somatosensory)	
Autonomic	Abdominal epilepsy
Psychic (déjà vu, fear, and others)	
Complex partial (consciousness impaired)	Psychomotor, temporal lobe
Impaired consciousness at onset	
Development of impaired consciousness	
2. Generalized seizures	
Absence (nonconvulsive)	Petit mal
Typical	
Atypical	
Tonic-clonic	Grand mal, major motor
Atonic	Akinetic, drop attacks
Myoclonic	Minor motor
Tonic	
Clonic	
3. Unclassified	Infantile spasms

Modified from The International League Against Epilepsy, Epilepsia, 1981.

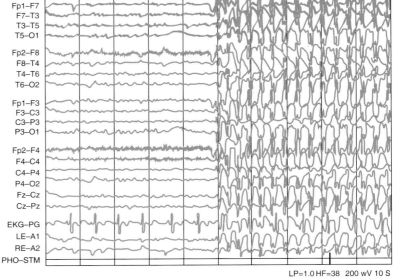

Figure 15-67. Absence seizure. This 8-year-old girl had a history of brief staring spells reported by teachers and family. Typical absence seizures were recorded during a video electroencephalogram with staring and ocular supraversion lasting under 10 seconds, which could be activated by hyperventilation.

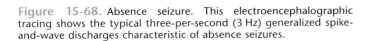

Figure 15-68. Absence seizure. This electroencephalographic tracing shows the typical three-per-second (3 Hz) generalized spike-and-wave discharges characteristic of absence seizures.

LP=1.0 HF=38 200 wV 10 S

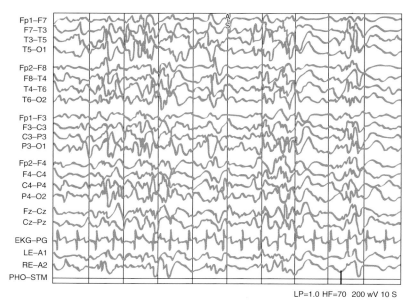

LP=1.0 HF=70 200 wV 10 S

Figure 15-69. Infantile spasms. This electroencephalograph tracing shows the hypsarrhythmia pattern consisting of markedly disorganized background and high-voltage multifocal epileptic spikes often found in patients with infantile spasms.

which can be activated by hyperventilation. Between 40% and 60% of patients with absence seizures go on to experience a generalized tonic-clonic convulsion.

Infantile spasms typically begin before age 2 with a peak age at onset between 4 and 6 months. They are classified as flexor, extensor, and mixed flexor-extensor types and are characterized by brief contractions of the neck, trunk, and extremities with the head thrown backward or forward in association with flexion and/or extension of the limbs. They often occur in clusters throughout the day, with greater frequency on awakening or falling asleep. Early in the course of the disorder, they may be mistaken for colic, hiccups, or gastroesophageal reflux. Etiologic origin of infantile spasms is varied and may include metabolic disorders, cerebral malformations, congenital infections, anoxic injury, and neurocutaneous disorders. However, up to 20% of cases are idiopathic or cryptogenic in origin. Tuberous sclerosis is the major single identifiable cause of infantile spasms, accounting for 7% to 25% of cases. Patients who have a known underlying disorder and infantile spasms have a higher incidence of developmental impairment than those of unknown cause. Neuroimaging is abnormal in 70% to 80% of affected children. The EEG in patients with infantile spasms often demonstrates a hypsarrhythmia pattern with markedly abnormal background features and multifocal high-voltage epileptic discharges, and it may show a burst-suppression pattern in sleep (Fig. 15-69). The triad of hypsarrhythmia, infantile spasms, and developmental delay is commonly referred to as *West syndrome.* More than 50% of patients with infantile spasms develop other forms of epilepsy later in life.

Paroxysmal Movement Disorders of Childhood

Paroxysmal (nonepileptic) movement disorders are relatively common in the pediatric population. They are manifest by excessive involuntary movement (dyskinesia) that is episodic and often stereotypic with preservation of consciousness.

Tic

Tics include a wide array of movements and sounds. They are involuntary, sudden, repetitive movements or vocalizations. They typically wax and wane, with old tics being replaced by new ones. Up to 25% of children may have a transient simple tic disorder lasting less than 1 year. The presence of multiple tics lasting longer than a year with both vocal and motor varieties fulfills diagnostic criteria for Tourette syndrome. Attention deficit hyperactivity disorder, obsessive-compulsive disorder, and learning disabilities are commonly seen in addition to tics in patients with Tourette syndrome.

Shuddering Attacks

Shuddering (shivering) spells are characterized by flexion of the head, trunk, elbows, and knees with adduction of the limbs and are often described as a "chill" or as having a sense of "ice water being poured down one's back." They represent a benign movement disorder often starting in infancy and usually abating in childhood.

Startle Disease

A startle response is a brief motor response to an unexpected stimulus (auditory, tactile, visual, or vestibular) that readily habituates (e.g., diminishes with repeated exposure). Hyperexplexia (startle disease) is characterized by a nonhabituating, exaggerated startle response to stimuli often followed by a tonic spasm. Affected children often have hypertonia in infancy, feeding difficulties, and apnea. The startle response can be elicited in hyperexplexic patients by tapping on the forehead, nose, glabella, or vertex of the skull. The course of the disease is variable, and cognitive abilities are not affected.

Head Bobbing

Head bobbing consists of jerky head movements at a frequency of two to three cycles per second and resembles that of a doll's head atop a spring. In childhood it may appear as part of spasmus nutans or the bobble-head doll syndrome. Spasmus nutans is a benign disorder of unknown etiology that occurs in early infancy and is characterized by nystagmus (binocular or monocular), head nodding, and head tilt. Neurologic examination is otherwise normal. The syndrome lasts 1 to 2 years and spontaneously resolves. The bobble-head doll syndrome consists of intermittent head nodding and is seen in association with an underlying CNS structural abnormality, often a third ventricular cyst or tumor.

Chorea or Choreoathetosis

Chorea consists of random, brief, rapid, purposeless jerking movements of the limbs, face, tongue, or trunk, whereas choreoathetosis is characterized by slow writhing movements that often are more prominent on one side of the body. Sydenham chorea (St. Vitus dance) is the most prevalent form of acquired chorea in childhood. It is a manifestation of poststreptococcal rheumatic fever and often begins insidiously weeks to months after a streptococcal infection that may or may not have been symptomatic. It is characterized by choreiform movements, emotional lability, and hypotonia. Behavior change, decline in school performance, and anxiety are common associated features. The disorder usually resolves after several months, although recurrences may be triggered by new episodes of streptococcal infection, pregnancy (chorea gravidarum), or oral contraceptive use. Other less common causes of chorea and/or choreoathetosis in childhood include Wilson disease, Huntington disease, systemic lupus erythematosus, and hyperthyroidism.

Bibliography

Bell WE, McCormick WF: Increased Intracranial Pressure in Children, 2nd ed. Philadelphia, WB Saunders, 1978.

Brooke MH: A Clinician's View of Neuromuscular Diseases, 2nd ed. Baltimore, Williams & Wilkins, 1987.

Chao DH: Congenital neurocutaneous syndromes of childhood. III: Sturge-Weber disease. J Pediatr 55:635-649, 1959.

Dubowitz V: The Floppy Infant, 2nd ed. Philadelphia, JB Lippincott, 1980.

Emery AEH: Duchenne Muscular Dystrophy, 2nd ed. Oxford, England, Oxford University Press, 1993.

Enjolras O, Riche MC, Merland JJ: Facial port-wine stains and Sturge-Weber syndrome. Pediatrics 76:48-52, 1985.

Fenichel GM: Clinical Pediatric Neurology: A Signs and Symptoms Approach, 5th ed. Philadelphia, WB Saunders, 2005.

Goldstein SM, Curless RG, Post JD, Quencer RM: A new sign of neurofibromatosis on magnetic resonance imaging of children. Arch Neurol 46:1222-1224, 1989.

Gomez MR (ed): Tuberous Sclerosis, 2nd ed. New York, Raven Press, 1998.

Hoffman EP, Fishbeck KH, Brown RH, et al: Characterization of dystrophin in muscle-biopsy specimens from patients with Duchenne's or Becker's muscular dystrophy. N Engl J Med 318:1363-1368, 1988.

International League Against Epilepsy, Commission on Classification and Terminology: Proposal for a revised classification of epilepsies and epileptic syndromes. Epilepsia 26:268-278, 1985.

Martuza RL, Eldridge R: Neurofibromatosis 2. N Engl J Med 318:684-688, 1988.

Menkes JH: Textbook of Child Neurology, 5th ed. Philadelphia, Lea & Febiger, 1995.

Mitchell WG: Current therapy in neurologic disease: Cerebral cysticercosis in North American children. Eur Neurol 37:126-129, 1997.

Osborne JP: Diagnosis of tuberous sclerosis. Arch Dis Child 63:1423-1425, 1988.

Paller AS: The Sturge-Weber syndrome. Pediatr Dermatol 4:300-304, 1987.

Riccardi VM: Von Recklinghausen neurofibromatosis. N Engl J Med 305:1617-1627, 1981.

Riccardi VM, Eichneer JE: Neurofibromatosis: Phenotypes-Natural History and Pathogenesis, 2nd ed. Baltimore, Johns Hopkins University Press, 1992.

Roach ES, Gometz MR, Northrup H: Tuberous Sclerosis Complex Consensus Conference: Revised clinical diagnostic criteria. J Child Neurol 13:624-628, 1998.

Roach ES, William DP, Laster DW: Magnetic resonance imaging in tuberous sclerosis. Arch Neurol 44:301-303, 1987.

Swaiman KF, Ashwal S: Pediatric Neurology: Principles and Practice, 3rd ed. St Louis, Mosby, 1999.

Warkany J, Lemire RJ, Cohen MM: Mental Retardation and Congenital Malformations of the Central Nervous System. St Louis, Mosby, 1981.

CHAPTER 16

Pulmonary Disorders

Jonathan D. Finder

Respiratory disease is one of the most common reasons that pediatric patients seek medical attention. Signs and symptoms can be subtle, and a careful history and physical examination are always useful in assessment of pediatric patients with respiratory complaints. Diseases of the chest can be divided into two major categories: acquired and congenital. Congenital chest diseases are often symptomatic at all times rather than episodically. A child who has chronic noisy breathing from a congenital vascular ring, for example, is not as likely as the patient with asthma to have intermittent periods of wheezing with long intervals of normal breathing. The spectrum of diseases involving the pediatric respiratory system is primarily dependent on the age of the patient; therefore age must be a primary consideration in the differential diagnosis.

History

Each pediatric history should include the obstetric history. A history of respiratory distress at birth or of intubation, however brief, is important. Noisy breathing starting early in life suggests congenital airway obstruction and should be evaluated. Regardless of cause, failure to thrive is a worrisome finding, whereas excellent weight gain in a child with noisy breathing is reassuring.

Distinguishing between constant and intermittent symptoms can be one of the most important means of diagnosing diseases of the pediatric chest. A good "cough history" and "wheeze history" are important and have similar elements. The clinician should inquire about the chronicity of the symptoms; association with feeding; upper respiratory infections; exposures (pets, dust, and especially cigarette smoking are important); and fevers. The effect—or lack thereof—of medications may give important diagnostic information. The nature of the cough is important: wet or dry, paroxysmal or continuous, and staccato (as seen in neonatal chlamydial pneumonia) are important descriptive terms. Post-tussive emesis is a "red flag" to the clinician. The cough that awakens the child at night or keeps the child up much of the night is another worrisome historical finding. Conversely, a persistent cough that disappears in sleep strongly suggests the diagnosis of habit (psychogenic) cough. In pursuing a history of wheeze, it is important to ask the parents or historians what they mean by the term; it may mean "noisy breathing," and it may even be applied to stridor.

In evaluating the infant with frequent episodes of cough and/or wheeze, the clinician should inquire about symptoms and signs of gastroesophageal reflux (GER): food refusal, arching, pain behaviors, frequent spitting, milk or formula found on the bed next to the infant's head in the morning, recurrent croup, hoarseness, and laryngomalacia. Because reflux is worse when the patient is lying down, symptoms tend to be more prominent at night and during naps.

A family history of atopy including eczema and environmental allergies should be investigated. In inquiring about cystic fibrosis, an autosomal recessive trait, an extended family medical history including grandparents and cousins should be taken. Frequent infections in parents or siblings, particularly those requiring hospitalization, suggest possible immunodeficiency in the family.

Immunization history is essential in identifying patients at risk for pertussis. Often, parents state that the immunizations are up to date, although the child has in fact not had any pertussis vaccinations. Immunization avoidance occurs commonly owing to publicity given to well-disproven theories of immunization-induced autism.

Exercise intolerance is one of the primary symptoms of respiratory disease. The neonate's main output of energy is in feeding, and thus difficulties with feedings should be monitored; toddlers are expected to keep up with peers and/or siblings in play; the school-age child's gym performance should be scrutinized. Wheezing or coughing fits following vigorous exercise can occur in asthma.

Physical Examination

Examination of the chest in any uncooperative patient is notoriously difficult, but it can be easily accomplished with patience and a few tricks. The infant or toddler is best examined with his or her shirt off while being held upright in the arms of a parent. The patient should face the parent; this maximizes contact with the parent and allows the patient to feel safe. The room should be at a comfortable temperature. The stethoscope head should be warmed in the clinician's hand or pocket for several minutes before use. The classic four steps in the physical examination—inspection, palpation, percussion, and auscultation—are well applied to the examination of the pediatric chest.

Inspection. Inspection should include evaluation for digital clubbing (see Fig. 16-39). Decreased subcutaneous adipose tissue as seen in a cystic fibrosis patient should be noted. The pattern of breathing should always be evaluated with the child disrobed. Any use of expiratory musculature is abnormal. Suprasternal and intercostal retractions reflect excessive negative pleural pressure and can be seen in normal children with thin chest walls after vigorous exercise. Subcostal retractions are always pathologic and are the result of a flattened diaphragm pulling inward on the chest wall. In advanced lung disease the use of accessory muscles of inspiration can be noted; the sternocleidomastoid muscle, for example, helps lift the chest (in a "bucket handle" fashion) and increase its anteroposterior diameter, thereby increasing intrathoracic volume. In respiratory muscle fatigue, a pattern of breathing can be observed in which the diaphragm alternates with the intercostal muscles to inflate the lungs. This is known as *respiratory alternans* and is seen as alternating abdominal and chest expansion instead of the usual pattern of simultaneous chest and abdominal expansion. Chest wall deformities such as pectus excavatum or pectus carinatum (see Chapter 17) should be noted.

Palpation. Palpation of the chest can reveal significant findings. The examiner places the hands on either side of the chest as the patient takes a deep breath. The chest should expand symmetrically; asymmetry can be seen in unilateral pulmonary hypoplasia, mainstem bronchial obstruction, and diaphragmatic paresis. Placing fingertips on the upper abdomen just over the insertion of the rectus muscles into the lower rib cage can reveal subtle use of expiratory muscles in children with obstructive lower airway disease. Similarly, the anterior lower ribs should be assessed with the fingertips. In infants with obstructive lung disease, the lower ribs can be felt to pull inwards on inspiration. This is the palpable aspect of a subcostal retraction. With the patient's head in the midline position, the trachea should be palpated at the sternal notch to evaluate for tracheal deviation, as is seen with mediastinal shift. Vocal fremitus should be assessed in patients with suspected pleural fluid accumulation; the vibrations transmitted from the larynx as the child says "99" are diminished when there is an accumulation of air or fluid in the pleural space. Infants and children with tracheomalacia and bronchomalacia often have a palpable vibration in the back. Palpable vibrations in only one hemithorax suggest a partial obstruction of the mainstem bronchus in that hemithorax as seen in bronchomalacia.

Percussion. Percussion of the chest can reveal much more than hyperresonance and dullness over an area of consolidation. Air trapping is the hallmark of small airway disease and results in a depressed position of the diaphragm. Ordinarily the diaphragm can be found just at or slightly below the tip of the scapula when the patient's arm is at his or her side in children 5 years and younger. In the patient with hyperinflation, the diaphragm is found several fingerbreadths below the scapular tips. This finding, even in the absence of wheezing on auscultation, suggests a lesion of the small airways. An area of consolidation or pleural effusion results in dullness to percussion. Another disorder causing asymmetry of percussion of the two hemithoraces is diaphragmatic eventration, a congenital lesion of the diaphragm in which the diaphragm is replaced with a thin fibrous membrane without contractile properties. Postoperative diaphragmatic paralysis (rarely found following cardiac surgery) can be diagnosed by percussion of the cooperative patient while holding his or her breath at maximal inspiration and at endexpiration.

Auscultation. Auscultation of the pediatric chest requires patience. One often must wait a minute or two for a deep breath in order to appreciate abnormal breath sounds that are not apparent on shallow breathing. Augmenting the expiratory phase with a gentle squeeze of the thorax while listening with the stethoscope may bring out expiratory wheezes.

Abnormal ("adventitial") breath sounds include crackles and wheezes. Wheezes are continuous sounds, whereas crackles (formerly referred to as rales) are discontinuous. Wheezes and crackles can be inspiratory or expiratory, although crackles are more commonly heard on inspiration and wheezes are more commonly heard on expiration.

Wheezes probably arise from the vibration of the walls of partially obstructed large and medium-sized airways. In a patient experiencing an acute exacerbation of asthma, the lungs have wheezes in a range of pitches (polyphonic) with substantial regional differences in auscultation. Patients with central airway obstruction such as tracheomalacia, on the other hand, have a single pitch of wheeze that sounds the same in all lung fields (monophonic) and is heard loudest over the central airway that is obstructed. Foreign bodies can cause a monophonic wheeze that can vary in pitch depending on the degree of obstruction.

Crackles are believed to arise from the popping open of fluid menisci within airways. The crackles heard in the lungs of patients with interstitial lung disease have yet to be explained adequately but may arise from popping open of small airways. Coarse crackles are often audible at the

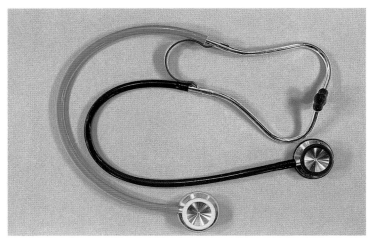

Figure 16-1. Differential stethoscope. A differential, or double-headed, stethoscope can be made from a Sprague-Rappaport type stethoscope by adding two chest pieces as shown. This allows for simultaneous auscultation of homologous lung segments. Certain findings can be found only with this stethoscope, including phase delay (typical of foreign body aspiration).

mouth and are a late finding in cystic fibrosis patients with advanced bronchiectasis. "Rhonchi" refers to the sound made by pooled secretions in the central airways, which can be categorized as harsh, low-pitched central wheezes or coarse, central crackles (depending on the nature of the sounds heard).

Other sounds that can be heard include friction rubs, which are creaking sounds heard during both phases of respiration as inflamed pleural surfaces rub over one another. One of the most important abnormal findings in children is the absence of breath sounds over an area of collapse or consolidation. Phase delay in air entry (such as in unilateral bronchial obstruction) can only be detected using the differential (double-headed) stethoscope (Fig. 16-1).

Radiology

The pediatric chest radiograph is unique in that normal findings may vary with age. The width of the chest on the lateral projection in the chest radiograph of a normal infant (Fig. 16-2) is about the same as the transverse dimension on a frontal projection, and the lungs may appear relatively radiolucent. Further, in contrast with the older child (>2 years of age), the cardiothoracic ratio in the infant normally may be as high as 0.65. The width of the superior mediastinum at this age may also be striking because the thymic shadow is particularly prominent during the first few months of life before the normal process of involution occurs. The normal chest radiograph of an older child (Fig. 16-3) shows the diaphragm on an inspiratory film at the eighth or ninth rib posteriorly (sixth rib anteriorly), a cardiothoracic ratio of 0.5, and pulmonary vessels extending two thirds of the way to the periphery. In most situations a lateral radiograph should accompany the posteroanterior (PA) view because some pathologic findings may be missed on a single projection. For example, a lateral x-ray examination yields the best information about the anterior mediastinum and the tracheal air column and may reveal a small pleural effusion that is unsuspected on the basis of a PA radiograph alone. In combination with the PA view, the lateral projection may help localize an abnormal finding to a particular lobe or segment. In most situations the chest x-ray film taken at full inspiration is most helpful. In the evaluation for bronchial foreign bodies, a comparison of inspiratory and expiratory views (or left and right lateral decubitus films in the younger patient) can help if one lung is unable to empty. In looking for a small pneumothorax, the expiratory film is more helpful because the smaller lung volume allows extrapulmonary air to expand to become more evident.

Cough

Persistent or recurrent cough represents one of the most common and vexing problems in pediatrics. In most circumstances the tracheobronchial tree is kept clean by

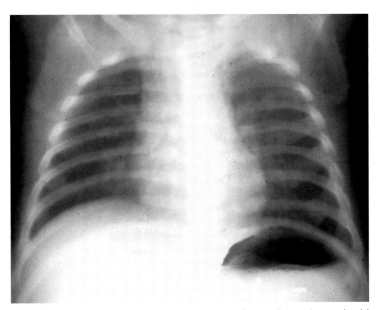

Figure 16-2. Normal posteroanterior chest radiograph in a 1-month-old infant. (Courtesy Beverly Newman, MD, Pittsburgh.)

airway macrophages and the mucociliary escalator, but cough becomes an important component of airway clearance when excessive or abnormal materials are present, or when mucociliary clearance is reduced, as during a viral respiratory illness. A cough clears airway secretions and inhaled particulate matter through a combination of the high airflow velocities generated during the expiratory phase of the cough and compression of smaller airways, which "milks" the secretions into larger bronchi where they can be eliminated by a subsequent cough. Cough is generally produced by a reflex response arising from irritant receptors located in ciliated epithelia in the lower respiratory tract, but it can be suppressed or initiated at higher cortical centers. One of the most common causes of cough in pediatric patients is the self-limited cough of an acute viral lower respiratory illness or bronchitis that lasts 1 to 2 weeks. The cough that persists longer than 2 weeks is potentially more worrisome. A diagnostic approach to chronic cough is best served by considering the age of the child (Table 16-1).

Several causes of persistent cough are common to all pediatric age groups, such as second-hand cigarette smoke exposure, recurrent viral bronchitis, asthma, gastroesophageal reflux (GER), cystic fibrosis, granulomatous lung disease (e.g., tuberculosis), foreign body aspiration, and pertussis.

Age and Cause

Infancy (Younger Than 1 Year)

Cough starting at birth or shortly afterward may be a sign of serious respiratory disease and must be evaluated assiduously. Cough beginning at this time raises the possibility of congenital infections, such as cytomegalovirus (Fig. 16-4) or rubella, which are often associated with other findings, such as hepatosplenomegaly, thrombocytopenia, or central nervous system disease. Pneumonia due to *Chlamydia trachomatis* (Fig. 16-5) generally develops after the first month of life and presents as an afebrile pneumonitis with congestion; wheezing; fine, diffuse

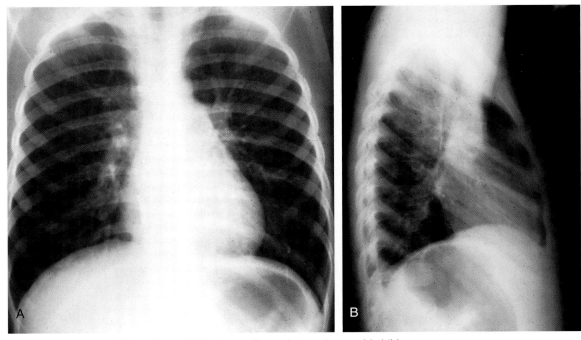

Figure 16-3. Normal posteroanterior **(A)** and lateral **(B)** chest radiographs in a 6-year-old child.

Table 16-1	Causes of Cough According to Age

Infancy (Younger Than 1 Year)
Congenital and Neonatal Infections
Chlamydia
Viral (e.g., RSV, CMV, rubella)
Bacterial (e.g., pertussis)
Pneumocystis jiroveci
Congenital Malformations
Tracheoesophageal fistula
Vascular ring
Airway malformations (e.g., laryngeal cleft)
Pulmonary sequestration
Other
Cystic fibrosis
Asthma
Recurrent viral bronchiolitis/bronchitis
Gastroesophageal reflux
Interstitial pneumonitides
Lymphoid interstitial pneumonitis
Diffuse interstitial pneumonitis

Preschool
Inhaled foreign body
Asthma
Suppurative lung disease
  Cystic fibrosis
  Bronchiectasis
Right middle lobe syndrome
Ciliary dyskinesia syndromes
Upper respiratory tract disease
Recurrent viral infection/bronchitis
Passive smoke inhalation
Gastroesophageal reflux
Interstitial pneumonitides
Pulmonary hemosiderosis

School Age to Adolescence
Asthma
Cystic fibrosis
Mycoplasma pneumoniae infection
Psychogenic or habit cough
Cigarette smoking
Pulmonary hemosiderosis
Interstitial pneumonitides
Ciliary dyskinesia syndromes

All Ages
Recurrent viral illness
Asthma
Cystic fibrosis
Granulomatous lung disease
Foreign body aspiration
Pertussis infection

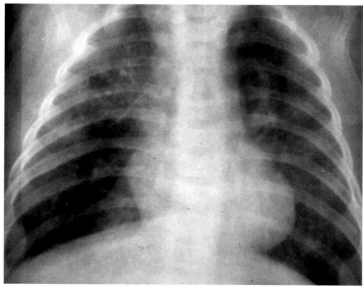

Figure 16-4. Pneumonia caused by cytomegalovirus in an infant. (Courtesy Beverly Newman, MD, Pittsburgh.)

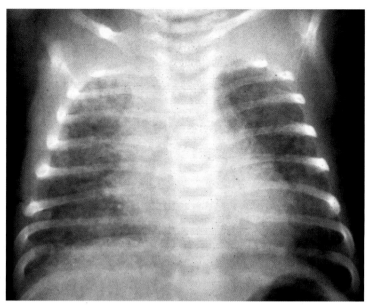

Figure 16-5. Pneumonia caused by *Chlamydia trachomatis* in a 3-month-old infant with inclusion conjunctivitis.

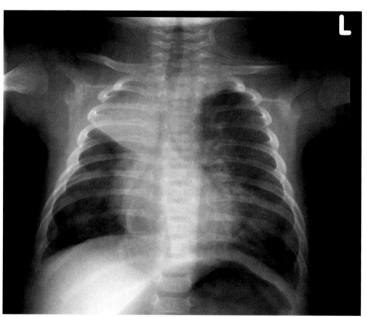

Figure 16-6. Pertussis in a 6-week-old infant demonstrates the typical radiographic pattern of perihilar involvement. This child also has right upper lobe atelectasis. (Courtesy Katie McPeak, MD, Pittsburgh.)

crackles; a paroxysmal cough; and, in approximately 50% of cases, a prior or concomitant inclusion conjunctivitis. Pneumonia caused by *Bordetella pertussis* is a potentially life-threatening illness characterized by severe paroxysmal coughing episodes followed by cyanosis and apnea and is often associated with an inspiratory "whoop." The latter finding may be missing in young infants or those weakened by the recurrent coughing spasms. Newborns and young infants may have apnea as the primary sign of a *B. pertussis* infection. The chest radiograph is nondiagnostic and can be normal or (Fig. 16-6) show perihilar infiltrates; atelectasis; hyperinflation; and, in some cases, interstitial or subcutaneous emphysema. A high white blood cell count with a predominance of lymphocytes supports the diagnosis, but unfortunately once the patient has passed through the usually innocent-appearing coryzal

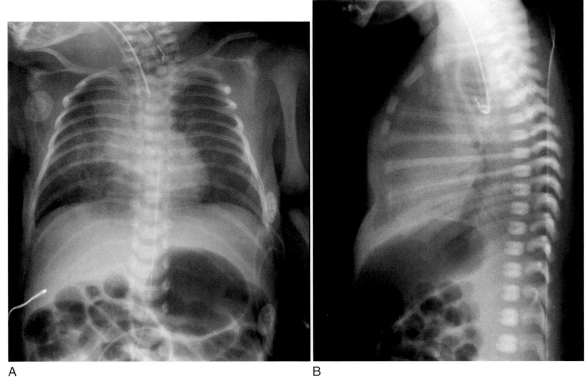

. A   B

Figure 16-7. Tracheoesophageal fistula. **A,** Anteroposterior chest radiograph shows feeding tube passing no farther than proximal esophagus; there is an aspiration pneumonitis present. **B,** Lateral view showing the feeding tube in the proximal esophageal pouch with air in the airway, distal esophagus, and intestine. (**A,** Courtesy Beverly Newman, MD, Pittsburgh; **B,** courtesy Katie McPeak, MD, Pittsburgh.)

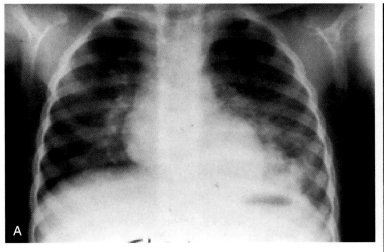

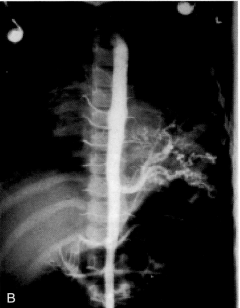

Figure 16-8. Pulmonary sequestration. **A,** Anteroposterior film shows left lower lobe infiltrate. **B,** Aortic angiogram demonstrates anomalous origin of pulmonary blood supply from abdominal aorta to the left lower lobe in a 7-year-old girl with extralobar sequestration. (Courtesy Geoffrey Kurland, MD, Pittsburgh.)

stage into the paroxysmal stage, diagnostic tests have a lower yield. Newer diagnostic approaches to whooping cough include detection of the *B. pertussis* DNA using the polymerase chain reaction (PCR) and serologic detection of *B. pertussis*-specific IgM or IgA. *Ureaplasma urealyticum* and *Pneumocystis jiroveci* (formerly known as *P. carinii*) have been recognized as causes of pneumonia and persistent cough in this age group.

Congenital malformations, such as tracheoesophageal fistula (Fig. 16-7) and laryngeal cleft or web, can produce cough via chronic aspiration of gastric contents, milk, or saliva. These anomalies are associated with feeding-related

coughing, choking, and occasional cyanosis. Infants with neurologic disorders may have incoordination of swallowing and sucking reflexes that lead to aspiration of milk or gastric contents into the lung. Pulmonary sequestration (in which a portion of the lung is perfused by systemic, not pulmonary arteries) (Fig. 16-8) and bronchogenic cysts (cystic structures arising from the pulmonary epithelium) are rare congenital anomalies that may compress the pulmonary tree or become infected, thereby producing a cough. Aberrant major blood vessels generally cause inspiratory stridor and expiratory wheezing from tracheal compression (Fig. 16-9; see also Fig. 16-23), but a brassy

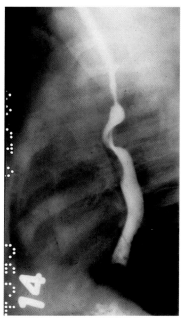

Figure 16-9. Vascular ring. Barium swallow in a toddler with posterior compression of esophagus and trachea from a vascular ring. (Courtesy Department of Radiology, Children's Hospital of Pittsburgh.)

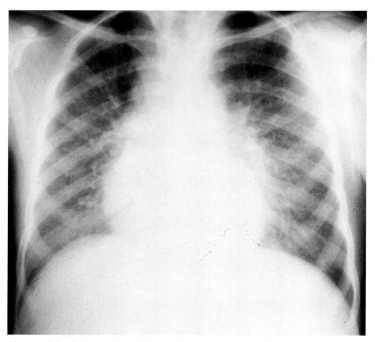

Figure 16-10. Lymphocytic interstitial pneumonitis. Posteroanterior chest radiograph of a 10-year-old boy shows a diffuse increase in interstitial markings.

cough may also be observed, as may dysphagia from the associated esophageal compression.

The triad of poor weight gain, steatorrhea, and chronic cough at this age makes cystic fibrosis a strong consideration, and a sweat test is mandatory. Asthma ("reactive airway disease") or bronchial hyperresponsiveness is a common and probably underdiagnosed cause of cough in infancy. Cough or persistent wheezing can be found in these infants, who may have a history of a previous viral lower respiratory illness with or without a family history of wheezing and/or asthma. Babies with GER may have a combination of effortless vomiting; nocturnal cough/wheeze; pain behaviors/arching; hoarseness; laryngomalacia; and, in some cases, poor weight gain. The absence of a history of vomiting ("spitting up") does not eliminate GER as a diagnostic consideration in infants with persistent coughing because occult reflux or microaspiration may induce bronchospasm.

Lymphocytic interstitial pneumonia (LIP) and the diffuse interstitial pneumonitides are rare causes of cough in children and are of unknown etiology. Usual interstitial pneumonitis (UIP) and desquamative interstitial pneumonitis (DIP) present with an insidious onset of cough, dyspnea, anorexia, weight loss, tachypnea, poor exercise tolerance, and scattered bibasilar crackles. Later, cyanosis and clubbing can occur. Both are chronic interstitial inflammatory lung diseases of unknown etiology, and both result in restrictive lung disease. LIP may present in a similar fashion, but it must also be suspected in those patients at risk for human immunodeficiency virus (HIV) infection. The diagnosis of interstitial pneumonitis depends on tissue obtained at lung biopsy. An interstitial pattern on chest radiograph (Fig. 16-10) is seen with varying degrees of hyperinflation or patchy atelectasis. High-resolution CT (HRCT) is a much more sensitive tool for the diagnosis of interstitial lung disease than routine chest radiograph or conventional CT.

Preschool

The two most common reasons for a persistent cough in this age group are recurrent viral infections and asthma.

The child with asthma may not manifest audible wheezing or dyspnea but rather may have persistent cough, especially with viral respiratory infections, following exposure to noxious inhalants, such as cigarette smoke, or following vigorous activity.

Upper respiratory tract disease and sinusitis have been implicated in the pathogenesis of chronic cough, presumably through the stimulation of pharyngeal cough receptors by upper airway secretions. Parental smoking (passive smoking) itself is a common cause of cough in preschool children. GER more commonly causes cough at a younger age but may appear at any age. The interstitial pneumonitides may also produce a chronic cough in this age group.

An inhaled foreign body in either the tracheobronchial tree or esophagus is an important cause of chronic cough, especially in toddlers. A history of gagging or choking may be absent at this age, physical examination may be unrevealing, and the plain chest radiograph may be normal. Subtle differences in air entry into homologous lung segments detected by the differential (double-headed) stethoscope (see Fig. 16-1) may be the only indication of a foreign body in the airway. Cough is present in more than 90% of cases; it is usually of abrupt onset, but a quiescent period may occur after inhalation and cough may disappear as irritant receptors adjust to the object's presence. A mobile foreign body may result in the recurrence of cough as new receptors are stimulated by the object. Although inspiratory and expiratory radiography and fluoroscopy are useful in the evaluation of a child with a possible bronchial foreign body, they may be normal and rigid bronchoscopy may be necessary to confirm or disprove the presence of a foreign object (Fig. 16-11). Unilateral air trapping demonstrated by inspiratory and expiratory radiographs (Fig. 16-12A and B) (or left and right lateral decubitus films in younger children) strongly suggests an inhaled foreign body.

Suppurative lung diseases, such as cystic fibrosis or bronchiectasis (Fig. 16-13), from any other causes (e.g., tuberculosis) characteristically result in a chronic cough producing purulent sputum. "Right middle lobe syndrome," commonly associated with enlargement of lymph nodes surrounding the right middle lobe bronchus in tuberculosis, has also been described in asthma and a number of other illnesses and may be associated with chronic cough. Recurrent infection of the middle lobe can ultimately lead to the development of bronchiectasis or fibrosis.

Disorders of ciliary motility (primary ciliary dyskinesia and acquired ciliary dyskinesia) may produce insidious symptoms of chronic productive cough, nasal drainage, recurrent middle ear infections, and fever. Clinical findings include basilar crackles (which can be expiratory) and, later, radiographic changes of recurrent lower lobe

infections and bronchiectasis. Repetitive infections occur unless measures such as chest physical therapy, postural drainage, and liberal use of antibiotics are employed. It is now recognized that the classic triad described by Kartagener of situs inversus, sinusitis, and bronchiectasis fits only a limited number of patients because situs inversus occurs in only about half of all patients with primary cilia dyskinesia. Far more common is an acquired ciliary dyskinesia that can follow certain lower respiratory infections (including adenovirus, *Mycoplasma*, respiratory syncytial virus, and influenza). Diagnosis can be made via biopsy of the respiratory epithelium, either from curettage of the nasal turbinate in the office or forceps biopsy of the bronchus via rigid bronchoscope under anesthesia.

Pulmonary hemosiderosis (Fig. 16-14) is a potentially fatal disorder that has been described in association with cardiac or panorganic disease, glomerulonephritis (Goodpasture syndrome), infantile hypersensitivity to cow's milk protein (Heiner syndrome), collagen vascular diseases, and as an idiopathic form. Idiopathic pulmonary hemosiderosis (IPH) is a disease of unknown etiology characterized by episodes of dyspnea, cough and/or hemoptysis, cyanosis, fever, and iron-deficiency anemia. Hematemesis or melena may be the only presenting complaint in some patients without symptoms referable to the respiratory tract. As a result of recurrent bleeding episodes, jaundice may be observed, and clubbing develops over time in some patients. Laboratory findings include iron-deficiency anemia and, in a small number of patients, peripheral eosinophilia. Radiographic findings (see Fig. 16-14) are quite variable, with some patients demonstrating scant transient infiltrates and others showing widespread parenchymal infiltrates that resemble miliary tuberculosis. Hemosiderin-laden macrophages obtained from sputum, gastric washings, or bronchoalveolar lavage suggest the diagnosis, but a lung biopsy is necessary and

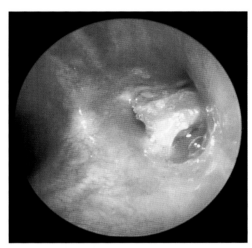

Figure 16-11. Foreign body. Portion of a carrot lodged in the right mainstem bronchus, as seen through a rigid bronchoscope. (Courtesy S. Stool, MD, Pittsburgh.)

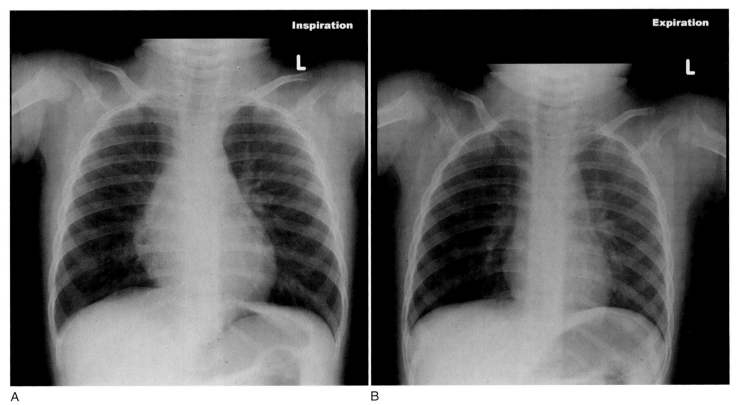

A   B

Figure 16-12. Foreign body. Inspiratory **(A)** and expiratory **(B)** radiograph in a child with an inhaled foreign body lodged in the right mainstem bronchus reveals hyperlucency of the right hemithorax and compensatory shift of the mediastinal structures to the left on expiration.

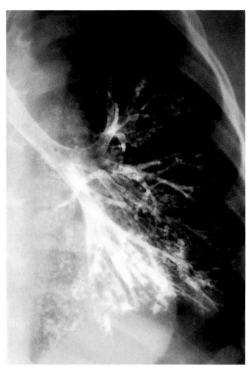

Figure 16-13. Bronchiectasis. Bronchogram shows cylindrical bronchiectasis of the left lower lobe in a 5-year-old girl with recurrent pneumonia and chronic cough.

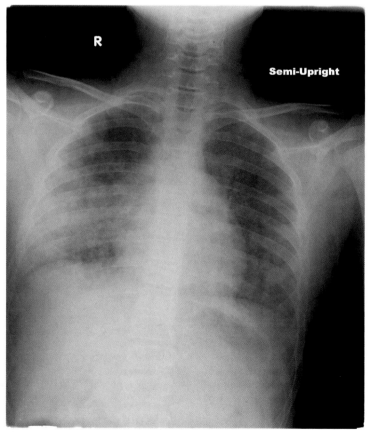

Figure 16-14. Idiopathic pulmonary hemosiderosis. Posteroanterior chest radiograph of a 15-year-old with idiopathic pulmonary hemosiderosis with an acute pulmonary hemorrhage in the right lower lobe shows alveolar space filling in the right lower lobe, as well as diffuse increase in interstitial markings.

will allow the clinician to differentiate vasculitis from capillaritis and assess for iron deposition. A percutaneous renal biopsy may help in cases of hemosiderosis associated with Goodpasture syndrome.

School Age to Adolescence

Because children are exposed to numerous respiratory viruses during the first several years of school, recurrent viral infection remains an important cause of chronic cough in this age group. Asthma continues to be a consideration in the patient with a chronic cough. Patients in this age group (older than 6) can perform pulmonary function tests including bronchodilator responsiveness or bronchial provocation studies to confirm the diagnosis. Other disorders may present with chronic cough at this age including allergic rhino-sinusitis, cystic fibrosis, pulmonary hemosiderosis, interstitial pneumonitis, and primary ciliary dyskinesia.

Mycoplasma pneumoniae infection is an important cause of chronic cough among school-age children. In its early stages, the disease is identical to a viral upper respiratory infection with coryza, sore throat, low-grade fever, and malaise. Gradually, the symptoms of lower respiratory involvement emerge and persist. Cough ranges from dry and hacking to one productive of mucoid sputum. Occasionally the disease progresses to lobar pneumonia (Fig. 16-15A and B) indistinguishable from typical bacterial pneumonia. The cough typically persists for 6 weeks, although it may last for 3 months. Physical findings tend to be minimal, although crackles and wheezing are often noted. The chest radiograph is not diagnostic, and the findings may be either interstitial or bronchopneumonic in character, with predilection for the lower lobes (see Fig. 16-15A and B). Often the chest radiograph is normal. Diagnosis of *M. pneumoniae* infection can be made most rapidly by PCR of throat swab. Serology is also commonly used, and either paired sera for IgG titer or a single elevated IgM titer can be diagnostic. *Mycoplasma* culture is performed, but the organism is difficult and slow to isolate (taking 60 to 90 days), making this test of little clinical utility.

A psychogenic or habit cough may be observed following a lower respiratory tract illness. Habit cough may persist for weeks or months after the acute process has subsided. A psychogenic cough tends to be loud and bizarre in nature and timing; it is often described as "honking" or "barking." This type of cough is short, nonproductive, and nonparoxysmal; it is quite disturbing to family members and classmates, to the point that the child may be excluded from school and other activities. It always disappears with sleep. The cough becomes more obvious with stressful situations or when parents (or physicians) express undue interest or anxiety regarding the cough. For this reason, extensive evaluations by medical personnel may merely exacerbate the problem when the diagnosis can be made on the basis of the characteristic quality of the cough and its disappearance in sleep. Demonstrating normal pulmonary function testing and a normal chest radiograph helps to reassure the parent that other disease has been excluded.

Cigarette smoking in this age group should also be a consideration, and, unless the rapport between physician and adolescent is particularly strong, the history will likely be unrevealing. Staining of the teeth or fingers or the presence of conjunctivitis may be indirect clues to the underlying cause of the cough.

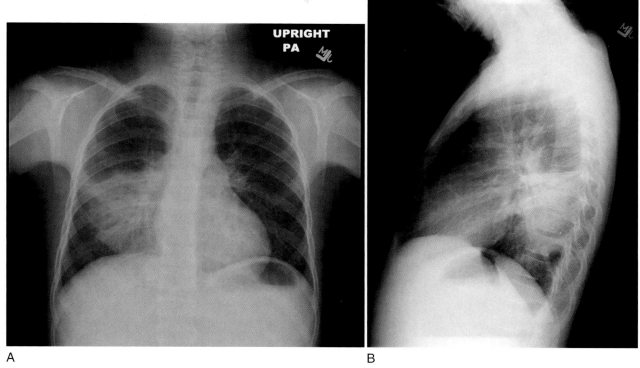

Figure 16-15. Pneumonia. **A,** Posteroanterior view. **B,** Lateral view of *Mycoplasma* pneumonia in a 10-year-old boy. Posteroanterior chest radiograph shows right lower lobe (apical segment) involvement of a lobar infiltrative process.

Table 16-2	Characteristics of Chronic Cough and Associated Conditions
CHARACTERISTIC	**ASSOCIATED CONDITION**
Loose, productive	Cystic fibrosis, bronchiectasis, ciliary dyskinesia
Croupy	Laryngotracheobronchitis
Paroxysmal	Cystic fibrosis, pertussis syndrome, foreign body inhalation, *Mycoplasma, Chlamydia*
Brassy	Tracheitis, upper airway drainage, psychogenic cough
After feedings	Pharyngeal incoordination, pharyngeal mass, tracheoesophageal fistula, gastroesophageal reflux
Nocturnal	Upper respiratory tract disease, sinusitis, asthma, cystic fibrosis, gastroesophageal reflux
Most severe in morning	Cystic fibrosis, bronchiectasis
With exercise	Asthma (including exercise induced), cystic fibrosis, bronchiectasis
Loud, honking, or bizarre	Psychogenic cough
Disappears with sleep	Psychogenic cough

Evaluation

The history may suggest the underlying cause of the cough (Table 16-2), and, perhaps more importantly, eliciting the cough during the physical examination can help. A loose or productive cough suggests suppurative lung disease, such as cystic fibrosis, other forms of bronchiectasis, or ciliary dyskinesia syndromes. The cough in these patients tends to be most severe in the morning because excessive secretions pool in the tracheobronchial tree during sleep. Increased morning cough is also common in patients with sinusitis or increased upper airway secretions from viral infection or allergic rhinitis. A croupy

cough may be observed in patients with acute laryngotracheobronchitis, and there may be associated wheezing. A dry or brassy cough is generally seen in patients with larger airway pathology, as in tracheitis or drainage from upper respiratory tract disease; a psychogenic cough may produce similar findings, but this type of cough may be distinguished from the others by its disappearance with sleep. As noted previously, a psychogenic cough is often (but not always) loud, honking, bizarre, and disruptive. A paroxysmal cough is seen in patients with pertussis syndrome, *Mycoplasma* or *Chlamydia* infection, foreign body inhalation, or cystic fibrosis. A coughing episode associated with feedings suggests pharyngeal incoordination or mass, tracheoesophageal fistula, or GER. Nighttime coughing is noted in cystic fibrosis, asthma, GER, sinusitis, and upper respiratory tract disease. Cough occurring during or shortly after activities suggests exercise-induced asthma, cystic fibrosis, or bronchiectasis.

Examination of the sputum may also be helpful in suggesting the diagnosis. Clear, mucoid sputum containing eosinophils is likely to represent asthma, whereas purulent green sputum is more suggestive of suppurative lung disease, such as cystic fibrosis. A yellow color can be imparted to the sputum by breakdown products of white blood cells; therefore yellow sputum can be seen with bacterial infection (polymorphonuclear leukocytes) or asthma (eosinophils). Bloody sputum can occur in cystic fibrosis, retained foreign body, idiopathic pulmonary hemosiderosis, tuberculosis, bronchiectasis, and some infections. Upper respiratory tract irritation with epistaxis may lead to the mistaken notion that hemoptysis is occurring. Hematemesis may also be mistaken for hemoptysis.

Clinical findings associated with a cough may also point to the nature of the problem. A cough occurring in the presence of poor weight gain and malabsorption makes cystic fibrosis a concern. Cough occurring with wheezing

Table 16-3	Diagnostic Approach to Cough

Complete history and physical examination
Chest and sinus radiographs
CBC with differential
Pulmonary function tests (including bronchoprovocation tests)
Sweat test (pilocarpine iontophoresis method)
Trial of bronchodilators
Sputum for Gram stain, AFB, bacterial, viral, and fungal cultures
Quantitative immunoglobulins
Tuberculin skin test/anergy panel
Serologic tests or PCR for *Mycoplasma pneumoniae*
Bronchoscopy
Barium swallow
pH probe or Bernstein test

AFB, acid-fast bacillus; CBC, complete blood count; PCR, polymerase chain reaction.

suggests asthma, and if evidence of rhinitis, conjunctivitis, or "allergic shiners" is present, allergic disease may also be a consideration (see Chapter 4). Cough that is worse in spring and summer months or that occurs only after exercise suggests asthma. Worsening of the cough in the winter is consistent with cold-induced bronchospasm or recurrent viral illnesses.

Diagnostic Approach

The approach to diagnosing a patient with persistent cough begins with a complete history in which some of the factors alluded to earlier (Table 16-3) are targeted. On physical examination, close attention to nutritional status, associated upper respiratory tract disease, or clubbing of the digits is as important as the examination of the chest. Clubbing of the fingers raises the possibility of cystic fibrosis; any patient with this finding requires a sweat test performed by quantitative pilocarpine iontophoresis. On auscultation of the chest, a localized wheeze, particularly if associated with delayed air entry, suggests a foreign body or focal airway lesion leading to narrowing. Inspiratory crackles may be noted in cystic fibrosis, bronchiectasis from other causes, interstitial lung disease, or pneumonia. Crackles are also present during one third to one half of untreated asthma exacerbations, even in the absence of infection.

Most patients with prolonged cough should have a chest x-ray examination and, if historical or physical findings are suggestive, a sinus x-ray examination as well. Inspiratory and expiratory radiographs and fluoroscopy may be indicated if inhalation of a foreign body is suspected. A complete blood count (CBC) with differential may suggest the diagnosis in some patients, with eosinophilia seen in allergic disease, lymphocytosis in pertussis and other viral diseases, and an increased proportion of neutrophils in bacterial infections.

In a child old enough to cooperate, pulmonary function testing can detect lower airway obstruction that may be inapparent on physical examination; improvement in airflow with bronchodilator administration supports a diagnosis of asthma. Certain abnormalities of the shape of the flow-volume loop (see Fig. 16-42) during spirometry can also suggest upper airway pathology (discussed later). In some cases an outpatient trial of inhaled corticosteroids lasting several months or an empirical brief course of oral corticosteroids may serve to confirm the suspicion of asthma. Failure to respond to this regimen suggests that asthma is not the problem, but it could be the result of noncompliance with the prescribed medications. The term *cough-variant asthma* is not used by pulmonologists. This phrase refers to asthma in which cough, rather than wheezing, is the primary symptom. Such patients always have other signs of small airway obstruction, ranging from hyperinflation evident on percussion of the chest to abnormalities on pulmonary function testing, and as such are diagnosed as having asthma on these grounds.

Examination of sputum with Wright or Gram stain or by cultures may lead to a diagnosis. Eosinophils suggest allergic disease, and polymorphonuclear leukocytes with organisms suggest a bacterial infection.

Quantitative immunoglobulins and immunoglobulin subclasses may be helpful in detecting some immunodeficiencies, and an elevated IgE suggests allergic disease. A purified protein derivative (PPD) intradermal skin test placed in conjunction with other antigens of known immunogenicity (e.g., *Candida* or mumps) may be important in some patients. In the appropriate clinical setting, PCR or serologic studies for *M. pneumoniae* are occasionally fruitful. Bronchoscopy may exclude the diagnosis of foreign body or airway malformation as the cause of chronic cough. If foreign body inhalation is likely (based on history and/or physical examination), bronchoscopy is essential and should be performed under general anesthesia with the rigid bronchoscope by a surgeon.

Chest CT may confirm the diagnosis of bronchiectasis and should be performed if surgical removal of the affected segment is contemplated. A barium swallow is useful in patients with suspected tracheoesophageal fistula or primary swallowing disorders. Diagnostic evaluation of suspected aspiration is discussed later. Prolonged monitoring of the pH ("pH probe") in the distal esophagus may confirm the suspicion of GER. In patients suspected of having ciliary dysmotility, a nasal or bronchial ciliary biopsy for examination by light and electron microscopy or a nuclear medicine scan measuring the movement of inhaled radiolabeled particles within the central airways may be indicated.

Stridor

A number of clinical entities can produce persistent or recurrent stridor (Table 16-4), and some of these may also be associated with a chronic cough, as described earlier. Stridor is characteristically a harsh inspiratory noise created by obstruction of the larynx or the extrathoracic trachea. With a mild degree of airway narrowing, breath sounds may be normal when the infant or child is at rest, but with any activity that increases tidal breathing (e.g., crying, feeding, agitation), inspiratory stridor may become noticeable.

The most common cause of inspiratory stridor in the pediatric population is infectious croup (acute laryngotracheobronchitis). This disease is most commonly caused by a respiratory virus (parainfluenza, respiratory syncytial, influenza, or rhinovirus), and the patient typically has coryza for 24 to 48 hours before the appearance of croupy cough, hoarseness, and stridor. Occasionally the inflammatory process may spread to the smaller airways and produce wheezing in addition to these symptoms. The "steeple sign" is a characteristic radiographic sign on anteroposterior projections (Fig. 16-16) that may be accompanied by marked dilation of supraglottic structures, particularly on lateral films. In the majority of patients, serious airway obstruction does not occur and the disease is self-limited. Acute angioneurotic edema is a less common cause of stridor. In most cases it results from an allergic reaction and is potentially fatal. Some children with anatomically normal airways suffer recurrent bouts of stridor, usually in the middle of the night, in the absence of signs of viral infection. Treatment for GER is often helpful in these patients, suggesting that for many, occult GER explains these bouts of recurrent airway obstruction.

The stridor associated with congenital laryngomalacia (Fig. 16-17) generally begins within the first week of life, varies with activity, may be expiratory, and is more noticeable in the supine position. Clinical symptoms may suggest the diagnosis, but bronchoscopic visualization of airway dynamics by flexible bronchoscopy is a safe and reliable method of confirming the suspicion of laryngomalacia. Parents can be reassured that this entity is self-limited, becomes less marked after 6 to 10 months of age, and rarely causes serious problems.

Narrowing of the subglottic region can be congenital or acquired, as in subglottic stenosis associated with endotracheal intubation. Congenital subglottic stenosis improves as the child grows older, but narrowing associated with tracheal intubation may require a tracheostomy, particularly if the infant remains dependent on ventilatory support.

Congenital laryngeal or pharyngeal masses can also produce stridor by obstructing airflow. Laryngeal papillomatosis (Fig. 16-18) is a rare and life-threatening illness that generally presents in the first decade of life. Papillomas can involve the vocal cords, but there may also be widespread involvement of the tracheobronchial tree. Although inspiratory stridor may be observed, hoarseness is a more common presenting feature. Hemangiomas of the larynx or trachea may also produce stridor or a brassy or dry cough. Cutaneous or mucosal hemangiomas noted during the physical examination suggest the diagnosis. Laryngeal webs (Fig. 16-19), cysts, and laryngoceles are quite uncommon and are accompanied by respiratory distress, stridor, feeding difficulties, and cyanosis. Diagnosis is made by bronchoscopy. A foreign body in the pharynx or larynx may also cause stridor.

Vocal cord paralysis, either unilateral or bilateral, may be present in the neonatal period, although in the case of

Table 16-4	Causes of Recurrent or Chronic Stridor

Croup
  Infectious
  Allergic/angioneurotic edema, GER
Laryngomalacia
Tracheomalacia
Subglottic stenosis
Extrinsic airway compression
  Vascular ring
  Mediastinal mass
  Lobar emphysema
  Bronchogenic cyst
  Foreign body in esophagus
  Thyromegaly
Pharyngeal or laryngeal masses
  Papilloma
  Hemangioma
  Laryngocele
  Web
  Foreign body
Tracheoesophageal fistula
Vocal cord paralysis
Hysterical or psychogenic

GER, gastroesophageal reflux.

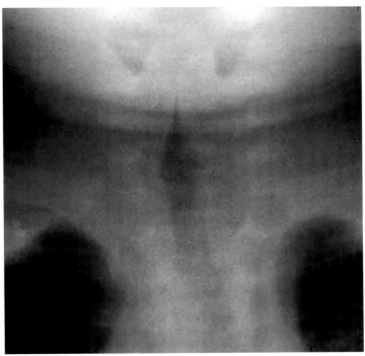

Figure 16-16. Croup (laryngotracheobronchitis). Radiograph of upper airway shows subglottic narrowing of the trachea, referred to as a "steeple sign." (Courtesy Beverly Newman, MD, Pittsburgh.)

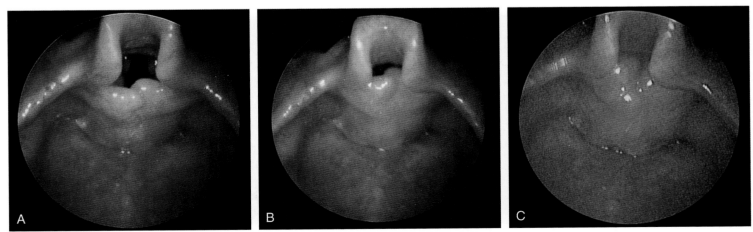

Figure 16-17. Laryngomalacia. A sequence of photographs demonstrates the degree of airway compromise occurring during inspiration in laryngomalacia. The epiglottis is supported by a laryngoscope blade, but the progressive collapse of the other laryngeal structures during inspiration, especially the arytenoid cartilages, is shown clearly. (From Benjamin B: Atlas of Paediatric Endoscopy. London, Oxford University Press, 1981.)

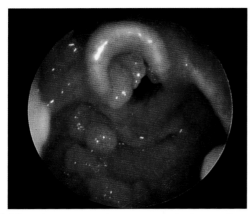

Figure 16-18. Laryngeal papillomatosis. Multiple papillomas involving the larynx are seen in this photograph taken during rigid bronchoscopy. (From Benjamin B: Atlas of Paediatric Endoscopy. London, Oxford University Press, 1981.)

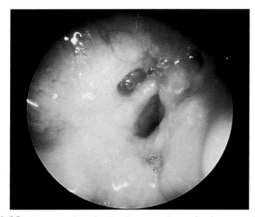

Figure 16-19. Laryngeal web. Expiratory view of a laryngeal web in an infant with inspiratory stridor that was exaggerated by crying noted at birth. The web is seen traversing the area of the glottis. (From Smalhout B, Hill-Baughan AB: The Suffocating Child. Bronchoscopy, A Guide to Diagnosis and Treatment. Ingelheim, Germany, Boehringer Ingelheim, 1980, p 86.)

unilateral paralysis several weeks may pass before the diagnosis is suspected. A weak or absent cry, hoarseness, inspiratory stridor with or without respiratory distress, and feeding difficulties are usual signs of vocal cord paralysis. Bilateral vocal cord paralysis may be seen with hydrocephalus, myelomeningocele, Arnold-Chiari malformation, or other malformations of the brain. Unilateral and bilateral cord paralyses are observed in patients with abnormalities of the cardiovascular system that are accompanied by cardiomegaly (e.g., ventricular septal defect, tetralogy of Fallot) or that cause abnormalities of the great vessels (e.g., vascular ring, transposition, patent ductus arteriosus). The diagnosis is best made by flexible bronchoscopy under minimal sedation so that vocal cord movement can be examined adequately.

A bronchogenic cyst (Fig. 16-20A and B) in the newborn can cause stridor, as the cyst fills with air after birth and compresses large airways. It can also cause tachypnea, dyspnea, cyanosis, and diminished breath sounds on the affected side. Later, the cyst may become infected, leading to recurrent bouts of fever, cough, and hemoptysis. Finally, an esophageal foreign body may compress the compliant posterior wall of the trachea and produce stridor, cough, and dysphagia.

The diagnosis of hysterical or psychogenic stridor is generally made during adolescence and is more common in girls. As in psychogenic cough, psychogenic stridor disappears with sleep and is more noticeable with anxiety or when excessive attention is given to the patient. It is the result of adduction of the vocal cords during inspiration.

Wheezing

Many diseases that produce chronic wheezing in pediatric patients overlap with entities that cause coughing or stridor (Table 16-5). Wheezing results from obstruction of airflow in intrathoracic airways. This obstruction can be at the lower trachea "downstream" to the small bronchi

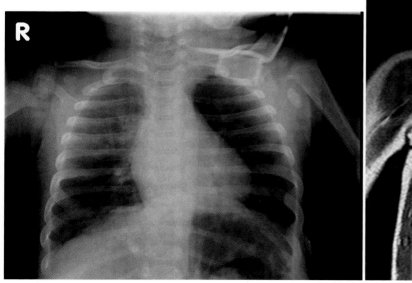
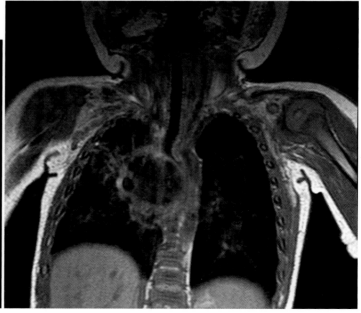

A   B

Figure 16-20. Bronchogenic cyst. **A,** Chest radiograph demonstrates hyperlucency of the left lung. **B,** MRI of chest demonstrates a large, centrally located cystic lesion of the left hilum with compression of adjacent airway. (Courtesy Beverly Newman, MD, Pittsburgh.)

Table 16-5	Causes of Chronic or Recurrent Wheezing

Asthma
   Exercise-induced asthma
Gastroesophageal reflux
Hypersensitivity reactions (e.g., ABPA)
Cystic fibrosis
Aspiration
   Tracheoesophageal fistula
   Foreign body
   Gastroesophageal reflux
   Laryngeal cleft
   Pharyngeal dysmotility
Extrinsic masses
   Vascular ring
   Cystic adenomatoid malformation
   Lymph nodes
   Tumors
Ciliary dyskinesia syndromes
Tracheomalacia and/or bronchomalacia
Congestive heart failure
Bronchopulmonary hemosiderosis or Heiner syndrome
Endobronchial lesions including localized stenosis
Interstitial pneumonitides
Bronchiolitis obliterans

ABPA, allergic bronchopulmonary aspergillosis.

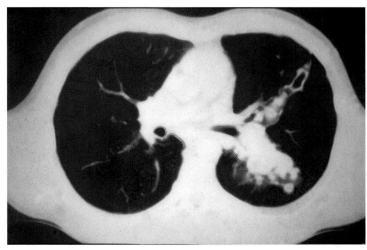

Figure 16-21. Allergic bronchopulmonary aspergillosis. Chest CT of a patient with asthma and allergic bronchopulmonary aspergillosis shows consolidation, atelectasis, and dilated bronchi radiating from the hilum.

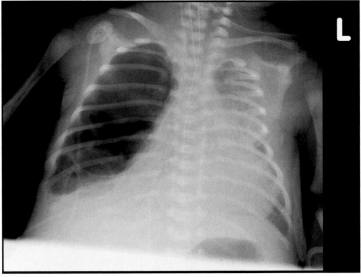

Figure 16-22. Congenital cystic adenomatoid malformation (CCAM). Anteroposterior chest radiograph of newborn shows a large air-filled cyst filling most of the right hemithorax. Smaller cysts on the right are apparent, although not as well delineated. The right lower lobe is compressed, and the mediastinum is shifted to the left. This infant had this diagnosis made by antenatal ultrasound. (Courtesy Beverly Newman, MD, Pittsburgh.)

and bronchioles. Wheezes can be heard on expiration or, less commonly, during both phases of respiration. The pitch of the wheeze, the variation in its pitch throughout the lung fields, and an association with hyperinflation as defined by percussion (described earlier) can help differentiate wheezing resulting from obstruction in the small airways from that in the large airways. Response to bronchodilator and/or steroids is a useful way of differentiating true asthma (which should improve with these treatments) from wheezing resulting from tracheomalacia or bronchomalacia (which does not improve and may even worsen with bronchodilators). Asthma is the most common cause of wheezing in pediatric patients. Asthma is usually associated with some degree of hyperinflation (air trapping) in the untreated patient younger than 5 years of age. Asthma may take many different forms including typical asthma, exercise-induced asthma, and wheezing associated with GER.

A disorder often mistaken for exercise-induced asthma is vocal cord dysfunction. In vocal cord dysfunction, the true vocal cords adduct during inspiration. The adduction of the cords is nearly always of a psychogenic origin. It results in a sensation of dyspnea, which the patient localizes to the throat—a history inconsistent with asthma. Often the stress of a competitive event brings out this reaction. This diagnosis is easily established in the exercise laboratory and is readily diagnosed by pulmonary function testing. The adduction of the vocal cords can also be demonstrated with flexible nasolaryngoscopy. Despite the psychogenic origin, this disorder is generally best treated by speech therapists; referral to a psychiatrist is rarely necessary.

Increased wheezing in a previously well-controlled asthmatic patient should raise the possibility of allergic bronchopulmonary aspergillosis (ABPA). These patients often have an insidious onset of low-grade fever, fatigue, weight loss, and productive cough. Physical findings include expiratory wheezes and bibasilar crackles and, later in the course, clubbing of the digits. Radiographic features of ABPA (Fig. 16-21) include areas of consolidation, atelectasis, and evidence of dilated bronchi radiating from the hila. Diagnosis can be made by positive skin test results with *Aspergillus fumigatus* antigens, elevated total serum

IgE levels, elevation of specific IgE, presence of serum precipitins to *Aspergillus* organisms, and isolation of *A. fumigatus* from the sputum culture. Pulmonary function studies may worsen considerably during episodes of ABPA with evidence of increased airway obstruction. A host of hypersensitivity reactions produce extrinsic allergic alveolitis with wheezing.

Other disorders that can provoke wheezing include cystic fibrosis, aspiration events from any cause, and extrinsic masses that compress the airways.

Congenital cystic adenomatoid malformation is a rare cause of extrinsic airway compression in which symptoms generally begin at birth or shortly afterward, as a normal lung is compressed by the lesion with the onset of tachypnea, respiratory distress, and cyanosis. Hydramnios is often noted at birth. Rarely, smaller cysts may be an incidental finding on chest radiography or symptoms may develop after infection of the cysts occurs. The radiographic appearance (Fig. 16-22) is that of single or multiple cystlike areas compressing normal lung, with mediastinal displacement. It is usually confined to a single lobe, and there is no apparent predilection for a particular lobe.

Extrinsic airway compression may produce wheezing or stridor, depending on the site of obstruction. A vascular ring (Fig. 16-23) is much more likely to cause expiratory wheezing than inspiratory stridor (see Chapter 5). Diagnosis can be made by MRI, echocardiography, barium swallow, or bronchoscopy; the last-mentioned may demonstrate a pulsatile lesion compressing the trachea. MRI, unlike the other diagnostic choices, delineates the vascular and airway anatomy simultaneously and has become the diagnostic test of choice. Barium swallow, which can demonstrate vascular compression, does not delineate vascular anatomy and is no longer routinely indicated for evaluation of vascular ring. Mediastinal masses or, occasionally, enlargement of the thyroid gland may produce tracheal compression and stridor.

Congenital or acquired lobar emphysema usually produces tachypnea and other respiratory symptoms, such as cough, wheeze, intermittent cyanosis, and occasionally stridor. The chest radiograph in lobar emphysema (Fig. 16-24) demonstrates a large, hyperlucent area with few bronchovascular markings and usually compression atelectasis of adjacent lobes. Left upper lobe involvement is most common, but right middle lobe emphysema is also seen. For the infant who is growing well and in whom tachypnea is the primary symptom, or in lobar emphysema associated with a mucus plug, conservative management is indicated. In the symptomatic infant with associated compression atelectasis and/or chronic respiratory distress, resection of the affected lobe is indicated.

Bronchopulmonary dysplasia (BPD), one of the sequelae of hyaline membrane disease and its treatment, is associated with recurrent episodes of wheezing, respiratory distress, and tachypnea (see Chapter 2). Otherwise mild respiratory illnesses in these infants with decreased respiratory reserve may progress to lower respiratory tract disease, necessitating frequent hospitalizations. Patients with BPD may develop chronic respiratory insufficiency, pulmonary hypertension, and cor pulmonale. The frequency of wheezing episodes may diminish with age, although it appears that these patients continue to have airway hyperreactivity that is triggered by any number of different insults. GER is common among patients with BPD, as is tracheobronchomalacia. Both of these entities can worsen wheezing in these patients.

Miscellaneous causes of wheezing include idiopathic pulmonary hemosiderosis; aspiration (acute or chronic, described later); endobronchial lesions associated with localized stenosis; and bronchiolitis obliterans. Obliterative bronchiolitis has been described in an idiopathic form, following adenoviral infections or inhalation of toxic agents and in conjunction with other diseases (including rheumatoid arthritis) in adults. Its most common current clinical setting in pediatrics is in the organ transplant recipient. Patients may present initially with fever, cough, or tachypnea and subsequently develop dyspnea and wheezing. Physical findings include wheezing, crackles, and diminished breath sounds. The radiographic pattern (Fig. 16-25) is that of hyperinflation, decreased vascularity, and increased interstitial markings (reflective primarily of increased airway marking) with areas of atelectasis and consolidation. Pulmonary function testing will reveal fixed lower airway obstruction. Complications of adenovirus-induced bronchiolitis obliterans include bronchiectasis, overinflation, recurrent ate-

lectasis, and pneumonia. In many patients the prognosis is poor.

Cystic Fibrosis

Cystic fibrosis (CF) is the most common life-shortening genetic disease among white North Americans, afflicting 1 in 3300 newborns in this group. The incidence in African Americans is approximately 1 in 17,000 and in people of Asian background, 1 in 35,000 to 1 in 50,000. The carrier frequency in whites is an estimated 1 in 30. CF is a generalized exocrinopathy characterized by the inspissation of abnormally thick and tenacious secretions, principally involving the pancreas and lungs. In the lungs, impaired airway clearance and increased secretions cause obstruction of the airways with retention of bacteria, resulting in chronic endobronchial infection and an inflammatory process that leads to bronchiolitis, bronchitis, bronchiectasis, and bronchiolectasis. The disease is characterized by a gradual decline in pulmonary function. Respiratory disease accounts for the vast majority of deaths in people with CF. In the pancreas, ducts become obstructed by the abnormal secretions, preventing pancreatic enzymes from entering the duodenum and therefore preventing breakdown of dietary fat and protein. The pancreas undergoes autodigestion and is replaced by scar tissue; lifetime deficiency of pancreatic exocrine function results. In 40% to 50% of newborns with CF, enough pancreatic function remains for normal digestion. By 4 to 8 years of age, the proportion of patients with pancreatic insufficiency rises to 85% to 90%, where it remains. The term "pancreatic sufficiency" is used to describe the minority (10% to 15%) of CF patients with enough pancreatic function to have normal absorption of nutrients (despite having diminished pancreatic function as compared with normal patients). The prognosis for patients with CF has improved dramatically over the past several decades. By 2004 the median age of survival had risen to 35.1 years of age.

The disease is inherited as an autosomal recessive trait. The protein product of the CF gene—cystic fibrosis transmembrane conductance regulator, or CFTR—functions as an epithelial chloride channel. Decreased chloride transport and hyperabsorption of sodium across various epithelia results in abnormally viscid and poorly hydrated secretions. Careful cell culture studies have demonstrated a decreased height of the airway surface liquid, which impairs ciliary beating. The most common mutation of the CFTR gene in North American whites is referred to as *delta-F508*. This mutation is the result of the deletion of three base pairs in the gene and results in a protein missing a phenylalanine residue at amino acid position 508. When genetic testing for CF became available, there was optimism that a small handful of mutations at the CF locus (located on the long arm of chromosome 7) would account for the vast majority of the patients with the disease and lead the way to population-wide screening. This, unfortunately, turns out not to be the case. At last count, more than 1500 mutations of this gene had been reported. The majority of these mutations, however, are isolated to a single patient or family; only 32 mutations account for 92% of CF alleles in white North Americans. In approximately 70% of CF genes delta-F508 is found, and half of CF patients in North America are homozygous for the delta-F508 mutation. Half of the remaining patients are compound heterozygotes with delta-F508 coupled with another CF allele; the remaining patients have other non-

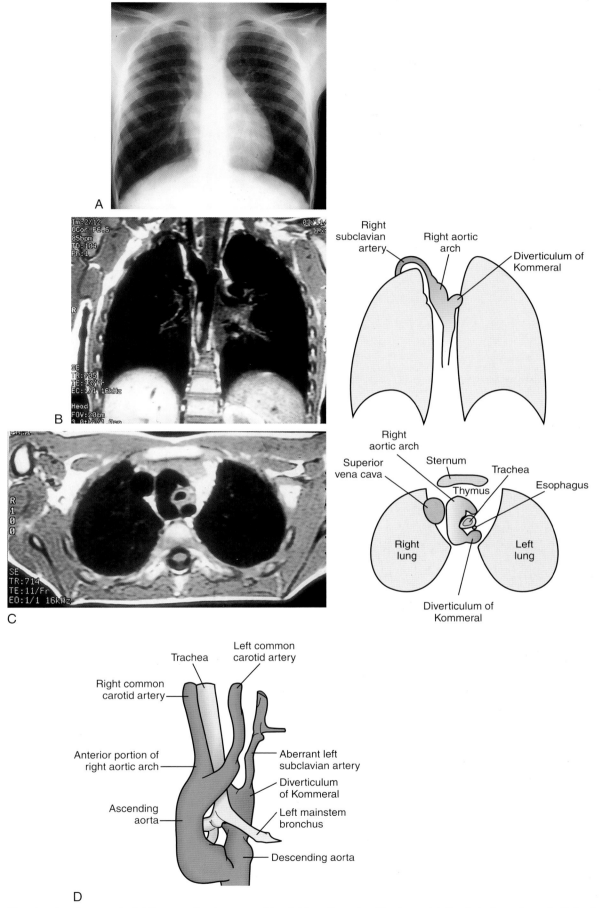

Figure 16-23. Vascular ring. Images depict the vascular ring caused by right aortic arch with aberrant left subclavian artery. **A,** Plain chest radiograph demonstrates a right-sided aortic arch, with tracheal deviation to the left. **B,** MRI in the sagittal plane shows the dominant right aortic arch and the remnant of the left aortic arch, called a diverticulum of Kommeral. The aberrant left subclavian artery arises posteriorly from the diverticulum of Kommeral. **C,** MRI of same patient in the axial plane, demonstrating the vascular ring incarcerating the trachea and esophagus. The ring is completed by the ductus arteriosus, not visible here. **D,** Three-dimensional reconstruction of the vascular anatomy shown in the MRI from the left anterior perspective. (Courtesy Beverly Newman, MD, Pittsburgh.)

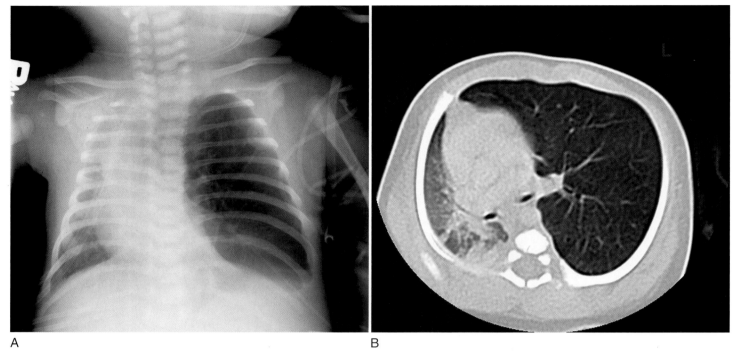

Figure 16-24. Congenital lobar emphysema. **A,** Anteroposterior chest radiograph. Left upper lobe shows hyperlucency of the affected globe, atelectasis of the lower lobe, and mediastinal shift. **B,** CT of same patient shows left upper lobe herniating across the midline with compression of structures on the right. (Courtesy Beverly Newman, MD, Pittsburgh.)

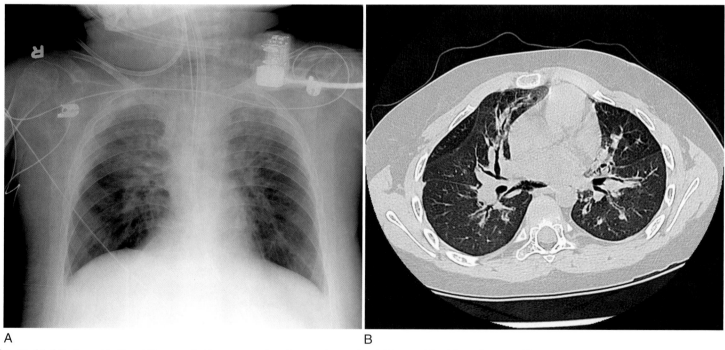

Figure 16-25. Bronchiolitis obliterans. **A,** Posteroanterior chest radiograph of 17-year-old with end-stage obliterative bronchiolitis as a complication of bone marrow transplantation for acute myelogenous leukemia. Film demonstrates increased interstitial and airway markings. **B,** CT of same patient demonstrates bronchiectatic changes. (Courtesy Beverly Newman, MD, Pittsburgh.)

delta-F508 mutations. A number of investigators have tried to discover genotype-phenotype correlations. The most reliable phenotypic correlate of genotype has been pancreatic function (the compound heterozygote delta-F508/R117H, for example, usually imparts a pancreatic-sufficient phenotype). Respiratory disease severity has not been well correlated to genotype, and on the basis of variability of disease within families, other modifier genes, as well as environmental factors, apparently play an important role in the clinical expression of CF.

Presentation

CF can present in any number of fashions (Table 16-6), but most symptoms are referable to respiratory or gastrointestinal involvement. Among CF patients, 5% to 10% present with meconium ileus, which is noted at or shortly after birth. Meconium ileus is a common cause of intestinal obstruction in the newborn; these infants present with abdominal distention, bilious vomiting, and failure

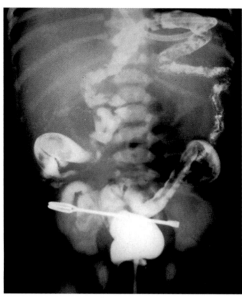

Figure 16-26. Meconium ileus. Barium enema in a newborn with meconium peritonitis and evidence of a small, unused distal colon (note small extraluminal calcifications).

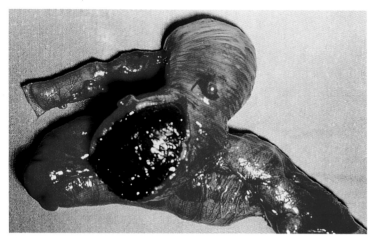

Figure 16-27. Meconium ileus. Gross appearance of the thick, tarlike meconium found at laparotomy in meconium ileus.

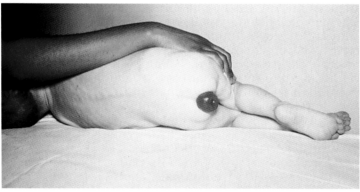

Figure 16-28. Rectal prolapse is shown in a toddler not previously recognized as having cystic fibrosis.

Table 16-6	Presentations of Cystic Fibrosis

General
  Failure to thrive
  Salty taste to skin
Gastrointestinal/nutritional
  Meconium ileus
  Foul-smelling stools, bloating, abdominal pain
  Rectal prolapse
  Intestinal impaction and obstruction
  Pancreatitis, acute and chronic
  Hypoproteinemia and edema
  Neonatal hyperbilirubinemia
  Cholelithiasis, cholecystitis
  Cirrhosis or portal hypertension
  Fat-soluble vitamin deficiency (A, D, E, K)
Metabolic
  Hyponatremic hypochloremic dehydration
  Heat stroke
  Metabolic alkalosis
  Diabetes mellitus
Respiratory
  Clubbing
  Asthma
  Chronic obstructive pulmonary disease
  Recurrent pulmonary infiltrates
  Chronic cough or sputum production
  Barrel chest
  Hemoptysis
  Pneumothorax
  Cor pulmonale
  Nasal polyps
Other
  Infertility (males)

to pass meconium stools. Abdominal radiographs show dilated loops of small bowel and a ground-glass appearance in the cecal region, signifying pockets of air within the thick meconium. A barium or water-soluble contrast enema may show a small distal colon (Fig. 16-26). In cases of meconium ileus associated with prenatal rupture and meconium peritonitis, abdominal calcifications may be noted on plain radiographs, and at laparotomy thick, tarlike meconium is found in the terminal ileum (Fig. 16-27). Prolonged neonatal jaundice, generalized edema in a breast-fed or soy formula–fed infant, or hypochloremia

with heat prostration are less common presentations of CF in early infancy.

A combination of poor weight gain; loose, foul-smelling, bulky stools; and a voracious appetite are signs and symptoms that most clinicians associate with CF and rarely present a diagnostic problem. Rectal prolapse (Fig. 16-28) may be the presenting feature of CF in about 5% of cases and may recur multiple times. Rarely, the patient may undergo a surgical procedure for the rectal prolapse before the underlying diagnosis is suspected. Rectal prolapse is thought to result from chronic malnutrition, reduced abdominal musculature, and voluminous stools. It does not generally pose problems once the diagnosis has been made and the patient started on supplemental pancreatic enzymes. Gastrointestinal complications of CF include biliary cirrhosis, portal hypertension, hypersplenism, esophageal varices, and clinical evidence of fat-soluble vitamin deficiency.

A chronic productive cough or wheezing in a patient with digital clubbing suggests the diagnosis of CF until proved otherwise. Patients may present with a history of recurrent pneumonia or sinus disease; it is worth noting that the large majority of patients with CF demonstrate pansinusitis radiographically. Nasal polyps (Fig. 16-29) may be a presenting manifestation of CF and are seen in about 20% of patients sometime during the course of the disease. Other initial respiratory presentations are listed in Table 16-6.

The clinical course and severity of the disease vary remarkably. Many patients do not develop signs or symptoms of respiratory disease other than an intermittent,

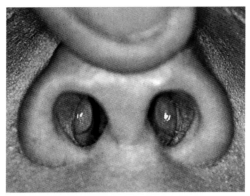

Figure 16-29. Cystic fibrosis. Nasal polyps in a patient with cystic fibrosis.

loose cough for years. Other patients have persistent symptoms from early infancy and are rarely without a cough. These patients tend to require frequent visits to the physician and frequent hospitalization and are more likely to have poor weight gain. Virtually all patients develop a loose, productive cough; the sputum may be blood-tinged during acute respiratory illnesses. Hemoptysis occurs in more than half of adult patients with CF and a considerable proportion of adolescents as well. Tachypnea, dyspnea, diffuse crackles, and digital clubbing will develop in most patients. Later, diffuse bronchiectasis, hyperinflation, and a barrel chest deformity are noted. The usual cause of death in patients with CF is respiratory failure, often in conjunction with cor pulmonale.

Complications

Complications of CF include hypochloremic metabolic alkalosis, hemoptysis, pneumothorax, pneumomediastinum, hypertrophic pulmonary osteoarthropathy, distal intestinal obstructive syndrome (meconium ileus equivalent), biliary cirrhosis, pancreatitis, cor pulmonale, and respiratory failure. Among the respiratory complications, massive hemoptysis and pneumothorax with or without pneumomediastinum are potentially life threatening. Blood streaking of sputum is not uncommon, and massive hemoptysis from rupture of dilated superficial bronchial arteries during chronic suppurative infections may occur in a small percentage of patients. Pneumothorax (see Fig. 16-31C) generally occurs from rupture of bullous lesions created from chronic airway obstruction and presents with acute onset of chest pain and shortness of breath with or without cyanosis. Pneumomediastinum and subcutaneous emphysema may result (Fig. 16-30). Hypertrophic pulmonary osteoarthropathy involving the knees and other major joints occurs in about 5% of patients and is characterized by pain, swelling, and limited mobility of the affected joint.

Acute or chronic pancreatitis occurs almost exclusively in patients with pancreatic sufficiency. These patients present with the acute onset of abdominal pain and vomiting and may have recurrent bouts of pancreatitis before the pancreas "burns itself out." Laboratory evaluations reveal elevations of serum lipase and amylase. The differential diagnosis in CF patients with acute abdominal pain and vomiting includes cholecystitis, appendicitis, and distal intestinal obstruction syndrome. The last is characterized by crampy abdominal pain; constipation; vomit-

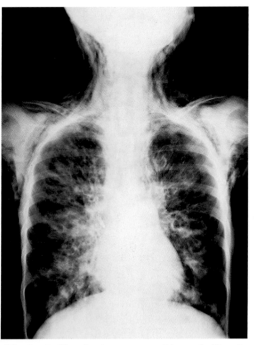

Figure 16-30. Cystic fibrosis. A teenager with cystic fibrosis, severe respiratory disease, pneumomediastinum, and massive subcutaneous emphysema.

ing; and, occasionally, a palpable mass in the right lower quadrant. A history of missed pancreatic enzyme supplements may exist, especially in adolescents.

Excessive loss of chloride and sodium from the salt can lead to hypochloremic metabolic alkalosis in infants who do not receive salt supplementation in their formula, especially during the summer months. This can occur even in the euvolemic state.

Right ventricular hypertrophy and cor pulmonale are findings in the terminal stages of many CF patients with severe pulmonary disease.

Radiographic Findings

The radiographic and CT findings in CF vary from early hyperinflation and patchy areas of atelectasis to a generalized increase in peribronchial markings with bronchiectasis, parenchymal densities, and large cystic areas noted in severe disease (Figs. 16-31 and 16-32). The Brasfield scoring system is widely used as a means of classifying chest radiographs of these patients. It is based on a point system for findings, such as hyperinflation, linear densities, cystic lesions, atelectasis, and right-sided cardiac enlargement or pneumothorax.

Diagnosis

Diagnosis of cystic fibrosis can be suggested by elevation in serum trypsinogen in the newborn. This test, immunoreactive trypsinogen (IRT), is used as a screening tool in most states as part of the extended newborn screen. Many laboratories will further analyze samples with elevated ITR for common genetic mutations of the CFTR gene. As a result, newborns may be referred to the local CF center having had a genetic diagnosis made before the first visit. Sensitivity of genetic testing for CF varies with ethnic group and remains approximately 92% for whites with the 87 mutation panel and 97% to 99% for a

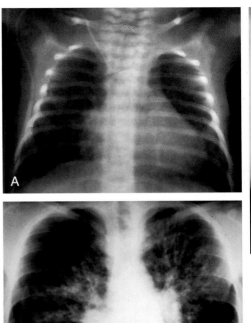
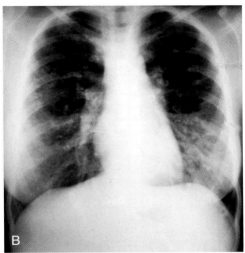
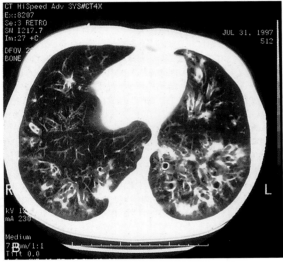

Figure 16-31. Cystic fibrosis. Typical progression of radiographic changes in cystic fibrosis. **A,** A 2-month-old child with hyperinflation and right middle lobe atelectasis. **B,** A 15-year-old girl with peribronchial cuffing, hyperinflation, and bronchiectatic changes, particularly of the lower lobes. **C,** A 21-year-old man with severe respiratory involvement and an unsuspected right pneumothorax.

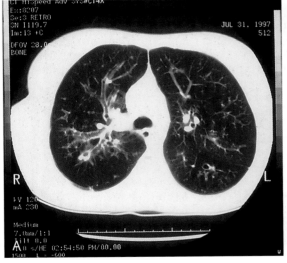

Figure 16-32. Cystic fibrosis. CT scans of a 19-year-old woman with severe bronchiectasis and cystic fibrosis. Thickened airways are seen in longitudinal section through the upper lobes **(A)** and in cross-section in an image from the lower lobes **(B).**

comprehensive (1300 mutation) screen. Still, the gold standard for initial diagnosis of CF remains the quantitative sweat test. Another advantage of the sweat test is that the results are available the same day, rather than the delay of several weeks with genetic testing. In sweat testing, pilocarpine is driven into the skin with a weak electrical charge (iontophoresis) and the resulting sweat is collected with a wristband containing a coiled capillary tube, which wicks the sweat and stores it for analysis. The sweat test must be performed in an experienced laboratory, such as those associated with one of the Cystic Fibrosis Foundation–approved CF centers. Both false-negative and false-positive results are alarmingly common in inexperienced hands. Sweat chloride values of 60 mEq/L or greater are

diagnostic of CF. A second sweat test is generally required for confirmation of diagnosis. Sweat chloride values of 40 to 60 mEq/L are considered borderline and generally require a second test. False-positive values can occasionally occur, but disorders that cause this are readily distinguished clinically from CF. Other entities that elevate sweat chloride include adrenal insufficiency, ectodermal dysplasia, nephrogenic diabetes insipidus, hypothyroidism, mucopolysaccharidoses, glucose-6-phosphatase deficiency, hypoproteinemia, and anemia associated with malnutrition. Patients with CF who present with severe malnutrition and edema may have false-negative values on initial sweat tests until their nutritional status improves.

Genetic testing is quite useful in the evaluation of the infant who produces too little sweat for analysis, the patient with borderline sweat chloride, or the patient with normal sweat chloride but clinical features characteristic of CF. Recently, broad testing of the CFTR gene has been offered. It includes all known mutations of both coding and noncoding DNA, which has greatly increased the sensitivity of genetic screening. Mutation-specific therapies have been proposed in CF, and therefore genetic testing of all patients with CF is recommended.

Sudden Infant Death Syndrome

Sudden infant death syndrome (SIDS) is defined as the unexpected death of an infant younger than 1 year of age who has been otherwise healthy and in whom there is no demonstrable pathologic basis for the death as determined by a thorough postmortem examination and death scene investigation. The annual incidence of SIDS in the United States is now approximately 0.5 per 1000 live births, a rate that has decreased 50% since 1992 (see later). SIDS is the leading cause of death after the neonatal period, with a peak at 2 to 4 months of life and rarely occurring after 6 months of age. Most of these infants die soundlessly during sleep, without any obvious sign of agitation. Occasionally, a history of the recent onset of a viral illness may be elicited. SIDS is not a single disease entity but a final common pathway for a number of diseases with early and fatal presentation. Diseases recognized to cause sudden death in infants include the long-QT syndrome (a cardiac conduction defect) and inborn errors of fatty acid oxidation. Accidental or intentional smothering of an infant is usually impossible to differentiate from SIDS at autopsy. The "apnea hypothesis" of SIDS (failure of infants to breathe sufficiently in sleep) has been discarded by the medical community, especially in face of those infants dying of SIDS on home monitors who did not have apnea. Thus the home apnea monitor is largely of no value in preventing SIDS in term infants (premature infants can have immature control of breathing and are thus at risk for apnea). The true cause of death in most SIDS victims remains unexplained. In SIDS there appears to be a vulnerable period, and other stressors (such as parental smoking, prone sleep position, and an overheated room) have been shown to increase the SIDS rate. No test can accurately predict which infant is at risk for SIDS. The sleep study (or pneumogram) is of no value in identifying infants at risk for SIDS. Screening electrocardiograms for newborns (looking to identify those with prolonged QTc) have not as yet been recommended by the American Academy of Pediatrics. One intervention that appears to have had an impact on SIDS incidence is the "back to sleep" campaign, in which parents are educated to keep their newborn in a supine position during sleep. The rate of SIDS in the United States has declined since the institution of this policy in 1992. Counseling parents to smoke outside the home and car is another important intervention that pediatricians can make.

The term *apparently life-threatening event* (ALTE) was coined to replace "near-miss SIDS." This term refers to an event, witnessed by a parent or caregiver, that is frightening to the observer and that is characterized by some combination of apnea, color change, marked change in muscle tone, choking, or gagging. The observer of an ALTE generally feels that the event would have resulted in the infant's death had he or she not intervened. The single most common cause of ALTE is GER. In these cases the infant has reflux, laryngospasm, and obstructive apnea. These events are usually associated with forceful respiratory efforts and a color change. Other disorders that can cause ALTE include sepsis/meningitis, inborn errors of metabolism, seizure, pertussis, respiratory syncytial virus infection, congenital cardiac disease, poisoning, and child abuse. Evaluation of an ALTE includes a careful history and physical examination (including funduscopy); electrocardiogram; serum electrolytes, glucose, calcium, and ammonia; blood cultures, CBC and white cell differential; blood gases; and toxicology screen. Evaluation for increased intracranial pressure may include a cranial CT and lumbar puncture when clinically indicated. Studies also include a sleep study that measures respiratory and abdominal wall movement, airflow at the mouth or nose, pulse oximetry and heart rate and, in some cases, pH monitoring of the distal esophagus. Of the above studies, the sleep study is usually the least revealing.

Apnea

Clinically meaningful apnea can be defined as the absence of airflow for at least 20 seconds or apnea accompanied by cyanosis or bradycardia. Apnea can be central, obstructive, or mixed. Absence of airflow accompanied by the cessation of chest and abdominal wall movement distinguishes central apnea. Obstructive apnea is the most common form of apnea and is characterized by the lack of airflow at the nose or mouth despite continued respiratory efforts. The first description of it in 1892 in Sir William Osler's *The Principles and Practice of Medicine* (under "chronic tonsillitis") remains the best one: "At night the child's sleep is greatly disturbed; the respirations are loud and snorting, and there are sometimes prolonged pauses, followed by deep, noisy inspirations." Patients with obstructive sleep apnea (OSA) fall into two categories: those with normal upper airway anatomy and those with abnormal upper airway anatomy. The former group includes those with obesity, GER, sickle cell anemia, severe laxity of the supraglottic structures, and marked adenoidal or tonsillar enlargement. The latter group includes patients with Crouzon syndrome, Apert syndrome, Down syndrome, Treacher Collins syndrome, the Pierre Robin sequence, Arnold-Chiari malformation, Prader-Willi, Möbius syndrome, and dwarfism. Children with OSA frequently do not have the adult pattern of obesity and daytime hypersomnolence; more often they fail to thrive and may have hyperactivity as a manifestation of inadequate sleep. Diagnosis of OSA requires a sleep study (polysomnogram) in which movement of the chest, movement of the abdomen, heart rate, arterial saturation, and end-tidal CO_2 is measured. Staging of sleep during these studies is important as multiple arousals and/or awakenings may occur in OSA. The arousal-plus-awakening index can quantify the severity of the effects of sleep-disordered breathing on the quality of sleep and help direct management. Cardiac echo and electrocardiogram are indicated in cases of severe OSA because pulmonary hypertension is a common complication. Home apnea monitoring is of no value in OSA because the chest will continue to move, despite absence of airflow. Management of OSA is directed at the underlying disorder (such as tonsillectomy in cases of tonsillar hypertrophy), but cases that result from collapse of the upper airway structures may require constant positive airway pressure administered via nasal mask.

Central apnea may occur in infants with seizure disorders or central nervous system pathology such as Arnold-Chiari syndrome, intraventricular hemorrhage, prematurity, and in congenital central hypoventilation syndrome (formerly known as Ondine's curse). Mixed apnea occurs when an obstructive apneic episode is followed by a central pattern of apnea (or vice versa).

Other studies that may be useful in apnea (all types) include ventilatory responses to hypercapnia or hypoxia, a chest radiograph, an electroencephalogram, CT of the brain, pH probe, and/or bronchoscopic evaluation of the airway, particularly in those patients with evidence of obstructive apnea. Laboratory evaluation may include any or all of the following: CBC, arterial or venous blood gases, chest radiography, and electrocardiogram.

Aspiration

Penetration of oral or gastric contents into the lungs is a common problem in patients with neurologic impairment. Aspiration can occur in patients with incoordination of swallowing and in neurologically normal patients with severe GER. The commonly used terms to describe these forms are "aspiration from above" and "aspiration from below." Patients with impaired mental status can have both forms of aspiration. Medical treatment of GER and feeding the patient via gastrostomy or gastrojejunal tube may not be sufficient to prevent progressive lung disease in patients who continue to aspirate oral secretions. Ongoing aspiration of saliva leads to a progressive injury to the lung and worsening respiratory impairment. Chronic inflammation leads to a mixed restrictive-obstructive pulmonary disease (Fig. 16-33) and difficult-to-control asthma. It is chronic aspiration that leads to the premature death that occurs in most children with profound neurologic impairment.

Aspiration can also be present in patients who are intellectually normal but who have delayed gastric emptying and GER. "Microaspiration," which refers to aspiration of tiny, essentially undetectable amounts of gastric contents, can cause intense bronchospasm due to the acidity of the aspirated material. In cats, just 50 µL of 0.1 N hydrochloric acid causes a fourfold increase in airway resistance. Patients with impaired clearance of food from the esophagus (achalasia) can also aspirate in sleep, despite having otherwise normal neurologic status. Aspiration should be suspected in patients with poorly controlled asthma despite aggressive management of asthma, especially in patients with neurologic impairment. Determination if aspiration exists in a patient remains challenging, as there is no gold standard for its diagnosis. For evaluation of swallowing, a barium contrast swallowing study using different consistencies of barium (thin liquid, paste, solid) can determine what consistency of food can be given safely to the patient (Fig. 16-34). It can document where in the swallowing cycle the main pathology resides. Parameters assessed during the modified barium swallow include all of the following: initiation of the swallow (timing and oral control); duration of the swallow; adequacy of the swallow to clear food bolus; presence, amount, and timing of aspiration; protective reactions in response to aspiration; and soft palate control during swallowing. In neurologically impaired individuals, particularly those fed via feeding tubes, the radionuclide "salivagram" is a rapid and sensitive means of determining whether the patient is aspirating his or her oral secretions. A small radioactive bolus is placed under the tongue, and the patient is then monitored under a gamma camera. The bolus is then traced: if it enters the lung it bifurcates at the carina; if it enters the esophagus it can be followed into the stomach (Fig. 16-35). The salivagram has the advantages of being physiologic (the patient is not held in an arbitrary position) and requiring no preparation. It results in a low-radiation dose to the patient, similar to that of the chest radiogram and a fraction of that used in a barium swallow. The radionuclide gastric emptying or "milk" scan, which uses the same radiation dose as the salivagram, can demonstrate reflux (Fig. 16-36) and delay in gastric emptying.

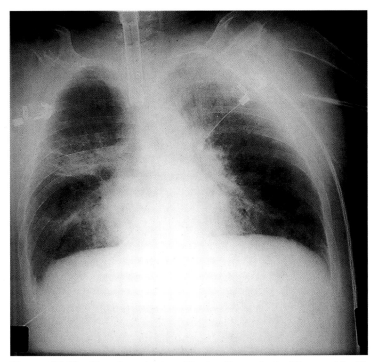

Figure 16-33. Chronic aspiration. Chest radiograph of a 20-year-old with lifelong chronic, severe aspiration shows increased interstitial markings and areas of consolidation-atelectasis.

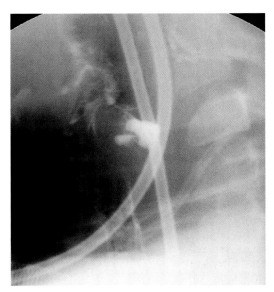

Figure 16-34. Aspiration. Barium swallow demonstrating aspiration. Barium has coated the upper airway, outlining the trachea. (Courtesy Avrum Pollack, MD, Pittsburgh.)

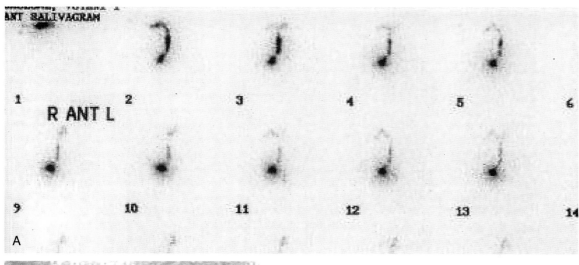

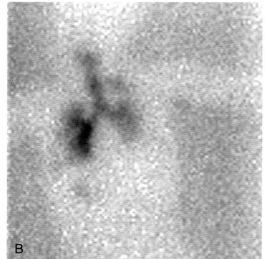

Figure 16-35. Salivagrams, both normal and abnormal. In the normal salivagram **(A)**, the bolus can be followed into the stomach in serial images taken over 5 minutes. **B** demonstrates severe aspiration into the lungs at the end of a study. (Courtesy Martin Charron, MD, Pittsburgh.)

Delayed gastric emptying is important to document because its treatment is essential to the successful treatment of GER. The milk scan is fairly insensitive for aspiration of refluxed gastric contents. When aspiration is strongly considered, flexible bronchoscopy with bronchoalveolar lavage (BAL) for assessment of lipid-laden macrophages (Fig. 16-37) is a useful test. Inspection of the upper airway may reveal edema and erythema of the aryepiglottic folds (Fig. 16-38). Alveolar macrophages from the BAL fluid are stained for fat. Globules of fat found in a predominance of the macrophages are concrete evidence of aspiration of food. The sensitivity of the test is unknown, but when moderate or high numbers of macrophages are found, it is believed to be specific for aspiration.

Diagnostic Techniques

The notion that the examination of the lungs begins at the fingertips is an important one, as digital clubbing may point to the presence of lung disease. Various stages of clubbing, from mild to severe, are depicted in Figures 16-39 and 16-40. Not all digital clubbing is associated with pulmonary disease (Table 16-7); nonpulmonary causes include cardiac, inflammatory, gastrointestinal, hepatic, and familial, as well as clubbing observed with thyrotoxicosis. Bronchiectasis from cystic fibrosis or from other chronic infectious causes is the major cause of clubbing among all pulmonary diseases. Digital clubbing in any child with a chronic cough or wheezing warrants a thorough evaluation and investigation to determine the underlying disorder.

Diagnosis and treatment of children with respiratory complaints may be assisted by the use of pulmonary function tests (PFTs). With appropriate training, and with the technician's patience and encouragement, most children 6 years of age or older can cooperate with simple spirometry and measurements of lung volumes (Fig. 16-41). Interpretation of PFT results in children must take into account variability in performance by children and differences in age, height, weight, sex, and race. In children, PFTs may be useful in establishing the severity of respiratory disease, in guiding the choice of therapy, and in measuring the response to a therapeutic regimen. In some diseases, such as cystic fibrosis or asthma, evidence of increasing airway obstruction may indicate the need to initiate or increase the aggressiveness of therapeutic intervention.

The inspection of the shape of flow-volume curves generated during forced expiratory maneuvers is critical for the appropriate interpretation of PFT results (Fig. 16-42). The initial portion of the flow-volume curve is effort dependent, while the terminal 25% of the expiratory maneuver is dependent on elastic recoil and airway resistance and is relatively independent of patient effort. A normal-appearing flow-volume curve is shown in Fig. 16-42A. With increased airway resistance distal to the central, large airways, the curve becomes concave toward

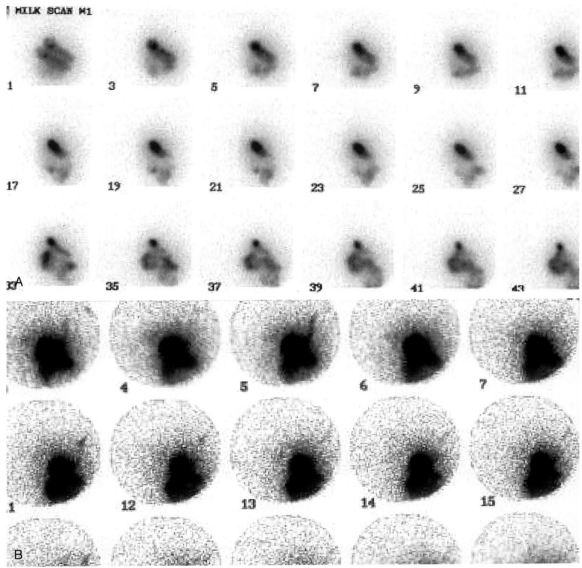

Figure 16-36. Milk scans. **A,** Normal scan demonstrates no evidence of reflux and normal gastric emptying. **B,** Abnormal scan shows repeated reflux of gastric contents into the esophagus. (Courtesy Martin Charrone, MD, Pittsburgh.)

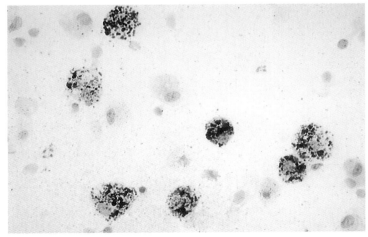

Figure 16-37. Lipid-laden macrophages obtained via bronchoalveolar lavage. If seen in moderate and high numbers, this finding is specific for aspiration of food, either the result of abnormal swallowing or from refluxed gastric contents. (Courtesy Paul Dickman, MD, Pittsburgh.)

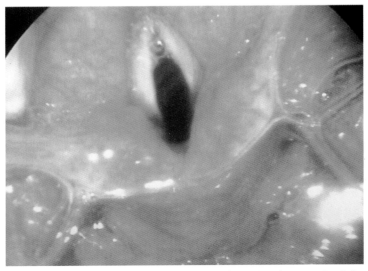

Figure 16-38. Gastroesophageal reflux. Endoscopic photograph of the larynx of a patient with severe gastroesophageal reflux. Erythema and edema of the aryepiglottic folds exists. (Courtesy Robert Yellon, MD, Pittsburgh.)

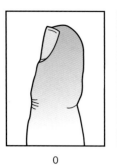 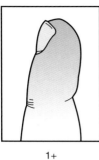 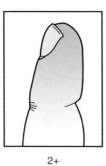 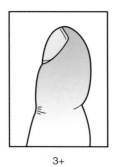 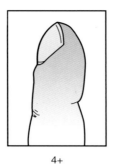

0   1+   2+   3+   4+

Figure 16-39. Digital clubbing. The 0-4 point scale describes the spectrum of digital clubbing as follows: 1+ very mild, 2+ mild, 3+ moderate, and 4+ severe.

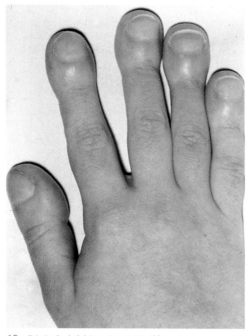

Figure 16-40. Digital clubbing in cystic fibrosis.

Table 16-7	Causes of Clubbing

Pulmonary
  Cystic fibrosis
  Other bronchiectasis
  Pulmonary abscess
  Empyema
  Neoplasms
  Interstitial fibrosis
  Pulmonary alveolar proteinosis
  Interstitial pneumonitis
  Chronic pneumonia
Cardiac
  Cyanotic congenital heart disease
  Subacute bacterial endocarditis
Gastrointestinal or hepatic
  Ulcerative colitis
  Crohn disease
  Polyposis
  Biliary cirrhosis/atresia
Familial
Thyrotoxicosis

Where:
TLC = IC + FRC
and
TLC = VC + RV

Figure 16-41. Schematic representation of lung volumes.

the abscissa (volume axis). This type of concavity therefore suggests obstruction to airflow (Fig. 16-42B). Patients with suspected asthma may develop this configuration of flow-volume curve after bronchoprovocation tests such as inhaled histamine, methacholine, cold air, or after exercise testing.

The restrictive pattern shown in Fig. 16-42C demonstrates preservation of expiratory flow function but a reduction in total lung volume. Interstitial lung diseases are among the entities that typically produce this pattern on pulmonary function testing.

The shape of the flow-volume curve may also be helpful in evaluating upper or central airway pathology (Fig. 16-43). Fixed obstruction of the upper airways, as in tracheal stenosis, produces a limitation and plateau of both the inspiratory and expiratory loops of the flow-volume

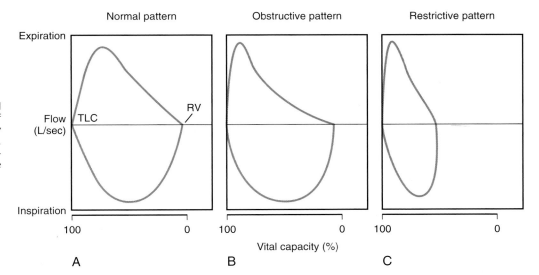

Figure 16-42. Flow-volume curves obtained by spirometry. **A,** Normal configuration of expiratory flow curve. **B,** Reduced expiratory flow rates suggest obstructive airway disease. **C,** Preservation of flow rates with a diminished vital capacity consistent with restrictive lung disease.

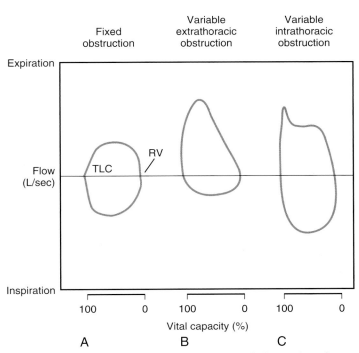

Figure 16-43. Pulmonary function tests. **A,** Fixed obstruction of upper airways with reduction in inspiratory and expiratory flow loops. **B,** Reduction in peak inspiratory flow observed in variable extrathoracic airway obstruction. **C,** Reduction and flattening of the expiratory limb in variable intrathoracic obstruction.

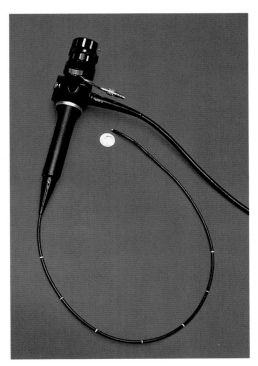

Figure 16-44. Flexible fiberoptic bronchoscope (Olympus BF3C10, 3.5-mm outer diameter) shown next to a dime, for size comparison.

curve. A reduced inspiratory flow and a plateau of the inspiratory loop are suggestive of variable extrathoracic obstruction seen in disorders such as laryngomalacia and vocal cord dysfunction. Chondromalacia of the intrathoracic trachea or major bronchi results in a picture of variable intrathoracic obstruction with reduction and flattening of the expiratory limb because with forceful expiration, pleural pressure exceeds that inside the airway lumen, and the weakened bronchial wall cannot withstand that pressure gradient.

Exercise testing can be a valuable tool to assess the cardiorespiratory fitness of a subject and may provide further information regarding a patient's respiratory reserve in addition to that found during routine PFTs. A progressive exercise study by bicycle ergometry can give important information regarding ventilatory effort, heart rate responses, oxygen delivery and uptake, and carbon dioxide

production. Evaluation of these parameters may provide information regarding exercise fitness and, if limited, identify whether the limiting factor is ventilatory or cardiac. Like PFTs, exercise testing can be used to assess the severity or progress of disease, evaluate effects of changes in treatment, and provide information about the safety or appropriateness of an exercise program in children with chronic lung disease.

Flexible fiberoptic bronchoscopy (Fig. 16-44) can be extremely useful in the diagnosis of lesions of the pulmonary tree and in isolating organisms from patients with pneumonia. Compared with traditional open-tube ("rigid") bronchoscopy, flexible bronchoscopy offers the advantage of better visualization of distal airway segments and upper lobes and allowing the study of airway dynamics during regular tidal breathing. Indications for pediatric flexible bronchoscopy include evaluation of stridor, unexplained or chronic cough or wheeze, suspected airway malformations or compression, atelectasis, or recurrent

| Table 16-8 | Range of Normal Arterial Blood Gas Values by Age |

	pH	Pco$_2$	Po$_2$
Newborn	7.33-7.49	27-41	>60
Infant (<1 year)	7.34-7.46	26-41	>75
Older child	7.35-7.45	35-45	>75

pneumonia. To obviate the need for open lung biopsy, flexible bronchoscopy and bronchoalveolar lavage may be particularly useful in immunosuppressed patients with unexplained pneumonia. Flexible bronchoscopy should not be attempted when there is a strong clinical or radiographic suggestion of inhaled foreign body. In these cases, rigid bronchoscopy is the procedure of choice to remove the object. Transbronchial biopsy is performed routinely in patients who have undergone lung transplantation in order to screen for rejection. This technique involves passing biopsy forceps via the suction channel of a bronchoscope under fluoroscopic guidance. It is of occasional usefulness in clinical situations in which the lesion is diffuse, such as interstitial lung disease. Tissue yield is low, and analysis requires an experienced pathologist. Risk of transbronchial biopsy is pneumothorax (approximately 1%) and bleeding.

Arterial blood gas measurements are the standard for assessing gas exchange in critically ill patients. Pulse oximetry and analysis of the CO_2 in exhaled air have become useful noninvasive means of assessing ventilatory status and have been used to avoid routine arterial puncture in both inpatient and outpatient settings. An example is the 16-year-old with Duchenne muscular dystrophy who presents with dyspnea and headache and is found to have an end-tidal CO_2 level of 90, prompting long-term institution of noninvasive ventilatory support. Venous or capillary blood gases can give accurate estimations of pH and Pco$_2$ but are not used for assessment of arterial Po$_2$. Normal arterial pH, Po$_2$, and Pco$_2$ values are provided in Table 16-8.

Sleep studies are still not widely available for the pediatric population, but they remain an important diagnostic tool. They are useful in diagnosis of obstructive and central apnea, hypoventilation, and hypoxemia during sleep, all of which can be inapparent on routine testing of the awake patient. Studies vary in complexity from a simple at-home overnight pulse oximetry study to full nocturnal polysomnography with assessment of sleep stage, movement of chest, abdomen, electromyogram of diaphragm, arterial saturation, heart rate, end-tidal CO_2, and eye movements. The "pneumogram" is an abbreviated form of the sleep study in which there is evaluation of chest wall movement, air flow by nasal thermistor (which measures temperature below the nostril), heart rate, and arterial saturation. The pneumogram is insensitive for obstructive apnea and does not assess ventilation (as it lacks CO_2 measurement), does not demonstrate sleep stage or changes in stage with respiratory events, but is sensitive for central apnea and bradycardia.

Acknowledgments

The author gratefully acknowledges Dr. Beverly Newman for her kind assistance with selection of radiographic images for this chapter.

Bibliography

American Academy of Pediatrics Task Force on Sudden Infant Death Syndrome. The Changing Concept of Sudden Infant Death Syndrome: Diagnostic Coding Shifts, Controversies Regarding the Sleeping Environment, and New Variables to Consider in Reducing Risk. Pediatrics 116:1245-1255, 2005.

Boucher RC: New concepts of the pathogenesis of cystic fibrosis lung disease. Eur Respir J 23:146-158, 2004.

Busse WW, Lemanske RF Jr: Asthma. N Engl J Med 344:350-362, 2001.

Chernick V, Boat T: Kendig's Disorders of the Respiratory Tract in Children, 6th ed. Philadelphia, WB Saunders, 1998.

Colombo JL, Hallberg TK: Pulmonary aspiration and lipid-laden macrophages: In search of gold (standards). Pediatr Pulmonol 28:79-82, 1999.

Daley KC: Update on sudden infant death syndrome. Curr Opin Pediatr 16:227-232, 2004.

Ferber R, Kyger M: Principles and Practice of Sleep Medicine in the Child, Philadelphia, WB Saunders, 1995.

Finder JD: Understanding airway disease in infants. Curr Probl Pediatr 29:65-81, 1999.

Hyatt R, Scanlon P, Nakamura M: Interpretation of Pulmonary Function Tests: A Practical Guide, 2nd ed. New York, Lippincott-Raven, 2003.

Martinez FD, Morgan WJ, Wright AL, et al: Diminished lung function as a predisposing factor for wheezing respiratory illness in infants, N Engl J Med 319:1112-1117, 1988.

Martinez FD, Wright AL, Taussig LM, et al: Asthma and wheezing in the first six years of life. The Group Health Medical Associates. N Engl J Med 332:133-138, 1995.

Orenstein SR: Update on gastroesophageal reflux and respiratory disease in children. Can Gastroenterol 14:131-135, 2000.

Orenstein D, Rosenstein B, Stern R: Cystic Fibrosis Medical Care. Philadelphia, Lippincott Williams & Wilkins, 2000.

Orenstein D, Stern R: Treatment of the Hospitalized Cystic Fibrosis Patient. New York, Marcel Dekker, 1998.

Taussig LM, Wright AL, Holberg CJ, et al: Tucson Children's Respiratory Study: 1980 to present. J Allergy Clin Immunol 111:661-675, 2003.

Vaucher YE: Bronchopulmonary dysplasia: an enduring challenge. Pediatr Rev 23:349-358, 2002.

CHAPTER 17

Surgery

EDWARD M. BARKSDALE, JR.

General pediatric surgery embraces a wide spectrum of disorders that overlap various other medical and surgical subspecialties. The focus of this chapter is on those common conditions that may be seen in the general pediatric primary care practice supplemented with the inclusion of unusual cases.

Respiratory Distress

Neonatal respiratory distress is rarely of surgical origin. Although medically related conditions such as transient tachypnea of the newborn and pneumonia may cause significant symptoms, severe dyspnea, hoarseness, or stridor requires urgent assessment and possible surgical intervention. These symptoms should alert the practitioner to the possibility of a surgical problem. If the plain radiographs rule out pneumothorax, atelectasis or pneumonia, the differential diagnosis of these conditions may include proximal obstructive airway lesions, intrathoracic masses, lung bud anomalies (bronchopulmonary foregut malformations), pneumothorax, or abdominal masses. An example is an infant with a lung bud anomaly such as a cystic adenomatoid malformation or congenital lobar emphysema. Alternatively, an infant with a diaphragmatic hernia may present in a similar manner. Second, a newborn who fails to respond to standard therapy for a presumed pulmonary disorder should be evaluated for a potential surgical etiology. Examples include a premature newborn with tracheoesophageal fistula and esophageal atresia or a neonate being treated for group B streptococcal sepsis who develops a right-sided diaphragmatic hernia.

The clinical evaluation of these patients should include both anteroposterior (AP) and lateral radiographs of the chest. Particular focus should be directed to the soft tissue views of the neck, mediastinum, and airway contour. Fluoroscopic examination provides critical insight into the airway contour and diaphragmatic mobility throughout the respiratory cycle. Esophagography with either barium or water-soluble contrast may be useful to delineate a vascular ring or mediastinal mass (Fig. 17-1). More invasive studies such as upper airway and esophageal endoscopy may be necessary to elucidate other surgical causes of respiratory distress. Surgical causes of respiratory distress may be subclassified into three major categories: upper airway, thoracic, and extrathoracic.

Upper Airway

The inability of the neonate to breathe orally at birth raises the possibility that an upper airway obstructive lesion may be the source of respiratory distress in this patient population. The newborn infant who is unable to nurse or has paroxysmal asphyxia (cyclic dyspnea) should undergo a thorough airway and cardiopulmonary evaluation. Lesions involving the upper airway create a characteristic "air hunger" that may progress to respiratory failure in the neonate. The respiratory difficulties are most marked during the inspiratory phase of the cycle, when the airway tends to collapse around the lesion. These infants may be asymptomatic during the expiratory component of the respiratory cycle, when the airway reaches its greatest diameter. The differential diagnosis for these symptoms should include choanal atresia, esophageal atresia, tracheoesophageal fistula, vocal cord paralysis, nasopharyngeal tumors, oropharyngeal masses, and foreign bodies.

The initial evaluation of infants with presumed airway obstruction should include the passage of a nasogastric tube. Signs of pharyngeal obstruction suggest choanal atresia. This obstruction may be membranous (90%) or bony (10%). Half of these patients may have other forms of associated craniofacial or remote congenital anomalies that require concurrent evaluation and management. Nasopharyngoscopy is diagnostic in most cases. The oral airway must be maintained, and the baby must be fed via gavage feedings until transpalatal repair. Oropharyngeal obstruction may be caused by macroglossia or jaw bony abnormalities. Beckwith-Wiedemann syndrome is associated with lingual hypertrophy and gigantism (Fig. 17-2). Presentation in the newborn should alert the practitioner to the possibility of hypoglycemia secondary to hyperinsulinism. Permanent neurologic sequelae may result from diagnostic delay. Sublingual or lingual lymphangiomas may be associated with massive macroglossia that leads to airway distress. The hypoplastic and recessed mandible associated with Pierre Robin syndrome may cause a normal-sized tongue to fall posteriorly and obstruct the airway (Fig. 17-3). The association of cleft palate and cardiac defects with Pierre Robin syndrome may further exacerbate respiratory distress. Prone positioning of the infant may assist breathing and avert the need for tracheostomy. Alternatively, tracheostomy placement may provide a safer temporizing measure to allow adequate mandibular growth and development and to prevent obstruction. Newer techniques of mandibular distraction may avoid the need for prophylactic tracheostomy.

Laryngeal lesions distinctively present with hoarseness, faint crying, or complete aphonia in association with dyspnea. The differential diagnosis for these patients includes laryngomalacia, laryngeal atresia, laryngeal webs, laryngeal clefts, subglottic stenosis, and vocal cord paralysis. Emergency tracheostomy is often indicated in these patients because of the inability to secure an airway, as occurs in laryngeal atresia. Direct airway contamination may occur with feeding in patients with laryngeal clefts due to the communication between the pharynx and the posterior laryngeal defect.

Pharyngeal masses may be another source of upper airway obstruction. These masses include branchial cleft remnants, dermoids, pharyngeal duplications, hemangiomas, lymphangiomas, lingual thyroids, sublingual teratomas, and Zenker diverticula. Large cervical masses such as a cystic hygroma (lymphangioma) (Fig. 17-4) and cervical teratoma (Fig. 17-5) may induce airway compression and cause dyspnea. Antenatal diagnosis of the lesions may indicate a potential airway emergency. The ex utero intrapartum treatment (EXIT) procedure allows time to secure airway control before division of the umbilical cord (Fig. 17-6).

Thoracic

Mediastinum and Diaphragm

Mediastinal masses are uncommon in the pediatric population. The limited space of the thoracic cavity pre-

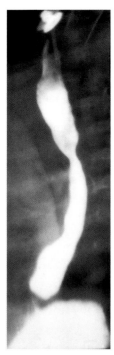

Figure 17-1. Midthoracic compressions into the esophageal barium column identify the presence of vascular ring anomalies (in this case, pulmonary artery sling).

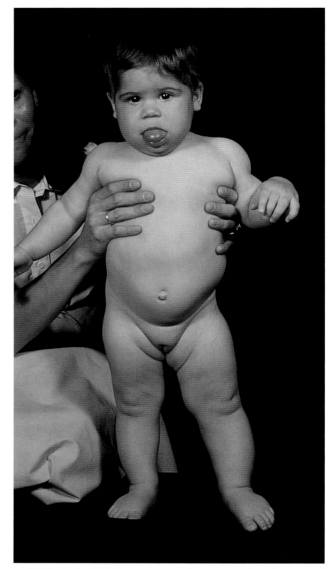

Figure 17-2. Beckwith-Wiedemann syndrome. Note hemihypertrophy on the left side, along with the prominence of the tongue. (Courtesy D. Becker, MD, Pittsburgh, Pa.)

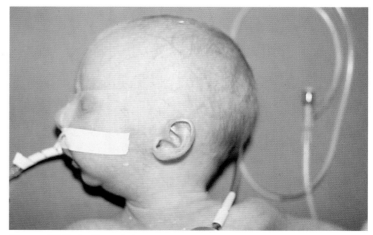

Figure 17-3. In Pierre Robin sequence, the hypoplastic mandible positions the tongue posteriorly, potentially obstructing the upper airway.

disposes normal structures to be compressed by space-occupying lesions. Masses in this anatomic region may lead to a host of symptoms including dysphagia, dyspnea, and superior vena cava syndrome. The mediastinal location and the patient's age provide the most critical insight into the diagnosis. The mediastinum may be divided into three major compartments: anterior-superior, medial, and posterior. The location of a mass in any one of these compartments is an important diagnostic feature (Table 17-1). The anatomic boundaries for these compartments include the sternum to the anterior aspect of the trachea and pericardium (anterior); the trachea, major bronchi, and paratracheal structures (middle); the posterior aspect of the trachea to the spine (posterior). Anterior mediastinal masses typically arise in tissues of thyroid, thymus, and lymphoid or are teratomatous in origin. Middle mediastinal masses are typically tumors or congenital anomalies arising from the tracheobronchial tree, lymph nodes, esophagus, or pulmonary parenchyma (Fig. 17-7). Posterior mediastinal masses are primarily neurogenic tumors or congenital enterogenous lesions (Fig. 17-8).

Esophageal atresia with or without tracheoesophageal fistula is a common cause of airway obstruction. The inability to pass a Replogle (nasogastric) tube into the stomach clarifies this diagnosis. This tube also serves as a sump catheter to drain the proximal pouch and limit upper airway contamination associated with this anomaly. Infants develop respiratory distress secondary to esophageal obstruction and the tracheoesophageal communication. Neonates with esophageal atresia characteristically have excessive salivation and coughing due to the pooling of secretions in the proximal pharyngeal pouch. Most patients are diagnosed by their inability to tolerate their initial feedings. The diagnosis of congenital esophageal obstruction secondary to esophageal atresia is frequently made on antenatal ultrasonography by the presence of microgastria, polyhydramnios, and frequent fetal hiccups. Although several major variants of this condition exist, the most common, a blind proximal pouch with the distal tracheoesophageal fistula, occurs in approximately 85% of all patients. Inspired air from the trachea communicates directly to the stomach via a fistulous connection (Fig. 17-9). This leads to gastric distention and retrograde gastroesophageal reflux into the lungs precipitating respiratory distress. Positive pressure ventilation either by mask or endotracheal tube should be avoided in these patients before surgery due to the risk of gastric distention and perforation, severe retrograde reflux, and pneumonia (Fig. 17-10). The second most common variant of this condition is pure esophageal atresia, which on plain radiography has a dilated proximal pouch and a gasless abdomen (Fig. 17-11). On physical examination these infants have scaphoid abdomens due to the lack of distal air passage into the bowels (Fig. 17-12). Isolated tracheoesophageal fistula without esophageal atresia is the third most common form of this anomaly. These children lack esophageal obstruction and may at times be diagnosed at later ages with symptoms of persistent cough or recurrent pneumonia. Although called an H-fistula, the appearance is more N-shaped with a more proximal communication with the trachea and distal communication into the esophagus. The diagnosis of this variant is made more challenging due to this acute angle of communication

between the esophagus and trachea, which inhibits reflux of orogastric contents into the airway (Fig. 17-13).

Congenital diaphragmatic hernia is a common cause of respiratory distress in newborns, occurring with an incidence of approximately 1 in every 4000 live births. Defects in the diaphragm may result from either abnormal fusion of the posterolateral pleuroperitoneal membrane (foramen of Bochdalek) or from defects in the central diaphragmatic muscle formation (foramen of Morgagni hernia). Diffuse muscular weakness may give rise to diaphragmatic eventration. Congenital diaphragmatic abnormalities of the foramen of Bochdalek are the most common form of lesion and are typically left sided in 85% of patients (Fig. 17-14). These defects occur early in gestation, allowing abdominal contents to migrate into the chest. This limits

Table 17-1	Mediastinal Masses in Childhood	
ANTERIOR AND SUPERIOR	**MIDDLE**	**POSTERIOR**
Teratoma including dermoid cyst	Bronchogenic cyst	Neurogenic tumor
Normal thymus	Pericardial cyst	Enterogenous cyst
Lymphoma		Pulmonary sequestration
Vascular malformation		
Thymic cyst		
Cystic hygroma		
Intrathoracic goiter		

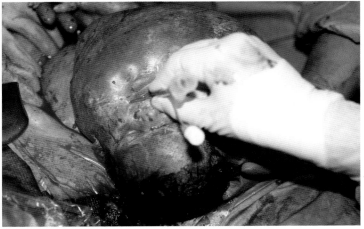

Figure 17-6. Ex utero intrapartum treatment (EXIT) procedure.

Figure 17-4. Large cervical masses like this cervical teratoma diagnosed by antenatal ultrasonography cause prenatal esophageal compression and polyhydramnios. Due to the high risk of upper airway compression at delivery, an ex utero intrapartum treatment (EXIT) procedure is indicated to avoid infant death.

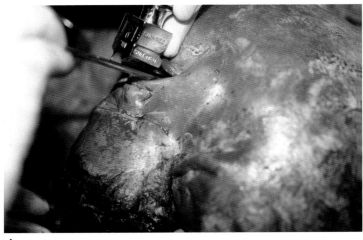

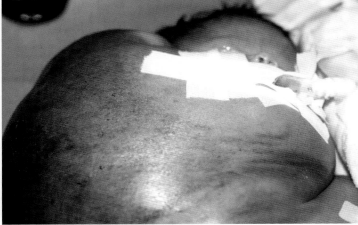

A   B

Figure 17-5. **A,** Cervical teratoma at delivery presents airway challenges **(B)** in the perinatal period.

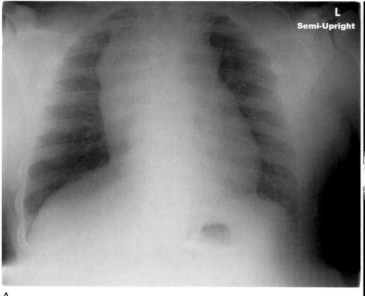

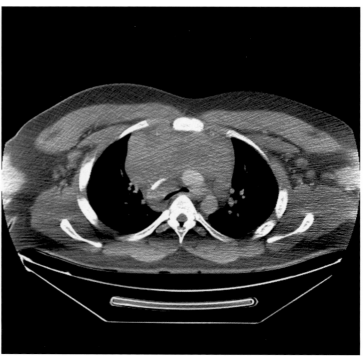

Figure 17-7. **A,** A large mediastinal thymic tumor seen on chest radiograph may induce dyspnea, orthopnea, and other pulmonary symptoms. **B,** CT scan demonstrating the anterior mediastinal thymic tumor.

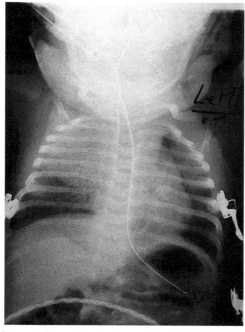

Figure 17-8. Posterior mediastinal masses include esophageal duplication (illustrated here), neurenteric cysts, extralobar sequestration, anterior myelomeningocele, and neural tumors. Vertebral anomalies coexist frequently.

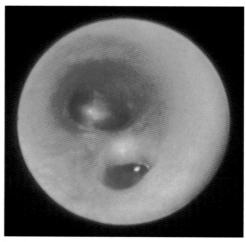

Figure 17-9. Bronchoscopy visualizes tracheoesophageal fistula, seen as a posteriorly positioned orifice *(bottom)* in the upper trachea. The carina, seen toward the top of the picture, lies distally.

lung expansion and growth, displacing the heart, resulting in pulmonary hypoplasia and persistent pulmonary hypertension. Many of these infants have severe respiratory distress that occurs shortly following umbilical cord division. On physical examination there is marked nasal flaring, chest wall asymmetry (larger contralateral hemithorax secondary to lung hyperplasia), displaced heart tones to the side opposite of the hernia, and ipsilateral absence of breath sounds with dullness to percussion due to the presence of abdominal viscera in that hemithorax. Plain chest radiography demonstrates intestinal loops within the hemithorax displacing the cardiomediastinal silhouette to the opposite side. Infants with foramen of Bochdalek congenital diaphragmatic hernias have severe respiratory failure secondary to both pulmonary hypoplasia and pulmonary hypertension. Despite aggressive efforts with nitric oxide, high-frequency oscillatory ventilation, and extracorporeal membrane oxygenation, mortality remains approximately 50% (Fig. 17-15).

Diaphragmatic eventration may have a radiographic appearance similar to that of diaphragmatic hernia but usually lacks acute neonatal presentation. Foramen of Morgagni diaphragmatic hernias represent less than 5% of all diaphragmatic hernias. Often they are incidental findings seen on routine radiography for other reasons. Morgagni hernias typically have a sac, which may include the transverse colon, liver, or small bowel (Fig. 17-16). Intestinal incarceration is a rare complication. Cystic adenomatoid malformations may be confused with diaphragmatic hernia on plain films and are usually distinguished by the location of the gastric air bubble (Fig. 17-17).

Vascular ring anomalies may be a source of tracheo-esophageal compression giving rise to varying degrees of dyspnea or dysphagia. These anomalies originate from persistence of the embryonic aortic arches. Plain film findings demonstrating narrowing of the mediastinal portion

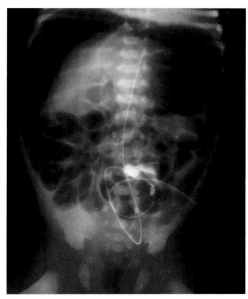

Figure 17-10. Tracheoesophageal fistula allows air to be forced into the stomach during positive pressure ventilation by bag and mask or through an endotracheal tube. The stomach may perforate or ventilation may become suddenly ineffective if a gastrotomy is placed initially during surgical repair.

of the tracheal air contour suggest the presence of the vascular ring. The diagnosis may be confirmed by nuclear magnetic resonance imaging (MRI), contrast barium swallow, or endoscopic evaluation of the airway. MRI has nearly replaced aortography for delineating the associated vascular anatomy (Fig. 17-18).

Lung
Lung Bud Anomalies (Bronchopulmonary Foregut Malformations). These cystic lung lesions may induce severe respiratory distress by direct compression of adjacent normal lung tissue. Acute expansion, which may often occur at the time of delivery, may require emergent surgical intervention or the use of high-frequency oscillatory ventilation. This ventilation technique serves as a temporizing means as the infant is prepared for surgery. Congenital cystic anomalies of the lung are the most common surgical cause of respiratory distress in infants and children. These bronchopulmonary foregut malformations have their origin during the stages of early fetal development between the 3rd and 16th weeks of gestation. Progressive enlargement during the first few months of life may lead to acute respiratory distress secondary to compression of normal lung tissue. Smaller or more slowly growing lesions may have a paucity of symptoms. They may go undetected for long periods, prior to diagnosis by routine chest radiography for infection, dyspnea, or tachypnea. Persistent cough, recurrent bouts of pneumonia, and paroxysmal dyspnea should prompt the primary care practitioner to investigate the diagnostic possibility of an occult congenital cystic lung lesion with plain chest radiography or CT.

Figure 17-11. A dilated blind proximal esophageal pouch **(A)** and a gasless abdomen **(B)** are the radiographic hallmarks of pure esophageal atresia.

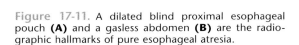
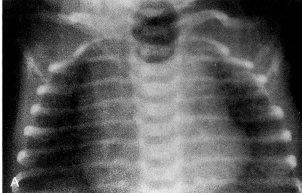
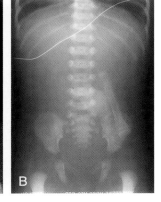

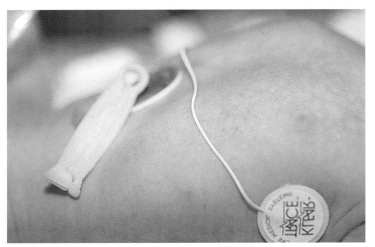

Figure 17-12. Pure esophageal atresia without distal tracheoesophageal fistula. Esophageal obstruction associated with scaphoid abdomen on physical examination is pathognomonic of pure esophageal atresia.

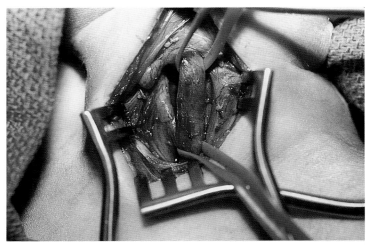

Figure 17-13. Isolated tracheoesophageal fistula (H-type) as seen here is typically accessed via a cervical approach. The patient's chin is to the left. Blue loops are around the esophagus with the fistula seen as a tubular structure immediately to the left of the esophagus.

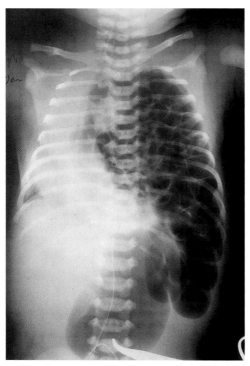

Figure 17-14. Congenital diaphragmatic hernia allows intestines to enter the chest in utero.

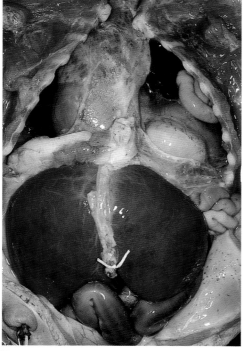

Figure 17-15. Autopsy specimen of a diaphragmatic hernia illustrates the right lung compression, cardiomediastinal shift, left lung hypoplasia, and visceral herniation through the diaphragmatic defect.

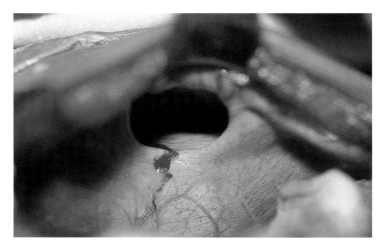

Figure 17-16. A foramen of Morgagni hernia, seen here as a central tendinous defect in the diaphragm, typically does not present as acute pulmonary distress in the newborn.

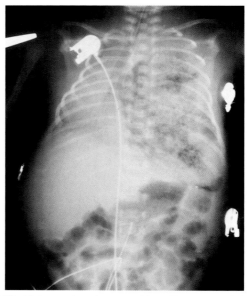

Figure 17-17. Macrocystic adenomatoid malformation of the left lung. Large cystic lesions can be mistaken for bowel loops herniating through a diaphragmatic hernia.

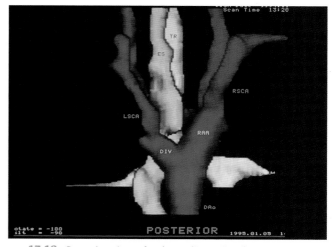

Figure 17-18. Posterior view of a three-dimensional reconstruction of an axial MRI scan of a right aortic arch with an anomalous left subclavian artery. Note the close proximity of the anomalous subclavian artery to the esophagus and its potential obstruction of the esophagus. ES, esophagus (yellow); DAo, descending aorta (red); DIV, diverticulum; LSCA, left subclavian artery (red); RAA, right aortic arch (red); TR, trachea (white). (Courtesy Beverly Newman, MD, Children's Hospital of Pittsburgh, Pa.)

Four major bronchopulmonary foregut malformations exist: congenital lobar emphysema (CLE), congenital cystic adenomatoid malformation (CAM), pulmonary sequestration, and bronchogenic cyst. The most common of these, CAM, is subclassified into one of three variants. Cystic adenomatoid malformation results from the proliferation of primordial bronchial structures in the absence of alveoli. The variants are classified on the basis of their size, shape, and pathologic appearance. Type I CAM comprises single or multiple cysts greater than 2 cm in diam-

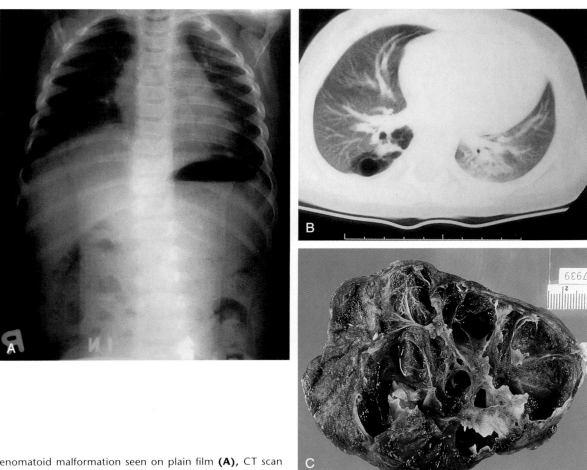

Figure 17-19. Macrocystic adenomatoid malformation seen on plain film **(A)**, CT scan **(B)**, and surgical specimen **(C)**.

eter lined by ciliated pseudostratified columnar epithelium. Type I lesions may be difficult to distinguish from diaphragmatic hernias (Fig. 17-19). Type II lesions are small with cysts and are less than 1 cm in diameter lined by cuboidal to columnar epithelium. These lesions are associated with a broad spectrum of congenital anomalies. Type III CAMs are large benign cysts lined by ciliated cuboidal epithelium or solid masses. These are often fatal and have a high incidence of associated anomalies.

Congenital lobar emphysema is a condition that results from a segment of poorly developed or absent cartilage in the tracheobronchial tree and leads to lung hyperexpansion secondary to a "check valve effect" and air trapping. Subsequent lung overdistention may lead to respiratory distress, pneumonia, and mediastinal shift. Many of these patients present with symptomatic lesions in the first few weeks of life; however, other patients have a more indolent progression of symptoms over the first 6 months of life. Other patients may remain entirely asymptomatic. The plain radiographic appearance of these patients demonstrates lung hyperlucency and hyperexpansion in the upper or middle lobes (Fig. 17-20). Acute cardiopulmonary decompensation may occur in otherwise healthy patients with this anomaly due to positive pressure ventilation such as that which might occur at the time of the induction of general anesthesia for surgery (Fig. 17-21).

Primary pulmonary blastoma is a stromal malignancy of the lung that may present with unilateral hyperinflation, mimicking and possibly confused with lobar emphysema (Fig. 17-22). Pulmonary sequestrations are accessory pulmonary parenchymal tissue that lacks direct tracheobronchial communication. These anomalies receive their

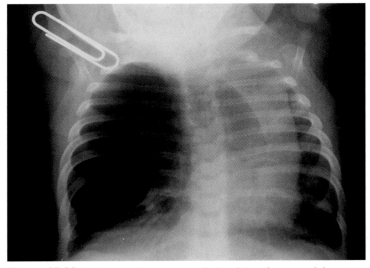

Figure 17-20. Lobar emphysema, usually involving the upper lobes, may become hugely distended and may cause life-threatening respiratory distress.

blood supply from the systemic circulation. They may arise from within the pulmonary parenchyma (intralobar) (Fig. 17-23) or reside separately from normal lung tissue (extralobar) (Fig. 17-24). Although commonly found in the left costophrenic sulcus, sequestrations may be located in either hemithorax or in the abdomen. They may also communicate with other foregut structures in the gastrointestinal tract owing to their shared embryonic origin. Usually asymptomatic and found on routine chest x-ray or noted as an incidental finding during another thoracic

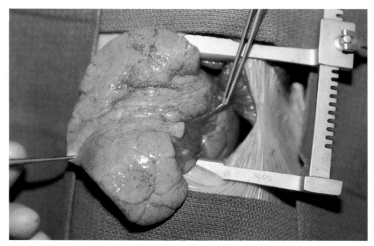

Figure 17-21. Lobar emphysema may acutely expand with positive pressure ventilation seen at the time of anesthesia induction. Hyperexpansion of the lobe is clearly apparent at thoracotomy when lung parenchyma "balloons" into field.

procedure, these lesions may be a source of recurrent intrathoracic infection and should undergo elective resection. Angiography; duplex ultrasonography; or, more commonly, MRI evaluation may be used in the diagnostic evaluation by demonstration of a systemic arterial blood supply (Fig. 17-25).

Pneumothorax may occur as a result of thoracic trauma, cystic fibrosis, or spontaneously (Fig. 17-26). Patients may develop acute severe pleuritic chest pain and associated dyspnea. Physical examination findings may demonstrate hyperresonance and diminished breath sounds over the ipsilateral hemithorax. Mediastinal shift, cervical venous distention, hypotension, and diaphragmatic flattening may result from the development of a tension pneumothorax. This requires emergent lifesaving needle decompression followed by a thoracostomy tube placement. A subpopulation of young patients, usually male and asthenic in build, may present with acute spontaneous pneumothorax. Spontaneous pneumothorax is typically

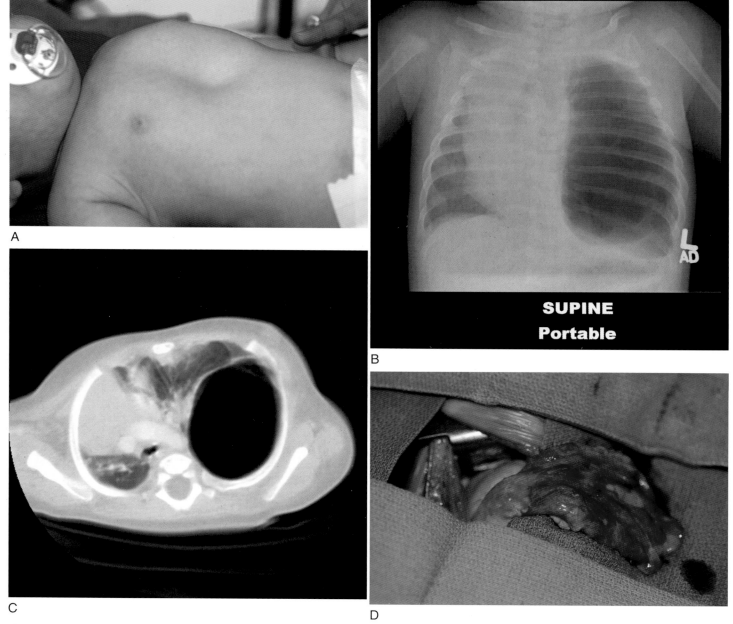

Figure 17-22. **A,** Clinical examination of an infant with primary pulmonary blastoma with thoracic asymmetry and hyperinflation. **B,** Anteroposterior chest radiograph demonstrating the unilateral hyperinflation of the left lung and mediastinal shift to the right. **C,** CT scan of the chest showing the pulmonary hyperinflation and tumor mass. **D,** Intraoperative tumor.

secondary to apical bullous lung disease (Fig. 17-27). The etiology of this condition is unknown. These patients usually require chest decompression by thoracostomy tube placement. Recurrent episodes of spontaneous pneumothorax are an indication for surgical exploration with resection of the apical bullae and either mechanical or chemical pleurodesis.

Occasionally, surgical intervention may be necessary in the treatment of pulmonary infections that persist despite aggressive antibiotic therapy (Fig. 17-28). The development of an intrathoracic empyema as the sequelae of streptococcal or staphylococcal pneumonia may restrict lung expansion. Surgical intervention may provide the means of diagnosis and the ability to rule out bronchial foreign body obstruction (Fig. 17-29); the capacity to

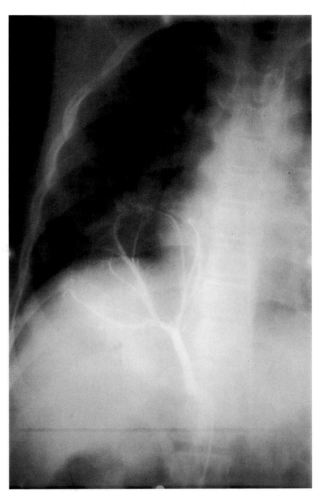

Figure 17-25. Extralobar sequestrations are characterized by the presence of pulmonary parenchyma that lacks tracheobronchial communication and has a systemic blood supply. Angiogram shows systemic blood supply. MRI has supplanted this technique.

Figure 17-23. Persistent infiltration of the lung parenchyma may indicate an intralobar sequestration, shown here involving the right lower lobe. Also shown is a right diaphragmatic hernia, a frequently associated malformation.

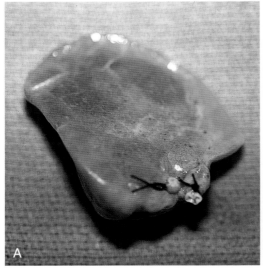

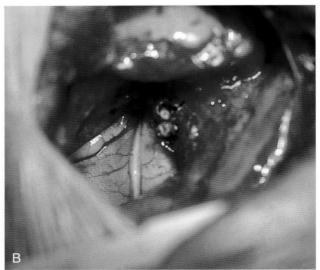

Figure 17-24. Resected extralobar sequestration shows the two systemic vessels **(A)**. Intrathoracic view shows the ligated vessels penetrating the posterior sulcus of the diaphragm **(B)**.

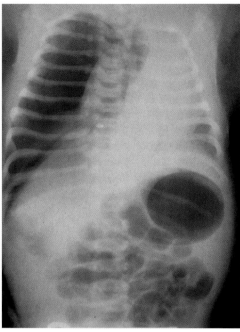

Figure 17-26. This chest film shows typical radiologic signs of tension pneumothorax: mediastinal shift, flattening of the diaphragm, and widening of the intercostal spaces.

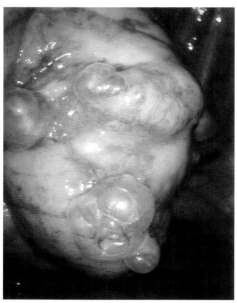

Figure 17-27. Thoracoscopic view of apical bullous lung disease. These bullae or blebs may rupture and give rise to spontaneous pneumothorax.

assess for evidence of malignancy; or allow treatment through providing adequate drainage or mechanical pleural clearance. In addition, surgery may provide a means of treatment of chest lesions that may become secondarily infected (Fig. 17-30). Thoracoscopy with video-assisted thoracic decortication may hasten the early recovery from pneumonia and these parapneumonic consequences.

Extrathoracic Causes

Intra-abdominal conditions are the most frequent causes of extrathoracic respiratory distress. These lesions decrease diaphragmatic excursion, limit intrathoracic volume, and precipitate respiratory embarrassment. Large upper abdom-

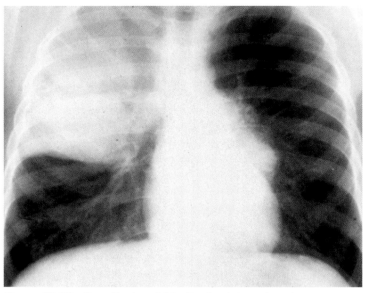

Figure 17-28. Chest film in a child with allergic bronchopulmonary aspergillosis of the right upper lobe, which ultimately required resection.

inal tumors, ascites, and gastrointestinal obstruction are common causes of respiratory distress. These are addressed in the section on abdominal disease.

Gastrointestinal Obstruction

Vomiting is the reflex-coordinated response of various stimuli to the central nervous system resulting in relaxation of the lower esophageal sphincter, increased gastric peristalsis, increased diaphragmatic contractions, and forceful expulsion of gastrointestinal contents. Vomiting is the primary presenting symptom of children with a wide range of conditions from benign responses to minor infectious diseases to the primary manifestation of life-threatening intra-abdominal disease. Although the vast majority of children who have this complaint do not have an obstructive lesion, vomiting is the principal symptom of major gastrointestinal obstructive diseases. Distinguishing between self-limited or medical conditions and those that require urgent surgical intervention may be challenging.

The first stage in the assessment is the differentiation of vomiting and regurgitation. Vomiting is the forceful expulsion of gastrointestinal contents, whereas regurgitation is the passive expulsion of enteric contents. The surgical causes of vomiting are typically extrinsic (serosal) inflammatory conditions or intrinsic (mucosal/structural) mechanical lesions. Diagnosis and management are best defined by the patient's age and level of gastrointestinal obstruction. Vomiting associated with fever, abdominal pain, and abdominal tenderness is highly suggestive of peritoneal irritation seen in conditions such as appendicitis. The presence of bilious emesis with or without abdominal distention should raise concern for a mechanical obstruction.

Bilious emesis is a critical finding in the pediatric population. Its presence should always raise a red flag in the evaluation of a vomiting child, especially the newborn or infant. The principal condition of concern is malrotation with midgut volvulus. This typically presents without abdominal distention because the level of obstruction is at or near the ligament of Treitz. Bilious emesis with asso-

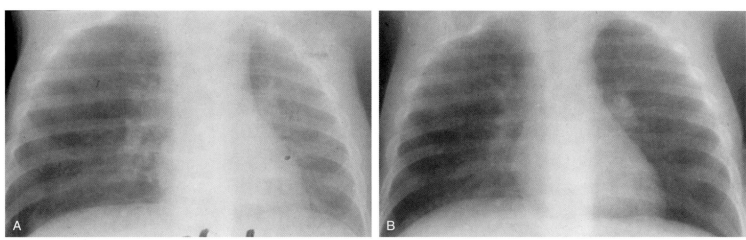

Figure 17-29. Signs of a radiolucent foreign body are often subtle. Persistent overdistention of the right lung during expiration **(A)** was due to right mainstem bronchial occlusion. Less marked changes are seen during inhalation **(B)**.

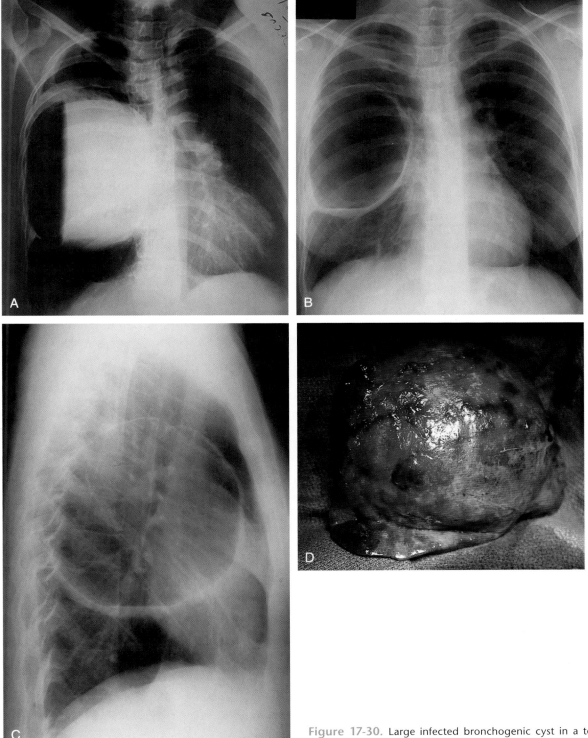

Figure 17-30. Large infected bronchogenic cyst in a teenager **(A)** who responded to aggressive antibiotic therapy (**B** and **C**), and surgical resection **(D)**.

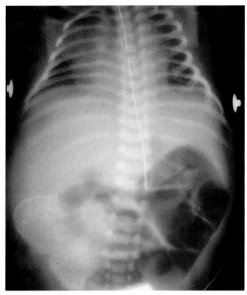

Figure 17-31. Calcification in an area of meconium peritonitis in the right iliac fossa.

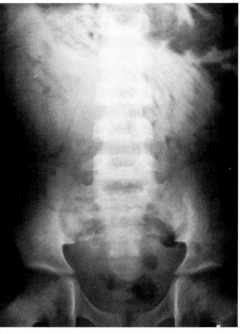

Figure 17-32. This plain film shows two signs indicative of meconium ileus: a "soap bubble" mass in the right iliac fossa, produced by the impacted meconium, and distended loops of different diameters, reflecting the gradual distention of the small bowel to the area of obstruction.

ciated abdominal distention is more characteristic of distal small bowel or colonic obstruction seen in conditions such as intestinal atresias, meconium disease, incarcerated hernias, or Hirschsprung disease. The presence of blood in the stool suggests an associated ischemic process as seen in midgut volvulus, necrotizing enterocolitis (NEC), internal hernia, or intussusception. Finally, the infant or child with a previous history of abdominal surgery, abdominal surgical scars, or abdominal trauma should be suspected of having adhesive small bowel obstruction.

Radiographic evaluation including AP and left lateral decubitus films of the abdomen is often sufficient to generate an adequate differential diagnosis. These studies help identify the presence of dilated bowel loops and/or intraperitoneal free air. In neonates, several common obstructive lesions such as esophageal atresia, pyloric atresia, and duodenal atresia may show no distention. Adjunctive techniques of gastric tube placement and air instillation may provide an air contrast upper gastrointestinal study in infants with proximal obstructions in which water-soluble or barium contrast instillation could be hazardous or contraindicated due to aspiration risks. Upper gastrointestinal contrast evaluation is indicated to rule out malrotation with midgut volvulus in those patients in whom the suspected level of obstruction is in the mid-duodenum or more distal. The presence of scattered abdominal calcifications in the newborn or a calcified pseudocyst indicates in utero bowel perforation and meconium peritonitis (Fig. 17-31).

Distal gastrointestinal obstructions in the newborn period are most indicative of Hirschsprung disease. Prior to rectal manipulation or examination, these children should undergo a contrast enema. Barium is the preferred contrast medium because of its greater density and improved retention. This is useful for delineating the transition zone on the initial images and retention of material on the postevacuation films. If the transition zone—the region of the bowel where there is a caliber change between proximally dilated and distally decompressed bowel—is not visualized, then consideration should be given to other conditions such as distal ileal atresia, small left colon syndrome, or meconium ileus. Water-soluble contrast may be useful in the latter two conditions by loosening the intraluminal concretions associated with these

entities. Meconium ileus is characterized by distal ileal narrowing and obstruction in association with inspissated meconium plugs ("rabbit pellets") and thick putty-like meconium in the more proximal ileum or bowel (Fig. 17-32). Contrast enema may be both diagnostic and therapeutic. Delayed abdominal radiographs in patients suspected of distal bowel obstructions may provide evidence for Hirschsprung disease.

The different surgical causes of gastrointestinal obstruction are organized by age and the level of obstruction. These have been subdivided into two age categories: neonates and infants to cover the first year of life and toddlers and older children.

Neonates and Infants

A systematic manner in which to subdivide the causes of vomiting is to categorize those with etiologies from the proximal gastrointestinal tract and those from the distal gastrointestinal tract.

Nonbilious Emesis

The most common cause of nonbilious emesis in neonates and infants is overfeeding. Gastroesophageal reflux is the second most common cause of vomiting in this group. This condition is associated with the immaturity of the lower esophageal sphincter mechanisms and delayed motility of the gastrointestinal tract. Age-related maturation of these sites leads to complete resolution of this process by 1 year of age in most children. Behaviors related to feeding including overfeeding, too-rapid feeding, inadequate burping, and infant overstimulation may exacerbate the symptoms.

A group of patients develop complications of their reflux related to esophageal or extraesophageal symptoms. These symptoms include pain, bleeding, dysphagia, and failure to thrive secondary to esophagitis. Recurrent pneumonias, otitis media, hoarseness, respiratory distress, and apneic

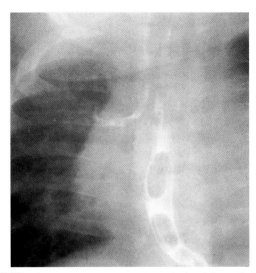

Figure 17-33. Fluoroscopic examination of the infant during barium swallow must be of sufficient duration to allow the identification of episodes of reflux (here associated with aspiration into the tracheobronchial tree).

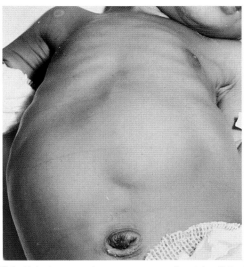

Figure 17-34. Pyloric stenosis may cause epigastric distention by the obstructed stomach. This patient also demonstrates a visible wave of peristalsis, which moves from left to right.

spells may also be related to reflux. Several studies are useful for diagnostic confirmation. Barium swallow with upper gastrointestinal series is quite useful for delineating the anatomy of the esophagus and stomach. It demonstrates pyloric stenosis, malrotation, and the presence of any webs, membranes, or stenoses in these structures. Although this study may show evidence of reflux, it is not a reliable means for the primary diagnosis of reflux (Fig. 17-33). The best methods for diagnosing reflux are esophageal pH probe testing or esophagoscopy with mucosal biopsy. Esophageal pH probe testing is usually performed as an overnight study with a nasoesophageal probe and monitor, which records the frequency and duration of reflux episodes. Distal esophageal mucosal biopsy may represent a more precise diagnostic criterion for clinically significant reflux and may better stratify those patients who would benefit from more aggressive therapies. Liquid-phase gastric radionuclide scintigraphy ("milk scan") may provide evidence of reflux; signal over the lung fields; and quantitative evidence of gastric emptying, an important factor in reflux (see Chapter 16).

Nonoperative and medical strategies are most often adequate to treat patients with reflux. Surgery is primarily reserved for those medically refractory patients with severe complications of reflux disease. The principal strategy of surgery is to strengthen the lower esophageal sphincter mechanism and to repair other associated pathologies that precipitate reflux including hiatal hernia, pylorospasm, or delayed gastric emptying. Fundoplication is the operation of choice and is highly effective at eliminating reflux. The principal side effects are the inability to vomit and a tendency toward the development of postprandial gastric bloating.

Hypertrophic pyloric stenosis is a common surgical condition of the newborn period with an incidence of approximately 1 in every 300 live births in the United States. The etiology is largely unknown. A genetic component to this disease, which occurs rarely in Asians relative to western European populations, is apparent. Furthermore, approximately 20% of the male infants and 7% of the female infants have a relative with pyloric stenosis. Vomiting typically begins during the first or second week of life and becomes progressively projectile. Many babies have undergone changes in formula due to concerns that emesis is formula related. Infants often present during the third week of life for surgical evaluation; however, the presentation may range from 1 week to 4 months of age. Physical examination findings show evidence of a distended abdomen. Peristalsis of the distended stomach may be visible (Fig. 17-34). The lesion itself is usually palpable in the epigastrium, between the midline and the right midclavicular line, and has the consistency of a small olive. An adequate examination requires a calm infant. Various maneuvers to relax the infant's abdominal musculature assist the physical examination. In the absence of a palpable "olive" on two serial examinations by an experienced examiner, the infant should undergo an abdominal ultrasound or upper gastrointestinal series (Fig. 17-35). The presence of a palpable olive requires no further imaging studies before surgery. The infant needs to be adequately hydrated and have any electrolyte abnormalities corrected before going to the operating room (Fig. 17-36).

Bilious Vomiting without Abdominal Distention

Malrotation is the failure of the midgut (small bowel, right colon, and one third of the transverse colon) to undergo adequate rotation and retroperitoneal fixation during embryonic development. Consequently, the bowel resides on a narrow pedicle (superior mesenteric artery) that is prone to undergo twisting and subsequent volvulus formation. The resulting proximal intestinal obstruction usually occurs in the distal duodenum or proximal jejunum presenting as bilious emesis. Abdominal distention may not be a component of the early presentation because of the location of the obstruction at the ligament of Treitz and the decompressive nature of the vomiting. The resulting superior mesenteric artery obstruction leads to midgut ischemia and subsequent infarction, if no surgical intervention occurs. Bloody rectal discharge and hematemesis may also occur as the ischemia time increases. Signs of intestinal necrosis may rapidly manifest as abdominal wall edema, cellulitis, distention, and crepitus. Severe short bowel syndrome or death may occur from delayed recognition, diagnosis, and treatment of this important pediatric condition.

Although most patients who present with bilious emesis do not have malrotation with volvulus, the ramifications of diagnostic delay mandate the prompt evaluation of infants who develop these symptoms (Fig. 17-37). Plain

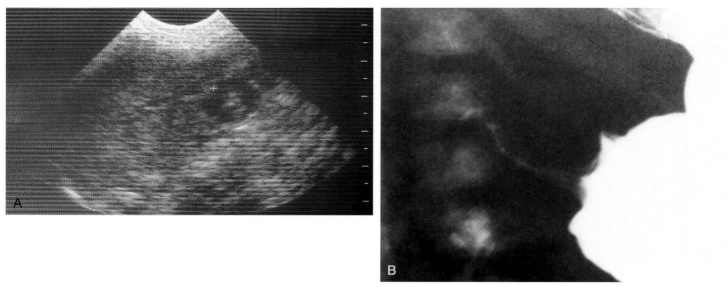

Figure 17-35. Hypertrophic pyloric stenosis. **A,** Ultrasonographic scan of the upper abdomen demonstrates the thickened pyloric muscle, indicated by the cursors. **B,** Barium study of the stomach *(right)* shows thin streaks of barium in the pyloric canal. The hypertrophic pyloric muscle bulged into the gastric antrum produces a "reversed 3" configuration.

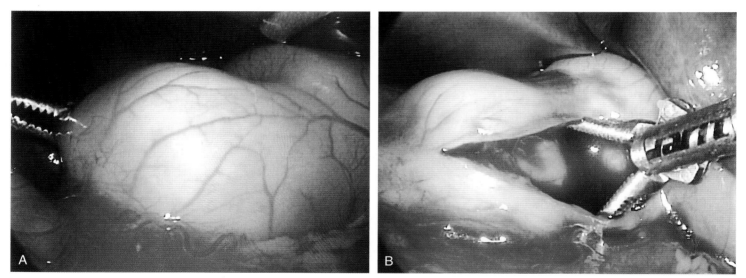

Figure 17-36. Laparoscopic view of pyloric stenosis viewing the hypertrophied pylorus **(A)** and pyloromyotomy, demonstrating the serosal incision **(B).**

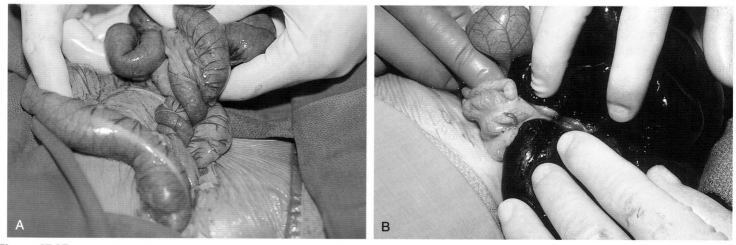

Figure 17-37. Malrotation with midgut volvulus without ischemia **(A).** Malrotation predisposes to volvulus and complete midgut infarction **(B).**

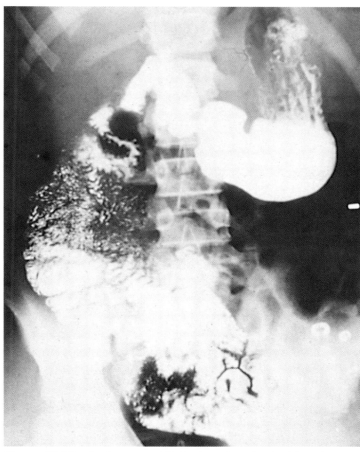

Figure 17-38. The ligament of Treitz in malrotation is either absent or abnormally located, and the duodenum and small intestine lie on the right side of the abdomen. Duodenal obstruction may be partial (caused by Ladd bands, as seen here) or complete (caused by volvulus).

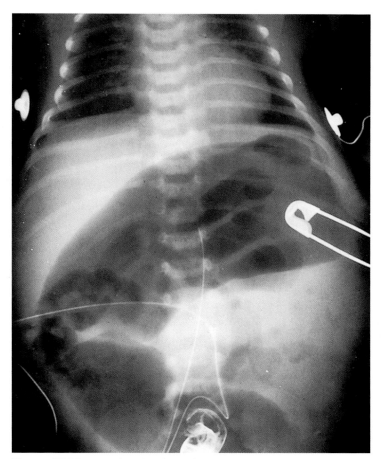

Figure 17-39. Complete duodenal obstruction from midgut volvulus. Air in the distal gastrointestinal tract fails to rule out complete obstruction from volvulus and distinguishes the diagnosis from duodenal atresia.

radiographs demonstrating gastric distention and duodenal dilatation in the setting of an otherwise nearly "gasless abdomen" should raise suspicions for this condition. The cornerstone of diagnosis is the upper gastrointestinal series, which identifies the contour of the duodenal sweep or C-loop, the location of the ligament of Treitz, and the unobstructed flow of contrast into the jejunum. The most critical of these is the position of the ligament of Treitz, which should be positioned to the left of midline on the AP view and above the level of the pylorus on the oblique view. An abnormally configured duodenal C-loop or a corkscrew appearance to the duodenum with small bowel loops positioned in the right side of the abdomen is diagnostic of disease (Fig. 17-38). Other findings on the upper gastrointestinal series such as duodenal dilatation imply obstruction from volvulus or Ladd bands (Fig. 17-39). Barium enema may demonstrate an abnormally placed cecum in the left upper abdomen; it is not an effective diagnostic tool in the acute setting.

Duodenal atresia and duodenal anomalies are important diagnostic considerations in the patient who presents with bilious emesis. Vomiting may occur shortly after birth or at a later time in the setting of annular pancreas, duodenal stenosis, and duodenal webs. Duodenal atresia is associated with Down syndrome and congenital heart disease in about 30% to 50% of patients. The radiographic appearance of a "double bubble" sign in the newborn is pathognomonic of duodenal obstruction usually secondary to duodenal atresia (Fig. 17-40). Malrotation without volvulus may be a source of bilious emesis secondary to Ladd bands (lateral peritoneal duodenal attachments), which may partially obstruct the duodenum.

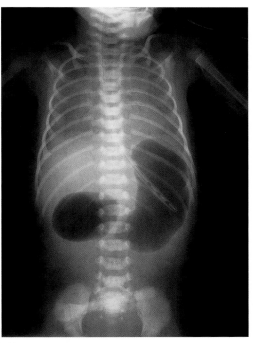

Figure 17-40. Swallowed air distends the stomach and proximal duodenum in duodenal atresia, producing the characteristic "double bubble" on plain film. Other contrast studies are unnecessary.

Bilious Vomiting with Abdominal Distention

Small bowel and colonic atresias are the sequelae of intrauterine vascular accidents. These are often late gestational events, and meconium may be present in the bowel distal to the atresia. Therefore early postnatal meconium passage does not rule out a coexisting atresia. Proximal

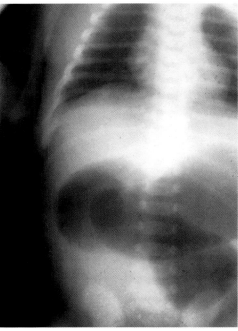

Figure 17-41. Jejunal atresia distends only a few bowel loops proximally, distinguishing it from duodenal and ileal atresia.

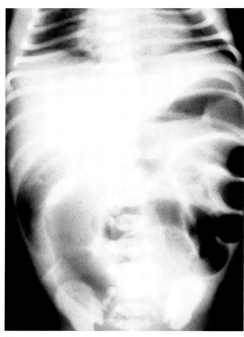

Figure 17-42. Many intestinal loops become distended in patients with ileal atresia (pictured here), making the distinction between this diagnosis and other causes of distal bowel obstruction difficult. Other signs (such as intraperitoneal calcification, indicating meconium peritonitis) and contrast enema are necessary to identify the cause of obstruction.

intestinal atresias are associated with abdominal distention with only a few dilated bowel loops on plain film (Fig. 17-41), whereas distal ileal and colonic atresias are characterized as having multiple dilated bowel loops (Fig. 17-42). The presence of a proximal bowel obstruction in the neonatal period requires no other diagnostic imaging studies before definitive surgery. Contrast studies are critical to differentiate ileal atresia from various other distal obstructions including Hirschsprung disease, meconium ileus, and small left colon syndrome.

Jejunoileal (small bowel) atresias are often isolated conditions, although they may be associated with gastroschisis and meconium disease. The major anatomic variants

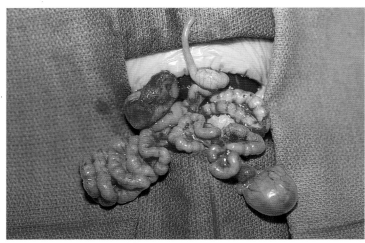

Figure 17-43. "Christmas tree" deformity results in proximal jejunoileal atresia secondary to an absent superior mesenteric artery beyond the middle colic branch. The helical appearance of the bowel around the remaining colic vessels gives the characteristic appearance.

are subdivided on the basis of whether the bowel and its mesentery are intact. The "Christmas tree" or "apple peel" deformity (type IIIb), named for the spiral appearance of the distal bowel around the ileocolic or right colic artery, may result in significant bowel loss (Fig. 17-43). Similarly, multiple atresias or the "string of sausages" defect (type IV) may involve an extensive amount of the jejunoileum, leaving little functional mucosal absorptive area. These two conditions put most infants at significant risk of developing short bowel syndrome and long-term, if not permanent, total parenteral nutrition (TPN) dependence.

Meconium disease is the initial presentation of cystic fibrosis in up to 20% of children. The thick viscous meconium in the distal bowel precipitates intraluminal intestinal obstruction. The distal ileum is small, and a microcolon is usually present. Marked proximal jejunoileal dilatation occurs, as does a "soap bubble" appearance of the abdomen on plain radiography (Fig. 17-44). Air-fluid levels are uncommon in this form of intestinal obstruction due to the dense concentration of meconium in the intestinal loops. Contrast enema reveals the presence of a microcolon and inspissated mucus or "rabbit pellets" in the distal ileum. Reflux of contrast proximal to these pellets into dilated bowel may be therapeutic, inducing evacuation of the thick meconium and relief of the obstruction. Occasionally, patients with meconium disease may develop an intestinal atresia, volvulus, or perforation with varying amounts of meconium peritonitis. These conditions are referred to as complicated meconium ileus and, unlike simple meconium ileus, they always require surgical intervention (Fig. 17-45). Evidence of complicated meconium ileus may be made on prenatal diagnosis or neonatal plain films by the presence of peritoneal calcifications and ascites. Unsuccessful attempts at contrast reduction of meconium ileus should raise the concern for an associated ileal atresia.

Hirschsprung disease, the absence of ganglion cells in the distal rectum, is a common cause of bilious emesis and abdominal distention. Although the classic presentation is that of failure to pass meconium, distal rectal obstruction may also induce vomiting. Plain radiographs of the abdomen in most patients demonstrate marked bowel dilatation. Barium enema studies show proximally dilated bowel (normal) and a nondilated segment (transition zone) juxtaposed to a distal decompressed segment of rectum (Fig. 17-46). Barium study, as outlined earlier, should precede rectal manipulation or enemas, as they

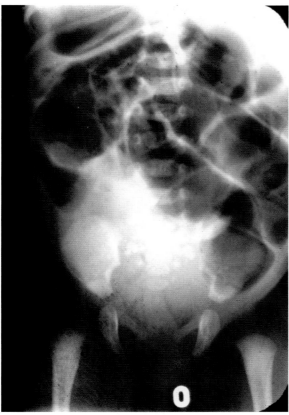

Figure 17-44. Meconium ileus presents as a distal small bowel obstruction in the newborn with few air-filled dilated loops due to the meconium-filled bowel loops.

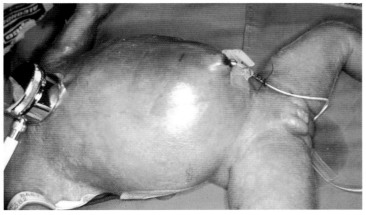

Figure 17-45. Intense inflammation resulting from free meconium in the peritoneal cavity (meconium peritonitis) may produce visible erythema and edema over the abdominal wall.

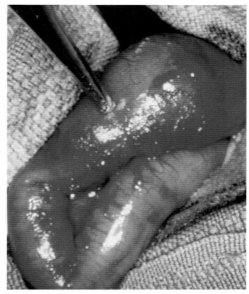

Figure 17-46. The absence of intramural ganglion cells prevents intestinal peristalsis through segments affected by Hirschsprung disease, causing a functional bowel obstruction. The involved segment appears narrow when compared with the distended, obstructed proximal bowel, which possesses normal ganglion cells.

may distort the radiographic findings typical of the transition zone and confuse the diagnosis. Suction rectal biopsy performed at the bedside without the need for anesthesia is diagnostic (Fig. 17-47).

Some children escape diagnosis in the first few days or months of life but are plagued by chronic constipation requiring rectal stimulation to evacuate. They may develop chronic symptoms of abdominal distention, growth failure, and constipation. These patients may also present with an acute life-threatening episode of Hirschsprung-related enterocolitis. These infants or young children develop severe explosive diarrhea, toxic megacolon, and systemic sepsis that may rapidly progress to death. Emergent laparotomy for bowel decompression is mandated (Fig. 17-48). Therapeutic delays secondary to attempts to perform preoperative suction rectal biopsy should be

avoided, due to the high attendant morbidity and mortality of this presentation.

Older Infants and Children

Age-specific considerations for the causes of vomiting should direct the diagnostic approaches for children outside of the neonatal and infancy period. Intussusception is a frequent cause of vomiting in toddlers from 6 months to 2 years of age. The etiology of this condition is idiopathic in the majority of children in this age group; however, the presence of mechanical lead points are more common in older children. These lead points include Meckel diverticula, intestinal polyps, Burkitt or non-Hodgkin lymphoma, intestinal duplication cysts, and seromuscular hematomas secondary to bleeding disorders such as hemophilia or Henoch-Schönlein purpura. Idiopathic intussusception occurs in the region of the distal ileum and ascending colon. The classic clinical presentation is that of an otherwise healthy infant who presents with paroxysmal bouts of severe colicky abdominal pain associated with drawing his or her legs to the chest followed by a period of sedation or somnolence. The presentation of this disease may be variable, however. Some children present with unexplained lethargy or seizure-like episodes, causing practitioners to suspect and work up potential neurologic diagnoses such as brain tumors and meningitis. Vomiting or the passage of a bowel movement may be associated with relief of these episodes. The child then resumes his or her typical behavior until another episode occurs. Initially vomiting episodes are nonbilious and likely related to a reflex response mediated by central nervous system mechanisms related to mesenteric traction. As time progresses, the bowel obstruction becomes more complete and the vomiting episodes may become progressively more bilious in nature. Bowel ischemia is typically a late finding in these cases (Fig. 17-49). Most infants are so violently ill that they are brought to medical attention earlier in their course. Mucosal sloughing may occur in the setting of bowel ischemia, producing "currant jelly" stools (Fig. 17-50). Physical examination findings may be notable for a palpable

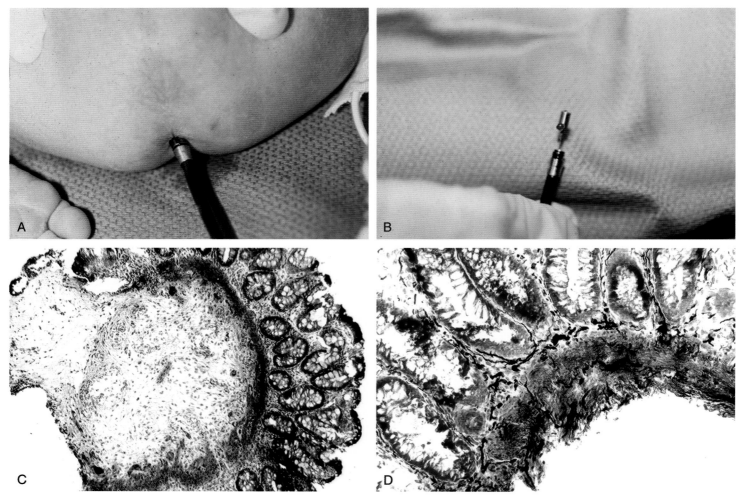

Figure 17-47. Suction rectal biopsy is a bedside procedure **(A)** that provides a small fragment of tissue for pathologic evaluation for ganglion cells **(B).** A normal suction rectal biopsy with an acetylcholinesterase stain demonstrates a normal band of staining and no giant nerve fibers between the muscular layers **(C).** Higher power view of a biopsy from a patient with Hirschsprung disease shows darkly staining giant nerve fibers in the muscularis layer (acetylcholinesterase stain) **(D).** (**C** and **D,** Courtesy Paul S. Dickman, MD, and Dan Galvis, BS.)

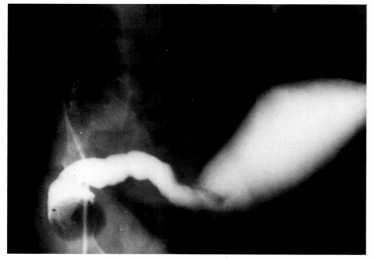

Figure 17-48. Barium enema outlines the transition zone between the contracted (aganglionic) rectosigmoid lying distal to the obstructed, but normally innervated, colon. To demonstrate this sign, the examination must be conducted in an unprepped patient who has undergone neither enemas nor digital rectal examination.

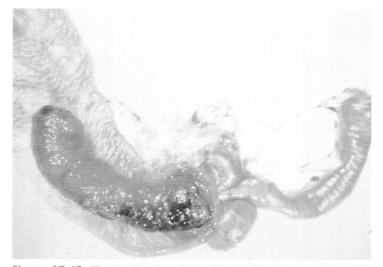

Figure 17-49. The intestine invaginates into itself in intussusception. The ileum is pulled through the ileocecal valve into the colon, the most common pattern seen in infancy, pictured here.

"sausage-shaped" mass located in the right upper quadrant or epigastrium. Consequently, the right lower quadrant may be empty (Dance sign).

The radiographic assessment of intussusception is initially performed with plain films, which in many instances

are not helpful. An intussusceptum visualized as a soft tissue cutoff sign or meniscus in the upper or mid abdomen is diagnostic (Fig. 17-51). Newer techniques using abdominal ultrasonography may have greater sensitivity and specificity than plain radiography. Contrast enema with either barium or air (preferred) may be both diagnostic

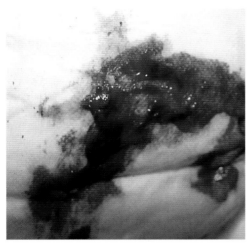

Figure 17-50. The intussusception—the invaginated portion of bowel—becomes congested and ischemic, leading to the passage of bloody stool mixed with mucus (currant jelly stool).

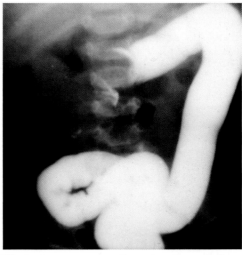

Figure 17-52. Barium enema confirms the diagnosis by outlining the intussusceptum. The column of contrast can then be used to push the invaginated bowel proximally. Free reflux of contrast into the bowel proximally signals complete reduction of the intussusception.

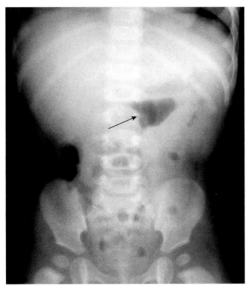

Figure 17-51. In some cases the intussusceptum can be seen as a meniscus-shaped mass outlined by air in the colon.

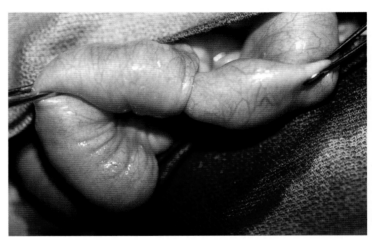

Figure 17-53. Small bowel intussusception typically has a lead point except in patients with postoperative intussusception as shown here. Upper gastrointestinal studies should be avoided in these patients secondary to aspiration risks.

and therapeutic (Fig. 17-52). Successful reduction is indicated by the prompt and free passage of barium or air into dilated loops of small bowel proximal to the obstruction. The inability to achieve this objective is indicative of a persistent obstruction either secondary to an incompletely reduced intussusception or a second site of intussusception. These techniques have a low incidence of failure (<10%). Those patients with an incomplete or failed reduction require emergent exploration and manual reduction or resection.

Intussusception may recur within the first 12 to 24 hours following radiographic reduction. Patients with recurrent symptoms should return promptly to the radiographic suite for repeat reduction attempts. Ileoileal or jejunoileal (small bowel) intussusceptions are generally too proximal to be amenable to radiographic reduction and typically are often due to mechanical lead points and require surgery. Postoperative intussusceptions are also small bowel in location and require operative reduction (Fig. 17-53). Controversy exists in regard to the older child who presents with intussusception. Due to the high frequency of surgical lead points, many favor only diagnostic and nontherapeutic contrast enemas. This is followed by surgical exploration and possible bowel resection.

Internal hernias around postoperative adhesions, amniotic bands, or omphalomesenteric (vitelline) remnants may produce intestinal obstruction. The most common cause of intestinal obstruction is related to adhesions from previous surgery or abdominal trauma. Often, early preemptive nasogastric decompression may alleviate the symptoms and halt the progression to complete obstruction. Failure of early resolution of the obstruction should prompt emergent exploration. Omphalomesenteric duct remnants, or vitelline bands, may attach to the umbilicus or mesentery producing a potential site of internal bowel herniation (Fig. 17-54). Rotational anomalies may leave spaces lateral to the duodenum, cecum, and sigmoid colon, giving rise to potential sites of bowel incarceration known as *paraduodenal* or *paracolic hernias*.

Gastrointestinal Bleeding

The evaluation of an infant or child with bleeding from the gastrointestinal tract involves a careful assessment of several important factors and the establishment of a management protocol (Table 17-2). Initially the practitioner must determine whether the episode of bleeding is hemodynamically significant. The next step in the evaluation is to confirm that what appears to be blood is truly blood. Subsequently, the physician should obtain a general idea of the location of blood loss (i.e., upper versus lower gas-

trointestinal tract) (Table 17-3). Those patients in acute or impending hypovolemic shock require urgent stabilization coincident with diagnostic studies. In cases of more chronic or subacute blood loss, symptoms of anemia, fatigue, and pallor are more common. A thorough history and physical examination in conjunction with serologic, radiologic, and endoscopic studies are critical to ascertain the etiology of the bleeding. The duration, severity (amount), and location of the episode of bleeding are among the most important historical factors. Drug ingestion, exposure to sick contacts, inherited coagulopathies, vitamin deficiencies, or a family history of chronic intestinal disorders may shed further light on the source of bleeding. Severe acute blood loss may be associated with both upper (hematemesis) and lower (hematochezia or melena) bleeding.

Infants

Swallowed maternal blood is a common source of bleeding in the newborn. Most infants have normal vital signs and stable hematocrits. The Apt-Downey test differentiates between maternal and fetal blood in the newborn. The mixture of 1 volume of gastric aspirate and 4 parts of water is centrifuged. The supernatant is removed and mixed in a 4 : 1 ratio with 1% sodium hydroxide. If the fluid remains pink, the blood has fetal hemoglobin; alternatively, if the mixture turns brown, the blood is from a maternal source. Hemorrhagic diseases of the newborn may lead to profound upper gastrointestinal bleeding, especially in those infants who fail to receive their perinatal vitamin K injection. This is a rare occurrence due to strict delivery room protocols; however, infants who are unstable or urgently transferred from the delivery room to other institutions may be at greatest risk. Hence the delivery room records should be examined in all newborns who present with upper gastrointestinal bleeding. Nasogastric tube placement or oropharyngeal suctioning shortly after birth may precipitate bleeding that enters the stomach and results in bloody emesis. This typically clears with gastric lavage. Anal fissures are a more benign cause of anorectal bleeding in infants. This may be associated with constipation, hard stools, and anal stenosis (Fig. 17-55).

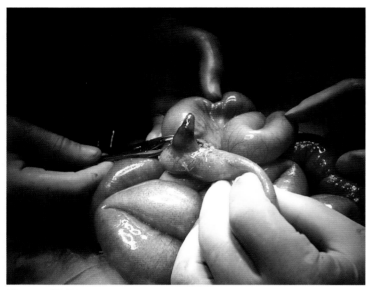

Figure 17-54. Omphalomesenteric remnants, also known as vitelline bands, may produce internal hernias that lead to obstruction.

Table 17-2	Common Causes of Gastrointestinal Hemorrhage

PATIENTS YOUNGER THAN 1 YEAR	PATIENTS OLDER THAN 1 YEAR
Upper	
Gastritis	Peptic ulcer
Swallowed maternal blood	Varices
Peptic ulcer (duodenal and gastric)	
Malrotation and volvulus	
Lower	
Anal fissure	Colonic polyps
Intussusception	Intussusception
Necrotizing enterocolitis	Meckel diverticulum
Meckel diverticulum	Infectious diarrhea
Malrotation and volvulus	Inflammatory bowel disease

Table 17-3	Causes of Gastrointestinal Bleeding

LOCATION	APPEARANCE	AGE		
		Newborn	*Infant*	*Child*
Upper	Well	Maternal blood	Nosebleeds	Nosebleeds
		Nasogastric tube	Nasogastric tube	Nasogastric tube
		Pyloric stenosis	Esophagitis	
		Esophagitis		
	Ill	Peptic ulcer disease	Varices	Varices
		Necrotizing enterocolitis	Peptic ulcer disease	Peptic ulcer disease
		Volvulus	Medications	Medications
Lower	Well	Anal fissure	Anal fissure	Anal fissure
		Maternal blood	Meckel diverticulum	Juvenile polyp
		Hemangioma	Duplication	Meckel diverticulum
		Duplication		Rectal prolapse
	Ill	Necrotizing enterocolitis	Intussusception	Infectious diarrhea
		Volvulus	Infectious diarrhea	Intussusception
		Infectious diarrhea	Medications	Trauma
			Henoch-Schönlein purpura	Medications
			Hemolytic uremic syndrome	Hemolytic uremic syndrome
				Henoch-Schönlein purpura
				Inflammatory bowel disease

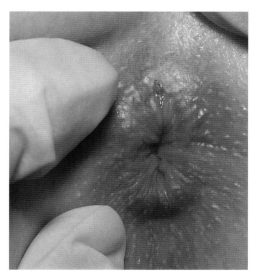

Figure 17-55. Small tears in the anoderm may bleed, producing small amounts of blood in the stool of healthy infants.

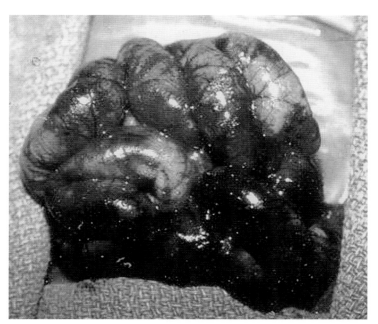

Figure 17-57. Diffuse necrotizing enterocolitis is associated with a patchy distribution of necrosis on the serosal surface of the bowel.

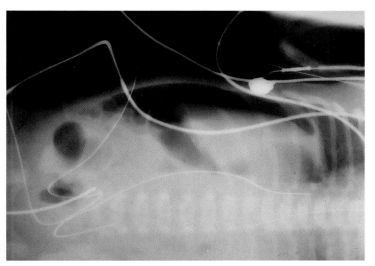

Figure 17-56. The large quantity of free air within the abdomen resulting from a gastric perforation (shown here outlining the edge of the liver) suggests its source.

Severe acute gastritis or gastric ulceration may occur in the newborn period and is associated with high morbidity and mortality. These infants often present with hypovolemic shock and free intraperitoneal air (Fig. 17-56). This typically occurs during the first 7 to 10 days of life. Malrotation with midgut volvulus may also present with severe upper gastrointestinal bleeding either secondary to bowel ischemia or sepsis-induced coagulopathy.

Necrotizing enterocolitis (NEC) is the most common abdominal surgical emergency of the newborn period. Although classically an inflammatory condition that presents with abdominal distention, NEC may also precipitate upper or lower gastrointestinal bleeding. Predominantly a condition of premature infants, nearly 15% of cases occur in term infants. The major risk factors in this group include sepsis, low birthweight, congenital heart disease, hyperviscosity syndromes, pulmonary insufficiency, drugs (indomethacin and methylxanthines), and maternal cocaine use. A variant may affect the entire small bowel. The associated pannecrosis of the small bowel is often referred to as "leopard skin" due to the patchy distribution of necrosis (Fig. 17-57). Numerous etiologic factors have been attributed to the onset of this

condition; however, none of them has been solely implicated in the onset of NEC. The patients may have vague symptoms including abdominal distention, vomiting, increased gastric residuals, and bloody stools. Constitutional symptoms consisting of temperature lability, apnea, and bradycardia, as well as inactivity, are quite common.

On physical examination patients often appear toxic with signs of abdominal distention, edema, and erythema. Apneic and bradycardiac episodes are common. Laboratory values may show neutropenia or leukocytosis, anemia, and metabolic acidosis. Plain radiographs demonstrate pneumatosis intestinalis, the pathognomonic hallmark of the disease. This radiographic finding suggests the subserosal dissection of air and may be linear or cystic (Fig. 17-58). Occasionally portal vein gas may be seen, but this may be evanescent. Small, localized collections of air or large amounts of free air that outline the falciform ligament are signs of free intraperitoneal perforation. Pneumoperitoneum, best visualized on the left lateral decubitus film, is an absolute indication for immediate surgical intervention. In general NEC is managed nonoperatively with intravenous hydration, parenteral antibiotics, nasogastric tube decompression, and suspension of feedings. In addition to perforation, deteriorating clinical status is the other major acute indication for surgery. Despite uneventful recovery from the initial acute-phase disease, some patients develop symptomatic strictures, which require surgical resection (Fig. 17-59).

Toddlers (1 to 5 Years)

Painless rectal bleeding in the toddler should raise concern for the presence of a Meckel diverticulum. Often the bleeding is massive with significant drops in the hematocrit requiring blood transfusion. The initial blood loss is variable and may present as a sentinel bleed that spontaneously resolves, followed by more massive bright red or maroon blood per rectum. Although spontaneous resolution may occur, subsequent episodes of bleeding may be life threatening. The bleeding results from the ulceration of the ileal mucosa located adjacent to the

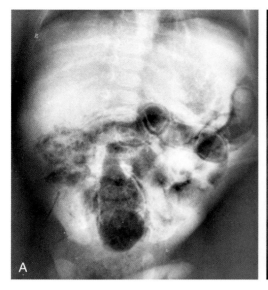

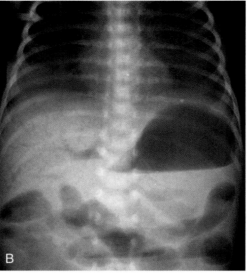

Figure 17-58. Pneumatosis intestinalis is seen most easily as linear streaks of air outlining the bowel and producing concentric rings when viewed on end. More common, however, is the bubbly pattern seen in the right iliac fossa in this patient, appearing like stool within the lumen **(A)**. In severely affected infants, gas may fill the portal system and produce visible streaks of air on abdominal plain film **(B)**.

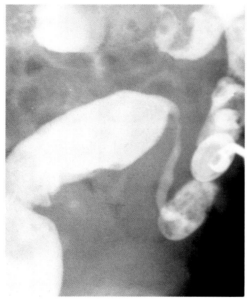

Figure 17-59. In a patient who develops intestinal obstruction during recovery from necrotizing enterocolitis, a colonic stricture must be suspected.

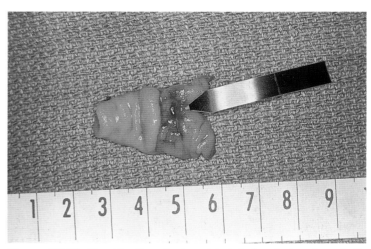

Figure 17-60. The bleeding site in a Meckel diverticulum is typically located on the mucosa of bowel adjacent to the ectopic gastric tissue.

ectopic gastric mucosa present at the base of the Meckel diverticulum (Fig. 17-60). A technetium-99m pertechnetate isotope scan, Meckel scan, identifies gastric mucosa and may be helpful in the diagnosis of disease (Fig. 17-61). During active bleeding the scan may be positive in 85% of patients. False-negative evaluations are common. The use of intravenous pentagastrin or cimetidine may improve the sensitivity of the study. Contrast studies of the distal small bowel (enteroclysis) or colon (barium enema) are of marginal diagnostic utility in this setting and may obscure the scan. Some children must undergo exploratory laparotomy or diagnostic laparoscopy (Fig. 17-62) to identify the presence of the diverticulum due to the presence of negative studies. Meckel diverticulum may present with obstruction (secondary to volvulus or internal hernia or intussusception) or acute inflammation (diverticulitis) similar to appendicitis.

Esophageal varices are a common source of massive upper gastrointestinal bleeding in children with portal hypertension. Other causes of portal hypertension in children include the presence of extrahepatic portal vein

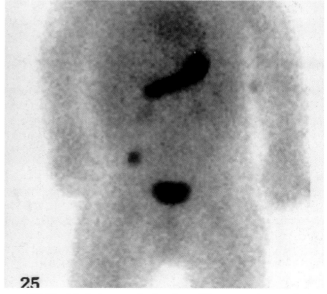

Figure 17-61. Meckel scan (technetium-99m pertechnetate) demonstrates a positive uptake in the right lower abdomen.

thrombosis or hepatic cirrhosis. Omphalitis, a complication of umbilical venous catheterization in newborns, may precipitate portal vein thrombosis. Children with short bowel syndrome or other chronic intestinal disorders such as intestinal pseudo-obstruction (Fig. 17-63) or microvillus inclusion disease may require chronic parenteral nutrition, which may induce TPN-related liver disease and hepatic failure. One third of patients who undergo a Kasai procedure (portoenterostomy) for biliary atresia develop progressive cirrhosis that leads to variceal bleeding secondary to portal hypertension. Cystic fibrosis, a_1-antitrypsin deficiency, and viral hepatitis are a few of the other common conditions that may induce a portal hypertension in children. Upper gastrointestinal endoscopy allows for direct visualization of the varices in cases of active bleeding and assists therapeutic banding or sclerosant techniques. Occasionally, angiography is useful to visualize the anatomy of the portal venous system and its branches. The advent of transjugular intracaval portosystemic shunting has almost eliminated the need for emergent surgical intervention in acutely bleeding esophageal varices.

Vasculitic conditions such as Henoch-Schönlein purpura (HSP) may be a source of lower gastrointestinal bleeding in children. Typically HSP occurs during the postinfectious stage of a major viral or streptococcal illness. Arthralgias and a macular purpuric skin rash in the lower extremities are characteristic of this entity. In both of these presentations, patients may develop intussusception due to the evolution of a subserosal mucosal hematoma, which functions as a lead point (Fig. 17-64). The presence of acute renal insufficiency, anemia, pain, and bloody diarrhea are suggestive of hemolytic uremic syndrome.

The triad of azotemia, anemia, and thrombocytopenia confirms the diagnosis. If a coexistent dysentery-like illness is present, then the pathogen should be determined by stool culture or analysis.

Older Children

Benign hamartomatous juvenile polyps most frequently affect children between 2 and 8 years of age. The incidence is approximately 1 in 1000 children. Bleeding is usually painless, low in volume, and found as streaks on the surface of the stool. Two thirds of the bleeding problems are found in the rectum, and 90% are found distal to the sigmoid colon. Many of these lesions undergo autonecrosis and slough into the stool, whereas others may prolapse through the anus (Fig. 17-65). Surgical or endoscopic resection is therapeutic. Patients with Peutz-Jeghers syndrome present with melanotic mucocutaneous pigmentation (Fig. 17-66) and gastrointestinal bleeding due to hamartomatous polyps (Fig. 17-67). These polyps may also cause recurrent episodes of abdominal pain and obstruction. Although most of these polyps are single and rarely present in numbers of more than 12, a life-threatening variant of this condition, diffuse juvenile polyposis, may present with severe bloody diarrhea, intussusception, rectal prolapse, and protein-losing enteropathy. Total abdominal colectomy is required in these patients.

In contrast with hamartomatous polyps, adenomatous polyps are quite rare as solitary colonic lesions. Children with familial adenomatous polyposis are usually asymptomatic until puberty or late adolescence, when they may develop diarrhea, hematochezia, and anemia. Diffuse adenomatous polyps blanket the colon and may have associated lesions throughout the intestinal tract from stomach to terminal ileum (Fig. 17-68). Surgery is frequently recommended to control recurrent bleeding and failure to thrive and to decrease the long-term high risk of malignancy in these patients.

Abdominal Pain

The most common surgical emergency of childhood is acute appendicitis. The pathogenesis arises from appendiceal obstruction usually secondary to hyperplasia of sub-

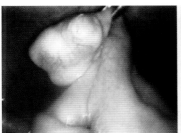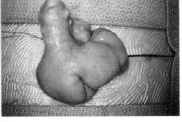

A   B

Figure 17-62. Laparoscopic view of a Meckel diverticulum with an apparent vitelline artery **(A).** Meckel diverticulum at surgery **(B).**

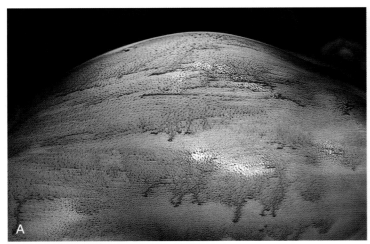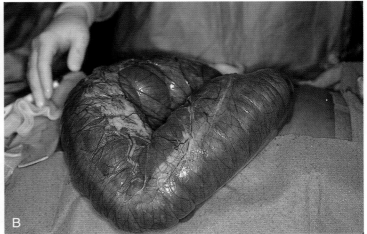

Figure 17-63. Massive abdominal distention **(A)** and colonic dilatation seen in intestinal pseudo-obstruction may mimic dilatation seen with mechanical obstruction or Hirschsprung disease **(B).**

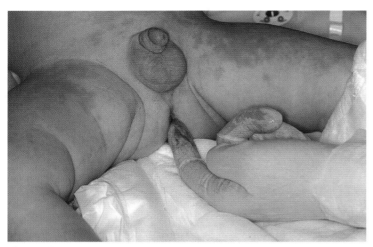

Figure 17-64. Henoch-Schönlein purpura causes submucosal and serosal hematomas that may act as a lead point. Note the presence of hematochezia and the diagnostic skin lesions.

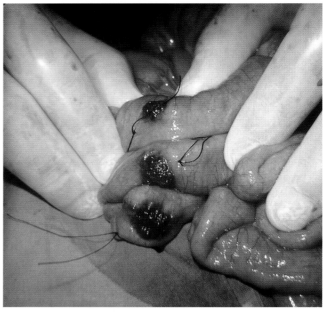

Figure 17-67. Melanotic small bowel polyps characteristic of Peutz-Jeghers syndrome are prone to bleeding or obstruction.

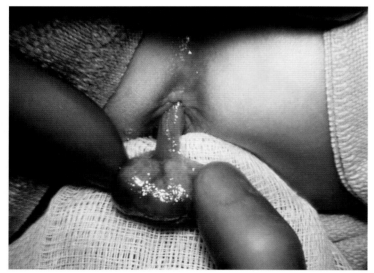

Figure 17-65. Juvenile polyps are found most often in the rectosigmoid colon. On occasion they may prolapse through the anus.

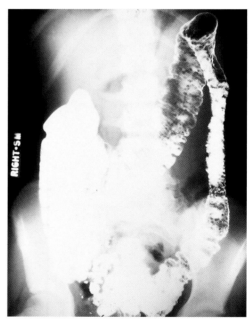

Figure 17-68. Familial adenomatous polyposis. A barium enema study demonstrates multiple small polyps throughout the colon.

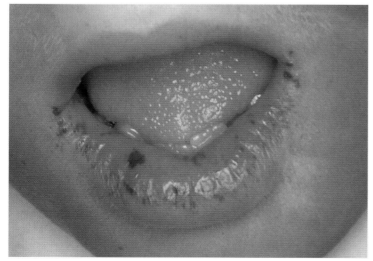

Figure 17-66. The characteristic melanotic spots of Peutz-Jeghers syndrome are seen on the lips, buccal mucosa, and anus.

mucosal lymphoid tissue or a fecalith. The subsequent development of appendiceal edema, ischemia, gangrene, and ultimately perforation will occur with the passage of time (Fig. 17-69). Despite the classic description of pain originating in the periumbilical region that progressively localizes to the right lower quadrant, the manifestations of appendicitis in childhood are protean. Although the symptom complex typically includes abdominal pain, low-grade fever, and anorexia, some children, particularly those with a retrocecal appendix, have few symptoms and may present days to weeks after their initial episode of appendicitis. These children may present with a localized abscess due to previous perforation and localization by host defense mechanisms. Physical examination findings in most pediatric patients demonstrate tenderness in the right lower quadrant, suprapubic, or lower flank regions

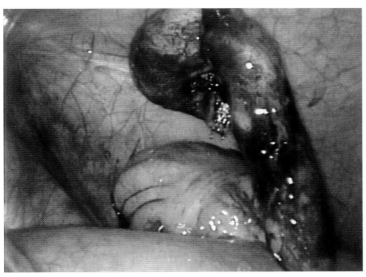

Figure 17-69. Laparoscopic view of appendicitis. Note the inflamed, swollen appendix.

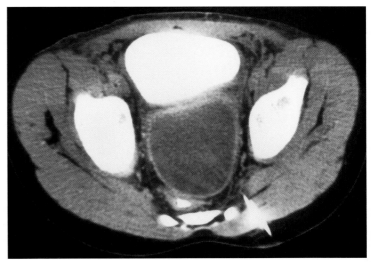

Figure 17-71. Perforated appendicitis with abscess seen on CT scan.

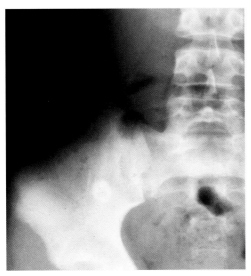

Figure 17-70. A fecalith, the round calcification in the iliac fossa, obstructs the appendiceal lumen and initiates inflammatory processes that produce appendicitis.

that persists or worsens despite hydration and cautious observation. Children with appendicitis are often found lying quietly in bed with their legs flexed at the hips resisting abdominal palpation. Maneuvers such as coughing, heel-tap, jumping, or even walking may exacerbate the symptoms and are suggestive of peritoneal irritation. Involuntary guarding or muscular spasm overlying the area of peritoneal irritation is a common examination finding that is not masked by mild forms of sedation. A positive psoas or obturator sign is indicative of retroperitoneal appendicitis, which may be associated with few anterior abdominal findings. In general the routine use of plain abdominal films is unnecessary in the evaluation of the child with abdominal pain. However, the presence of a fecalith in a child with abdominal pain warrants appendectomy (Fig. 17-70). Children with fecaliths in the absence of abdominal pain do not need surgery and should be followed. Operative intervention is indicated at this point to avoid progression to perforation.

Perforation occurs due to diagnostic delay that may be related to the nonclassical presentation of acute appendicitis. Symptoms may be confused with gastroenteritis or other nonsurgical intestinal illnesses. Perforation leads to either free peritoneal soilage or the development of a localized abscess (Fig. 17-71). Initially, perforation may be associated with the relief of symptoms, which is usually followed by diffuse abdominal tenderness, distention, and rigidity. Patients often appear quite toxic. Alternatively, isolation of the inflammatory process by the omentum and adjacent bowel loops may lead to abscess formation. Patients with localization may appear surprisingly well. Perforation associated with diffuse peritoneal soilage requires surgical exploration for drainage and appendectomy. Localized perforation may be initially managed by the use of intravenous antibiotics with or without percutaneous drainage followed by an interval appendectomy at approximately 6 to 8 weeks following the original presentation. This management approach is associated with fewer perioperative complications and improved outcomes.

Acute appendicitis in the preschool-aged child is a clinical challenge for even the most experienced practitioner. Acute abdominal pain is a common presentation of other conditions including otitis media, pneumonia, urinary tract infections, diabetes, sickle cell disease, vasculitis, or enteritis (bacterial or viral). The difficulties in obtaining a history in this age group, the poor understanding of time, and the challenges of obtaining a reliable physical examination may all contribute to the diagnostic delay. The incidence of perforation exceeds 50%. Unlike older children, these preschoolers seldom wall off their perforation and commonly present with severe peritonitis requiring urgent operative intervention.

The differential diagnosis for appendicitis includes several nonsurgical problems such as gastroenteritis, mesenteric adenitis, constipation, and urinary tract infections, as well as surgical conditions such as Meckel diverticulitis, inflammatory bowel disease (particularly Crohn disease) (Fig. 17-72), and intussusception. Pelvic pathology including ovarian cysts, ovarian torsion (Fig. 17-73), or acute salpingitis with or without associated tubo-ovarian abscess may be readily confused with acute appendicitis, making the negative appendectomy rate much higher in girls than boys. Advancements in radiographic imaging techniques and the increased use of laparoscopy have helped with improving diagnostic accuracy. Cystic ovarian masses represent a wide spectrum of conditions from the simple follicular cyst (see Fig. 17-73) to hormonally active cystic tumors (Fig. 17-74). Large ovarian cysts (>5 cm)

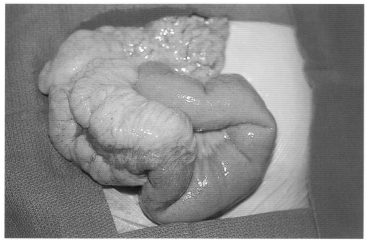

Figure 17-72. Findings at laparotomy in Crohn disease reveal petechiae over the serosa of thickened small bowel, which has mesenteric "creeping fat."

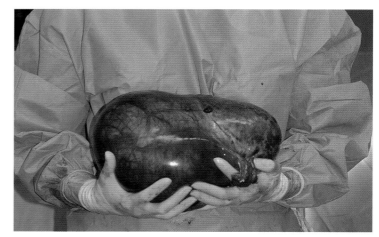

Figure 17-74. A large cystic ovarian tumor removed from a teenage girl with a slowly increasing abdominal girth.

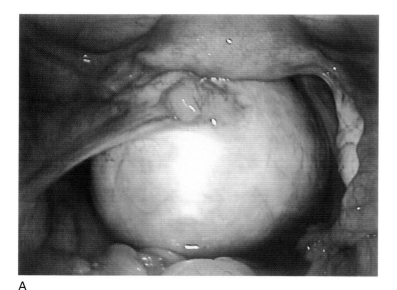

A

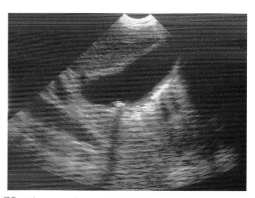

Figure 17-75. Ultrasound examination of the right upper quadrant easily demonstrates stones within the gallbladder. An acoustic shadow extends beneath the stone.

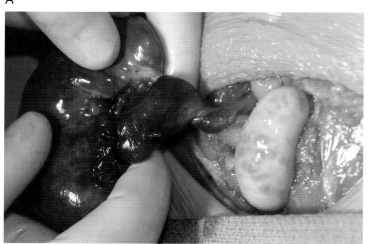

B

Figure 17-73. **A,** Simple follicular cysts may grow to very large sizes that may fill the cul-de-sac. **B,** Ovarian torsion.

that persist for more than 2 to 4 weeks should undergo ultrasonographic-guided aspiration or laparoscopic fenestration due to their risk of undergoing torsion (Fig. 17-75). Ovarian torsion classically presents with pain out of proportion to the physical examination findings, and typically these patients lack significant gastrointestinal symptoms. Other pelvic masses related to uterine congenital pathology may be a source of abdominal pain (see earlier discussion).

Less common causes of abdominal pain in childhood include symptomatic biliary tract disease related to gallstones or choledochal cyst. Children who have a history of hemoglobinopathy (sickle cell disease), chronic hemolysis (spherocytosis), or strong family incidence of cholelithiasis and who develop colicky right upper quadrant discomfort, epigastric pain, unexplained jaundice, or pancreatitis should undergo ultrasound evaluation for the presence of cholecystitis, cholelithiasis, choledocholithiasis, and pancreatitis (Fig. 17-76). Choledochal cyst is a congenital condition, more common in young girls than boys, that typically presents around 4 years of age with fusiform to cystic dilatation of the common bile duct. Pain from common duct obstruction or acute pancreatitis may be the initial presenting symptom. Surgical excision of the abnormal common duct is indicated in the short term to prevent episodes of pancreatitis and over the long term to eliminate the risk of malignancy. Pancreatitis, most often secondary to idiopathic causes in children, may cause abdominal pain in children that may have surgical implications. Initial presentation with hyperamylasemia and hyperlipasemia may progress to the development of a midabdominal mass. These patients should be evaluated for the presence of a pancreatic pseudocyst. Many of these lesions resolve spontaneously and do not require surgical drainage.

Abdominal Masses

The presence of an abdominal mass in an infant or child mandates a systematic assessment of various factors including the age of the patient, the location of the mass, characteristics of the mass (e.g., firm, cystic, mobile, fixed), and initial diagnostic imaging studies. Although important in other conditions, the history is rarely of major clinical significance in children with abdominal masses because of the protracted presentation of these lesions. Occasionally, children may present with acute gastrointestinal or genitourinary tract obstruction. Typically, the physical examination and initial radiographic studies lead to the development of a differential diagnosis that will focus efforts at diagnosis. This serves as a framework from which to further define the nature of the disease.

Location is the most important factor for determining the tissue of origin and behavior of an abdominal mass (Fig. 17-77). Retroperitoneal masses are often solid in nature and fixed to adjacent structures. Intraperitoneal masses that arise from the bowel, mesentery, or omentum are usually cystic and mobile. Dense fibrous adhesions encasing inflammatory lesions may also restrict mobility. Cystic intra-abdominal lesions arising from the gastrointestinal or genitourinary tract are usually benign in

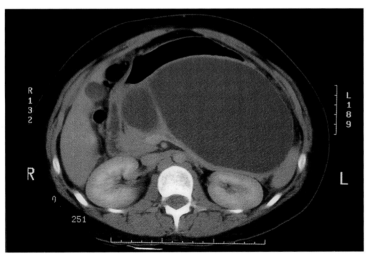

Figure 17-76. Pancreatic pseudocysts in the pediatric population most commonly result from blunt traumatic injuries to the abdomen, as occurred in this patient with a handlebar injury.

nature. In contrast, solid intra-abdominal lesions are predominantly malignant. Extra-abdominal manifestations (metastases and associated congenital anomalies) should always be investigated. Age is the second most important factor in determining the differential diagnosis of abdominal masses. Table 17-4 summarizes the causes of abdominal masses by age and location.

Plain abdominal radiography often provides basic information in determining the location and potential differential diagnosis of an abdominal mass. Bowel displacement from the pelvis suggests the presence of a pelvic extraluminal mass. In contrast, intraluminal lesions may lead to a small bowel obstruction pattern as seen in meconium ileus, intussusception, or constipation. Calcification seen within the mass on plain film suggests the presence of a malignant lesion such as a neuroblastoma, rhabdomyosarcoma, or teratoma. Ultrasonography is traditionally the initial diagnostic tool of choice in patients with abdominal masses. This modality allows the differentiation of solid versus cystic lesions, a critical first stage of evaluation. Ultrasonography may characterize the lesion as arising within the kidney or in the juxtarenal location. Alternatively, pelvic lesions may also be determined as being cystic or solid in nature (Fig. 17-78). CT allows precise anatomic differentiation of abdominal lesions and the assessment of extra-abdominal disease.

CT has become the study of choice by surgeons and other interventionalists in the evaluation of patients with abdominal masses. Because of its utility for assessing extent of local disease, the sites of distant metastases and the character of the lesion, the use of the upper and lower gastrointestinal contrast, in conjunction with intravenous contrast, allows for careful analysis of abdominal and pelvic structures. The presence of bilateral nephrograms and caliceal excretion of contrast is a critical factor if the patient is to undergo a nephrectomy as part of his or her surgical therapy. MRI may be of some utility in patients with abdominal masses; however, in infants this is a somewhat cumbersome study because it is relatively slower and mandates intravenous sedation.

Neonates

Neonatal abdominal masses are benign genitourinary lesions in 75% to 80% of cases. The most common abdominal masses are congenital obstructive hydronephrosis and multicystic dysplastic kidney. Congenital hydrone-

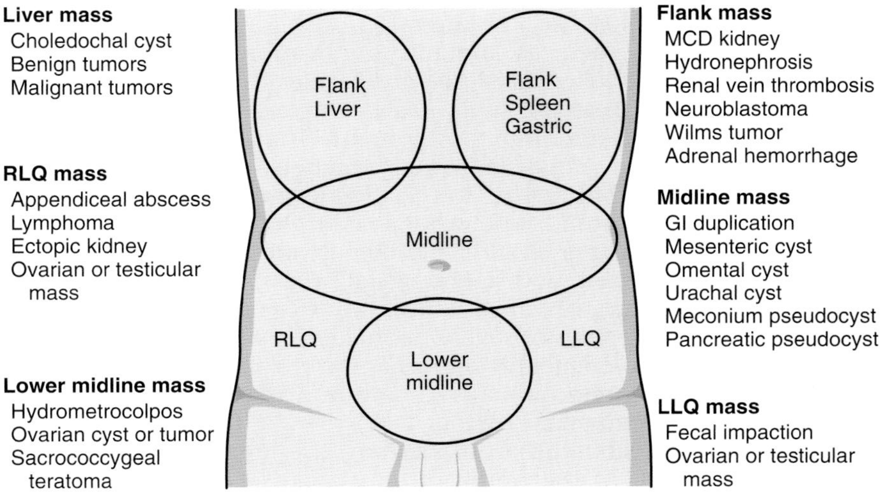

Liver mass
Choledochal cyst
Benign tumors
Malignant tumors

RLQ mass
Appendiceal abscess
Lymphoma
Ectopic kidney
Ovarian or testicular mass

Figure 17-77. Location of commonly found abdominal masses in children.

Lower midline mass
Hydrometrocolpos
Ovarian cyst or tumor
Sacrococcygeal teratoma

Flank Liver | Flank Spleen Gastric
Midline
RLQ | LLQ
Lower midline

Flank mass
MCD kidney
Hydronephrosis
Renal vein thrombosis
Neuroblastoma
Wilms tumor
Adrenal hemorrhage

Midline mass
GI duplication
Mesenteric cyst
Omental cyst
Urachal cyst
Meconium pseudocyst
Pancreatic pseudocyst

LLQ mass
Fecal impaction
Ovarian or testicular mass

Table 17-4	Possible Diagnoses of Abdominal Masses in Infancy and Childhood	
REGION	**ORGAN**	**DIAGNOSIS**
Epigastrium	Stomach	Distended stomach from pyloric stenosis, duplication
	Pancreas	Pseudocyst
Flank	Kidney	Hydronephrosis, Wilms tumor, dysplastic kidney, ureteral duplication
	Adrenal	Neuroblastoma, ganglioneuroblastoma, ganglioneuroma
	Retroperitoneum	Neuroblastoma, ganglioneuroblastoma, ganglioneuroma, teratoma
Lower abdomen	Ovary	Dermoid, teratoma, ovarian tumors, torsion of ovary
	Kidney	Pelvic kidney
	Urachus	Urachal cyst
	Omentum, mesentery	Omental, mesenteric, peritoneal cysts
Pelvis	Bladder, prostate	Obstructed bladder, rhabdomyosarcoma
	Uterus, vagina	Hydrometrocolpos, hydrocolpos, rhabdomyosarcoma
Right upper quadrant	Biliary tract	Cholecystitis, choledochal cyst
	Liver	Hepatomegaly resulting from congestion, hepatitis, or tumor; mesenchymal hamartoma; hemangioendothelioma; hepatoblastoma; hepatocellular carcinoma; hepatic abscess; hydatid cyst
	Intestine	Intussusception, duplication
Left upper quadrant	Spleen	Splenomegaly resulting from congestion, infectious mononucleosis, leukemic infiltration or lymphoma; splenic abscess; cyst
Right lower quadrant	Appendix	Appendiceal abscess
	Ileum	Meconium ileus, inflammatory mass (complicated Crohn disease), intestinal duplication
	Lymphatics	Lymphoma, lymphangioma
Left lower quadrant	Colon	Fecal impaction
	Lymphatics	Lymphoma, lymphangioma

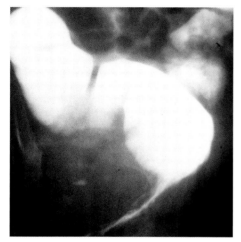

Figure 17-78. A pelvic neuroblastoma causes compression of the rectum on barium enema study.

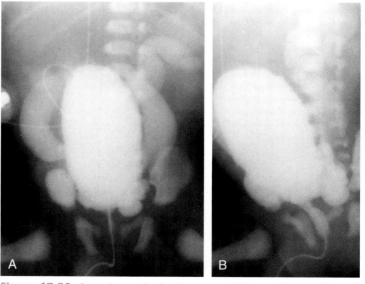

Figure 17-79. The dashed line indicates the extent of a flank mass in an infant with ureteropelvic junction obstruction.

phrosis (Fig. 17-79) usually develops from a ureteropelvic junction obstruction. They are bulky, smooth, flank masses on physical examination that are usually secondary to ureteropelvic junction obstruction. These are treated with pyeloplasty to prevent further loss of renal parenchyma or the development of infection. Other genitourinary anomalies such as ureteral duplications and ureteroceles may produce obstructive uropathies that lead to palpable masses. Bilateral flank masses with hydroureteronephrosis may result from posterior urethral valves, the most common cause of distal urinary tract obstruction in boys (Fig. 17-80). Multicystic dysplastic kidney disease often occurs as a unilateral, soft, cystic mass in more than three quarters of the cases (Fig. 17-81). Renal vein thrombosis may also present as an abdominal mass in the neonate. This condition is most commonly the result of hyperviscosity syndromes or severe neonatal dehydration (Fig. 17-82). Mesoblastic nephroma, a benign renal tumor that mimics Wilms tumor, is also a common mass that may present in the neonatal period.

Other common abdominal masses in the neonatal period may arise from other genitourinary organs, gastro-

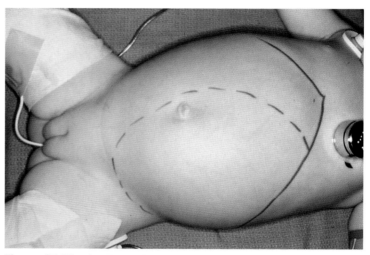

Figure 17-80. Posterior urethral valves cause dilation of the bladder and both upper tracts, shown here on anteroposterior **(A)** and lateral **(B)** views of a retrograde contrast study.

intestinal structures, or other intra-abdominal sites. Ovarian cysts are quite common in the neonatal period. Maternal hormonal stimulation in utero promotes their development, and subsequent withdrawal of this stimulus following delivery leads to their resolution. Congenital vaginal obstruction may also lead to development of a large abdominal mass. Gastrointestinal duplication cysts are often present at birth, but the diagnosis is often not made until later in childhood (Fig. 17-83). Mesenteric and omental cysts are soft, diffuse, and multiloculated lesions that may arise from the omentum or mesenteric. These lesions are due to congenital lymphatic obstruction and may be a source of intra-abdominal pain secondary to acute hemorrhage (Fig. 17-84). Adrenal masses are common in the newborn and in infancy. These masses may range from the benign mass associated with spontaneous adrenal hemorrhage, perinatal stress, or birth trauma to the malignant neuroblastoma (Fig. 17-85). Occasionally, intra-abdominal extra lobar sequestration may be adjacent to the adrenal gland, suggesting the presence of a malignancy. The most common malignancy of infancy is malignant sacrococcygeal teratoma (Fig. 17-86).

Toddlers and Young Children

In stark contrast with the neonate, the presence of an abdominal mass in a toddler or young child is almost equally as likely to be malignant as benign. Neuroblastoma, Wilms tumor, rhabdomyosarcoma, hepatoblastoma, and lymphoma are the most common pediatric solid malignancies. Although each may have histologic similarities, they all have distinct differences in behavior and prognosis that are described later.

Neuroblastoma is the most common extracranial malignancy of childhood. The vast majority of patients present before their fifth birthday with extensive locoregional disease (stage 3) or widespread metastases (stage 4). These tumors occur along the embryonic tract of neural crest cell migration and may arise anywhere from the neck to the pelvis. They are typically multilobular and firm retroperitoneal masses that encase vessels and cross the abdominal midline. More than half occur in the adrenal or juxtarenal location (Fig. 17-87). Presenting symptoms may include local pain, abdominal distention, failure to thrive, or paralysis. Several major extra-abdominal symptoms

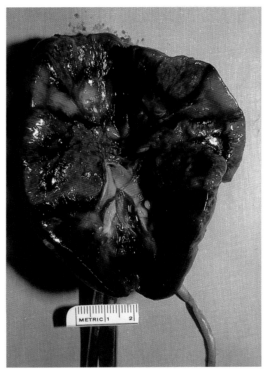

Figure 17-82. Renal vein thrombosis may occur as the result of hyperviscosity syndromes or severe neonatal dehydration.

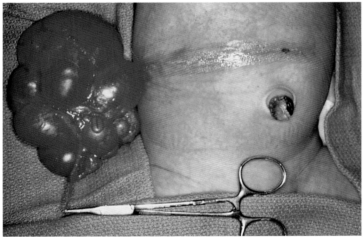

Figure 17-81. A multicystic kidney produces a knobby flank mass.

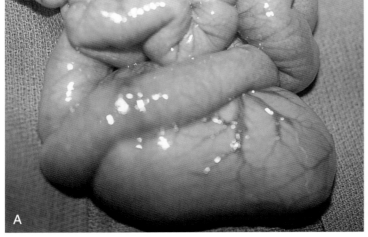
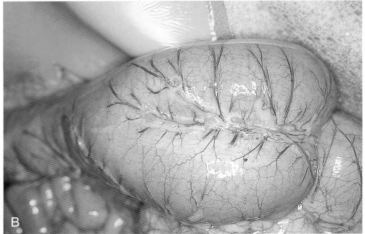

Figure 17-83. Duplications of the gastrointestinal tract usually arise from the mesenteric border of the bowel and may be cystic **(A)** or tubular **(B)**.

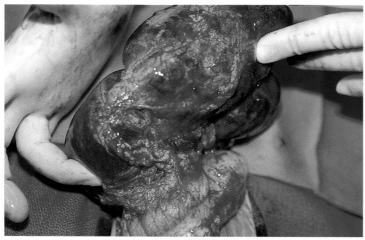

Figure 17-84. Omental cyst may cause ill-defined episodic abdominal pain.

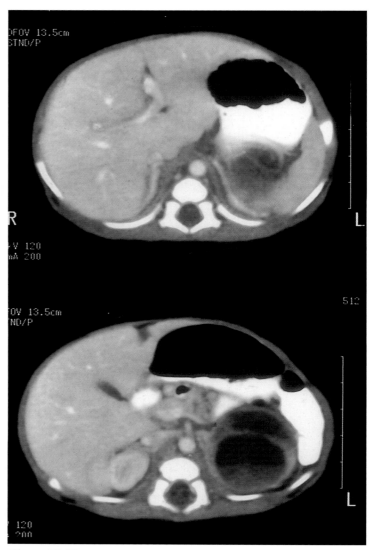

Figure 17-85. Adrenal hemorrhage often results from perinatal stress or birth trauma. The radiographic appearance showing a left suprarenal heterogeneous mass is suspicious for neuroblastoma.

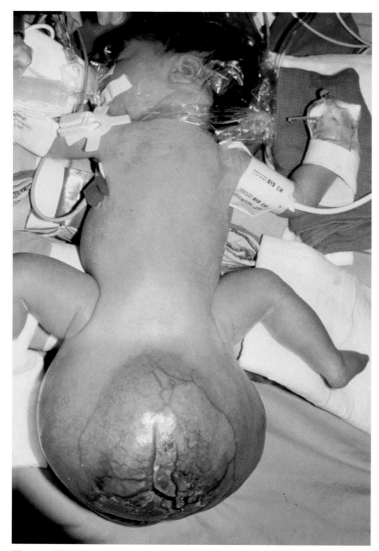

Figure 17-86. Sacrococcygeal teratoma may grow to be fairly large in size, causing in utero growth retardation and/or hydrops fetalis.

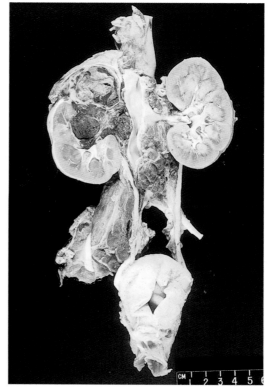

Figure 17-87. Adrenal neuroblastoma with signs of local metastasis to retroperitoneal lymph nodes.

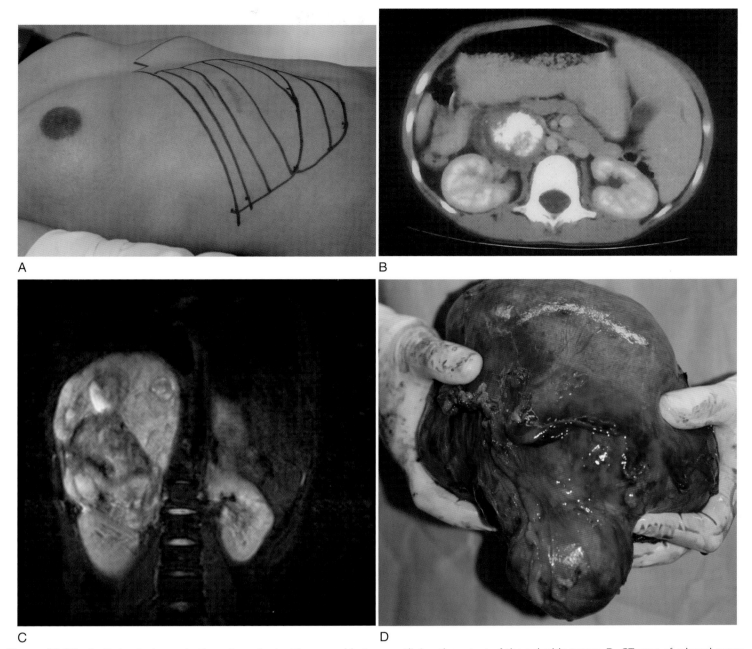

A

B

C

D

Figure 17-88. **A,** Abdominal examination of a patient with a neuroblastoma outlining the extent of the palpable tumor. **B,** CT scan of adrenal neuroblastoma with stippled calcifications. **C,** MRI demonstrating inferior displacement of the kidney by the large tumor. The tumor also has calcifications. **D,** Pathological specimen of the patient's tumor at surgery.

including cerebellar ataxia; opsoclonus-myoclonus, also known as *dancing eyes and feet syndrome;* and diffuse, watery diarrhea may be present. Patients may also present with remote neurologic symptoms of paralysis and weakness due to spinal cord invasion or peripheral nerve compression. The prognosis is generally poor (<25% survival). A rare variant of this malignancy known as stage IV-S disease presents with extensive local disease and widespread metastases to bone, skin, and liver in children younger than 1 year of age. Many of these patients will ultimately undergo spontaneous regression with minimal or no therapy.

The radiographic appearance of an intra-abdominal neuroblastoma may reveal evidence of an upper abdominal mass with areas of stippled calcifications (Fig. 17-88). CT shows a retroperitoneal mass that crosses the midline with intimate involvement of adjacent vascular structures including the aorta, vena cava and renal vessels, and mesenteric artery. Before CT scanning, intravenous pyelogra-

phy was the most frequently used modality for diagnosing retroperitoneal masses in children. This has largely been supplanted by the use of ultrasonography and CT scan imaging. Large adrenal or juxta-adrenal neuroblastoma may cause displacement of the kidney, giving a characteristic "drooping lily" sign on intravenous pyelography (Fig. 17-89). The workup of these masses includes an evaluation of the urine for the dopaminergic metabolites vanillylmandelic and homovanillic acid, abdominal and chest CT, technetium scintigraphy (bone scan), and metaiodobenzylguanidine (MIBG) scan. Serologic studies including ferritin, neuron-specific enolase, and lactate dehydrogenase have prognostic significance and should be measured in all patients. Newer markers including TRK-A expression and ganglioside GD_2 expression may also be useful in determining long-term prognosis.

Wilms tumor is the second most common abdominal malignancy in childhood. Approximately 450 new cases are diagnosed annually in the United States. Most children present before their fifth birthday with a bulky abdominal mass, hematuria, and/or hypertension. Although most children are healthy and asymptomatic at presentation, some children present with severe pain secondary to intratumor bleeding or, rarely, rupture. The physical examination reveals a large bulky tumor in the subcostal region that is usually firm, smooth, immobile, and nontender. Unlike neuroblastoma, at presentation these tumors usually do not cross the midline, nor are there usually signs of metastatic disease. The role of diagnostic imaging is to assess the nature of the tumor, site of origin, contralateral renal function, presence of bilateral disease, extent of local disease (involvement of the renal vessels and/or inferior vena cava), and evidence of metastases. Plain film studies in most tumors may show calcifications, but unlike neuroblastomas these tend to be more linear in appearance than stippled. CT of the chest and abdomen may answer most of the critical questions important to clinical staging (Fig. 17-90). Signs of tumor extending into the renal veins are of major surgical significance and mandate careful evaluation of the inferior vena cava and right atrium by ultrasound and echocardiography. Evidence of intracaval and right atrial thrombus requires chemotherapy before surgical resection. Lungs, lymph nodes, and the liver are the most common sites of metastasis. Formerly, clear cell sarcoma was considered to be a variant of Wilms tumor but is now believed to be a distinct pathologic entity. Bony metastases are common with this malignancy, and these patients should be evaluated by bone scan.

Rhabdomyosarcoma is the most common soft tissue sarcoma of childhood. Although these tumors have histologic features of striated skeletal muscle, they may arise anywhere in the body (Fig. 17-91). Lesions arising in pelvic locations (bladder, vagina, or paratesticular regions) have a nonalveolar histology and a more favorable prognosis (Fig. 17-92). Primary lesions are not confined to the abdominal location but may appear throughout the body. Prognosis depends on the site of occurrence and the histologic characteristics.

Non-Hodgkin lymphoma may present with abdominal involvement in 25% to 50% of all cases. The peak incidence of occurrence is between 5 and 8 years of age. Most children present with abdominal pain and a palpable mass. These are rapidly growing tumors that may arise from bowel, mesentery, or retroperitoneal structures. Some children may develop an irreducible intussusception requiring surgical resection. These tumors are usually quite responsive to chemotherapy.

Hepatic lesions often present in this age group. They may range from benign conditions such as hemangioendothelioma, arteriovenous malformations, mesenchymal hamartoma, and choledochal cysts (Fig. 17-93). Hepatic tumors may present as bulky masses present in the right upper quadrant or midline that are fixed to the adjacent liver and poorly mobile (Fig. 17-94). Splenomegaly occurs from underlying hematologic diseases such as immunodeficiencies and lymphoproliferation (Fig. 17-95). Splenic cyst may also mimic splenomegaly before radiographic evaluation. These may be congenital in nature or the result of previous trauma (Fig. 17-96).

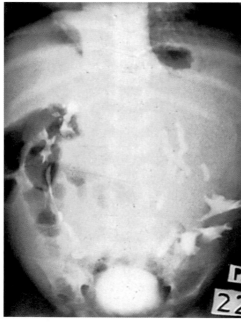

Figure 17-89. Downward displacement of the entire kidney by a left adrenal neuroblastoma leaves the intrarenal collecting system anatomically intact but gives it a "drooping lily" appearance.

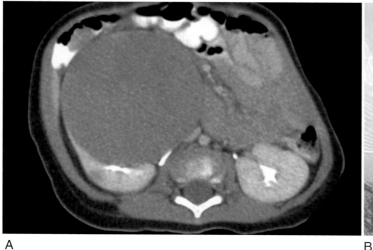

A

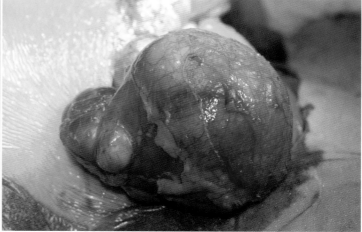

B

Figure 17-90. A, Abdominal CT scan of Wilms tumor shows a bulky mass to the right of midline. **B,** Intraoperative Wilms tumor with a large tumor mass involving the kidney.

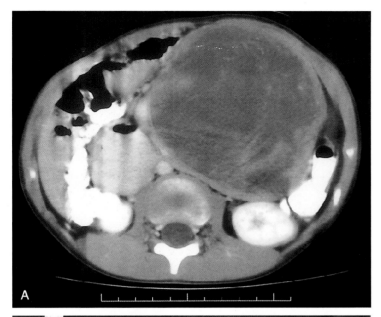

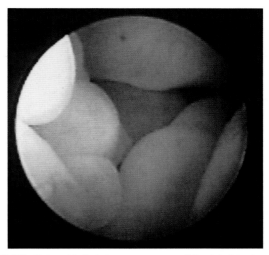

Figure 17-92. Botryoid rhabdomyosarcoma of the bladder has the characteristic "clustered grape" appearance on cystoscopy. Prognosis is usually favorable.

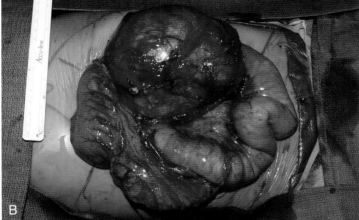

Figure 17-91. **A,** Abdominal CT scan showing a large retroperitoneal rhabdomyosarcoma. **B,** Intraoperative view of retroperitoneal rhabdomyosarcoma extending through the mesentery, displacing small bowel and colon.

Older Children and Teenagers

Pelvic tumors in children may also present as lower abdominal masses due to the small, shallow nature of the pediatric pelvis. The differential diagnosis of midline pelvic masses includes ovarian cysts and tumors, hydrocolpos, hydrometrocolpos, and sacrococcygeal teratoma. Ovarian masses may occur in all age groups but are most commonly seen in adolescence. More than 75% of ovarian masses are cystic and benign in nature. Twenty-five percent are solid and may have evidence of malignant changes. Ovarian cysts commonly occur in newborn infants and may be diagnosed prenatally. Many of these resolve spontaneously in the early neonatal period. Large cysts of more than 5 cm in infants are prone to undergo torsion and should be aspirated. Obstruction of the female genital tract by vaginal atresia or imperforate hymen may cause hydrocolpos in infancy that may manifest as a large abdominal mass with respiratory embarrassment secondary to diaphragmatic compression. Alternatively, these girls may present at puberty with cyclic abdominal pain, a large pelvic or lower abdominal mass, and the absence of menses (Fig. 17-97). This occurs due to the uterine retention of menstrual products. They may also develop

hydronephrosis due to extrinsic vesicoureteral obstruction and coexisting genitourinary tract anomalies, which are quite common in this population.

Inflammatory Masses

Numerous inflammatory conditions that involve intra-abdominal organs may lead to masses. Following bowel perforations associated with appendicitis, Meckel diverticulitis, or Crohn disease, the omentum and adjacent bowel loops migrate to the area in an attempt to localize the process. Development of an abscess cavity with a dense fibrous capsule may mimic a lower abdominal or pelvic tumor. Typically, inflammatory masses are tender and associated with systemic symptoms. Early institution of intravenous antibiotics and percutaneous drainage may lead to prompt resolution of the mass. Children with ventriculoperitoneal shunts may develop inflammatory pseudocysts at the tips of these catheters that may become secondarily infected. This is often associated with symptoms of abdominal pain or fever. Prompt shunt exteriorization and intravenous antibiotic therapy may allow catheter salvage. Persistent symptoms of sepsis suggest the possibility of an abscess formation or bowel perforation that requires surgical exploration and catheter removal.

Crohn disease may present with inflammatory lower abdominal masses or abscesses (Fig. 17-98). These usually respond to aggressive medical management and resolve without surgery. Failure to respond to medical therapies suggests the presence of a fistula formation to an adjacent bowel loop or bladder. Upper gastrointestinal contrast studies with small bowel follow-through and barium enema with reflux into the terminal ileum help delineate the extent of bowel involvement and the presence of fistulas.

Head and Neck

Most lesions of the head and neck are benign in nature. Location provides essential insight into the likely diagnosis. Table 17-5 provides a summary of the common pediatric head and neck lesions by anatomic location. Physical examination and diagnostic imaging studies are impor-

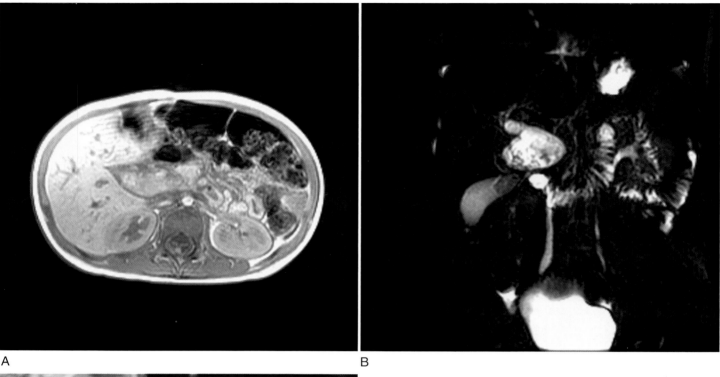

A

B

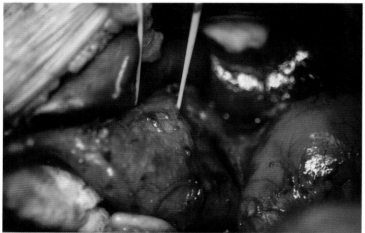

C

Figure 17-93. **A,** Magnetic resonance cholangiopancreatography of a choledochal cyst demonstrating a large cystic mass within the hilum of the liver. **B,** Contrast MRI of a choledochal cyst demonstrating the same irregular mass in the hilum of the liver. **C,** In situ choledochal cyst with fusiform dilation extending from the hilum to the ampulla. The duodenum is the southwest corner of the photo, the liver hilum is in the northwest corner, and the triangular dilated cyst has the yellow tape around it.

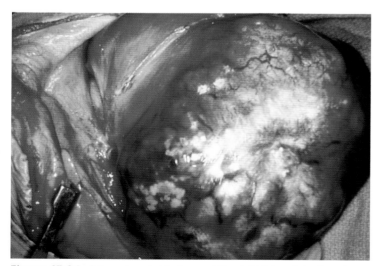

Figure 17-94. A large hepatoblastoma of the right lobe of the liver. Intravenous urography, CT, and ultrasonography all identify it as a hepatic tumor instead of one arising from the kidney or an adrenal gland.

tant to generate a differential diagnosis and further determine the nature and extent of the lesion. Critical physical examination findings include determination of size, evidence of airway compromise, signs of inflammation, presence of sinus tracts, or ocular involvement.

CT and MRI have almost completely eliminated plain radiography in the evaluation of lesions of the head and neck. These modalities may better demonstrate details of the bony and vascular structures of the skull base and the cervical spine. Furthermore, underlying brain involvement as either primary or secondary site may be visualized. Skull and facial films are of limited utility at present. Children with disorders of breathing, swallowing, or phonation require adjunctive endoscopic procedures (nasopharyngoscopy, laryngoscopy, and esophagoscopy) to assist with the diagnosis.

Surgery is frequently necessary in head and neck lesions for both diagnostic and therapeutic reasons. Incision and drainage of a cervical abscess may provide a specimen for culture and a means of drainage for resolution. Excisional biopsy is critical to determine the precise pathology of the

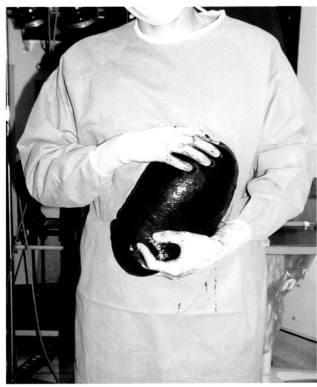

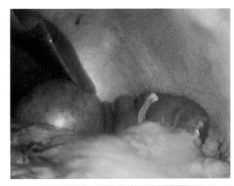

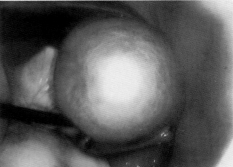

Figure 17-96. Laparoscopic view of a symptomatic splenic cyst in an active teenager caused disabling left upper quadrant pain.

Figure 17-95. Massive splenomegaly in a patient with a lymphoproliferative disorder. This patient had early satiety and vomiting.

Figure 17-97. **A,** Imperforate hymen. Accumulated secretions in the vagina and uterus caused bulging of the hymen and a pelvic mass in this newborn. **B,** A pelvic mass arising at the expected time of menarche suggests the presence of an obstructed uterine anomaly, here demonstrated by pelvic ultrasound as an oval mass compressing the bladder anteriorly. Urinary anomalies commonly coexist.

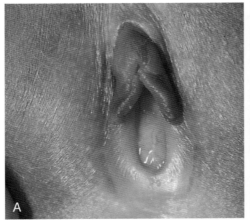

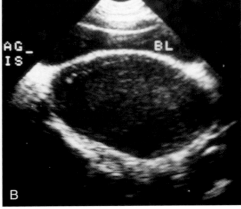

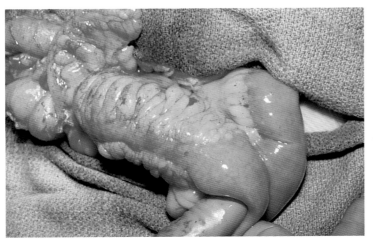

Figure 17-98. Findings at laparotomy in Crohn disease reveal petechiae over the serosa of thickened small bowel, which has mesenteric fat "creeping" over its surface.

Table 17-5		Common Lesions of the Head and Neck in Infancy and Childhood
REGION	**LOCATION**	**COMMON LESIONS**
Head	Scalp	Hemangioma, dermoid cyst
	Ear	Preauricular sinus, tag
	Eyebrow	Dermoid cyst
	Base of nose	Meningocele, encephalocele
	Parotid gland	Hemangioma, lymphangioma, rhabdomyosarcoma, lymphoma, mixed tumor, parotitis
Mouth	Tongue	Tongue-tie, macroglossia, lingual thyroid
	Floor of mouth	Ranula
	Cheek and lip	Papilloma, mucocele
	Alveolar ridge	Tooth bud, epignathus
Neck	Midline	Thyroglossal duct cyst, dermoid cyst, submental lymph node, goiter
	Lateral	Branchial cleft cyst or sinus, lymphadenitis, lymphoma, lymphangioma, torticollis

lesion and assist with determining the need for further therapies. Several important conditions of the head and neck exist in which surgery is unnecessary or may unduly create complications. These include hemangioma, torticollis, and benign reactive adenopathy.

Scalp

Hemangiomas are benign, congenital, vascular tumors that most frequently arise in the head and neck. These lesions are typically raised above the skin level and may be red or somewhat purple in color. They may blanch on contact. Often hemangiomas may not be present at birth but develop in the first few months of life. Rapid growth and expansion may occur, leading to platelet sequestration and coagulopathy, known as the *Kasabach-Merritt syndrome*. This condition may be refractory to various medical maneuvers including steroids, radiation therapy, and chemotherapy. Recent progress in the use of various angiogenic agents such as α-interferon and angiostatin has shown some promise. Despite significant growth in size during the first year of life, most hemangiomas have a benign course and undergo spontaneous resolution over the first 7 years of life (Fig. 17-99). Surgical intervention is rarely necessary and should be reserved for those patients with impending airway compromise or periorbital involvement. Special consideration must be given to those patients with lesions extending toward the eye or impinging on the airway. Subsequent blindness or airway compromise may be the consequences if intervention is inordinately delayed.

Dermoid cysts are congenital lesions that are composed of sequestered hair, skin, and sebaceous structures that occur in areas of embryonic fusion. These lesions are most frequent in the head and neck, but they may arise in other midline sites including the sacral, perineal, and sternal region. They are typically located in the head and neck along the lateral palpebral fissure, occipital scalp, and midline of the neck. Scalp dermoids are often well-circumscribed, firm, and fixed to underlying deep structures such as bone, typically arising from the outer bony table of the bone. Midline scalp or back dermoids may

have intracranial or intraspinal extension, respectively. They should always be evaluated by MRI before surgical intervention. Dural or central nervous system extension mandates neurosurgical consultation before resection. Treatment for these conditions is surgical (Fig. 17-100).

Face

Several benign remnants of congenital structures may persist at birth, and they raise numerous management considerations. Preauricular skin tags are vestigial cartilaginous remnants that are primarily lesions for cosmetic consideration. In contrast, preauricular pits or sinuses are prone to infectious complications. These anomalies represent epidermal inclusion structures that are related to the embryologic formation of the ear. The sinus may be lined by pilosebaceous structures and exude a sebaceous-like fluid. Complete surgical excision of the sinus and subcutaneous cystic elements is curative. Because most of these lesions are asymptomatic, routine excision should be reserved for those patients who have had infectious complications.

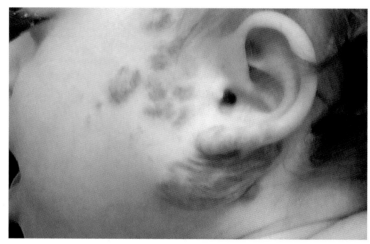

Figure 17-99. Involuting parotid and neck hemangioma. Note the grayish discoloration indicative of resolution.

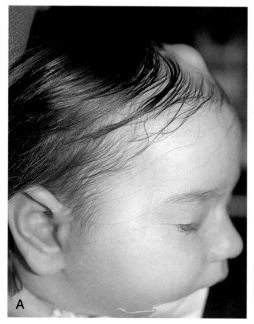

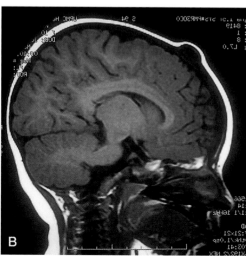

Figure 17-100. A, Midline scalp dermoid cysts may have intracranial extension and should always be evaluated by MRI before surgery. **B,** The dermoid in this 2-year-old child extends to but not through the dura.

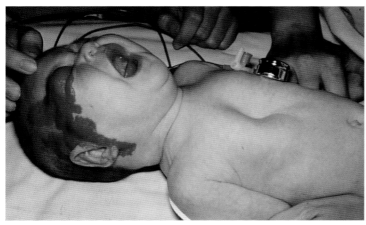

Figure 17-101. Facial hemangioma covering the eye requires intervention with prednisone to hasten resolution and avoid loss of sight from amblyopia.

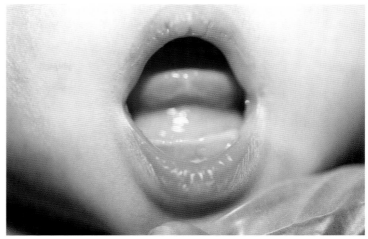

Figure 17-102. A ranula arises in the floor of the mouth, caused by congenital obstruction of the sublingual duct.

Surgically significant salivary gland pathology is uncommon in the pediatric population. Hemangiomas are the most common benign lesions of the parotid gland in children. As with hemangiomas in other sites, these may not be entirely visualized at birth and may occur over the first few months of life. A small cutaneous birthmark may be the only initial presentation. Rapid growth and significant asymmetry may be apparent (Fig. 17-101). These lesions spontaneously involute with time. In the absence of early complications, surgery, sclerotherapy, or intralesional injection techniques should be reserved until the period after involution. Other causes of parotid enlargement in children include viral (mumps), bacterial (staphylococcal), and mycobacterial (atypical mycobacterial infection or tuberculosis) infections, as well as chronic inflammatory conditions. Treatment specific to these conditions is implemented.

Various intraoral lesions may arise that have surgical significance primarily due to their effects on swallowing, speech, and breathing. Tongue-tie (ankyloglossia inferior) occurs commonly in infancy, usually resolving spontaneously. Some cases persist, and these children may have impaired speech development. Usually a thin membranous structure, the frenulum regresses with feeding. A persistent frenulum may impair speech and feeding. Simple division is therapeutic. Similarly, ranulas may form as pseudocysts in the floor of the mouth. Some spontaneously resolve, whereas a few may become quite large and impair lingual mobility, feeding, speech, and most significantly, breathing. Marsupialization or complete excision is curative (Fig. 17-102).

Lymphangiomas of the floor of the mouth may pose especially challenging management problems (Fig. 17-103). These lesions may cause significant macroglossia that obstructs the airway, requiring tracheostomy. Small vesicular lesions may occur on the lingual surface and exude fluid that may become purulent. Suppurative glossitis may require systemic antibiotic therapy. In addition to the airway complications, problems with speech development and mandibular growth may occur. Some authors have proposed partial glossectomy as a therapy.

Lingual thyroid is a rare developmental anomaly of the thyroid. Congenital failure of thyroid descent results in persistence of thyroid tissue at the base of the foramen cecum, giving rise to this problem. At birth infants may present with acute airway obstruction, whereas older children may describe feeling a lump in the throat with swallowing. This condition is often associated with hypo-

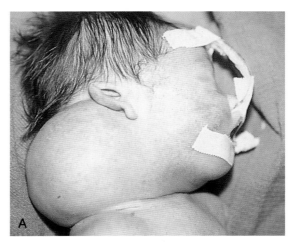

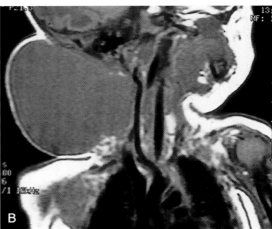

Figure 17-103. Cervical cystic hygroma **(A)**. MRI demonstrates its juxtaposition to the airway structures and vessels in the neck **(B)**. Acute enlargement at birth secondary to hemorrhage may lead to airway compression.

thyroidism. Transoral excision requires permanent thyroid replacement because these lesions typically represent the only functioning thyroid tissue in these children.

Neck—Midline

The differential diagnosis for midline neck masses includes thyroglossal duct remnants, dermoid cysts, and lymphadenopathy. During fetal development, the thyroid gland originates at the base of the foramen cecum and descends in the midline along the course of the thyroglossal duct close to the hyoid bone until it reaches its final destination in the base of the neck. Failure of regression of the thyroglossal duct may lead to cyst formation (Fig. 17-104). These lesions are quite prone to infectious complications and require surgical excision. This excision requires resection of the midportion of the hyoid bone and ligation of the tract leading to the foramen cecum to prevent future recurrence (Fig. 17-105). Thyroid nodules are common in the pediatric population (Fig. 17-106). A greater incidence of malignancy occurs within these lesions in children, however.

A relatively high incidence of associated cancer occurs in children. Thorough evaluation and management of these lesions is critical to a favorable outcome. These nodules are twice as common in girls as boys. They typically present with a midline anterior cervical mass that moves with the thyroid gland. Initial physical examination should thoroughly assess the location of the lesion, as well as the presence of associated lymphadenopathy. In general, clinical findings are unreliable in distinguishing between benign and malignant disease. Although thyroid imaging studies are often indicated, they are rarely helpful in assisting with the diagnosis, unless there is evidence of multiple nodules. A multinodular goiter would suggest nodular Hashimoto disease, which is the most common benign lesion of the thyroid (Fig. 17-107). The utility of

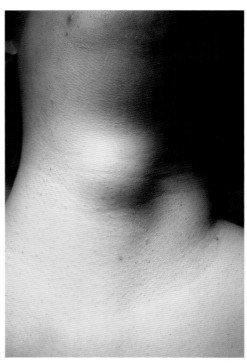

Figure 17-104. Thyroglossal duct cyst produces a firm swelling in the midline of the neck. Its initial manifestation is sometimes a midline cervical abscess.

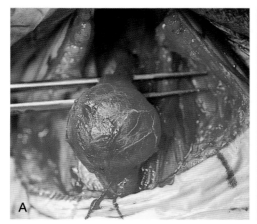
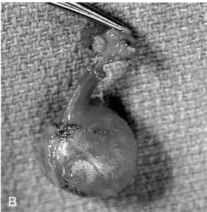

Figure 17-105. The surgical specimen shows the thyroglossal duct as it courses from the lesion to the hyoid bone (the thicker transverse piece of tissue) **(A)**. The hyoid must be resected to gain access to the tissue that extends to the base of the tongue (foramen cecum), which must be ligated to prevent recurrence **(B)**.

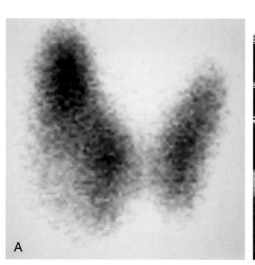
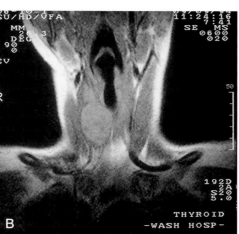

Figure 17-106. Nonfunctioning or "cold" thyroid nodule visualized by thyroid scan **(A)** and MRI **(B)** at surgery was found to be a benign follicular adenoma.

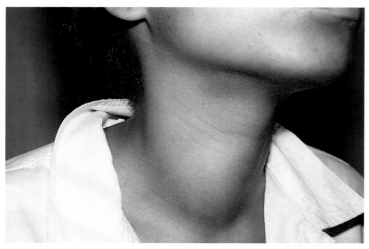

Figure 17-107. Goiter in a 15-year-old girl, resulting from Hashimoto thyroiditis.

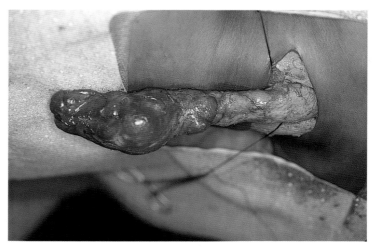

Figure 17-109. Thymic cyst extending from the anterior mediastinum on the right into the neck on the left of the photo.

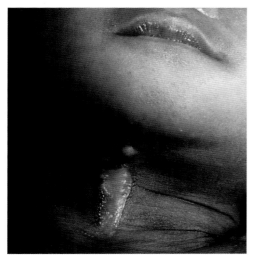

Figure 17-108. Midline cervical cleft.

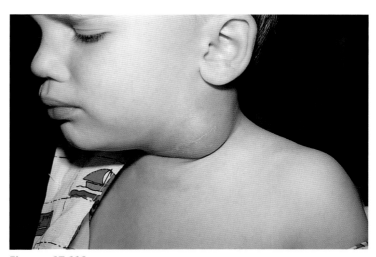

Figure 17-110. Erythema and fluctuance identify the presence of an abscess. An abscess may be present without fluctuance, however, the result of induration from surrounding inflammation.

ultrasound in distinguishing benign from malignant disease on the basis of a cystic appearance of the lesions is also not helpful. Furthermore, the utility of fine-needle aspiration cytology in the pediatric population remains an area of considerable debate. Reports in the older medical literature suggested a much higher incidence of malignancy in thyroid nodules in children than current studies. Consequently, there was a much stronger recommendation for surgical excision as the diagnostic procedure of choice. Recent reports have shown that the incidence of benign disease is approximately 20%. Therefore needle aspiration may offer considerable savings in unnecessary surgical resections for benign disease. Needle aspiration cytology that shows a true malignancy or has indeterminate pathology should undergo surgical resection. Total thyroidectomy is recommended for malignant primary lesions; lobectomy and isthmusectomy are recommended for benign lesions in which cancer cannot be completely ruled out.

Other miscellaneous conditions may occur in this location, such as midline branchial (cervical) cleft, a linear tract of epithelialized tissue in the anterior midline of the neck that occurs due to aberrant fusion of the branchial arches (Fig. 17-108). In addition, mediastinal lesions such as thymic cyst may present as midline cervical masses (Fig. 17-109).

Neck—Lateral

Benign reactive cervical lymphadenopathy is the most common mass in the lateral triangle of the neck. These lesions arise as nonspecific hyperplastic responses to infection of the upper respiratory tract (nose, sinuses, ears, mouth, and pharynx) or skin (face and scalp). Typically these nodes are less than 2 cm in size and are rubbery, oval, and isolated. They characteristically occur in children between 2 and 10 years of age. *Streptococcus pyogenes* and *Staphylococcus aureus* are the most common organisms that lead to this adenopathy. The nodes spontaneously regress following the resolution of the inciting infection in most cases. Bacterial infection of the node may lead to more significant enlargement with increased tenderness, erythema, and ultimately suppuration (Fig. 17-110). Aggressive antibiotic therapy in the early stages of infection may prevent the development of the late suppurative stages that require surgical intervention. Fluctuant masses should be aspirated or incised and drained.

The differential diagnosis of chronic cervical lymphadenopathy (i.e., nodes that persist beyond 4 weeks) includes cat-scratch disease; atypical mycobacterial infection (*Mycobacterium avium-intracellulare scrofulaceum,* or MAIS); and tuberculosis. Cat-scratch disease is a common cause of lymphadenopathy in children that usually develops as

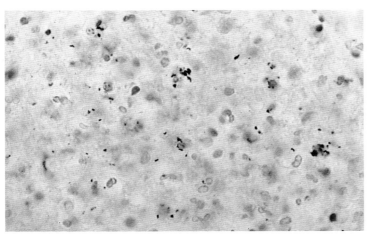

Figure 17-111. Warthin-Starry silver stain identifies the black-staining organisms associated with cat-scratch disease, seen on examination of an enlarged lymph node.

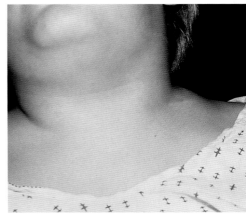

Figure 17-113. Enlarged lymph nodes in unusual locations, such as in this patient with supraclavicular lymphadenopathy from non-Hodgkin lymphoma, require excisional biopsy to rule out malignancy.

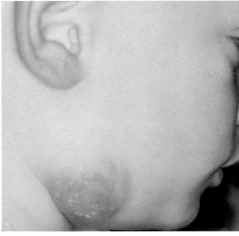

Figure 17-112. The skin overlying a tuberculous lymph node is often discolored and may break down into a chronically draining sinus.

regional nodal enlargement 2 to 4 weeks following inoculation by either a dog or cat. There may be a local reaction to the scratch followed by the evolution of lymphadenopathy that may persist for several months. Occasionally these nodes become suppurative and fluctuant and require surgical drainage. The diagnosis may be made by serologic testing for the antigen or polymerase chain reaction of nodal tissue. Alternatively, Warthin-Starry, an immunohistochemical silver stain specific for cat scratch, may identify the *Bartonella* organisms in tissue specimens (Fig. 17-111).

Various clinical presentations may occur with mycobacterial infections including local cervical adenopathy, pulmonary infection, and disseminated disease. The most common form is caused by one of the MAIS complex, which consists of approximately 15 organisms. These mycobacterial organisms typically produce local cervical disease. Mycobacterial tuberculosis usually presents with pulmonary infection but may rarely have supraclavicular or cervical lymphadenopathy (Fig. 17-112). In contrast, atypical mycobacterial infection usually involves the submandibular, submaxillary, or preauricular lymph nodal regions. Large, firm immobile and nontender lymph nodes may arise following inoculation. These may undergo spontaneous breakdown with the development of an abscess and sinus formation. Incision and drainage of fluctuant nodes may lead to a chronically draining sinus.

Complete resection of the node and any tracts is usually curative. Antimycobacterial therapy is not indicated in most cases of MAIS.

Cervical adenitis secondary to *Mycobacterium tuberculosis* infection is usually a manifestation of significant intrathoracic disease and requires aggressive antimycobacterial drug therapy. Surgery is usually unnecessary and should be avoided because of the risk of developing a chronically draining sinus (cervical tuberculosis). Lymphoma may present as painless cervical adenopathy. The absence of antecedent upper respiratory or cutaneous infections, the persistence of nodes beyond 6 weeks, size greater than 2 cm, and firm consistency should raise concern for malignancy. Although cervical adenopathy is more common in Hodgkin disease, non-Hodgkin lymphoma may also present with a cervical mass (Fig. 17-113). Incisional biopsy is diagnostic and mandated when these criteria are met. Other primary malignancies such as neuroblastoma and rhabdomyosarcoma may present as lateral neck masses. Secondary metastases from intra-abdominal or head and neck tumors may also occur.

Cysts and Sinuses

Branchial cleft anomalies give rise to the cysts and sinuses in the lateral triangle of the neck. Second branchial cleft anomalies are the most common and typically present as an opening along the lower anterior border of the sternocleidomastoid muscle. These sinuses have their origin in the tonsillar fossa and may travel between the carotid sheath to exit along the border of the sternocleidomastoid muscle. A complete fistula drains through a sinus opening (Fig. 17-114), while an incomplete fistula may present as a simple cystic structure in the subcutaneous tissue in the region (Fig. 17-115). Secondary infection of these lesions is common. Excision of the tract to the site of origin in the peritonsillar region prevents recurrence. Other branchial cleft and arch anomalies are less common (Fig. 17-116).

Fibromatosis coli, or fibrous dysplasia of the sternocleidomastoid muscle, is commonly seen in infants and young children (Fig. 17-117). These children present with a mass in the lower neck with tilting of the head and face to the side of the lesion (Fig. 17-118). Parents most often bring their infants in due to concerns with the possibility of a malignant tumor, whereas older children may present with hemifacial hypoplasia and asymmetry. Early recognition of this condition in infancy and the institution of daily physical therapy may avert surgery and long-term cosmetic deformity. Plagiocephaly and facial asymmetry are the sequelae of untreated deformities.

Chest Wall

Pectus excavatum ("funnel chest") is the most common congenital chest wall deformity (Fig. 17-119). This condition is characterized by the posterior angulation of the sternum toward the spine and abnormalities of the costal cartilages. Pectus excavatum has a 3 : 1 male predominance. Although not impressive during infancy, this deformity increases during early childhood and adolescence. This chest wall malformation typically causes no cardiopulmonary symptoms or disability. However, a small subpopulation of patients have exercise intolerance, mitral valve prolapse, or gastroesophageal reflux that may be attributed to the deformity. Debate remains as to the relationship of these symptoms to the defect. The psychological implications of this deformity for teenagers relative to their self-esteem may be a more compelling indication for surgical repair. The resulting withdrawal from social settings by these children may be devastating. New, minimally invasive techniques (Nuss procedure) may make the repair of pectus excavatum more appealing to many patients and their families.

Pectus carinatum, "pigeon chest," is a protrusion deformity of the chest wall (Fig. 17-120). This condition represents a spectrum of sternal and midchest anomalies that may give rise to this malformation. Pectus carinatum occurs more commonly in males than females and is usually asymptomatic. Marfan syndrome must be considered in pectus carinatum deformity. The coexistence of other conditions such as aortic root abnormalities and lens subluxation should be evaluated in these patients. Poland syndrome is an uncommon chest wall anomaly that consists of a constellation of abnormalities including

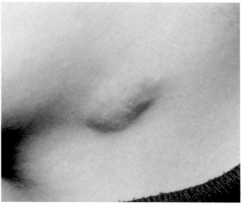

Figure 17-116. First branchial arch fistula, previously diagnosed as an infected lymph node. The location of the secondary opening is near the angle of the mandible.

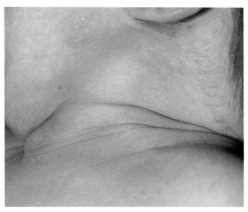

Figure 17-117. The sternocleidomastoid in a newborn with torticollis may exist as a tight tendon-like cord or may swell and appear as a discrete tumor in the midportion of the muscle, pictured here.

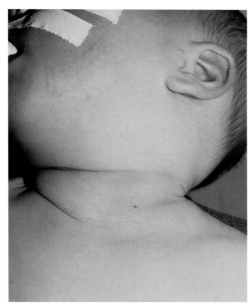

Figure 17-114. Mucus may drain from a small punctum at the anterior border of the sternocleidomastoid, identifying it as the secondary opening of a second branchial cleft fistula. The primary opening lies in the tonsillar fossa.

Figure 17-115. Cartilaginous remnants from the second branchial cleft present as a mobile cyst beneath the anterior border of the sternocleido-mastoid **(A)**. In another patient the cyst was infected, producing redness of the overlying skin **(B)**.

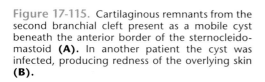

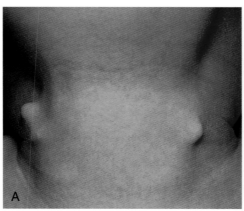

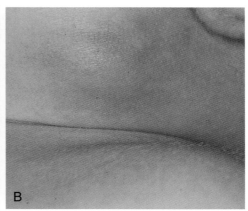

A

B

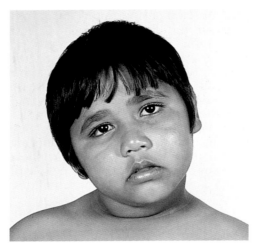

Figure 17-118. Long-standing torticollis may cause permanent "wry-neck," facial shortening of the affected side of the face, and plagiocephaly.

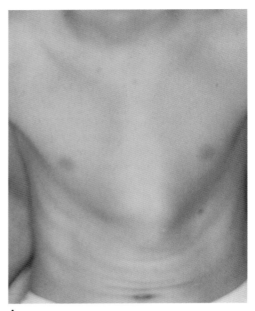

A

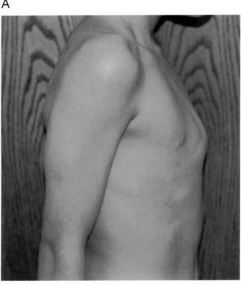

B

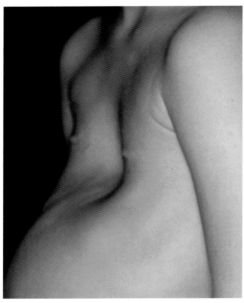

Figure 17-119. Pectus excavatum (funnel chest) seldom creates cardio-respiratory symptoms, but psychological consequences may be severe.

Figure 17-120. **A,** The sternum projects like a keel in front of the anterior chest wall in pectus carinatum (pigeon chest). Like pectus excavatum, pectus carinatum produces no symptoms. **B,** Lateral view of a pectus carinatum.

unilateral agenesis or dysplasia of the rib cage and chondral cartilages, absence of pectoralis major and minor muscles, hand deformities, and breast and areolar defects (Fig. 17-121). Other chest wall deformities include sternal cleft, ectopia cordis, and asphyxiating thoracic dystrophy (Jeune syndrome). Sternal cleft may be associated with ectopia cordis or as a component of the superior abdominal wall defect, pentalogy of Cantrell, discussed in the section on abdominal wall defects. Ectopia cordis is often complicated by the presence of severe congenital heart disease.

Axilla

Axillary lesions are most often lymphatic in origin. Benign reactive lymphadenopathy secondary to viral or bacterial infections is the most common mass. Cystic hygromas or lymphangiomas, also common in the lateral neck, may frequently appear in the axilla. These lesions may exist in continuity with cervical lesions or, more importantly, extend into the mediastinum. Plain chest

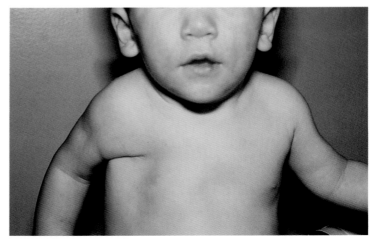

Figure 17-121. Congenital unilateral absence of the anterior ribs, muscle, and soft tissues characterize Poland syndrome, producing its typical appearance pictured here.

films or CT scan imaging (preferred) assist in delineating the anatomy. Hidradenitis, a condition related to the obstruction of sebaceous and sweat glands, commonly presents as an axillary or inguinal mass that may become superinfected and require surgical drainage.

Breast

Mastitis is a common breast problem of infancy. The evolution of fluctuance or purulence is diagnostic of a breast abscess (see Chapter 12). The presence of the condition requires aggressive antibiotic therapy (sometimes intravenous) and warm compresses. Antibiotics with broad staphylococcal and streptococcal coverage are usually adequate; however, in some cases the addition of gram-negative coverage is necessary. Restraint relative to invasive procedures, particularly incision, drainage, and debridement, should be maintained to allow spontaneous resolution with medical therapies. Damage to the breast bud may lead to permanent breast asymmetry and deformity in the future. Needle aspiration may be judiciously performed in cases in which there is significant concern about the possibility of pus. True abscess formation requires incision and drainage, and families should be warned of the potential long-term ramifications.

Localized breast masses in children are typically benign. In the preadolescent, as early as 6 or 7 years, the development of a firm mobile mass under one areola or both areolae may represent precocious thelarche. This condition may be asynchronous with a pseudotumor appearing several months ahead of the opposite side. Biopsy is never indicated in this scenario because unilateral iatrogenic amastia will result. In adolescents and teenagers, fibroadenomas account for approximately 90% of the reported masses. These smooth and mobile masses are approximately 1 to 2 cm in size. The juvenile variant of this condition may be associated with much larger lesions that cause significant breast asymmetry. The malignant potential of these lesions is low; however, excision is strongly advised because these lesions do not spontaneously resolve. Cosmetic periareolar incisions should be used to excise most tumors. Fibrocystic disease, occurring primarily in older teens and young women, is a breast condition associated with one or multiple firm, fixed, and ill-defined masses. These masses result from the hyperplasia of the fibrous parenchymal tissue of the breast. Variation in the associated symptoms and even size of these lesions with the phases of the menstrual cycle is distinctive of fibrocystic disease. This is also a benign condition. Breast malignancies are rare in the pediatric population. Phyllodes tumors, formerly cystosarcoma phyllodes, are rare fibroepithelial tumors that may be benign with aggressive local behavior leading to malignancy with the propensity for distant metastases. These tumors may be associated with significant asymmetrical gynecomastia and reach up to 40 cm in size. Surgical evaluation should be sought early. Routine monthly breast self-examination should be encouraged at puberty in all girls to aid in the detection of significant disease and to avoid undue intervention in benign conditions.

Breast masses in children should be evaluated in a systematic manner. History including details regarding medications, age of menarche, and family history of breast diseases is essential. Mammography is of limited utility in the evaluation of the dense breast tissue of children and teenagers and is strongly discouraged. Breast ultrasound

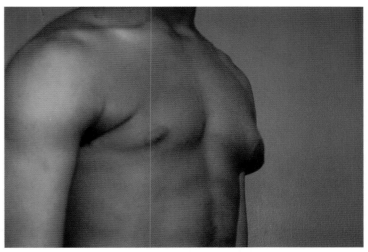

Figure 17-122. Unilateral adolescent male gynecomastia.

for cystic lesions is quite helpful and may assist with decisions to attempt needle aspiration. Larger lesions in which there are concerns regarding chest wall involvement should be evaluated by MRI. Fine-needle aspiration cytology may be necessary to further assist with diagnosis. Most breast lesions in children can be serially monitored without intervention. Excisional biopsy may then be indicated in a select group of postpubertal girls with solid discrete lesions that are increasing in size. Precautions regarding the breast biopsy in prepubertal girls have been outlined previously.

Nipple discharge is not a common complaint in the pediatric population but usually indicates the presence of a parenchymal breast lesion, ductal abnormality, or hormonal stimulation. Purulence signifies infection that usually responds to antibiotic therapy. Green or brown serous drainage is typical of a draining simple cyst. Bloody drainage in pediatric populations is most commonly due to an intraductal papilloma; however, in adults malignancy should be strongly considered. Excision of the duct is curative. Galactorrhea may be the result of endogenous hormonal stimulation from a pituitary tumor or pregnancy.

Breast lesions do occur in young men. Pubertal gynecomastia, a benign overgrowth of the glandular breast tissue, is common in the early years following the onset of puberty. The psychosocial implications of this condition are significant and justify the performance of bilateral subcutaneous mastectomy (Fig. 17-122).

Abdominal Wall

Gastroschisis and omphalocele are the two principal congenital abdominal wall defects. Omphalocele arises as a consequence of the embryonic extrusion of the developing midgut from the coelomic cavity into the yolk sac to allow midgut elongation as the abdominal wall expands to accommodate the rapidly growing viscera. Resulting central defects in the medial and lateral wall folds and umbilical ring result in a central abdominal wall deformity. This defect is covered by a sac that has an outer amniotic and inner peritoneal layers. The umbilical cord inserts into the sac. This midline defect may be of various sizes from so-called "umbilical cord hernias" to "giant omphaloceles" greater than 10 cm and may exist in the central, epigastric, and hypogastric regions (Figs. 17-123,

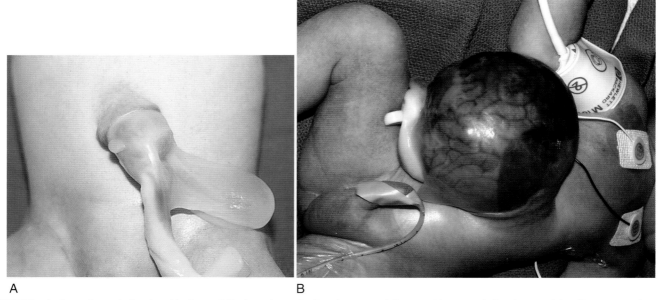

A   B

Figure 17-123. A, A small omphalocele with the umbilical cord attached to the apex of the sac. Giant omphalocele containing liver, stomach, and bowel **(B).** Chromosomal and other anomalies, particularly cardiac, are common and should be evaluated in both conditions.

17-124, and 17-125). Coexisting anomalies of other midline structures including the heart, sternum, diaphragm, and bladder may occur in 30% to 50% of all patients. Chromosomal anomalies may also be common in this population.

In contrast with omphalocele, gastroschisis is a defect of the right lateral abdominal wall. Although controversy exists as to the distinct etiology, most believe this deformity results from a vascular accident that leads to occlusion of the right umbilical vein with subsequent disruption of the end of the abdominal wall and mild evisceration. The defect is usually small in term infants; however, large amounts of bowel may lie in the amniotic cavity. This anomaly occurs early in gestation, and the bowel is left in contact with the amniotic fluid, which produces an intense inflammatory response or "peel" (Fig. 17-126). This peel is believed to alter bowel motility in the postoperative period, leading to long delays in the return of bowel function. Recent efforts have focused on earlier delivery in the 32- to 34-week gestational age range in order to diminish these deleterious effects on bowel function.

In contrast with omphalocele, gastroschisis is generally not associated with other congenital anomalies. Only 7% to 10% of patients have associated conditions, the most common of which are intestinal atresias. Ischemia due to in utero volvulus, malrotation, or incarceration through the narrow defect may lead to vascular compromise that causes an atresia (Fig. 17-127).

The surgical management of these conditions is similar. In both conditions the goal is the safe primary closure of the defect without creating an abdominal compartment syndrome that leads to pulmonary embarrassment, renal insufficiency, intestinal ischemia, or necrotizing enterocolitis either due to the size of the defect or the rigidity of the bowel. Gastroschisis constitutes a surgical emergency because the exposed bowel may become desiccated or injured. Omphaloceles, which have a protective peritoneal covering, may be managed in a more elective manner. A staged closure must be performed in some patients; this may include placement of a prosthetic Silastic silo with daily reductions (Fig. 17-128), topical desiccants such as silver sulfasalazine (Silvadene), povidone-iodine (Betadine), or merbromine. Placement of a prosthetic material

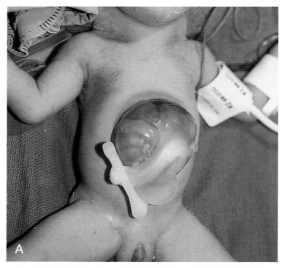

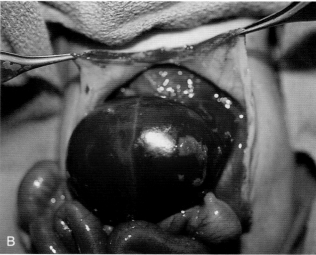

Figure 17-124. Pentalogy of Cantrell is a midline abdominal wall defect (epigastric omphalocele) **(A)** associated with anterior diaphragmatic defect, sternal cleft, ectopia cordis, and congenital heart disease (usually a ventricular septal defect) **(B).**

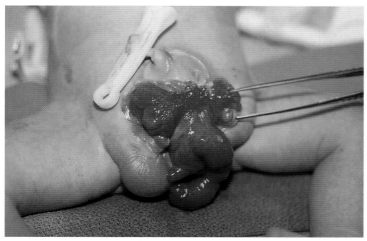

Figure 17-125. Cloacal exstrophy consists of an infraumbilical omphalocele with exstrophy of the bladder, in which the bladder is separated into halves by the exposed intestine. Both the proximal and distal loops have prolapsed, producing the "elephant trunk" appearance.

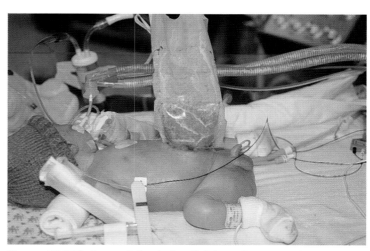

Figure 17-128. Large abdominal wall defects that cannot be closed primarily may undergo a staged closure with silo placement and daily reductions until the bowel rests comfortably in the abdominal cavity.

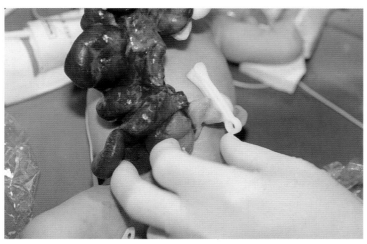

Figure 17-126. The abdominal defect lies to the right of an intact umbilical cord without a sac, and the intestines are exposed to the amniotic fluid. An inflammatory "peel" develops, which may affect motility.

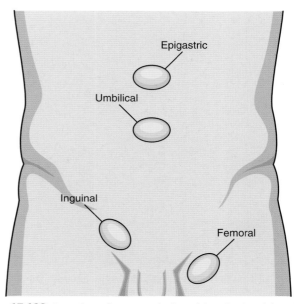

Figure 17-129. Location of commonly found hernias involving the abdominal wall.

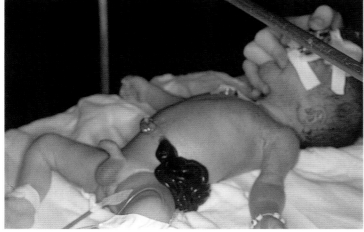

Figure 17-127. In utero volvulus may complicate gastroschisis. Occurrence of this event early in gestation may lead to intestinal atresia. Extraintestinal anomalies are rare in gastroschisis.

such as Gore-Tex (W. L. Gore & Associates, Flagstaff, Ariz.) or Surgisis (Cook Surgical, Bloomington, Ind.) may provide coverage. These infants have significant postoperative delays in the return of intestinal function and require TPN support for survival.

Umbilicus

The most common condition of the abdominal wall is an umbilical hernia (Figs. 17-129 and 17-130). This results from the failed closure of the fascial ring during the first few years of life. Following desiccation of the umbilical vessels and urachus and separation of the umbilical remnant in the first month of life, the umbilical ring typically undergoes closure in the next 2 to 3 years. In some patients this process never occurs. For unclear reasons there appears to be a strong familial and racial predilection for hernia development. This condition has been described as being up to 50 times more common in African Americans than in white populations. Since most of these lesions resolve spontaneously, repair is typically deferred

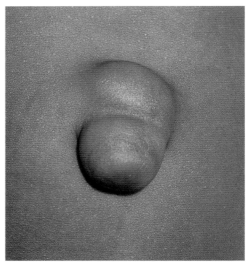

Figure 17-130. Most infants with umbilical hernia undergo spontaneous closure by age 3 to 4 years. Those that persist require repair.

Figure 17-131. Supraumbilical hernia, shown here as a crescent-shaped defect above an umbilical hernia, does not close spontaneously and requires repair.

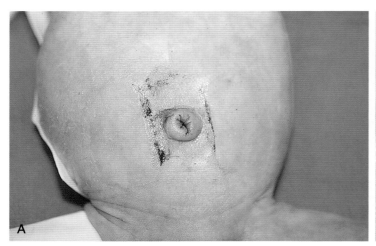

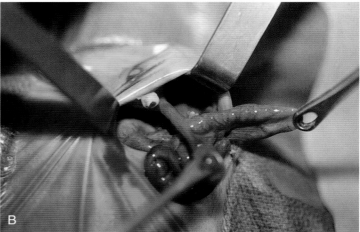

Figure 17-132. Omphalomesenteric duct remnant with communication to the umbilicus with meconium exuding from the umbilicus and meconium staining of the abdominal wall **(A)**. Intraoperative view showing omphalomesenteric duct leading from the bowel to the umbilicus **(B)**.

until the fifth birthday. Hernias that are larger than 2 cm in diameter, have a proboscoid or "elephant's trunk" appearance (usually due to a supraumbilical component) (Fig. 17-131), or have a history of incarceration should not have their surgery delayed.

Following the desiccation of the umbilical remnant there may be the persistence of a polypoid mucosal-appearing lesion at the base of the umbilicus. These are most often umbilical granulomas and represent residual hypertrophic granulation tissue at the base of the cord. These are typically managed with topical treatments including alcohol or silver nitrate sticks. Yellow serous or feculent brown drainage from an apparent umbilical granuloma should raise concerns for a patent urachus or persistence of an omphalomesenteric duct sinus. Drainage of yellow serous fluid is suspicious for urine and in the presence of a patent urachus represents the precordial connection between the allantois and the fetal bladder. The persistence of these anomalies raises concern for bladder outlet obstruction and mandates a urologic workup consisting of ultrasound of the bladder and kidney for signs of obstructive uropathy and voiding cystourethrogram. Persistence of an omphalomesenteric sinus may lead to the development of an internal hernia or volvulus (Fig.

17-132). Surgical exploration to ligate the fistula and resect the omphalomesenteric duct remnant is indicated.

Inguinal Disorders

Aberrant descent of the gonads and processus vaginalis gives rise to numerous disorders including hernias, hydroceles, undescended testicles, and testicular torsion (Fig. 17-133). During embryonic development the testicles have their origin at the base of the kidney. Testicular descent leads to an outpouching or evagination of the peritoneal cavity, the processus vaginalis, which follows the gubernaculum into the scrotum. Following completion of testicular descent, the processus vaginalis obliterates, separating the scrotum from the peritoneal cavity. Failure of obliteration results in a persistent patent processus that may allow fluid (hydrocele) or intraperitoneal viscera (intestine, bladder, or ovary) to enter the sac (Figs. 17-134 and 17-135). In girls, fusion of the processus vaginalis occurs earlier in embryonic development, which explains their markedly decreased incidence of inguinal hernias. The ovary is typically found in the hernia sac in girls (Fig. 17-136). Clinically, hernias present as bulges in the groin

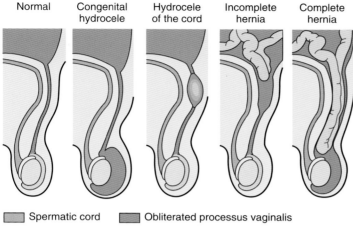

Normal   Congenital   Hydrocele   Incomplete   Complete
          hydrocele   of the cord   hernia   hernia

☐ Spermatic cord   ☐ Obliterated processus vaginalis

Figure 17-133. Abnormalities of the processus vaginalis.

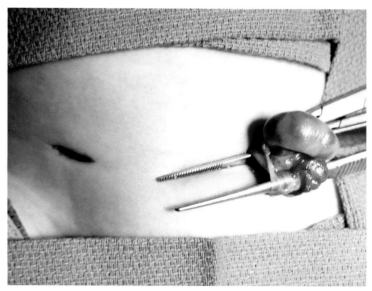

Figure 17-136. Ovaries are frequently found in the hernia sac of young girls.

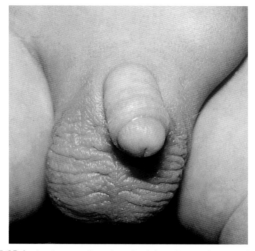

Figure 17-134. An incomplete inguinal hernia produces a bulge in the left groin but does not extend into the scrotum.

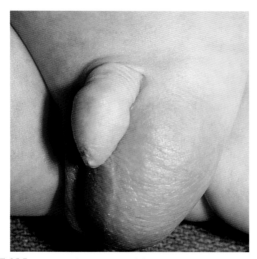

Figure 17-135. A complete inguinal hernia extends into the scrotum, obscuring the testis.

and scrotum (upper labia majora) that increase in size with Valsalva maneuvers including coughing, straining, or crying. Usually the mass reduces spontaneously or with gentle upward manual pressure on the hernia and downward testicular traction. The inability to reduce the mass should raise concerns for incarceration. Alternatively, persistent inguinoscrotal swelling may represent a nonreducible hydrocele or undescended or retractile testicle.

Identification of pediatric hernias on routine physical examination is sometimes difficult. Several provocative maneuvers including induced crying, coughing, gentle abdominal pressure, or other forced Valsalva maneuvers may be helpful. Patients should be examined in both supine and upright positions. Despite these attempts, the hernia may not be visualized. The presence of a reliable history and the palpation of a thickened processus vaginalis or "silk glove" sign are adequate evidence to proceed with herniorrhaphy. The "silk glove" sign is the sensation on direct palpation of the spermatic cord as it gently glides between two layers of tissue—"silk." This represents the layers of processus vaginalis or hernia sac. Alternatively, parents may be asked to take a picture of the inguinal region and return when a definite bulge appears. Formerly, herniograms were used to assist in the diagnosis of these difficult cases. However, the attendant complications and risk of pelvic and gonadal radiation have diminished the utility of this study. Occasionally other noninvasive studies such as ultrasound have been suggested in these difficult cases.

The presence of an inguinal hernia is an indication for prompt repair. These hernias do not resolve spontaneously and have a high risk of incarceration (up to 30%), the inability to reduce the inguinal hernia into the peritoneal cavity, in the first few months of life. Incarceration may be due to strangulation. Strangulated hernias develop intestinal and/or testicular ischemia with subsequent infarction due to vascular entrapment. Incarceration is associated with severe irritability and emesis. The groin hernia becomes erythematous, edematous, and tender. Signs of complete intestinal obstruction may occur with associated ileus, emesis, and bloody stools. Systemic sepsis from bowel ischemia may occur.

Acute scrotal inflammation is often a surgical emergency (Fig. 17-137). This may occur not only with incarcerated inguinal hernias but also with other important conditions such as torsion of the testicle, torsion of the appendix testis, testicular trauma, and epididymoorchitis. Testicular torsion is associated with an acutely tender testicle that may be retracted toward the inguinal region and lie in a somewhat transverse orientation in the scrotum (Fig. 17-138). Torsion of the appendix testis is associated with the "blue dot" sign, which may be seen

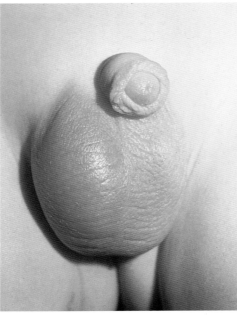

Figure 17-137. A red, tender hemiscrotum may be due to torsion of the testis with gangrene, a surgical emergency.

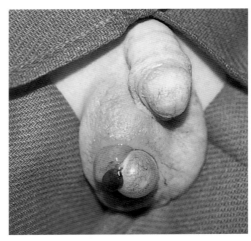

Figure 17-139. The congested, twisted appendix testis contrasts with the normal pale pink testis. If the appendix testis can be identified through the scrotum, scrotal exploration is unnecessary. This torsed appendix testis may appear through the translucent skin as a "blue dot" sign.

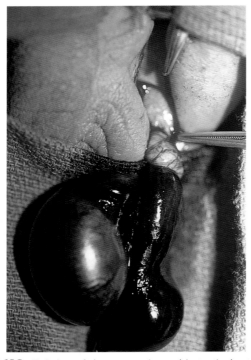

Figure 17-138. Twisting of the spermatic cord in testicular torsion pulls the testis proximally, making it lie in a transverse axis. The dark, congested epididymis is seen overlying and to the left of the testis.

through the translucent scrotal skin of infants and young children (Fig. 17-139). This condition does not require surgery if an accurate diagnosis can be made. An antecedent history of testicular injury may assist in distinguishing testicular trauma from an incarcerated hernia. A digital rectal examination is one of the most reliable means of determining whether there is incarcerated hernia in an infant. Transrectal palpation of the internal inguinal ring for the presence of a mass or fullness suggests incarceration. Trans-scrotal transillumination is not always a reliable means of distinguishing between a hydrocele and incarcerated hernia. Occasionally the thin-walled dilated

bowel may transilluminate, giving the misleading impression that a hydrocele is present. Epididymo-orchitis may be associated with urinary tract symptoms or previous viral or bacterial urinary tract infection.

Hydroceles are most common in infancy and diminish significantly during childhood. They appear as scrotal swellings that may have a diurnal variation in size, often largest in the evening and smaller or absent in the morning. Most hydroceles are isolated to the scrotal region. However, occasionally an isolated inguinal hydrocele may exist that mimics an incarcerated hernia. The classic means of diagnosing hydrocele is by transillumination. Hydroceles that appear at birth are usually noncommunicating and undergo spontaneous resolution over the first year of life. Those that persist beyond 12 to 18 months of age typically have a persistent communication with the peritoneal cavity and need surgical care (Fig. 17-140). Hydroceles may also develop in older children in response to infection or trauma. Persistent hydroceles also require surgical repair. Femoral hernias are uncommon in children (Fig. 17-141).

Anus and Rectum

Most congenital anorectal anomalies are clinically apparent at birth. Bilious emesis, poor feeding, abdominal distention, and delayed or absent passage of meconium may herald the presence of a distal obstruction. Imperforate anus is the general category assigned to these patients and may present in one of three principal anatomic groups. These rectal anomalies are classified on the basis of the position of the rectum and the levator ani muscle complex. Low imperforate anus is associated with the passage of the rectum through the levator ani, and a fistulous tract extends to the perineal region ending in the center of a ridge of tissue on the anus ("bucket handle" deformity) (Fig. 17-142) or anterior to these structures as a perineal fistula (Fig. 17-143). In male infants the fistula may travel in the median raphe of the scrotum, and the meconium may be seen as a string of white or black beads (Fig. 17-144). The prognosis is generally favorable for low lesions because they lie within the levator ani complex. In contrast, high lesions do not pass through the levator ani. A visible fistula does not exist. Most commonly the rectal fistula ends in the prostatic urethra, bulbar urethra, or

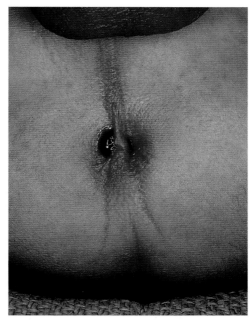

Figure 17-142. A spot of meconium is visible beneath a "bucket handle" bridge of skin in an infant with a low imperforate anus.

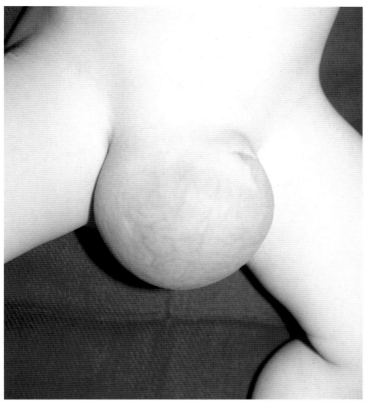

Figure 17-140. Bilateral congenital hydroceles with buried penis. Groin swellings are absent, distinguishing them from hernias. The fluid collections may fluctuate in size, filling and emptying through a patent processus vaginalis. Spontaneous closure of the processus and absorption of fluid around the testis generally occurs, reserving hydrocelectomy for those that persist after age 2 years.

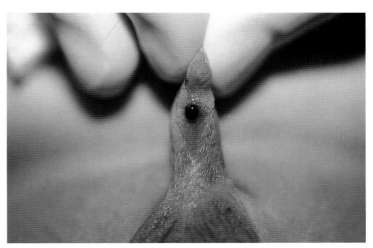

Figure 17-143. In male infants, white mucus or black meconium may extend through a low perineal fistula to the midline scrotal raphe to the level of the penis.

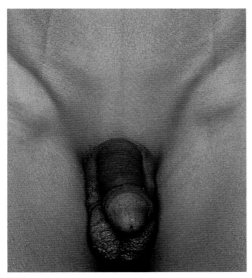

Figure 17-141. Swelling lying below the inguinal ligament identifies femoral hernias, extremely rare in childhood.

bladder neck in males or above the hymen in girls. Meconium is passed with urine via the urethra in males (Fig. 17-145) or transvaginally in females (Fig. 17-146). A variant of high imperforate anus is a cloacal anomaly, which is a complex congenital anomaly in which the urethra, vagina, and rectum share a single perineal opening (Fig. 17-147). The third variant represents intermediate lesions that are partially within the levator ani complex (Fig. 17-148). The surgical management of these lesions is currently undergoing major reevaluation. However, the classic approach

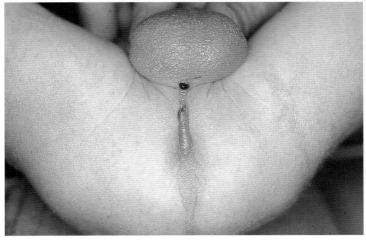

Figure 17-144. Low imperforate anus in a male infant. White mucus or black meconium may pass through a perineal fistula from a low imperforate anus into the scrotal raphe.

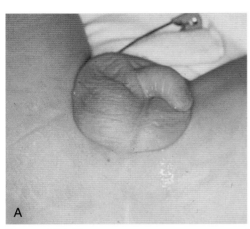
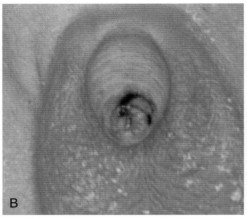
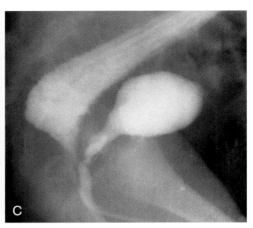

Figure 17-145. **A,** No visible external opening forms in high imperforate anus. Absence of the intergluteal cleft is also common, frequently associated with sacral agenesis. **B,** Meconium passes into the bladder or urethra through a rectal fistula and appears in the urine. **C,** Retrograde urethrography demonstrates the rectourethral fistula.

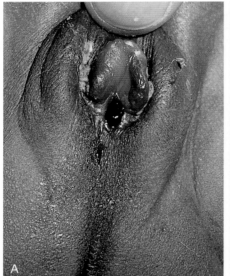
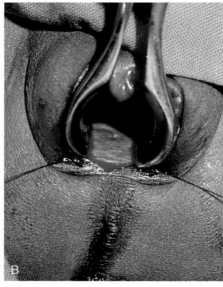

Figure 17-146. A high imperforate anus communicates into the vagina. Meconium is passed through the vagina **(A).** Vaginoscopy reveals the fistula on the posterior wall of the vagina well above the hymen **(B).** A bicornuate uterus accompanies rectovaginal fistula in high lesions in girls.

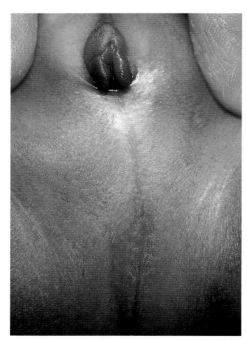
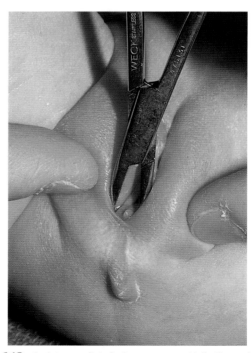

Figure 17-147. Cloacal anomaly is the most complete expression of imperforate anus in girls, with urinary, genital, and intestinal tracts converging into a single cloacal channel that exists as the sole perineal opening.

Figure 17-148. An intermediate lesion passes partially through the levator ani but fails to approach the perineum as closely as low lesions.

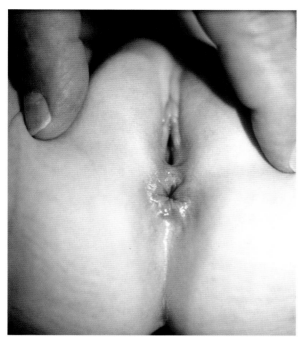

Figure 17-149. Anteriorly displaced anus partially within the anal sphincter complex.

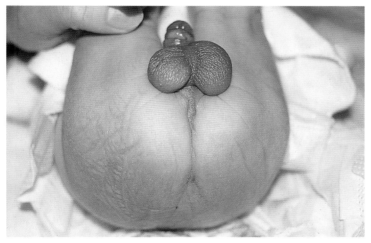

Figure 17-150. Bifid scrotum in an infant with imperforate anus is indicative of a high lesion and the likely presence of other anomalies.

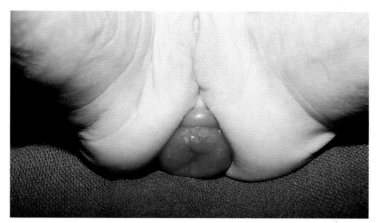

Figure 17-151. Although the cause of rectal prolapse is unknown in the majority of cases, all infants should be evaluated for cystic fibrosis.

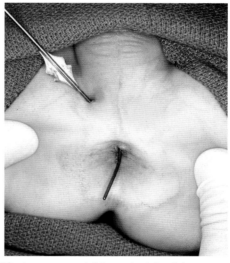

Figure 17-152. A punctum visible to the left of the anus with a lacrimal duct probe communicates to a crypt in the anal canal by a fistulous tract. Recurrent abscesses arise from a well-formed fistula like this one, an indication for fistulectomy.

to the care for patients with low lesions is a one-stage repair, or perineal anoplasty (Fig. 17-149). Patients with high and intermediate lesions classically undergo staged repairs with a primary colostomy at birth followed by a perineal pull-through at a later age. Several months following the pull-through they return for their colostomy closure. The prognosis for fecal continence is excellent in patients with low lesions. Because they partially extend into the levator, intermediate lesions also tend to have good outcomes. The prognosis for high lesions is more guarded due in part to the presence of associated congenital anomalies and the quality of the reconstruction (Fig. 17-150).

Rectal prolapse is an uncommon condition that is most often idiopathic in children (Fig. 17-151). The peak incidence of idiopathic rectal prolapse occurs in the second year of life, often precipitated by episodes of diarrheal illnesses, efforts to toilet train or severe constipation. This process responds spontaneously after the resolution of the acute illness or with dietary and medical manipulations

to treat the constipation. Nonidiopathic cases are often related to neurologic conditions or chronic diseases. Abnormalities in the development of the muscles of the pelvic floor or the innervation occur in patients with spina bifida and related spinal cord abnormalities. Refractory cases should be evaluated for chronic hookworm infestation with stool evaluations for ova and parasites, which may cause severe tenesmus and straining. Rectal polyps may precipitate prolapse by acting as a lead point for this form of rectal intussusception. Evaluation by contrast enema and sigmoidoscopy are important components of the assessment of children with recurrent episodes. Cystic fibrosis is another common cause of prolapse and should be evaluated in patients with this condition. Surgery is rarely indicated. Circumferential submucosal injections with concentrated dextrose functions as a sclerosant that prevents prolapse from recurring.

Anorectal abscess is a common condition in the first 6 to 10 months of life. The lesions arise from infections of the submucosal crypt glands found along the dentate line. Significant fluctuance requires incision and drainage followed by warm soaks or sitz baths. Recurrent episodes of infection, although rare, may give rise to a fistula-in-ano or chronically draining sinus (Fig. 17-152). Anal fistulectomy with debridement of the tract is usually curative.

Minor degrees of incontinence may complicate this procedure. Chronic recurrent anal fistulas may indicate the presence of Crohn disease, chronic granulomatous disease, or immunodeficiency. Patients with a persistent or refractory condition should be thoroughly evaluated for these entities.

Anal fissure, discussed previously as a cause of gastrointestinal bleeding, is common in young infants. Hemorrhoids are less common in children and typically respond to nonoperative maneuvers.

Acknowledgment

I would like to thank Nancy Van Balen, RN, and Nathaniel Cook for their patience and assistance in the operating room while taking many of these photographs.

Bibliography

Ashcraft KW, Murphy JP, Sharp RL, et al: Pediatric Surgery, 3rd ed. Philadelphia, WB Saunders, 1999.

O'Neil JA Jr, Rowe MI: Pediatric Surgery, 5th ed. St Louis, Mosby–Year Book, 1998.

Rowe MI, O'Neil JA Jr, Grosfeld JL, et al: Essentials of Pediatric Surgery. St Louis, Mosby–Year Book, 1994.

CHAPTER 18

Pediatric and Adolescent Gynecology

Pamela J. Murray and Holly W. Davis

Pediatricians and other primary care physicians who treat children and adolescents are regularly confronted with patients with gynecologic complaints. This trend stems in part from earlier onset of puberty and of sexual activity and consequent concerns about pregnancy prevention and sexually transmitted diseases (STDs). In addition, there is increased media interest in and consequently greater public and family discussion of sexual and gynecologic subjects. Today, young women and their mothers are more inclined to seek medical attention for reproductive system problems including dysmenorrhea, abnormal uterine bleeding, and vaginal discharges. The increased survival of children with chronic illnesses creates another patient group in need of skilled and sensitive attention to the psychological and physiologic aspects of their sexual development.

Among primary care physicians there is a growing interest in gynecologic pediatrics and adolescent medicine. Many are increasing their understanding of the gynecologic conditions affecting children and adolescents including vulvovaginitis, STDs, menstrual disorders, and sexual abuse. In the current practice environment there are pressures and incentives to evaluate and treat problems without referral, incorporating gynecologic health concerns into primary care. Hence, an adolescent's first pelvic examination may no longer require transferring "well-child care" to a gynecologist. Accordingly, this chapter emphasizes normal anatomy, techniques of examination, and the pathologic conditions most commonly encountered: obstructive anatomic abnormalities, gynecologic trauma, inflammation, and infections.

Chapter 6 provides a more detailed description of the approach to sexual abuse and an outline of specimen collection in the prepubertal girl. Chapter 9 illustrates Tanner staging and discusses normal, delayed, and precocious pubertal development.

Normal Female Genitalia

Newborn and Prepubertal Periods

In the newborn girl the physical appearance of the genitalia reflects stimulation by maternal sex hormones. The labia majora appear puffy, and the thickened labia minora protrude between them (Fig. 18-1). Separation of the labia minora reveals thick, redundant hymenal folds that often hide the small central vaginal opening and urethral meatus. The mucosa is pink and moist, vaginal pH is acidic, and a milky discharge (physiologic leukorrhea) is seen often. Vaginal bleeding during the first week of life is common. It is caused by withdrawal of maternal estrogen following delivery, and parents can be reassured that this is normal. Breast development with palpable breast tissue, engorgement, and less commonly a clear or cloudy discharge is observed in full-term neonates of both genders (see Chapter 2). Without ongoing estrogen stimulation, these findings gradually subside over several months as maternal estrogen levels fall. During this period, infants are at increased risk for developing breast inflammation and infection (see Chapter 12). Local trauma including squeezing may increase the likelihood of infection.

Similarly, the effect of maternal hormones on the female genitalia gradually disappears; the labia majora lose their fullness, and the labia minora and hymen become thinner and flatter. Separation of the labia minora usually exposes the vaginal opening (Fig. 18-2). As the young infant matures, the labia cover less of the vaginal vestibule, particularly when the infant or child is sitting, and thus offer incomplete protection from external sources of irritation. The mucosa is thin and relatively atrophic and has a glistening, reddish-pink hue. On first inspection this normal red vascular appearance is sometimes mistaken for inflammation by observers unaccustomed to examining prepubertal genitalia. Vaginal pH is now neutral or alkaline, and secretions are minimal.

Physiologic changes also cause variations in the appearance of the hymenal tissues during childhood. During early infancy the tissues remain relatively thick and often are redundant (Fig. 18-3A and B), but in the first months of life, the hymen becomes thin and translucent, with smooth edges (see Figs. 18-2 and 18-3C to D). When the child enters puberty, the hymen again thickens under the influence of estrogen.

The shape of the vaginal orifice also varies. *Annular* (see Fig. 18-3C), *crescentic* (see Fig. 18-3D and E), and *fimbriated* (which has fingerlike projections around the hymenal rim) hymens are all normal variations. Other irregular shapes occur, such as a teardrop with the narrow portion formed by an anterior notch to one side of the clitoris (see Fig. 18-6A and D). On rare occasions a complete septum (see Fig. 18-3E) or a fenestrated hymen with small perforations is seen.

From about 6 to 8 weeks of age until puberty the perineum, perivaginal tissues, and pelvic supporting structures are relatively rigid and inelastic. This factor increases the likelihood of tearing as a result of trauma. In addition, before the onset of puberty, the ovaries are positioned above the pelvic brim. This intra-abdominal location accounts for the fact that ovarian disorders in childhood frequently present with abdominal rather than pelvic signs and symptoms.

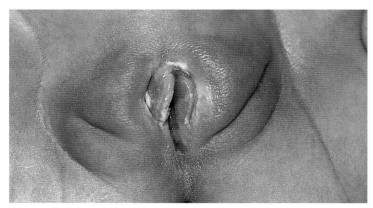

Figure 18-1. Normal appearance of the genitalia in a newborn girl. The labia majora are full, and the thickened labia minora protrude between them. The mucosa is pink, and a milky white discharge is seen, reflecting stimulation by maternal hormones. (Courtesy Ian Holzman, MD, Mt. Sinai Medical Center, New York.)

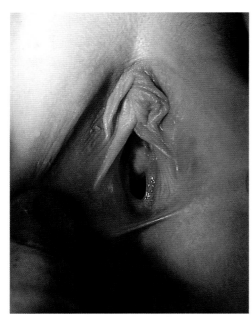

Figure 18-2. Normal appearance of the genitalia of a 2-year-old girl. The labia majora are flattened, and the labia minora and hymen are thin and flat. The vaginal orifice is easily seen, and the mucosa is thin, relatively atrophic, and red in color. Visualization was assisted by use of the labial traction technique with the patient in the semisupine lithotomy position.

Peripubertal Period

With the onset of puberty the mons pubis begins to thicken and midline hair begins to grow. Fat deposition fills out the labia majora. The labia minora thicken, become softer and more rounded, and asymmetry and variations in size and shape become more evident. The clitoris enlarges slightly, and the estrogen-responsive urethral mucosa is altered, becoming more prominent. The hymen also thickens as its central orifice enlarges. The vaginal mucosa thickens and softens and becomes moist and pink as secretions increase and pH levels drop. Perineal and pelvic tissues become more elastic, and the ovaries gradually descend into the pelvis. In the months preceding menarche, physiologic leukorrhea increases and becomes noticeable. It consists of a white discharge containing mature epithelial cells and vaginal secretions stimulated by estrogen (Fig. 18-4). In some girls the unopposed estrogen secretion of puberty stimulates leukorrhea so profuse that it becomes concerning and irritating because the perineum is constantly moist. The developmental aspects of gynecologic anatomy and physiology are summarized in Table 18-1. The Tanner stages of pubertal development are presented in Chapter 9.

Gynecologic Evaluation

Examination of the Prepubertal Patient

Indications

Inspection of the external genitalia should be a part of each general physical examination. Careful perineal inspection of girls during the first several well-child visits enables early identification of congenital anomalies of the labia and hymen. Anomalies of these external structures are relatively uncommon and, with the exception of distal or complete vaginal agenesis, are not associated with malformations of the upper genital or urinary tract.

Evidence of virilization noted in the newborn, especially when accompanied by hyperpigmentation, should prompt immediate laboratory investigation for evidence of salt-losing adrenal hyperplasia and warrants urgent endocrinology referral.

The proximal vagina, uterus, cervix, and fallopian tubes are derived from the müllerian or paramesonephric ducts and develop concurrently with the urinary tract. Thus girls with renal or urinary tract abnormalities are at greater risk for having associated anomalies of internal genital structures. During puberty, if menarche is delayed or menstrual periods are unusually problematic (e.g., excessive pain, unusually irregular flow patterns), ultrasound evaluation should be considered. Ultrasonography has also proved useful in evaluating neonates for suspected upper genital tract anomalies because these structures are relatively large during the neonatal period due to the influence of maternal hormones and higher levels of gonadotrophins. Later in infancy and during childhood before puberty they may be difficult to detect because of their small size, although this is less of a problem with skilled pediatric technicians and radiologists and more sensitive contemporary equipment. Hence failure to visualize internal genital structures in prepubertal girls does not equate with agenesis and, in such cases, magnetic resonance imaging can clarify the presence or absence of pelvic organs.

Continuing the practice of routine inspection of the external genitalia at each well-child visit beyond infancy is recommended because it assists early diagnosis of any new problems that may arise. This practice also creates an opportunity to discuss normal anatomy and behaviors including masturbation; to distinguish acceptable from unacceptable (exploitative or abusive) forms of touching; and to help overcome the reluctance of some parents and children to express concerns about the genitalia. Ultimately, making assessment and counseling a routine part of well-child care may help reduce anxiety and embarrassment for the child when genital or pelvic examinations are recommended after puberty.

Patients who have specific complaints at acute care visits warrant inspection of the genitalia and, on occasion, colposcopic, radiologic, or internal examination. These complaints include abdominal pain; dysuria, urinary frequency, urgency, incontinence, or enuresis; constipation or encopresis; perineal pruritus and/or pain; vaginal discharge or bleeding before menarche; and suspected or acknowledged sexual abuse.

Technique

Whether the patient is being seen for a routine checkup or for a specific problem, the gynecologic portion of the assessment should occur only after establishing rapport to avoid frightening the child. Because parents and health care providers communicate their own comfort levels to their children both verbally and nonverbally, a discussion of any parental anxieties and the clinician's self-awareness of his or her own attitudes can assist successful examination. The use of pictures and terms or language familiar to the child may further enhance cooperation, but interspersing anatomically correct vocabulary also can be educational. Careful evaluation of physical growth and secondary sex characteristics is important for patients in the peripubertal and pubertal periods, and all children with potential gynecologic problems deserve a thorough

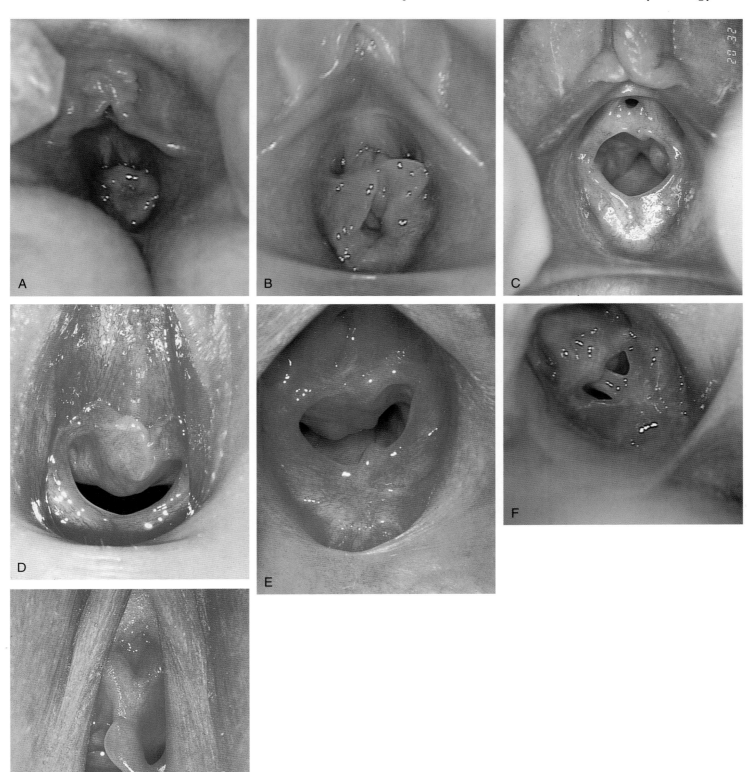

Figure 18-3. Normal variations in hymenal configuration. **A,** In this young infant the redundant hymen totally obscures the vaginal orifice. **B,** In a 23-month-old, although hymenal folds are redundant, the central orifice is visible. **C,** Annular orifice of a 2-year-old. Note the thin, sharp edges of the hymenal membrane. **D,** Crescentic hymenal orifice. **E,** Crescentic orifice with septal remnants at 1 and 5 o'clock. **F** and **G,** Two variations of a septate hymen are seen, one in an infant and another in an older child. See also Figure 18-6. (**A** and **B,** Courtesy Janet Squires, MD, Children's Hospital of Pittsburgh; **C,** Courtesy John McCann, MD, University of California at Davis; **D, E,** and **G,** Courtesy Pat Bruno, MD, Sunbury Community Hospital Center for Child Protection, Sunbury, Pa; **F,** Courtesy Carol Byers, CRNP, Children's Hospital of Pittsburgh.)

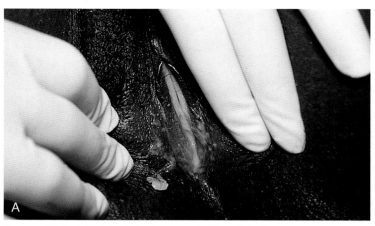
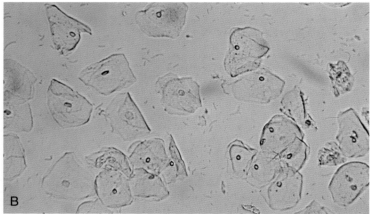

Figure 18-4. Physiologic leukorrhea. **A,** The clinical appearance of this milky discharge is seen on the perineum of this normal adolescent. It consists of cervical and vaginal secretions produced in response to estrogen stimulation and is evident in the newborn, peripubertal, and postpubertal periods. **B,** On microscopy the discharge is found to contain sheets of estrogenized vaginal epithelial cells. Leukocytes are not increased, and lactobacilli are the predominant flora.

Table 18-1	Developmental Gynecologic Anatomy and Physiology			
	NEWBORN	**EARLY CHILDHOOD**	**PERIPUBERTY (8-13 YR)**	**POSTMENARCHE (>13 YR)**
Ovary	Not palpable 0.1-0.2 cc	Pelvic brim 0.7-0.9 cc	Within pelvis 2-10 cc	$1.5 \times 2.5 \times 4$ cm 15 cc
Uterine length (cm)	2.5-4.0	2.0-3.0	3.2-5.4	8.0 (nulliparous) ($8 \times 5 \times 2.5$)
Corpus-cervix ratio	3 : 1	2 : 1	1 : 1	2-3 : 1
Vaginal length (cm)	4	4-5	7-8.5	10-12
Hymen				
Orifice diameter (mm)	1-4	1-6	5-10	10
Thickness	Thick	Thin	Thickening	—
Clitoris				
Width (mm)	5	2-5	2-5	≤10
Length (mm)	10-15			15-20
Labia minora	Smooth	Smooth, flat	Progressive increase in size and texture	Tanner stages IV-V completed
Labia majora	Hairless, prominent	Hairless, thin	Hair growth, vulval growth	Separation and differentiation of labia minora and majora
Vaginal secretions	Whitish-clear, copious	Minimal	Physiologic leukorrhea	Physiologic leukorrhea may decrease
pH	5.5-7.0	6.5-7.5	4.5-5.5	3.5-5.0
Normal flora	Maternal enteric	Nonpathogenic flora including staphylococci and coliforms	Mixed vaginal flora	Lactobacilli dominant
Hormonal influence	Maternal hormones	Minimal sex steroids	Low and variable levels of endogenous estrogen and androgens	High levels of endogenous cyclic hormones
Maturation index of vaginal epithelium			Proliferative phase*	Secretory phase[†]
Parabasal (%)	0	90-100	20-70	0 0
Intermediate (%)	95	0-10	25-50	70 95
Superficial (%)	5	10	10-20	30 5

*First half of cycle.
[†]Second half of cycle.

abdominal and inguinal examination and may warrant a rectal examination as well.

For routine checkups the task is simple external inspection. In such instances, after abdominal and inguinal examination, the clinician generally can say to patients old enough to understand, "Now, I need to take a look at your bottom, and you can help me." The desired position for examination can be explained or demonstrated, and the patient shown how to maneuver into it. Drapes are generally unnecessary for toddlers and preschoolers because they are isolating and often perceived as threatening. However, school-age children may find drapes helpful in reducing embarrassment, as do some adolescents.

Young infants can be assessed easily on an examination table after being positioned by the examiner. Older infants,

toddlers, and preschool children tend to be more relaxed when examined on their mother's lap, with the mother assisting by gently holding the child in either the frog-leg or lithotomy position (Fig. 18-5). School-age children can usually be examined on the table in the frog-leg, lithotomy, or knee-chest position (see Chapter 6). Knee-chest positioning enables the best visualization of the hymen and the distal vagina and may even permit inspection of the cervix because on deep breathing the vaginal orifice tends to open widely (Fig. 18-6A). This phenomenon also assists specimen collection. Although the knee-chest position is unacceptable to some patients who feel threatened by examination from behind, it can be useful for many school-age patients and even for younger children with careful preparation and with use of a combination of

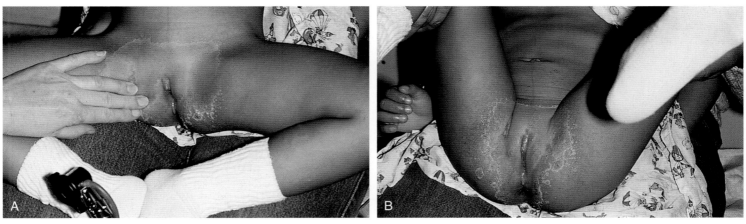

Figure 18-5. Optimal positions for perineal inspection of the young prepubertal girl. **A,** Frog-leg position on the mother's lap. **B,** Lithotomy position on the mother's lap.

Figure 18-6. Perineal visualization in various positions and with different techniques of parting the labia. **A,** Knee-chest position. **B,** Semisupine lithotomy position with labial separation. To assist visualization of the introitus and lower third of the vagina, the examiner can either press down and laterally on the labia majora with the index and middle fingers of both hands as shown here or gently grasp the labia majora between thumbs and index fingers and pull forward and laterally—labial traction. **C,** Supine frog-leg position with labial separation. **D,** Supine frog-leg position with labial traction. **A, C,** and **D** are views of the same child, taken on the same day, and clearly show the variations in appearance using different positions and different techniques. **B** and Figure 18-2 are two views of another child. (**A, C,** and **D,** Courtesy Mary Carrasco, MD, Mercy Hospital, Pittsburgh.)

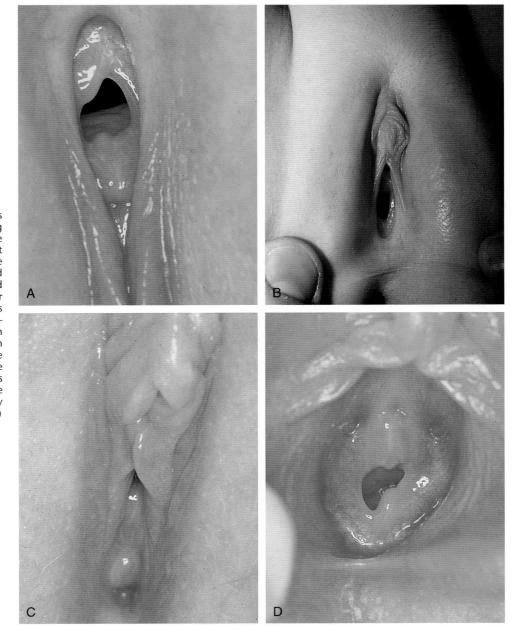

support and distraction during the assessment. An alternative means of achieving visualization of the distal vagina is with the patient supine and use of the Valsalva maneuver (i.e., asking the child to push down as if she is going to have a stool). This often produces distention of the distal vagina and hymenal orifice, assisting visualization and atraumatic collection of specimens.

Use of good focused lighting is essential. In the office setting the otoscope provides excellent focused light and low magnification, which is sufficient for most examinations. Because some young children fear otoscopy due to prior painful experiences, the patient should be reassured ahead of time that no speculum will be attached and that she will not be forcibly restrained. Preliminary "examination" of the umbilicus (belly button) may help allay anxiety. Colposcopes and hand-held lenses also provide excellent magnification when available.

Once the patient is in position, visualization of the introitus, hymen, and lower portion of the vagina is assisted by maneuvers that separate the labia. These maneuvers should be explained first, and the child reassured that the examiner is just going to look. If the patient desires or is mildly anxious, she may place her hands beneath the examiner's, or the mother may be enlisted to perform the maneuver. Some girls prefer to separate their labia themselves. The maneuvers include *labial separation,* which is achieved by pressing down and laterally with the index and middle fingers of both hands on the lower portion of the labia majora (see Fig. 18-6B), and *labial traction,* which involves grasping the labia majora between the thumbs and index fingers and gently pulling them down, laterally and slightly toward the examiner (see Fig. 18-6D). When using hand-held light (otoscope), a second set of hands (parent or nurse) may be necessary to maximize labial separation and focus the light. Care must be taken to ensure that excess traction is not applied during these maneuvers because it can result in painful tearing of labial adhesions, if present.

If the patient is unusually anxious about the procedure and cannot be reassured, the examination should be deferred to a later date. Occasionally conscious sedation of the patient or anesthesia may be necessary for an adequate evaluation. At no time should a frightened, struggling child be physically restrained and forced to undergo examination; the yield is minimal, and the experience physically and emotionally traumatic.

On inspection the physician can readily ascertain the presence or absence of pubic hair; note the appearance and configuration of the labia majora, labia minora, clitoris, urethra, hymen, and vaginal orifice; observe the color of the mucosa and the presence or absence of rash or discharge; and often visualize the distal vagina. Vaginoscopy is required only occasionally in the prepubertal child and then only in those with specific problems. Such problems include vaginal bleeding with or without evidence of trauma, discharges resistant to routine therapy, a suspected vaginal foreign body, and suspected vaginal tumors. Because of the high potential for inflicting pain, especially if the patient moves suddenly, vaginoscopy generally is best performed under anesthesia or sedation. Some older school-age children may tolerate internal examination by a highly skilled examiner without sedation if preparation is careful. Again, a traumatic experience should be avoided.

If a prepubertal child with vaginal discharge or perineal or urinary complaints is to be evaluated, it is advisable to ask the family not to bathe the patient or apply any creams for at least 12 hours before the examination. Similarly, adolescents should be advised never to douche or use tampons or feminine hygiene products before an examination. The patient should always be prepared for the procedure with simple and truthful explanations.

Specimen Collection

When specimens of vaginal secretions are required for cultures, wet mounts, cytology, or maturation index, they can be collected easily and with little or no discomfort by use of Dacron wire swabs premoistened with sterile nonbacteriostatic saline. Before starting, it is often helpful to allow the patient to handle a moistened swab and touch herself with it. However, if collection is likely to be difficult because of pain or anxiety or because the hymenal orifice is small, application of a topical anesthetic ointment to the perineal and hymenal area beforehand can be beneficial. Although topical lidocaine preparations work within 5 to 10 minutes, they can produce transient discomfort before onset of anesthetic action, reducing cooperation in some patients. When time permits, use of lidocaine-prilocaine (EMLA) cream is an excellent alternative. It also provides effective local anesthesia for minor elective surgical procedures such as removal of skin tags and hymenal septae.

Routine bacterial cultures including those for gonococci can be collected from any visible discharge on the perineum in the prepubertal child. *Chlamydia* cultures, however, must contain superficial epithelial cells from the vaginal wall. Herpes cultures should be obtained from the base of unroofed fresh vesicles or ulcers. When a patient presenting with a complaint of vaginal discharge has no discharge visible on the perineum at the time of examination, having her perform a Valsalva maneuver may bring some discharge down to the introitus. If this fails and specimens must be collected because of a history of discharge or suspicion of sexual abuse, a small premoistened Dacron swab is inserted gently through the vaginal opening with care taken to avoid contact with the hymen, which is exquisitely sensitive unless preanesthetized, as described earlier. This is most easily accomplished with the patient in the knee-chest position or with use of the Valsalva maneuver. Dry cotton-tipped swabs should be avoided because they tend to abrade the thin vaginal mucosa of the prepubertal child. Table 18-2 lists the specimens that may be considered in evaluating patients with symptoms of vulvitis, vaginitis, or vaginal discharge.

The newer nucleic acid amplification tests (NAATs) are highly sensitive and specific in detecting *Neisseria gonorrhoeae* and *Chlamydia trachomatis* and offer the advantage that specimens may be collected from a variety of sites (e.g., vaginal wall, urine, urethra, cervix). Product variations necessitate careful adherence to the manufacturer's instructions regarding acceptable collection sites or specimens to ensure optimal results; some permit urine, others require vaginal secretions. Although these tests can obviate some of the difficulties in specimen collection, they are still not accepted as best evidence in court cases. Hence obtaining specimens for gonorrhea and *Chlamydia* cultures is advised when forensic evidence is necessary. In addition, in cases of symptomatic gonococcal infection in which there are concerns about antibiotic resistance, a culture with sensitivities may also be desirable to ensure proper antibiotic selection because sensitivities are not part of NAATs. When suspicious of infection with *Trichomonas* in a prepubertal patient, because of a history of sexual abuse, or wet preparation findings, a confirmation by culture incubated in Diamond's medium or with the In-pouch system is recommended. In a few settings the Affirm VP III system that uses a DNA probe may be available; PCR confirmation exists but is not commercially available.

Table 18-2 Laboratory Investigations Contributing to the Diagnosis of Vulvovaginitis with Vaginal Discharge

LABORATORY STUDY	INDICATION
Saline wet mount	Inflammatory cells, yeast, *Trichomonas,* clue cells, lactobacilli, mature and immature epithelial cells, pinworms, sperm
Gram stain	Inflammatory cells, gram-negative intracellular diplococci (gonorrhea), other bacteria, clue cells
KOH	Yeast, "whiff test" for bacterial vaginosis (also can be positive for *Trichomonas*)
Vaginal pH	Bacterial vaginosis, *Trichomonas* (lateral or anterior wall, not pooled secretions)
Cervical/vaginal cultures	Routine culture for normal flora, nonvenereal pathogens; gonorrhea culture; culture in stool transport media for enteric bacteria, especially *Shigella;* anaerobic cultures; viral culture for HSV; *Chlamydia* culture (for forensic evidence); *Mycoplasma* and *Ureaplasma* cultures; *Trichomonas* culture
Urethral cultures	*Chlamydia,* gonorrhea, *Trichomonas*
Pap smear—conventional or liquid preparation	Squamous intraepithelial lesions; precancerous and cancerous cervical lesions: nonspecific inflammation or evidence suggestive of HPV (koilocytes), HSV, fungi,* *Trichomonas,** or *Chlamydia;* cell maturation index (estrogenization), HPV typing
Tzanck smear (Giemsa stain)	HSV (multinucleated giant cells)
Perianal Scotch tape test	Pinworms and eggs
Serologic tests	RPR and other serologic tests for syphilis, HIV titers, hepatitis serology, HSV typing
Urine tests	Urinalysis, urine culture, *Trichomonas*
Nucleic acid amplification tests	*Chlamydia,* gonorrhea
Antigen-detection assays	*Chlamydia* (Chlamydiazyme)
Biopsy	Dysplastic, atrophic, and unusual lesions of vulva, vagina, and cervix

*See text; do not treat on the basis of Pap results alone.
HPV, human papillomavirus; HSV, herpes simplex virus; RPR, rapid plasma reagin.

Patients with precocious puberty, suspected abdominal masses, suspected vaginal foreign body, and/or abdominal pain should undergo rectal bimanual examination (vaginal bimanual examination is rarely, if ever, necessary). Use of adequate lubricant, having the child perform a Valsalva maneuver as the finger is inserted into the rectum, and gentle technique reduce discomfort. In most cases this can be accomplished readily in the office. If the patient is unable to cooperate, the procedure should be deferred and an examination under anesthesia considered, when warranted on the basis of clinical circumstances or the results of ancillary studies such as sonography, computed tomography, or magnetic resonance imaging.

Examination of the Adolescent or Pubertal Patient

Indications

A pelvic examination should be considered part of the evaluation of any adolescent with a variety of specific complaints and concerns (Table 18-3). These include abnormal vaginal discharge; pelvic, abdominal, or perineal pain or dysuria; severe dysmenorrhea, amenorrhea, oligomenorrhea, polymenorrhea, or abnormal uterine bleeding; sexual contact with a partner with a suspected or confirmed STD; and suspected sexual abuse. Certain concerns with pubertal development require inspection of the external genitalia and assessment of internal pelvic structures either by internal examination or by radiologic imaging. These include absence of menarche in a girl with mature secondary sex characteristics 2 years after the onset of puberty; hirsutism and/or masculinization; abnormal sequence of pubertal development; anatomic genital anomalies; lack of secondary sex characteristics by age 14; and absence of menarche by age 16. Furthermore, the pelvic examination is an important part of routine health care for sexually active adolescent girls (Table 18-4) and should be given serious consideration when requested by the patient. In the absence of the above complaints or sexual activity, the first pelvic examination should be considered at age 18 and performed sometime between the ages of 18 and 21 years. Currently, the American College of Obstetrics and Gynecology recommends a first Papanicolaou (Pap) smear in healthy adolescents 3 years

Table 18-3 Indications for Pelvic Examination of Adolescent Patients

Abnormal Vaginal Discharge

Pain
Pelvic
Perineal
Dysuria
Abdominal (unexplained)

Sexual Activity
Routine sexual health care (i.e., routine health care for sexually active individual)
Sexual contact with partner with a suspected or confirmed sexually transmitted disease or related genital symptoms

Suspected Sexual Abuse (see Chapter 6)

Concerns with Pubertal Development (see Chapter 9)
No secondary sexual development by age 14
No menarche by age 16; earlier if start of puberty more than 2 years ago and no menarche
Abnormal sequence or plateau of pubertal development
Anatomic abnormalities on genital inspection
Increased body hair, severe acne, or masculinization

Menstrual Disturbances
Severe dysmenorrhea
Amenorrhea or oligomenorrhea
Abnormal uterine bleeding or polymenorrhea

Patient Request (with Support from History)

after the initiation of vaginal intercourse, or by age 21, whichever is sooner.

The nature of the initial experience with pelvic examination may greatly affect a young woman's comfort with her body and the ease with which she experiences routine gynecologic care and sexual relations throughout her adult life. Hence the examiner's approach should be sympathetic, unhurried, and sensitive to the modesty of the patient. When patients have had pelvic examinations in the past, it is helpful to ask them about their prior experience to avoid repeating any previous emotional or physical trauma.

A thorough and directed history precedes the examination. A comprehensive outline is suggested in Table 18-5. Adequate time should be devoted to interviewing the patient alone, which provides an opportunity to ask questions about voluntary and involuntary sexual activity and explore other concerns that may be difficult to discuss in

Table 18-4 Sexual Health Care Guidelines for Sexually Active Adolescent Girls at Medical Visits

PROCEDURE	INITIAL	6-MO	ANNUAL	3-MO* PILL-CHECK	STD FOLLOW-UP
Complete H&P	✓				
Update H&P			✓		
Problem-focused H&P		✓		✓	✓
Pelvic examination	✓	✓	✓		✓
Weight	✓	✓	✓	✓	
Blood pressure	✓	✓	✓	✓	
Breast examination and SBE education	✓		✓		
Pap smear†	✓	H&P‡	✓		
Gonorrhea culture or NAAT	✓	✓§	✓		H&P‖
Chlamydia determination	✓	✓	✓		H&P‖
Oral & rectal STD specimens	H&P	H&P	H&P	H&P	H&P‖
Wet mount (saline/KOH)	✓	✓§	✓	H&P	H&P
RPR or STS	H&P		H&P§		
Rubella titer or 2nd MMR	✓				
Pregnancy prevention	✓	✓	✓	✓	✓
STD/AIDS prevention	✓	✓	✓	✓	✓
HIV risk assessment	✓	✓	✓	✓	✓
HIV counseling and titer¶	H&P	H&P	H&P		
CBC or hematocrit	✓ (and then every 2 yr)				
UA or dipstick	✓	H&P	✓		
Cholesterol	H&P				
Pregnancy test	✓	H&P	H&P	✓	H&P
Hepatitis B and HPV immunization status	✓**				

*Patients starting oral contraceptives should be seen after 3 cycles, then at 6 months from the initial visit, then every 6 months for routine care.
†Current ACOG and American Society for Colposcopy and Cervical Pathology (ASCCP) recommendations are to perform a Pap smear within 3 years of onset of sexual activity or by age 21 (whichever comes first) in healthy young adult women. Initiate earlier in patients with HIV, those who are immunosuppressed, or when other clinical concerns arise.
‡If recommended as follow-up to previously abnormal Pap, or colposcopy results.
§The frequency of these studies is related to the STD prevalence in a given community and the individual's behaviors.
‖STD tests of cure are not current CDC recommendations. However, because of the high rate of noncompliance with medication regimens and recommended abstinence during treatment, a test for reinfection may be indicated by interim history.
¶HIV determinations should be done in the context of documented pretest and post-test counseling protocols.
**Hepatitis and HPV immunization series require 3 shots at prescribed intervals. Most teenagers will have been immunized as infants or at school entry for hepatitis B.
H&P, history and physical; HPV, human papillomavirus; MMR, measles, mumps, rubella shot; RPR/STS, rapid plasma reagin/serologic test for syphilis; SBE, breast self-examination; STD, sexually transmitted disease; UA, urinalysis.

Table 18-5 Complete History of an Adolescent with Gynecologic Concerns

LABORATORY STUDY	INDICATION
General	
Home	Who lives there and quality of relationships; sources of conflict and support
Education/employment	School, grades, curriculum, repeated grades, goals, behavioral or learning difficulties; if working—type, occupational hazards, hours, literacy/numeracy
Activities	Exercise; nutritional content (specifically calcium, iron, fat, fiber, folate); body image; eating behaviors/patterns; peer activities; friends; hobbies
Drugs	Caffeine, tobacco, alcohol, marijuana, crack, cocaine, heroin, hallucinogens, pills, injectable drugs; rehabilitation or treatment history
Suicide	Depression, anxiety, psychiatric treatment, medications, major losses or disruptions, counseling history
Abuse	Physical, sexual, or emotional; family, relationship, peer, school and community violence or exploitation
Obstetric and Gynecologic History	
Menstrual	Menarche (age); cycles (length, duration, quantity of flow, use of pads or tampons); LMP—first day of; dysmenorrhea, associated disability; PMS; abnormal bleeding and other irregularities; mittelschmerz, midcycle spotting; douching; feminine hygiene product use (including scented products and deodorants)
STD	Herpes, gonorrhea, chlamydia, syphilis, PID, pubic lice ("crabs"), HPV (venereal warts), *Trichomonas*, HIV, hepatitis B and C
Pap	Abnormal results, colposcopy, biopsies, treatments, follow-up
Vaginitis	Yeast, bacterial vaginosis, trichomoniasis
Urologic	Urinary tract infection or kidney problems, enuresis, incontinence, dysuria, urgency, frequency
Vaginal discharge	Color, odor, quantity, duration, abnormal bleeding, pelvic pain, pruritus
Obstetric	Previous pregnancies and outcomes, future plans, fertility, concerns
Sexual	Last and other recent intercourse and protection; specific HIV risk of self and partners; sexual experience and age of onset; sexual practices, condom use; gender of partners, sexual orientation; number of partners, lifetime and recent; satisfaction with sexual experience; sexual problems with self or partner
Contraceptive	Current and past methods, satisfaction, consistency of use, problems
Past Medical History	Prior sources of care (routine, episodic, and emergency); hepatitis B immunization; rubella and varicella status; hypertension, migraines with aura or neurologic signs
Family History	Thromboembolic events at an early age or associated with pregnancy or with hormonal contraceptives; disease or death caused by alcohol, drugs, tobacco; gynecologic or obstetric problems; age of childbearing; endocrine problems (especially thyroid); bleeding problems (especially ob-gyn related); congenital malformations; mental retardation; reproductive loss

HIV, human immunodeficiency virus; HPV, human papillomavirus; LMP, last menstrual period; PID, pelvic inflammatory disease; PMS, premenstrual symptoms; STD, sexually transmitted disease.

the presence of a parent. A similar opportunity should be given to the parent to express any particular concerns or worries that he or she has been reluctant to share in the daughter's presence.

Young women should be given the choice of being examined with or without an accompanying adult in the room. The older teenager generally prefers to undergo pelvic examination without her mother present; but if she wishes her to remain, this wish should be respected. Early adolescents may be conflicted between their desire for support and their extreme modesty. On occasion an accompanying friend or partner can provide the support necessary. Setting a guideline that the support person must stay at the head of the table and using drapes that allow visual (eye) contact between patient and examiner is often the most comfortable compromise for younger adolescents. A chaperone (such as a nurse or an aide) is recommended for propriety and to assist handling of specimens. This practice is desirable for all examinations and is considered standard when the examiner is male, is a trainee, or when there is a history of sexual abuse.

At times, patient anxiety and/or other factors make it impossible to do a full pelvic examination. In such cases a partial, less invasive examination can still provide valuable information. This may include inspection of the external genitalia, obtaining vaginal specimens with swabs for a wet preparation and cultures, and performing a rectal bimanual examination if indicated. Although testing of vaginal specimens for gonorrhea and *C. trachomatis* may not match the cervical specimen gold standard, these tests can contribute useful diagnostic information, especially with NAATs. Some girls who initially refuse an "internal examination" can be persuaded by additional counseling after visible discharge or an abnormal microscopic wet preparation is found. A pelvic ultrasound is a more costly alternative to an internal examination, and its costs and benefits should be weighed carefully, assessing each patient and complaint individually.

Examination Technique and Specimen Collection

Successful examination depends on adequate patient preparation and use of appropriate instruments. For virginal adolescents, the narrow-bladed Huffman speculum ($\frac{1}{2} \times 4\frac{1}{2}$ inches) is recommended. Though long enough to expose the cervix, its narrow blades are inserted easily through the virginal introitus. Most sexually active adolescents can be examined with the straight-sided Pedersen speculum ($1 \times 4\frac{1}{2}$ inches); however, the Huffman speculum should be considered as an alternative for a first pelvic examination or for particularly anxious patients. The duck-billed Graves speculum ($1 \times 3\frac{3}{4}$ inches) is useful in parous patients (Fig. 18-7). Gloves should be available in the examining room and worn by the practitioner for both external and internal examinations. Metal speculums are preferred because they are easier to manipulate and are available in a greater range of lengths and widths. If only a single size of disposable plastic speculum is routinely used at a facility, it is important to have a backup supply of smaller metal speculums.

Before beginning, the examiner should carefully explain the various parts of the examination: inspection of the external genitalia, speculum examination of the vagina and cervix (with specimen collection), and bimanual palpation. Use of anatomic drawings and/or models can be helpful and educational (Fig. 18-8).

The patient should be shown the speculum and allowed to touch it if she so desires. Patients experiencing their first pelvic examination should be reassured that only the

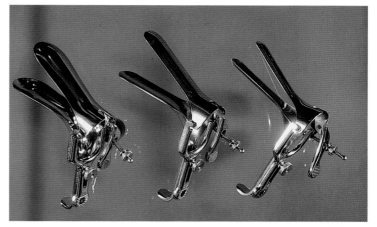

Figure 18-7. Equipment needed for pelvic examination of adolescent patients. From left to right, a Graves speculum, a Pedersen speculum, and a narrow-bladed Huffman speculum are shown. The Graves and Pedersen speculums are useful for examining sexually active patients, and the Huffman is ideal for virginal adolescents.

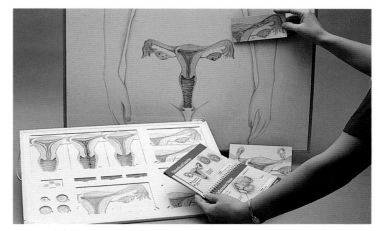

Figure 18-8. Anatomic drawings are useful in preparation of the adolescent patient for examination and in gynecologic education.

blades of the speculum will be inserted. Comparing the size of an open speculum to a finger or tampon often is reassuring. Both plastic and metal speculums should be moistened with warm water to increase comfort and ease of insertion. Lubricant should not be used because it can compromise specimen collection.

During the examination, the examiner should talk to the patient to explain what she or he is seeing and to provide reassurance and education. Maintaining a dialogue throughout the procedure also usually helps the patient relax. Conversation can confirm normal anatomic findings and provide the patient with examples of a correct and comfortable vocabulary describing her reproductive anatomy and function. A hand mirror held by the patient is often useful for similar reasons. The patient should be told that she will feel "a sense of pressure," not pain, during speculum insertion and should be reminded to breathe at a regular rate because tensing abdominal or pelvic muscles can produce discomfort and make the examination more difficult to perform.

The pelvic examination is done after other components of the physical examination. The patient should empty her bladder beforehand, and a urine specimen can be collected at this time for urinalysis; urine human chorionic gonadotropin (hCG); and, when indicated, culture and/or NAATs. Raising the head of the examining table 20 to 45 degrees helps relax abdominal muscles and assists maintenance of visual contact with the patient. She is then assisted into the lithotomy position at the end of the examination table. Her comfort with being touched may be increased by identifying and then touching distal areas first and moving proximally (e.g., knees, thighs, groin, labia, introitus). Next, the external genitalia are inspected. Pubic hair pattern and clitoral size are assessed. The presence of vulvar lesions or vaginal discharge on the perineum should be noted. The introital opening is examined, and its edges palpated for any swellings in the regions of the Bartholin glands. The urethral opening is then inspected, and if erythema or discharge is noted, the urethra can be gently stripped with a gloved finger along the vaginal roof. Any purulent material obtained should be cultured for gonorrhea, but swabs used to obtain *C. trachomatis* cultures from the urethra and any other sites must have direct contact with the mucosal surface, rather than the discharge itself.

The examiner may then gently insert the index finger into the vagina to assess the size of the introital opening and to locate the cervix. Vaginal muscle tone can be assessed by asking the patient to "tighten her muscles" around the examiner's finger. Conscious relaxation can be practiced by asking the patient to relax those same muscles and to push her buttocks onto the examining table. With the index finger partially withdrawn but gently pressing on the vaginal floor, the speculum (premoistened with warm water, not lubricant) is inserted over the finger into the vagina. This is done at an oblique angle along the posterior wall to accommodate the vertical introitus and avoid traumatizing the urethra, which lies above the anterior vaginal wall. Another technique that effectively assists insertion involves using the thumb and index fingers to stretch the posterior labial folds down and out before inserting the speculum. Care must be taken to avoid catching pubic hairs or the labia in the mechanism of the speculum.

With the speculum in place, the vaginal walls are inspected for erythema, lesions, and quality and quantity of discharge. The vaginal pH level is measured by holding pH paper (with an appropriate range of 3.6 to 6.1) against the lateral vaginal wall, away from pooled secretions. This is useful because vaginal pH levels are elevated in bacterial vaginosis and tend to be increased with trichomonal and decreased with candidal infections, respectively. Visible vaginal secretions from the posterior vaginal pool should be sampled with a cotton or Dacron swab and placed in a small amount of nonbacteriostatic normal saline for wet mount and potassium hydroxide (KOH) examination. The cervix is then examined. Cervical mucus should be gently removed from the cervical surface with cotton swabs before inspection of the cervix or sampling of cervical secretions. Purulent secretions (mucopus) typically turn the swab yellow and may be saved for microscopic examination. The normal nulliparous cervix usually has a small round os and is covered with squamous epithelium that is pink and uniform in consistency (Fig. 18-9). Any cervical lesions seen, such as cysts, warts, polyps, or vesicles, should be noted. An ectropion (or eversion) of the endocervical columnar epithelium onto the cervical surface is common and normal in adolescents (Fig. 18-10). Ectropion should be distinguished from cervicitis, the latter being suggested by erythema, friability, and/or mucopurulent cervical discharge (see Fig. 18-36B).

Cervical specimens are then collected. First, to check for cervical dysplasia (a precursor of cervical cancer), a traditional slide or liquid media Pap smear is obtained by rotating a wooden or plastic Ayre spatula circumferentially

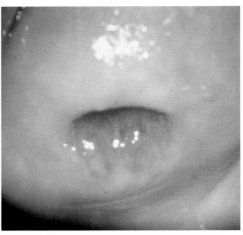

Figure 18-9. Normal nulliparous cervix. The surface is covered with pink squamous epithelium that is uniform in consistency. The os is small and round. A small area of ectropion is visible inferior to the os. (Courtesy C. Stevens.)

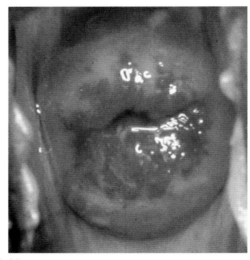

Figure 18-10. Ectropion. Columnar mucosal cells usually found in the endocervical canal have extended to the surface of the cervix, creating a circular, raised, erythematous appearance. Note the normal nonpurulent cervical mucus. This normal variant is not to be confused with cervicitis. (Courtesy E. Jerome, MD.)

(360°) around the cervical os. The entire squamocolumnar junction should be gently scraped. A sample from the endocervical canal is collected with a Cytobrush (or a cotton swab if the patient is pregnant). Each sample is smeared onto a labeled glass slide and treated immediately with fixative or swished in thin-prep solution according to laboratory protocol to ensure adequate fixation. Because Pap smear results can be uninterpretable in the presence of inflammation and bleeding, ideally collection should be deferred until infections are treated and menstrual bleeding has finished. However, concerns about patient compliance and follow-up or urgent clinical needs can justify collection of Pap specimens at less optimal times. Occasionally, Pap smear results contribute to identification of the source of abnormal bleeding or chronic cervicitis (i.e., when these problems are caused by infection with human papillomavirus [HPV] or herpes simplex virus). In response to increased understanding of the nature of HPV infection in young women, current recommendations from the American College of Obstetrics and Gynecology and the American College of Physicians advises that a first Pap smear be collected 3 years after the first intercourse or by 21 years of age, whichever comes first.

Experts have identified a number of HPV strains as causative in cervical cancer and genital warts. This has spurred development of new vaccines that immunize against some of the most common strains associated with cervical cancer. One of the vaccines also immunizes against two of the most common strains associated with genital warts. Currently, one vaccine is approved and recommended for girls/women between the ages of 9 and 26. Because these vaccines do not cover all strains associated with cervical cancer, Pap smears are still necessary.

Once the Pap smear has been collected, specimens should be obtained to determine the presence of infection as part of routine sexual health care and evaluation of pain, bleeding, or cervical discharge. A saline wet mount for microscopic evaluation in the office can be prepared by placing a sample of cervical discharge into a small amount (1 mL) of saline or by placement directly onto a slide with a drop of saline. Gonorrhea cultures are obtained by inserting a sterile swab into the endocervical canal and rotating it for at least 10 seconds. The swab is then placed immediately into a selective transport or culture medium. Either medium must be at room temperature before inoculation. Gonorrhea-specific media prevent bacterial overgrowth by other species and allow a longer transport time. *C. trachomatis* cultures and enzyme-linked immunosorbent assays (ELISA) (e.g., Chlamydiazyme [Abbott, Abbott Park, Ill.]) require mucosal surface cells because the pathogen is an obligate intracellular organism. Dacron swabs are placed in the endocervical canal and thoroughly rotated to obtain the necessary cellular material. Wooden swabs are not acceptable for *C. trachomatis* tests. NAATs, because of their ability to detect minute quantities of pathogen DNA/RNA, do not require obtaining mucosal cells.

After specimens have been collected, the speculum is removed and the bimanual (vaginal-abdominal) examination is performed. Water-based lubricant is placed on the two gloved fingers to be used before inserting them carefully through the introitus into the vagina. The examiner should note the size, consistency, position, and mobility of the uterus and check for tenderness on cervical or fundal motion. The adnexa should be palpated for evidence of enlargement or tenderness. After changing the glove on the examining hand, a rectovaginal examination using the index and middle finger may be performed to confirm an abnormal or uncertain finding on vaginal-abdominal examination, palpate the cul-de-sac, and examine a retroflexed uterus.

Once the examination is completed, the patient should be helped out of the lithotomy position, given tissues to wipe away any lubricant or discharge, and allowed privacy to get dressed. During this time the examiner can review the wet mount and KOH preparations. A drop of the saline solution of vaginal secretions is examined under low (×10) and high (×40) power for distribution of epithelial cells, leukocytes, yeast forms, *Trichomonas* organisms, and clue cells. A drop of 10% KOH is added to a second drop of the saline solution. This preparation is immediately "whiffed" for the presence of the acrid odor associated with amines that is found in bacterial vaginosis and often in patients with trichomoniasis. Following this, microscopic scanning of the KOH preparation assists identification of yeast forms that may be obscured by epithelial cells on the wet mount.

With this additional information, the practitioner can then review the presenting problems and subsequent findings with the patient. Use of handouts, printed pictures, or line drawings can enhance the patient's understanding of the results (see Fig. 18-8). This is also an opportunity to encourage communication between the young woman and her parent, as appropriate to the circumstance.

Genital Tract Obstruction

Labial Adhesions

The most common form of "vaginal obstruction" in prepubertal patients is really a pseudo-obstruction or partial obstruction produced by "fusion" of the labia minora as a result of labial adhesions. On inspection the clinician finds a smooth, flat membrane with a thin lucent central line overlying the introitus. It is postulated that inflammation and erosion of the superficial layers of the mucosa—whether caused by infection, dermatitis, or mechanical trauma—result in agglutination of the apposed labia minora by fibrous tissue on healing. The process typically begins posteriorly and extends forward. In most cases the fused portion is less than 1 cm in length, but on occasion it can extend to cover the vaginal vestibule and rarely the urethra (Fig. 18-11A and B). Even when fusion is extensive, urine flow and vaginal secretions are able to exit through the opening anteriorly. However, some urine may become trapped behind the adhesions after toileting. This may cause further irritation, perpetuating the condition or fostering extension of the adhesions. Although most labial adhesions are asymptomatic, some patients have symptoms of lower urinary tract and vulval inflammation.

If resolution of the fused labia is desired, the condition readily responds to application of estrogen cream along the line of fusion twice daily for 2 weeks, followed by nightly application for an additional week. Occasionally the course needs to be extended for an additional 2 weeks, or an increased volume of estrogen cream is advised. After the labia have separated, a zinc oxide–based cream should be applied nightly for several months to prevent recurrence. The patient's parent should be informed that topical estrogen may cause transient hyperpigmentation of the labia and the areolae and an increase in breast tissue, but that these changes regress once therapy is completed. An estrogen withdrawal bleed (similar to that seen in the neonate) occasionally occurs. Removal of irritants, treatment of infections, and instructions on good perineal hygiene help prevent recurrence. Nonetheless, refusion can occur, although repeated treatment is not necessary if the child is asymptomatic.

Manual separation of fused labia is painful, traumatic, and frequently followed by a recurrence. Hence this practice should be abandoned. True fusion—adhesions present in the first months of life or adhesions that do not respond to the prescribed therapy—requires further evaluation for abnormalities in gender differentiation or androgen production.

Imperforate Hymen

The congenital anomaly referred to as *imperforate hymen* consists of a thick imperforate membrane located just inside the hymenal ring. This is the most common truly obstructive abnormality. It is frequently missed on the newborn examination because of the redundancy of hymenal folds. However, it may become evident by 8 to

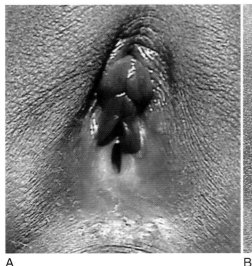

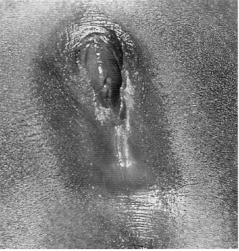

A   B

Figure 18-11. Labial adhesions. Agglutination and adhesion of the labia minora, as a result of healing after inflammation, produce the appearance of a smooth, flat surface overlying the introitus, divided centrally by a thin lucent line. **A,** In this infant the fused portion involves the posterior half of the introitus. **B,** In another, the fused area has extended much farther anteriorly. (**A,** Courtesy Carol Byers, CRNP, Children's Hospital of Pittsburgh; **B,** Courtesy D. Lloyd, MD.)

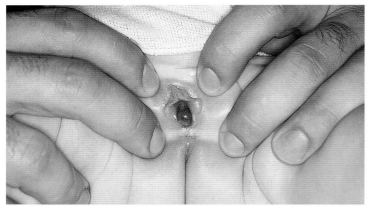

Figure 18-12. Imperforate hymen with neonatal hematocolpos. A dark, purplish bulge at the introitus was noted by the mother during a diaper change.

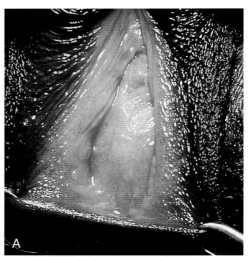

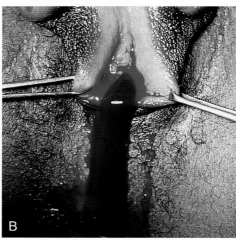

Figure 18-13. Imperforate hymen with hematocolpos. This adolescent presented with a 2-month history of intermittent crampy lower abdominal pain, which had acutely worsened. She had well-developed secondary sex characteristics but was premenarchal by history. **A,** Examination revealed midline fullness and tenderness of the lower abdomen and a smooth bulging mass at the introitus. **B,** Incision of the imperforate membrane just inside the hymenal ring allowed the accumulated menstrual blood and vaginal secretions to drain. (Courtesy D. Lloyd, MD.)

12 weeks of age on careful perineal inspection, appearing as a thin, transparent hymenal membrane that bulges when the infant cries or strains. Occasionally, young infants with this anomaly have copious vaginal secretions secondary to stimulation by maternal hormones and, as a result, they develop hydrocolpos. In such cases the infant may have midline swelling of the lower abdomen (especially noticeable when the bladder is full) that feels cystic on palpation. Perineal inspection reveals a whitish, bulging membrane at the introitus. The cystic mass may also be palpable on rectal examination. In the presence of a neonatal withdrawal bleed or trauma, a hematocolpos may develop. This presents as a red or purplish bulge (Fig. 18-12). Treatment consists of incision of the membrane to allow drainage, followed by excision of redundant tissue.

If her condition goes undetected, the patient with an imperforate hymen usually develops hematocolpos in late puberty. The major complaints are intermittent lower abdominal and low back pain, which rapidly progress in severity and duration. Over time, difficulty in urination and defecation may develop and a lower abdominal swelling may become noticeable. The patient has well-developed secondary sex characteristics but has had no menstrual periods. Perineal inspection reveals a thick, tense, bulging membrane, often bluish in color, at the introitus (Fig. 18-13A). A low cystic swelling is palpable anteriorly on rectal examination. Operative incision allows drainage of the accumulated blood and vaginal secretions (see Fig. 18-13B) and is followed by excision of the mem-

brane. Other partially obstructive hymenal abnormalities may allow menstrual blood to flow but later cause difficulty inserting tampons or initiating intercourse. Because hymens are not of müllerian origin, imperforate hymens are not associated with other genitourinary abnormalities.

Table 18-6	Causes of Genital Tract Obstruction

Labial fusion (underlying endocrine pathology)
Imperforate hymen
Vaginal atresia (failure to canalize the vaginal plate)
Vaginal (with or without uterine) agenesis including Mayer-Rokitansky-Küster-Hauser syndrome (müllerian aplasia); congenital absence of the vagina and uterus
Transverse vaginal septum at the junction of the upper one third and lower two thirds of the vagina
Longitudinal vaginal septum
Androgen insensitivity (testicular feminization syndrome)
Absence of the cervix and/or uterus
Obstructing müllerian malformations, with elements of duplication, agenesis, and/or incomplete fusion
Tumors of the upper and lower genital tracts; other pelvic masses
Labial adhesions (partial obstruction)
Genital mutilation, scarification

Table 18-7	Symptoms and Signs Associated with Genital Tract Obstructions

Symptoms
Vaginal, pelvic, or abdominal pain (especially cyclic)
Dysmenorrhea
Urinary tract symptoms
Primary amenorrhea
Irregular vaginal bleeding
Purulent vaginal discharge
Difficulty initiating intercourse
Dyspareunia

Signs
Vaginal, pelvic, or abdominal mass
Hydrocolpos (mucus in vagina)
Hematocolpos (blood in vagina)
Pyohematocolpos (pus and blood in vagina)
Hematometra (blood within the uterus)

Other forms of genital tract obstruction (Table 18-6) are rare. In most cases early routine genital inspection reveals the absence of a vaginal orifice, enabling early delineation of the anomaly and thus facilitating treatment. If missed in infancy or childhood, partial or complete obstruction can present with a wide range of signs and symptoms (Table 18-7). These may include cyclic or persistent vaginal, pelvic, or abdominal pain; primary amenorrhea or irregular vaginal bleeding; urinary tract symptoms; and difficulty inserting tampons and initiating intercourse, or dyspareunia. Clinically, a vaginal, pelvic, or abdominal mass may be found, reflecting hydrocolpos, hematocolpos, pyohematocolpos, or hematometra.

As noted earlier, ultrasonography is a valuable screening tool in evaluating girls suspected of having genital tract obstruction, bearing in mind its limitations in visualization of internal structures after the neonatal period and before puberty, because they are small in the absence of normal stimulation. When structures are not seen or when further anatomic detail is required, consultation with a radiologist regarding magnetic resonance imaging is recommended.

Genital Trauma

As mentioned earlier, the genital structures and pelvic supporting tissues of the prepubescent girl are smaller and considerably more rigid than those of adolescent or adult women. This inelasticity significantly increases the risks of tearing with either blunt or penetrating trauma, and of internal extension of injury, especially in cases of pene-

trating trauma. Appropriate assessment and management necessitate appreciation of these differences because serious internal injuries of the vagina, rectum, urethra, bladder, and peritoneal structures may underlie deceptively mild external abnormalities. Careful attention must be given to vital signs; abdominal examination; and evaluation of the urethra, hymen, lower vagina, perineal body, and rectum.

Clues to internal extension of injury include hymenal tears, vaginal bleeding and/or vaginal hematoma, tears of the perineal body, inability to urinate or gross hematuria, and abnormal sphincter tone or rectal bleeding. When injuries have extended to involve peritoneal structures, lower abdominal tenderness is seen and, at times, is associated with signs of hypovolemia. Direct tenderness may range from mild to marked and may or may not be accompanied by rebound tenderness. Occasionally a palpable mass is present. Adolescents, in contrast, are more likely to have contusions than tears and are less likely to have internal extension of injury unless the applied force is great.

The role of the primary care or emergency physician is to assess the patient's general status and determine the likely extent and cause of the injury. This can be accomplished largely with a good general examination, careful perineal and perianal inspection, rectal examination, and urinalysis. Rectal examination should be deferred in cases of possible anal rape and when anal lacerations are evident on inspection, to prevent further physical and emotional trauma. The physician must be sensitive to the patient's physical discomfort and emotional distress at all times, providing emotional support and appropriate pain control whenever possible. Patients should also be protected from having to undergo multiple examinations, a particular risk with consultation of multiple subspecialists, transfer to other institutions, or in teaching hospitals.

When external inspection suggests that the prepubertal patient's perineal or perianal injuries are more than superficial, internal examination under anesthesia (by a pediatric surgeon or gynecologist) should be arranged. This enables meticulous inspection, wound exploration, and repair under optimal conditions without further traumatizing the child.

Some adolescents may be able to tolerate inspection and internal examination as outpatients. However, if injuries are severe or if the postmenarchal patient is too anxious to undergo pelvic examination when indicated, examination under anesthesia is the better course.

Superficial Perineal Injuries

The majority of superficial perineal trauma cases are the result of mild, blunt force incurred via straddle injury, minor falls, or sexual abuse. Patients with accidental injuries that result in pain, swelling, or bleeding are rapidly brought to medical attention. A clear history of the preceding incident (often witnessed) is usually given, and findings fit the reported mechanism of injury. However, accidentally incurred superficial abrasions may not be noticed by parents until the child cries on urination, complains of dysuria, or a small amount of blood is noticed on the child's underwear or toilet paper. As noted in Chapter 6, victims of sexual abuse may complain of abuse but more often complain of unexplained bleeding or pain with no history of trauma, and the time of presentation is often significantly delayed.

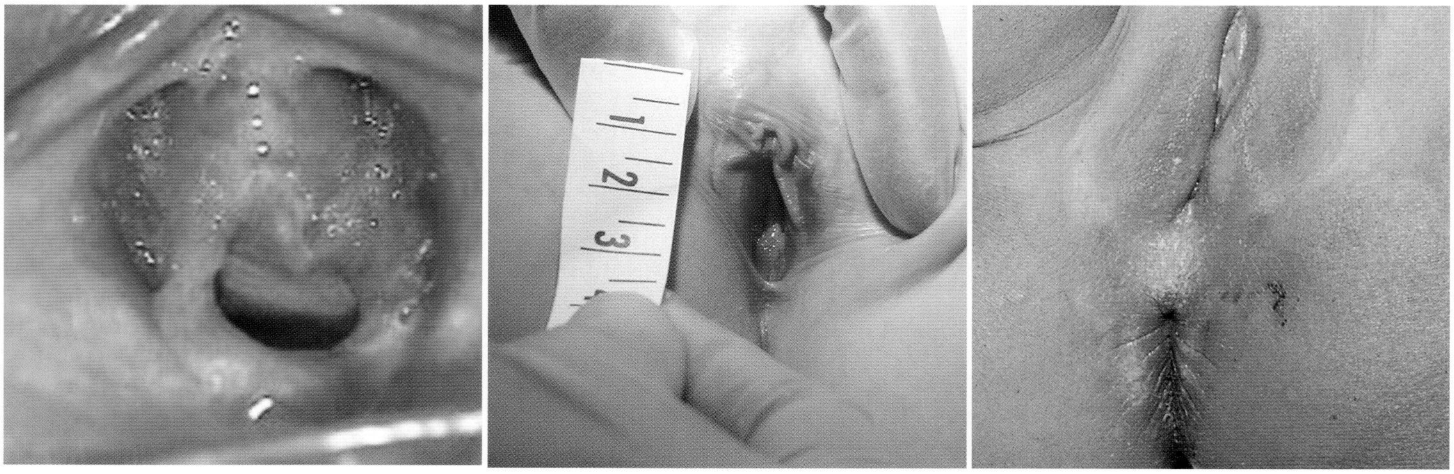

A　　　　　　　　　　B　　　　　　　　　　C

Figure 18-14. Superficial blunt trauma. **A,** Superficial abrasions and bruising are seen anteriorly on either side of the clitoris and urethra in a 3-year-old who presented with dysuria. **B,** In another toddler a superficial abrasion/laceration is seen between the left labia minora and majora following a straddle injury. **C,** These healing superficial abrasions involving the posterior fourchette and perianal area were the result of sexual abuse. (**A** and **B,** Courtesy Janet Squires, MD, Children's Hospital of Pittsburgh.)

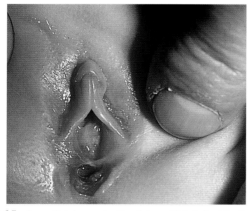

Figure 18-15. Superficial penetrating injury. This infant had a chief complaint of blood spotting on the diaper. Inspection revealed a perineal tear just posterior to the hymenal ring. There was no evidence of internal extension on vaginoscopy under anesthesia. Sexual abuse was suspected.

Typical lesions include superficial abrasions, mild contusions, and occasionally superficial lacerations (Fig. 18-14A-C). The latter are found most frequently at the junction of the labia majora and minora and usually are only 1 to 3 mm deep. Accidental straddle injuries result in the crushing of the perineal soft tissues between the pubis and the object on which the patient falls or bumps herself. Hence these tend to produce abrasions, contusions, or tears in and around the area of the clitoris and the anterior portions of the labia majora and minora (Fig. 18-14A and B and see Fig. 18-16). Minor falls onto or scrapes against sharp objects tend to produce simple perineal and vulval lacerations. As in cases of mild blunt trauma, the junction of the labia minora and majora is the site most frequently involved; however, tears of the labia majora or perineal body are not uncommon. In contrast to accidental injuries, those that result from sexual abuse tend to be more posteriorly located and typically involve tears of the posterior portion of the hymen, the posterior fourchette, or perineal body (Fig. 18-14C and Fig. 18-15 and see Chapter 6).

Whether blunt or penetrating, when injuries are truly superficial, bleeding, if present at all, tends to be scant. The exception to this is a penetrating injury involving the corpus cavernosum of the labia majora, in which case hemorrhage may be profuse. Patients with superficial injuries may experience mild perineal discomfort and pain on urination but are otherwise asymptomatic. Most of these injuries can be managed supportively with analgesia, topical bacteriostatic and/or anesthetic ointments, sitz baths, and careful perineal cleansing. Application of the ointment before urinating reduces the severity of dysuria, as does urinating in a tub of water. If urinary retention continues to be a problem, use of a topical anesthetic ointment for a few days may be necessary. Deeper tears of the labia majora necessitate control of bleeding vessels and suturing under anesthesia.

Urethral prolapse and lichen sclerosus et atrophicus may cause bleeding that mimics superficial perineal injury, and the edematous friable appearance of the prolapsed urethra often has been mistakenly attributed to trauma. Knowledge of the clinical appearance of these conditions is important to avoid misdiagnosis (see Figs. 18-25 and 18-26).

Moderate Genital Trauma

Moderately forceful blunt trauma often results in perineal tears and in venous disruption and hematoma formation. Hematomas of the perineum appear as tense, round swellings with purplish discoloration that are tender on palpation (Fig. 18-16). When large, these may cause intense perineal pain. Those located in the periurethral area may interfere with urination. Moderate blunt force can also produce submucosal tears of the vagina and even mucosal separation with resultant vaginal bleeding or vaginal hematoma formation (Figs. 18-16 and 18-17). In some cases the associated external injuries can be deceptively mild (see Fig. 18-17). Vaginal hematomas are the source of significant pain that is usually perceived as perineal and/or vaginal but at times is referred to the rectum or buttocks. Inspection through the vaginal orifice reveals a bluish swelling involving one of the lateral walls. This may also be evident as a tender swelling anterolaterally on rectal examination.

Moderate penetrating injuries result primarily from falls onto sharp objects ("picket fence injury"), rape, sexual

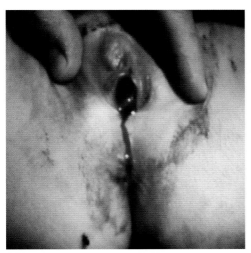

Figure 18-16. Moderate genital trauma. After a straddle injury on a diving board, this 9-year-old girl had vaginal bleeding. Inspection disclosed a hematoma of the anterior portion of the right labia majora, contusions of the clitoris and anterior labia minora, and a hematoma protruding through the vaginal opening. A small superficial laceration is present on the left, between the labia majora and minora. At vaginoscopy under anesthesia a vaginal tear involving the right lateral wall was found. (Courtesy K. Sukarochana, MD, Pittsburgh, Pa.)

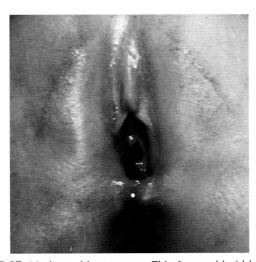

Figure 18-17. Moderate blunt trauma. This 6-year-old girl had painless vaginal bleeding, which had soaked three sanitary pads in 2 hours. External inspection revealed a superficial tear of the anterior portion of the perineal body, a small hematoma to the right of the introitus, and blood trickling through the vaginal orifice. Examination under anesthesia disclosed a tear of the lateral vaginal wall. Sexual abuse was strongly suspected. (Courtesy K. Sukarochana, MD, Pittsburgh, Pa.)

molestation with phallic-shaped objects, and occasionally auto accidents. Lesions include perineal tears that extend into the vagina, rectum, or bladder but do not breach the peritoneum. Although many patients have external lacerations that obviously are extensive on inspection (Fig. 18-18; see also Chapter 6 and Fig. 6-90C), a significant proportion have deceptively minor external injuries. In the absence of associated hematomas, extensive tears may produce little pain. Furthermore, although most such injuries result in moderate bleeding, some patients have remarkably little blood loss.

Whether the mechanism of injury involves blunt force or penetration, when physical findings include bleeding through the vaginal orifice; a vaginal hematoma; rectal bleeding, rectal tenderness, or abnormal sphincter tone; gross hematuria; or inability to urinate, internal extension of injury is probable. All such patients warrant exploration

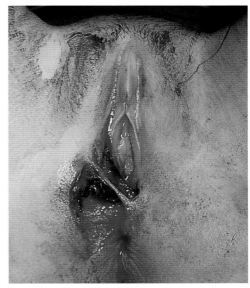

Figure 18-18. Moderately severe penetrating genital trauma. This youngster fell while roller skating downhill and slid on her bottom for several feet over the sidewalk, tearing her perineum on an object projecting up between two of the cement plates. A laceration involving the right labia majora and minora, extending through the perineal body to the anus, is evident on inspection. The patient complained of only minor discomfort. Examination under anesthesia revealed vaginal and rectal extension of the tear with complete transection of the external anal sphincter. The peritoneum was intact.

and repair in the operating room. This obviates the need for extensive examination in the office or emergency department.

Severe Genital Trauma

Severe falls from heights onto flat surfaces can produce major perineal lacerations simulating penetrating injury. In addition, they occasionally disrupt the pelvic vessels, mesentery, and intestine, with or without pelvic fracture (Fig. 18-19). Similarly, severe penetrating injury may produce tears that extend through the cul-de-sac, rupturing pelvic vessels and tearing intra-abdominal structures. External injuries in these cases are usually extensive and associated with significant bleeding, but on occasion can be deceptively minor in appearance. Children with peritoneal extension of injury complain of lower abdominal and perineal pain, which may radiate down one leg. Abdominal examination should reveal at least mild direct tenderness early on. Later, guarding and rebound tenderness may be noted. Patients with pelvic bleeding ultimately tend to develop signs of hypovolemia, although this may not be evident immediately after the injury. Any patient with clinical signs of peritoneal extension of genital trauma warrants prompt hemodynamic stabilization followed by appropriate imaging, surgical exploration, and repair.

Nontraumatic Vulvovaginal Disorders

Prepubertal "Vulvovaginitis"

Strictly defined, the term *vulvovaginitis* denotes an inflammatory process involving both the vulva and the vagina. In practice, however, the term is used less precisely

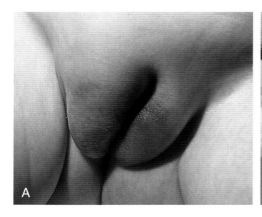
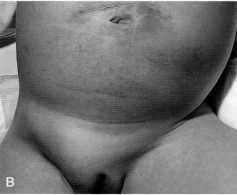

Figure 18-19. Severe blunt perineal trauma. **A,** Following a fall from a second-story window in which she had landed on her bottom, this young child had labial contusions and hematomas, lower abdominal tenderness, and signs of hypovolemia. **B,** The force of the fall ruptured pelvic vessels, resulting in retroperitoneal bleeding that ultimately extended along the anterior abdominal wall. These photographs were taken several days after the injury. (Courtesy Marc Rowe, MD, Sanibel, Fla.)

Table 18-8	Causes of Noninfectious Vulvovaginitis and Dysuria

CONDITION	HISTORICAL CLUES
Poor hygiene	Infrequent bathing, hand washing, and clothing changes; soiled underwear, toilet independence
Poor perineal aeration	Tight clothing, nylon underwear, tights, and leotards; wet bathing suits; hot tubs; obesity
Frictional trauma	Tight clothing, sports, sand from sandbox or beach play, excessive masturbation or sexual abuse, obesity
Chemical irritants	Bubble bath, harsh or perfumed soaps or detergents, powder, water softeners, perfumed and dyed toilet paper; ammonia; perfumed sanitary pads and panty liners; douches and feminine hygiene products in adolescents
Contact dermatitis	Poison ivy, topical creams or ointments
Vaginal foreign bodies	Wiping habits, excessive masturbation or self-exploration, sexual abuse
Parasites, insect bites, infestations	Home environment, pets, sandboxes, travel, camping, exposure to woods or beach
Medication-related	Topical steroid or hormone creams, antibiotics, chemotherapy
Generalized skin disorders	History of pruritus, chronic skin lesions, prior diagnosis
Anatomic anomalies	Vesicovaginal or rectovaginal fistula, ectopic ureter, spina bifida, cloacal anomalies, urogenital anomalies
Neoplasms	Discharge, bleeding, bulging abdomen, change in bowel or bladder function, premature puberty
Systemic illness (Stevens-Johnson syndrome, Crohn disease with perineal fistulas and ulcers, toxic shock syndrome)	Prior infection or medication use; tampon use; evidence from other physical findings including rash, failure to gain weight or height, abdominal pain, diarrhea
Pelvic appendiceal abscess	History of fever, anorexia, vomiting, progression of periumbilical to right lower quadrant pain

to refer to prepubertal patients who describe symptoms of dysuria, vulvar pain or itching, or vaginal discharge but who often lack signs of inflammation or who have evidence of vulvar inflammation without vaginal involvement. Given this caveat, vulvovaginitis is relatively common in prepubertal girls and accounts for a majority of genital complaints before menarche. Its frequent occurrence is explained in part by the fact that the labia do not fully cover and thus do not completely protect the vaginal vestibule from friction and external irritants, especially when the child is sitting or squatting. Additionally, the unestrogenized vaginal epithelium is thin, relatively friable, and more easily traumatized. Transient irritation without discharge is common in the young child as a result of exposure to chemical irritants, inconsistent hygiene, and poor aeration. Finally, young children are less careful than older children and adults about cleansing their perineum after toileting and avoiding contamination with stool.

Causes of vulvovaginitis are most easily classified into noninfectious and infectious subgroups, with the latter subclassified into nonsexually and sexually transmitted infections. Table 18-8 presents the most common causes of noninfectious vulvovaginitis with specific historic clues suggestive of each condition. Table 18-9 presents the infectious causes. Nonsexually transmitted bacterial pathogens and the herpes simplex viruses are often spread to the

Table 18-9	Infectious Causes of Prepubertal and Postpubertal Vulvovaginitis

NONSEXUALLY TRANSMITTED PATHOGENS	SEXUALLY TRANSMITTED PATHOGENS
Bacterial Respiratory and/or Skin Pathogens Group A β-hemolytic streptococci* *Streptococcus pneumoniae** *Haemophilus influenzae** *Neisseria* species Staphylococci	**Bacterial Pathogens** *Chlamydia trachomatis** *Neisseria gonorrhoeae** *Treponema pallidum* *Mycoplasma genitalis** *Ureaplasma* species*
Viral Pathogens Varicella-zoster virus Herpes simplex viruses types 1 and 2* Adenoviruses* Echoviruses* Measles virus Epstein-Barr virus	**Protozoa** *Trichomonas vaginalis** **Viral Pathogens** Herpes simplex viruses types 1 and 2* Human papillomavirus Human immunodeficiency virus
Gastrointestinal Pathogens *Candida* species† *Escherichia coli** *Shigella* species* *Enterobius vermicularis* *Yersinia* species	**Parasites** *Phthirus pubis* (lice) *Sarcoptes scabiei*

*Conditions in which vaginal discharge is prominent.
†Discharge prominent only after puberty.

vulvovaginal area from another site (e.g., nose, mouth, throat, skin, gastrointestinal tract) by the patient's hands, whereas involvement with nonherpetic viral organisms is more often a part of systemic infection. Although a common cause of diaper dermatitis, *Candida* organisms rarely cause vulvovaginitis in the prepubertal child who is no longer wearing diapers. However, children who are receiving systemic antibiotics or steroids, using topical steroid hormone creams, or have underlying diabetes mellitus may develop dysuria and vulvar discomfort, which responds to topical (azole) antifungals. In the prepubertal child, vulvovaginitis caused by sexually transmitted pathogens is almost always acquired through sexual contact (see Chapter 6).

In contrast to adolescents and adults, prepubertal girls are at little risk for internal extension of vulvovaginal infections (cervicitis and pelvic inflammatory disease) because the unestrogenized genital tract does not support the ascent of infection through the uterus and fallopian tubes.

The evaluation of these patients must include questions related to symptoms experienced (including any associated abdominal pain; dysuria, frequency, or urgency; or perianal pruritus); their duration; a history of any recent respiratory, gastrointestinal, and urinary tract infections; exposure to irritants such as bath additives, laundry detergents, fabric softeners, bubble bath, and harsh soaps; hygienic practices; bowel and bladder habits; type of clothing worn; recent activities (such as daily swimming); medications; and topical agents. When sexual abuse is suspected, a list of the child's caretakers should be obtained, along with any history of possible sexual contact (Chapter 6). Developmental, behavioral, environmental, and medical histories all may contribute to a definitive diagnosis and aid in the formulation of a therapeutic plan.

Physical assessment must include determination of the degree of pubertal development; inguinal and abdominal examination; and careful rectal, perineal, and vaginal inspection. The degree and extent of inflammation and excoriation should be documented. Parents should be encouraged to bring in any available soiled or discolored underwear, which should be checked for fit, cleanliness, and signs of blood, discharge, stool, and urine. When patients are seen by appointment for vulvovaginal complaints, parents should be asked not to bathe or apply creams to the child for 12 to 24 hours before the evaluation; otherwise, many children with a history of discharge have none when examined.

The presence of a vaginal discharge necessitates specimen collection (see Table 18-2 and "Examination of the Prepubertal Patient" earlier). Urine should be collected for urinalysis and culture, and possibly for NAATs. If a vaginal foreign body is suspected, rectal examination and vaginoscopy are indicated in consultation with a practitioner experienced in such procedures. Ultrasonography can be helpful in confirming the presence of some foreign objects. Radiographs of the pelvic area should be ordered selectively when benefit outweighs the risk, and information cannot be obtained without radiographic exposure.

Vulvovaginal Complaints in Adolescents

Among sexually active adolescent girls, infectious processes are the major source of vulvovaginal inflammation, and sexually transmitted pathogens are the predominant offending organisms. Estrogenization and maturation of the genital tract alter its pathophysiological response, favoring upward spread of some infectious processes, particularly those caused by gonorrhea and *C. trachomatis*. As a result, asymptomatic or subclinical upper tract infection, endometritis, cervicitis, and pelvic inflammatory disease are significant concerns, in addition to vulvovaginitis after menarche.

Vulvar lesions, vaginal discharge, odor, pruritus, and dysuria are common complaints in adolescents. Irregular or postcoital bleeding, dyspareunia, pelvic pain, and fever may be reported as well. These symptoms are relatively nonspecific and may represent the final common pathway of different causes of irritation, infection, or infestation.

In addition to identification of specific etiologic agents, a major goal of evaluation is to differentiate vulvovaginal or cervical processes from pregnancy (normal or ectopic); upper tract disease (e.g., pelvic inflammatory disease, adnexal torsion, cysts); urinary tract problems; and intra-abdominal processes (e.g., appendicitis, endometriosis, chronic constipation, tumors). Hence a complete pelvic examination is necessary when evaluating sexually active adolescents with vulvovaginal complaints and should be considered for symptomatic, non–sexually active teens. Systemic signs and symptoms and abnormalities on bimanual pelvic examination suggest processes involving the uterus and adnexal and/or peritoneal structures. In contrast, isolated vulvovaginal disorders are rarely accompanied by such findings. In most cases careful history, inspection, "bench" or bedside laboratory tests (e.g., wet mount, KOH preparation, Gram stain, pregnancy test, urine dipstick, vaginal pH), and selected cultures and other tests for infectious etiologic agents provide a specific diagnosis on which to base treatment decisions. Some clinical and laboratory features of various etiologic agents of vaginal discharge are presented in Table 18-10.

Physiologic Leukorrhea

Physiologic leukorrhea, though often perceived as a vaginal discharge, is (in actuality) a normal phenomenon and not a form of vulvovaginitis. These normal secretions are produced in response to estrogen stimulation and thus are seen in the newborn period and return during the months preceding menarche. Physiologic leukorrhea is clear or milky, relatively thin, odorless, and (usually) nonirritating (see Fig. 18-4A). When dried on underwear, it may appear yellow. Girls near menarche often complain of discharge because they and their mothers are not aware that these new secretions are normal. Furthermore, some girls experience a period of excessive leukorrhea that can be irritating due to the unopposed influence of estrogen.

Examination reveals normal pubertal development including findings of breast development, presence of pubic hair, and evidence of estrogenization of the labia and distal vaginal mucosa along with the typical discharge. Diagnosis is confirmed by findings on wet preparation microscopy, which discloses estrogenized epithelial cells with no increase in leukocytes (see Fig. 18-4B). As a general guide, there should be no more than one polymorphonuclear leukocyte for each vaginal epithelial cell. Neither bimanual nor speculum examinations are necessary, unless concurrent symptoms or findings suggest other problems. Treatment consists of reassurance and education.

Noninfectious Vulvovaginitis

Clinical findings of noninfectious vulvovaginitis vary considerably depending on cause. Although the physical

Table 18-10 Clinical and Laboratory Features of Disorders Causing Vaginal Discharge in Adolescents

	PHYSIOLOGIC	CANDIDA	CHLAMYDIA	GONORRHEA	TRICHOMONAS	BACTERIAL VAGINOSIS	HPV	HSV
Appearance of discharge	White, gray, or clear; mucoid	White, curdlike, with adherent plaques	Mucopus at cervix; friable cervix with bloody discharge	Mucopus at cervix; yellow or greenish discharge	Gray, yellow, or green; sometimes frothy; malodorous	Gray, white; homogeneous, thin	White or clear, generalized or localized inflammation	Serosanguineous
Amount	Variable	Variable	Variable	Variable	Profuse	Variable	Scant	Varies widely
Vulvar and vaginal inflammation	None or mild with copious leukorrhea	Usual	Not usual, with or without Bartholin gland abscess	Variable, with or without Bartholin gland abscess	Common	Rare	Common, evidence of HPV with acetic acid wash or overt condylomata	Common with a few to many ulcers
pH of vaginal discharge	≤ 4.5	≤ 4.5	≤ 4.5	≤ 4.5	≥ 4.5	≥ 4.5	≤ 4.5	≤ 4.5
Microscopy	Epithelial cells, few WBCs, lactobacilli	↑WBCs, + KOH with pseudohyphae and budding yeast in 50% of symptomatic patients	↑WBCs	↑↑WBCs	↑↑WBCs, motile trichomonads (in saline prep) in 40%-60% of symptomatic patients; trichomonads in urine	Few WBCs, + clue cells in saline prep, + Gram stain	↑WBCs (usually)	↑↑WBCs
Predisposing or concurrent factors	Secretion of estrogen	Menstruation, broad-spectrum antibiotics, diabetes, local heat and moisture, pregnancy, OCPs, HIV, topical steroid or hormone creams, immune deficiencies	Sexual activity, gonorrhea	Often accompanied by chlamydial infection; symptoms often develop toward the end of a menstrual period	Other STDs	Previous BV, sexual activity, douching	Abnormal Pap smear, other STDs; history of genital warts or recurrent, unexplained vulvovaginitis	Stress and local trauma (including shaving)
Other clinical signs and symptoms	None	Itching prominent, may have dysuria or dyspareunia	Urethritis, PID, perihepatitis	Pharyngitis, with or without PID, proctitis, urethritis, systemic illness, arthritis, tenosynovitis, perihepatitis, skin lesions	Vulvar itching and burning prominent, dysuria, pelvic discomfort	Fishy odor, odor ↑ after unprotected intercourse	Visible external or flat warts, chronic low-grade vulvovaginitis, fissures, failure of other therapies	Regional adenopathy with primary infection, prodromal and intercurrent itching and pain
Whiff test (acrid amine odor on addition of 10% KOH)	Negative	Negative	Negative	Negative	Sometimes positive	Positive	Negative	Negative

BV, bacterial vaginosis; HIV, human immunodeficiency virus; HPV, human papillomavirus; HSV, herpes simplex virus; OCP, oral contraceptive pill; PID, pelvic inflammatory disease; +, positive; ↑, increased; ↑↑, markedly increased.

Table 18-11	Organisms Thought to Constitute Normal or Nonpathogenic Vaginal Flora

Aerobes and Facultative Anaerobes	Anaerobes
Branhamella catarrhalis	*Bacteroides* species
Candida albicans and other yeasts*	*Clostridium* species
Corynebacterium species	*Peptococcus* species
Diphtheroids	*Peptostreptococcus* species
Enterococcus species	
Escherichia coli	
Haemophilus species	
Lactobacillus species	
Klebsiella species	
Mycoplasma species*	
Neisseria sicca	
Proteus species	
Pseudomonas species	
Staphylococcus species	
Streptococcus species	

*Mycoplasma hominis, Ureaplasma urealyticum, and *Candida* species can constitute normal flora in asymptomatic women; however, they may be responsible for genital tract infections as well.

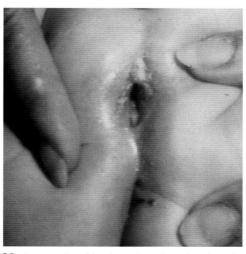

Figure 18-20. Poor perineal hygiene. Despite prior cleansing by a nurse for "a clean-catch" urine, the initial specimen contained numerous white cells and debris. When the perineum was rechecked, the infant was found to have copious amounts of smegma adhering to the clitoris and labia minora and stool on the posterior perineum. Urine obtained after thorough recleansing was normal.

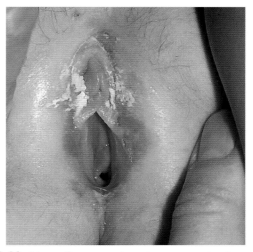

Figure 18-21. Maceration secondary to poor perineal aeration. This child's chief complaint was one of dysuria. On examination the inner surfaces of the labia were found to be macerated and mildly inflamed. Adherent smegma is also visible. The child had been wearing tights over nylon underwear.

findings are often unimpressive, patient and parental concern with the symptoms may be great. In some patients the vulva and vagina appear normal, whereas in others varying degrees of inflammation or irritation are present, at times accompanied by signs of excoriation. Vaginal discharge is unusual, however, and vaginal cultures grow normal or nonspecific flora (Table 18-11). These disorders are common in prepubertal children but are relatively infrequent after menarche. Individuals with underlying dermatologic disorders may be more susceptible to noninfectious causes of vulvovaginitis. Symptoms are similar for most etiologies: perineal itching or pain; external or contact dysuria; and, occasionally, vaginal discharge.

Treatment consists of removal of the offending agent or causative circumstance along with symptomatic measures. Recommended hygienic practices include providing a sufficient number of opportunities to urinate, use of a front-to-back wiping technique, and regular washing with mild soap without excessive scrubbing. Products to avoid include skin and vaginal cosmetics, scented pads and feminine hygiene products, bubble bath and other bath additives, fabric softeners and dryer sheets, and douches. Patients with vulvovaginal inflammation are encouraged to wear loose-fitting clothes and white cotton underwear that is well rinsed after regular washing. Failure to improve should lead to consideration of other etiologies, the possibility of noncompliance with treatment, or sexual abuse.

In prepubertal girls, chronic irritation from any cause may predispose the labia minora to agglutinate, resulting in labial adhesions (see Fig. 18-11). Urine trapped behind the adhesions after toileting may cause further irritation, helping to perpetuate the condition or causing adhesions to extend.

Noninfectious Vulvovaginitis Secondary to External Factors

Irritation Secondary to Poor Hygiene. Poor perineal hygiene is one of the most common causes of irritation. Examination typically reveals mild, nonspecific vulvar inflammation. Pieces of stool and toilet paper may be seen adhering to the perineum and perianal areas, and smegma may be found around the clitoris and labia (Fig. 18-20). Underwear is often soiled. Coliforms tend to predominate on vaginal culture when there is associated vaginal inflammation. In the majority of cases the search for other causes

is unrewarding, and symptoms resolve with a regimen of sitz baths and careful cleansing after urination and defecation. Finding a frankly feculent vaginal discharge should lead to the consideration of a rectovaginal fistula.

Maceration Secondary to Poor Perineal Aeration. Moisture, whether from normal secretions, perspiration, or swimming, when unable to evaporate, promotes maceration and inflammation of perineal tissues. Obesity, wearing tight clothing or tights over nylon underwear, and sitting for long periods in a wet bathing suit or leotard are common predisposing factors to this form of vulvar irritation. Nonspecific inflammation, often with frank maceration, is the predominant physical finding (Fig. 18-21). Patients with urinary incontinence, a vesicovaginal fistula, or ectopic ureter can also have these findings. A history of a chronically wet perineum and the smell of urine on the child's underclothes should lead the clinician to consider these possibilities.

When maceration occurs, secondary infection is common, and some patients have associated intertrigo.

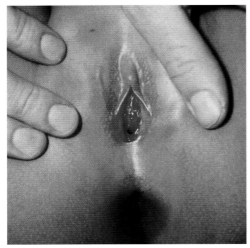

Figure 18-22. Nonspecific inflammation characteristic of chemical irritant vulvovaginitis.

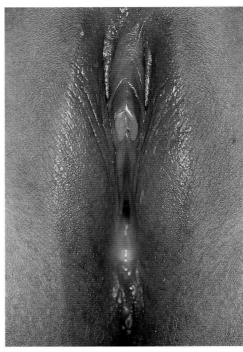

Figure 18-23. Frictional trauma (nonspecific thickening of the vulvar skin). This patient's labial skin is thickened and mildly irritated. She had a history of recurrent vaginal foreign bodies and was strongly suspected to be a victim of chronic sexual abuse. (Courtesy K. Sukarochana, MD, Pittsburgh, Pa.)

Attention to perineal hygiene and drying, weight loss (when appropriate), avoidance of tight clothing, and treatment of secondary infection are the mainstays of management.

Contact Dermatitis, Allergic Vulvitis. Allergic vulvitis should be considered in patients whose most prominent symptom is pruritus, although scratching and excoriation may result in secondary burning and dysuria. When patients are seen in the acute phase, inspection of the labia and vestibule reveals a microvesicular papular eruption that tends to be intensely erythematous and may be somewhat edematous. Excoriated scratch marks are common. When the process has become chronic, the vulvar skin has an eczematoid appearance with cracks, fissures, and lichenification. Over-the-counter and prescribed topical ointments, creams, and lotions; perfumed soaps and toilet paper; and poison ivy are common causative factors in prepubertal children. In adolescents, feminine hygiene products, cosmetics, spermicides, douches, and perfumed sanitary pads or tampons may be responsible.

Chemical Irritant Vulvovaginitis. Many of the agents capable of causing allergic vulvitis can also act as chemical irritants. Bubble bath, harsh soaps, laundry and dish detergents, fabric and water softeners, feminine hygiene products, spermicides, and perfumed or dyed toilet paper are common offenders. Before toilet training, children whose diapers are changed infrequently may develop irritation caused by ammonia produced when the organisms in stool split the urea in urine. Itching and dysuria are prominent symptoms, and examination usually discloses mild, nonspecific inflammation (Fig. 18-22), at times associated with signs of scratching. On occasion, findings are normal. Diagnosis is dependent on a thorough history (see Table 18-8).

Frictional Trauma. Frictional trauma may be the source of superficial abrasive changes and, when chronic, may result in lichenification or even atrophic skin changes (Fig. 18-23). Wearing tight clothing, certain sporting activities (especially gymnastics, long-distance cycling, and running), sand from sandboxes, and excessive masturbation are the major predisposing factors.

The practice of shaving pubic hair can result in local skin irritation and abrasions and often precipitates development of folliculitis. It can also precipitate reactivation of herpes simplex.

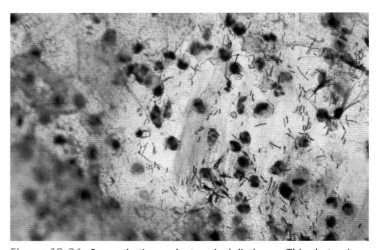

Figure 18-24. Sympathetic purulent vaginal discharge. This photomicrograph shows numerous leukocytes and epithelial cells, with mixed flora. The 4-year-old patient had a history of vomiting, anorexia, abdominal pain with marked right lower quadrant and pelvic tenderness, and a purulent vaginal discharge and was found to have a pelvic appendiceal abscess. The vaginal discharge was the result of sympathetic inflammation.

Other Inflammatory Conditions
Sympathetic Inflammation and Fistulas
Appendicitis with Pelvic Appendiceal Abscess. Preschool and young school-age children with appendicitis often do not come to medical attention until after appendiceal rupture has occurred. Girls with a pelvic appendix who wall off the rupture in a periappendiceal abscess may develop a copious purulent vaginal discharge caused by sympathetic inflammation of the vaginal wall. On microscopy the discharge contains numerous leukocytes, epithelial cells, and mixed flora (Fig. 18-24). The antecedent clinical course consisting of anorexia, nausea, vomiting, and abdominal pain along with findings on examination suggest the diagnosis. The latter may include abdominal

distention, direct and percussion tenderness (especially in the right lower quadrant), and a tender cystic mass palpable on rectal examination. The fact that the unestrogenized genital tract of the prepubertal girl does not promote the ascent of sexually transmitted infections eliminates pelvic inflammatory disease from the differential diagnosis.

Fistulas. Because patients with vesicovaginal fistulas and ectopic ureters have a history of a constantly wet perineum, they frequently have symptoms of vulvovaginitis. Nonspecific inflammation and maceration are the predominant physical findings (see Fig. 18-21).

Rectovaginal fistulas can also cause vulvovaginal inflammation, but the presence of a grossly feculent vaginal discharge usually makes diagnosis relatively easy. When rectovaginal fistulas are neither congenital nor post-traumatic in origin or when a perianal fistula is found, inflammatory bowel disease should be considered (see Chapter 10).

Vaginal Foreign Body. The hallmark of a vaginal foreign body is the presence of a profuse, foul-smelling, brownish or blood-streaked vaginal discharge. However, some children have a less dramatic presentation with a yellow, mildly purulent discharge. The majority of patients are in the 3- to 8-year-old age group. Some have developmental delay or other psychosocial and behavioral problems. Although wads of toilet tissue, paper, cotton, crayons, and small toys are the materials found most often, all types of small objects have been retrieved. A long non-inflammatory latency period may exist for inert materials. The objects most commonly found in adolescents are forgotten tampons or retained condoms. Suppositories or substances inserted for therapeutic purposes or objects used in sexual activity may also cause problems. Objects made of hard materials may be palpable on rectal examination.

Radiographs are rarely necessary because direct vaginoscopy is almost always required. Results of wet preparation, Gram stain, and culture are nonspecific. Vaginoscopy is diagnostic and, when tolerated, it provides access for extraction, which is curative. In the prepubertal age group, it is best accomplished under general anesthesia or conscious sedation.

When a prepubertal patient is found to have a vaginal foreign body, it is important to obtain a detailed behavioral history of the child in addition to a family psychosocial history because the problem is often recurrent and may be the result of disturbed behavior by the patient or of chronic sexual abuse.

Major differential diagnostic considerations for a brownish/bloody vaginal discharge are *Shigella* vaginitis, seen in prepubertal patients, and necrotic tumors, which can produce a discharge that is clinically indistinguishable from that of a vaginal foreign body.

Vulvovaginal Conditions Sometimes Mistaken for Vulvovaginitis

Urethral Prolapse

Urethral prolapse is often mistaken for vulvovaginitis or perineal trauma. Dysuria, perineal pain, and bleeding are the most frequent symptoms. The phenomenon is more prevalent among African-American and obese prepubertal school-age girls. Increased intra-abdominal pressure often precipitates the prolapse of the urethra through the urethral meatus. Constipation, especially when chronic; coughing; and crying may all contribute. The classic phys-

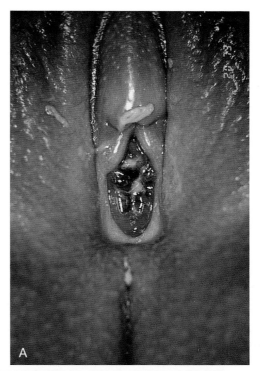

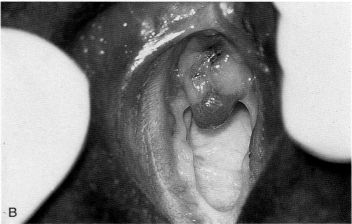

Figure 18-25. Urethral prolapse. **A,** This child had acute complaints of bleeding and dysuria. The prolapsed urethral mucosa is red and friable and has a doughnut shape encircling the urethra. **B,** In another patient the prolapsed mucosal tissue is thickened, and erythema is less prominent. (**A,** Courtesy John McCann, MD, University of California at Davis; **B,** courtesy Carole Jenny, MD, Hasbro Children's Hospital, Providence, RI.)

ical finding is a red or purplish red, swollen, and friable piece of tissue lying over the anterior introitus (Fig. 18-25). It often has a doughnut shape and is tender. With optimal positioning and careful visualization, the clinician can see that it encircles the urethral meatus. Because the urethral mucosa is responsive to estrogen, application of estrogen cream twice daily usually results in resolution. Oral analgesics and topical antibacterial and/or anesthetic creams provide symptomatic relief. Treatment of underlying causes reduces the risk of recurrence.

Lichen Sclerosus

Lichen sclerosus is a chronic dermatologic disorder of unknown etiology that primarily involves the perineum and perianal area in prepubertal girls. It begins insidiously, sometimes preceded by perineal itching and occasionally by a mild watery discharge. Initially there may be no readily visible signs, and symptomatic treatment is often prescribed to no effect. Eventually small pink or

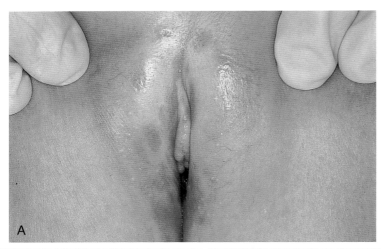

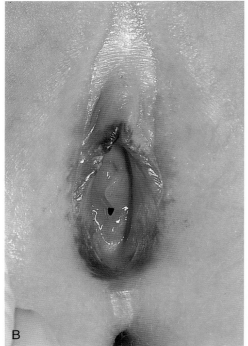

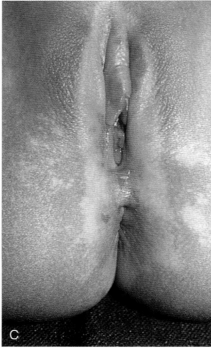

Figure 18-26. Lichen sclerosus. **A,** The skin overlying the labia majora has become atrophic and appears pale and thin. It is dotted with small, superficial ulcerations. **B,** In this child with complaints of bleeding and pruritus, skin breakdown is evident along with petechial hemorrhages. **C,** A pruritic, atrophic, eroded, hypopigmented patch involving the anogenital skin and mucous membranes in this 5-year-old girl has an hourglass configuration. (**C,** From Cohen BA: Pediatric Dermatology, 2nd ed. London, Mosby, 1999.)

white, flat-topped papular lesions appear on both cutaneous and mucosal surfaces, and these coalesce to form larger plaquelike lesions that may have scaly surfaces. Vesiculation may occur, followed by superficial ulceration or excoriation with increased erythema, maceration, and punctate bleeding (Fig. 18-26A). The latter occurs especially when pruritus incites rubbing or scratching (Fig. 18-26B). With progression, the involved epithelium becomes thin, atrophic, and hypopigmented. When both the vulvar and perianal areas are affected, the distribution has been likened to an hourglass or a figure-eight (Fig. 18-26C). On resolution of active lesions, the involved area is characterized by confluent, white, atrophic patches with a shiny surface.

The disorder tends to wax and wane over one to several years, often resolving around puberty. Acute exacerbations, which are often precipitated by local irritation or trauma, respond best to short-term treatment with ultra-high-potency topical steroids. Diagnosis generally can be made on clinical grounds, although some atypical cases may require dermatologic consultation and possibly a biopsy. When ulcerations and bleeding are present, concerns regarding sexual abuse may arise. The pattern and distribution of lesions, their failure to heal rapidly, and

the chronicity of the disorder help distinguish it from abrasions and lacerations due to abuse. In vitiligo, which may have a similar distribution when present in the anogenital area, the involved skin is totally devoid of pigment but is otherwise normal (i.e., not atrophic or inflamed) in appearance. In the adolescent, lichen planus may present with similar features.

Infectious Vulvovaginitis

In contrast to most of the primarily noninfectious forms of vulvovaginitis, vaginal discharge is usually a prominent part of the clinical picture of infectious vulvovaginitis in all age groups. Although a few pathogens produce a fairly characteristic clinical picture, most do not, the symptoms and discharge seen with many pathogens being relatively nonspecific. Furthermore, in the case of sexually transmitted infections, more than one pathogen may be present. For these reasons, careful attention to specimen collection technique is important.

Two major subgroups of vulvovaginal infection exist. In the first subgroup genital involvement is secondary to a systemic infection or the result of transfer of the pathogen

| Table 18-12 | Major Characteristics of the Most Common Sexually Transmitted Diseases and Diagnostic Measures |

	HSV	HPV	HIV	TRICHOMONAS	GONORRHEA	CHLAMYDIA	SYPHILIS
Possible clinical findings	Vulvar skin lesions, vulvitis, vaginitis, cervicitis; may be normal	Nonspecific vulvovaginal inflammation; subclinical lesions revealed by acid wash; vulvar, vaginal, and/or cervical condylomata and flat warts	Unusually severe presentation of Candida, HPV, HSV, or molluscum contagiosum; often resistant to treatment	Vaginitis, vulvitis, vaginal and/or cervical petechiae, profuse watery discharge	May be normal, cervicitis, salpingitis, urethritis, occasionally proctitis, pharyngitis; vaginitis and vulvitis in prepubertal girls	Often normal, cervicitis, salpingitis, urethritis, proctitis; vaginitis, and vulvitis in prepubertal girls	Primary—vulvar, vaginal, or cervical chancre; secondary—condylomata lata involving vulva with or without generalized exanthem
Incubation period	3-14 days	On average 1-3 months (up to 9 mo)	Acute flulike viral illness (several weeks); AIDS (variable—up to 10 yr)	3-30 days	2-7 days	7-21 days	Primary (15-90 days); secondary (6 wk-6 mo); tertiary (2-20 yr)
Infectivity	75%-80% (with active infection)	60%-70%	Varies with infecting behavior	70%-90% for M/F transmission, less for F/M	100% M/F; 25% F/M	45% M/F	10% single encounter; 30% after 1 mo of sexual activity with an infected partner
Duration	Primary (2-3 wk); secondary (7-12 days)	Variable; often, persistent clinical lesions and subclinical infection	Acute infection (2-3 wk); asymptomatic phase (months); symptomatic HIV (months-years); AIDS (months-years)	Self-limiting in many males; persistent in most females until treated	Until treated	Until treated	Primary (2-6 wk); secondary (2-6 wk) may recur; tertiary persists until treated
Recurrence	60% (HSV-1); 90% (HSV-2) within 1 yr	Variable	Persistence	With reinfection	With reinfection	With reinfection	With reinfection
Routine diagnostic techniques	Culture, Tzanck prep, Pap smear, antigen testing, serology	Inspection, Pap smear, acetic acid wash, colposcopy, HPV typing	ELISA, Western blot, viral culture become + within 6 wk-6 mo of infection	Wet prep, urinalysis, culture	Cervical culture,* pharyngeal or rectal culture, Gram stain, NAATs	NAATs, antigen detection by immunoassay, cervical swab for tissue culture*	Dark-field microscopy, serologic tests including VDRL, RPR, and FTA
Antenatal or perinatal transmission	Yes—can cause skin, CNS, and disseminated infection	Yes—can cause laryngeal papillomas and perineal lesions	Yes, and postpartum via breast milk	Yes—may have neonatal vaginal discharge or asymptomatic colonization	Yes—can cause conjunctivitis, septicemia, meningitis	Yes—can cause conjunctivitis and/or pneumonia	Yes, and postpartum via breast milk
Partner evaluation	Inspection	Inspection	Antibody test	Antimicrobial Rx	Diagnostic tests as above and antimicrobial Rx	Diagnostic tests as above and antimicrobial Rx	Serologic and clinical, antimicrobial Rx

*In prepubertal girls, culture discharge for gonorrhea, vaginal wall for C. trachomatis.
CNS, central nervous system; ELISA, enzyme-linked immunosorbent assay; F/M, female to male; FTA, fluorescent treponemal antibody; HIV, human immunodeficiency virus; HPV, human papillomavirus; HSV, herpes simplex virus; M/F, male to female; NAATs, nucleic acid amplification tests; RPR, rapid plasma reagin (test); VDRL, Venereal Disease Research Laboratory (test for syphilis); +, positive.

from another primary site such as the skin or the respiratory, gastrointestinal, or urinary tracts via contaminated fingers or proximity (see Table 18-9). Infection at the primary site may precede or coexist with the genital infection and, in some cases, colonization of another site, without overt infection, appears to predispose. This nonvenereal infectious vulvovaginitis is common in prepubertal patients but rare in adolescents because the mature female genital tract does not support growth of most of these pathogens.

The second subgroup of infectious vulvovaginitis consists of those infections caused by venereal or sexually transmitted pathogens (see Tables 18-9 and 18-10). Both prepubertal and postmenarchal patients can have vulvovaginitis when infected with these organisms. After puberty, however, patients can have other clinical pictures as well including cervicitis (with or without vulvovaginal inflammation) and salpingitis. Table 18-12 enumerates the possible clinical features seen in adolescent girls with sexually transmitted infections and summarizes other major epidemiologic characteristics and appropriate diagnostic measures.

Regardless of age, the most frequent mode of transmission of venereal infection is sexual contact. The majority

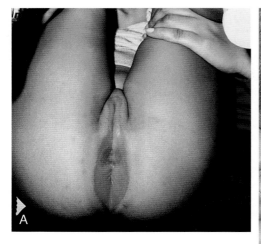

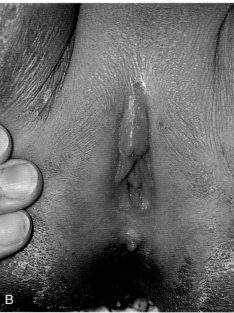

Figure 18-27. Streptococcal vulvovaginitis. **A,** In this child who had acute vulvar pain, dysuria, and discharge, the area of inflammation is sharply circumscribed and extends from the vulva to the perianal area. **B,** In another patient, who presented late in the course of a case of scarlet fever, vulvar inflammation is still evident and desquamation has begun.

of these infections in prepubertal patients are the result of sexual abuse, although in a small minority of cases transmission occurs perinatally or as a result of sex play with other children who have been abused (see Chapter 6). Hence when venereal disease is found in the prepubertal child, the possibility of sexual abuse *must* be investigated. In adolescence, consensual sexual activity is the major mode of infection by sexually transmitted pathogens, although sexual exploitation and abuse remain significant possibilities. These factors necessitate obtaining a confidential history of sexual activity and case finding of sexual partners. *The presence of one venereal pathogen in any child or adolescent should prompt investigation for others because infection with multiple organisms is common* (see "Genital Infections Caused by Sexually Transmitted Pathogens" later).

Infectious Vulvovaginitis Caused by Nonsexually Transmitted Pathogens

Vulvovaginitis Caused by Respiratory and/or Skin Pathogens. Bacterial respiratory pathogens can cause vulvovaginitis in prepubertal patients, presumably as a result of orodigital transmission. *Streptococcus pneumoniae* and *Haemophilus influenzae* cause purulent vaginal discharge, with associated vulvitis and vaginitis, either following or concurrent with upper respiratory tract infection. The most common and dramatic form of bacterial vulvovaginitis caused by a primary respiratory pathogen is that caused by group-A β-hemolytic streptococci. This infection may be associated with streptococcal nasopharyngitis or scarlet fever, or it may occur in apparent isolation, although a throat culture is often positive for streptococci even in the absence of pharyngeal or upper respiratory symptoms. The onset of vulvovaginal symptoms is abrupt, with severe perineal burning and dysuria. Inspection reveals a sharply circumscribed area of intense erythema involving the vulva, distal vagina, and perianal area (Fig. 18-27A). The involved skin may weep serous fluid. Most patients have a serosanguineous or grayish-white vaginal discharge, and about one third have vaginal petechiae. Culture of perineal skin and/or discharge is positive. Desquamation ensues with recovery (Fig. 18-27B and see Fig. 18-5).

Viral pathogens have also been linked to vulvovaginitis in young children. Varicella is perhaps the most common,

with pruritus and dysuria as its most prominent symptoms. Inspection reveals typical lesions involving the perineum and/or vagina (see Chapter 12) in addition to other skin and mucous membrane involvement. Adenovirus is reported to cause vulvovaginitis with a serous discharge in association with pharyngitis, conjunctivitis, and an exanthem, whereas echovirus causes a thick, clear vaginal discharge concurrent with gastroenteritis.

Impetigo and folliculitis may occur in the vulvar area of patients of any age and is generally secondary to poor hygiene, excessive sweating, shaving, or mechanical irritation. Simultaneous involvement of the buttocks or other skin sites is common (see Chapter 12). Some young women with increased androgens, children with a familial predisposition to keratosis pilaris, and patients with Down syndrome may be especially prone to developing folliculitis and/or impetigo.

Vulvovaginitis Caused by Gastrointestinal Pathogens

Shigella. A distinct form of vulvovaginitis caused by *Shigella* species has been recognized in prepubertal patients. The majority have no overt gastrointestinal symptoms, although approximately one third have had associated diarrhea.

The predominant complaint is one of an acute or chronic vaginal discharge. Most patients are otherwise asymptomatic, although some have dysuria. A greenish brown, often blood-streaked, purulent, and foul-smelling vaginal discharge is seen on inspection, along with vulvar and vaginal erythema. The clinical appearance of the discharge may be indistinguishable from that seen with a vaginal foreign body. Gram stain reveals large numbers of polymorphonuclear leukocytes and a predominance of gram-negative rods. A positive culture is diagnostic, but enteric-specific bacteriologic transport and culture media must be used. Antibiotic sensitivities may demonstrate broad resistance. Without proper treatment the discharge may persist for months. A high rate of coinfection with pinworms has been reported.

Pinworms. Intestinal infestation with pinworms (*Enterobius vermicularis*) is primarily associated with perianal pruritus. However, the worms may crawl forward into the vagina, bringing enteric flora with them and depositing eggs. In some cases vaginal infection and discharge may

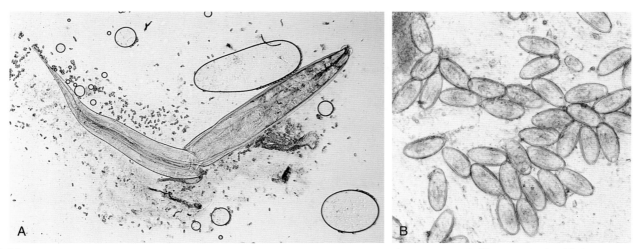

Figure 18-28. Pinworms *(Enterobius vermicularis)*. **A,** On this wet mount a mature worm is shown surrounded by eggs. **B,** Ovoid pinworm eggs at higher power. Patients with intestinal infestation may have vulvovaginal symptoms as a result of scratching and excoriation or migration of the worms into the vagina.

result. Scratching may produce excoriation and secondary dysuria. A history of preceding perianal pruritus generally is elicited. Inflammatory changes are nonspecific. Pinworm ova and/or adult worms may be found on wet mount examination of vaginal secretions (Fig. 18-28). In the occasional patient with associated vaginal discharge, culture is positive for enteric pathogens. When pinworm infestation is suspected despite negative vaginal smears, the perianal sticky tape test should be obtained by the mother during the night to increase the likelihood of detection. Alternatively, empirical treatment may be instituted.

***Candida* Vulvovaginitis.** *Candida* species are one of the more common sources of nonvenereal infectious vulvovaginitis after puberty. This is rare in the healthy prepubertal child. Predisposing factors include recent antibiotic intake, poor perineal ventilation, diabetes mellitus, immunodeficiency, pregnancy, and the use of combined hormonal or estrogen-containing oral contraceptives. Pruritus, contact dysuria, and dyspareunia are the most prominent complaints. Symptoms are most likely to develop in the perimenstrual phase of the patient's cycle. Examination usually discloses diffuse erythema of the vulva associated with a thick cheesy vaginal discharge (Fig. 18-29A). With chronic involvement, white or pink cobblestone plaques on an erythematous base may be seen over the vulva. Excoriations from scratching may also be noted, and satellite lesions on the perineum are common. In some cases, signs of perianal dermatitis and intertrigo are found in association with vulvovaginal involvement.

Inspection of the lower third of the vagina in young patients and speculum examination in adolescents may reveal a thick white discharge of creamy or cheesy consistency. Whitish plaques may adhere to the vaginal mucosa or to the cervix in adolescents (Fig. 18-29B). A KOH or wet preparation confirms the presence of budding yeast and pseudohyphae in 50% to 60% of cases and may demonstrate a modest increase in inflammatory cells (see Fig. 18-29C and D). Vaginal pH is low (3.5 to 5).

Topical application of an azole antifungal cream into the lower vagina or single-dose oral fluconazole are the treatments of choice. Single-dose oral regimens are less efficacious but are simple and may be more reliable when problems with compliance are an issue. In sexually active adolescents, careful consideration must be given to the possibility of pregnancy before prescribing antimicrobials

or any other medication. In patients with recurrences, predisposing factors such as medications and human immunodeficiency virus (HIV) infection should be considered. An infected male partner with subacute or chronic monilial balanitis rarely may be the source of recurrences in sexually active patients. This infection is generally not transmitted sexually, and treatment of the partner does not decrease recurrence rates.

Other fungi such as *Torulopsis* may also cause vulvovaginitis. Clinical presentation tends to be similar to that of *Candida*, but under microscopy these organisms do not demonstrate the classic branching morphology seen with *Candida*. They are often more resistant to first-line antifungal agents, and this should be suspected in the patient who appears to have persistent or recurrent *Candida* infection and a fungal culture obtained. This will provide diagnostic specificity and guide the choice of antifungal treatment.

Genital Infections Caused by Sexually Transmitted Pathogens

The rise in prevalence of sexually transmitted diseases and the recognition of an increasing array of pathogens (see Table 18-9) have prompted research that has produced a better understanding of their pathophysiology and the clinical pictures they produce (see Table 18-12). It has also made the evaluation of patients with STDs considerably more specific and complex. The majority of symptomatic infections are manifest by external lesions and/or vulvovaginal inflammation with vaginal discharge. Although some infections produce relatively specific clinical findings, many are characterized by nonspecific signs and symptoms that appear to represent a final common pathway of a number of different etiologic agents of irritation, infection, or infestation. Several pathogens can induce two or three different clinical pictures (or a mixed picture) in adolescents. Furthermore, the high frequency of multiple simultaneous infections adds to the complexity and necessitates more extensive laboratory evaluation. The clinical approach to these patients must be sensitive and individualized but also must differ considerably depending on whether or not the patient is prepubertal or postpubertal.

Approach to Sexually Transmitted Diseases in Prepubertal Patients. Before menarche, lack of estrogenization inhibits ascent of infection to the upper genital tract,

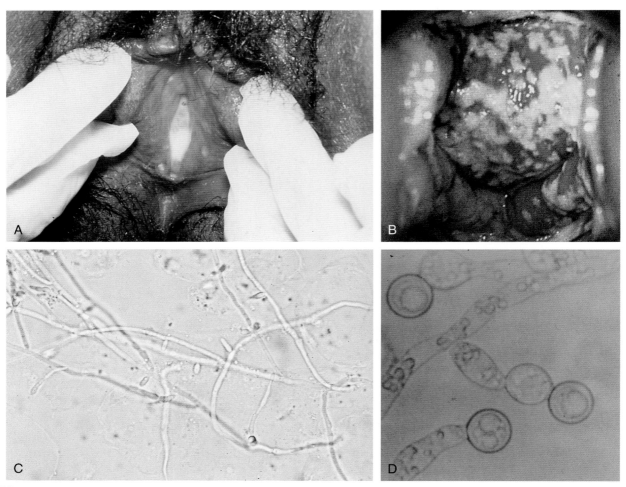

Figure 18-29. *Candida* vulvovaginitis and cervicitis. **A,** The vulva is intensely hyperemic, and a thick, cheesy, white discharge covers the urethra, introitus, and hymenal area. **B,** Whitish plaques may be seen on the perineum and vaginal mucosa and occasionally on the cervix in adolescents. A whitish cheesy or creamy vaginal discharge may be noted as well. **C** and **D,** These low- and high-power wet mount specimens contain pseudohyphae and budding yeast. (**A,** Courtesy B. Cohen, MD, Johns Hopkins Hospital, Baltimore; **B** and **D,** courtesy Ellen Wald, MD, University of Wisconsin Children's Hospital.)

and subclinical lower tract infection is probably unusual if not rare. Hence manifestations of venereal infection are primarily confined to the vulva and lower vagina. As a result, external inspection of the perineum and lower vagina and laboratory evaluation of vaginal discharge samples are sufficient for identification of most pathogens and for institution of therapy, with the exception of *Chlamydia*, which necessitates swabbing the vaginal wall to obtain mucosal cells. This does not complete the assessment, however, because whenever an STD is identified in a prepubertal patient, *sexual abuse must be considered as the probable source.* This necessitates obtaining an extensive psychosocial history and initiating a thorough investigation to find the person responsible for transmitting the infection to the child (see Chapter 6).

Complaints of pubertal patients with vulvovaginitis include vulvar lesions, vaginal discharge, odor, pruritus or perineal discomfort, and dysuria. These symptoms may also be associated with pelvic pain, dyspareunia, fever, and irregular bleeding. A number of pathogens cause inflammation of not only the vulva and vagina but the cervix as well. Herpes simplex, *Trichomonas vaginalis,* and human papillomaviruses are prime examples. Patients infected with *N. gonorrhoeae* or *C. trachomatis* may be asymptomatic even in the presence of cervicitis. When symptomatic, they may have bleeding and/or dysuria; vaginal discharge; or, with ascent of infection to the upper tract, signs of salpingitis, although this, too, can be clinically silent (see Tables 18-10 and 18-12). *N. gonorrhoeae* and

C. trachomatis also infect the columnar epithelium of other genital sites including the Bartholin glands, Skene ducts, the urethra, and the rectum.

Hence a complete pelvic examination is desirable when evaluating adolescents for vulvovaginal complaints and possible STDs. After inspection of the perineum, the vaginal mucosa and the cervix must be visualized and their appearance assessed for signs of erythema, friability, focal lesions, and mucopurulent discharge. To differentiate a true cervical discharge from normal pooled vaginal secretions adhering to the cervix, visible discharge should be removed gently with cotton swabs before inspection. Some clinicians advocate collection of a urethral specimen that can be pooled with the cervical specimen as a way to enhance detection. Cervical secretions should be sampled (for wet preparation and cultures) by insertion of swabs into the os. The finding of cervicitis with a mucopurulent cervical discharge suggests gonorrheal and/or chlamydial infection and necessitates an attempt to identify or rule out upper tract involvement via bimanual examination. Cervical motion and uterine tenderness and/or a tender, palpable adnexal mass with or without systemic signs and symptoms suggest this possibility (see "Pelvic Inflammatory Disease" later). The recent advent of Food and Drug Administration–approved nucleic acid amplification tests (NAATs) using urine or vaginal swabs for detection of *N. gonorrhoeae* and *C. trachomatis* is transforming practice and may ultimately reduce the need for speculum examinations.

A number of additional considerations are important in evaluating postpubertal patients suspected of having an STD. A sexual history obtained in confidence is essential, and although consensual activity is common in adolescence, these patients may be victims of sexual abuse including incest, sexual exploitation, and date rape. Sexual partners should be evaluated and treated whenever an STD is identified; otherwise, reinfection is probable.

Adolescent girls with asymptomatic cervical infections may serve as silent reservoirs of venereal pathogens. This phenomenon is quite significant in the epidemiology of STDs. Hence women partners of men known to have gonococcal, chlamydial, or nonspecific urethritis should be evaluated and treated appropriately. The patient and partner(s) must be advised to abstain from sexual intercourse until the course of treatment is completed by all. In the case of single-dose regimens, abstinence should be practiced for 7 days after the partner (or partners) begins treatment. They also should be seen in follow-up to test for reinfection, and thereafter at least every 6 months for STD surveillance because of the significant incidence of (often subclinical) reinfection.

The importance of aggressive case finding, diagnosis, and treatment cannot be overemphasized because of the potential for spread to others and of major sequelae that include ectopic pregnancy and infertility as a result of smoldering or recurrent acute upper genital tract disease. Finally, it is the clinician's responsibility to provide education regarding STDs. Patients should clearly understand how the disease was contracted and how to prevent recurrence. Use of condoms should be emphasized at each opportunity. Education includes discussion of responsible sexuality including abstinence, use of contraceptives and safer sex practices, as appropriate to the patient.

Surface Infestations and Perineal Lesions

Parasitic Infestations. Two parasitic infestations—scabies and pubic lice—may be transmitted via sexual contact. Both produce symptoms of vulvar and inguinal pruritus and irritation accompanied by finding dark specks of parasite feces on underwear or blood caused by excoriation from scratching. Sexual transmission is more likely in adolescents than in young children, who may acquire the parasites by close, nonsexual contact. Development of pubic hair is necessary for acquisition of pubic lice. Meticulous inspection of the pubic area for nits and adult lice ("crabs") may be necessary to discover early infestations. The clinical findings of both disorders are presented in Chapter 8.

Human Papillomavirus. HPV has emerged as the most prevalent sexually transmitted pathogen found in adolescent girls. Genital or venereal warts, also called *condylomata acuminata,* are no longer regarded as an isolated nuisance, being recognized as but one manifestation of a spectrum of lower genital tract diseases caused by HPV. The virus has been identified as causative in the development of cervical intraepithelial neoplasia and dysplasia (atypical squamous cells of undetermined significance, low-grade squamous intraepithelial lesions, or high-grade squamous intraepithelial lesions) and, similarly, carcinoma of the cervix and of other genital tissues in both men and women.

Transmission is usually via sexual contact in adolescents. Passage to neonates during delivery has also been documented and can result in subsequent development of laryngeal papillomata and perineal lesions. Vaginal involvement is uncommon in the prepubertal child but, when present, is often accompanied by a vaginal discharge. The incubation period is variable and ranges from 1 to 9 months (see Table 18-12).

Condylomata may emerge after subclinical, acute, or chronic nonspecific vulvovaginal inflammation incited by the virus. In most cases the lesions are asymptomatic, although pruritus is reported by some patients. However, when the warts are traumatized or become secondarily infected, pain may be a complaint. A rapid increase in warty tissue may be associated with diabetes, pregnancy, or HIV infection.

Generally the warts appear as fleshy, rounded, or ragged papules often located at the posterior edge of the introitus and/or in the perianal region. Lesions may be discrete early on (Fig. 18-30A), but with evolution they tend to become confluent (Fig. 18-30B). The warts can also be flat or even clinically unapparent to the naked eye. Although most lesions involve the perineum and perianal areas, vaginal and cervical involvement is also common in adolescents (Fig. 18-30C). Hence when vulvar condylomata are found in postpubertal patients, inspection of the vagina and cervix should be undertaken and a Pap smear

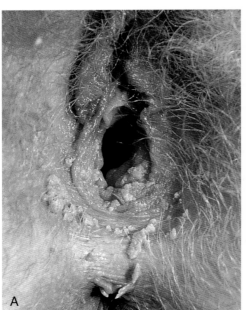
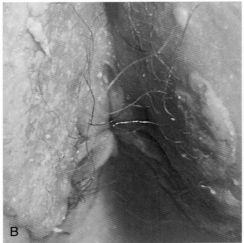
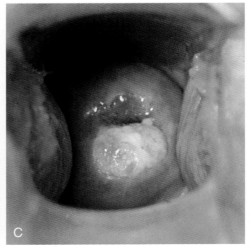

Figure 18-30. Condylomata acuminata. These sexually transmitted viral warts **(A)** tend to be discrete early on, but with evolution become confluent **(B)**. Adolescents have a significant risk of developing vaginal and cervical lesions **(C)**. (**A** and **C**, Courtesy E. Jerome, MD; **B**, courtesy M. Sherlock, MD, Lutherville, Md.)

obtained. The virus can also infect other mucous membranes including the anus, urethra, mouth, larynx, and conjunctiva.

Clinical diagnosis is made by careful inspection of the external genitalia, vagina, cervix (in adolescents), and perianal areas for visible warts. Examination of genital tissue after washing or soaking with 5% acetic acid (household vinegar) for up to 5 minutes reveals subclinical lesions because it causes proliferating and immature epithelium to turn white due to disordered orientation of intracellular fibers. Most normal tissues retain a pink color. Other disorders that damage the epithelium produce aceto-white changes as well. These include injury, contact dermatitis, candidiasis, folliculitis, and allergic excoriation.

HPV infection is identified cytologically on Pap smear or thin prep by characteristic changes, including koilocytosis, which is pathognomonic for HPV infection. DNA hybridization has identified more than 100 subtypes of the virus, many of which are site- and pattern-specific in their disease expression. Identification of subtypes is possible, and guidelines have been published by the American College of Obstetrics and Gynecology and American Society for Colposcopy and Cervical Pathology (ASCCP) to assist the clinician in further evaluation and treatment of abnormal Pap and thin preps (see Web sites—in bibliography). A negative VDRL or RPR helps differentiate HPV disease from the condylomata lata of secondary syphilis. Patients with cervical lesions merit gynecologic referral for HPV typing, colposcopy, biopsy, and definitive treatment (as indicated) because of the potential of these lesions to undergo malignant transformation.

Molluscum Contagiosum. These sharply circumscribed, waxy, papular, umbilicated lesions caused by a poxvirus can be spread as a result of sexual contact, in which case lesions are found predominantly on the labia, mons pubis, buttocks, and lower abdomen. This mode of spread is much more likely in the adolescent than in the young child. The clinical characteristics of molluscum lesions are presented in Chapter 8.

Syphilis
Syphilitic Chancre. Primary syphilis should be considered in any patient with a genital ulcer. The typical syphilitic chancre is painless and indurated with rolled margins and a smooth base (Fig. 18-31). It begins as an erythematous papule that erodes centrally. Most involve the genitalia, and in women they tend to be found more often on the cervix or vaginal walls than on the labia. Both external and internal lesions are painless and tend to go unnoticed unless a young woman happens to undergo pelvic examination while they are present. Hence active syphilis in women often goes undiagnosed until the secondary stage of the disease. Although a single lesion is typical, multiple chancres are seen in some cases. The chancre usually appears 3 to 4 weeks (up to 3 months) after inoculation with *Treponema pallidum* and is accompanied by inguinal adenopathy. Involved nodes are firm, mobile, and nontender. Because atypical lesions are common, all suspicious ulcers should prompt investigation by dark-field examination of scrapings from the base of the ulcer or of material aspirated from an enlarged regional node. Prior application of topical antibiotic ointment to a chancre can give false-negative results with ulcer scrapings. Reagin serologic tests (Venereal Disease Research Laboratory or rapid plasma reagin) usually become positive within 1 to 2 weeks after the appearance of the chancre and are uniformly elevated after a month. Positive reagin tests should always be confirmed by a fluorescent treponemal antibody test. Left untreated, chancres heal spontaneously in 3 to 8 weeks, but the infection persists.

Secondary Syphilis. In the absence of early diagnosis and treatment, hematogenous spread occurs approximately 1 to 3 months after the appearance of the primary chancre whereupon the lesions of secondary syphilis appear. These are accompanied or preceded by generalized adenopathy and are often associated with systemic flulike symptoms of fever, headache, malaise, arthralgia, sore throat, and rhinorrhea. The rash generalizes rapidly, has a symmetrical distribution, and involves the palms and soles. The lesions usually take the form of reddish-brown maculopapules, although commonly they are papulosquamous (Fig. 18-32A). Follicular and pustular lesions may also be seen, making secondary syphilis the "great mimicker." They range in size from a few millimeters to 1 cm and can be round or oval. Occasionally they clear centrally, becoming annular. As in pityriasis rosea, for which the rash is often mistaken, they are frequently oriented along lines of skin cleavage. Moist papules, called *condylomata lata,* are found in the genital folds, gluteal cleft, and over the medial surfaces of the upper thighs (Fig. 18-32B). These papules often resemble small mushroom caps or have a warty appearance with a pinkish-gray color and range in size from 1 to 3 cm. Many patients develop an associated patchy alopecia.

Mucosal lesions, termed *mucous patches* (Fig. 18-32C), appear as centrally eroded, grayish-white plaques 0.5 to 1 cm in diameter and can be found on all mucosal surfaces. Condylomata lata and mucosal lesions teem with organisms and are thus highly infectious. They are ideal sites for obtaining specimens for dark-field examination. Serologic tests are positive at this stage. The rash persists for 1 to 3 months if untreated, then clears spontaneously, marking the beginning of a period of latency in which the organism persists in multiple tissues with the potential for causing tertiary disease years later.

Bartholin Gland Abscess. This problem presents as a unilateral red, hot, tender mass at the posterior margin of the introitus at the base of a labia majorum (see Fig. 18-36A). It is generally seen in adolescents with gonorrhea, but it can occur in younger patients infected with gonococci, and it is increasingly associated with *C. trachomatis.* When such a mass is encountered, material expressed from the abscess should be cultured because other agents such as streptococci and vaginal anaerobes

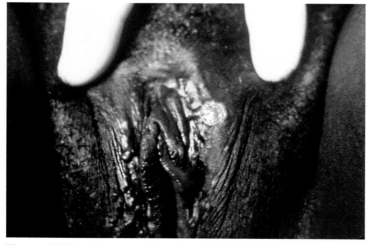

Figure 18-31. Primary syphilis. This syphilitic chancre was painless and indurated on palpation. The base is smooth, and the margins are rolled. (Courtesy Centers for Disease Control and Prevention Public Health Image Library.)

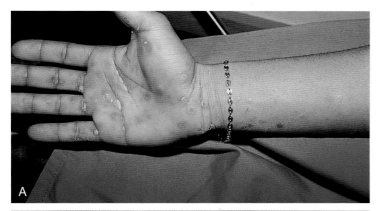
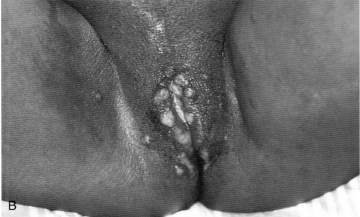
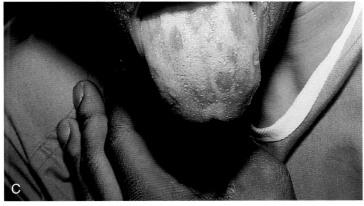

Figure 18-32. Secondary syphilis. **A,** This adolescent had flulike symptoms and a generalized papulosquamous eruption involving the palms and soles. **B,** In another patient, the characteristic moist papules of condylomata lata are seen over the vulva and the medial thighs. **C,** Mucosal lesions were also prominent. The systemic symptoms, mucosal lesions, and involvement of palms and soles helped distinguish the eruption from that of pityriasis rosea, with which it is commonly confused. (**A** and **C,** Courtesy Robert Hickey, MD, Children's Hospital of Pittsburgh; **B,** Courtesy J. Pledger, Centers for Disease Control and Prevention.)

have also been documented as pathogens. A full evaluation for STDs including cervical swabs may be necessary for organism identification. Treatment is based on Gram stain and culture results. Often, incision drainage and packing are required.

Lower Tract Disease. A number of sexually transmitted infections that are manifest as vulvovaginitis in the prepubertal patient produce findings limited to the lower genital tract (e.g., vaginitis, cervicitis) in the adolescent. A discussion of these infections follows. Upper tract manifestations are discussed later in "Pelvic Inflammatory Disease."

Genital Herpes. Type 2 and, less commonly, type 1 herpes simplex viruses have been confirmed as genital

pathogens in both pubertal and prepubertal girls. In adolescents, genital infection is acquired almost exclusively by sexual or intimate contact with infected mucosal surfaces. In prepubertal children, vulvar involvement can also result from sexual contact but more often results from spread from another infected site such as the lip, mouth, or a herpetic whitlow. It has also been acquired from parents with herpes labialis who fail to wash their hands properly before changing diapers or before assisting young children with toileting. Following exposure to the virus, 75% to 80% of susceptible individuals develop signs of infection after an incubation period of 3 to 14 days. Most infections are symptomatic, but occasionally infected individuals have no symptoms. An antibody response, with or without symptoms, can be produced within a few days.

Patients with primary infection frequently have systemic symptoms of fever, malaise, and myalgia, in addition to severe perineal pain and dysuria. Tender inguinal adenopathy is usually prominent but may not develop for several days. Perineal inspection reveals single or clustered vesicular lesions and/or ulcers on erythematous and edematous bases (Fig. 18-33A). Acute ulcerations are typically covered by yellow exudate and may be extensive (Fig. 18-33B). A copious, foul-smelling, watery yellow vaginal discharge may be seen as well. Associated sterile pyuria may be a feature. Dysuria may be so severe as to cause acute urinary retention. The ulcerative phase gradually resolves as lesions heal within a period of 14 to 21 days. Following primary infection, a persistent subclinical infection is established in the lumbosacral ganglia.

Diagnosis can usually be made on the basis of clinical appearance and can be confirmed in the laboratory by finding multinucleated giant cells on cytologic smears obtained by scraping the base of a lesion, smearing the specimen on a glass slide, and staining it with Wright-Giemsa stain (Fig. 18-33C). Viral culture of a fresh and ideally vesicular lesion is usually confirmatory within a few days and is the diagnostic test of choice. Serum confirmation of type I or II infection is possible but does not influence treatment decisions. Clinical suspicion is the usual indication for initiating antiviral therapy because the earlier it is begun, the more efficacious it is likely to be.

Recurrences are common and generally milder, of shorter duration, and only locally symptomatic. Possible triggers of recurrence include fever, menstruation, emotional stress, and friction. Occasionally, prodromal tingling, pain, burning, or hyperesthesia is noticed in the area where vesicles ultimately recur. The interval between episodes varies widely.

In postpubertal patients with vulvar herpetic lesions, speculum examination should be considered to look for the presence of other STDs and of herpes cervicitis, which is characterized by ulceration, friability, and a serosanguineous discharge. Herpetic ulcers are often found on the vaginal mucosa as well. However, severe local pain may preclude internal examination. In such cases obtaining distal vaginal swabs for NAATs for gonorrhea and *C. trachomatis* is clearly the better course, and early presumptive antibiotic treatment should be offered.

Trichomonas Infection. *Trichomonas vaginalis* is a flagellated protozoan. It has been found in the vaginal discharge of neonates delivered of mothers infected at the time of delivery, but thereafter it tends to be an unusual finding until the peripubertal period. This is thought to be due to the alkaline environment of the unestrogenized vaginal mucosa, which is unfavorable for growth of the

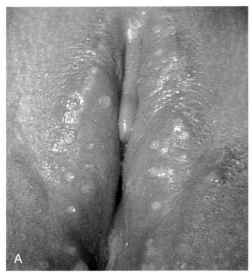
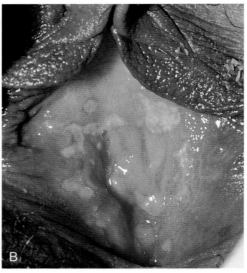
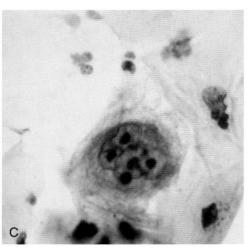

Figure 18-33. Herpes simplex. **A,** This prepubertal child had intense dysuria, perineal pain, and numerous thick-walled vesicular lesions, a few of which have ulcerated, over her perineum. **B,** The full-blown ulcerative phase of herpetic vulvitis is seen in this adolescent patient. **C,** Wright-Giemsa stain of scrapings from the base of a herpetic ulcer demonstrates a typical multinucleated giant cell with viral inclusions. (**C,** Courtesy Ellen Wald, MD, University of Wisconsin Children's Hospital.)

organism. Beyond the neonatal period it is acquired almost exclusively by sexual contact, often in concert with other sexually transmitted pathogens. However, trichomonads can live on warm, moist surfaces outside a living host for up to 45 minutes. Hence transmission via fomites is possible though infrequent. Although infection is occasionally asymptomatic in adolescents, the majority of patients have vulvar pruritus, burning, and dysuria, in association with a profuse vaginal discharge. The latter may be watery, yellowish gray, or green. In some cases it is bubbly; in others it is homogeneous. Frequently the discharge has a foul, acrid odor. Some affected adolescents may complain of pelvic pain or heaviness.

On inspection the vulva may be hyperemic and edematous, but the degree of inflammation is highly variable. Because the discharge is profuse, it may be present on the perineum (Fig. 18-34A). It pools in dependent portions of the vagina and coats the vaginal walls. The vaginal mucosa is erythematous, and punctate petechial lesions may be noted. In the adolescent these hemorrhagic areas may involve the cervical mucosa, producing the pathognomonic, albeit relatively uncommon, strawberry cervix (Fig. 18-34B). This organism does not routinely ascend to infect the upper genital tract.

Diagnosis is usually confirmed by finding motile trichomonads on microscopic examination of a saline wet mount (Fig. 18-34C), but this may be positive in only 50% to 60% of infections. On close observation, whiplike flagellar movements are noted. Leukocytes are usually present in increased numbers and may surround the organisms, making detection more difficult. Test yield may be increased by warming the saline solution to body temperature, and diluting a densely cellular discharge may make it easier to see the organisms moving. The slide must be examined soon after preparation because drying makes it uninterpretable. A mildly positive whiff test (release of amine odor on addition of 10% KOH to a drop of discharge) is also common. Trichomonads may also be found in urine specimens. Reports of trichomonads on Pap smears have a high rate of false-positives and false-negatives. Positive reports in symptomatic patients warrant treatment. Finding an elevated vaginal pH may also support diagnosis. *Trichomonas* cultures, the gold standard

of diagnosis, are generally not available in clinical laboratories. An office test, the InPouch TV test, a contained culture system, and several other FDA-cleared rapid assays are available but not commonly used in clinical settings.

Oral metronidazole is effective for treatment but should be avoided in pregnant patients because of its teratogenic potential. Intravaginal metronidazole does not have sufficient absorption to reach the multiple sites of trichomonal infection including the urethra and Skene glands. Tinidazole is used when metronidazole fails or organisms are known to be resistant. Sexual partners are usually asymptomatic carriers of small numbers of organisms but occasionally have symptoms of urethritis. Whether symptomatic or not, they should be treated to avoid subsequent transmission.

Bacterial Vaginosis. Bacterial vaginosis (BV), formerly called *Gardnerella vaginalis,* is a noninflammatory condition that represents a disturbance in the vaginal ecosystem. Women with BV have an overgrowth of multiple species of anaerobic bacteria and a corresponding decrease in their population of lactobacilli. The overall concentration of bacteria increases 100-fold. The condition is associated with an increased frequency of preterm labor, and data suggest an association with increased incidence of pelvic inflammatory disease. The major symptom in all age groups is a vaginal discharge with a noticeable fishy odor. Adolescents with BV have little vulvovaginal irritation, and the cervix and upper genital tract are spared.

On inspection, discharge is frequently present on the perineum (Fig. 18-35A) and may be seen adhering to the vaginal walls, which do not appear to be inflamed. Generally the discharge is thin and homogeneous in consistency, grayish white in color, and malodorous. Addition of 10% KOH to a sample of the discharge produces a noticeable amine odor (positive whiff test). A saline wet preparation usually reveals characteristic "clue cells," vaginal epithelial cells whose cell membranes are stippled with adherent refractile bacteria (Fig. 18-35B). On Gram stain the cells appear studded with gram-negative or gram-variable rods.

The diagnosis is made clinically by meeting three of the following four criteria: homogeneous white discharge, a positive whiff test, clue cells representing more than 20%

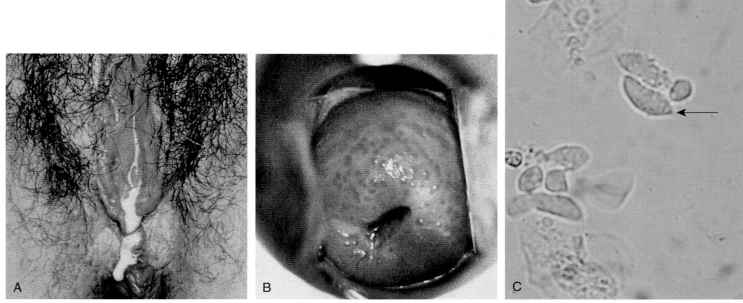

Figure 18-34. *Trichomonas* infection. **A,** *Trichomonas vaginalis* produces a profuse, acrid-smelling, thin discharge that often is visible on perineal inspection. In some cases it is homogeneous, and in others it is bubbly. Vulvar pruritus is often intense. **B,** The vaginal mucosa is inflamed and often speckled with petechial lesions. In adolescents, petechial hemorrhages may also be found on the cervix, resulting in the so-called strawberry cervix. **C,** Microscopic examination of a wet mount reveals multiple motile trichomonads. A sperm is seen in the upper portion of the picture (*arrow*). (**A** and **B,** Courtesy Ellen Wald, MD, University of Wisconsin Children's Hospital.)

Figure 18-35. Bacterial vaginosis (previously called *Gardnerella vaginalis*). Overgrowth of multiple anaerobes produces this form of vaginosis. **A,** The major symptom is one of a malodorous homogeneous vaginal discharge. **B,** Characteristic "clue cells" are seen on wet mount and consist of vaginal epithelial cells covered with adherent refractile bacteria. Because the organisms are non-invasive, leukocytes are not increased and mucosal changes are not present. (**A,** Courtesy Ellen Wald, MD, University of Wisconsin Children's Hospital.)

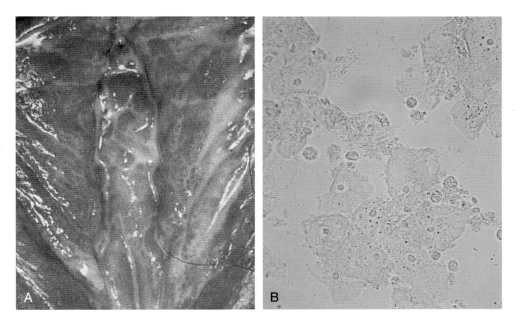

of the epithelial cells on a saline wet mount preparation, and vaginal secretions with a pH greater than 4.5. Because BV alone is rarely associated with evidence of tissue invasion, leukocytes should not be seen in increased numbers. If they are, additional pathogens should be sought and are often found. Both oral and intravaginal metronidazole and intravaginal clindamycin are acceptable forms of treatment in the nonpregnant patient.

Gonorrhea. Gonococci are still a common cause of treatable bacterial cervicitis in the adolescent and vulvovaginitis in the prepubertal child. The major complaint is of a purulent vaginal discharge. Before menarche the child may be otherwise asymptomatic, but most experience some degree of vulvar discomfort, pruritus, and/or dysuria. Symptomatic adolescents without upper genital tract extension can have a similar picture. Inspection reveals a profuse purulent discharge that usually is greenish yellow but also can be creamy, yellow, green, or white (Fig. 18-36A). Inspection of the distal vaginal mucosa in younger children reveals prominent inflammation. In adolescents the vaginal mucosa can appear normal, but the cervix is usually erythematous and friable, with purulent material seen draining through the os (Fig. 18-36B). Patients in this age group may also have objective evidence of urethritis as manifested by erythema, edema, and tenderness of the urethra. When the latter findings are present, purulent material can sometimes be expressed by pressing along the length of the urethra through the anterior vaginal wall. A sample of this material should be sent for culture along with a cervical swab. Other sites

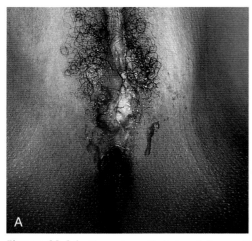
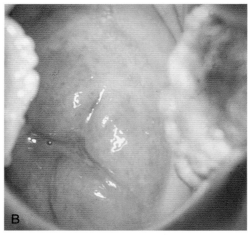
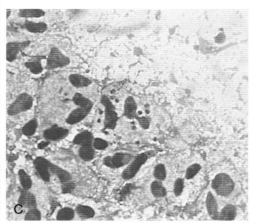

Figure 18-36. Gonorrhea. **A,** Vulvar inflammation, edema, and a purulent vaginal discharge are seen in this peripubertal child who was a victim of sexual abuse. She also has a unilateral Bartholin gland abscess. **B,** Adolescents are vulnerable to ascent of infection and usually have findings of cervical inflammation with mucopurulent discharge. **C,** On Gram stain the vaginal discharge from the patient in **A** is found to contain sheets of leukocytes, many of which contain gram-negative intracellular diplococci. This test is highly reliable for prepubertal girls and for boys with a urethral discharge, but adolescent girls have a significant incidence of false-negatives and false-positives. (**B,** Courtesy L. Vontver, MD.)

with columnar epithelium are similarly vulnerable to infection. These include the Bartholin and Skene glands and the rectum.

Laboratory studies are essential for accurate diagnosis. In prepubertal patients a Gram-stained smear of the vaginal discharge is reliably positive for large numbers of leukocytes and gram-negative intracellular diplococci and is adequate for initiation of treatment (Fig. 18-36C). Culture is important to detect the few cases with a false-negative Gram stain and determine antimicrobial sensitivity, and it is essential for medicolegal confirmation. Because simultaneous throat and anal cultures commonly are positive (despite the absence of anorectal or pharyngeal symptoms) in the prepubertal child who is likely to be a victim of sexual abuse, these sites should also be cultured when gonorrhea is suspected or confirmed. They may even be positive when the perineal or vaginal culture is negative. Both tonsils and the posterior pharyngeal wall should be swabbed in obtaining the throat specimen, and the rectal swab should be inserted no more than 1 to 2 cm past the anal orifice to avoid fecal contamination. Culture swabs should be placed immediately in appropriate transport medium or plated promptly on Thayer-Martin culture plates and incubated under appropriate exacting conditions to maximize the chance for positive results. An exception can be made when an abuse victim has made a clear disclosure, whereupon site-specific cultures may be obtained.

In adolescents with symptomatic gonorrhea, Gram stain of the mucopurulent cervical discharge reveals a predominance of leukocytes that may contain gram-negative intracellular diplococci. When results are positive, this is specific and treatment may be instituted. The incidence of false-negative Gram stains is significant, however. False-positives may also be encountered in asymptomatic women colonized by other *Neisseria* species. Cultures or NAATs are thus essential to confirm infection. Cultures are also necessary to identify antibiotic resistance. Recent studies of women with culture-proven gonococcal cervicitis have shown concurrent chlamydial infection is present in up to one third. Thus when purulent cervicitis is found, specific specimens for detection of *C. trachomatis* should also be obtained and treatment for both pathogens begun empirically.

Knowledge of local patterns of bacterial resistance dictates antibiotic choices. Several single-dose oral therapies are usually acceptable for cervicitis. Pharyngeal and anal infection with *N. gonorrhoeae* may also influence antibiotic choice, and current Centers for Disease Control and Prevention (CDC) guidelines should be consulted. Because current treatment regimens no longer include penicillin, serologic tests for syphilis should be obtained when other STDs are suspected, especially if the patient has had sexual contact with an individual who is likely to be at high risk for having syphilis and/or lives in an area where syphilis is endemic.

On occasion, patients with gonorrhea may develop disseminated gonococcal infection via hematogenous spread. This phenomenon may occur at any age. It is more common in adolescent girls with asymptomatic (and therefore untreated) endocervical infection, in men with asymptomatic urethral infection, and in patients of both genders and all ages with silent anal or pharyngeal infections. It can also be seen in patients with symptomatic vulvovaginitis, cervicitis, or urethritis. In postmenarchal women, systemic symptoms are more likely to develop during a menstrual period.

The clinical picture often has two stages. Initially fever and chills are prominent, and the patient is intermittently bacteremic. During this stage, which lasts 2 to 5 days, polyarthralgias are experienced (involving the knees, wrists, ankles, elbows, and hands) and characteristic skin lesions often appear. The latter begin as small erythematous papules or petechiae that usually evolve to form pustules surrounded by red halos (Fig. 18-37A and B). Later, these may necrose centrally. Lesions often contain gram-negative diplococci, which can be seen on a Gram stain but usually fail to grow on culture. If not diagnosed and treated promptly, patients progress to a second phase, characterized by monarticular arthritis with effusion or tenosynovitis (Fig. 18-37C and D). In up to 50% of these cases, culture of joint aspirates is positive. Specialized techniques to isolate cell wall–deficient organisms further increase culture yield. Myocarditis, pericarditis, endocarditis, and meningitis are other complications of hematogenous seeding.

Chlamydia Infection. *C. trachomatis* is the most prevalent treatable STD, and has replaced *N. gonorrhoeae* as the most common sexually transmitted pathogen causing cervicitis and upper genital tract disease. Its high prevalence (up to 25%) in adolescent populations and its serious

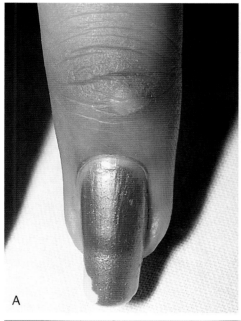
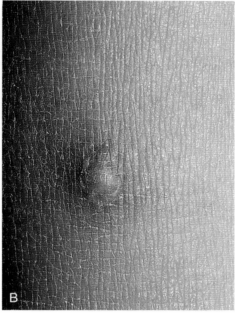
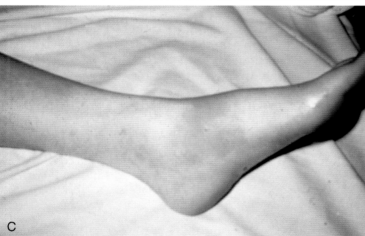
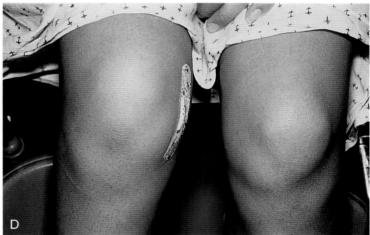

Figure 18-37. Disseminated gonococcal infection. **A** and **B,** These pustular skin lesions with red halos are characteristic of disseminated gonorrhea, which can occur at any age. **C** and **D,** Tenosynovitis and monarticular arthritis are commonly seen in association with skin lesions in disseminated disease. Note the signs of effusion in the right knee of the girl shown in **D.** (**D,** Courtesy Robert Hickey, MD, Children's Hospital of Pittsburgh.)

sequelae make its proper diagnosis and treatment an important aspect of adolescent sexual health care. When compared with gonococcal infection, its transmission rate for a single episode of intercourse is lower, but its prevalence is greater and infection persists longer.

Chlamydiae are unique microorganisms. They are slowly replicating obligate intracellular organisms that cannot be cultivated on artificial media and depend on their cellular hosts for high-energy ATP and other nutrients. Identification has become more accessible with sensitive and specific NAATs and other laboratory techniques in addition to tissue culture, but all are still relatively expensive laboratory procedures. Specimens must be appropriately collected and transported. Cultures are the gold standard for forensic evidence and currently must be used for prepubertal, medicolegal, and rectal specimens. With the exception of NAATs, cell scrapings are necessary rather than secretions or discharge because of the intracellular nature of the organism. External mucus and debris should be removed first. A Dacron swab with a plastic or metal shaft should be used for culture because cotton swabs may interfere with recovery of the organism from tissue culture. Care must be taken to follow specimen collection directions exactly including type of swab, duration of contact, and whether or not to leave the swab in the specimen container. Serologic tests are not useful, except for confir-

mation of lymphogranuloma venereum caused by specific immunotypes. Tests of cure are not reliable for several weeks after treatment and are not recommended by the CDC. Reinfection is common.

Although some prepubertal girls are asymptomatic, most of those infected with *C. trachomatis* tend to have vaginal discharge and/or bleeding, vulvar pruritus or pain, and vulvar erythema. Symptoms may be intermittent or persistent, and coinfection with *N. gonorrhoeae* is common.

Adolescent girls may have symptoms of both cervical and urethral infection. Pelvic or abdominal pain, spotting or irregular vaginal bleeding, dysuria, and/or vaginal discharge may accompany infection. A picture indistinguishable from that of symptomatic gonorrhea (purulent vaginal discharge, perineal irritation, and findings of cervicitis with mucopurulent discharge) can also be seen (see Fig. 18-36B). Endometritis is common with cervicitis, even in the absence of classic symptoms of pelvic inflammatory disease, and Bartholin duct infections also occur. Importantly, asymptomatic chlamydial infection in both females and males is common.

On examination of the cervix, the presence of yellowish green mucopus, cervical ectopy, and erythema are all associated with chlamydial infection. Often the cervix is friable, bleeding during the minimal manipulation necessary to obtain specimens. When seen as an isolated infection, the cervical discharge contains increased numbers of leukocytes without intracellular organisms. Microscopic evidence of other infections does not decrease the likelihood of chlamydial coinfection and should not deter the practitioner from testing and treating for *C. trachomatis* if its presence is suggested by the history or physical findings. As noted earlier, patients commonly have simultaneous infection with gonococci and chlamydia—hence the rationale for culturing for both organisms and covering for both with treatment, when purulent cervicitis is found on examination.

Chlamydia can also produce an acute urethral syndrome in postpubertal patients. Dysuria, urgency, and frequency may be accompanied by physical signs of urethral discharge, meatal redness, and swelling. Pyuria may exist in the absence of bacteriuria. Urethral specimens for chlamydia culture must be collected by inserting a thin Dacron swab 2 cm into the urethra and rotating it 360 degrees before withdrawal. A NAAT for *C. trachomatis* using a urine specimen is now available as well. Rectal infection exists in both heterosexual and homosexual populations. Pharyngeal infection is rarely detected. A careful sexual history may reveal extragenital sites of infection, but treatment for infection at these other sites is not known to differ.

Genital Mycoplasmas. *Mycoplasma hominis, Mycoplasma genitalium,* and *Ureaplasma urealyticum* are the three species of mycoplasma implicated in genital infections. The organisms may be cultured from vaginal specimens of neonates and sexually active women in the absence of disease, but colonization in the prepubertal girl is rare. Mycoplasmas have also been cultured from polymicrobial upper genital tract infections, but it remains unclear whether they are initiators of ascending infections or if they behave as normal bacterial flora accompanying the primary ascending infection of gonorrheal or chlamydial organisms, becoming pathogenic once relocated in the fallopian tubes. Mycoplasmas have also been found causative in some cases of acute urethral syndrome.

The currently widespread practice of broad-spectrum antimicrobial treatment of STDs to include *C. trachomatis* and the general unavailability of laboratory confirmation of *Mycoplasma* organism involvement in infection have made it difficult to further understand the role of these organisms. This broad-spectrum therapy, however, has provided treatment for problems that might have persisted because of an inability to establish a precise diagnosis. Although routine cultures for mycoplasmas are not justified, they should be considered for infections resistant to documented therapy in the absence of reinfection by an untreated partner.

Human Immunodeficiency Virus. Acquired immunodeficiency syndrome (AIDS) and other manifestations of HIV infection are discussed in Chapter 12. The adolescent history outlined previously (see Table 18-5) should identify teenagers at risk of acquiring HIV infection. In an attempt to reduce subsequent transmission and treat infection early, confidential HIV testing is encouraged for teens at risk of exposure to the virus. The definition of moderate to high risk has been regularly changing as our understanding of the disease, its epidemiology, and treatment opportunities evolve. Reliable sources of such information (e.g., the CDC) should be consulted regularly.

From the gynecologic perspective, a number of infections may present differently in the HIV-infected individual. These include infections with *Candida* organisms, human papillomaviruses, herpes simplex viruses, and molluscum contagiosum. In such cases the disease may be unusually severe, may present atypically, or may be resistant to treatment.

Upper Tract Disease

Pelvic Inflammatory Disease. An important complication of lower genital tract infection in the postmenarchal female is pelvic inflammatory disease (PID). PID results from ascending spread of a cervical infection that may or may not have been symptomatic. PID is now recognized as a polymicrobial infection. Initiating pathogens implicated include *N. gonorrhoeae, C. trachomatis,* and *M. hominis.* Other organisms, usually considered normal vaginal or enteric flora, are potentially pathogenic when introduced into the upper genital tract. Among these are *Bacteroides* species; other anaerobic gram-positive bacilli and cocci, such as those found in bacterial vaginosis; and aerobes including streptococcal species, *E. coli, Klebsiella* and *Proteus* species, and *Trichomonas* (see Table 18-11). The majority of cases of salpingitis are due to mixed anaerobic and aerobic infections, although the classically recognized venereal pathogens play a critical initiating role.

Risk factors for developing upper genital tract infection include being an adolescent, having multiple sexual partners, use of an IUD, and previous PID. Because menstruation assists ascent of pathogenic organisms from the cervix to the uterus and fallopian tubes, the onset of symptoms often occurs during or shortly after a menstrual period. Long-term morbidity includes an increased incidence of ectopic pregnancy, decreased fertility, and chronic pelvic pain. These sequelae are secondary to tubal occlusion and scarring of pelvic structures. Adverse clinical outcomes and long-term morbidity may be more severe among the *C. trachomatis*–positive or culture-negative patents with PID. Delay in diagnosis and treatment, unusually severe PID, and repeated infection are associated with more severe long-term sequelae. For each episode of PID there is an estimated additional 15% chance of subsequent fertility problems.

The classic picture of acute PID is one of a sexually active female who abruptly develops a high fever and shaking chills in association with intense lower abdominal pain. Nausea and vomiting are common. The patient appears acutely ill and uncomfortable and walks with an antalgic gait. On abdominal examination there is prominent lower abdominal tenderness and guarding. Cervical visualization discloses signs of cervicitis with mucopurulent discharge. Bimanual palpation elicits extreme pain on cervical motion and reveals marked tenderness of the fundus and adnexa. Adnexal enlargement, if present, suggests abscess formation. The erythrocyte sedimentation rate is markedly elevated, and there is a pronounced leukocytosis with a left shift on CBC and differential. This classic picture has the highest likelihood of being associated with positive cultures for *N. gonorrhoeae.* It is not the most typical scenario, however. More commonly the onset of symptoms is insidious, and the clinical picture more subtle. This is particularly likely with nongonococcal PID. Fever may be absent or low grade; abdominal pain is mild; and blood work is frequently normal. In such cases diagnosis can be particularly difficult, requiring considerable suspicion and a low threshold for obtaining cultures or other tests on the part of the clinician. Lower abdominal, pelvic, and/or cervical motion tenderness and some evidence of lower genital tract inflammation are usually present even in clinically mild cases. A low-grade tubal infection may produce more in the way of adnexal findings and few, if any, uterine signs.

Diagnosis is complicated by the fact that not only is there a wide range in severity of the clinical picture but also a lack of clear, quantifiable diagnostic guidelines for PID. Furthermore, acute salpingitis may mimic a number of other disorders (Table 18-13). The adolescent girl with right lower quadrant (RLQ) abdominal pain is particularly challenging diagnostically. Table 18-14 summarizes clinical findings that may aid in distinguishing among the many potential causes. Ultrasonography has proved to be a useful diagnostic tool in many such cases. Optimal imaging of the pelvis and adnexae is achieved with a transvaginal probe. Most of the time, an abdominal probe will be sufficient to provide diagnostic information. Figure 18-38 illustrates some of the ultrasound findings in disorders that may cause pelvic or right lower quadrant abdominal pain. When appendicitis is suspected, a computed tomography scan with contrast of the right lower quadrant is the preferred radiologic test.

Given the variability of the clinical picture in PID, minimal diagnostic criteria have been developed. These include lower abdominal or pelvic pain, cervical motion, and adnexal tenderness. Although adding criteria such as fever, leukocytosis, and abnormal vaginal microscopy may increase specificity of diagnosis, it also increases the risk of missing the diagnosis and delaying treatment. Because of the potentially devastating long-term sequelae of PID, aggressive, empirical broad-spectrum antimicrobial therapy is warranted. Treatment should include antibiotics that cover the common organisms in accordance with current CDC recommendations.

Indications for hospitalization and parenteral therapy from the outset include: suspected abscess, toxicity, inability to take and retain oral medication, and concurrent pregnancy. Admission is also advisable in cases in which the exact diagnosis is unclear and when poor compliance is likely. When initial outpatient treatment is elected, it is mandatory that the patient be reexamined within 24 to 48 hours to document clinical improvement and confirm compliance with antibiotic use. If on follow-up it is found that there has been no significant clinical improvement, she should be considered to have failed outpatient therapy and be admitted for parenteral medication. In addition to antibiotic resistance, failure to improve promptly on therapy, whether oral or parenteral, raises the possibility of complications such as abscess formation; development of a tubo-ovarian complex; or a missed diagnosis of ectopic pregnancy, miscarriage, or appendicitis. As noted earlier, sonography is useful in evaluating masses and suspected tubo-ovarian complexes. Laparoscopy may be necessary when surgical conditions are suspected or parenteral medical treatment fails.

Perihepatitis (Fitz-Hugh-Curtis Syndrome). One complication of PID, seen in 5% to 20% of cases, presents as right-upper-quadrant (RUQ) pain caused by perihepatitis. In these instances the inflammatory process probably ascends from the fallopian tubes along the paracolic gutters to the right upper quadrant, resulting in inflammation of the liver capsule and adjacent peritoneum.

The clinical picture is one of moderate to severe pleuritic RUQ pain, which may be referred to the right shoulder, and is associated with fever, chills, nausea, and vomiting. Although the pain can develop simultaneously with pelvic symptoms of PID, in the majority of cases it may have its onset in the course of an asymptomatic ascending lower genital tract infection or later in the course of a partially treated infection. In many of these patients upper abdominal pain is so severe that the patient is relatively unconcerned about milder degrees of lower abdominal and pelvic discomfort.

On examination RUQ tenderness and guarding are the major physical findings, and peritoneal signs may be present. Gynecologic examination in most instances discloses findings of purulent cervicitis and PID. *N. gonorrhoeae* and *C. trachomatis* are the major pathogens associated with this syndrome. When nongonococcal in origin, the predisposing salpingitis may be silent.

Patients with Fitz-Hugh-Curtis syndrome have minimal if any abnormalities of liver function tests. Although usually not necessary, ultrasound examination of the right upper quadrant should demonstrate a normal liver, biliary tree, and gallbladder. Laparoscopic findings of purulent and fibrinous inflammation of the capsule and hemor-

Table 18-13	Medical Conditions Manifesting as Acute Right-Sided Abdominal Pain in Adolescent Girls

Gynecologic
Pelvic inflammatory disease
Ovarian cyst, torsion, rupture, hemorrhage
Dysmenorrhea
Ectopic pregnancy

Hepatic
Fitz-Hugh-Curtis syndrome
Viral hepatitis (A, B, C, etc.)
Drug-induced hepatitis
Autoimmune hepatitis
Alcoholic hepatitis
Hepatitis secondary to bacteremia
Epstein-Barr virus hepatitis

Biliary
Acute cholecystitis
Cholelithiasis

Intestinal
Inflammatory bowel disease
Irritable bowel syndrome
Constipation
Lactose intolerance

Other Gastrointestinal
Subphrenic abscess
Appendicitis
Perforated gastric or duodenal ulcer

Pulmonary
Pneumonia, pleuritis, pleurodynia

Renal
Acute pyelonephritis or perinephric abscess

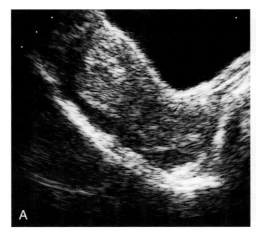 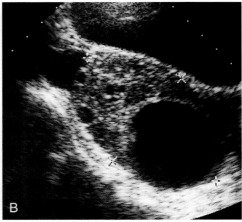

Figure 18-38. Ultrasound findings in the diagnosis of pelvic or abdominal pain. **A,** This image shows an abnormal amount of fluid in the cul-de-sac released from a ruptured ovarian cyst in a 15-year-old with left-lower-quadrant and midline pelvic pain. **B,** In a 12-year-old girl with a 4-day history of colicky right-lower-quadrant pain, ultrasound demonstrates a single, large, abnormal cyst and multiple small physiologic cysts. Operative diagnosis was right ovarian torsion.

Table 18-14	Pertinent Clinical Characteristics of Disorders Causing Right-Sided or Lower Abdominal Pain in Adolescent Girls			
	PID	**OVARIAN TORSION**	**OVARIAN CYST**	**ECTOPIC PREGNANCY**
Location and Quality of Pain	Mid and lateral pelvis, usually bilateral; can be vague, dull, crampy, or sharp	Unilateral RLQ or LLQ pain, colicky	Usually asymptomatic but may have colicky RLQ or LLQ pain	Lateral pain, colicky, ± uterine cramping
Onset	With GC, rapid, immediately postmenstrual. With *Chlamydia,* gradual over days to months	Sudden	Gradual, though rupture or hemorrhage is associated with acutely increased pain	Gradual with sudden exacerbation
History	Unprotected sexual intercourse, previous PID or STDs, multiple partners	± History of previous episodes of similar pain with resolution, increased ovarian size (anatomic variation predisposes)	Midcycle or luteal phase, physiologic rupture causes mittelschmerz of 24-48 hrs' duration	Amenorrhea (75%), ± early symptoms of pregnancy, unilateral pelvic pain
GI Symptoms	Nausea, vomiting, anorexia may be present	Vomiting with onset of pain (25%)	Rare	GI symptoms secondary to pregnancy or severe vomiting secondary to rupture and peritonitis
Masses	Occasional; if present, consider tubo-ovarian complex or ectopic pregnancy	Usually present, increased size secondary to edema	Often palpable if not physiologic cyst	Unilateral doughy adnexal mass palpable in 50% of cases
Physical Examination and Laboratory Findings	Cervical motion and adnexal tenderness, clinical and lab evidence of cervicitis; vaginal bleeding; ± discharge; ± RUQ pain; perihepatitis; + cervical cultures for gonorrhea and/or *C. trachomatis*	Tender adnexa, ± guarding or peritoneal signs	Unilateral cystic adnexal mass, radiograph rules out dermoid	Normal or soft uterus may be slightly enlarged; unilateral or bilateral adnexal tenderness; pregnancy test positive in most but inadequate β-HCG rise on 48-hr retest; drop in Hct, hypotension, and signs of peritoneal irritation with rupture
Ultrasound Findings	Usually normal, tubo-ovarian complex seen in 10%-15%	Usually solid ovarian mass, ± compromised blood supply on Doppler	Cyst >3 cm, ± fluid in cul-de-sac (a frequent incidental finding on ultrasound)	Tubal mass, vaginal probe enhances detection

rhagic areas of adjacent parietal peritoneum are diagnostic, but laparoscopy is rarely indicated for this condition. Major differential diagnostic considerations are listed in Tables 18-13 and 18-14.

Pregnancy

Sexual activity among teenagers has dramatically increased since the early 1970s, with a greater percentage of young women of all ages reporting having had sexual intercourse. The pregnancy rate for adolescents in the United States is approximately 49 per 1000 for 15- to 19-year-old girls per year. Although this represents a greater than 50% drop over the past several years, it remains one of the highest among industrialized countries, as does the rate of pregnancies and births among younger adolescents (younger than 15 years of age). These pregnancies are usually unintended and unplanned, and many occur within 6 months after first intercourse. A number of factors contribute to this problem including social and cultural factors and values and misconceptions about reproductive functioning and regarding contraceptive use and its risks and effectiveness. Misconceptions stem in part from lack of access to early comprehensive sex education and counseling and reluctance to seek and use professional services. This explains to some extent the fact that the average adolescent seeks contraceptive counseling almost 1 year after initiating sexual activity.

Some of the forces that delay education, counseling, and medical care needed to effectively prevent pregnancy also contribute to delayed pregnancy diagnosis and failure to seek and obtain good antenatal care. Furthermore, in many instances of unplanned pregnancy, adolescents deny their condition for extended periods to themselves, their parents, and others. This delay is associated with increases in complications of pregnancy and neonatal morbidity. Vaginal bleeding or spotting in early pregnancy may falsely reassure a young woman that she is not pregnant, and minimal weight gain (whether voluntary or involuntary) may further assist denial. Some such patients may present with substitute (non–pregnancy related) or peripheral chief complaints. Among these are pelvic, abdominal, or back pain; vomiting and dehydration; constipation; urinary complaints; and urinary tract infection. Phlebitis; rupture of membranes; symptoms of gestational diabetes; or secondary problems of fatigue, insomnia, or headache ultimately bring some of these patients to medical attention.

With or without denial, at the time of presentation the teenager or her parent may suspect pregnancy. Interviewing the patient and parent separately and sensitively addressing underlying concerns is usually the best way to get a complete and honest history.

Considering the frequency of teenage pregnancy and the tendency of individuals to have alternate chief complaints, practitioners who care for adolescents should be familiar with the signs, symptoms, and methods of diagnosing pregnancy.

	INFLAMMATORY BOWEL DISEASE	APPENDICITIS	IRRITABLE BOWEL/ CONSTIPATION	DYSMENORRHEA
Location and Quality of Pain	LLQ pain, crampy	Periumbilical cramping changing to RLQ cramping or sharp pain	LLQ pain, crampy or colicky	Suprapubic, midabdominal, lower back, dull cramping
Onset	Gradual over weeks to months with exacerbations	Gradual over hours to days	Long history of GI problems over months to years	Periodic, evolving over hours; close to onset of flow
History (Hx)	Weight loss or growth failure, fatigue, rashes, arthritis, fever	Usually no prior pain	± Constipation or diarrhea, distention common, + family Hx, symptoms increase with stress	Increasing severity 1-3 yr after menarche
GI Symptoms	Increased stool frequency, nocturnal stools, sometimes bloody diarrhea	Vomiting may follow onset of pain, anorexia	Long intermittent history of constipation, ± diarrhea	Diarrhea, flatulence, vomiting not uncommon with start of menses
Masses	Unusual, except with chronic complicated disease	Rare	Feces	None
Physical Examination and Laboratory Findings	Rectoabdominal tenderness, hematologic abnormalities, stool heme +	↑WBCs, fever, evolving peritoneal signs	Occasional tender colon, usually normal	Normal
Ultrasound Findings	Normal	Appendix frequently visible	Normal	Normal

GC, gonococcus; GI, gastrointestinal; HCG, human chorionic gonadotropin; Hct, hematocrit; LLQ, left lower quadrant; PID, pelvic inflammatory disease; RLQ, right lower quadrant; RUQ, right upper quadrant; STD, sexually transmitted disease; ↑, increased; +, positive; ±, with or without.
NOTE: This table is designed not only to aid the clinician in distinguishing among disorders that present with abdominal pain in adolescent girls but to enhance recognition of the fact that a complaint of abdominal pain must be taken seriously and evaluated carefully. One must remember that the diagnosis of functional abdominal pain is and must be a diagnosis of exclusion.

In the first trimester, patients often experience fatigue and mood swings. At about 5 weeks' gestation, breast tenderness and swelling, along with darkening and increased sensitivity of the nipples, develop. Nausea and vomiting, especially in the morning, tend to begin at about 6 weeks' gestation. Weight changes, food cravings, and increased facial oil gland activity and chloasma (darkening of facial pigmentation) may be noted. If a pregnant adolescent is examined between the sixth and eighth weeks, the Hegar sign (softening of the lower corpus), Chadwick sign (bluish discoloration of the cervix), and Goodell sign (softening of the cervix) may be noted. Ultrasonography can detect the fetus by the fifth or sixth week of pregnancy.

In the second and third trimesters, breast enlargement increases, as do abdominal girth and weight. Normal vaginal discharge increases as well. On examination, congestion of the vaginal mucosa is seen. The uterus is palpable as a midline mass, with its dome at the pelvic brim at about 12 weeks; midway between the pelvic brim and the umbilicus at 16 weeks; and at the level of the umbilicus at 20 weeks. Fetal heart tones become detectable with Doppler between 12 and 14 weeks, and fetal movements are perceptible between 16 and 20 weeks' gestation. Signs and symptoms of pregnancy are outlined in Table 18-15.

Current laboratory pregnancy tests give us the opportunity to diagnose pregnancy earlier and with greater reliability. Serum radioimmune assay for β-hCG is positive 24

Table 18-15	Signs and Symptoms of Pregnancy
FIRST TRIMESTER (6-12 WK)	**SECOND TRIMESTER (12+ WK)**
Amenorrhea	Increased size of breasts, abdomen, waist
Light, irregular vaginal bleeding	Increased weight and clothing size
Syncope or fainting	Increased vaginal discharge
Fatigue	Increased skin pigmentation
Urinary frequency	Congestion of vaginal mucosa
Mood swings	
"Morning" sickness	
Nausea and vomiting	
Food cravings	
Increased facial oil gland activity ("glow")	
Elevated body temperature	
Chloasma (dark facial pigmentation)	
Nasal stuffiness or mucous membrane congestion	

to 48 hours after implantation (about 7 days after conception). A urine specimen gives a positive result on a sensitive urine ELISA assay for an intrauterine pregnancy 10 days after conception or 1 week after implantation. Most home tests have similar sensitivity to the commonly used clinic tests; many of the sensitive immunometric tests are sold to both medical offices and consumers. A chronology of laboratory and clinical findings during pregnancy is presented in Table 18-16.

Table 18-16	Clinical and Laboratory Correlations of Pregnancy			
GESTATION (WK)	**PREGNANCY DETECTION BY LABORATORY TEST**	**FUNDAL HEIGHT**	**URINE hCG (MIU/mL)**	**SIGNS, SYMPTOMS, AND SIGNIFICANT EVENTS**
1				LMP
2			5	Conception
3	Serum ELISA		(24 hr postimplantation)	Implantation
4	Urine ELISA assay		70-100	Missed period, vaginal ultrasound detects pregnancy
5	Urine β-hCG assay, other methods		>250	Pelvic ultrasound detects pregnancy; breast changes—tender, swollen; nipples—sensitive, dark
6			>1000	Nausea, morning sickness; **Hegar sign**—softening of lower corpus; **Chadwick sign**—bluish color of cervix; **Goodell sign**—softening of cervix
7				
8			>10,000	
10			100,000 (peak)	
12		Pelvic brim		Uterine enlargement; fetal heart tones detectable with Doppler
14				Decrease in early signs and symptoms
16		Midway between pelvic brim and umbilicus	10,000; false-negatives may occur in second and third trimesters	Fetus visualized by radiograph; perception of fetal movement
20		Umbilicus		

ELISA, enzyme-linked immunosorbent assay; hCG, human chorionic gonadotropin; LMP, last menstrual period.

Table 18-17	Causes of False-Positive and False-Negative Pregnancy Tests

FALSE-NEGATIVE TEST	**FALSE-POSITIVE TEST**
Too early (commonly) or too late (rarely)	Hydatidiform mole
Adulterated urine	Malignancies
Ectopic pregnancy (occasionally negative, most are positive)	Postabortion (up to 4 wk)
Impending or missed abortion	Midcycle LH surge
Dilute urine	Perimenopausal (LH elevation)
	Premature ovarian failure (LH elevation)

LH, luteinizing hormone.

Home pregnancy tests are variable in sensitivity. Some are identical to and as sensitive as office laboratory ELISA assays, and others may not give a positive result on a first-morning specimen until 14 to 21 days after conception. False-positive and false-negative results are encountered infrequently and are most often caused by errors of timing and dilution. In particular, false-positives are not caused by foods, drugs, and other medical conditions (Table 18-17). They can occur in adolescents with hydatidiform moles or malignancies, after abortion or miscarriage, or during a midcycle luteinizing hormone surge. Causes of false-negative findings include testing too early (mentioned earlier) or too late (after 16 to 20 weeks), dilute urine (specific gravity <1.010), adulterated urine (another person's urine substituted for the patient's), ectopic pregnancy, or an impending or missed abortion (see Table 18-17).

Pregnancies are dated from the last normal menstrual period and not from conception, which occurs 2 weeks later. This is not well known by the public and should be explained to minimize confusion, assist decision making, and clarify paternity.

Bibliography

American Academy of Pediatrics: Red Book: Report of the Committee on Infectious Diseases, 27th ed. Pickering LK (ed). Elk Grove Village, Ill, AAP, 2006.

Berenson AB, Heger AH, Hayes JM, et al: Appearance of the hymen in prepubertal girls. Pediatrics 89:387-394, 1992.

Berenson AB: Appearance of the hymen at birth and one year of age: A longitudinal study. Pediatrics 91:820-825, 1993.

Centers for Disease Control and Prevention: 2006 Guidelines for treatment of sexually transmitted diseases. MMWR 55:1-94, 2006.

Emans SJ, Laufer MR, Goldstein DP: Pediatric and Adolescent Gynecology, 5th ed. Boston, Lippincott-Raven, 2005.

Hatcher RA, Trussell J, Stewart F, et al (eds): Contraceptive Technology, 18th ed. New York, Ardent Media, 2004.

Holmes KK, Sparling PF, Mårdh P-A, et al (eds): Sexually Transmitted Diseases. 4th ed. New York, McGraw-Hill, 2006.

McCann J, Wells R, Simon M, Voris J: Genital findings in prepubertal girls selected for non-abuse: A descriptive study. Pediatrics 86:428-439, 1990.

McCann J, Voris J, Simon M, Wells R: Comparison of genital examination techniques in prepubertal girls. Pediatrics 85:182-187, 1990.

Muram D, Dewhurst J, Lee PA, Sanfilippo JS (eds): Pediatric and Adolescent Gynecology, 2nd ed. Philadelphia, WB Saunders, 2001.

Paradise JE, Campos JM, Friedman HM, Frishmuth G: Vulvovaginitis in premenarchal girls: Clinical features and diagnostic evaluation. Pediatrics 70:193-198, 1982.

Perlman SE, Nakajima ST, Hertweck SP (eds): Clinical Protocols in Pediatric and Adolescent Gynecology. New York, The Parthenon Publishing Group, 2004.

Pokorny SF, Kozinetz CA: Configuration and other anatomic details of the prepubertal hymen. Adolesc Pediatr Gynecol 1:97-103, 1988.

Pokorny SF, Stormer J: Atraumatic removal of secretions from the prepubertal vagina. Am J Obstet Gynecol 156:581-582, 1987.

Web Sites

www.acog.org
www.youngwomenshealth.org
www.asccp.org
www.adolescenthealth.org
http://phil.cdc.gov/phil/home.asp

CHAPTER 19

Ophthalmology

Kenneth P. Cheng and Albert W. Biglan

Infants and children may be affected by conditions not seen in adults, and the examination techniques and treatments that they may need frequently require subspecialty care. Since the 1960s pediatric ophthalmology has become established as a distinct subspecialty of ophthalmology. Common problems include refractive errors, strabismus, amblyopia, infections, and trauma. Other problems encountered include ocular complications of systemic disease, developmental and genetic conditions, and neoplasms affecting the globe and orbits.

Anatomy of the Visual System

The visual system is conveniently separated into three principal parts: the globe and surrounding structures (Fig. 19-1), the visual pathways, and the visual or calcarine cortex.

The eyelids provide protection for the globe and assist in even distribution of the tear film over the cornea to provide a clear, undistorted optical system for focusing light. The crystalline lens complements the cornea's refracting power with its ability to adjust the focal length of the optical system so that incoming light from objects at any distance may be clearly imaged on the retina. During the first 2 to 3 months of life, children develop the ability to focus on images at any range (accommodation). Light is focused on the macula, the portion of the retina responsible for the central field of vision (Fig. 19-2). The retina contains the sensory receptors: the rods and cones. The fovea centralis is the center of the macula; it has the greatest concentration of cones and is responsible for detailed, central visual acuity.

Light falling on the fovea and peripheral retina is converted into nerve impulses by the rods and cones. Nerve fibers emanate from the ganglion cell layer of the retina, coalesce to form the optic nerve, and synapse in the lateral geniculate body. The right and left optic nerves pass from the orbits and join together to form the optic chiasm. Fibers from the temporal retina travel without crossing at the chiasm to the ipsilateral visual cortex (Fig. 19-3). Nerve fibers from the nasal retina decussate at the chiasm and are directed toward the contralateral visual cortex. This decussation of nerve fibers causes portions of each retina to image a different part of the visual field. For example, if an object is seen off to the person's left, the image is received by the nasal retina of the left eye and the temporal retina of the right eye. Similarly, if the object is off to the person's right, the image falls on the nasal retina of the right eye and the temporal retina of the left eye. The temporal retina images objects in the contralateral visual field, and the nasal retina images objects in the ipsilateral visual field. Because of the decussation of nasal retinal fibers, the right visual cortex receives images from the left side of the visual field and the left visual cortex receives images from the right side of the visual field.

Lesions of the visual pathways produce predictable patterns of visual field loss; for example, a left homonymous hemianopsia (loss of the left side of the visual field) is produced by a lesion of the right occipital cortex. Detection of a visual field defect that respects or does not extend across the vertical midline of the visual field indicates pathology posterior to the optic chiasm (within the intracranial portion of the visual system). Visual field defects that involve both the right and left sides of the visual field in one or both eyes indicate either retinal or optic nerve pathology or lesions to both sides of the intracranial visual system. Because of the anatomy of the optic chiasm, compressive lesions of the chiasm (e.g., pituitary tumors) produce visual field defects involving the left side of the visual field of the left eye and the right side of the visual field of the right eye (bitemporal defects).

The visual field can be arbitrarily divided into the central field of vision and the peripheral field. The macula is responsible for the central field. A physiologic blind spot is found about 10 to 15 degrees temporal to central fixation (the fovea) and represents the area of the visual field that corresponds to the optic nerve head (optic disc). Precise measurement of the visual field of each eye can be obtained in a cooperative child or adult using a Goldmann visual field perimeter or an automated visual field device. This test requires steady fixation and concentration. In young children, it is impractical to attempt this tedious measurement. In a patient unable to cooperate for a formal visual field test, the fields are assessed by observation of the child's eyes fixating on small targets brought into the peripheral field of vision in each quadrant of the visual field. Visual fields may also be assessed using a confrontation method in which the child fixates on the examiner's nose and is asked to identify or count the examiner's fingers as they are presented in each quadrant of the visual field.

Evaluation of Vision

Selection of a test to measure a patient's visual acuity depends on the patient's age, cooperation, and level of development. The evaluation of vision in a young infant or nonverbal patient requires the use of the fixation reflex. This reflex develops during the first month or two of life. Although almost all 2- to 3-month-old infants can fixate and follow a face or bright object quite well into all fields of gaze, it is not necessarily abnormal for this milestone to not be present until 6 months of age. The level of vision can be estimated by the quality and intensity of the fixation response. If the visual acuity is normal, central fixation is steady and maintained on objects. If visual acuity is profoundly decreased, the quality of fixation may be wandering in nature, poorly maintained, or eccentric. Central, steady, maintained fixation equates to visual acuity of 20/200 or better. Eyes with unsteady or wandering fixation usually have visual acuity decreased to the 20/800 range (Fig. 19-4).

The visual pathways coalesce in the visual cortex. Electrical impulses in the visual cortex produced by light stimulation of the retina can be measured by placement of sensitive electrodes on the overlying scalp. This is termed the *visual evoked potential* or *response* (VEP or VER). The pattern visual evoked potential is generated with a CRT monitor that produces an alternating checkerboard stimulus, which can be controlled to produce a pattern of checks that may be increased or decreased in size. This test can be used to estimate visual acuity in preverbal or nonverbal children. Caution must be used in interpreting

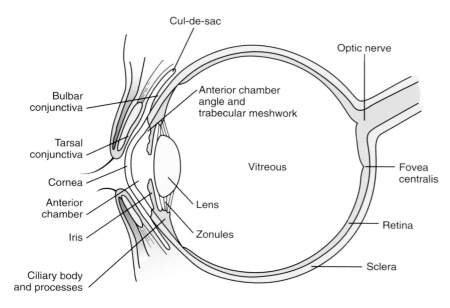

Figure 19-1. Globe and surrounding structures.

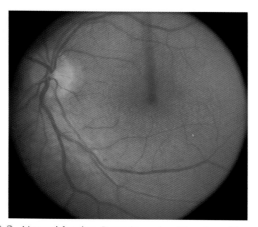

Figure 19-2. Normal fundus. Posterior pole of fundus with normal optic disc and retinal vasculature. The macula is visualized as an area of increased pigmentation surrounded by retinal vessels. The fovea centralis or center of the macula is maintaining fixation on the end of a vertical fixation target.

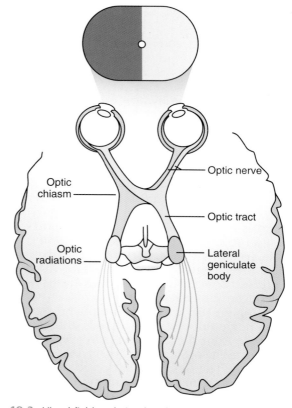

Figure 19-3. Visual field and visual pathways.

this test, however, because children and adults with known 20/20 vision can suppress the visual evoked response. Additionally, children who have significant decreases in their visual acuity may have a visual evoked response that overestimates the visual acuity.

Nonverbal infants or children may have their grating visual acuity measured with Teller Acuity Cards. This test is based on a child's reflex to move the eyes or head toward a pattern of alternating black-and-white stripes of increasing frequency rather than neutral gray of the same brightness.

The Allen object recognition cards, simple pictures of common objects, are useful for assessing visual acuity in a 2- to 3½-year-old child who cannot comprehend the illiterate or tumbling E game or recognize Snellen letters. To perform this test, the child is taught what the pictures are, and then one eye is occluded and picture cards are individually presented at increasing distances until the patient recognizes the cards at 20 feet or fails to recognize the cards (Fig. 19-5). Recognition of the cards at a distance of 20 feet equates to a visual acuity of 20/30. The farthest distance at which the cards can be recognized is noted, and the visual acuity is quantitated as that distance over the denominator of 30 (e.g., 5/30, 15/30, 20/30). This is a measurement of recognition visual acuity. Although use

of isolated targets is not ideal for detection of amblyopia, the test can be quickly and easily taught to apprehensive or shy young children and comparison of vision between the eyes detects most cases of amblyopia and other defects in visual acuity.

The Sheridan-Gardiner or HOTV visual acuity tests are easy to administer and more accurately measure visual acuity in 4- to 6-year-old children who are beginning to read letters. In the HOTV test the letters H, O, T, and V are individually presented on cards, and the child matches the letter with a corresponding letter on a card that is held on the lap (Fig. 19-6).

Another commonly used test to measure the visual acuity in 3½-year-old children is the "E game." The letter E in decreasing size is presented to the child rotated in an

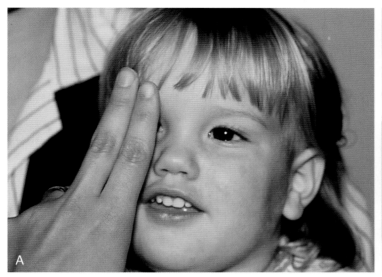
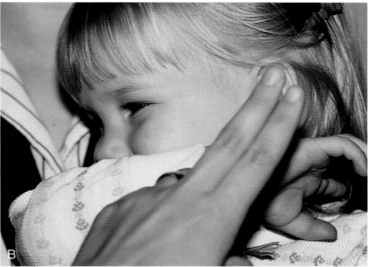

Figure 19-4. Test for central fixation. **A,** An alert child seated on her mother's lap with one eye covered. The child is content to fix and follow with the normal left eye. **B,** The cover (in this case, fingers) is then transferred to the normal eye. The child becomes disturbed, pushes the hand away, and moves her head to see. This suggests that the visual acuity in the right eye is not as good as the acuity in the left eye.

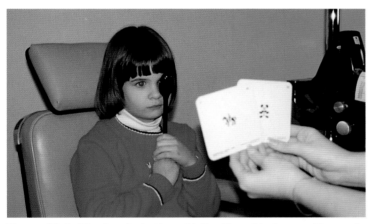

Figure 19-5. Visual acuity testing with the Allen object recognition cards. Recognition of each figure at a distance of 20 feet is equivalent to a visual acuity of 20/30. The visual acuity is quantitated as the number of feet at which each figure may be recognized over 30 (e.g., 5/30, 15/30, 20/30).

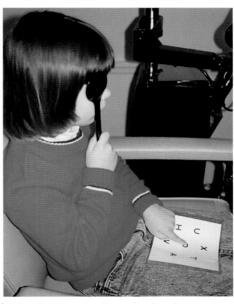

Figure 19-6. The Sheridan-Gardiner visual acuity test presents letters of decreasing size to a child who matches the figure presented to one on a card held on his or her lap. This test provides an accurate assessment of visual acuity for children who have not yet mastered reading the alphabet.

up, down, right, or left orientation, and the child indicates the direction of the crossbars of the E by pointing.

The gold standard for measurement of visual acuity is the presentation of a full line of letter optotypes. This presentation is best achieved with a wall chart or by projection of the letters onto a standardized reflective surface. Presentation of several letters at a time is a more accurate measurement of visual acuity due to a phenomenon termed *crowding.* Amblyopic eyes recognize letters or symbols better if they are presented in isolation or one at a time than if four or more are presented together on lines above and below one another. The difference may be as much as one or two lines of visual acuity (e.g., 20/30 isolated symbol visual acuity reducing to 20/40 or 20/50 when measured with a Snellen letter chart). Many different visual acuity tests are calibrated using different letters and symbols or groups of symbols.

Discussion of visual acuity measurements should include whether the visual acuity has been measured without correction of refractive errors or whether any refractive error has been corrected with glasses or contact lenses (best corrected visual acuity). To differentiate an organic problem of the visual system from simple refractive error,

it is the best corrected visual acuity that provides the most useful information.

Normal values for best corrected visual acuity depend on the patient's age. A child at 6 months of age should have a visual acuity of 20/60 to 20/100. A child who is 3 years old can be expected to have an acuity in the range of 20/25 or 20/30 using the E game or a recognition target test. With further maturation, a 5- to 7-year-old child should have visual acuity of 20/20 to 20/25 as tested with a full-line presentation of Snellen letters. If the best corrected visual acuity is less than 20/20 in a child older than 8 years of age, investigation for the cause of the decrease in visual acuity should be made.

It is recommended that vision screening be conducted as part of well-child care at regularly scheduled intervals in the pediatrician's or family practitioner's office. In infancy the response of each eye to a fixation target should be recorded. Beginning at age 3, quantitation of the visual acuity using Allen cards, the E game, an HOTV chart, or other preliterate vision test should be completed. Later a Snellen or letter chart visual acuity test should be performed by the office staff or physician, and the results should be recorded as part of the patient's medical record. Most importantly, the visual acuity should appear to be equal in both eyes. Further evaluation in a young child is prompted if the patient is cooperating well and the visual acuity is less than 20/40 with letters or less than 15/30 measured with the Allen visual acuity cards in either or both eyes.

Some state laws require that vision screenings be performed in school at 1- to 2-year intervals. In a child 6 or more years of age, referral to an ophthalmologist is indicated if the vision is less than 20/30 in either eye.

Refractive Errors

Subnormal visual acuity may be the result of an error in the refractive power of the eye. This may be due to variation in the curvature of the cornea or lens or variation in the axial length of the eye. If visual acuity is improved by looking through a pinhole held in front of an eye, a refractive error is the cause of the decrease in visual acuity. The pinhole eliminates the off-central rays of light that require refraction. Patients demonstrate the pinhole effect by squinting to compensate for refractive errors. Those patients who do not have an improvement in visual acuity with a pinhole usually have some other cause for the decrease in visual acuity present.

Determination of the refractive state of the eye is part of a comprehensive ophthalmic evaluation. In children, an objective measurement of the refractive error may be obtained by using drugs that temporarily inhibit accommodation and cause pupillary dilation. Cycloplegic-mydriatic agents such as cyclopentolate or tropicamide are instilled, and 30 minutes later accommodation is temporarily paralyzed and the pupil is dilated. A retinoscope is used to project a beam of light into the eye and illuminate the retina. The light is then reflected back to the examiner through the patient's pupil and optical system.

The focus of the reflected light is neutralized by placement of appropriate lenses in front of the eye, and the refractive error of the eye is accurately and objectively measured (Fig. 19-7).

Low levels of hyperopia (farsightedness) in the range of +1.50 to +2.00 diopters are normal during childhood and are easily compensated for by the focusing mechanism of the lens (accommodation) so glasses are not necessary. The amount of hyperopia normally increases until 6 years of age and then decreases. Under normal circumstances, emmetropia, or no refractive error, is achieved around adolescence. If excessive axial growth of the eye occurs, myopia (nearsightedness) develops. A patient's refractive error is for the most part genetically predetermined. The effect that environment has on refractive error remains unclear.

The optical image formed by a hyperopic eye is in focus behind the retina (Fig. 19-8C). By changing the shape of the lens with accommodation, the image can be brought into focus on the retina and glasses may not be required. If a large amount of hyperopia is present (+4.00 diopters

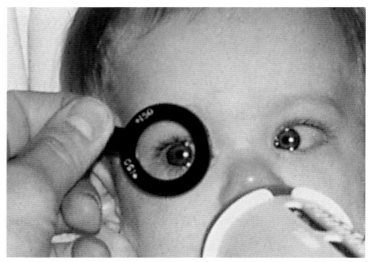

Figure 19-7. The examiner is viewing light emanating from the retina through the retinoscope. A lens is held in front of the patient's eye to neutralize refractive errors.

REFRACTIVE ERRORS

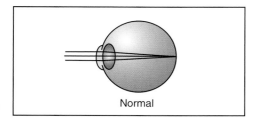

Normal

A

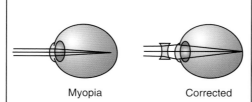

Myopia   Corrected

B

Hyperopia   Corrected

C

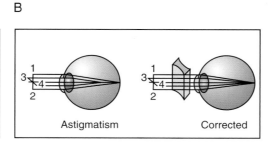

Astigmatism   Corrected

D

Figure 19-8. In the normal or emmetropic eye **(A)**, light from a distant object is focused on the retina. In a myopic eye **(B)**, it is focused in front of the retina; in a hyperopic eye **(C)**, it is focused behind the retina; and in an astigmatic eye **(D)**, light in different meridians is brought to focus either in front of or behind the retina.

or more), fatigue; headaches; asthenopia; and blurring of vision, especially at near, may occur. Hyperopia greater than +5.00 or +6.00 diopters may cause ametropic amblyopia. When this occurs, glasses are prescribed to correct the child's refractive error so that focused images stimulate the development of normal vision. If large hyperopic refractive errors are not treated by 6 to 8 years of age, the resultant amblyopia may be irreversible. The optic discs in eyes with large degrees of hyperopia may have an appearance simulating papilledema (pseudopapilledema) (Fig. 19-9).

Myopia is most commonly caused by an increase in axial length of the eye with respect to the optical power of the eye (see Fig. 19-8B). Children who are myopic can see near objects clearly; objects at distance are blurred and cannot be brought into focus without the aid of glasses or a contact lens. Wearing glasses for myopia does not change the growth pattern of the eye and, as such, does not promote the resolution or progression of the myopia. No treatment has proved effective to modify the progression of childhood myopia.

Myopia may be present at birth but usually develops with growth spurts that occur between 8 and 10 years of age. The amount of myopia present usually increases until growth is completed after adolescence.

High degrees of myopia ranging from −8.00 to −20.00 diopters may be associated with systemic conditions such as Stickler and Ehlers-Danlos syndromes, conditions associated with increased axial length of the eye. Myopia is inherited as a multifactorial trait. High myopia with

extreme lengthening of the globe may be associated with retinal thinning, peripapillary pigment crescents, staphylomas (a focal area of bulging of the posterior globe wall), and decreased macular function with poor visual acuity. The optic nerve may appear to enter the eye at an angle (Fig. 19-10).

In astigmatism the refractive power of the eye is different in different meridians (see Fig. 19-8D). This produces a blurred retinal image for objects at any distance. Astigmatism occurs when the cornea, lens, or retinal surface has a toric shape rather than a spherical one. This may be likened to the two different radii of curvature that give a football its characteristic shape. Bulky masses in the lids such as chalazions or hemangiomas may compress the cornea and induce astigmatic refractive errors.

Anisometropia refers to the condition in which one eye has a different refractive error than the other. Usually the eye with the least amount of hyperopia or refractive error is the dominant or preferred eye. The fellow eye may be suppressed and develop amblyopia because the development of the visual system is being stimulated by a sharp focused image from one eye and a less focused image from the other eye. The magnitude of the amblyopia depends on the magnitude of the anisometropia and age at which it developed. Anisometropia may occur with hyperopia, myopia, astigmatism, or a combination of these refractive errors. If the degree of anisometropia is large, the optical properties of the required correcting lenses produce a difference in image size between the two eyes that may be difficult for the patient to tolerate. This is called *aniseikonia*.

Strabismus

Misalignment of the visual axes is referred to as *strabismus*. Strabismus occurs in 1% to 4% of the population and may be congenital or acquired. It may occur on a hereditary basis, most commonly without a clearly defined inheritance pattern. In the majority of childhood strabismus the misalignment of the eyes is not caused by a specific cranial nerve or extraocular muscle dysfunction. In some cases, strabismus may be caused by cranial nerve paralysis or neuromuscular disorders (myasthenia gravis).

Voluntary and reflex movement of the eyes is mediated via the extraocular muscles. These muscles are coordinated in their saccadic and pursuit movements by centers in the frontal and occipital areas of the cerebral cortex with modification by the cerebellum. Saccades are volun-

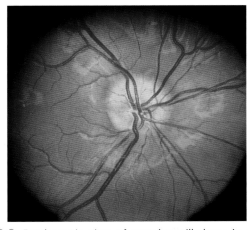

Figure 19-9. Funduscopic view of pseudopapilledema in a hyperopic child. Vessels are normal sized; small vessels are continuously visible at the disc margins. No hemorrhages or exudates exist.

Figure 19-10. Ophthalmoscopic view of an eye with high myopia. Thinning of the retinal pigment epithelium produces a tessellated fundus appearance. A temporal crescent adjacent to the optic disc is present, and the optic disc has an anomalous tilted appearance.

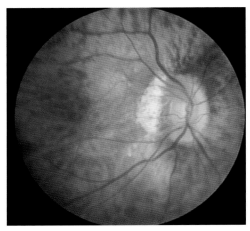

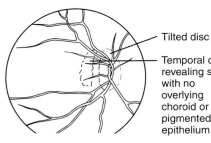

Tilted disc

Temporal crescent revealing sclera with no overlying choroid or pigmented epithelium

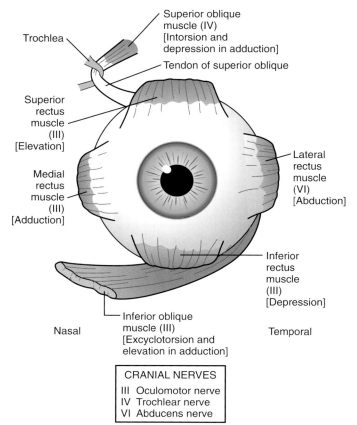

Trochlea

Superior oblique
muscle (IV)
[Intorsion and
depression in adduction]

Tendon of superior oblique

Superior
rectus
muscle
(III)
[Elevation]

Medial
rectus
muscle
(III)
[Adduction]

Lateral
rectus
muscle
(VI)
[Abduction]

Inferior
rectus
muscle
(III)
[Depression]

Nasal

Inferior oblique
muscle (III)
[Excyclotorsion and
elevation in adduction]

Temporal

CRANIAL NERVES
III Oculomotor nerve
IV Trochlear nerve
VI Abducens nerve

Figure 19-11. Innervation (in parentheses) of extraocular muscles and their primary actions [in brackets].

tary movements used to move the eyes to the object of regard. These are rapid eye movements. Pursuit or following movements are used to track or follow moving objects. These are slow eye movements.

The third, fourth, and sixth cranial nerve nuclei, located in the brainstem, are the centers responsible for innervating the extraocular muscles. In addition to innervation of the inferior oblique, medial, inferior, and superior recti, the third cranial nerve is responsible for innervation of the levator muscle, pupillary constriction, and accommodation of the lens. The fourth cranial nerve provides innervation to the superior oblique muscle, and the sixth cranial nerve supplies the lateral rectus muscle (Fig. 19-11). When one or more of the cranial nerves are paretic, the action of the innervated muscle is decreased, leading to a deficit in the duction or movement of the eye into the field of action of the muscle. The muscle having a function of movement in the opposite direction is no longer balanced, producing strabismus.

An abnormal head posture may be a sign of strabismus. These postures are usually observed in children who have good binocular function. Head postures are used to compensate for double vision caused by horizontal, vertical, or cyclovertical muscle palsies. For example, in a patient with a right sixth nerve palsy the abduction of the right eye is deficient. The adducting force of the medial rectus is not balanced, and the eye is in a relatively adducted or esotropic position. The patient then manifests a head turn to the right to allow the right eye to be in a position where less abducting force is required to allow both eyes to fixate together. In a patient with nystagmus, a head posture may be used to place the eyes in the null point or direction of gaze where the amplitude of nystagmus is the least. In cases of torticollis, if the head posture is present while the

patient is sleeping, the cause of the head posture is unlikely to be ophthalmologic in nature. Conversely, if a patient's head posture goes away when either eye is occluded, it suggests that the cause of the head tilt or turn may be related to a problem of ocular alignment or strabismus.

Versions

Eye movements are tested by moving the eyes right, left, up, down, up and right, down and right, up and left, and down and left. This tests the function of each of the extraocular muscles and its counterpart or yoke muscle in the fellow eye. A duction is the movement of a single eye. Versions refer to movement of both eyes together in conjugate gaze. Normal version movements should be present by 4 months of age.

Vergence movements consist of convergence or divergence of the eyes. Vergences are well established by 6 months of age. Convergence of the eyes, coupled with accommodation and miosis of the pupil, is referred to as the *near response*. Convergence assists alignment of the eyes at near.

A strabismus deviation that changes in size in different gaze positions is termed *incomitant*. Strabismus deviations that remain the same in all gaze positions are termed *comitant*. Strabismus caused by cranial nerve paralysis is incomitant.

Phorias and Tropias

If strabismus is present, it may be manifest (i.e., a tropia) or held latent by sensory fusion (i.e., a phoria). When the fusion of a patient with a phoria is interrupted by placing an occluder in front of one eye, the eye seeks its position of rest and deviates so that the visual axes of the two eyes are no longer both aligned on the point of fixation. When the eye is uncovered and binocular vision is reestablished, the fusion response assists in the realignment of the eyes on the object of regard. A phoria may produce symptoms of fatigue, blurring, or movement of objects. When a phoria breaks down into an intermittent tropia, there may be a symptom of intermittent double vision or *diplopia*. Phorias become symptomatic at times of fatigue, stress, or illness.

A tropia is a constant or intermittently present ocular deviation. The fusion mechanism is unable to maintain alignment of the eyes on an object of fixation. Young children with tropias develop suppression of the tropic eye as a response to avoid the symptom of diplopia. Older children or adults who acquire a tropia (e.g., from an acquired cranial nerve palsy) have diplopia as a symptom of the misalignment of their visual axes. The deviation present in a tropia may occur in one or all positions of gaze, depending on the cause of the tropia.

Phorias and tropias are classified according to the pattern of the eye deviation. The prefixes *eso-* and *exo-* classify horizontal strabismus. *Hyper-* and *hypo-* are used for vertical deviations, and *incyclo-* and *excyclo-* for torsional deviations.

Esodeviations

An esodeviation is a convergent deviation of the eyes. The deviation may be latent, a phoria (esophoria), or it

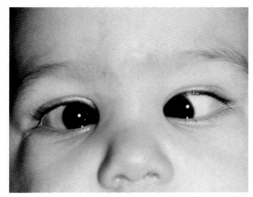

Figure 19-12. Infantile esotropia with asymmetrical corneal light reflexes.

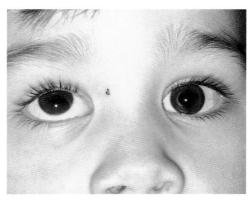

Figure 19-13. Dissociative vertical deviation, an upward and outward drifting of the right eye. Covering the fixating left eye in the cover-uncover test causes the deviating right eye to move into alignment with the left eye.

may occur as a manifest deviation, a tropia (esotropia). Common esodeviations seen in children are infantile esotropia, accommodative esotropia, esotropia resulting from sixth cranial nerve palsy, and Duane syndrome.

Infantile Esotropia

The most common cause for an esodeviation presenting in infancy is infantile, or congenital, esotropia (Fig. 19-12). Occasionally a family history of infantile esotropia exists, and the child's eyes are crossed at birth or shortly thereafter. The angle of esodeviation is large and constant. Defects in abduction may appear to be present, and differentiation from sixth cranial nerve palsy may be difficult. Cross-fixation is usually present, with the adducted right eye used for vision to the left and the adducted left eye used for vision to the right. Abduction of an eye is checked by occluding the contralateral eye. Children with this condition usually maintain good visual acuity in both eyes, without the development of much amblyopia, whether they are treated or not. They are otherwise systemically normal.

The esodeviation present in infantile esotropia requires surgical correction. After correction, the ocular alignment is frequently unstable, with further surgery commonly required later in life. Inferior oblique overaction or dissociated vertical deviations frequently develop later in childhood or adolescence. Inferior oblique overaction is seen as an elevation of one or both eyes in adduction. Dissociated vertical deviation (DVD) (Fig. 19-13) is an upward and outward "floating" movement of one or both eyes that becomes more prominent with fatigue or inattention. A DVD may be elicited on examination by covering one eye and watching its position as the eye is covered. These patients do not experience diplopia. Patients with infantile esotropia also commonly develop accommodative esotropia, with a need for glasses later in childhood.

Accommodative Esotropia

Accommodative esotropia most commonly presents as an acquired strabismus at $2\frac{1}{2}$ to 5 years of age. Family histories of esotropia and amblyopia are common. The presence of uncorrected hyperopia causes the patient to accommodate or focus to obtain clear visual acuity. With accommodation, the synkinetic near response, which includes miosis, accommodation, and convergence of the eyes, occurs. If the fusion mechanism is unable to diverge the eyes to compensate for the excessive convergence accompanying the need to accommodate to correct for the patient's hyperopia, esotropia results.

If an esodeviation is associated with a modest degree of farsightedness, treatment of the hyperopia optically with glasses is indicated. In patients with purely accommodative esotropia, this measure alone may completely correct the deviation (Fig. 19-14). Frequently, especially if the esodeviation has been left untreated for a long period of time, a residual esodeviation will remain. This is a partially accommodative esotropia. Surgical correction may be recommended for these patients. Some patients have straight eyes for some time with their glasses in place and decompensate to nonaccommodative esodeviations later.

In patients with accommodative esotropia, the eyes are straight with their glasses on and esotropic when they are removed. Frequently, if the patient is only moderately hyperopic in the preferred fixating eye, the patient will say that he or she can see just as well or perhaps better with his or her glasses off than on because the glasses are not prescribed to necessarily improve visual acuity; rather, the glasses are intended to decrease the accommodative effort and decrease the esotropia.

In another form of accommodative esotropia, the ratio between accommodative convergence and accommodation (AC/A ratio) may be abnormally high, producing excessive convergence when focusing on near objects. In high AC/A ratio accommodative esotropia, the esodeviation with near vision is greater in magnitude than it is with distance vision (Fig. 19-15). These patients may be treated with a bifocal, which gives them additional hyperopic correction for near, decreasing their accommodative effort at near and decreasing the near esodeviation.

Nonaccommodative Esotropia

Children may develop an esodeviation that is present without any relationship to the patient's refractive error (Fig. 19-16). These nonaccommodative esodeviations may be associated with poor vision, trauma, prematurity, aphakia, or high myopia. Nonaccommodative esotropia may also develop when accommodative esotropias are left untreated.

Other Causes of Esotropia

Unilateral or bilateral sixth cranial nerve palsy causes deficient abduction and an esodeviation. In sixth nerve palsy the esotropia increases with gaze directed toward the side of the palsy. This finding of gaze incomitance may be easier to detect than other signs of the nerve paralysis, including the extent or speed of abduction of the eye. Patients may display a head turn toward the side of the palsy to hold the involved eye in adduction and maintain

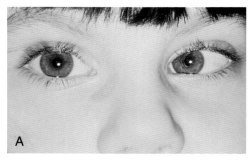
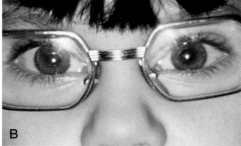

Figure 19-14. The child in **A** has esotropia with a high degree of hyperopia. In **B** we see that corrective glasses have reduced the hypertropia, and the esotropic eye has returned to orthophoria.

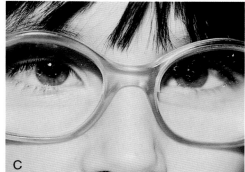
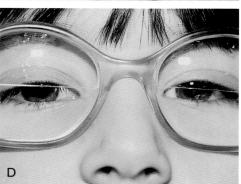

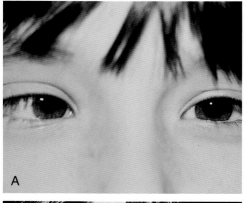
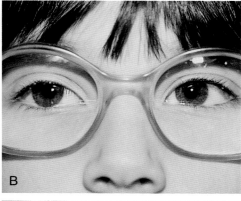

Figure 19-15. **A,** This child with hyperopia has an esotropia when fixing at distance, and even greater esotropia in the near range. **B,** When glasses are prescribed, correction of the hyperopia occurs and her eyes straighten at distances. **C,** However, the near esotropia remains. **D,** When bifocals are used, the near esotropia is corrected.

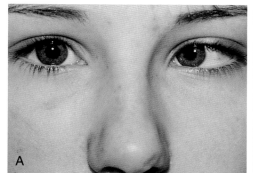
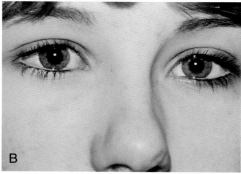

Figure 19-16. The girl in **A** shows nonaccommodative esotropia, an esotropia that could not be corrected with glasses or miotics. Surgery was performed, and the 1-week postoperative photograph in **B** shows normal ocular alignment with symmetrical corneal light reflexes.

binocular vision. Sixth cranial nerve palsies in children may be associated with increased intracranial pressure, trauma, tumor, or antecedent viral illness. In benign or "postviral" and traumatic cases the lateral rectus function may return fully over a 6-month period. In idiopathic cases if improvement does not occur, if the deviation increases, or if a gaze palsy develops, suspicion should be raised that a pontine glioma is the cause for the sixth nerve paralysis.

Duane syndrome is a congenital unilateral or bilateral defect characterized by inability to abduct an eye. This may be accompanied by an up or down shoot of the eye and narrowing of the lid fissure on attempted adduction. In attempted abduction the palpebral fissure widens. Duane syndrome is caused by a malformation of the cranial nerve nuclei producing coinnervation of the medial and lateral rectus muscles. The lateral rectus muscle does not contract with abduction and paradoxically co-contracts along with the medial rectus on adduction. Patients with Duane syndrome may be esotropic and have a head turn toward the involved side analogous to those seen with a sixth cranial nerve palsy. The changes in lid position and vertical deviations help to differentiate the two conditions (Fig. 19-17).

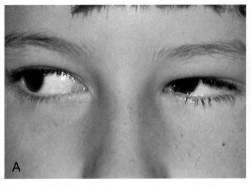 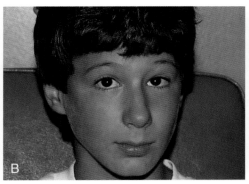 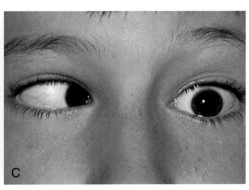

Figure 19-17. Left Duane syndrome. **A,** Right gaze. While the left eye is noted to move into adduction, retraction of the globe is noted along with narrowing of the palpebral fissure. The globe retraction and lid changes are due to co-contraction of the medial rectus and lateral rectus muscles on the involved side. **B,** Fixation target directly in front of patient. The patient is noted to maintain a slight left head turn to maintain normal alignment of the eyes with the affected left eye held slightly in adduction. If the patient's head is forced out of the slight left head turn, the left eye would become slightly esotropic. **C,** Left gaze. The affected left eye is seen to have an absence of abduction resulting from aberrant innervation of the lateral rectus muscle.

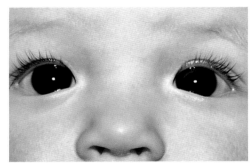

Figure 19-18. This infant has pseudostrabismus, caused by a flat nasal bridge, wide epicanthal folds, and closely placed eyes.

Pseudostrabismus

Pseudostrabismus is seen in infants with prominent epicanthal folds, closely placed eyes, and flat nasal bridges. Asymmetry of the lids or nasal bridge may also produce pseudostrabismus. When these facial features are present, the white of the sclera between the cornea and inner canthus frequently may be obscured, giving the optical illusion that the eyes are esotropic (Figs. 19-18 and 19-19). Parents and caretakers frequently report subtle esodeviations that worsen with gaze to the right or left. This is frequently pointed out in photographs in which careful examination shows the eyes to be in slight right or left gaze. Observation of symmetrical corneal light reflexes or cover testing confirms or excludes the presence of a true deviation.

Exodeviations

When the visual axes are divergent, an exodeviation is present (Fig. 19-20). Many children with exodeviations have family histories of strabismus. Exodeviations may also occur with vision loss in one eye (sensory exotropia) and cranial nerve paralysis (third nerve palsy). An exodeviation may be controlled by fusion (exophoria), be manifest intermittently (intermittent exotropia), or be constant (exotropia). Intermittent exodeviations become manifest with fatigue, daydreaming, or illness. Patients with exodeviations frequently squint one eye in bright light and may complain of discomfort at night or when tired.

If there is a defect in visual acuity, the decreased visual stimulation may produce a sensory deviation. Generally speaking, if the onset of decreased vision occurs after the age of 4 years, an exodeviation will occur; however, if

PSEUDOSTRABISMUS

The eyes appear to be esotropic but they are not. The appearance of esotropia is due to the presence of a wide and flat nasal bridge, prominent epicanthal folds, and decreased intraorbital distance.

The pupillary light is centered. Cover testing shows no movement of eyes.

In left gaze, the white of the sclera is covered by the inner canthal tissue. It appears as if the right eye is esotropic but the light reflex remains centered in the pupil.

The same may be true for right gaze.

Figure 19-19. The characteristics of pseudostrabismus are illustrated.

sensory input to the eye is decreased before the age of 2 years, an esodeviation usually occurs. Because young children do not complain of monocular vision loss, especially if congenital or with onset during infancy, sensory strabismus is frequently the presenting sign of vision-limiting pathology of the retina or optic nerve.

Exodeviations may be simulated in patients with widely spaced eyes (hypertelorism) or in those whose maculae are temporally displaced, as may occur in retinopathy of prematurity. When the macula is displaced temporally, the eye rotates outward to align its visual axis on the fixation target. This simulates an exodeviation. The term *positive angle kappa* is used to describe this condition (Fig. 19-21).

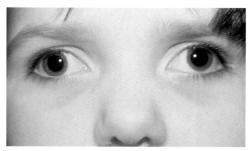

Figure 19-20. Exotropia, a divergent deviation of the eyes.

ANGLE KAPPA

Positive angle kappa produces an appearance of exotropia. This appearance is caused by a temporal displacement of the fovea, usually due to cicatricial changes of the retina after retinopathy of prematurity.

The left eye appears exotropic.
Cover testing shows no movement of the eyes.

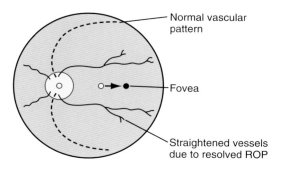

Normal vascular pattern

Fovea

Straightened vessels due to resolved ROP

Temporal retinal cicatricial changes after resolution of stage 3 ROP have caused the fovea to be displaced temporalward.

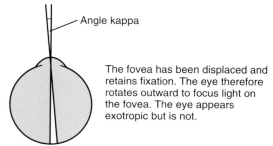

Angle kappa

The fovea has been displaced and retains fixation. The eye therefore rotates outward to focus light on the fovea. The eye appears exotropic but is not.

Figure 19-21. Angle kappa.

Convergence Insufficiency

Convergence insufficiency describes an exodeviation in which the size of the deviation is greater in the near range than at distance. Most frequently, there is an exodeviation at near only and no distance deviation. This may cause symptoms of discomfort while reading and possibly intermittent double vision at near range. To test for convergence insufficiency, the child is asked to fixate on a target with detail as it is brought progressively closer. Normally the child should be able to converge to a point 10 cm from the nose. If the eyes converge, and then break their alignment and diverge at a distance greater than 10 cm from

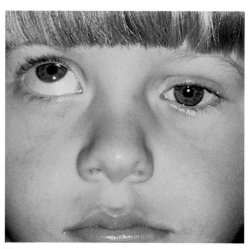

Figure 19-22. Left third nerve palsy with ptosis and an inability to elevate and adduct the eye.

THIRD CRANIAL NERVE PALSY

A patient with left third cranial nerve palsy will not have a Bell's phenomenon on the affected side. The forced opening of tightly closed eyelids will reveal an upward, slightly outward movement of the eye under the closed eyelids (normal Bell's response). The patient with a third cranial nerve palsy cannot elevate or adduct the eye. The eye, when opened or under forced eyelid closure, is not elevated.

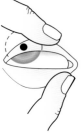 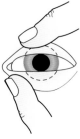

Figure 19-23. Third cranial nerve palsy.

the eyes, the patient should be evaluated for convergence insufficiency.

Third (Oculomotor) Cranial Nerve Palsy

The third cranial nerve innervates the medial rectus muscle. In third nerve paralysis the action of the lateral rectus muscle, innervated by the sixth cranial nerve, is unopposed and produces an exodeviation. The third nerve also innervates the superior and inferior recti; the inferior oblique muscles; the levator palpebrae superioris, which elevates the lid; the ciliary muscle, which is responsible for accommodation of the lens; and the iris sphincter muscle, which produces miosis of the pupil. In the presence of a complete third cranial nerve palsy, the eye assumes a down and outward position, the eyelid is ptotic, and the pupil is enlarged (Fig. 19-22). Elevation of the eye with forced eyelid closure (the Bell phenomenon) is typically absent in patients with a third cranial nerve palsy (Fig. 19-23). The most common causes for acquired third nerve paralysis in children are trauma and tumor. A third nerve palsy may also occur as a congenital defect.

Vertical Deviations

Isolated vertical misalignment of the eyes is uncommon. Vertical deviations may occur in only one field of

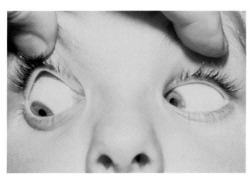

Figure 19-24. Left fourth nerve palsy with an inability to depress the involved eye in adduction. Abnormal head posture is common, as is overaction of the direct antagonistic inferior oblique muscle.

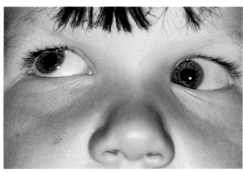

Figure 19-26. Brown syndrome, an inability to elevate an eye in adduction resulting from a tight superior oblique tendon.

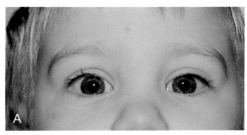

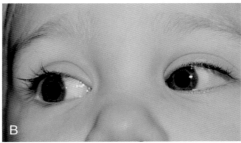

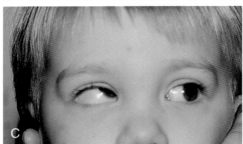

Figure 19-25. Right inferior oblique overaction. In primary (straight ahead) **(A)** and right gaze **(B)** the eyes are well aligned. In left gaze **(C)** the right eye is elevated or hypertropic because of overaction of the right inferior oblique.

Brown syndrome describes an isolated motility disorder in which there is an inability to elevate the eye when it is adducted (Fig. 19-26). This may be caused by a congenital anomaly of the superior oblique tendon, or it may be acquired as an idiopathic inflammation or tenosynovitis of the superior oblique tendon. Acquired cases may be persistent, resolve spontaneously, or respond to nonsteroidal anti-inflammatory drugs.

Abnormalities of extraocular muscle innervation rarely cause vertical deviations. Double elevator palsy is an inherited unilateral or bilateral condition in which there is hypotropia and limitation of elevation of the involved eye. To achieve binocularity, patients tilt their chins up and position their heads back. Ptosis is frequently present.

Additional causes of vertical deviations include myasthenia gravis, thyroid ophthalmopathy, chronic progressive external ophthalmoplegia, orbital fractures with muscle entrapment (most commonly the inferior rectus entrapped within a blowout fracture of the orbital floor), and orbital disease with intraorbital masses.

Tests for Strabismus

Although gross observation may detect the majority of cases of strabismus, pseudostrabismus will lead frequently to unnecessary referrals or, more significantly, many smaller angle deviations may be missed, leading to delays in treatment if further tests for strabismus are not employed by the primary care physician.

The type and degree of ocular misalignment may be estimated using the corneal light reflex test, or Hirschberg method. The patient fixates on a penlight held at 1 m. Using the pupil edge as a point of reference, the light reflections between the two eyes are compared for symmetry; if the light reflex is displaced temporally, an esotropia is present. If the light reflex is displaced nasally in comparison with the other eye, an exodeviation is present (Fig. 19-27). This test only estimates ocular alignment. The most accurate method of detecting misalignment of the eyes is cover and uncover testing.

The cover test requires vision in each eye and use of a target that stimulates accommodation. Cover testing is performed while the patient maintains fixation on targets at 6 m and at 1 m because some types of strabismus produce misalignment of the eyes that is present only at either distance or near. The cover-uncover test is used to detect phorias. This test is performed by placing a cover over one eye to disrupt fusion or binocularity. As the cover is removed, the previously covered eye is observed. If the eye does not move, both eyes are aligned on the object at

gaze, or they may be comitant and equal in all fields of gaze. Vertical deviations may have a cyclotorsional component and be associated with a head tilt or head posture to eliminate double vision. All patients with torticollis should be evaluated for cyclovertical muscle palsies.

The most common cyclovertical deviation is due to a palsy of the fourth cranial (trochlear) nerve (Fig. 19-24). Fourth nerve palsies in children occur congenitally and secondary to trauma. The eye is excyclorotated, and the head is tilted to the shoulder opposite the side of the paretic superior oblique muscle. Other features are elevation of the eye and difficulty depressing the eye in adduction (Fig. 19-25). Patients with fourth nerve palsies have diplopia in the contralateral field of gaze. Patients with congenital palsies may not always recognize this diplopia, however.

HIRSCHBERG TEST
FOR OCULAR ALIGNMENT

A penlight is held 1 meter from the eyes.
The pupillary light reflex is observed and its
relationship to the center of the pupil is noted.

Normal corneal light reflex
The reflexes are symmetrical and slightly
displaced nasally to the center of the pupils.

Left esotropia
The reflex is displaced temporally to
the center of the pupil.

Left exotropia
The corneal light reflex is displaced
nasally to the center of the pupil.

Figure 19-27. Hirschberg test for ocular alignment.

HETEROPHORIAS

Normally, both eyes appear to be aligned and centrally fixed.

Exophoria

Cover one eye—that eye deviates away from the other eye.

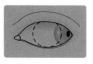

The cover is then removed—the now uncovered eye returns
to a central position.

The same procedure is then performed on the other eye.

Esophoria

Cover one eye—that eye deviates toward the other eye.

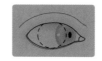

The cover is then removed—the now uncovered eye returns
to a central position.

The same procedure is then performed on the other eye.

Hyperphoria

Cover one eye—that eye deviates superiorly.

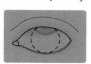

The cover is then removed—the now uncovered eye returns
to a central position.

The same procedure is then performed on the other eye.

Figure 19-28. The cover-uncover test for heterophorias.

that distance; orthophoria is present. If the eye deviates while covered and then moves to regain fusion and assumes fixation as the cover is removed, a phoria exists. The test is then repeated, covering and uncovering the other eye (Fig. 19-28).

The second component of the cover test is performed by covering one eye and observing the movement of the other eye. If neither eye moves as the eyes are alternately covered, the eyes are both aligned on the fixation target and the term *orthophoria* is used. No deviation is present in this case. If a tropia and a fixation preference are present, a fixation movement of the deviating uncovered eye occurs when the preferred fixating eye is covered; when the cover is transferred back, the previously deviating eye again deviates behind the cover (Fig. 19-29). If a deviation is well controlled by fusion (a phoria) and is small in size, it may be safely observed if there are no symptoms and the fundus is normal. When a tropia is present, either constantly or intermittently, after 3 months of age, the patient should be referred to an ophthalmologist. Ophthalmologists use prisms along with cover testing to measure the size of strabismic deviations.

Amblyopia

Amblyopia is present when there is a decrease in vision in one or both eyes and all potential organic causes (refractive errors, media opacities, structural abnormalities) for the decrease in vision have been corrected or excluded. Amblyopia is caused by the absence of stimulation of the immature visual system by a focused retinal image or by strabismus and the resultant suppression of one eye. Visual deprivation amblyopia may be caused by a corneal opacity, a dense cataract, vitreous opacity (hemorrhage or inflammation), or high refractive error (Fig. 19-30).

In anisometropic amblyopia an image is clearly focused on the fovea of one eye, but in the other eye the image is out of focus. The blurred retinal image is suppressed by the child's immature visual system, and that eye is affected

HETEROTROPIAS

In esotropia, one eye is deviated toward the other. Note that the corneal light reflex is not centrally placed.

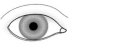

Cover the esotropic eye—there is no movement of either eye.

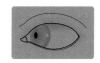

The cover is then removed—again, there is no movement of either eye—no proof of tropia.

The other eye is now covered—as a result, that eye becomes esotropic and the formerly esotropic eye moves to a central position to take up fixation.

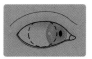

If the cover is removed and no eye movement occurs, this indicates that the eyes have equal visual acuity or fixation. This also indicates a relative absence of amblyopia.

If the cover is removed and both eyes move so that the original fixing eye is again centrally fixed and the originally esotropic eye is again esotropic, this indicates that there is amblyopia present. In this case, the patient's left eye is amblyopic.

The same maneuvers can be used to determine the presence of exotropia (outward deviation), hyper- and hypotropia (upward and downward deviation), and cyclotropia (rotary displacement)

Figure 19-29. The cover-uncover test for heterotropias.

by amblyopia. In anisometropic amblyopia, most commonly one eye is more hyperopic than the other. Because both eyes must accommodate the same amount, the less hyperopic eye is preferred and the more hyperopic eye has the blurred image and develops the amblyopia. With high hyperopia or astigmatism affecting both eyes, bilateral ametropic amblyopia may occur if the child does not or cannot accommodate to produce a focused retinal image to stimulate the visual system with either eye. These patients have decreased vision in both eyes. In children with strabismus, the image from the deviating eye is suppressed by the brain as an adaptation to avoid diplopia, and the deviating eye develops strabismic amblyopia. Patients often have both strabismus and anisometropia simultaneously as causes for their amblyopia.

The severity of the visual loss produced by amblyopia is determined by the nature of the visual deprivation; the age of onset; and its consistency, severity, and duration. If a patient is suspected of having amblyopia, careful measurement of visual acuity is performed in a well-illuminated room. Suspicion is heightened if there is a coexistent strabismus, anisometropia, or if there is evidence of an opacity that interferes with visualization of the fundus. Patients who are suspected of having amblyopia should be referred promptly to an ophthalmologist.

Amblyopia is treated by removing the cause of the amblyopia, if possible, and by forcing use of the affected eye to stimulate the development of the vision from that eye. In bilateral ametropic amblyopia, the appropriate glasses are given as treatment. In strabismic or anisometropic amblyopia, appropriate glasses are given, and the preferred, nonamblyopic eye is penalized to force the use of the amblyopic eye. An occlusion patch placed over the preferred fixating eye is commonly used as treatment.

Other methods of treatment are optical via the eyeglass prescription and pharmacological, with atropine drops placed in the nonamblyopic eye, which prevents accommodation in the nonambylopic eye. This forces the use of the amblyopic eye for reading and near vision.

Amblyopia responds most rapidly and completely to treatment begun early in life. The visual system has developmental phases, and if certain levels of visual acuity are not reached early in life the amblyopia present is unlikely to respond completely to treatment. Treatment has less effect after 8 years of age.

Diseases of the Eyes and Surrounding Structures

Eyelids and Adnexae—Anatomy of the Eyelid

The eyelid is comprised of skin and its related appendages, glands that contribute to the tear film, and muscular structures permitting the eyelid to open and close (Fig. 19-31). Conditions affecting the eyelid are related to these anatomic structures.

Telecanthus refers to an increase in the distance between the inner canthus of each eye (Fig. 19-32). Telecanthus can be due to the hereditary transmission of facial features or midline embryonic defects, or it can be related to a syndrome such as the blepharophimosis, or Komoto syndrome (Fig. 19-33). This inherited syndrome consists of telecanthus, epicanthus inversus (a skinfold projecting over the inner angle of the eye and covering part of the canthus, arising from the lower lid skin), blepharophimosis (horizontal shortening of the lid fissure), and ptosis. *Hypertelorism* refers to an increase in the distance between the nasal walls of the orbits. This is usually associated with telecanthus.

Blepharoptosis, or ptosis, is a unilateral or bilateral decrease in the vertical distance between the upper and lower eyelids (palpebral fissure) because of dysfunction of the levator muscle (Fig. 19-34). Congenital blepharoptosis is frequently transmitted as an autosomal dominant trait with variable penetrance. Congenital ptosis may be either unilateral or bilateral. Other causes for blepharoptosis include ocular inflammation, chronic irritation of the anterior segment of the eye, chronic use of topical steroid eye drops, third nerve palsy, and trauma. Ptosis may be severe enough to cause visual deprivation and amblyopia if the visual axis is occluded. Children with even mild degrees of congenital ptosis should be referred for evaluation because they have a higher than normal incidence of

AMBLYOPIA

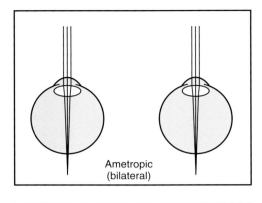

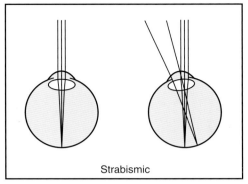

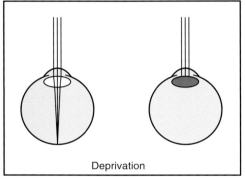

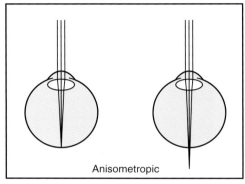

Figure 19-30. Amblyopia is produced either by the absence of a focused retinal image (ametropic, deprivation, or anisometropic) or by suppression (strabismic).

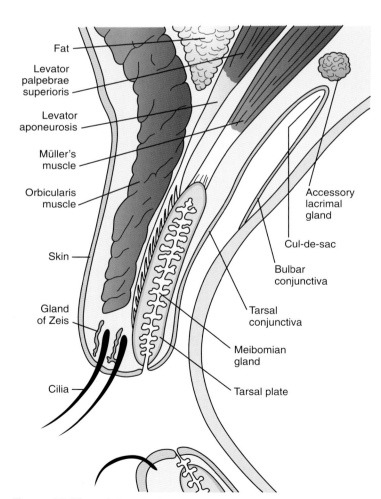

Figure 19-31. Eyelids and adnexae. Cross-section of the eyelid.

strabismus and anisometropic amblyopia than the general population.

The Marcus Gunn, or jaw-winking, phenomenon is caused by a misdirection of the motor division of the fifth cranial nerve to the ipsilateral levator muscle of the eyelid (Fig. 19-35). With jaw movement to the ipsilateral side the eyelid droops, and when the jaw is moved to the contralateral side, the eyelid elevates. The eyelid winks with chewing or feeding. This is a benign phenomenon and no further evaluation is required. Surgical treatment is not indicated unless the associated ptosis warrants it. Most patients learn to control the winking by avoiding the inciting jaw movement.

Trichiasis is the term used to describe misdirected eyelashes that irritate the cornea or conjunctiva. It can be caused by chronic inflammation of the eyelids, entropion (inturning of the eyelid), eyelid trauma, or inflammatory conditions with scarring of the conjunctiva such as Stevens-Johnson syndrome.

Districhiasis describes a condition where there is an accessory row of eyelashes (cilia) along the posterior border of the eyelid (Fig. 19-36). Eyelid eversion or ectropion frequently coexists because of defects in the tarsal plate. This condition is inherited as an autosomal dominant condition, but it may also be a sequela of severe ocular inflammation.

Entropion is an inverted eyelid with the lashes rubbing against the conjunctiva or cornea. This may be present at birth or occur with severe blepharospasm, inflammation, or trauma. If severe, the abrasion of the cornea by the lashes can cause permanent corneal scarring (Fig. 19-37).

In epiblepharon a skinfold extends over the lid margin and presses the lashes against the globe. It is commonly observed during the first year of life (Fig. 19-38). The lower lid is more commonly affected in Caucasians, and both the upper and lower lid may be affected in Asian infants. This defect usually corrects itself spontaneously by 1 year

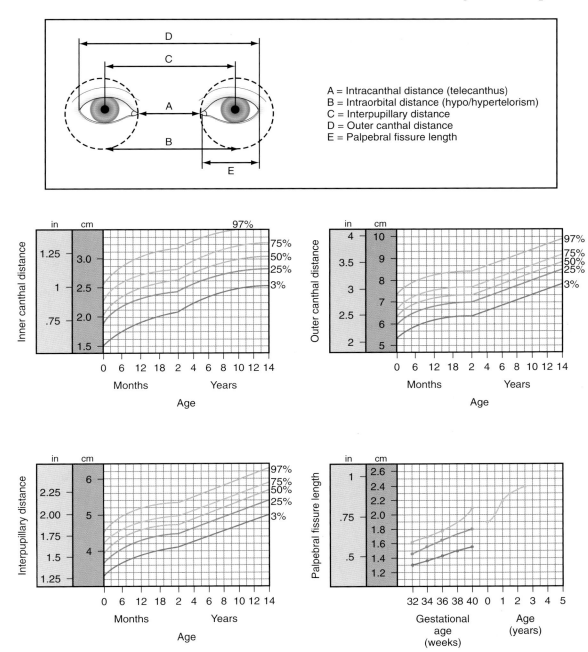

A = Intracanthal distance (telecanthus)
B = Intraorbital distance (hypo/hypertelorism)
C = Interpupillary distance
D = Outer canthal distance
E = Palpebral fissure length

Figure 19-32. Normal adnexal measurements.

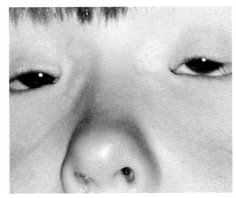

Figure 19-33. Komoto syndrome, a combination of blepharophimosis, ptosis, epicanthus inversus, and telecanthus.

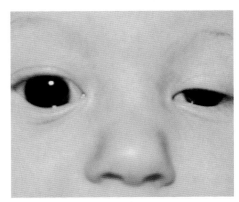

Figure 19-34. Unilateral congenital ptosis with lid covering pupil.

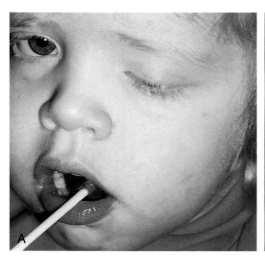

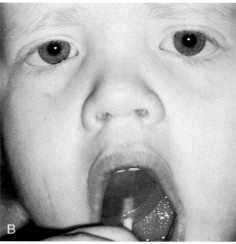

Figure 19-35. **A,** The toddler exhibits the Marcus Gunn jaw-winking phenomenon with ptosis, whereas in **B,** he shows a wide-open lid with movement of the jaw.

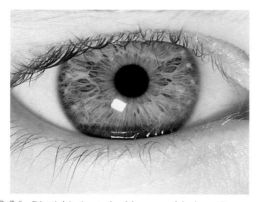

Figure 19-36. Districhiasis, a double row of lashes. One row, directed toward the cornea, arises from the meibomian gland orifices. The second row is directed outward in the normal position.

of age. In Asians the problem may be persistent. Corneal abrasion usually does not occur because of the soft texture of the infant's eyelashes or when it is the shaft of the eyelash rather than the tip of the lash that touches the cornea. However, surgical correction may be required if it is persistent and causing corneal abrasion with conjunctival injection, epiphora, and photosensitivity.

Ectropion is an outward rotation of the eyelid margin. If severe, ectropion can lead to problems of corneal exposure. Ectropion may be congenital or caused by any condition (trauma, scleroderma), causing the eyelid skin to contract and evert the eyelid (Fig. 19-39). Ectropion may occur after seventh cranial nerve palsy with paralysis of the facial musculature.

Congenital eyelid colobomas are defects or notches in the eyelid margin caused by failed fusion of embryonic fissures early in development. These may be isolated defects or associated with conditions such as Goldenhar syndrome (Fig. 19-40). Goldenhar syndrome consists of eyelid colobomas, corneal limbal dermoids, vertebral anomalies, and preauricular skin tags.

Ankyloblepharon is a fusion of the upper and lower eyelid margins. This may range from a few thin strands of tissue to complete fusion of the lids. The majority of cases are mild, isolated anomalies and no further evaluation is required. Treatment is by separating the lids, by simple eyelid opening if only threadlike strands are present, or with scissors if necessary.

Children frequently have a low-grade inflammation of the eyelid margin, chronic blepharitis, caused by staphylococcus infection. Blepharitis may be associated with

seborrhea or allergies and occurs commonly in children with Down syndrome. Symptoms include itching, light sensitivity, and irritation of the lids. The lashes may be matted and adherent in the morning. If the condition is chronic and severe, thickening of the eyelid and misdirection of the eyelashes to the point where they may invert and irritate the cornea or conjunctiva may occur (Fig. 19-41). Complications include ulceration of the lid margin, abscess or hordeolum formation, chronic conjunctivitis, and keratitis (corneal irritation and inflammation).

A hordeolum is an inflamed gland of Zeis at the base of the cilia (Fig. 19-42). This produces painful swelling and erythema of the eyelid. These lesions are commonly called styes. Infection, frequently with *Staphylococcus,* may occur. Some discharge may be seen. Rarely, preseptal cellulitis may occur as a complication.

A chalazion is a chronic granulomatous inflammation of the meibomian glands within the tarsal plate. Painless swelling and redness of the eyelid results from distention of the gland and the inflammatory response caused by the retained glandular secretions. The gland may spontaneously rupture either to the conjunctival surface or externally to the skin (Figs. 19-43 and 19-44). Spontaneous resolution may occur; however, tissue reaction may persist and leave a firm mass within the lid.

The mainstay of treatment of hordeolums and chalazions is frequent application of warm compresses. Topical antibiotics may be used, as well as systemic antibiotics if secondary infection or cellulitis appears to be present. Some patients may be affected by multiple, recurring lesions. Surgical excision of the lesions may be required if chronic or inflamed in order to prevent drainage through the skin surface with skin scarring.

Primary herpes simplex infection may affect the periocular skin (Fig. 19-45). This is characterized by small skin vesicles, frequently unilateral, with an associated mild conjunctivitis and punctate keratitis. Although self-limited, herpes simplex should be treated with topical antivirals to prevent scarring from keratitis. Systemic antivirals may also be used, and if given early, they may reduce the number and duration of lesions. Recurrence or reactivation unfortunately is not prevented. Varicella produces eyelid swelling and vesicular skin eruptions, usually without scarring. Conjunctival vesicles and keratitis may also occur, and topical antibiotics are indicated to prevent secondary bacterial infection. Herpes zoster is uncommon in children. If present, zoster should be treated as early in its course as possible in order to promote healing and to prevent zoster-associated hyperesthesias. A lesion on the

Figure 19-37. Congenital entropion of the right upper lid. The lid is inverted, and the lashes and skin rest on the corneal surface. **A,** The eyelid is propped up with a cotton-tipped applicator displaying the area of skin inverted against the eye. The povidone-iodine prep solution has not coated the affected area of the lid. **B,** With the upper lid everted and the lids held widely open, extensive corneal scarring caused by the abrasion from the inverted skin and lashes is seen.

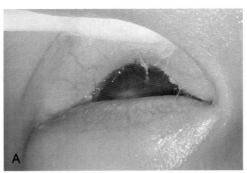
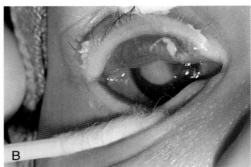

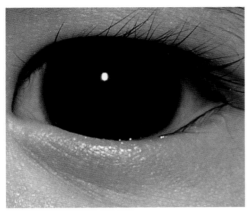

Figure 19-38. In epiblepharon the eyelashes are rotated upward against the globe in the medial third of the eyelid.

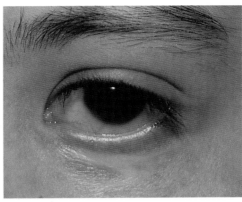

Figure 19-39. Ectropion of the left lower lid resulting from scleroderma. The lower eyelid skin has become contracted, causing eversion of the lower eyelid.

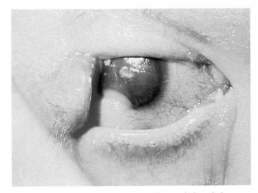

Figure 19-40. Goldenhar syndrome with eyelid coloboma and corneal limbal dermoid.

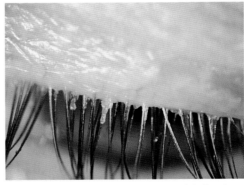

Figure 19-41. Thickened lids with crusts around lashes in a patient with blepharitis.

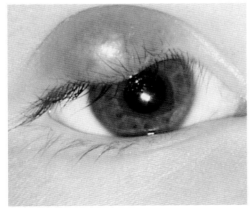

Figure 19-42. Acute hordeolum of the eyelid (pointing externally) with swelling, induration, and purulent contents.

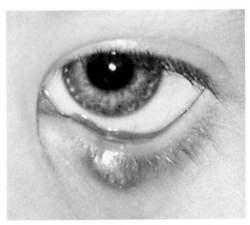

Figure 19-43. Chalazion, a painless lid mass pointing externally or internally.

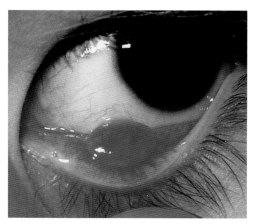

Figure 19-44. Chalazion of the left lower lid pointed internally. A pyogenic granuloma consisting of a vascularized mound of conjunctival tissue has developed over the chalazion because of spontaneous rupture of the chalazion under the palpebral conjunctiva.

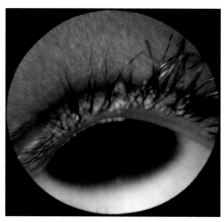

Figure 19-46. Infestation of the eyelashes with the crab louse *Phthirus pubis*. The lid margin has a crusty appearance because of the presence of adult organisms and eggs adherent to the eyelashes. The salivary material of the parasites results in toxic and immunologic reactions that cause itching and burning of the eyes.

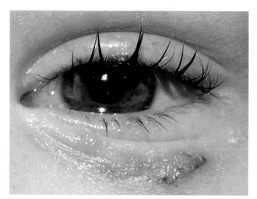

Figure 19-45. Primary herpes simplex infection involving the periocular area. Primary infection is frequently associated with a mild diffuse keratoconjunctivitis; dendritic corneal lesions are uncommon in primary infections.

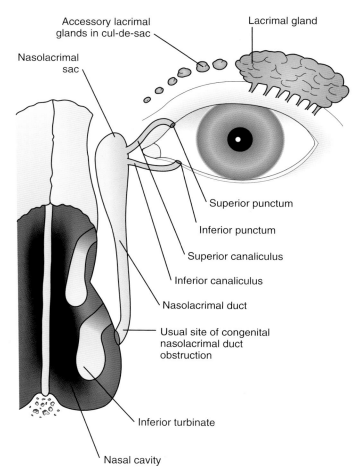

Figure 19-47. Lacrimal secretory and collecting system.

tip of the nose indicates involvement of the ophthalmic division of the maxillary nerve and possible involvement of the eye with keratitis, uveitis, and glaucoma. Another common eyelid lesion found in children is caused by *molluscum contagiosum* (see Chapter 8). Molluscum is characterized by elevated, 1- to 2-mm umbilicated lesions of the eyelid skin. If the lesions involve the eyelid margin, they may cause an associated keratoconjunctivitis. Molluscum is included in the differential diagnosis of chronic conjunctivitis.

Phthiriasis—infestation of the lashes with the crab louse *Phthirus pubis*—manifests as a crusty appearance of the lid margin. Closer inspection reveals egg cases and the adult louse (Fig. 19-46). Ophthalmic ointment, almost any type, suffocates the organisms. Phthiriasis may also produce chronic conjunctivitis.

Lacrimal Gland and Nasolacrimal Drainage System

Reflex tears are produced by the lacrimal gland, whereas the basal secretion of tears comes from the accessory lacrimal glands (Fig. 19-47). The secretions from the glands of Zeis and the meibomian glands contribute to the tear film. During the first month of life the eye remains moist, but reflex tearing or tearing resulting from emotion does not occur until the second month of life.

Disorders of the lacrimal gland are rare in children. Acute dacryoadenitis may occur with viral infections, most frequently mumps (Fig. 19-48). Chronic diseases such as sarcoid, Hodgkin disease, leukemia, and mononucleosis may produce lacrimal gland swelling with a palpable mass in the upper outer portion of the orbit.

The tears are drained from the eye by the superior and inferior puncta, which connect to the superior and inferior canaliculi (see Fig. 19-47). The canaliculi may unite into a common canaliculus before they enter the nasolacrimal sac, or they may enter the sac separately. The medial

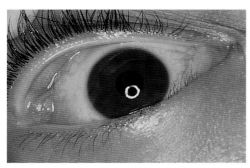

Figure 19-48. Dacryoadenitis. The lacrimal gland has become swollen and inflamed and is visible beneath the lateral aspect of the upper eyelid. The swelling is frequently accompanied by symptoms of pain and tenderness.

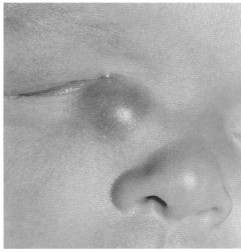

Figure 19-50. Congenital nasolacrimal sac mucocele presents shortly after birth as a bluish mass below the medial canthal tendon.

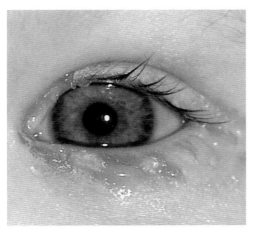

Figure 19-49. Obstruction of the left nasolacrimal duct has led to the development of mucopurulent discharge and tearing.

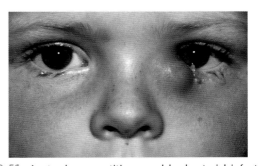

Figure 19-51. Acute dacryocystitis caused by bacterial infection of the nasolacrimal sac associated with nasolacrimal duct obstruction. The infection of the nasolacrimal sac has spread to the surrounding tissues, producing a cellulitis.

canthal tendon is anterior and superior to the nasolacrimal sac. Disorders of the lacrimal sac are then seen primarily inferior to the medial canthus unless there is an overlying cellulitis. The sac is connected to the nasolacrimal duct, which is located in the nasal bone. The distal portion of the nasolacrimal duct enters the nasal antrum beneath the inferior turbinate.

Stenosis or obstruction of the nasolacrimal duct is present in 30% of newborns (Fig. 19-49). The obstruction is usually caused by a membranous obstruction of the nasolacrimal duct. Obstruction may also be caused by the inferior turbinate within the nose. Signs include tearing and mucopurulent discharge, which usually begins 3 to 5 weeks after birth. The absence of conjunctival injection differentiates this condition from conjunctivitis. A helpful diagnostic technique is to apply gentle pressure over the nasolacrimal sac to cause reflux of tears and mucopurulent material from the sac. Spontaneous resolution of the obstruction is common before 6 to 8 months of age. If the obstruction has not cleared by this age, spontaneous resolution is much less likely and the patient should be referred for probing of the nasolacrimal duct. If left past 13 months of age, the recurring infections may cause scarring and stenosis of the nasolacrimal duct, which may require more complicated procedures for treatment.

If both the nasolacrimal duct and the canaliculi entering the sac are obstructed at birth, a bluish firm mass may be present or develop in the area of the nasolacrimal sac (congenital nasolacrimal sac mucocele or dacryocele) (Fig. 19-50). These patients should be referred promptly because of the risk for development of infection and cellulitis. Other congenital defects of the nasolacrimal collecting

system include absence of the puncta or accessory puncta with fistulas from the nasolacrimal sac to the overlying skin.

Obstruction of the nasolacrimal system may also occur secondary to infections such as viral conjunctivitis, trachoma, tuberculosis, or fungal infections. Dacryocystitis, an infection and inflammation of the lacrimal sac and passages, may spread to the surrounding tissues, producing a periorbital cellulitis. Acute dacryocystitis is usually due to bacterial infection (Fig. 19-51).

Conjunctiva

The conjunctiva is a mucous membrane that covers the posterior aspect of the eyelids. It is reflected into the cul-de-sac and extends onto the globe, where it fuses to the sclera at the corneal scleral limbus. The conjunctiva has goblet cells that contribute mucin to the tear film. When the eyelids are closed, the oxygen supplied by the blood vessels of the conjunctiva is responsible for maintaining oxygenation of the cornea. *Conjunctivitis* refers to inflammation of the conjunctiva. Infections of the conjunctiva may be bacterial or viral.

The etiology of neonatal conjunctivitis is related to the time of onset. Neonatal conjunctivitis occurring within the first day or two of life is usually due to the use of Credé prophylaxis. One percent silver nitrate solution may cause a mild chemical conjunctivitis that spontaneously resolves within 1 or 2 days. This is becoming less common as

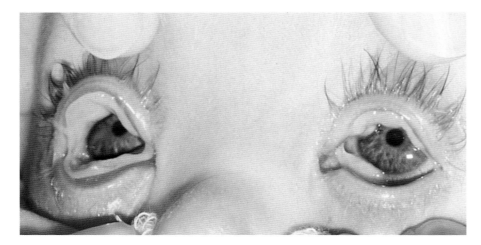

Figure 19-52. Ophthalmia neonatorum, a hyperacute bacterial conjunctivitis, with thick purulent discharge and red swollen lids.

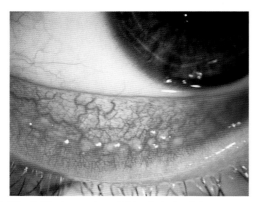

Figure 19-53. Follicular conjunctivitis of viral origin.

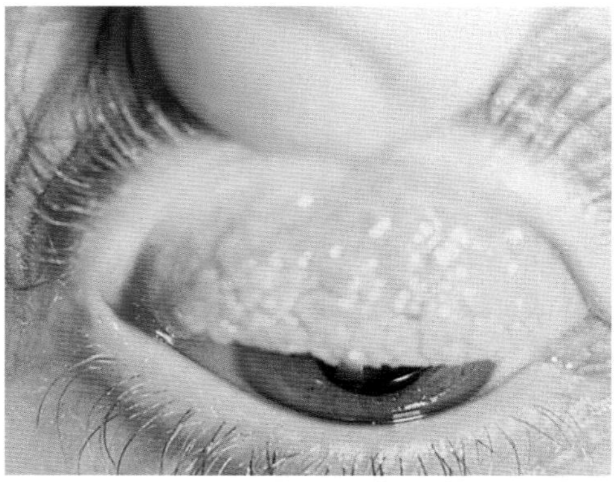

Figure 19-54. Papillary conjunctivitis of bacterial or allergic origin.

erythromycin ointment replaces the use of silver nitrate. Neonatal conjunctivitis occurring 2 to 4 days after birth and accompanied by a copious purulent discharge, either with or without corneal involvement, may be caused by gonococci (Fig. 19-52). All cases of neonatal conjunctivitis are emergencies and must be evaluated by an ophthalmologist. Aerobic, anaerobic, and viral cultures must be obtained because corneal involvement, particularly with gonorrhea, may lead to corneal scarring or perforation. With *Pseudomonas* infection corneal perforation may occur within hours of presentation. Infectious neonatal conjunctivitis occurring after 8 days (but before 2 weeks) and accompanied by a watery discharge is often due to chlamydiae. Other common pathogens include *Staphylococcus, Streptococcus,* and *Enterococcus.* Conjunctivitis is usually contracted after early rupture of membranes or during passage through the birth canal.

The conjunctiva has a limited variety of responses to infection or inflammation. Inflammation of the conjunctiva results in the formation of follicles or papillae. A follicle is an aggregate of lymphocytes with an avascular center and a peripheral vascular network (Fig. 19-53). Newborns seldom develop follicles because lymphoid tissues have not yet developed. Viral infections frequently lead to follicular reaction.

Papillae are small, raised nodules with a central vascular core (Fig. 19-54). They may be located on the tarsal surface of the upper and lower eyelids. Papillae may become large, measuring 1 to 2 mm in diameter if inflammation is chronic. Papillae are the conjunctiva's response to bacterial or allergic conjunctivitis. Giant papillae may be produced by the continuous irritation caused by a contact lens. Differentiation of a follicular response from a papil-

lary response is frequently difficult, and differentiating viral conjunctivitis from bacterial conjunctivitis without cultures is not always definite.

Bacterial conjunctivitis may be acute or chronic. Acute conjunctivitis is painful, with lid edema and keratitis. The bulbar conjunctiva swells (chemosis) and becomes hyperemic (injection). Corneal ulceration may occur as a complication. Children with viral conjunctivitis frequently develop secondary bacterial conjunctivitis. Acute bacterial conjunctivitis is usually due to staphylococcal, pneumococcal, or *Haemophilus* infections. Mucopurulent discharge is associated with tearing, and the eyelids may be stuck together on awakening (Fig. 19-55).

Chronic bacterial conjunctivitis results from bacterial toxins of *Staphylococcus aureus; Proteus* organisms; *Moraxella* organisms; or, in Third World countries, trachomata. A foreign body sensation may be experienced, and the eyes may be hyperemic with a chronic, mucopurulent or watery discharge. Papillary hyperplasia and thickening of the conjunctiva may also occur.

Viral conjunctivitis is usually caused by various strains of adenovirus (Fig. 19-56). Signs include copious tearing with a watery or thin mucopurulent discharge, conjunctival redness, and preauricular lymph node enlargement. Viral conjunctivitis is self-limited and usually resolves in 7 to 10 days depending on the viral strain. Viral conjunctivitis is highly contagious. Certain strains of adenoviral conjunctivitis may cause epidemic keratoconjunctivitis (EKC), which produces corneal involvement with a punctate keratitis that progresses to subepithelial infiltrates (Fig. 19-57) as an immunologic reaction. Patients are only contagious early in their course. Because of the corneal involvement, symptoms of photophobia are more pro-

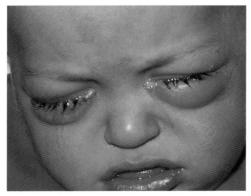

Figure 19-55. Acute bacterial conjunctivitis. Copious amounts of muco-purulent discharge have made the upper and lower eyelids adherent to each other. Chemosis of the upper and lower lids may also make opening of the eyelids difficult.

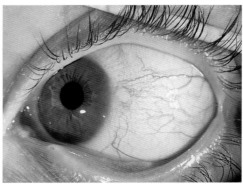

Figure 19-58. Conjunctival phlyctenule. A raised area of conjunctival infiltration and localized infection is commonly seen at the corneal-scleral limbus. The center of the lesion is clear or white and may ulcerate. Phlyctenules may also occur elsewhere on the bulbar or tarsal conjunctiva or on the cornea. (Courtesy Robert Arffa, MD, Pittsburgh, Pa.)

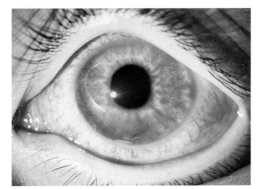

Figure 19-56. Viral conjunctivitis with hyperemia and a watery discharge.

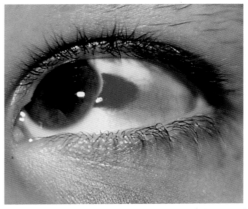

Figure 19-59. Subconjunctival hemorrhage secondary to blunt ocular trauma.

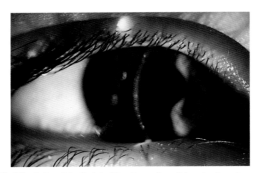

Figure 19-57. Subepithelial infiltrates of epidemic keratoconjunctivitis caused by adenovirus. The beam of the slit lamp is used to demonstrate corneal subepithelial infiltrates (small white opacities). Only severe adeno-viral keratoconjunctivitis produces subepithelial infiltrates. These may persist for months, causing symptoms of glare and blurring of vision.

nounced, and when subepithelial infiltrates are present patients complain of glare and decreased visual acuity. Symptoms in EKC may last from weeks to months. The infiltrates eventually resolve spontaneously. Steroids may alleviate symptoms; however, they prolong the overall course.

Allergic conjunctivitis occurs as a hypersensitivity response to dust, pollen, animal dander, or other airborne allergens. The eyes exhibit copious tearing, itching, and photophobia. The eyelids and palpebral conjunctiva are hyperemic and edematous (see Chapter 4). The development of extensive chemosis of the conjunctiva may be sudden and rapid. The conjunctiva may swell to protrude between the eyelids or obscure part of the cornea over the course of hours. A similar rapid development of chemosis

may occur with viral conjunctivitis. Simple treatment with cold compresses usually leads to improvement over several hours, and there are no significant sequelae. If the symptoms produced by allergic conjunctivitis are mild, no treatment is required because the child may object more to the use of the drops than to the discomfort of the disease. Allergic conjunctivitis may become chronic with repeated exposure to the allergen. In cases of chronic allergic conjunctivitis, the conjunctiva becomes pale and boggy and demonstrates a papillary reaction. Rare complications include keratitis and iritis.

Phlyctenular conjunctivitis is the result of a cell-mediated hypersensitivity reaction (Fig. 19-58). Phlyctenular lesions are small, pinkish-white vesicles or pustules in the center of hyperemic areas of the conjunctiva. These lesions may occur at the limbus; on the conjunctiva; or, more rarely, on the cornea. Phlyctenulosis most commonly occurs in association with chronic staphylococcal infection. Symptoms consist of itching, tearing, and irritation. A mucopurulent discharge may occur if secondary infection is present. Patients with corneal phlyctenulosis have more severe symptoms of pain, light sensitivity, and tearing.

Subconjunctival hemorrhages may occur spontaneously, or they may be secondary to trauma (Fig. 19-59). Such a hemorrhage presents as a striking bright red discoloration underneath the bulbar conjunctiva. The size and configuration of the hemorrhage depend on the amount and location of the blood between the conjunctiva and the globe. The size of the hemorrhage is not indicative of the

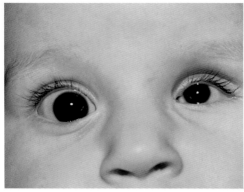

Figure 19-60. Unilateral microcornea and microphthalmos.

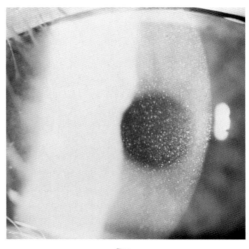

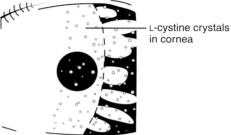

L-cystine crystals in cornea

Figure 19-62. Cystinosis of the cornea with deposition of L-cystine crystals in the corneal stroma.

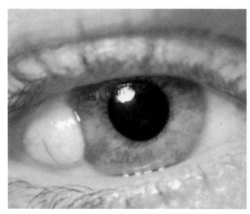

Figure 19-61. Corneal-limbal dermoid, often associated with Goldenhar syndrome.

severity of an injury, and the hemorrhage itself does not have any visual significance. Spontaneous resolution occurs over the course of several weeks.

Cornea

Developmental anomalies of the cornea include sclerocornea, Rieger syndrome, microcornea, and corneal dermoid.

Sclerocornea, present at birth, is a rare condition in which the cornea is white and resembles sclera. Rieger syndrome, a variant of anterior segment dysgenesis, is a dominant hereditary disorder that affects development of the anterior segment of the eye. Features include hyperplasia of the iris stroma, pupillary anomalies, anomalies of the trabecular meshwork, and early-onset glaucoma. Microcornea, whether an isolated anomaly or associated with glaucoma, cataracts, iris abnormalities, or anterior segment dysgenesis, is present when the corneal diameter is 9 mm or less (Fig. 19-60).

The developmental abnormalities mentioned necessitate further tests to exclude glaucoma. If the anterior segment of the eye is severely disorganized, the cornea is opaque, or glaucoma exists, surgical reconstruction and repair are indicated. The prognosis for vision is guarded for severe cases.

Corneal dermoids occur at the limbus (junction between the cornea and sclera); grow slowly, if at all; and may encroach on the visual axis or cause high degrees of astigmatism (Fig. 19-61). They are composed of fibrolipid tissue containing hair follicles and sebaceous glands. Corneal dermoids may occur as isolated anomalies or they may

be associated with syndromes such as Goldenhar syndrome.

The cornea is also involved in many systemic diseases. Hurler syndrome, a mucopolysaccharidosis, produces clouding of the cornea. The cornea, clear at birth, develops an opacification by 2 to 3 years of age. Pigmentary retinopathy and optic atrophy coexist.

Cystinosis, seen in the early months of life, involves the deposition of L-cystine in the cornea. This may be seen as a subtle haze of the cornea. Slit lamp examination is necessary to clearly visualize the corneal deposits (Fig. 19-62).

Corneal inflammations are associated with bacterial, viral, mycotic, and allergic diseases. Infectious corneal ulcers usually occur only in the setting of some compromise of the corneal epithelium (e.g., with traumatic corneal abrasion; foreign bodies; exposure keratitis; or contact lens wear, especially sleeping with lenses in place). In the abusive contact lens patient a corneal ulcer may be sterile and caused by the improper use of the lenses. Infectious corneal ulcers are caused by the invasion of bacterial organisms into the corneal stroma (Fig. 19-63). If the visual axis is involved, scar formation may affect visual acuity. If corneal perforation occurs, a loss of the eye may occur. Bacteria commonly involved include staphylococci, pneumococci, *Moraxella* organisms, *Pseudomonas aeruginosa*, *Escherichia coli*, and *Klebsiella pneumoniae*. Acanthamoeba and Fusarium infectious corneal ulcers in contact lens patients have been recognized and frequently lead to severe vision loss and the need for corneal transplantation. Appropriate smears and cultures are obtained, and treatment is started as soon as the diagnosis is suspected.

Herpes simplex may be transmitted from active herpes in the maternal birth canal, or it may result from direct contact with infected individuals. Primary herpes is a unilateral lesion that occurs as a blepharoconjunctivitis or

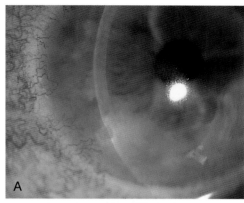

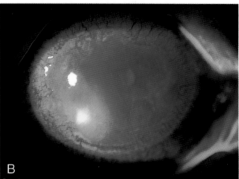

Figure 19-63. Bacterial corneal ulcer. **A,** The conjunctiva displays a marked inflammatory response with injection, most prominent in the quadrant nearest the corneal ulcer. The ulcer is visualized in the slit beam as a small white infiltrate of the corneal stroma. There is an overlying epithelial defect. **B,** The epithelial defect is easier to visualize after the application of fluorescein dye. The dye is taken up by the corneal stroma in the area of the epithelial defect. The areas fluoresce with cobalt blue light illumination.

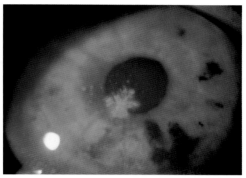

Figure 19-64. Herpes simplex keratitis. Infection of the corneal epithelium with herpes simplex virus produces a pattern of fluorescein staining that resembles a neuronal dendrite. The surrounding area may be hazy because of epithelial and stromal edema and infiltration. Conjunctival infection is typically present.

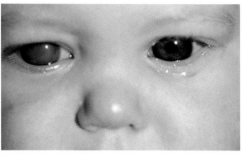

Figure 19-65. Congenital glaucoma. The right cornea is hazy and opaque resulting from corneal edema. Breakdown of the corneal epithelium has caused ocular irritation, and the conjunctiva is slightly infected. Epiphora is present because of reflex tearing caused by the pain of epithelial breakdown and increased intraocular pressure.

as vesicular lesions of the eyelids with regional lymphadenopathy. A few weeks after infection, half of all patients develop a punctate or typical dendritic keratitis (Fig. 19-64). This is best seen using fluorescein stain and a cobalt blue filter over a penlight.

Recurrent herpes keratitis occurs in 25% of infected individuals. The lesions may have a typical appearance of branching dendrites. Recurrences may be complicated by stromal keratitis, keratouveitis, and anesthesia of the cornea. Stromal disease is a serious complication that reduces visual recovery because of corneal vascularization and scarring. Patients with a history of herpes keratitis must be evaluated by an ophthalmologist for any episode of conjunctivitis.

Anterior Chamber

The term *anterior chamber* refers to the fluid-filled space between the cornea and the iris diaphragm. The aqueous fluid is optically clear, and it provides nutrition for the corneal endothelial surface. The aqueous fluid is secreted by the ciliary processes, reaches the anterior chamber by passing through the pupillary space, and leaves via the trabecular meshwork in the periphery of the anterior chamber angle.

Glaucoma

The incidence of infantile or congenital glaucoma is approximately 1 in 12,500 births. The inheritance of congenital glaucoma is multifactorial; parents of an affected child have a 5% chance of having another child with

glaucoma, and an affected parent has a 5% chance of having an affected child. Two thirds of all patients are male. Glaucoma can present at birth, but more commonly, clinical signs develop during the first several weeks or months of life. An embryonic defect in the development of the trabecular meshwork or filtration area of the eye has been hypothesized as the cause.

Infants with glaucoma have corneal edema, which gives the cornea a hazy or cloudy appearance. Corneal edema may produce an irregular corneal light reflex or dull the red reflex. Initially, the edema may be limited to the epithelium, but stromal edema may follow (Fig. 19-65). As this increases, Descemet membrane may rupture and produce Haab striae (Fig. 19-66).

A break in Descemet membrane may produce a corneal opacity, or, if edema is not present, it may be visualized against the red reflex when viewed with a slit lamp or direct ophthalmoscope. Breaks in Descemet membrane can produce irregular astigmatism. Glare from the scatter of light produced by the epithelial and stromal edema is responsible for photophobia and blinking. Breakdown of the corneal epithelium may produce pain, squinting, and blepharospasm.

In children younger than 2 years of age, an increase in corneal diameter frequently accompanies increased intraocular pressure (Fig. 19-67). An infant's horizontal corneal diameter is normally 9.5 mm; this increases over the first 2 years of life to a normal corneal diameter of 11.5 mm. Small increases in corneal diameter may be recognized first as asymmetries in the corneal diameter between the two eyes. In addition to enlargement of the corneal diameter, chronic elevated intraocular pressure may also enlarge

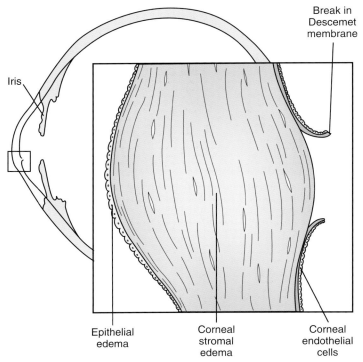

Figure 19-66. Haab striae (break in Descemet membrane).

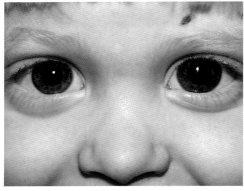

Figure 19-67. Congenital glaucoma. This patient has corneal asymmetry resulting from glaucoma in the left eye. The horizontal corneal diameter is 11 mm in the right eye and 13.5 mm in the left eye. The entire left eye has become enlarged, and the axial length is greater than normal. The increase in axial length of the left eye has produced a myopic refractive error.

the entire eye. This produces an increase in axial length and a myopic refractive error. A rapid increase in myopia may be a sign of glaucoma. The anterior chamber in infancy is shallow when compared with that of older children. An anterior chamber that is deeper than normal is a sign of congenital glaucoma.

Epiphora, or tearing, is a sign of glaucoma and is differentiated from nasolacrimal duct obstruction by the presence of rhinorrhea. When the nasolacrimal duct is obstructed, rhinorrhea is absent.

The optic nerve damage caused by elevated intraocular pressure is reflected in the degree of enlargement of the optic cup (Fig. 19-68). Asymmetry of the cup-to-disc ratio between the eyes or an increase in the cup-to-disc ratio to greater than 0.5 is a possible sign of glaucoma. In infants and young children the intraocular pressure may be elevated for a prolonged period of time before optic disc cupping occurs. Enlargement of the optic cup is reversible to an extent in infants and young children but is usually permanent in adults. Enlargement of the optic

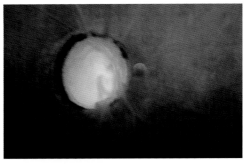

Figure 19-68. Glaucomatous optic atrophy. In glaucoma, excavation extends to the disc edge in contrast to the cupped disc seen in myopia where a normal rim of tissue exists. Retinal vessels emerge from under the disc edge.

cups without glaucoma may be inherited; examination of family members may be of value.

Elevation of intraocular pressure (IOP) is the hallmark of congenital glaucoma. Normal IOP in infants and young children is less than 20 mm Hg. Pressures greater than 25 mm Hg strongly suggest glaucoma.

Precise measurement of pressure is difficult in children. An estimate of the IOP may be obtained by palpating the globes with the fingertips over closed eyelids. More precise measurements are obtained with instruments that require anesthetizing and coming in contact with the cornea. These procedures and decisions regarding the management of IOP may require an examination that is conducted with sedation or under general anesthesia. Unfortunately, some anesthetic agents alter IOP.

Glaucoma may occur with congenital ocular malformations such as aniridia or mesodermal (iridocorneal) dysgenesis, in systemic syndromes, or after trauma. Sturge-Weber syndrome, neurofibromatosis, Lowe syndrome, Rubinstein-Taybi syndrome, and congenital rubella syndrome are associated with congenital glaucoma. Patients with chronic uveitis frequently develop glaucoma, and 8% to 25% of children with congenital cataracts, especially those with microcornea or microphthalmia, develop glaucoma at some point in life.

Iris

A coloboma results from failed fusion of the embryonic fissure of the optic cup (Fig. 19-69). The defect is usually inferior and nasal in location, and it may involve any ocular structure, most commonly the iris.

Colobomas occur either as isolated defects or in association with systemic syndromes. Iris colobomas occur in the CHARGE association, cat-eye syndrome, Rieger syndrome, and the facioauriculovertebral anomalies. Isolated colobomas may be inherited as a dominant trait.

Aniridia, an apparent absence of the iris, is caused by failure of the mesoderm to grow outward from the iris root during the fourth month of gestation. The pupil appears the same size as the cornea, and iris structures are present as only rudimentary findings (Fig. 19-70). A fibrovascular membrane can form between the rudimentary iris and the trabecular meshwork and cause glaucoma. Hypoplasia of the macula occurs in patients with aniridia, and visual acuity may be decreased to the 20/400 level. Associated defects include corneal opacities, lens dislocations, and cataracts. Affected patients have photophobia and nystagmus.

An autosomal dominant inheritance pattern is present in two thirds of all patients with aniridia. An estimated 1

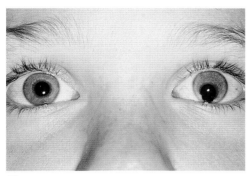

Figure 19-69. Typical unilateral iris coloboma in an otherwise normal left eye.

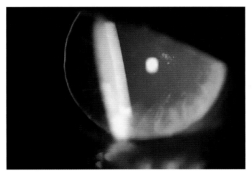

Figure 19-70. Aniridia. Iris structures are present only as rudimentary findings, and the red reflex fills the entire corneal diameter. The edge of the lens is visible peripherally, and early cataractous lens changes are present centrally.

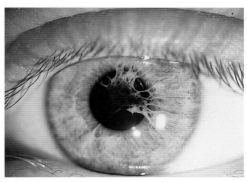

Figure 19-71. Persistent pupillary membranes. Hyperplasia of the mesoderm of the anterior layer of the iris has caused iris strands to become adherent to the anterior lens surface. The lens is clear, and these are visually insignificant.

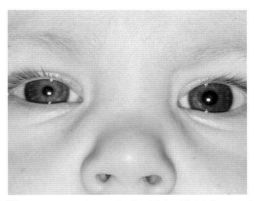

Figure 19-72. Horner syndrome (right side) with iris heterochromia. The right upper lid is slightly ptotic, and the right lower lid is slightly higher than its mate. Anisocoria is present. The right pupil is smaller than the left. The iris on the side affected by Horner syndrome is lighter in color than the iris of the fellow eye.

to 70 patients with sporadic aniridia will have Wilms tumor, and 90% of these will occur before age 3. Other genitourinary defects and mental retardation may occur, and many of these patients have chromosomal abnormalities (11p-).

Persistent pupillary membranes are caused by hyperplasia of the mesoderm of the anterior layer of the iris and are a frequent finding in children born prematurely (Fig. 19-71). Instead of terminating at the pupillary margin, iris strands with accompanying blood vessels encroach on the pupillary space or adhere to the anterior lens surface. They are rarely visually significant and, especially in the premature infant, the iris strands frequently spontaneously release from the lens surface with pupil dilation.

Heterochromia iridis, or asymmetry in the color of the iris, if isolated, is visually insignificant. Heterochromia may occur in congenital Horner syndrome, the eye with Horner syndrome being lighter in color. Heterochromia may also occur secondary to inflammation or after intraocular surgery or ocular trauma. Trauma may cause the affected iris to become darker than the fellow iris as late as many years after the incident (Fig. 19-72).

The iris may provide signs that aid in the diagnosis of systemic conditions. Patients with neurofibromatosis may have multiple small melanocytic iris nevi, called Lisch nodules, on the surface of the iris (see Chapter 15). These may be identified with magnification provided by the direct ophthalmoscope or by slit lamp examination. Other ocular findings associated with neurofibromatosis include plexiform neurofibromas of the lids, thickened corneal nerves, congenital glaucoma, and optic nerve gliomas producing optic atrophy.

In chronic anterior uveitis or iritis, for example, in association with sarcoidosis or juvenile rheumatoid arthritis, the iris may be affected by adhesions between the papil-

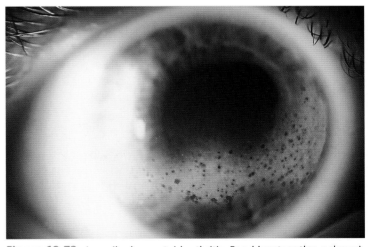

Figure 19-73. Juvenile rheumatoid arthritis. Band keratopathy, a deposition of calcium, is seen as white scalelike deposits present on the anterior corneal surface. The pupil is not round due to the presence of posterior synechiae and adhesions between the iris and lens; a cataract is present.

lary border and the lens (posterior synechiae) or between the peripheral iris and the cornea (anterior synechiae). Posterior synechiae cause the pupil to be less reactive in the area of the synechiae and cause the pupil to lose its round shape (corectopia) (Fig. 19-73).

Patients with juvenile xanthogranuloma, usually younger than 1 year of age, may develop unilateral asymptomatic fleshy, yellowish-brown tumors on the surface of

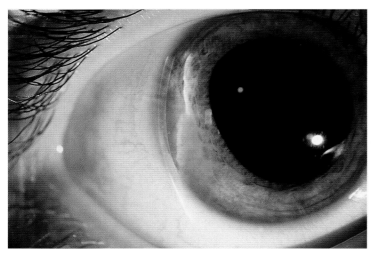

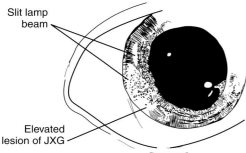

Figure 19-74. Juvenile xanthogranuloma (JXG). The ocular lesion of JXG is visualized as a fleshy, yellowish-brown tumor on the surface of the iris. The lesions are vascular, bleed easily, and can cause spontaneous hyphemas.

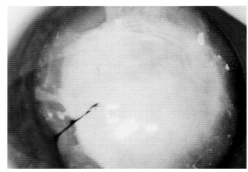

Figure 19-75. Total cataract with no view of the red reflex or retina.

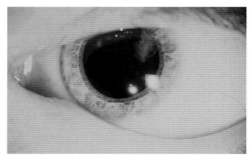

Figure 19-76. Spokelike cortical cataract of Down syndrome. The lens opacification does not affect the visual axis and is visually insignificant. Lens opacification such as this may rapidly progress and produce visual loss, or it may remain unchanged for years.

Table 19-1	Differential Diagnosis of Leukocoria
Angiomatosis retinae	Persistent hyperplastic primary vitreous
Cataracts	Retinal detachment
Coats disease	Retinal dysplasia
Colobomas	Retinoblastoma
Congenital retinal fold	Retinopathy of prematurity
High myopia	Toxocariasis
Incontinentia pigmenti	Uveitis
Medulloepithelioma	Vitreous hemorrhage
Myelinated nerve fibers	

the iris (Fig. 19-74). These vascular lesions bleed easily and may produce a spontaneous hyphema.

Brushfield spots are found in patients with Down syndrome. The spots consist of tiny areas of normal iris stroma that are surrounded by rings of mild iris hypoplasia. Brushfield spots give the iris a speckled appearance.

Lens

The lens may be affected by developmental, hereditary, syndrome-related, inflammatory, metabolic, or traumatic conditions. This can result in the development of a cataract, an opacification of the crystalline lens that may be either partial or complete. The lens may also be dislocated from its supporting zonulae or subluxated.

Cataracts

Leukocoria refers to the white pupillary reflex produced by reflection of light from a light-colored intraocular mass or structure. Many conditions of variable severity and prognosis produce leukocoria (Table 19-1). Examination

with a penlight, the plus lens of a direct ophthalmoscope, or slit lamp biomicroscopy helps to differentiate lens opacification (cataract) from other forms of leukocoria.

Congenital or infantile cataracts may be unilateral or bilateral, and the extent of opacification may be complete or partial (Fig. 19-75). Bilateral cataracts usually arise early in infancy and, if not treated early, may produce severe visual deprivation accompanied by poor fixation and nystagmus. Visually significant unilateral cataracts are associated with severe deprivation amblyopia and strabismus. Early referral for treatment prompted by detection of abnormalities of the red reflex is critical for successful visual rehabilitation. Although visually significant bilateral cataracts have gross signs of poor visual reflex development, monocular cataracts may not have grossly visible signs for many months or years until the cataract is obvious or a sensory strabismus develops.

Opacification of a child's lens may be due to heredity (autosomal dominant), chromosomal disorders (trisomy 13, 18, and 21) (Fig. 19-76), inflammation (iritis and uveitis), infection (TORCH), metabolic disorders (galactosemia and disorders of calcium and phosphorus metabolism), exposure to toxins, vitamin deficiencies (vitamins A and D), systemic syndromes with cataracts (Table 19-2), ocular conditions producing retinal detachment, radiation exposure, and trauma. Roughly one third of pediatric cataracts are hereditary, one third are syndrome or disease related, and one third are attributed to other or undetermined causes.

The presence of ocular anomalies frequently identifies a developmental defect as being the cause for the cataract. Microphthalmia, the globe being smaller than normal, may be caused by ocular disease or inflammation, or it may be present as a developmental defect (see Fig. 19-60). Eyes with persistent hyperplastic primary vitreous (PHPV) are usually microphthalmic, sometimes only mildly so, and frequently have visually significant cata-

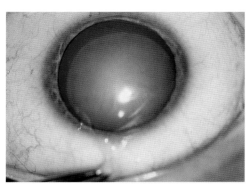

Figure 19-77. A microspherophakic cataractous lens in rubella syndrome.

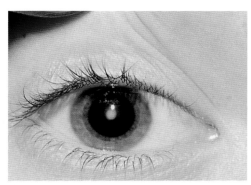

Figure 19-78. Anterior polar cataract. This type of lens opacity is a developmental abnormality that in most cases remains stable and rarely affects vision.

Table 19-2	Syndromes Associated with Cataracts

Albright hereditary osteodystrophy
Alport syndrome
Cat-eye syndrome
Cerebro-oculo-facial-skeletal syndrome
Chondrodysplasia punctata (Conradi-Hünermann syndrome)
Cockayne syndrome
Congenital ichthyosis
Conradi syndrome
Craniofacial syndromes (Apert and Crouzon syndromes)
Down syndrome (trisomy 21)
Edward syndrome (trisomy 18)
Hallgren syndrome
Hallermann-Streiff syndrome
Ichthyosis
Incontinentia pigmenti
Kniest syndrome
Lanzieri syndrome
Laurence-Moon-Bardet-Biedl syndrome
Lowe syndrome
Marinesco-Sjögren syndrome
Marshall syndrome
Myotonic dystrophy
Osteogenesis imperfecta
Patau syndrome (trisomy 13)
Progeria
Roberts syndrome
Rothman-Thomson syndrome
Rubinstein-Taybi syndrome
Smith-Lemli-Opitz syndrome
Stickler syndrome
Turner syndrome
Zellweger syndrome

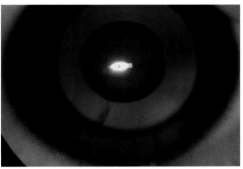

Figure 19-79. Lamellar cataract with riders, surrounded by a clear cortex.

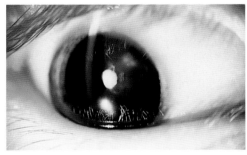

Figure 19-80. Cataract of galactosemia. Early lens changes cause the nucleus of the lens to have an "oil droplet" configuration resulting from the accumulation of dulcitol, a metabolic product of galactose, within the lens. The resultant osmotic gradient draws water into the lens, producing the opacification. Early lens changes in galactosemia are reversible.

racts, as well as vision-limiting retinal or optic nerve abnormalities.

The morphology of the lens opacification may provide a clue to the cause of a congenital cataract if opacification is not complete. During development, the lens cells lay down fibers that grow out from the peripheral lens to the anterior and posterior lens surfaces. These form sutures. Because of this, the gestational age at the time of cataract development determines the location of the opacity. For example, the nuclear cataracts of rubella syndrome (Fig. 19-77) indicate infection early in gestation, whereas a zonular or lamellar cataract represents an insult to the lens occurring later in lens development.

Small central opacities on the anterior or posterior poles of the lens, termed *polar cataracts,* are developmental abnormalities that remain stable and rarely affect vision (Fig. 19-78). Lamellar or zonular cataracts have a normal, transparent central nucleus; an affected lamellar zone; and a clear outer layer of cortex. Riders or radial extensions are frequently present (Fig. 19-79). Zonular cataracts may be autosomal dominant, associated with vitamin A

and D deficiency, or follow hypocalcemia. Multicolored flecks may be seen in hypoparathyroidism or myotonic dystrophy, and an oil droplet configuration is seen in galactosemia (Fig. 19-80).

If a child has no history of trauma, the family history is unremarkable, the general physical examination fails to uncover a systemic syndrome or chromosomal abnormality, and ocular examination does not help to determine the cause of a cataract, then a focused laboratory evaluation to determine the cause of the cataract may be undertaken. The most common metabolic disorders causing congenital cataracts are hypoglycemia and hypocalcemia. Laboratory evaluation for galactosemia and galactokinase deficiency should include blood tests for galactose and galactose-1-phosphate, as well as examination of the urine for reducing substances. Examination of the urine for protein and amino acids identifies patients with Lowe (oculocerebrorenal) syndrome, and a urine nitroprusside

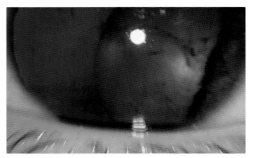

Figure 19-81. A traumatic, dislocated cataractous lens.

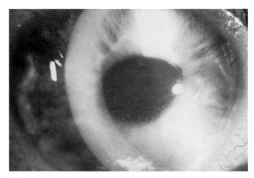

Figure 19-82. Iritis with circumcorneal ciliary flush.

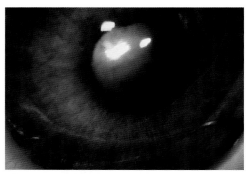

Figure 19-83. Yellow cyclitic membrane behind a clear lens in a soft phthisic eye.

test diagnoses homocystinuria. Screening tests for congenital TORCH infections and syphilis should also be performed.

Positional abnormalities of the lens may occur. A partial dislocation of the lens is referred to as *subluxation.* A dislocated lens, called *ectopia lentis,* may cause a profound decrease in vision by producing a large refractive error and amblyopia. Ectopia lentis may be unilateral, bilateral, inherited or sporadic, or it may be due to trauma (Fig. 19-81).

Simple ectopia lentis is a bilateral, symmetrical condition with an autosomal dominant inheritance pattern. Bilateral superotemporal lens dislocation is present in 50% to 80% of patients with Marfan syndrome. Ninety percent of patients with homocystinuria have an inferior lens dislocation, and patients with Weill-Marchesani syndrome may have dislocation of their microspherophakic lenses.

Uvea

Inflammation of the uveal tract (iris, ciliary body, and choroid) has many potential causes including infections (toxoplasmosis, herpes zoster and simplex, and Lyme disease); collagen vascular disease (most frequently juvenile rheumatoid arthritis and sarcoidosis); and trauma. In the majority of children the etiologic agent cannot be determined. Advanced retinoblastoma may also present with signs that suggest uveitis.

Involvement of the iris alone (iritis or anterior uveitis) produces pain, ciliary injection (conjunctival redness in the circumlimbal area), tearing, photophobia, and decreased vision. Synechiae, adhesions between the iris and lens or peripheral cornea, may produce corectopia, an abnormally shaped pupil. Inflammatory reaction in the anterior chamber may be viewed with the aid of a slit lamp as inflammatory cells and fibrin or protein (flare) in the aqueous fluid. With the high magnification of the slit lamp, inflammatory cells may be seen floating in the aqueous fluid much like dust is seen in bright sunlight shining through a window. If marked, this may give the eye a dull or glassy appearance (Fig. 19-82). Clumps of inflammatory cells may adhere to the posterior corneal surface, forming keratic precipitates (KPs). Inflammatory nodules may also be seen on the surface of the iris or at the border (Busacca and Koeppe nodules) in chronic uveitis.

Because iritis may be present without signs and symptoms, children with juvenile rheumatoid arthritis should have periodic screening ophthalmic examinations. Children with polyarticular disease should be examined annually, and those with positive antinuclear antibodies and pauciarticular disease, who are more likely to develop ocular complications, should be examined three to four times a year to detect and treat the uveitis before complications of cataracts, glaucoma, and macular edema develop (see Chapter 7).

Pars planitis, or intermediate uveitis, is an idiopathic, bilateral inflammation of the pars plana or pars ciliaris portions of the ciliary body. Symptoms include light sensitivity, "floaters," and blurring of vision. Inflammatory cells in the anterior vitreous can make visualization of the retina with the direct ophthalmoscope difficult. If the inflammation is severe, it may produce leukocoria. No laboratory findings are available in pars planitis, and the diagnosis is made on the basis of characteristic findings and by exclusion. Most cases are self-limited; however, chronic courses with exacerbations and remissions may produce visual loss resulting from cataracts, glaucoma, optic nerve inflammation, and cystoid macular edema. Retinal detachment because of membrane formation and phthisis bulbi may occur in advanced cases (Fig. 19-83).

Posterior uveitis (inflammation of the posterior vitreous, retina, and/or choroid) can be caused by infection, but frequently the precise cause is undetermined. Infection of the retina by protozoa, fungi, and viruses may produce an intense inflammatory response in the vitreous, rendering it hazy or opaque. Leukocoria may be produced if the vitreous is cloudy or if extensive retinal involvement is present.

Vitreous

Vitreous Hemorrhage

Trauma, be it penetrating, concussive, or the result of shaken baby syndrome, is the most common cause of vitreous hemorrhage. Vitreous hemorrhage may occur with hemorrhagic disease of the newborn (hypoprothrombinemia), thrombocytopenia, or in advanced stages of retinopathy of prematurity. Patients with a subarachnoid

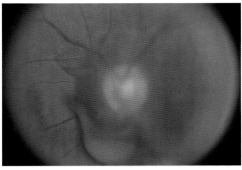

Figure 19-84. Vitreous hemorrhage. Dispersed red blood cells in the vitreous have made it hazy. The diffraction of light causes blurred vision. Fluid levels are often visible, and collections of blood may appear to float within the eye.

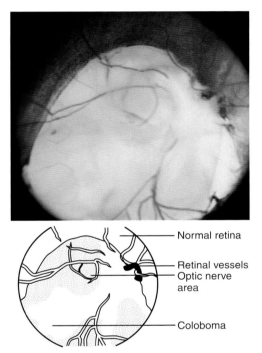

— Normal retina

— Retinal vessels
Optic nerve
area

— Coloboma

Figure 19-85. Coloboma of optic nerve, retina, and choroid. Yellowish-white sclera is visible, and retinal vessels can be seen coursing through the coloboma.

hemorrhage may develop vitreous hemorrhage (Terson syndrome), and vitreous hemorrhage may also occur in patients with leukemia.

Blood in the vitreous, if located centrally or posteriorly, may be visible with the direct ophthalmoscope. If the vitreous is liquid, the hemorrhage may appear to float inside the eye (Fig. 19-84). Blood in the vitreous may produce leukocoria as it organizes and becomes yellow and then gray in color. Vitreous hemorrhages may resolve simultaneously or, if extensive, require surgery.

Retina

Developmental Abnormalities

Colobomas. Retinal colobomas are caused by a defect in closure of the embryonal fissure of the optic cup. They may occur unilaterally or bilaterally. Large colobomas are manifest as an absence of the retina and choroid with or without marked excavation of the optic disc (Fig. 19-85). A ring of pigment usually exists around the coloboma. Leukocoria may be produced by the yellowish-white reflec-

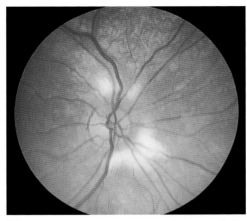

Figure 19-86. Myelinated nerve fibers. Myelination of the optic nerve fibers may continue beyond the optic disc to include the retinal nerve fibers. This is visible as yellowish-white, flame-shaped patches oriented with the retinal nerve fibers. Myelinated nerve fibers may produce the clinical sign of leukocoria.

tion of the underlying sclera, and the red reflex may be seen as flashing from red to white as the eye moves to produce a reflex from normal areas of retina to the area of the coloboma. Using a direct ophthalmoscope, an occasional vessel may be seen bridging the area of the coloboma. The coloboma and retina are at a different plane of focus when visualized with the ophthalmoscope.

Colobomas may occur in otherwise normal eyes or in association with microphthalmia or retinal detachment. If the optic disc and macula are not involved, central visual acuity may be normal. In these eyes there is a peripheral visual field defect corresponding to the area of retinal involvement. Usually the patient is asymptomatic if the optic disc and macula are not involved. Colobomas may be inherited as isolated anomalies, or they may be associated with chromosomal defects (trisomy 13) or other syndrome-related entities (CHARGE association).

Myelinated Nerve Fibers. Before birth, myelination of the optic nerve begins in the central nervous system, progresses peripherally, and usually stops at the optic disc before birth. Myelination may continue beyond the optic disc to include the retinal nerve fiber layer as a relatively benign, isolated, congenital abnormality. Once present, the changes are permanent; however, there is no progression or worsening of the condition. Myelinated fibers are oriented with the retinal nerve fibers and are easily seen with the direct ophthalmoscope as yellowish-white, flame-shaped patches overlying the sensory retina and choroid (Fig. 19-86). The macula is rarely involved, and normal vision is usually present, although scotomas corresponding to the areas of myelination may be found on visual field examination.

Persistent Hyperplastic Primary Vitreous. PHPV occurs as a unilateral defect in the involution of the primary vitreous during the seventh month of gestation. No systemic associations exist. Eyes with PHPV are usually microphthalmic. PHPV may be associated with cataracts, intraocular hemorrhage, glaucoma, and retinal detachment. Many eyes with mild changes of PHPV may have good visual acuity following cataract surgery and visual rehabilitation; however, retinal or optic nerve abnormalities, if present, may limit vision. These rehabilitated eyes remain at risk for the development of glaucoma later in life. Eyes with advanced PHPV can become phthisical (Figs. 19-87 and 19-88).

Albinism. *Albinism* refers to conditions involving deficiencies of melanin in the skin or eye (Fig. 19-89). The

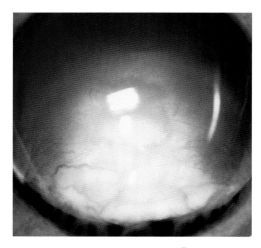

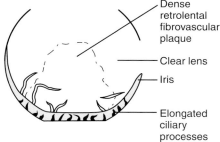

Dense
retrolental
fibrovascular
plaque

Clear lens

Iris

Elongated
ciliary
processes

Figure 19-87. Persistent hyperplastic primary vitreous presenting as a dense fibrovascular retrolental mass with microspherophakia, microphthalmia, and elongated ciliary processes.

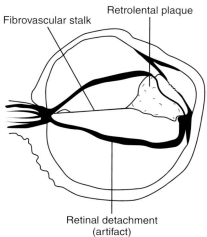

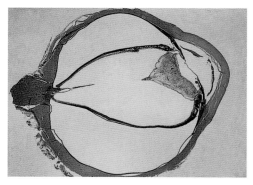

Retrolental plaque

Fibrovascular stalk

Retinal detachment
(artifact)

Figure 19-88. Pathologic section of persistent hypoplastic primary vitreous. (Courtesy B. L. Johnson, MD, Pittsburgh, Pa.)

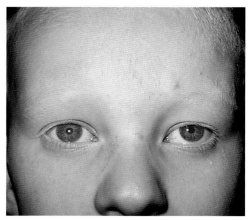

Figure 19-89. Albinism, characterized by white hair, pale skin, and translucent irides.

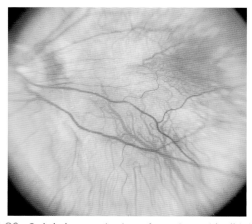

Figure 19-90. Ophthalmoscopic view of a patient with albinism demonstrates a pale fundus, poor macular development, and prominent choroidal vasculature.

loss of pigmentation may predominantly affect the eye (ocular albinism), be generalized to the skin and eye (oculocutaneous albinism), or occur in conjunction with a systemic syndrome such as Chédiak-Higashi or Hermansky-Pudlak syndrome.

Ocular albinism occurs as an X-linked or autosomal recessive trait. Photophobia is frequently a symptom. The loss of cutaneous pigmentation may be mild. Patients have iris transillumination defects in which the red reflex is seen through multiple punctate defects in the iris. Absence of pigment in the retinal pigment epithelium layer of the retina makes the fundus appear a lighter yellowish-orange color than usual. The choroidal vasculature, usually hidden by the retinal pigment epithelium, is visible. The macula and fovea are hypoplastic, and visual acuity is decreased to a degree dependent on the absence of pigment and development of the macula and fovea. The visual acuity may be only mildly affected or, in patients with marked nystagmus, the vision may be severely limited (Fig. 19-90). Ocular albinism is a frequent cause of sensory nystagmus in infancy.

Ocular pigmentary abnormalities may also occur in a milder form, albinoidism. Such patients have iris transillumination defects, fundus hypopigmentation, and photophobia. Their maculae, however, are less severely affected or are normal. Because of this, nystagmus is uncommon and visual acuity is normal or only minimally reduced. Albinoidism is inherited as an autosomal dominant trait with incomplete penetrance.

Coats Disease (Retinal Telangiectasis). Coats disease occurs unilaterally in boys younger than 18 years of age. The most common age at diagnosis is between 8 and 10 years. Peripheral retinal vessel telangiectasis and aneurysmal dilation lead to extensive areas of exudation, giving the retina a yellowish-white appearance, which may produce leukocoria (Fig. 19-91). The macula is a common site for exudate to collect, and when this is present, visual loss is profound. Treatment is with cryotherapy or laser photocoagulation of the retina; success depends on the degree of macular damage present.

Retinitis Pigmentosa. Retinitis pigmentosa (RP) is a pigmentary retinopathy characterized by visual field loss, night blindness, and a depressed or extinct electroretinogram. Symptoms of visual loss may be present in childhood but usually do not become apparent until the second or third decade of life. Poor night vision is the earliest symptom, followed by progressive loss of peripheral visual field and, finally, loss of central vision. Many different diseases are characterized by pigmentary retinopathy, and the presentation, progression, and extent of visual loss vary widely. In general, disease within pedigrees has similar clinical characteristics. Unfortunately, treatment for the overwhelming majority of patients is not available at this time.

The retinal pigment epithelial changes include deposition of pigment in a perivascular pattern. Pigment deposition in the midperipheral retina gives a characteristic "bone spicule" pattern late in the course of the disease

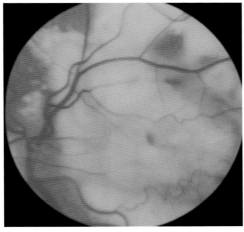

Figure 19-91. Ophthalmoscopic manifestations of Coats disease. Peripheral telangiectasis along the course of the retinal veins leads to exudation, giving the retina a yellowish-white appearance.

(Fig. 19-92A). Early in the disease, the optic nerve may have a waxy pallor and the retinal arteries may be attenuated (see Fig. 19-92B).

Systemic disease entities are associated with RP. Patients with sensorineural hearing loss should be examined for the associated presence of retinitis pigmentosa (Usher syndrome and Hallgren syndrome). Renal diseases including Fanconi syndrome, cystinuria, cystinosis, and oxalosis may be associated with pigmentary retinal changes, as may the mucopolysaccharidoses, Refsum disease, and syphilis.

Retinal Detachment

Trauma is the most common cause of retinal detachment in children. Leukocoria occurs when the detached retina is in apposition to the lens. Retinal detachments, if large and located posteriorly, may be viewed with the direct ophthalmoscope as elevations of the retina (Fig. 19-93). The detached retina may move or undulate with eye movement. Symptoms of retinal detachment, which all patients with a history of blunt trauma to the eye should be advised of, include photopsia (flashing lights), floaters (potentially caused by vitreous hemorrhage), or changes in vision including blurring of vision or the sensation of a veil or curtain obscuring part of their vision.

Retinopathy of Prematurity

Retinopathy of prematurity (ROP) is characterized by abnormalities in the developing retinal vascular system. Mild forms affect the peripheral retina at the junction between the vascularized and immature avascular retina. These changes can be observed only with an indirect ophthalmoscope and scleral depression. Severe forms produce fibrovascular proliferations that extend into the vitreous (stage 3 disease), which may lead to traction resulting in poor macular development (temporal macular drag) or detachment of the retina (stage 4 and 5 disease) (Fig. 19-94). A white fibrovascular mass may occupy the retrolental space (retrolental fibroplasia) and produce leukocoria.

In 75% of patients, ROP is bilateral and symmetrical. The majority of patients have only mild forms of the disease (stages 1 and 2 disease), and these patients do not have significant visual sequelae. Advanced ROP primarily affects the ill, premature infant whose birthweight is less than 1250 g. Treatment with laser photocoagulation to reduce the progression of the disease and the risk of visual loss is indicated when advanced disease is present and programs to screen neonates at risk for developing this condition are necessary.

Figure 19-92. **A,** Retinitis pigmentosa, characterized by retinal pigment disposition, narrow arterioles, and a pale disc. **B,** Early fundus signs of retinitis pigmentosa. The optic disc has a waxy pallor, and the retinal arterial system is sclerotic. In children, pigmentary changes may not be as advanced or as noticeable as in adults.

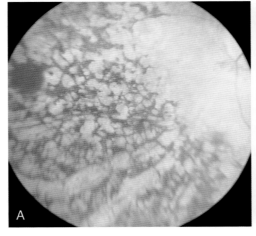
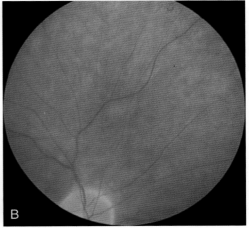

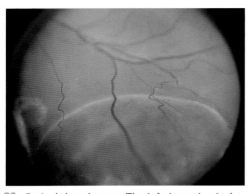

Figure 19-93. Retinal detachment. The inferior retina is detached, and a demarcation line between the attached and detached retina is visible. Fluid beneath the detached sensory retina shifts with movement of the eye and causes the detached retina to move or undulate.

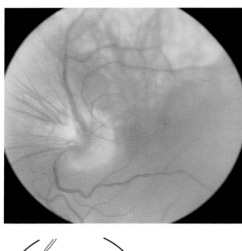

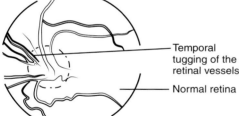

Temporal tugging of the retinal vessels

Normal retina

Figure 19-94. Retrolental fibroplasia with temporal tugging of the disc.

Retinitis and Retinochoroiditis

Inflammation of the retina and choroid is most commonly the result of viral, protozoal, fungal, or bacterial infection. The final common pathway for recovery or resolution of retinal inflammation is the production of a pigmented chorioretinal scar. The characteristics and location of these scars are frequently diagnostic for the infecting agent. In many cases, however, isolated chorioretinal scars do not suggest any particular disease.

A rare cause of retinochoroiditis is sympathetic ophthalmia. Sympathetic ophthalmia occurs after a severe injury of one eye, the "exciting" eye, followed by a latent period and the development of uveitis in the uninjured eye, the "sympathizing" eye. Sympathetic ophthalmia may occur as early as 10 days after the original injury but may also have a delayed onset years after the incident. Sympathetic ophthalmia is an autoimmune disorder, and treatment is with immunosuppression, both topically and systemically.

TORCH Infection
Toxoplasmosis. Toxoplasmosis, a protozoal infection, causes disease in several forms, depending on whether the

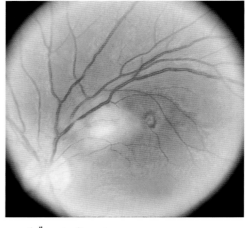

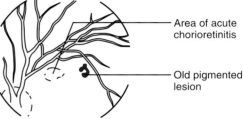

Area of acute chorioretinitis

Old pigmented lesion

Figure 19-95. Acute, recurrent, toxoplasmic chorioretinal inflammation adjacent to a healed pigmented lesion.

infection is congenital and when it is acquired during pregnancy, or acquired. Infants congenitally infected may have widespread involvement resulting in fetal death if maternal infection is in the first or early in the second trimester. If infection occurs in the third trimester effects may include chorioretinitis and encephalomyelitis but a viable pregnancy. Of neonates severely affected by toxoplasmosis, 80% have retinochoroiditis. Congenital disease may also occur in inactive and recurrent forms whose effects may be limited to retinitis alone. Toxoplasmosis may also be acquired, the incidence worldwide being extremely high with increasing age. Ocular involvement includes papillitis, retinitis, and iritis and is usually bilateral. The retinal lesions are frequently asymptomatic and are found incidentally as inactive pigmented chorioretinal scars.

Inactive lesions may reactivate anytime throughout life, with active inflammation developing adjacent to areas of scarring. This is seen as a white fluffy response that may extend into the vitreous overlying the lesion (Fig. 19-95). Patients with lesions close to the macula or optic nerve should be wary of any visual changes and should be screened for reactivation of their disease.

Rubella. Exposure to rubella virus during the first trimester of pregnancy results in an intrauterine infection manifested as congenital rubella syndrome. Ocular findings include microphthalmia, microcornea, anterior uveitis, iris hypoplasia, nuclear or complete cataracts, corneal opacification, and glaucoma. The retinopathy of rubella syndrome is a diffuse "salt and pepper" retinopathy that develops early in childhood and does not affect vision. The pigmentary changes may be similar in appearance to those of syphilis, retinitis pigmentosa, and Leber congenital amaurosis (Fig. 19-96).

Cytomegalovirus. Cytomegalovirus (CMV) infection produces a bilateral retinochoroiditis manifested as multiple, yellowish-white, fluffy retinal lesions (Fig. 19-97). Hemorrhage is a prominent feature. Other ophthalmic manifestations include microphthalmia, uveitis, cataracts, optic disc atrophy, strabismus, and nystagmus.

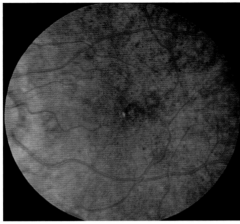

Figure 19-96. Pigmentary retinopathy in rubella syndrome.

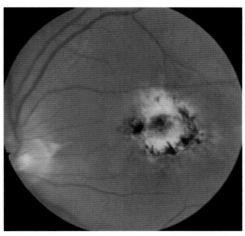

Figure 19-98. A retinal toxocariasis lesion appears as a white elevated mass with surrounding pigmentation.

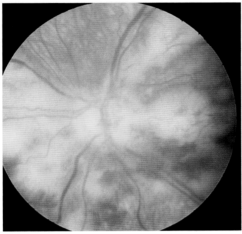

Figure 19-97. Retinitis, with obvious hemorrhages and perivascular yellowish-white exudates secondary to cytomegalic inclusion disease.

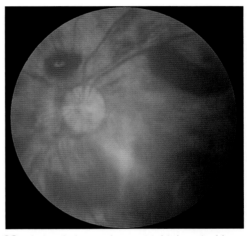

Figure 19-99. Shaken baby syndrome. Multiple retinal hemorrhages are present in the posterior fundus. There are small flame-shaped hemorrhages within the nerve fiber layer that follow the pattern of the retinal vessels. More extensive areas of hemorrhage have broken through to the preretinal space and are seen as areas of blood that obscure the retina. A Roth spot, a hemorrhage with a white center, is visible just above the optic disc. The white reflection from the camera flash is visible because of dispersed red blood cells within the vitreous.

CMV retinitis may be an opportunistic infection occurring in patients who are immunosuppressed because of immunodeficiency disorders or who are receiving immunosuppressive drugs. Retinal inflammation, edema, and hemorrhage may be extensive and rapidly progressive in these patients.

Herpes Simplex Virus. Herpes simplex virus infection may involve the anterior segment of the eye, with conjunctivitis, keratitis, and iritis or, when disseminated in the perinatal period, retinochoroiditis. Retinal involvement with disseminated herpes simplex virus is severe, with extensive inflammatory reaction producing yellowish-white exudates and retinal necrosis. Ocular involvement occurs in roughly 13% of herpetic infections in newborns.

Syphilis. Congenital syphilis may cause bilateral chorioretinitis, resulting in a salt and pepper fundus appearance. Differentiation of the retinopathy of congenital syphilis from retinitis pigmentosa may be difficult. Syphilis may also cause interstitial keratitis, anterior uveitis, glaucoma, and optic nerve atrophy.

Toxocariasis. *Toxocara canis* larvae infect children from 2 to 9 years of age. When the eye is involved, a white, elevated chorioretinal granuloma develops (Fig. 19-98). Chronic unilateral uveitis with opacification of the vitreous overlying the granuloma may occur. Inflammation in ocular toxocariasis occurs only after the organism dies. Externally, the eye does not appear to be inflamed. With extensive inflammation, fibrotic preretinal membranes

may develop and produce retinal detachment. Differentiation from retinoblastoma may be difficult. Calcification of the lesion is rare in toxocariasis as opposed to retinoblastoma. The diagnosis is confirmed by enzyme-linked immunosorbent assay for *T. canis* on blood or intraocular fluid.

Bacterial Endocarditis

Cotton-wool spots frequently develop in patients with bacterial endocarditis and septic emboli. These represent infarction of the nerve fiber layer of the retina and appear as white, irregular lesions with indistinct borders. Cotton-wool spots may be seen in any condition that produces retinal ischemia, such as hypertension and diabetes, or in patients with acquired immunodeficiency syndrome. Intraretinal hemorrhages occur with septic emboli and are flame shaped or dot-blot in nature. If the hemorrhage has a white center from the accumulation of leukocytes, the term *Roth spot* is used. Roth spots are not specific for bacterial endocarditis. They may occur in leukemia or shaken baby syndrome (Fig. 19-99). Conjunctival petechiae may be present as a sign of septic emboli.

Emboli to the eye may cause a central or branch retinal artery obstruction. Occlusion of the central retinal artery causes a sudden profound loss in vision, loss of the pupillary direct light reflex, absence of venous pulsations, and the development of a cherry-red spot in the fovea. Edema and opacification of the ganglion cell layer surrounding the fovea make the fovea stand out as red to produce this sign (Fig. 19-100). Treatment must be provided virtually immediately with the episode and is therefore of limited effectiveness.

Leukemia

Patients with acute lymphoblastic, myelogenous, or monocytic leukemia may develop flame-shaped intraretinal hemorrhages. These are usually extensive and visible with the direct ophthalmoscope. The presence of hemorrhage is not correlated with anemia or thrombocytopenia. Leukemic infiltration may also occur in the retina as a perivascular infiltrate in the choroid or in the optic disc, producing disc swelling and a papilledema-like appearance. Leukemic involvement of the orbit may be difficult to distinguish from bacterial orbital cellulitis.

Diabetes

The most common ocular finding in young diabetic patients is lenticular myopia. This occurs in patients who have had a rapid rise in blood glucose level. Sorbitol accumulates within the lens as a metabolic product. This increases the lens osmolarity and causes the lens to swell, producing myopia. After the blood sugar level returns to normal, myopia may continue to persist for several days or even weeks with gradual spontaneous resolution. Children with diabetes rarely develop cataracts.

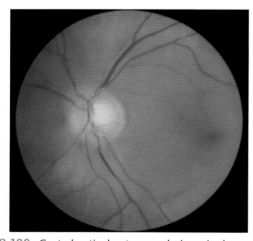

Figure 19-100. Central retinal artery occlusion. A cherry-red spot is visible in the fovea. This sign is due to edema and opacification of the ganglion cell layer of the retina surrounding the fovea.

The earliest sign of background diabetic retinopathy is the presence of microaneurysms (tiny discrete red spots). Small retinal hemorrhages, cotton-wool spots, venous dilation, and hard exudates (small, discrete, yellow lesions) may also be seen. The occurrence of background diabetic retinopathy is related to the duration and control of the diabetes. Young children appear to have a protective effect from diabetic retinopathy, and changes are seldom diagnosed until years after puberty; however, yearly screening examinations are recommended for juvenile diabetics. Proliferative diabetic retinopathy seen in adults essentially does not occur until after puberty.

Sickle Cell Retinopathy

The ocular abnormalities of the sickle hemoglobinopathies are caused by intravascular sickling, hemostasis, and thrombosis. Retinal findings occur in the peripheral fundus and cannot be visualized with a direct ophthalmoscope, necessitating detection by an ophthalmologist. Retinal vascular complications occur most frequently in patients with Hgb SC and S-thalassemia disease. Patients with sickle cell disease (Hgb SS) are less frequently affected, their decreased hematocrit providing protection to the retinal vasculature. Rarely, patients with the milder hemoglobinopathies, AS and AC, may have retinal findings.

Retinal findings may be divided into nonproliferative and proliferative changes. Proliferative changes include arteriolar occlusions that lead to arteriovenous anastomosis, causing areas of retinal nonperfusion. Neovascularization occurs at the edge of these areas of nonperfusion, in the form of a gossamer vascular network (a sea fan) and often leads to vitreous hemorrhage, traction, and retinal detachment (Fig. 19-101A). The disease process is similar to that seen in retinopathy of prematurity. Proliferative changes of sickle retinopathy should be treated with laser photocoagulation.

Nonproliferative changes include refractile or iridescent deposits, black sunburst lesions, and salmon patch hemorrhages. Refractile deposits are sequelae of old reabsorbed hemorrhages. Sunburst lesions are areas of perivascular retinal pigment epithelial hypertrophy and pigment migration (see Fig. 19-101B). Salmon patch lesions represent areas of intraretinal hemorrhage. Parafoveal capillaries and arterioles may become occluded and produce decreased visual acuity in sickle cell retinopathy. Segmentation of the conjunctival blood vessels produces comma-shaped capillaries ("comma sign").

Permanent vision loss from sickle cell retinopathy is rare in the pediatric age group.

Metabolic Diseases

The mucopolysaccharidoses are syndromes caused by inherited defects in the lysosomal enzymes that degrade

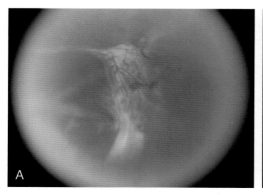

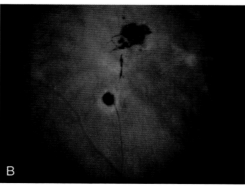

Figure 19-101. Sickle cell retinopathy. **A,** Neovascularization or growth of fragile blood vessels into the vitreous in the midperipheral retina. The white fibrous tissue present is due to the proliferation of fibroglial elements. This produces traction on the retina, which may subsequently lead to retinal detachment. **B,** The black sunburst lesions are areas of perivascular retinal pigment epithelial hypertrophy with pigment migration. This finding is an example of nonproliferative change.

A   B

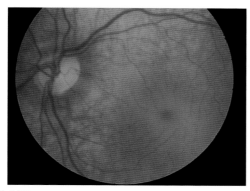

Figure 19-102. Tay-Sachs disease. Because the parafoveal area has many retinal ganglion cells and the fovea has none, the fovea retains its orangish-red color but is surrounded by retina that is whitish in color. This produces the cherry-red spot in the macula.

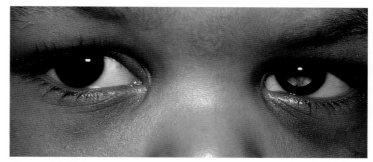

Figure 19-103. Leukocoria. The patient's left eye has a white pupillary reflex produced by reflection of light from a retinoblastoma. Leukocoria is the most common presenting sign (60%) of retinoblastoma.

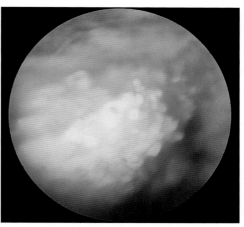

Figure 19-104. Retinoblastoma. The tumor mass of retinoblastoma is usually elevated and yellow or white in color. Dilated feeding vessels of the tumor may be visible. Seeding into the vitreous from the tumor may produce a cloudy vitreous.

acid mucopolysaccharide. All of the mucopolysaccharidoses are transmitted as autosomal recessive traits except type II (Hunter), which is X-linked recessive. A common ocular finding is retinal pigmentary degeneration, which closely resembles retinitis pigmentosa. Optic atrophy also occurs, as does corneal clouding resulting from stromal infiltration.

The sphingolipidoses are caused by a deficiency of the lysosomal enzymes responsible for the degeneration of sphingolipids. Tay-Sachs disease (GM_2 type I gangliosidosis) and Niemann-Pick disease are the two most common sphingolipidoses. Sphingolipids accumulate in the retinal ganglion cells, giving a whitish appearance to the retina. Because the parafoveal area has many retinal ganglion cells and the fovea none, the fovea has its normal orangish-red color, whereas the retina peripheral to the fovea is white. This produces a "cherry-red spot" in the macula (Fig. 19-102).

The mucolipidoses are caused by abnormal glycoprotein metabolism. Mucolipidoses have clinical findings of some of the sphingolipidoses and some of the mucopolysaccharidoses. The ocular findings include corneal epithelial edema, retinal pigmentary degeneration, macular cherry-red spots, and optic atrophy.

Cystinosis represents a defective transport mechanism for cystine within the lysosomes, which causes intralysosomal accumulation of cystine. Only patients with the nephritic type of cystinosis develop retinal changes, which include salt and pepper changes of the retinal pigment epithelium and areas of patchy depigmentation with irregularly distributed pigment clumps. These changes do not produce loss of vision. Photophobia is due to the accumulation of corneal crystals, which may occur in all types of cystinosis and may be extreme, producing a functional blindness. Treatment of the corneal crystallization with topical cysteamine drops is effective if used on a frequent and long-term basis.

Retinoblastoma

Retinoblastoma is the most common intraocular malignancy of childhood. It occurs with a frequency of between 1 in 14,000 and 1 in 20,000 births. The most common age of diagnosis is between 1 and $1\frac{1}{2}$ years, with 90% of cases presenting before 3 years of age. The most common presenting signs of retinoblastoma are leukocoria (60%) and strabismus (22%) (Fig. 19-103). One third of cases are bilateral. The tumor may present as an elevated, round, white, or yellow mass (Fig. 19-104). Retinoblastoma may be multicentric, with several tumor masses arising within the same eye. Seeding into the vitreous may occur, pro-

ducing a cloudy vitreous. A frequent feature of retinoblastoma is the presence of calcification within the mass.

Great advances have occurred in the understanding of the genetics of retinoblastoma. Retinoblastoma may be transmitted in an autosomal dominant inheritance pattern. Of patients with the disease, 60% have a family history of retinoblastoma. Penetrance is high (60% to 90%) but incomplete. Sporadic cases occur as either somatic mutations in 75% of patients or as germinal mutations that may be passed on to offspring. These sporadic cases are almost always unilateral, and the hereditary forms are usually bilateral; however, a patient with a unilateral tumor may have heritable disease. The gene for retinoblastoma has been identified, and it is possible to determine which patients with unilateral tumors have the hereditary form of the disease and which patients do not. Patients who have the heritable form of the disease, with the deletion of the retinoblastoma gene, may develop tumors of the pineal gland (trilateral retinoblastoma) and have a markedly increased risk of secondary tumors (osteogenic sarcoma).

Untreated, retinoblastoma is virtually 100% fatal. The treatment of retinoblastoma is advancing rapidly, and many eyes, even those with extensive tumor that were previously enucleated, may be saved with combinations of local treatment (laser, thermal, and plaque radiation) and chemotherapy.

Optic Nerve

The optic nerve relays information from each eye to the brain. Its function is assessed by measuring visual acuity, visual fields, color vision, and the pupillary response. Visualization and assessment of the morphology of the optic disc with a direct ophthalmoscope can provide valuable information regarding the function of the nerve.

Color Vision

Change in color vision, particularly the ability to perceive red, is an early feature seen in disorders that compromise the function of the optic nerve. Patients may complain of subjective changes in color perception, or they may demonstrate defects in color vision on objective tests.

An easy test to assess color vision is to compare color perception between the two eyes. The patient is asked to look at a red object first with one eye, then with the other, and is asked whether it is more red with one eye or the other. A subjective desaturation of red in one eye is an indication of dyschromatopsia and a potential optic nerve disorder. If the patient reports that the object is only 50% as red with one eye compared with the other, the results would be recorded as a red desaturation of 50%. In children it is valuable to present the object to the "normal eye" first with the question "If this is $1 of red, how much red is it now?" and offering a comparison with the fellow eye. A similar comparison may be performed for brightness by shining a light first into one eye and then into the other. The sense of brightness is also decreased in the presence of optic nerve disease. Formal assessment of color vision is performed using color plates such as the Hardy-Rand-Rittler or Ishihara color plates. Patients with heritable congenital color vision defects are equally affected in both eyes. Patients with asymmetrical optic nerve disease (optic neuritis, tumor, toxic optic neuropathy) have asymmetrically decreased color vision, especially for the red hues.

Pupils

Assessment of the pupils for size, shape, position, and reactivity is an important part of the neurologic and ophthalmic evaluation. Neurologic abnormalities that affect the pupil include defects of the afferent pathway (the optic nerve and visual system), the parasympathetic pathway (for pupillary constriction), and the sympathetic pathway (for pupillary dilation).

Afferent Pupillary Defects. In a normal patient, shining a penlight into one eye causes both pupils to constrict. Pupillary constriction in the illuminated eye is the direct response, and the constriction in the fellow eye is the consensual response. The pupils are normally equal in size even if one eye is blind; each eye receives equal pupillary innervation.

The swinging flashlight test is used to assess optic nerve function (Fig. 19-105). If an afferent pupillary defect (APD) is present, the term *Marcus Gunn pupil* is used. A penlight is used to illuminate one eye and then the other. The pupil of the illuminated eye is observed. If both eyes have equal afferent input, then illumination of either eye should produce equal constriction of the pupils. Normally, after shining a light into one eye, the response is initial constriction of both pupils followed by a small dilation. If the light is then swung quickly to the fellow eye, the response is the same. When there is a decrease in afferent input for pupillary constriction on one side (e.g., a monocular optic neuritis with one optic nerve acutely affected), constriction is either absent or decreased and the pupils do not constrict as much when the light is shown into the affected eye (i.e., both eyes display a relative dilation compared with their size when the normal side was stimulated).

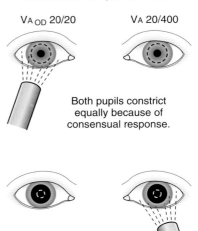

MARCUS GUNN PUPIL

To perform test:
Shine a bright light into each pupil for about 3–4 seconds. Alternate back and forth. Look for pupil to dilate, instead of constrict, with light.

Left eye has decreased vision due to retinal lesion or optic nerve lesion.

VA$_{OD}$ 20/20   VA 20/400

Both pupils constrict equally because of consensual response.

Both pupils dilate on illumination of eye with afferent defect.

Figure 19-105. Swinging flashlight test.

The critical observation is that when the affected eye is illuminated, a gradual dilation of the pupils occurs as compared with the response when the normal eye is illuminated. Having the patient maintain fixation on a distant object is important because accommodation causes constriction of the pupils and may lead to misinterpretation of the findings. This test is applicable even if one iris and pupil are of abnormal size or shape or nonreactive (e.g., following intraocular surgery, trauma, or synechiae from uveitis). The normal pupil is observed when the light is shown into either eye, and if there is a greater constriction of it when the light is shown into one side compared with the other, an APD is present.

An APD indicates disease affecting the optic nerve. Unilaterally or bilaterally asymmetrical optic nerve disease always causes a relative APD. Mild optic nerve disease producing minimal or no objectively measurable decrease in visual acuity still produces an APD, whereas a retinal defect must be profound to produce an APD. Afferent pupillary defects are not seen with dense cataracts, refractive errors, cortical lesions, or functional visual loss. Amblyopia may produce a subtle APD.

Anisocoria. Lesions of the parasympathetic or sympathetic system, if unilateral or asymmetrical, cause pupillary constriction or dilation and produce pupils that are unequal in size, termed *anisocoria*. Pupillary involvement in third nerve palsy is usually accompanied by ptosis and disturbances in ocular motility. In cases of brainstem herniation and basilar meningitis, however, pupillary dilation may be the only sign of the third nerve palsy. Pharmacologic mydriasis may occur with minimal exposure to atropine, cyclopentolate, or other parasympatholytic agents (e.g., accidental exposure to some pesticides). Pharmacologic testing with 1% pilocarpine is useful for differentiating pharmacologic mydriasis from third cranial nerve palsy; pupillary constriction occurs in third nerve palsy and does not occur with pharmacologic mydriasis. Pharmacologic miosis occurs with echothiophate iodide or pilocarpine.

A lesion at any point along the sympathetic pathway for pupillary constriction results in Horner syndrome. The classic triad of findings includes ptosis, miosis, and anhidrosis on the affected side. The anisocoria of Horner syndrome is more apparent in dim illumination, and the affected pupil shows a lag in dilation on dimming of the lights. The light and near pupillary reactions are intact. Paresis of Müller muscle of the lid leads to the mild upper lid ptosis. The lower eyelid on the affected side may rest 1 mm higher than the fellow lid, and the narrowed palpebral fissure gives the appearance of enophthalmos (see Fig. 19-72). Anhidrosis of the ipsilateral side of the body, side of the face, or forehead may be present, depending on the site of the innervation defect. Anhidrosis of the forehead may be assessed by lightly rubbing a smooth plastic ruler across the forehead skin. If the ruler moves smoothly, anhidrosis is present because small amounts of perspiration will cause the ruler to stick and have a jerking motion. A characteristic of congenital Horner syndrome is the development in later childhood or adolescence of iris heterochromia with the affected iris being lighter in color.

The sympathetic pathway for pupillary constriction involves three neurons. The location of first-order neuron lesions is in the brainstem and spinal cord, examples being cervical trauma or demyelinating disease. Preganglionic or second-order neuron lesions occur within the chest or neck (e.g., neuroblastoma arising in the sympathetic chain). Congenital Horner syndrome caused by birth trauma to the brachial plexus is another cause for a second-order neuron lesion. Third-order neuron lesions, postganglionic in reference to the superior cervical ganglion, are usually benign; however, extracranial or intracranial tumors of the nasopharynx or cavernous sinus may produce such lesions. More common causes for a postganglionic Horner syndrome are migraine variants such as cluster headache. Pharmacologic testing with hydroxyamphetamine drops can differentiate a third-order lesion from a first- or second-order lesion. With a third-order lesion the pupil does not dilate because the nerve's norepinephrine stores are depleted. With a first- or second-order lesion the nerve's norepinephrine stores are normal and pupillary dilation occurs with instillation of the drops.

Physiologic Anisocoria. Approximately 10-20% of the population has a perceptible anisocoria. The degree of anisocoria may vary from day to day, but usually the difference in pupil size is 1 mm or less. The magnitude of anisocoria remains the same in bright or dim illumination; however, in some cases the anisocoria may be more apparent in dim light than in bright light, thereby simulating Horner syndrome. Differentiating physiologic anisocoria from Horner syndrome may be difficult, especially in a moving infant. In physiologic anisocoria, there is no dilation lag. Pupils with physiologic anisocoria dilate after the instillation of 4% cocaine drops, whereas a Horner pupil fails to dilate.

Optic Neuritis. Inflammation of the optic nerve may occur either as a papillitis, referring to the intraocular form in which optic disc swelling is present, or as a retrobulbar neuritis, in which the optic disc appears normal and inflammation of the optic nerve occurs posterior to the globe. Vision loss may be sudden, profound, and accompanied by complaints of pain in or behind the eye, which may be accentuated by movement of the eyes. An

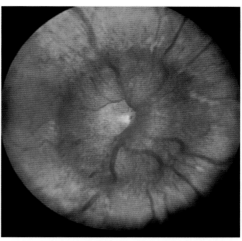

Figure 19-106. Acute papilledema, characterized by blurred disc edges, an absent physiologic cup, and intraretinal exudates.

afferent pupillary defect is present if the condition is unilateral or if it is bilateral and asymmetrical. Visual fields usually show a cecocentral scotoma, an area of vision loss located in the central visual field.

The optic disc, if affected, may show swelling of the peripapillary nerve fiber layer and elevation. Small vessels at the optic disc margin may hemorrhage or become obscured by edema. The appearance in bilateral disease cannot be differentiated from the optic disc swelling present with increased intracranial pressure.

Optic neuritis in children is frequently bilateral and may follow infection with mumps, measles, chickenpox, or meningoencephalitis. Collagen vascular disease, particularly systemic lupus erythematosus and sarcoidosis, may be associated with optic neuritis. Syphilis and tuberculosis also cause optic neuritis. Visual acuity in idiopathic optic neuritis gradually improves 1 to 4 weeks after onset and usually returns to normal over several months.

Papilledema
Increased intracranial pressure is transmitted to the optic nerves via the cerebrospinal fluid within the subarachnoid space and causes papilledema. The axoplasmic flow from the retinal ganglion cells to the cells in the lateral geniculate nucleus is blocked and causes the optic disc to swell. The degree of disc swelling may be asymmetrical; however, increased intracranial pressure rarely causes papilledema in only one eye. Ophthalmoscopic signs include blurring of the disc margin and disc edema. The disc may be hyperemic because of telangiectasia of the superficial capillaries on the disc, and small hemorrhages may appear on the disc margin (Fig. 19-106). Visual acuity is normal unless hemorrhage and edema involve the macula. Patients complain of transient obscurations of vision. The visual fields may show an enlarged blind spot, and the pupillary response and color vision are normal.

If increased intracranial pressure is chronic, elevation of the optic disc may persist but the hemorrhages and exudates seen in the acute phase resolve. When the condition is prolonged, optic nerve atrophy and vision loss occur. If intracranial pressure is normalized, it may take 6 weeks for papilledema to resolve and the optic disc to normalize.

Pseudopapilledema
Pseudopapilledema occurs in eyes with high hyperopia or optic disc drusen (see Fig. 19-9). The disc is not hyper-

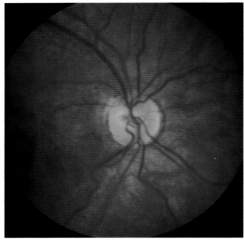

Figure 19-107. Optic atrophy, characterized by a sharply demarcated, pale, yellowish-white disc, with an absence of small vessels and disc substance.

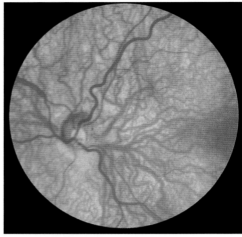

Figure 19-108. Optic nerve hypoplasia. A pigment crescent surrounds the hypoplastic nerve. This corresponds to the scleral opening for a normal-sized optic nerve and is termed the *double ring sign*. In this patient the pattern of the retinal vasculature is also abnormal, as is the retinal pigmentation.

emic, the vessels at the disc margin remain visible, and there is no nerve fiber layer swelling. There may be anomalous branching and tortuosity of the retinal vessels, and the physiologic cup is usually absent. The disc borders may be irregular. Hemorrhages, exudate, cotton-wool spots, and venous congestion do not occur. Spontaneous venous pulsations are an indication that the disc swelling is pseudopapilledema and not caused by increased intracranial pressure; however, they are not present in 20% of the normal population, so their absence does not indicate that the disc swelling is necessarily true papilledema. Central visual acuity is normal.

Optic Disc Atrophy

Optic nerve atrophy is present if the optic disc does not have its typical reddish-orange color. Initially the disc becomes more yellow in color, gradually developing more pallor. The lamina cribrosa may become visible with enlargement of the optic cup, leaving a "pinholed" appearance (Fig. 19-107). As the disease process continues, the disc eventually becomes white in color, visual acuity decreases, and visual field defects emerge.

Optic atrophy may occur as a sequela of papilledema, optic neuritis, compressive lesions of the optic nerve or chiasm, trauma, hereditary retinal disease, or glaucoma. Optic atrophy may also be inherited as a recessive or dominant trait. Atrophy may occur as a component of a generalized neurologic condition, such as Behr optic atrophy with cerebellar ataxia, hypotonia, and mental retardation. Leber optic atrophy occurs in late adolescence or early adulthood, with acute disc edema being rapidly followed by progressive bilateral optic atrophy.

Developmental Anomalies of the Optic Nerve

Developmental anomalies of the optic nerve include colobomas, tilted discs, and optic nerve hypoplasia (see Figs. 19-9 and 19-85). The level of visual acuity is related to the type and extent of the defect. Although profound abnormalities certainly have a significant effect on visual acuity, it is difficult to estimate the effect that more minor anomalies, especially optic nerve hypoplasia, may have on vision.

Hypoplasia of the optic nerve occurs either unilaterally or bilaterally. The optic disc is smaller than normal and has a surrounding yellowish-white ring that corresponds to the scleral opening for a normal-sized optic nerve. The

term *double ring sign* is used to describe the ring with its surrounding pigment crescent. The retinal vessels are normal in size but may appear crowded as they leave the optic disc (Fig. 19-108). Visual acuity is related to the degree of hypoplasia, and an afferent pupillary defect may be present if the degree of involvement is asymmetrical. Optic nerve hypoplasia is associated with midline central nervous system abnormalities including absence of the septum pellucidum (de Morsier syndrome). Children with optic nerve hypoplasia should be examined for abnormalities in pituitary and hypothalamic function. Optic disc hypoplasia is frequently seen in patients with fetal alcohol syndrome (FAS) (48%). Increased tortuosity of the retinal vasculature may also exist in FAS patients.

Orbit

Clinical signs of orbital disease are proptosis and restriction in ocular motility, compression of the optic nerve producing optic disc swelling, changes in refraction, and retinal striae. Retinal striae appear as radial lines on the retinal surface and are caused by compression of the posterior portion of the globe.

Orbital disease or trauma may cause orbital asymmetry with displacement of the globe (Fig. 19-109). Posterior (enophthalmos) or anterior (exophthalmos) displacement of the globe in orbital disease may be subtle. Comparison of the position of the globes in relation to the lateral orbital rims, looking especially for asymmetry, is a valuable clinical test, with subtle differences most easily visualized by viewing the patient from above. The Hertel exophthalmometer is an instrument used to compare the position of the globes in relation to the lateral orbital rim (Fig. 19-110). Palpation of the globes over closed eyelids, gently retropulsing the globe into the orbit, may reveal the character of an orbital mass and is helpful in assessing proptosis caused by orbital cellulitis. Ocular rotations are tested looking for restrictions in motility. Other adjuncts to the clinical examination include B scan ultrasonography, CT, and MRI of the orbit.

The most common orbital disease in childhood is cellulitis (see Chapter 23). Capillary hemangioma and lymphangioma are the most common benign primary orbital tumors of childhood. Orbital capillary hemangiomas

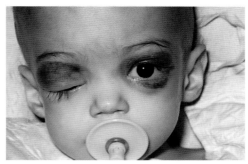

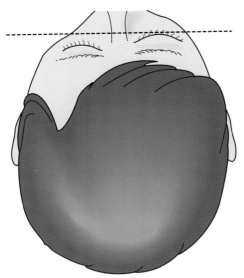

Figure 19-109. Blowout fracture of inferior orbital wall and dislocation of zygoma.

Figure 19-111. Neuroblastoma. Neuroblastoma metastatic to the orbit may present with an abrupt onset of unilateral or bilateral proptosis and ecchymosis of the eyelids. Neuroblastoma is the most common lesion to metastasize to the orbit in childhood.

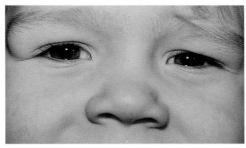

Figure 19-110. The Hertel exophthalmometer measures the anterior-to-posterior distance from the corneal surface to the lateral orbital rim. A base measurement, the distance between the two lateral orbital rims, is recorded to ensure repeatable instrument placement. Progression or regression can be determined with serial measurements.

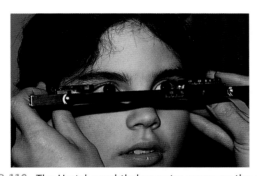

Figure 19-112. Dermoid cyst. These cysts present as smooth, painless, mobile, subcutaneous, round or oval masses. Dermoid cysts are most frequently located in the lateral brow area adjacent to the zygomaticofrontal suture. Although benign, if they are ruptured by trauma, an intense inflammatory reaction with scarring in the area may occur.

present shortly after birth, enlarge over the first 6 to 12 months of life, have a period of stability between 1 and 2 years of age, and then begin to regress. Intralesional and systemic steroids may be used to promote regression. Lymphangiomas may involve the conjunctiva, lids, or orbit. These tumors may rapidly enlarge during upper respiratory tract infections. Sudden enlargement may occur after hemorrhage within the lesion.

Rhabdomyosarcoma is the most common primary orbital malignancy in childhood. This tumor should be a consideration in any child between the ages of 7 and 8 years who has rapidly progressing unilateral proptosis. The tumor mass may be palpable in the upper eyelid area, or it may be located deeper in the orbit.

The most common metastatic lesion to the orbit in childhood is neuroblastoma. This tumor presents with an abrupt onset of proptosis and ecchymosis that may be bilateral (Fig. 19-111). Metastasis in neuroblastoma typically occurs late in the course of the disease when the primary tumor can easily be detected in the abdomen.

Dermoid and epidermoid cysts are relatively common. These benign masses are usually located anterior to the orbital septum but may extend posteriorly into the orbit. These cysts present as smooth, painless, freely movable round or oval masses and are usually located in the lateral brow area, adjacent to the zygomaticofrontal suture (Fig. 19-112). They may, however, be found near any bony suture. If these lesions can be palpated around their entire

extent, no neuroimaging studies may be necessary; however, if they are palpated as extending posterior to the orbital rim, imaging is indicated to exclude extension into the intracranial space or a diagnosis of encephalocele. These cysts contain dermal and epidermal elements that have become isolated from the skin during the course of embryonic development. If ruptured by trauma, an intense inflammatory reaction occurs. Because of this reaction, surgical excision of these lesions is indicated before potential trauma when the child learns to walk.

Optic nerve gliomas are tumors that occur in children younger than 10 years of age. At least one third of children have a history of neurofibromatosis. The presenting sign may be loss of vision or painless proptosis. An afferent pupillary defect and optic atrophy are usually present. Papilledema may also occur. Strabismus may be present because of decreased visual acuity (Fig. 19-113).

Plexiform neurofibromas are also seen in association with neurofibromatosis. They occur within the orbit or within the upper lid tissue and cause a fullness and ptosis of the lateral portion of the eyelid, leading to S-shaped upper lid deformity.

Orbital pseudotumor is a unilateral or bilateral orbital inflammatory process affecting the structures within the orbit. Children with pseudotumor have signs of headache, fever, lethargy, orbital pain, proptosis, lid erythema, conjunctival injection, and restricted ocular motility causing diplopia. The extraocular muscles and their tendons may be thickened. Orbital pseudotumor is a benign condition; however, recurrent tumor with scarring and fibrosis may cause restriction of ocular motility and optic nerve atrophy. Orbital pseudotumor must be differentiated from leukemia. The most common form of leukemia that affects the orbit is acute lymphoblastic leukemia.

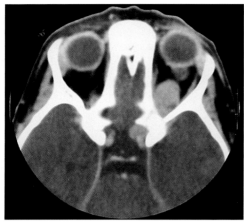

Figure 19-113. Optic nerve glioma. Its presence may cause a gradual onset of painless proptosis. Children seldom complain of monocular visual loss, and the discovery of a profound loss of vision may be the presenting sign of an optic nerve glioma. In children, optic nerve gliomas are benign lesions that may, however, extend to the optic chiasm or intracranially.

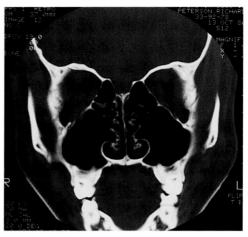

Figure 19-115. Blowout fracture of the right orbit (coronal CT scan). Protruding through the fracture in the orbital floor into the maxillary sinus is orbital fat. The inferior rectus muscle is potentially entrapped within the fracture site.

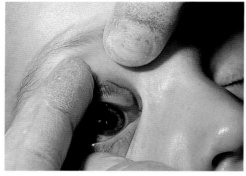

Figure 19-114. Canalicular laceration. This patient experienced a laceration of the upper canaliculus. Simple apposition of the wound edges in this case will not approximate the cut ends of the canaliculus. Silastic tubes are used to splint the canaliculus during the healing process.

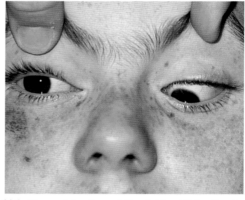

Figure 19-116. Blowout fracture of the right orbit leading to the inability to depress the right eye.

Ocular Trauma

In the evaluation of children with orbital or periocular trauma, serious ocular injury must be presumed even if only minimal external signs exist. Before any evaluation or manipulation of the patient, an assessment of visual acuity must be performed if possible. This provides information regarding the severity and nature of the trauma, and records data that may be of medicolegal importance.

The anatomy of a laceration of the eyelid dictates the measures required for repair. The presence of orbital fat indicates penetration of the septum and entrance into the orbit. Additionally, evaluation of the laceration must include the degree of involvement of the lid margin, loss of tissue, injury to the medial and lateral canthal tendons, and injury to the canaliculi of the nasolacrimal drainage system (Fig. 19-114). Each of these injuries requires a special technique for repair.

Patients who have sustained blunt orbital trauma should be evaluated for a fracture of the orbital floor or the medial wall of the orbit. Signs of a fracture with entrapment of one of the extraocular muscles include enophthalmos, diplopia, restricted gaze, and paresthesias in the distribution of the infraorbital nerve. Exophthalmos may occur if there is significant orbital swelling or hemorrhage. Fractures may be isolated to the floor, or they may extend to the orbital rim (Fig. 19-115). If subcutaneous air or orbital

emphysema is present, the fracture has permitted communication with the sinuses. Intraorbital edema or hemorrhage within the extraocular muscles may also restrict ocular motility. The most commonly involved muscles are the inferior and medial rectus muscles (Fig. 19-116).

Conjunctival lacerations may appear greatly disproportionate to their degree of severity. On the other hand, a small laceration of the conjunctiva may be present in association with a penetrating injury to the globe. The history and circumstances of the injury must be considered in determining the likelihood of serious injury and the extent of the evaluation necessary because traumatized uncooperative young children may need to be sedated for complete evaluation.

The use of a topical anesthetic such as tetracaine or proparacaine anesthetizes the cornea and conjunctiva and permits a close examination for foreign bodies. A Desmarres lid retractor may help exert gentle pressure to open the lids of uncooperative children or if swelling of the lids makes examination difficult (Fig. 19-117). The lids may also be everted over a cotton swab to inspect the underside of the eyelid (Fig. 19-118). The presence of a foreign body under the upper eyelid causes vertical epithelial abrasions on the underlying corneal surface (Fig. 19-119). Corneal abrasions cause extreme pain and photophobia. The use of sodium fluorescein dye applied to the conjunctival cul-de-sac and examination with a cobalt blue filtered light aid in the detection of a superficial epi-

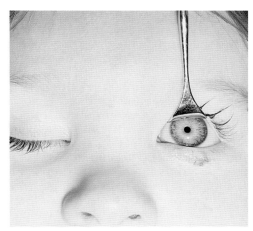

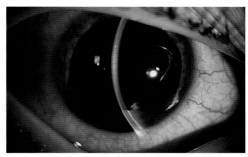

Figure 19-120. Hyphema. Red blood cells within the anterior chamber have settled into the inferior anterior chamber angle.

Figure 19-117. A Desmarres lid retractor may be used to gently open the eyelids of an uncooperative child, or in cases of trauma or preseptal cellulitis in which lid swelling makes opening of the lids for globe examination difficult.

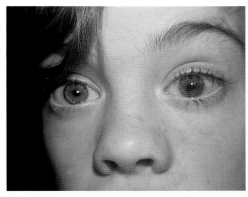

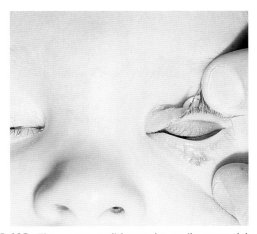

Figure 19-121. A complication of hyphema is corneal blood staining. This patient's left cornea has an area of brown staining inferiorly because of prolonged presence of blood within the anterior chamber.

Figure 19-118. The upper eyelid may be easily everted by placing a cotton swab at the upper edge of the tarsal plate. The lashes are then gently grasped and pulled anteriorly and upward to evert the lid over the cotton swab. The tarsal conjunctiva may be inspected for the presence of a foreign body.

for further evaluation. Such lesions may be treated with topical antibiotic drops or ointment, observing significant improvement in signs and symptoms in 24 hours and complete resolution in 48 hours. Patching of the eye to keep the lid completely closed promotes healing of the epithelium and may make the eye more comfortable.

Blunt trauma to the eye may cause iritis or an anterior uveitis. Patients complain of dull eye pain and light sensitivity. Signs of iritis include miosis of the pupil, tearing, and ciliary injection. With severe blunt trauma, the iris may be avulsed from its insertion (iridodialysis) or the iris and ciliary body may be avulsed (cyclodialysis). Tears of the pupillary sphincter may also occur, enlarging the pupil, and are a sign that further evaluation should be conducted. Eyes that receive blunt trauma may develop traumatic angle recession and glaucoma years after the incident.

An injury to the globe may cause bleeding from the small vessels of the peripheral portion of the iris or the ciliary body. Blood, which is heavier than aqueous fluid, usually settles out in the inferior portion of the eye, causing a hyphema (Fig. 19-120). While the red blood cells are dispersed throughout the aqueous fluid, vision may be dramatically decreased. The blood may remain fluid and shift with changes in head position, or it may clot. Complications after a hyphema include rebleeding, glaucoma, and blood staining of the cornea (Fig. 19-121). Increased intraocular pressure increases the risk of developing blood staining. The opacification of the cornea may resolve over several months. In children, this may cause amblyopia. Hyphemas are serious injuries that require evaluation by an ophthalmologist. The majority of hyphemas resolve over 4 to 5 days with only observation and reduced activity.

Immediate or delayed opacification of the lens, cataract formation, may occur with penetration of the lens

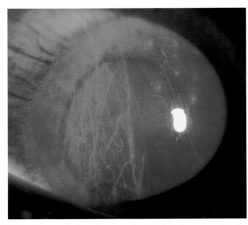

Figure 19-119. Corneal abrasions stained with fluorescein dye and viewed under blue light. The abrasions appear green in the area of corneal epithelial loss.

thelial abrasion. The dye stains areas that are missing epithelium. When possible, examination should be conducted with magnification as provided by a slit lamp or magnifying glass. If the history and examination do not prompt significant concern for a retained foreign body, small corneal abrasions do not necessarily require referral

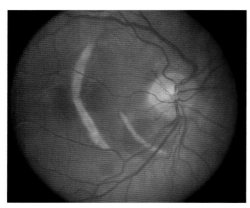

Figure 19-122. Blunt trauma to the eye has caused a rupture of the choroid. This is visualized as white concentric rings around the optic disc where, beneath the retina, the choroid has separated, making the underlying sclera visible.

capsule or with blunt trauma alone. Blunt trauma may disrupt the lens zonules and dislocate the lens (see Fig. 19-81).

All eyes receiving significant trauma must have an examination of the fundus. Blunt trauma may cause a macular hole or a rupture of the choroid. A choroidal rupture is visualized as a white concentric ring around the optic disc where the underlying sclera has become visible (Fig. 19-122). Retinal tears or detachment may follow trauma, and the clinician's index of suspicion should take into account the history of the trauma and presence of symptoms (photopsia, floaters, and visual changes). Patients with high myopia are at a greater risk for retinal detachment following blunt trauma.

Trauma may produce retinal hemorrhages that are limited to the retina or that extend into the vitreous. Crushing injury to the chest may raise intrathoracic pressure, with transmission to the retina causing hemorrhages. Purtscher retinopathy includes retinal hemorrhages, cotton-wool spots, retinal edema, and fat emboli. Terson syndrome is the transmission of subarachnoid hemorrhage to the optic nerve and disc and results in vitreous

and retinal hemorrhages. Infants with shaken baby syndrome may have extensive intraretinal hemorrhages accompanying their intracranial injuries, and the severity of intraocular hemorrhage may correlate with the severity of intracranial injury.

In cases of penetrating injury to the eye, the key to examination is to be brief and gentle so as not to complicate the injury by causing expulsion of intraocular contents. Immediately after identifying an ocular injury as penetrating, further examination should be limited and conducted in the operating room under general anesthesia. Topical medications should not be applied to the eye, and the eye should be protected at all times with a shield. Penetrating injuries caused by projectiles or foreign bodies may produce subtle findings. In cases in which the index of suspicion is high, appropriate evaluation may include plain film x-rays or imaging studies including CT or MRI. If the potential intraocular foreign body is metallic, MRI scanning is contraindicated.

Bibliography

Eye examination and vision screening in infants, children and young adults. Pediatrics 98:153-157, 1996.

Fraunfelder FT, Roy FH: Current Ocular Therapy, 5th ed. Philadelphia, WB Saunders, 2000.

Helveston EM, Ellis FD: Pediatric Ophthalmology Practice, 2nd ed. St Louis, Mosby, 1989.

Isenberg SJ: The Eye in Infancy, 2nd ed. St Louis, Mosby, 1993.

Margo CE, Hamed LF, Mames RN (eds): Diagnostic Problems in Clinical Ophthalmology. Philadelphia, WB Saunders, 1994.

Miller NR: Walsh Hoyt's Clinical Neuro-ophthalmology, 5th ed. Baltimore, Williams & Wilkins, 1998.

Nelson LB: Harley's Pediatric Ophthalmology, 4th ed. Philadelphia, WB Saunders, 1998.

Renie WA: Goldberg's Genetic and Metabolic Eye Disease, 2nd ed. Boston, Little, Brown, 1986.

Tasman W, Jaeger EA: Duane's Clinical Ophthalmology. Philadelphia, JB Lippincott, 1996.

Taylor D (ed): Pediatric Ophthalmology, 2nd ed. Boston, Blackwell Scientific Publications, 1997.

von Noorden GK: Binocular Vision and Ocular Motility: Theory and Management of Strabismus, 6th ed. St Louis, Mosby, 2001.

Yanoff M, Fine BS: Ocular Pathology, 4th ed. Philadelphia, JB Lippincott, 1995.

CHAPTER 20

Oral Disorders

MAMOUN M. NAZIF, BRIAN S. MARTIN,
DAVID H. MCKIBBEN, AND
HOLLY W. DAVIS

Assessment Techniques

Because oral and oropharyngeal problems and disorders are common and cause a wide variety of symptoms, a thorough oral examination is an essential component of a complete physical examination, enabling the practitioner to make appropriate diagnoses without undue delay.

Key elements of the oral/dental history include the following:

1. Timing of eruption and exfoliation of primary teeth, timing of eruption of permanent teeth, and any problems encountered
2. Brushing and flossing frequency and technique
3. Dietary habits including frequency of bottle-feeding and breastfeeding in infancy; whether infants and toddlers are put to bed with a bottle; time of weaning; frequency of carbohydrate intake; and possible symptoms of eating disorders in adolescence
4. Current source of dental care and frequency of visits
5. Current history of symptoms: oral pain, redness, swelling, drainage, headaches, abdominal pain, decreased appetite (especially for chewy foods)
6. Problems with bite or occlusion
7. History of dental problems and/or orofacial trauma and their treatment
8. Family history of dental problems or disorders

A systematic approach to the examination of a child's dentition is essential and should include assessment of the following:

1. Facial symmetry and balance
2. Lip seal at rest position
3. Occlusion (bite) and tooth alignment
4. Mandibular excursion in lateral, vertical, and anterior/posterior planes
5. Integrity of enamel, presence of caries
6. Appearance of gingivae from both labial-buccal and lingual sides
7. Condition of the other oral soft tissues: tongue, palate, mucobuccal folds, and sublingual spaces

Successful examination requires close visual inspection of the face; palpation of suspected areas of abnormality; and systematic inspection of the dentition, its supporting structures, and the oral soft tissues. This can be challenging with young children, but patience and a gentle, even playful manner can be of great help. At least initially, young children should be allowed to sit on the parent's lap. Toys, puppets, and a rubber glove blown up into a balloon can serve as useful distractions. Drawing a face on a tongue depressor and giving it to the child to hold, as well as letting the child look in the dental mirror are good ways to introduce these basic instruments and make them less threatening (Fig. 20-1A and B). If an otoscope is being used as a light source in a medical office setting, letting the child "blow out the light" is another good introductory game, as is demonstrating the examination on the parent or examiner. Then the examiner can gradually begin the hands-on assessment. If cooperation cannot be achieved despite these measures, immobilization in a papoose board may be necessary. With older children, examination of the patient in the supine or semirecumbent position with good lighting assists visualization and may be more practical.

Use of a tongue depressor is necessary to ensure direct visual access to all intraoral areas, and a dental mirror can be quite helpful, especially in assessing the lingual surfaces of the anterior teeth and gingivae and the buccal surfaces of rear molars (Fig. 20-1C). Extra effort and patience may be required to ensure that the mucobuccal folds, sublingual space, lingual surface of the anterior teeth, and anterior palate are adequately visualized.

The special aspects of the history and physical assessment of dental and orofacial trauma are detailed in the trauma section of this chapter.

Normal Oral Structures

The oral cavity, including the teeth, gingivae, and periodontal ligaments, is in a constant state of evolution during infancy and childhood. From the early teething stage, through the eruption and exfoliation of the primary dentition, and finally to the eruption of all permanent teeth, the oral cavity provides one of the most visible signs of development.

To assist understanding of this chapter and communication when consulting dentists, a review of basic terminology is in order. Each tooth is composed of an outer protective enamel layer; an inner layer of dentin consisting of tubules, which are thought to serve a nutritional function; and a central neurovascular core termed the *pulp*. The roots of the teeth are anchored in the sockets of the alveolar processes of the mandible and maxilla by an encompassing periodontal membrane or ligament. The neurovascular supply to the root apex also passes through this structure. The bony processes between the teeth are referred to as the *interdental septae* (Fig. 20-2).

After eruption, the visible portions of teeth are referred to as the *crowns,* and the interface between them and the gingivae is termed the *gingival crevice.* Finally, the portions of the gingivae located between teeth are called *interdental papillae.*

Oral Cavity in the Newborn

The lips of an infant reveal a prominent line of demarcation at the vermilion border. The mucosa may look wrinkled and slightly purple at birth, but within a few days it exhibits a drier appearance, with the outer layer forming crusty "sucking calluses." This callus formation affects the central portion of the mucosa and persists for only a few weeks.

The maxillary alveolar arch is separated from the lip by a shallow sulcus. In the midline the labial frenulum extends posteriorly across the alveolar ridge to the palatine incisive papilla. Two lateral miniature frenulae are also evident. The alveolar ridge peaks anteriorly and gradually flattens as the ridge extends posteriorly, forming a pseudoalveolar groove medial to the ridge along its palatal side. This flattened appearance is seen in young infants and gradually disappears with the growth of the alveolar process and the formation and calcification of posterior

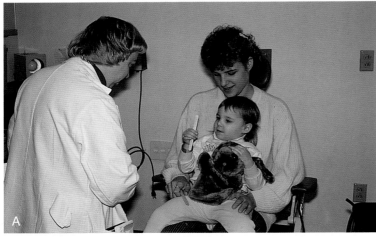

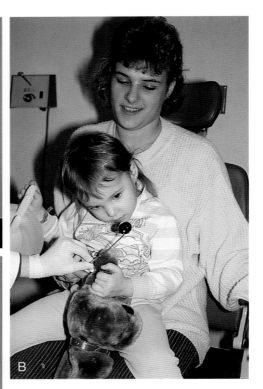

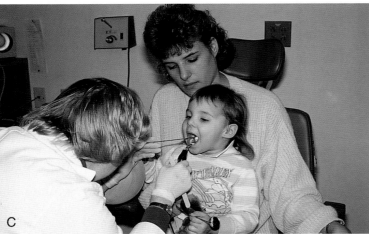

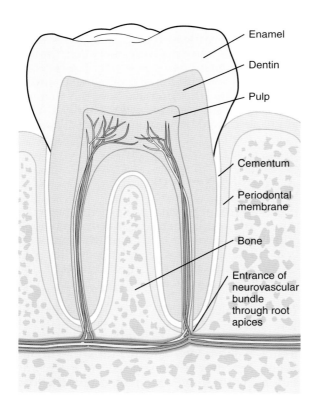

Figure 20-1. Oral examination of a toddler. **A** and **B,** Use of toys and puppets as distracters, introduction of nonthreatening instruments by drawing a face on the tongue depressor, and letting the child look at herself in the dental mirror assist cooperation. **C,** The dental mirror is useful for visualizing the lingual surfaces of the anterior dentition and gingivae and the buccal surfaces of rear molars.

Figure 20-2. Diagrammatic representation of a molar shows the enamel, dentin, and pulp; the cementum; the periodontal membrane; the entrance of the neurovascular bundle through the root apices; and the bony supporting structures.

tooth buds. The mandibular alveolar ridges also peak anteriorly and flatten posteriorly. The mandibular labial frenulum connects the lower lip to the labial aspect of the alveolar ridge. Careful visual inspection and palpation of the ridges should confirm the presence and location of tooth buds. Anterior tooth buds are located on the labial side of the alveolar ridges, whereas posterior tooth buds are often located closer to the crests of the alveolar ridges. Palatal morphology and color are variable. The tongue and the floor of the mouth differ only slightly from those of older children.

Primary Dentition

Development of the alveolar bone is directly related to the formation and eruption of teeth, and normal patterns of dental development occur symmetrically. At approximately 6 months of age, the mandibular central incisors erupt. This stage is often preceded by a period of increased salivation, local gingival irritation, and irritability. These symptoms may vary in intensity, but they respond well to oral analgesics and usually subside when the primary tooth erupts into the oral cavity. Other symptoms such as fever or diarrhea have never been proved to be directly related to teething. The lower incisors are soon followed by the maxillary central incisors and the maxillary and mandibular lateral incisors (Fig. 20-3). By the end of the first year, all eight anterior teeth are usually visible. At 2 years, all primary teeth have erupted with the exception

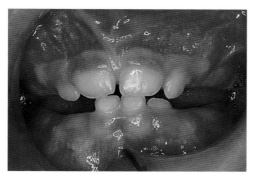

Figure 20-3. Early primary dentition. The mandibular and maxillary central and lateral incisors are the first to erupt.

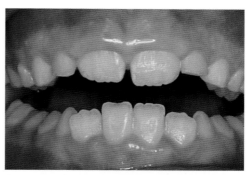

Figure 20-5. Mixed dentition. This transitional stage from primary to permanent dentition begins at age 6 and lasts for about 6 years.

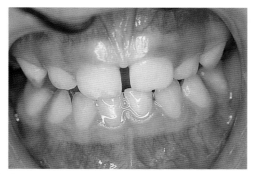

Figure 20-4. Full primary dentition. By age 3, all 20 primary teeth have erupted.

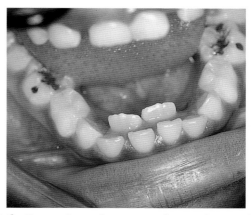

Figure 20-6. Abnormal eruption patterns frequently occur in the early mixed dentition phase. One example is shown here, with eruption of the permanent central incisors behind the primary teeth.

of the second primary molars, which erupt shortly thereafter. By the age of 3 years, the primary dentition is fully present and functional (Fig. 20-4).

Any variation in the time and sequence of eruption in an otherwise normal infant may call for early dental referral. In most instances, careful observation is the best course of action. For example, delayed eruption of primary teeth for up to 8 months is occasionally observed, and if seen in the absence of other abnormalities may be a normal variation. Delayed dentition can be a feature of moderate to severe cases of failure to thrive, where it is seen in association with and is a visible reflection of delayed bone age. More rarely, retarded eruption is associated with Down syndrome, hypothyroidism, hypopituitarism, achondroplastic dwarfism, osteopetrosis, rickets, or chondroectodermal dysplasia. A significant variation affecting a single tooth or only a few teeth should be carefully investigated as well.

Spacing (extra space between teeth) during this stage is normal and desirable and often indicates that more space is available for the larger permanent teeth. The completed primary dentition establishes a baseline that dictates to a great extent the future alignment of permanent teeth and the future relationship between the maxillary and mandibular arches.

During most of the primary dentition stage, the gingiva appears pink, is firm, and is not readily retractable. A well-defined zone of firmly attached keratinized gingiva is present, extending from the bottom of the gingival sulcus to the junction of the alveolar mucosa. Rarely, local irritation may develop into acute or subacute pericoronitis, with elevated temperature and associated lymphadenopathy (see Fig. 20-50). Topical and/or systemic therapy may be required for treatment; however, lancing the gingiva to relieve such symptoms is not usually indicated.

Mixed Dentition

This stage of development begins with the eruption of the first permanent molars at about 6 years of age and continues for approximately 6 years. During this period, the following teeth erupt from the gums in sequence: mandibular central incisors, maxillary central incisors, mandibular lateral incisors, maxillary lateral incisors, mandibular cuspids, maxillary and mandibular first premolars, maxillary and mandibular second premolars, maxillary cuspids, and mandibular and maxillary second molars (Fig. 20-5).

The mixed dentition during this stage undergoes certain physiologic changes including root resorption followed by exfoliation of primary teeth, eruption of their successors, and eruption of the posterior permanent teeth. During the period of root resorption of primary teeth, and for several months after the eruption of permanent teeth, the teeth are relatively loosely embedded in the alveolar bone and more vulnerable to displacement with trauma. Other minor complications may occur during resorption and exfoliation of primary teeth and eruption of permanent teeth. Gingival irritation can occur as a result of increased mobility of primary teeth but usually disappears spontaneously when the tooth is lost or extracted. Two transient deviations of eruption pattern may occur: the mandibular incisors may erupt in a lingual position behind the primary incisors ("double teeth") (Fig. 20-6), and the maxillary incisors may assume a widely spaced and labially inclined position ("ugly duckling" stage). Finally, the occlusal surfaces of newly erupted permanent teeth are relatively "rough" (see Figs. 20-5 and 20-43), assisting plaque accumulation that increases the risk of staining, gingivitis, and formation of caries.

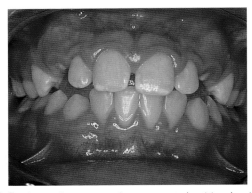

Figure 20-7. The earliest stage of permanent dentition begins with the eruption of the 6-year molars and central incisors. The cuspids and second molars are the last to erupt.

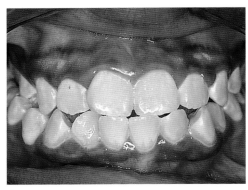

Figure 20-8. Gingivitis during puberty. The gingival tissues are mildly erythematous and edematous, and they tend to bleed easily with brushing. Hormonal changes and inattention to careful dental hygiene are thought to be contributory.

Early Permanent Dentition

This stage marks the beginning of a relatively quiescent period in dental development. Activities are limited to root formation of a few permanent teeth and the calcification of the third molars. By this time the length and width of the dental arches are well established (Fig. 20-7); however, the jaws undergo a major growth spurt during puberty that alters their size and relative position. The gingiva begins to assume adult characteristics, becoming firm and pink in color, with an uneven, stippled surface texture and a thin gingival margin. Puberty is occasionally associated with gingivitis, thought to be secondary in part to hormonal changes (Fig. 20-8). The gingivae become mildly edematous and erythematous and bleed with brushing (the common chief complaint). Inattention to careful dental hygiene may also contribute to development of this disorder, which necessitates good oral hygiene for control.

In Figure 20-9 the primary and permanent dentition are presented diagrammatically.

Harmful Oral Habits

Thumb and Finger Sucking

Children often develop sucking habits, using the thumb, finger(s), or objects. Thumb and finger sucking begins antenatally and is considered a normal behavior pattern. However, if the habit persists beyond the late primary dentition stage of dental arch development (5 years), the extrinsic forces applied by the sucking action can produce pathologic changes in the child's normal arch growth. These deviations range from minor, reversible changes to gross malformations in the dental arches that produce significant anterior open bites and/or posterior crossbites. The degree of change depends on the duration, frequency, and intensity of the sucking habit (Fig. 20-10).

Bottle and Pacifier Habits

The forces produced by prolonged use of bottles and pacifiers can first cause dental malocclusions and may, if the habit persists, worsen the resulting deformity with the involvement of adjacent jaw structures. Usually, if the child is weaned from the bottle and pacifier by the age of 18 months, no permanent changes in bite development can be expected. The longer any force is applied, however, the greater the risk that the distortion in the dental arches and adjacent bony structures will not self-correct (Fig. 20-11).

Thus the use of bottles and pacifiers should be discouraged by the age of 18 months. After this age, changes in the oral structures have been noted and are more likely to be permanent. Counseling parents during the neonatal period not to put their infants to bed with a bottle, but rather to hold them during all feedings, is probably one of the best ways to prevent later difficulties with weaning. Such practices also prevent the development of nursing bottle caries (see Fig. 20-42).

Therapy

Clinical management of harmful oral habits should be customized to the child's age. Obviously, harsh measures to discourage digit sucking in a 2-year-old are not justified and may be counterproductive. Children who receive frequent criticism for thumb sucking are probably more likely to cling to the habit than are those whose families ignore it. However, when the habit persists beyond a reasonable age, calm discussions with the child concerning feelings related to the sucking and the physical damage possible if it continues often produce the desired results. When a child has expressed a strong will to cease sucking but is unable to accomplish this goal without help, appliance therapy by a dental professional may be indicated. Referral for oral evaluation and consultation is appropriate after the child has passed the appropriate age of the behavior pattern involved (e.g., older than 5 years of age for digit-sucking habits or 18 months for pacifiers).

Natal and Neonatal Abnormalities

Teeth

Teeth that are present in the oral cavity at birth are called *natal teeth*, whereas those erupting during the neonatal period are called *neonatal teeth*. The incidence of natal teeth has been reported to be approximately 1 in 2000 births. Although seen in normal infants, this anomaly is more frequent in patients with cleft palate (Fig. 20-12) and is often associated with the following syndromes: Ellis-van Creveld, Hallermann-Streiff, and pachyonychia congenita. The majority of such teeth are true primary teeth, but occasionally they are supernumerary. Some are abnormal, with either hypoplastic defects or poor crown or root development. Natal teeth may cause feeding problems for both the infant and mother. Ulceration

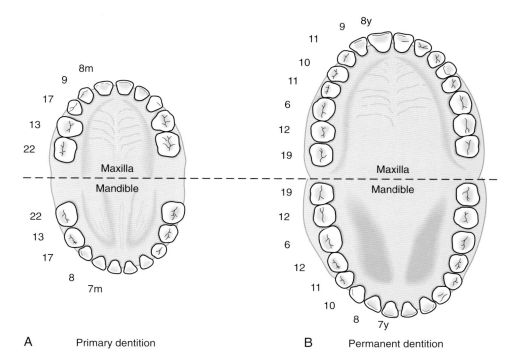

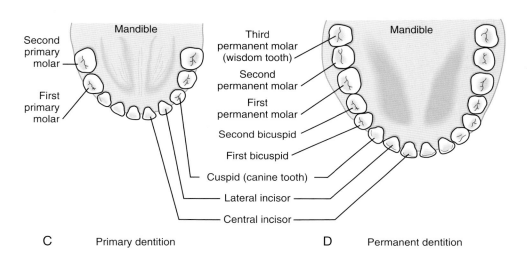

Figure 20-9. Artist's illustrations of the primary and permanent dentition. **A** and **B**, The numbers represent the average age of eruption for the teeth, indicated in months for the primary teeth and years for the permanent dentition. **C** and **D**, The names of specific teeth in the primary and permanent dentition are shown.

A   Primary dentition

B   Permanent dentition

C — Primary dentition

Second primary molar
First primary molar
Mandible

D — Permanent dentition

Third permanent molar (wisdom tooth)
Second permanent molar
First permanent molar
Second bicuspid
First bicuspid
Cuspid (canine tooth)
Lateral incisor
Central incisor
Mandible

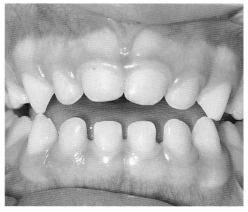

Figure 20-10. Changes in the bite often occur as the result of prolonged digit sucking. This child's upper arch has been narrowed, and an anterior open bite is developing.

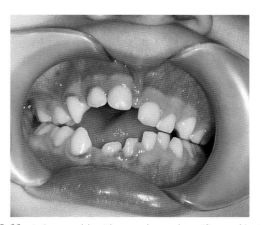

Figure 20-11. A 2-year-old with a prolonged pacifier-sucking habit has severe deformity of the alveolar arches and teeth caused by the extrinsic force of the pacifier-sucking action.

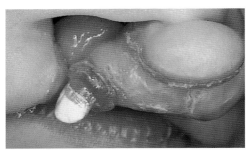

Figure 20-12. A natal tooth associated with cleft palate. Extraction is necessary only if it is of abnormal morphology or causes feeding difficulties.

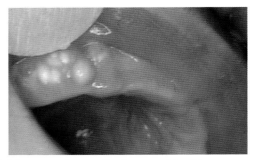

Figure 20-14. Gingival cysts. The firm, grayish-white mucous gland cysts on the buccal aspect of the alveolar ridges are called *Bohn nodules.*

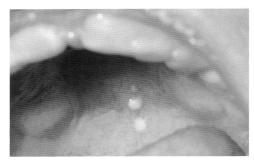

Figure 20-13. Gingival cysts. The small, whitish cystic lesions seen along the midpalatine raphe are called *Epstein pearls.*

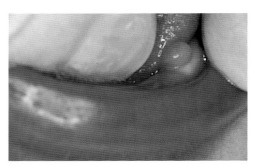

Figure 20-15. Dental lamina cyst. These cysts are found on the alveolar ridge and usually occur singly.

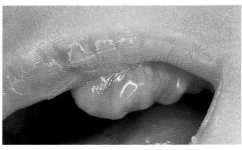

Figure 20-16. Congenital epulis. This 4-day-old patient has a benign tumor of the anterior maxilla.

of the ventral surface of the tongue by sharp tooth edges (Riga-Fede disease) may develop if natal teeth remain in the oral cavity. This condition is usually transient, but in persistent cases symptomatic treatment or extraction of such teeth may be indicated. Most normal-appearing natal teeth can be retained, but those that are supernumerary, abnormal, or very loose may have to be removed.

Gingival Cysts in the Newborn

Gingival cysts of the oral cavity are small, single or multiple superficial lesions that are formed by tissues trapped during embryologic growth and occur in about 80% of newborns. They are asymptomatic, do not enlarge, seldom interfere with feeding, and usually exfoliate within a few weeks.

Three types of cysts exist:
1. *Epstein pearls* are keratin-filled cystic lesions lined with stratified squamous epithelium. They appear as small, whitish lesions along the midpalatine raphe and contain no mucous glands (Fig. 20-13).
2. *Bohn nodules* are mucous gland cysts, often found on the buccal or lingual aspects of the alveolar ridges and occasionally on the palate. They are multiple, firm, and grayish white in appearance. Histologically they show mucous glands and ducts (Fig. 20-14).
3. *Dental lamina cysts* are found only on the crest of the alveolar mucosa. Histologically, these lesions are different because they are formed by remnants of dental lamina epithelium. They may be larger, more lucent, and fluctuant than Epstein pearls or Bohn nodules and are more likely to occur singly (Fig. 20-15).

Congenital Epulis in the Newborn

This benign, soft tissue tumor is seen on the alveolar mucosa at birth or shortly after. It is usually found on the anterior maxilla as a pedunculated swelling (Fig. 20-16) but may appear on the mandible or occasionally on both

jaws. The mass is firm on palpation, and the overlying mucosa appears normal. Histologically, sheets of large granular cells are seen. Differential diagnosis should include rhabdomyoma and melanotic neuroectodermal tumor of infancy. The lesion is amenable to conservative surgical excision, and recurrence is infrequent.

Melanotic Neuroectodermal Tumor of Infancy

This benign yet aggressive tumor develops during the first year of life and is often found on the anterior maxilla in association with unerupted or erupted teeth. It often bulges and destroys the alveolar bone, thus displacing the associated primary tooth. The tumor mass is grayish blue, firm on palpation, and spherical in shape (Fig. 20-17). Careful surgical removal is effective, and recurrence is unusual.

Developmental Abnormalities

Soft Tissue Abnormalities

Geographic Tongue (Benign Migratory Glossitis)
This painless condition is characterized by inflamed, irregularly shaped areas on the dorsum of the tongue that

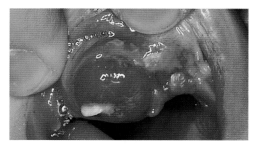

Figure 20-17. Melanotic neuroectodermal tumor. This benign but locally aggressive tumor of the anterior maxilla has produced elevation of the lip and displaced a primary tooth.

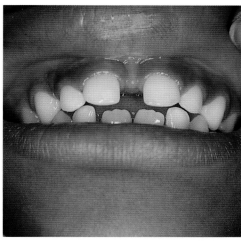

Figure 20-19. Large diastema (excessive spacing) between the front teeth secondary to an inferiorly positioned maxillary frenum.

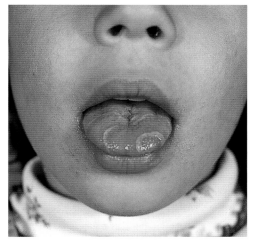

Figure 20-18. Characteristics of benign migratory glossitis (geographic tongue), which is a chronic and often recurring condition affecting the filiform papillae of the tongue. Lesions are red, slightly depressed, and bordered by a whitish band.

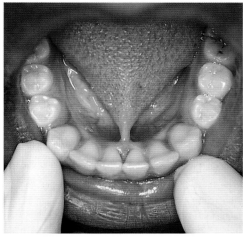

Figure 20-20. Ankyloglossia. This extremely short lingual frenulum with a high insertion point on the gingival margin is an indication for surgical intervention.

are devoid of filiform papillae. Lesions are red, slightly depressed, and bordered by a whitish band (Fig. 20-18). Spontaneous healing followed by the formation of similar lesions elsewhere on the tongue results in a migrating appearance. Etiology is unknown; however, strong association with stress and allergies is suspected. Although benign, the course of this disorder may be prolonged for months, and it may recur.

Abnormalities of the Frenula

During embryonic life, the maxillary labial frenulum extends as a band of tissue from the upper lip over and across the alveolar ridge and into the incisive (palatine) papilla. Postnatally, as the alveolar process increases in size, the labial frenulum separates from the incisive papilla and becomes relatively smaller. With the eruption of primary and later permanent teeth, the frenulum attachment moves apically and further atrophies as a result of vertical growth of the alveolar process. The developmental gap (diastema) between the maxillary central incisors tends to close with the full eruption of the maxillary permanent canines. Occasionally the maxillary frenulum fails to atrophy and the diastema persists (Fig. 20-19). The mandibular midline frenulum only rarely maintains a lingual extension and therefore only rarely causes a diastema between the mandibular central incisors.

The lingual frenulum extends almost to the tip of the tongue in early infancy and then gradually recedes. Occasionally, ankyloglossia (tongue tie) is seen (Fig. 20-20), but this is rarely associated with feeding or speech difficulties. Various surgical procedures have been advocated to correct this condition. In general, frenulectomy is seldom indi-

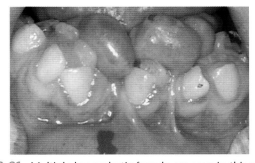

Figure 20-21. Multiple hyperplastic frenula are seen in this patient with orofaciodigital syndrome. These frenula interfered with the eruption of teeth, causing rotation and crowding.

cated and should be recommended only after appropriate justification. Congenital anomalies may include an enlarged frenulum, labiolingual frenulum extensions, or supernumerary frenula as seen in orofaciodigital syndrome (Fig. 20-21).

Gingival Hyperplasia

Generalized gingival hyperplasia is a fairly common nonspecific pathologic entity. This disorder is frequently a complication of drug therapy, as is seen with phenytoin and cyclosporine. Gingival hyperplasia may also be idiopathic or genetically transmitted as in familial fibromato-

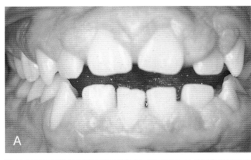

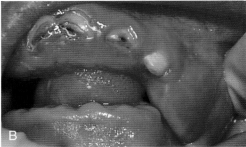

Figure 20-22. Phenytoin-induced gingival overgrowth. **A,** A typical gingival response (hyperplasia) to chronic phenytoin ingestion. Similar gum changes can result from cyclosporine therapy. **B,** Severe overgrowth. The firm, hyperplastic gingival tissues have completely covered the posterior teeth and are interfering with mastication.

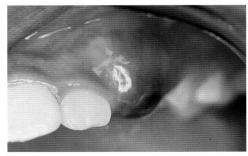

Figure 20-23. Eruption hematoma. A bluish, fluid-filled, fluctuant swelling can be seen over the crown of an erupting maxillary cuspid. The lesion resolved without treatment when the tooth erupted.

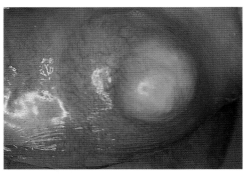

Figure 20-24. A mucocele on the lower lip with the characteristic translucent coloration secondary to fluid retention.

sis. Differentiation of various types of hyperplasia must be based on thorough physical evaluation and appropriate medical history. Histopathologically, it is impossible to differentiate among these various disorders; therefore the final diagnosis and recommendations for therapy should be based on all available clinical data and an appropriate dental consultation.

Phenytoin-Induced Gingival Hyperplasia. The administration of phenytoin over a period of time frequently causes generalized hyperplasia of the gingivae (Fig. 20-22A and B). The gingiva may become secondarily inflamed, edematous, and boggy, especially if proper oral hygiene is not practiced. The severity is often related to the degree of local irritation, stemming from poor oral hygiene, mouth breathing, caries, or poor occlusion (alignment). Because hyperplasia tends to recur after surgical excision, gingivectomy is usually reserved for those patients whose overgrowth interferes with function and for those whose therapy has been discontinued.

Cyclosporine-Induced Gingival Hyperplasia. Cyclosporine has been used primarily in treating patients after organ transplants. The drug has been demonstrated to directly increase cellular growth of gingival fibroblasts. It also increases the production and retention of collagen. Further, this agent's immunosuppressive action may predispose gingival tissues to invasion by microorganisms, thereby increasing inflammatory changes. Although meticulous oral hygiene reduces inflammation, it has no significant effect on the degree of hyperplasia.

Fibromatosis Gingivae. This rare, genetically determined condition may be clinically evident at birth and in such instances may prevent or slow subsequent dental eruption. The clinical manifestations include the generalized presence of firm fibrous tissue that extends around the crowns of involved teeth. Inflammation, when present, is usually secondary.

Surgical excision of excessive tissues is usually indicated, but recurrence is a distinct possibility.

Idiopathic Gingival Hyperplasia. Different types of patients, often with significant systemic illnesses or syn-

dromes, may manifest generalized gingival enlargements. These may primarily involve the gingival tissues or may sometimes be related to underlying thickening of cortical bone, which causes gingival hyperplasia by impeding dental eruption. Each of these cases must be evaluated individually for possible etiology and appropriate treatment.

Eruption Cysts (Eruption Hematoma)

An eruption cyst is a fluid-filled swelling, nontender in the majority of cases, over the crown of an erupting tooth. When the follicle is dilated with blood, the lesion takes on a bluish color and is termed an *eruption hematoma* (Fig. 20-23). Although the eruption cyst is a superficial form of dentigerous cyst, it rarely impedes eruption. Surgical exposure of the crown is seldom necessary. Rarely, such a cyst may become secondarily infected. In such cases, patients complain of headache or facial pain and the cyst is tender on palpation. Incision and drainage are required when infection has developed.

Mucocele and Ranula

A mucocele is a painless, translucent or bluish lesion of traumatic origin, most often involving minor salivary glands of the lower lip (Fig. 20-24). The lesion may alternately enlarge and shrink. The treatment of choice is surgical excision of the lesion and the associated minor salivary gland.

A simple ranula is a retention cyst in the floor of the mouth that is confined to sublingual tissues superior to the mylohyoid muscle. It appears clinically as a bluish, transparent, thin-walled, fluctuant swelling (Fig. 20-25). Herniation of the ranula through the mylohyoid muscle results in a cervical or plunging ranula that becomes more apparent in the oral cavity with the muscle contraction associated with jaw opening. Simple incision and drainage of the ranula is not an acceptable treatment because healing is followed by recurrence. Marsupialization by

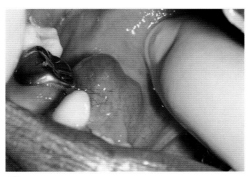

Figure 20-25. Ranula. The bluish, fluctuant swelling in the floor of the mouth is a retention cyst associated with trauma to a salivary duct.

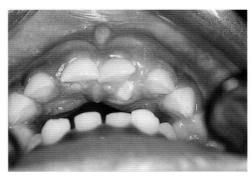

Figure 20-27. Hyperdontia. Erupted supernumerary tooth lingual to the maxillary central incisor in the deciduous dentition.

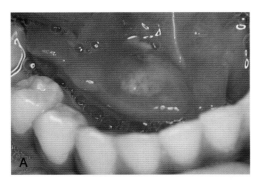

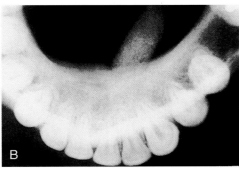

Figure 20-26. Salivary calculus. **A,** This sialolith obstructing a salivary duct is observed in the floor of the mouth. **B,** A dental radiograph of the sublingual space reveals the size and location of the salivary calculus.

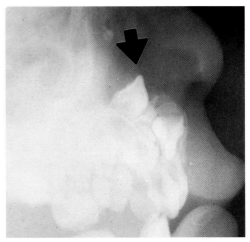

Figure 20-28. Supernumerary nasal tooth. A lateral radiograph of the maxilla shows a supernumerary tooth *(arrow)* erupting through the floor of the nasal cavity in a child with cleft palate who had recurrent epistaxis.

suturing the edges of the opened cystic wall to the mucous membrane is the recommended treatment. The plunging ranula must be removed in its entirety along with the associated salivary gland to avoid recurrence.

Salivary Calculus (Sialolithiasis)

Formation of a salivary calculus is rare in the pediatric population, but when it does occur it may affect either the Wharton or Stenson duct (Fig. 20-26A). Partial obstruction of the duct results in pain and enlargement of the gland, especially at mealtime. Although palpation of the stone may be possible, dental radiographs confirm the diagnosis and give appropriate information about its size and location (Fig. 20-26B). Larger salivary stones wedged within the ducts may cause localized irritation and secondary infection. If the calculus cannot be manipulated through the duct, surgical intervention may be necessary.

Hard Tissue Abnormalities

Hyperdontia and Hypodontia

Variations in tooth number include both hyperdontia and hypodontia. Supernumerary teeth occur in about 3%

of the normal population, but patients with cleft lip and/ or cleft palate and cleidocranial dysostosis have a significantly higher incidence. The most common site is the anterior palate (Fig. 20-27). Supernumerary teeth may have the size and morphology of adjacent teeth or may be small and atypical in shape. They may erupt spontaneously or remain impacted. Early consideration of removal is justified because of complications such as impeded eruption, crowding, or resorption of permanent teeth; cystic changes; or ectopic eruption into the nasal cavity, the maxillary sinus, or other sites (Fig. 20-28).

Congenital absence of teeth is more often seen in the permanent dentition than in the primary. Most frequently missing are third molars, second premolars, and lateral incisors. Hypodontia is frequently associated with several ectodermal syndromes such as anhidrotic ectodermal dysplasia and chondroectodermal dysplasia (Fig. 20-29).

Alterations in Tooth Size and Shape

Teeth that are smaller or larger than normal are termed *microdonts* and *macrodonts,* respectively. These teeth are genetic anomalies. They are clinically significant when a discrepancy in tooth size and dental arch length results in severe crowding or spacing of the teeth. Size abnormalities are often localized to one tooth or to a small group of teeth (Fig. 20-30).

Variations in shape also result from the joining of teeth or tooth buds. Fusion is the joining of two tooth buds by the dentin. Concrescence is the joining of the roots of two or more teeth by cementum. Gemination (twinning) results from the incomplete division of one tooth bud,

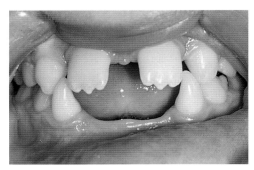

Figure 20-29. Hypodontia. The congenital absence of teeth is seen in this patient with hereditary ectodermal dysplasia. This phenomenon may be an isolated anomaly or a manifestation of several syndromes.

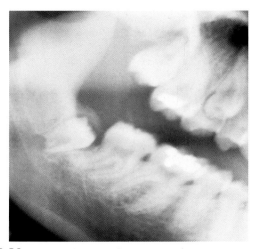

Figure 20-30. A microdont can be seen on this panoramic radiograph near the second molar. Microdonts are often seen in the maxillary lateral incisor region.

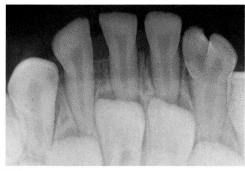

Figure 20-31. Radiograph demonstrates gemination (twinning), the incomplete division of a tooth bud resulting in a tooth with a large, notched crown and a single root.

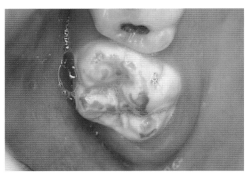

Figure 20-32. Hypocalcification. This 6-year-old patient exhibits early signs of hypocalcification of his permanent molars. Chalky white spots indicate poor calcification of the enamel.

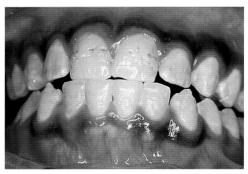

Figure 20-33. Amelogenesis imperfecta, hypoplastic type. This process results in generalized pitting of the enamel.

resulting in a large crown with a notched incisal edge and a single root (Fig. 20-31).

Hypoplasia and Hypocalcification

Numerous local and systemic insults are capable of causing the enamel defects of hypoplasia and hypocalcification. The most common etiologic factors are local infection such as an abscessed primary tooth, which, when not diagnosed and treated promptly, may damage the enamel of its developing permanent counterpart. Other causes include systemic infections with associated high fever; trauma such as intrusion of the primary tooth; and chemical injury, of which excessive ingestion of fluoride is an example. Other etiologic factors include nutri-

tional deficiencies, allergies, rubella, cerebral palsy, embryopathy, prematurity, and radiation therapy. Hypoplasia results from an insult during active matrix formation of the enamel and clinically manifests as pitting, furrowing, or thinning of the enamel (see Fig. 20-33). Hypocalcification results from an insult during mineralization of the tooth and is seen as opaque, chalky, or white lesions (Fig. 20-32).

Heritable Defects of Enamel and Dentin

Amelogenesis Imperfecta. *Amelogenesis imperfecta* is the term used to describe a group of genetically determined defects that involve the enamel of primary and permanent teeth without affecting dentin, *pulp*, or cementum. Although the types of amelogenesis imperfecta are numerous, the major defect in each is hypoplasia, hypomaturation, or hypocalcification. The hypoplastic type results in thin, pitted, or fissured enamel (Fig. 20-33). Hypomaturation manifests as discolored enamel of full thickness but decreased hardness that tends to chip away slowly, exposing underlying dentin. Radiographic evaluation demonstrates the decreased density of enamel. In the hypocalcified form the enamel is chalky, variable in color, and quickly erodes (Fig. 20-34). Depending on the type of amelogenesis imperfecta, inheritance may be autosomal dominant, autosomal recessive, or X-linked.

Dentinogenesis Imperfecta. Dentinogenesis imperfecta results in dentin defects and is usually inherited as an autosomal dominant trait. The most common manifestation is opalescent dentin, which may be associated with osteogenesis imperfecta (see Chapter 21). Due to variable phenotypic expression, teeth may be blue, pinkish-brown, or yellowish brown in color and have an opalescent sheen (Fig. 20-35). In any given patient, individual teeth may be variably affected. Despite normal enamel morphology, patients tend to have relatively rapid attrition or

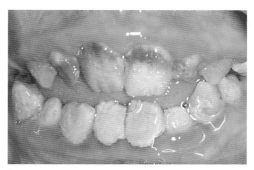

Figure 20-34. Amelogenesis imperfecta, hypocalcified type. The enamel defects result in discoloration and erosion caused by errors in the mineralization stage of tooth development and secondary staining.

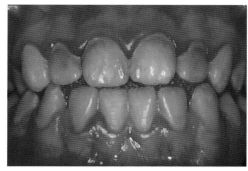

Figure 20-36. Extrinsic discoloration. The green stain seen on the gingival third of the incisors is associated with poor oral hygiene.

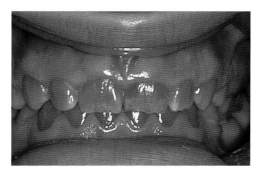

Figure 20-35. Dentinogenesis imperfecta. The bluish, opalescent sheen on several of these teeth results from genetically defective dentin. This condition may be associated with osteogenesis imperfecta.

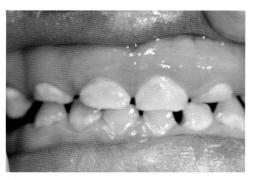

Figure 20-37. Hepatic discoloration. Generalized intrinsic discoloration of the primary teeth is seen in this patient with biliary atresia.

wearing down of the crowns, although the rate of wear can be quite variable. The roots are shortened, and the *pulp* cavities are calcified. Primary teeth are more severely affected than the permanent, although permanent teeth are prone to develop enamel fractures, which can chip or flake off.

Discoloration

Three major types of tooth discoloration are frequently observed: (1) discoloration from stains that adhere externally to the surfaces of the teeth (extrinsic); (2) discoloration from various pigments that are incorporated into the tooth structure during development (intrinsic); and (3) intrinsic discoloration secondary to hereditary defects, which was discussed previously.

Extrinsic Discoloration

Extrinsic discoloration is primarily limited to patients with poor oral hygiene, those receiving certain medications, those who heavily consume stain-containing foods or drinks, or those who smoke or chew tobacco or other substances. It occurs more often at certain locations, especially on the gingival third of the exposed crown. Diagnosis requires appropriate medical, dental, and dietary histories with emphasis on oral hygiene, food and drug intake, and tobacco habits. Treatment includes scaling, dental prophylaxis and polishing, and the practice of regular oral hygiene. The use of abrasive toothpaste can cause excessive wear of the enamel and should be avoided.

Brownish-black stain on the lingual surfaces of anterior and posterior teeth is most common among young children who are taking liquid oral iron supplements and

among adolescents who are smokers and tea drinkers. Green stain on the labial surfaces of the anterior maxillary teeth is common among children with poor oral hygiene. The source is usually chromogenic bacteria and fungi (Fig. 20-36). Orangeish-red stain is unusual, but when it does occur it can be found around the gingival third of the exposed crown. This stain often results from antibiotic intake, which causes a temporary shift in the oral flora.

Intrinsic Discoloration

Intrinsic discoloration is usually induced during the calcification of dentin and enamel by excessive levels of the body's natural pigments such as hemoglobin and bile or by pigments introduced by the intake of chemicals such as fluorides or tetracyclines. Occasionally, isolated intrinsic discoloration occurs as a result of pulpal necrosis, pulpal calcification, or internal resorption.

Hepatic Discoloration

Generalized intrinsic discoloration of primary teeth is seen in patients with advanced hepatic disease associated with persistent or recurrent jaundice and hyperbilirubinemia (Fig. 20-37). The intensity of discoloration varies and may be related to the severity of the disease. Color ranges from brown to grayish-brown and usually has no clinical significance unless it is associated with significant hypoplasia of the dentition.

Discoloration due to Tetracycline

Teeth stained as a result of tetracycline therapy may vary in color from yellow to brown to dark gray. Staining

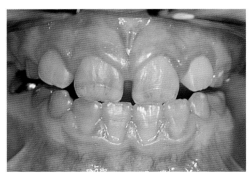

Figure 20-38. Tetracycline discoloration. The severe discoloration seen in this patient is the result of tetracycline administration at a time when calcification of the permanent teeth is occurring.

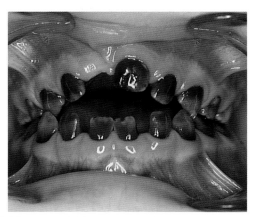

Figure 20-39. The reddish-brown tooth discoloration associated with porphyria.

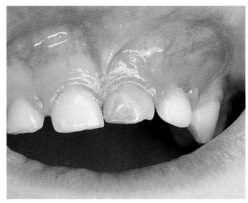

Figure 20-40. Isolated intrinsic discoloration. The central incisor is discolored secondary to trauma. Often, such a change is a manifestation of pulpal necrosis.

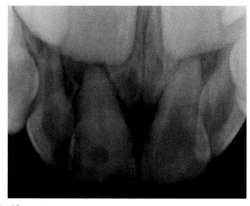

Figure 20-41. Radiographic evidence of dystrophic calcification of the pulp and root canal of the upper right primary central incisor.

occurs when the tetracycline is incorporated into calcifying teeth and bone. The enamel and to a greater degree the dentin that are calcifying at the time of intake incorporate tetracycline into their chemical structures. The severity of discoloration depends on the dose, duration, and type of tetracycline administered. The initial yellow or light brown pigmentation tends to darken with age (Fig. 20-38). Tetracyclines readily cross the placenta, so staining of primary teeth is possible if tetracycline is taken during pregnancy. Therefore tetracycline should not be prescribed to pregnant women or to children younger than 10 years of age.

Discoloration due to Erythroblastosis Fetalis

Children born with congenital hemolytic anemia caused by Rh incompatibility may exhibit distinct discoloration of their primary teeth as a result of the deposition of bilirubin in the dentin and enamel during primary tooth development. The color ranges from green to blue to orange. No treatment is indicated unless discoloration is associated with significant hypoplasia or hypocalcification. The permanent dentition is usually not affected.

Discoloration due to Porphyria

This hereditary disturbance of porphyrin metabolism may produce a distinct reddish or brownish discoloration of the primary and permanent teeth secondary to deposition of porphyrin in developing teeth (Fig. 20-39).

Isolated Intrinsic Discoloration

Teeth with necrotic *pulps* develop an opaque appearance with discoloration ranging from light yellow to gray (Fig. 20-40; see Fig. 20-47B). Such teeth may develop abscesses, periapical cystic lesions, or chronic fistulas. Pulpal calcification (Fig. 20-41) is often associated with a localized yellow discoloration. Internal resorption manifests clinically as a pink discoloration secondary to loss of dentin thickness.

Caries

The interaction of microorganisms, especially *Streptococcus mutans,* and fermentable carbohydrates results in acid demineralization of susceptible enamel. Caries are seen as yellowish-brown to gray defects in the enamel surfaces of affected teeth (Fig. 20-42). Untreated, carious destruction progresses through the enamel and dentin and with bacterial contamination of the *pulp* ultimately renders the *pulp* necrotic. The deep pits, fissures, and grooves characteristic of the surfaces of newly erupted teeth are at increased risk for developing carious lesions (Fig. 20-43; see Fig. 20-5). Sealing these defects with plastic bonding agents may prevent the initiation of caries. Other preventive methods include brushing and flossing on a daily basis (beginning with eruption of the first tooth) to remove bacteria-containing plaque; implementation of systemic fluoride via the water supply or prescribed supplements; and control of the frequency of intake of fer-

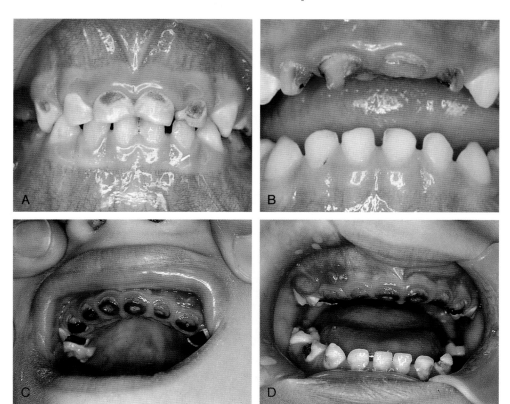

Figure 20-42. Caries. **A,** The typical pattern of nursing bottle caries, with the upper incisors being the first involved. **B,** When badly neglected, severe tooth erosion occurs and periapical abscesses may develop. **C** and **D,** This 3-year-old victim of medical and dental neglect represents the extreme end of the spectrum of nursing bottle caries. When placed in foster care, she was still drinking from a bottle and had never had her teeth brushed or seen a dentist. **C,** Marked discoloration, extreme wear, and carious destruction of her entire maxillary dentition are evident. **D,** All of her upper teeth were abscessed, and her mandibular teeth were severely decayed as well.

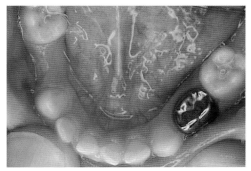

Figure 20-43. The occlusal surfaces of newly erupted molars exhibit varying degrees of pit and fissure depth. The morphology of these patterns makes these teeth more prone to early decay.

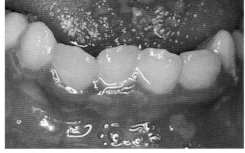

Figure 20-44. Herpetic gingivostomatitis. The ulcerations seen on the oral mucosa were preceded by fever, headache, and lymphadenopathy. Note the erythematous halos around the ulcerations.

mentable carbohydrates, especially those high in sugar and adhesiveness.

Nursing bottle caries involve the primary dentition of the child who is habitually put to bed with a bottle containing milk or another cariogenic (sugar-containing) liquid. This form of caries was originally associated with bottle-feeding only; however, an association with frequent and prolonged nocturnal breastfeeding has become apparent. Carious lesions initially develop on the maxillary incisors and later on the molars and cuspids (see Fig. 20-42A and B). The mandibular incisors are spared by the protective position of the tongue during nursing. The particularly deleterious effect of nocturnal nursing is due to the fact that the rates of salivation and swallowing are decreased during sleep. Hence the liquid ingested has more prolonged contact with dental surfaces and oral flora. Brushing before bedtime and after any nocturnal feedings is especially important in prevention.

An especially severe variant of nursing bottle caries is seen in toddlers whose parents have deferred weaning until well after 1 year of age, continued to provide them with nighttime bottles, and failed to ensure regular brushing and to seek dental care for their children. In such cases

decay is extensive and deep, the teeth show signs of wearing down, and numerous abscesses are found (see Fig. 20-42C and D). This constitutes significant dental neglect, and these children often must undergo multiple dental extractions.

Infections

Viral Infections

Herpetic Gingivostomatitis

Primary herpetic gingivostomatitis, caused by herpes simplex type 1 virus, is an extremely painful disease that affects children, especially those between the ages of 6 months and 3 years. The vesicular lesions of the lips, tongue, gingivae, and oral mucosa are preceded by fever, headache, regional lymphadenopathy, and gingival hyperemia and edema. These lesions tend to rupture quickly, leaving shallow ulcerations covered by a gray membrane and surrounded by an erythematous halo (Fig. 20-44; see also Fig. 12-10). The inflamed gingivae are friable and

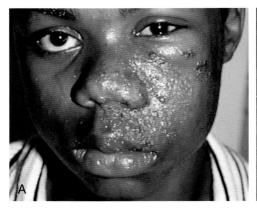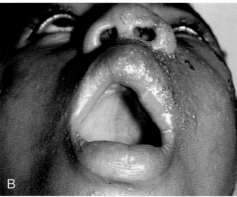

Figure 20-45. Herpes zoster. This patient's infection involved the trigeminal nerve including the nasociliary branch. The extraoral **(A)** and the intraoral **(B)** lesions stop at the midline.

bleed easily. Lesions heal spontaneously in 1 to 2 weeks without scarring. Because inflammation makes brushing too painful, oral hygiene should be maintained using a preparation such as chlorhexidine or glycerin and peroxide (in very young children) to decrease the incidence of secondary infection. A bland diet and rinsing with viscous lidocaine (in children older than 6 or 7 years) or a solution of equal parts of Benadryl and Maalox, in addition to use of oral analgesics, are indicated to minimize and control pain. In some severe cases, codeine may be required. The use of systemic acyclovir may be indicated in cases with moderate to severe involvement. Topical application of the same drug can be helpful in milder cases.

Recurrent infections caused by reactivation of latent herpes simplex virus are fairly common. Lesions are few in number, and more localized; systemic symptoms are absent unless the host is immunocompromised. Lesions are usually located on the lips, with prodromal symptoms of itching and burning preceding the development of thin-walled vesicles that rupture and become crusty in appearance (see Fig. 12-14). When intraoral lesions occur, they manifest as small vesicles in a localized group on mucosa that is tightly bound to periosteum.

Herpes Zoster (Shingles)

Herpes zoster results from reactivation of the varicella-zoster virus and inflammation of a dorsal root or extramedullary cranial nerve ganglion. Although the disease is seen in otherwise healthy children, it is more likely to occur in the severely debilitated or immunosuppressed child. The patient exhibits a prodrome of malaise, fever, headache, and tenderness along the affected dermatome that may last 3 or more days. This is followed by the extraoral formation of painful, grouped vesicular lesions that rupture to form ulcerations. The oral cavity also may be affected with erosions when maxillary and mandibular divisions of the trigeminal nerve are involved (Fig. 20-45).

Recurrent Aphthous Ulcers (Canker Sores)

Aphthous ulcers are similar in appearance to herpetic ulcers. Precipitating factors include trauma, stress, sunlight, endocrine disturbances, hematologic disorders, and allergies. Infection with viruses and L-forms; immunologic dysfunction or dysregulation; deficiency of iron, trace elements, vitamin B_{12} and folate; and genetic factors have all been postulated as causative but have not been proved so by scientific study. Most likely, etiology is multifactorial. Alternatively, the lesions may represent a final common pathway of a number of different and separate etiologies. Onset is usually during adolescence or young adulthood, and between 5% and 25% of the population

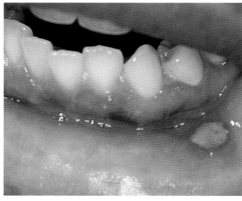

Figure 20-46. Recurrent aphthous ulcers. The ulceration seen on the labial mucosa is surrounded by a characteristic erythematous halo.

is affected at some time during their lives by recurrent ulcers. Unlike herpetic lesions, these ulcerations are not preceded by vesicle formation. They are extremely painful and have a pseudomembrane and an erythematous halo (Fig. 20-46). They can vary in size, number, and distribution. Small aphthae may coalesce into larger lesions. Although any oral mucosal surface may be involved, freely movable mucosa is more frequently involved than tightly bound. Lesions heal in 1 to 2 weeks without scarring. Recurrences have no regular periodicity and are not accompanied by fever or other systemic symptoms. Absent a recognized etiology, treatment is symptomatic, usually with a topical anesthetic/antiseptic preparation. More recently, use of immunomodulating agents is being studied.

A much less common disorder, seen only in children, in which recurrent aphthous ulcers are a feature is Marshall syndrome (also known as *periodic fever, aphthous stomatitis, pharyngitis,* and *cervical adenitis* [PFAPA], first described in 1987. Affected patients have onset before 5 years of age and recurring episodes with a distinct periodicity in both duration of symptoms and asymptomatic interval for each given patient. The average duration of episodes is 5 days (range, 3 to 6 days), and the average interval 28 days (range, 2 to 9 weeks). Episodes tend to begin abruptly with a rapid rise in temperature to 39° C or 40° C accompanied by malaise, chills (not rigors), and often headache with cervical adenitis (seen in 88%) and/or nonexudative pharyngitis (seen in 72%) and/or aphthous ulcers (seen in 70% but thought to be possibly overlooked in some cases). Oral aphthae are three or more in number, shallow, less than 5 mm in diameter and not described as remarkably painful. Cervical nodes rapidly enlarge bilaterally and, although tender, are not warm,

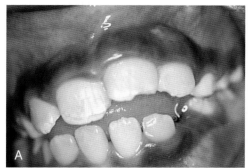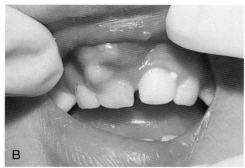

Figure 20-47. Dental abscesses. **A,** An abscess above the left upper lateral incisor developed after an injury in which the patient had chipped that tooth and his central incisor. **B,** This abscess above the right central incisor has ruptured through the gingiva and begun to drain. The tooth is discolored as a result of pulp necrosis stemming from an injury 2 years earlier.

and no overlying erythema, edema, or fluctuance is present. Rhinorrhea, cough arthralgias, and myalgias are not seen. Signs and symptoms tend to clear just as abruptly as they appear, although the aphthous ulcers may take 5 to 10 days to resolve (without scarring). During episodes, affected children look relatively well and between episodes they are not only healthy with normal growth and development but appear less susceptible to the common cold and other infections their siblings develop. The only associated laboratory abnormalities are mild leukocytosis and an elevated erythrocyte sedimentation rate. Cultures are negative, and antibiotics and antiviral agents have no ameliorative effect. Of note, early administration of one to two doses of 1 to 2 mg/kg of prednisone promptly aborts episodes, although its use may shorten the asymptomatic intervals between bouts. Daily administration of cimetidine (used for its immunomodulating properties) for 6 months has stopped episodes in up to 30% of patients; however, they may resume when treatment is discontinued. Tonsillectomy and adenoidectomy has been reported curative in up to 70% of children so treated, and tonsillectomy alone in 50%. Spontaneous resolution has been seen in about 40% after an average of 5 years, but some patients continue to experience recurrences for 15 years or more.

Currently, infection with periodic flares and some form of immune dysregulation are considered the major etiologic possibilities. The disorder is distinguished from cyclic neutropenia by finding normal neutrophil counts at 2-week intervals for 6 weeks and by the absence of unusual and serious bacterial infections. In Behçet disease, the periodicity is not so exact; fever is not so prominent; oral aphthous ulcers are large and heal with scarring; and genital ulcers, arthritis, and uveitis are typical features.

Bacterial Infections

Odontogenic infections are caused by both aerobic and anaerobic microorganisms. Streptococci and staphylococci are isolated most frequently; however, any oral flora or opportunistic microorganism may be involved.

Dental Abscesses

Abscesses are most common in children with neglected dental caries as a result of poor dental hygiene and irregular dental care. Once caries extend to the *pulp*, infection and pulpal necrosis ensue, setting the stage for formation of a periapical abscess. Children with traumatized teeth may go on to develop abscesses if the resulting pulpal hyperemia is so extreme that it causes pressure necrosis, if the neurovascular bundle is severed, or if *pulp* is exposed by a crown fracture.

Periapical abscesses require endodontic therapy or extraction of the offending tooth. The potential for complications makes early diagnosis important, yet frequently this does not occur because often symptoms are insidious in onset and progression and nonspecific in nature. This is in part because the alveolar processes of the mandible and maxilla in young children are fenestrated anteriorly, assisting early decompression of the abscess through the alveolus and gingiva. Patients may complain of headaches as the abscess enlarges and pressure builds up, then of abdominal pain after decompression as the draining pus is swallowed, causing gastric irritation. Later in childhood, abscessed maxillary teeth may intermittently decompress through the floor of a maxillary sinus, producing recurrent sinus infections. Other symptoms may include anorexia, avoidance of chewy foods, halitosis, toothache, a sensitive tooth, or facial swelling. Nonspecific complaints and complaints of referred pain are more common than a toothache in children, some of whom have no overt symptoms but report feeling better after treatment.

On physical examination the examiner may find localized gingival swelling and/or erythema, a gingival abscess, a fistula, or a granuloma (Figs. 20-47 and 20-48A). On occasion there is increased sensitivity to percussion. Left untreated, a periapical abscess of a primary tooth may damage the underlying developing tooth bud. Abscesses may also result in formation of an apical granuloma or a radicular cyst, or they may rupture and spread through the adjacent soft tissues to create a fistula, which drains through the skin (see Fig. 20-48B). In some instances infection can spread into adjacent facial soft tissues, resulting in facial cellulitis (Fig. 20-49). More ominously, the infection may track through lateral pharyngeal, retropharyngeal, or sublingual spaces, threatening the airway and causing sepsis and/or mediastinitis. Rarely, septic thrombosis of the cavernous sinus may result from badly neglected infections.

Pericoronitis

Pericoronitis is a bacterial infection of the gingival soft tissue surrounding the crown of a partially erupted tooth. This occurs when food particles and plaque become trapped under the residual gingiva, stimulating bacterial growth and abscess formation. The third molars are most commonly involved. Symptoms include localized pain and tenderness and occasionally fever and malaise. Erythema and edema are readily apparent on examination (Fig. 20-50A), and an enlarged tender submandibular node

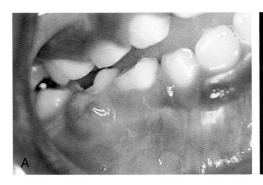

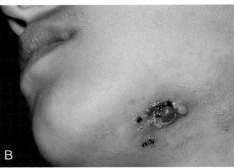

Figure 20-48. A, A deep, neglected cavity in this mandibular molar predisposed to development of a periapical abscess that, after rupture, resulted in formation of a gingival granuloma. **B,** Left untreated, such abscesses can be responsible for this type of extraoral lesion in which infection has spread by way of a fistulous tract to the skin. Extraction of the offending tooth is necessary for resolution of the extraoral lesion.

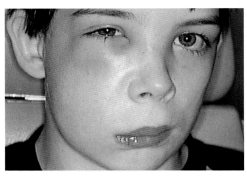

Figure 20-49. Facial cellulitis associated with an abscessed maxillary tooth. Hospital admission for intravenous antibiotics, incision and drainage, and extraction of the abscessed tooth was necessary.

is often found. Figure 20-50B demonstrates the presence of both partially impacted and erupted teeth. The maxillary third molars and right mandibular third molar have erupted into a favorable position. The left mandibular third molar is partially erupted; however, it has been unable to erupt into occlusion. Partially erupted mandibular third molars are often associated with pericoronitis and/or periodontal defects distal to the second molar.

Acute Necrotizing Ulcerative Gingivitis (Vincent Infection, Trench Mouth)

This is a fusospirochetal infection caused by fusiform bacilli and *Borrelia vincentii,* which is seldom seen before the age of 10. Patients experience abrupt onset of fever, malaise, severe mouth pain, and anorexia. The gingivae are reddened, edematous, and friable with necrotic punched-out craters in the interdental papillae. Occasionally the palate and tongue are affected as well. Involved areas bleed readily and become covered with a pseudomembrane (Fig. 20-51). The breath is fetid, and cervical and submandibular nodes are enlarged and tender. Treatment generally consists of gentle dental prophylaxis followed by improved oral hygiene measures and topical peroxide applications. In most cases resolution occurs within several days without the use of antibiotics. Occasionally, secondary infection or severe involvement may necessitate the use of antibiotics; penicillin is then the antibiotic of choice.

Fungal Infections

Candidiasis (Moniliasis, Thrush)
Oral candidiasis results from infection with the opportunistic pathogen *Candida albicans.* This is seen most commonly as a relatively benign infection in infants and in young children who may be on or may have recently completed a course of antibiotic treatment. Less frequently,

it may be seen in immunocompromised or immunosuppressed children or in those with serious underlying systemic diseases. In the latter the infection is likely to be more extensive and severe. Common sites of involvement are the buccal mucosa, tongue, palate, and commissures of the lips (Fig. 20-52). The intraoral lesions of acute infection are soft, elevated, creamy white plaques that do not scrape off easily. Chronic candidiasis, usually seen in the immunocompromised host, can result in marked hypertrophy and fissuring of the tongue mucosa. Although culturing is difficult and not reliable, diagnosis may be made on the basis of clinical findings or examination of a potassium hydroxide (KOH) preparation. Treatment consists of local application of nystatin (miconazole or other antifungal agents for severe or chronic cases) and control of the underlying causes including sterilization of nipples used for formula feedings.

Trauma

Assessment of Patients with Orofacial and Dental Injuries

In evaluating patients with orofacial and dental trauma, key elements of the history include when, where, and how the injury occurred; the child's subsequent behavior; any prior treatment; and general health and tetanus immunization status. In asking about the mechanism of injury, the examiner must determine the forces involved. Did the child trip and fall while walking, or was he or she running; if riding a bike, how fast was he or she going; in the case of falls, from what height, onto what kind of surface? This gives the examiner a better idea of the potential severity of injury and risk of associated injuries. If the mechanism of injury reported is minor and significant injuries are found, if the mechanism does not fit the injuries seen, and/or if a parent tries to prevent an older child from giving a history, the possibility of abuse should be considered.

Physical examination is first directed at determining the adequacy and stability of airway, breathing, and circulation followed by evaluation for associated head and neck injury. When these areas have been cleared and/or stabilized, then the examiner may proceed with the orofacial examination, assessing the extent and nature of injuries. Because the presence of underlying injuries is often belied by the degree and nature of overlying soft tissue trauma, assessment begins with external inspection of facial structures for swelling, deformity, contusions, abrasions, and lacerations. The presence of associated periorbital ecchymoses or swelling; subconjunctival hemorrhage or edema; diplopia; and nasal bleeding should raise suspicion of frontal skull and midface fractures. Meticulous examination of cranial nerve function is essential. This is followed

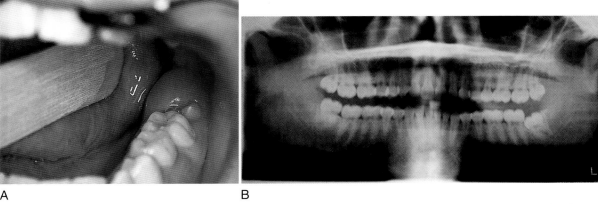

Figure 20-50. A, Pericoronitis involving a partially erupted third molar. Food particles and bacteria have become trapped under the residual overlying gingiva, resulting in inflammation and abscess formation. This condition can occur with eruption of any molar but is most common with partially erupted third molars (wisdom teeth). **B,** Panoramic radiograph demonstrating the presence of erupted maxillary third molars and mandibular right third molar but only partial eruption of the left mandibular third molar.

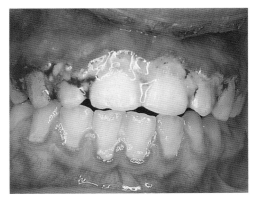

Figure 20-51. Acute necrotizing ulcerative gingivitis. The infected gingiva exhibits localized necrosis and hemorrhage and is covered with pseudomembranes.

by observation of occlusion and jaw motion on opening and closing, checking for deviation or trismus. Older patients can be asked if it feels normal when they bite down; parents of young children can report if the child's occlusion looks normal. The temporomandibular joint should be palpated while the child's facial expression is observed, assessing for tenderness, snap, or pain on opening and closing.

Next, intraoral soft tissues are inspected for evidence of swelling, hematoma, abrasions, and lacerations. Displacement, loosening, and fractures of teeth are noted. Palpation of facial bones and the labial and lingual surfaces of the dental arches and assessment of abnormal maxillary mobility may be best left until last because resulting pain may reduce cooperation. All internal and external lacerations must be carefully inspected to check for injury to underlying neural and ductal structures.

Recommended radiographs include apical and occlusal views for displacement or loosening of a permanent tooth, panoramic and facial bone radiographs for possible mandibular fractures, and a CT scan for suspected maxillary and midface fractures.

Soft Tissue Injuries

A variety of soft tissue injuries including lacerations, contusions, abrasions, perforations, avulsions, and burns may occur. Although soft tissue injuries may occur in isolation, they are often associated with injuries of teeth and supporting bones. Thus any assessment of a soft tissue

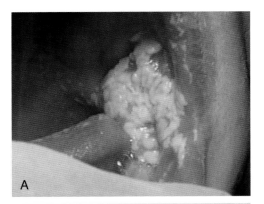

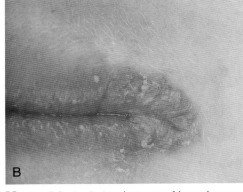

Figure 20-52. Candidiasis. **A,** Involvement of buccal mucosa with white plaque. **B,** Mucocutaneous infection of the commissures of the lips.

injury must include careful attention to the teeth and underlying structures. The injured area should be cleansed of blood clots, debris, and foreign material, then carefully examined to determine the extent of tissue involvement. Mechanical debridement of any ragged, necrotic, or beveled margins may be necessary. Appropriate tetanus prophylaxis should also be considered. Saline rinses, careful attention to oral hygiene, penicillin prophylaxis, and soft diet are mainstays of management of all intraoral soft tissue injuries.

Abrasions

Superficial abrasions usually heal without complications. Extensive abrasions should be covered with a water-soluble, medicated gauze after irrigation. Extensive deep abrasions may require skin grafting.

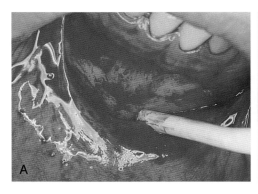

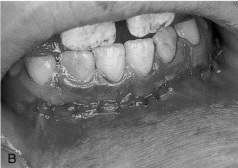

Figure 20-53. Degloving injury, before **(A)** and after **(B)** repair. Such an injury to the oral mucosa requires immediate inspection, irrigation, approximation, and suturing.

Contusions

A contusion, or bruise, usually requires no treatment, and healing proceeds favorably in most instances. However, contusions are often associated with underlying injuries; therefore a careful examination of adjacent structures is indicated.

Perforations

These small, deep wounds caused by sharp objects are fairly common in children, especially as a result of falls with such an object in the mouth. Careful examination of the wound and the object is essential. Following careful inspection and irrigation, larger wounds should be closed in layers; smaller wounds may not require closure. If doubt exists concerning foreign bodies and/or contamination, a drain should be left in place and proper antibiotics prescribed. The possibility of damage to large vessels should be recognized, especially when the perforation involves the posterolateral palate or a tonsillar pillar (see Chapter 23).

Avulsions (Degloving Injuries)

Avulsions of oral soft tissues are uncommon injuries, yet when they occur they may involve deep and superficial tissues (Fig. 20-53A and B). Small avulsions can be treated by undermining and suturing surrounding tissues. Larger avulsions can be treated by reattaching the avulsed tissues or by use of a graft.

Lacerations

Lacerations of facial and oral tissues are common in children. Small intraoral lacerations with well-approximated margins do not require suturing. Bleeding usually subsides spontaneously, and healing proceeds satisfactorily. Large lacerations, through-and-through lacerations, and those associated with extensive, recurrent, or uncontrolled bleeding require careful assessment and surgical closure (Fig. 20-54). To reduce risk of infection, saline irrigation and antimicrobial prophylaxis are indicated for all intraoral lacerations, regardless of whether sutures are required.

Lip lacerations are often caused by penetration of teeth through the labial soft tissues (Fig. 20-55). Thus the adjacent dentition must be carefully inspected for evidence of chipping and for signs of loosening or displacement. If chipping is found, embedded tooth particles should be suspected. These may be difficult to palpate but are easily detected radiographically. If present, they must be removed to prevent infection.

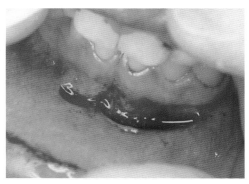

Figure 20-54. This laceration of the oral mucosa—deep and not well approximated—requires immediate treatment and surgical closure.

Because the trauma that results in chin lacerations commonly involves forced occlusion of the dentition with transfer of impact forces to the underlying bone and condyles, these cases warrant assessment of underlying dental and bony structures (see Figs. 20-55, 20-65, and 20-66). Forced occlusion injuries can also produce tongue lacerations. Closure is required for large, gaping wounds with persistent bleeding (Fig. 20-56A), but conservative management is best for smaller lesions (Fig. 20-56B).

Soft palate lacerations require a thorough pharyngeal inspection. The possibility of foreign body entrapment, immediate or delayed vascular injury (particularly when the laceration involves posterolateral structures), or formation of pharyngeal abscesses should be seriously considered. Lacerations involving the labial frenulum of infants are common and require only restriction of lip manipulation and a soft diet.

Burns

Burns involving the oral cavity usually heal rapidly but, when deep, may do so with contracture and scarring. Burns at the angle of the mouth incurred by chewing on an electrical cord (Fig. 20-57) are particularly problematic. After the injury an eschar forms over the necrotic tissue. This tends to separate approximately 10 days later, at which time profuse bleeding from the labial artery may occur. Parents need to be informed of this possibility and instructed on what action to take if it should occur. Splints fabricated from dental materials are important in long-term management to prevent or minimize contracture by maintaining proper anatomic relationships during healing.

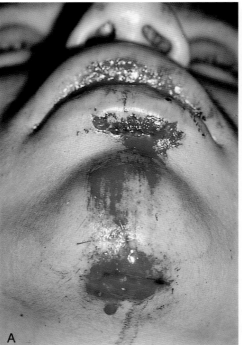

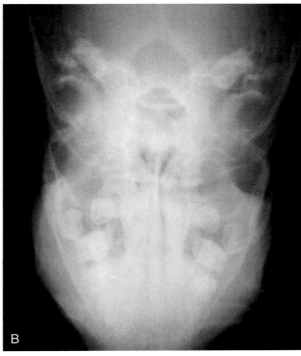

Figure 20-55. **A,** This boy incurred a forced occlusion injury when hit by a car and thrown from his bike. Note the chin laceration and through-and-through lip laceration. **B,** He also had bilateral condylar neck fractures of the mandible. In this radiograph the condyles bend inward at nearly 90 degrees above the fracture lines.

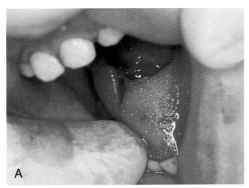

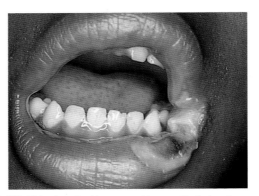

Figure 20-57. This electrical burn was the result of chewing on an extension cord. In this site, delayed hemorrhage after separation of the eschar and deformity with scarring are particular problems.

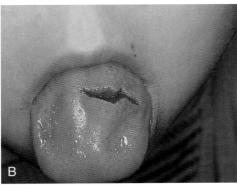

Figure 20-56. Tongue lacerations. **A,** A large gaping tongue laceration in a toddler produced by the upper front teeth being forced through the tissue by a fall with the tongue protruded. This type of injury requires suturing. **B,** This small laceration, though gaping slightly, does not require surgical closure.

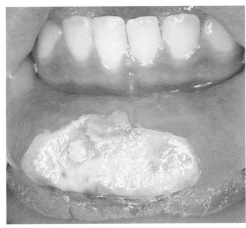

Figure 20-58. Traumatic lip ulceration caused by lip biting after administration of local anesthesia.

Traumatic Ulcers

These painful ulcerations result from mechanical, chemical, or thermal trauma. Injury may be secondary to irritation by objects, trauma during mastication, toothbrush trauma, or abnormal habits. Large ulcerations involving the buccal mucosa or lower lip may be associated with cheek or lip biting after inferior alveolar nerve block (Fig. 20-58). Topical peroxide application (Gly-

Oxide) is useful in cleansing the area. Lesions usually heal without scarring, but secondarily infected lesions may require antibiotic therapy. Identification and elimination of the habit is necessary for resolution of habit-related lesions.

Trauma to the Dentition

As noted earlier, facial injuries in childhood frequently involve the dentition and supporting bones. One prospective study showed that 50% of children had suffered at least one dental injury by age 14. Although falls are the major source in early childhood, bicycle and skateboard accidents, contact sports, fights, and motor vehicle accidents become more prevalent with advancing age. The possibility of child abuse must be considered for all age groups. The risk of facial injuries is relatively high in (1) children with neurologic disorders that impair coordination; (2) children with protruding maxillary anterior teeth; and (3) children with a deviant anatomic relationship, such as an anterior open bite or a hypoplastic upper lip. Preventive measures, such as use of helmets, mouthguards, and seat belts, significantly reduce the incidence and severity of such injuries.

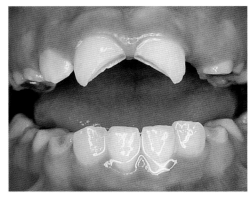

Figure 20-59. These crown fractures demonstrate involvement of enamel and dentin, without exposure of the pulp. Immediate dental referral is necessary to prevent contamination of the pulp through the dentinal tubules.

Potential Complications

Pulp hemorrhage and/or vasodilation of the *pulp* vessels are a common response to concussive injury to a tooth and can lead to development of permanent discoloration within 10 to 14 days. Excessive pulpal vasodilation can actually result in pressure necrosis of the *pulp*. Injuries that produce loosening or displacement of a tooth disrupt the anchoring periodontal ligament. If disruption is mild, there may be no sequelae, although in some cases it stimulates overactive bony repair, ankylosing the tooth in place. When disruption is more severe, the neurovascular bundle can be torn, resulting in *pulp* necrosis, which then predisposes to abscess formation. Finally, dental fractures in which dentin and/or *pulp* are exposed open a pathway for bacteria and predispose to abscess formation. The fracture surface must be sealed and the crown restored emergently.

Several extensive classifications of tooth injuries have been suggested, but for the purpose of this text a more simplified descriptive classification is presented.

Crown Craze or Crack

A significant number of children are discovered during routine physical examination to have "cracks" in the enamel of their teeth. Such cracks are presumably caused by relatively minor trauma or temperature changes. The majority of such teeth are asymptomatic and require no treatment.

Crown Fractures without Pulpal Exposure

Fractures that traverse only the enamel layer often require no treatment other than smoothing down rough edges and ensuring close follow-up (see Fig. 20-47A). However, any fracture of the crown that results in exposure of the dentin requires emergent treatment to prevent infection and subsequent *pulp* necrosis (Fig. 20-59) because oral flora enter the dentinal tubules and rapidly migrate to the pulp. The treatment of choice is to seal the exposed dentin with calcium hydroxide and protect it with an acid-etched resin bandage for a minimum of 2 to 3 months to enhance healing. This procedure should be performed as soon as possible after the injury. As noted earlier, dental fragments are occasionally embedded in the soft tissues of the lip or tongue; therefore appropriate examination

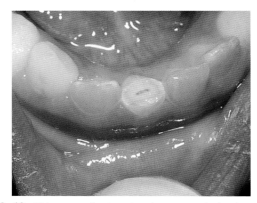

Figure 20-60. This crown fracture involves enamel, dentin, and the soft tissue of the pulp as well. Immediate dental referral is mandatory to save the tooth.

and palpation of these areas are indicated. The presence of such fragments may be confirmed by radiographic examination.

Crown Fractures with Pulpal Exposure

Fractures that traverse all three tooth layers to expose the *pulp* usually involve a significant loss of tooth structure. On physical examination, the fracture surface reveals the pink central *pulp* surrounded by the brown or beige dentinal layer (Fig. 20-60). Severe vertical or diagonal fractures may also result in *pulp* exposure and can at times extend to involve the root (Fig. 20-61). Such teeth must be treated emergently with *pulp* capping, pulpotomy, or root canal therapy, depending on severity.

Root Fractures

Root fractures are less common in the primary dentition, and when they occur they usually require no therapy. Root fractures of permanent teeth may occur with or without loss of crown structure and may be asymptomatic (Fig. 20-62). If a seemingly normal tooth is tender or exhibits increased mobility after trauma, root fracture should be suspected and radiographs obtained. Generally the prognosis is good, and treatment may include splint-

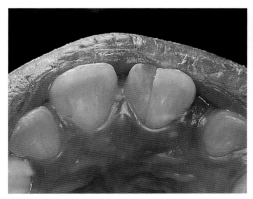

Figure 20-61. A vertical fracture of the upper central incisor extending below the gum line resulted in pulp exposure.

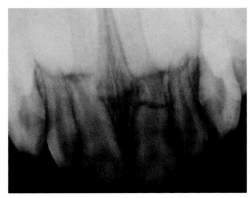

Figure 20-62. This radiograph reveals a root fracture in the apical third of an upper primary incisor. This was suspected clinically because of tenderness and increased mobility.

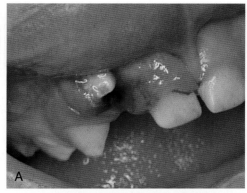

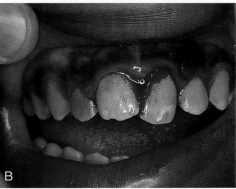

Figure 20-63. Displacement injuries. **A,** This primary lateral incisor was traumatically intruded. Such intrusions usually spontaneously reerupt. **B,** Lateral displacement. The left upper central incisor is lingually displaced, and its crown appears elongated as a result of partial extrusion. This would require repositioning and splinting.

ing the involved segment for 6 to 10 weeks, with or without root canal therapy.

Displacement Injuries

Displacement injuries result in extrusion, intrusion, or lateral displacement (labially or lingually) and are most commonly seen in the primary dentition where the combination of a short root length and a "pliable" bony structure seem to permit displacement to occur (Fig. 20-63A and B). Displacement injuries are often the cause of significant discomfort, bleeding, and possible interference with mastication and occlusion. All result in some degree of disruption of the periodontal ligament. Further, being the result of moderate to severe mechanisms of injury, fractures of underlying bony structures are common associated findings. Because the primary teeth are most vulnerable to these types of injury, there is always a risk of damage to and interference with normal development of permanent tooth buds; therefore immediate care is advised. Treatment may include observation with or without prophylactic antibiotic coverage, immediate correction in cases of lingual displacement that is likely to interfere with mastication, or extraction of the displaced tooth in cases of severe labial or vertical displacement. Most intruded primary teeth reerupt within 6 to 8 weeks with antibiotic coverage, sensible oral hygiene, and an appropriate diet. In general, displaced permanent teeth should be surgically repositioned and splinted, with close follow-up. It is not uncommon for these teeth to require root canal therapy.

Avulsion and Reimplantation

Avulsion is the complete displacement of a tooth from its socket and is seen mostly in preschool and early school-age children. Reimplantation of primary teeth is still experimental and should be done only under selective conditions. However, the prognosis is usually poor, and splinting is not easily carried out.

On the other hand, reimplantation of permanent teeth is an acceptable technique with a relatively good prognosis (Fig. 20-64A and B). The major factors in improving prognosis are as follows:

1. A short period between avulsion and reimplantation, preferably less than half an hour.
2. Appropriate storage of the avulsed tooth (the most desirable "medium" would be the socket itself, followed by saliva and milk).
3. Appropriate irrigation of the surgical site, replacing the tooth into the socket without pressure, and stabilizing it with the use of a resin-bonded splint.
4. Appropriate removal of the *pulp* within 2 weeks as a first step in completing root canal treatment, unless the tooth was immature with incomplete root formation.
5. Removal of the splint within 2 weeks.

It is generally accepted that scraping of the root or the socket is contraindicated because preservation of adherent shreds of periodontal membrane appears to improve prognosis.

Trauma to Supporting Structures

The developing facial bones in the young child are small relative to the calvarium and thus somewhat pro-

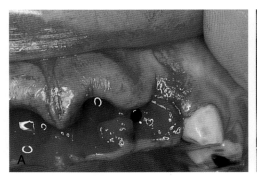
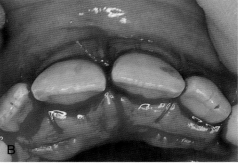

Figure 20-64. **A,** Four permanent incisors have been avulsed. **B,** The teeth have been reimplanted successfully.

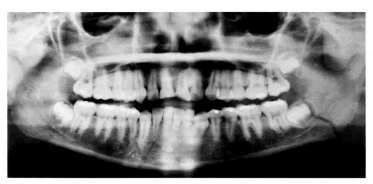

Figure 20-65. A panoramic radiograph reveals a nondisplaced mandibular fracture extending through the wall of the third molar tooth bud. An associated hairline fracture exists near the midline on the patient's right.

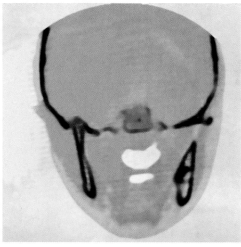

Figure 20-66. CT scan reveals the intrusion of the mandibular condyle into the middle cranial fossa as a result of an extremely severe forced occlusion injury. Careful "pull back" and splinting is a common treatment for this type of injury.

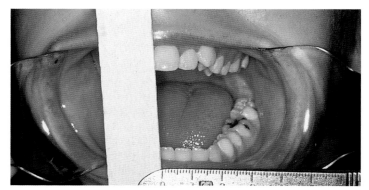

Figure 20-67. A method of measuring deviation of the mandible on opening, showing a shift to the fracture side the width of one lower central incisor.

tected by it. They are compact, spongy, and have greater elasticity, which tends to reduce the risk of fractures. However, the relatively thin outer cortices make alveolar process fractures somewhat more likely with dental displacement injuries, and their growth centers and developing tooth buds serve as weak points and thus are major sites of fractures when they do occur (Fig. 20-65). Finally, their thick periosteum has remarkable osteogenic potential, which speeds healing remarkably. Injuries to these bony supporting structures of the dentition may result from birth trauma (rarely), bicycle accidents, car accidents, various physical and sporting activities, child abuse, and animal bites. Because major forces are required to produce jaw fractures in children, the examiner must carefully search for evidence of associated head and neck injuries (Fig. 20-66) and be vigilant in observing for evidence of expanding hematomas that may later compromise the airway.

Fractures of the Mandible

Excluding nasal fractures, the most common facial fractures in children involve the mandible. The two major mechanisms are forced occlusion and lateral or frontolateral impact. Forced occlusion can produce hemarthrosis of the temporomandibular joint, a compression fracture of the condylar process, or a greenstick condylar fracture (see Fig. 20-55). These injuries can be associated with fractures of the molar crowns. Lateral and frontolateral blows tend to produce fractures of the mandibular body, usually through the wall of a developing tooth bud (see Fig. 20-65). Because the mandible is an arch through which the force of the impact is transmitted, these injuries are often associated with a contralateral fracture of the mandibular body or condyle (see Fig. 20-65). Important diagnostic clues may include ecchymosis, facial swelling, deviation on opening or closing (Fig. 20-67), trismus, and

malocclusion that may be apparent visibly or only subjectively evident to the patient. Severe bilateral mandibular fractures can result in posterior displacement of the mandible and tongue with secondary airway obstruction. Palpation may reveal localized tenderness and hematoma formation, a stepoff, or abnormal mobility with or without gingival tears. Examination of the child with a temporomandibular joint injury may reveal tenderness and decreased motion, clicking, or crepitus when the examiner's fingers are pressed just anterior to the external auditory canal as the child opens and closes the mouth. A panoramic radiograph and a mandibular series should be ordered if there is clinical suspicion of a fracture. If routine views are unrevealing, CT may be called for in certain unusual, difficult, or complex cases.

Management requires careful assessment of the stability and type of erupted dentition, as well as the location of the tooth buds. Nondisplaced fractures with no occlusal abnormalities may require no treatment other than a soft diet. Most displaced fractures can be treated conservatively: first by appropriate reduction, followed by simple intermaxillary fixation or intraoral splints and circumferential wiring (closed reduction). Seldom is open reduction indicated; however, if this technique is used, careful placement of intraosseous holes is essential to avoid damaging the developing tooth buds.

Fractures of the Maxilla and Midface

Other than minor fractures of the alveolar process seen with dental displacement injuries, fractures of the maxilla and midface are uncommon in infants and young children. This is because the relatively large cranial vault provides protection, with the forehead bearing the brunt of most frontal impacts. The elasticity of the facial bones further reduces the risk of fracture. When such injuries do occur in older children and adolescents, they are generally the result of major impacts and are often associated with injuries to the nose, ethmoid sinuses and orbits, and the frontal portion of the skull. As noted earlier, careful attention must be given to the airway, breathing, and circulation, along with assessment for associated head and neck injuries. Exact diagnosis of the location and extent of maxillary fractures is challenging and necessitates a thorough and detailed examination and specialized imaging techniques. CT scan of the midface in both sagittal and coronal planes is the most reliable diagnostic tool.

The LeFort classification of midfacial fractures, devised in 1901, divides them into three groups (Fig. 20-68) as follows:

1. LeFort I primarily involves the maxilla, separating it from the pterygoid plates and the nasal and zygomatic struts (Fig. 20-69).
2. LeFort II, in which the maxilla and nasal complex are separated from the orbits and the zygoma (Fig. 20-70).
3. LeFort III, in which there is complete separation of the midface from the cranial vault at the level of the naso-orbital ethmoid complex and the zygomaticofrontal suture area with extension through the orbits (Fig. 20-71).

Often these fractures occur in combination, and the involved maxilla may be further fragmented. It is not unusual to encounter the combination of a LeFort II on one side and a LeFort III on the other. Sagittal splitting of the palate, often accompanied by palatal laceration, is seen in about 10% of patients. Associated mandibular fractures are common.

The diagnosis of LeFort I fracture is often made by finding abnormal mobility of the maxilla when the maxillary dental arch is grasped anteriorly and a vertical "pull-push" maneuver performed, although on occasion the fracture may be impacted or incomplete and malocclusion without mobility is found. Associated findings may include midfacial swelling or ecchymosis (Fig. 20-72; see Fig. 20-70), epistaxis, malocclusion, and apparent elongation or shortening of the midface.

LeFort II fractures should be suspected when both the maxilla and nasal complex are mobile. Physical findings are similar to those noted in LeFort I fractures,

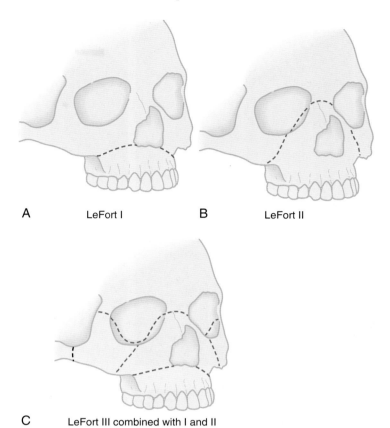

A LeFort I   B LeFort II

C LeFort III combined with I and II

Figure 20-68. Diagrammatic representation of fracture patterns of LeFort fractures. **A,** LeFort I: the fracture separates the maxilla from the pterygoid plates and the nasal complex. **B,** LeFort II: the fracture line separates the maxilla and nasal complex from the orbits and the zygoma. **C,** LeFort III: the fracture line separates the midface from the cranial vault, traversing the zygomaticofrontal sutures and extending through the orbits and the naso-orbital ethmoid complex. Fracture lines of types I and II are shown as well because they are commonly present with the LeFort III.

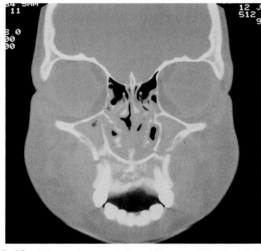

Figure 20-69. CT scan shows a LeFort I fracture. The maxilla is separated from the midface. The degree is greater on the right.

but wrinkling of the skin above the nose may also be seen.

Beyond these findings, patients with LeFort III fractures tend to have prominent periorbital hematomas and swelling and may have subconjunctival hemorrhage, disconjugate gaze, and limited extraocular motion, any of which should prompt careful assessment for associated orbital rim and frontal bone fractures. Up to 25% of patients with LeFort II and III fractures have cerebrospinal fluid rhinor-

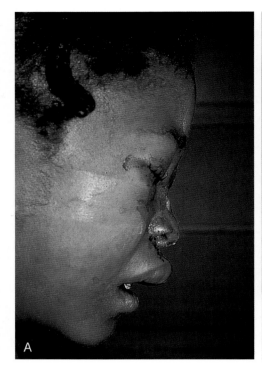
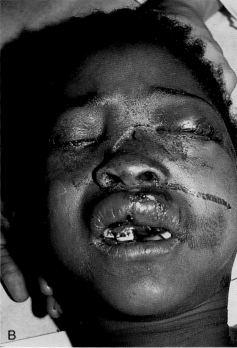

Figure 20-70. LeFort II fracture. This adolescent boy sustained multiple midfacial and naso-orbital injuries in a motor vehicle accident. **A** and **B**, He has a collapsed midface with marked swelling of the upper lip, deviation of the nose, and prominent periorbital swelling and ecchymosis. (Courtesy Joseph Andrews, MD.)

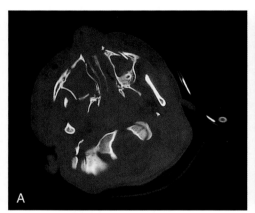
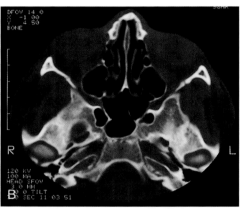

Figure 20-71. LeFort III fracture. This 10-year-old girl was hit by a car while sledding. Clinically, she had bilateral raccoon eyes; severe facial edema with a mobile maxilla; and bleeding from the nose, mouth, and eyes. She had the constellation of fractures that constitutes a LeFort III fracture and numerous other facial and skull fractures. **A**, CT cut shows multiple fractures involving the anterior, posterior, and medial walls of the maxillary sinuses. **B**, Bilateral zygoma fractures are evident in another cut.

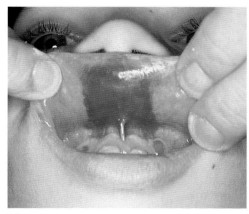

Figure 20-72. Delineated ecchymosis with hematoma formation on the mucosa of the upper lip is a common sign associated with underlying fractures, in this case a fracture of the anterior nasal spine of the maxilla.

rhea and pneumocephaly. Injury to the naso-orbital ethmoid complex can also cause detachment of the medial canthal ligaments, with resultant widening of the intercanthal distance.

Progression of edema and often profuse nasopharyngeal bleeding necessitate frequent reassessment of the patient's airway and circulatory status. The airway may need to be stabilized via orotracheal intubation (or rarely tracheotomy) to protect the patient from aspiration of blood or airway narrowing from edema or an expanding hematoma. Total blood loss must be monitored carefully, the patient typed and crossmatched, and blood replacement initiated when necessary.

Once airway, circulatory status, and head and neck injuries have been stabilized or ruled out, appropriate imaging can be performed and treatment initiated. Primary objectives include control of hemorrhage; reestablishing normal occlusion, vertical dimension, and width of the midface; and immobilization of fractures and restoration of normal fronto-orbital architecture. This often necessitates a team approach. It is preferable to plan and carry out the repair as soon as possible after more serious injuries are stabilized because delays increase infection risk and can make repair more difficult as edema worsens and the bones begin to knit over the first 2 to 3 days postinjury.

Craniomandibular Dysfunction (Temporomandibular Joint Disease)

The term *craniomandibular dysfunction* (CMD) is used to define a set of signs and symptoms that involve the masticatory musculature, the temporomandibular joint (TMJ), or both. Most clinicians and investigators agree that signs and symptoms of CMD may include the following: tenderness or pain of the masticatory muscles, TMJ tenderness, limited or asymmetrical mandibular movements, clicking or crepitation of the joint, and secondary headaches. Reported signs and symptoms are generally mild, fluctuate over time, and exhibit no sex predilection. Their prevalence ranges from 9.8% to 85% of subjects surveyed, with results varying with patient selection, subject age, sample size, and definition of diagnostic criteria. Prevalence has been shown to increase with age. Despite the high frequency of CMD signs and symptoms, it is estimated that only 5% of children and adolescents are in need of treatment. The discrepancy can be attributed to the subclinical nature of many of the signs and symptoms recorded in epidemiologic studies.

The etiology of CMD is multifactorial. Oral parafunctional habits such as bruxism (grinding), bite deviations (malocclusion), trauma to the TMJ or mandible, orthodontic treatments, and history of stress are often cited as etiologic factors. Of these, bruxism and stress (possibly with attendant jaw clenching) are most significantly associated with symptomatic CMD. Trauma, the next most common factor, has been reported to be responsible for TMJ pain in 26% of pediatric CMD patients. We have also encountered a number of young musicians, especially violinists who practice for long periods daily, who have CMD symptoms. Both cross-sectional and longitudinal studies have failed to show a one-to-one relationship between signs and symptoms of CMD and morphologic and functional malocclusion. Hence malocclusion alone is not a primary etiologic factor. Similarly, orthodontic treatment has not been shown to significantly increase or decrease the frequency of signs and symptoms.

Patients presenting with symptoms of CMD should undergo a comprehensive history and examination. The history should include present illness and time of onset of symptoms, their nature, exacerbating and ameliorating factors, and prior therapy; a complete medical history; and a detailed dental history. The latter should note whether there has been a history of treatment under general anesthesia; trauma to the TMJ or mandible; oral parafunctions such as bruxism, thumb sucking, nail biting, or gum chewing; headaches related to clenching of the teeth; and unusually diligent practice with a musical instrument such as the violin, horn, or reed instrument. In addition, family and social history with emphasis on recent changes and potential sources of emotional stress should be obtained. Clinical examination includes inspection of the head and neck; intraoral examination; palpation of the TMJ and masticatory musculature; auscultation of the TMJ during opening and closing; and observation of mandibular movements in all planes (opening, protrusive, and lateral). Significant deviations from normal mandibular motion, tenderness, clicking or crepitus of the joint, or generalized TMJ pain all suggest the need for further evaluation.

Identification and elimination of etiologic factors is of paramount importance in treatment of CMD. Studies on children and young adults suggest that conservative or reversible types of treatment are most appropriate. Such modalities may include physical or behavioral modification therapy, bite splints, and judicious use of analgesics. The application of irreversible treatment modalities such as bite adjustment (selective grinding of the teeth), orthognathic surgical intervention, and orthodontics to correct CMD are not supported scientifically.

Bibliography

American Academy of Craniomandibular Disorders: Guidelines for evaluation, diagnosis and management. In McNeil C (ed): Craniomandibular Disorders. Chicago, Quintessence Publishing, 1990.

Bhaskar SN: Oral lesions of infants and newborns. Dent Clin North Am July: 421-435, 1966.

Christensen RE Jr: Soft tissue lesions of the head and neck. In Sanders B (ed): Pediatric Oral and Maxillofacial Surgery. St Louis, Mosby, 1979.

Long SS: Syndrome of periodic fever, aphthous stomatitis, pharyngitis, adenitis (PFAPA)—what it isn't. What is it? J Pediatr 135:1-5, 1999.

Martin B, Armanazi Y, Bouquot J, Nazif MM: Dental and gingival disorders. In Bluestone CD, Stool SE (eds): Pediatric Otolaryngology, 4th ed. Philadelphia, Saunders, 2002.

Nazif MM, Ruffalo RC: The interaction between dentistry and otolaryngology. Pediatr Clin North Am 28:977-1010, 1981.

Sanders B et al: Injuries. In Sanders B (ed): Pediatric Oral and Maxillofacial Surgery. St Louis, Mosby, 1979.

Schuit KE, Johnson JT: Infections of the head and neck. Pediatr Clin North Am 28:965-971, 1981.

Sonis A, Zaragoza S: Dental health for the pediatrician. Curr Opin Pediatrics 13:289-295, 2001.

Vanderas AP: Prevalence of craniomandibular dysfunction in children and adolescents: A review. Pediatr Dent 9:312-316, 1987.

Walund K, List T, Dworkin SF: Temporomandibular disorders in children and adolescents: Reliability of a questionnaire, clinical examination, and diagnosis. J Orofac Pain 12:42-51, 1998.

CHAPTER 21

Orthopedics

Vincent F. Deeney, Morey S. Moreland,
W. Timothy Ward, and Holly W. Davis

Children with musculoskeletal injuries and afflictions are brought for care because of pain, deformity, or loss of function. Often the clinical challenge lies not so much in recognizing the impaired or injured part, which in most cases is readily accessible to inspection and examination, but in making an accurate diagnosis in order to plan and initiate appropriate treatment. Because of their rapid physical growth and the special properties of their developing bones, children often pose special problems for the clinician.

Musculoskeletal problems in children fall into several general categories:
1. Trauma (discussed here and in Chapter 6).
2. Congenital problems—malformations resulting from genetic factors and from exposure to teratogens during the first trimester, as well as deformations stemming from insults later in pregnancy, many of which are associated with anomalies of other organ systems (discussed here and in Chapters 1, 2, and 15).
3. Infections (see Chapter 12).
4. Inflammatory processes such as the collagen vascular diseases, the vasculitides, rheumatoid arthritis, and inflammatory bowel disease (see Chapters 7 and 10).
5. Metabolic diseases (see Chapters 9, 10, and 13).
6. Neoplastic disorders (see Chapter 11).

This chapter focuses on primary musculoskeletal problems, and the discussion is divided into eight sections: (1) development of the skeletal system, (2) physical assessment, (3) musculoskeletal trauma, (4) disorders of the neck and spine, (5) disorders of the upper extremity, (6) disorders of the lower extremity, (7) generalized musculoskeletal disorders, and (8) sports medicine.

Development of the Skeletal System

The assessment, diagnosis, and management of pediatric orthopedic problems necessitate a clear understanding of the physiology of the growing musculoskeletal system and especially of the unique properties of growing bone. The process of growth begins in utero and continues until the end of puberty. Linear growth occurs as the result of multiplication of chondrocytes in the epiphyses, which align themselves vertically, forming a transitional zone of endochondral ossification in the metaphyses. The shafts of long bones widen, and flat bones enlarge through the deposition and mineralization of osteoid by the periosteum. Hence genetic and congenital disorders that affect connective tissue (and thus the skeleton) tend to cause abnormal growth. Most commonly this results in dwarfism, with varying degrees of deformity. However, in some conditions such as Marfan syndrome, excessive linear growth occurs, resulting in an abnormally tall stature and unusually long fingers and toes.

The terminal arterial loops and sinusoidal veins that form the vascular bed of growing metaphyses have slug-gish blood flow, which increases the risk of thrombosis and of the deposition of bacteria during periods of bacteremia. As a result, there is a greater risk of developing hematogenous osteomyelitis in pediatric patients than in adults. Furthermore, the epiphyseal plates, which are incompletely formed in infancy, are a less effective barrier to extension of infection into adjacent joints, and the relatively thin diaphyseal cortices tend to permit rupture outward under the overlying periosteum. Similarly, penetration of vascular channels through the vertebral endplates into the intervertebral disks makes diskitis more likely than vertebral osteomyelitis in early childhood (see Chapter 12).

A thorough understanding of musculoskeletal development and of the radiographic findings at differing stages is particularly important in the diagnosis and management of orthopedic injuries. At birth only a few epiphyses have begun to ossify; the remainder are cartilaginous and thus are invisible radiographically. With development, other epiphyses begin to ossify, enlarge, and mature in such an orderly fashion that one can estimate a child's age from the number and configuration of ossification centers (Figs. 21-1 and 21-2). The epiphyseal plates (physes), which are sites of cartilaginous proliferation and growth, do not begin to ossify and thereby close until puberty (Fig. 21-3). This process starts and ends earlier in girls than in boys. When skeletal injuries involve sites where ossification has not begun or is incomplete, radiographic findings may appear normal or may not reflect the full extent of the injury. This necessitates greater reliance on clinical findings. MRI can be of assistance in defining unossified or incompletely ossified structures.

Before closure of the physis during puberty, the growth plate is actually weaker than nearby ligaments. As a result, injuries that occur near joints are more likely to result in physeal disruption than in ligamentous tearing (i.e., sprains and dislocations are seen less commonly in prepubescent children than in adolescents and adults). Similarly, avulsion fractures at sites where strong muscular attachments join secondary ossification centers are unique to children and adolescents. When there is displacement of an epiphyseal fracture and the fragments are not anatomically reduced, growth disturbances may occur. Because the epiphysis may not be ossified, radiographs often fail to reveal the injury, and for this reason children with injuries at or near joints must be examined with meticulous care so that epiphyseal fractures are not missed. Clinically, pain and swelling may be detected over the epiphyseal plate region and, less notably, over the joint itself.

The periosteum of a child is much thicker than that of an adult, strips more easily from the bone, and is rarely disrupted completely when the underlying bone is fractured. Because of the immature elements in the rapidly growing skeleton of the child, the bone has more viscoelasticity and can sustain plastic deformation more easily than the adult skeleton. Consequently, a given compressive force that would produce a comminuted fracture in an adult tends to be dissipated in a child in part by the bending that occurs in the more flexible bone of the child. Such a force is thus more likely to result in plastic deformation or to produce an incomplete fracture, such as a torus fracture or a greenstick fracture, in a child.

Thus fracture patterns in children often differ from those in adults. Their fractures can be considerably more difficult to detect clinically and radiographically, and because the growing cells in the epiphyseal plate may be injured, growth disturbances may occur. Children do have advantages, however, in that their actively growing

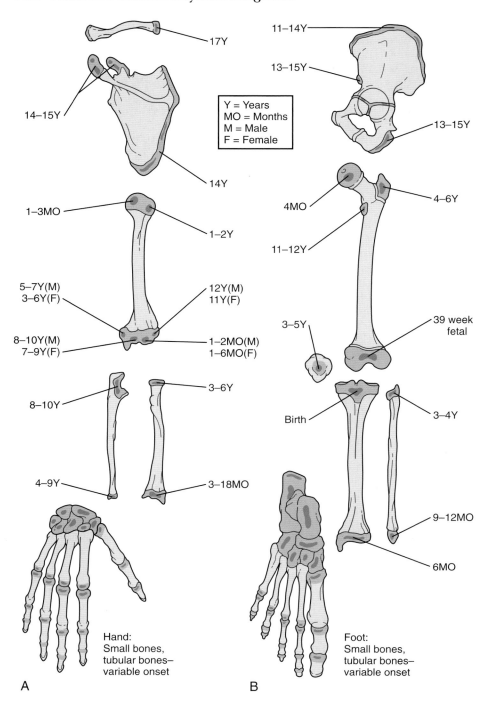

Y = Years
MO = Months
M = Male
F = Female

17Y

14–15Y

14Y

1–3MO

1–2Y

5–7Y(M)
3–6Y(F)

12Y(M)
11Y(F)

8–10Y(M)
7–9Y(F)

1–2MO(M)
1–6MO(F)

8–10Y

3–6Y

4–9Y

3–18MO

Hand:
Small bones,
tubular bones—
variable onset

A

11–14Y

13–15Y

13–15Y

4MO

4–6Y

11–12Y

3–5Y

39 week fetal

Birth

3–4Y

9–12MO

6MO

Foot:
Small bones,
tubular bones—
variable onset

B

Figure 21-1. Ages at onset of ossification. At birth only a few epiphyses have begun to ossify. The remainder are cartilaginous and therefore invisible radiographically. With development, other epiphyses begin to ossify, enlarge, and mature in an orderly fashion, making it possible to estimate a child's age from the number and configuration of ossification centers. This forms the basis for the use of bone age as part of the evaluation of children with growth disorders. When evaluating the radiographs of injured children, it is of crucial importance to bear in mind that fractures involving nonossified epiphyses are radiographically invisible until healing begins (see Fig. 21-56).

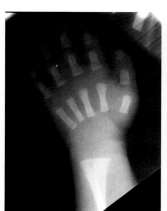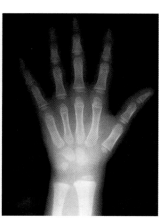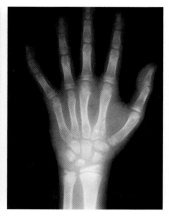

Figure 21-2. Increasing numbers of ossification centers become radiographically visible with age. From left, the hands shown are those of a toddler, a young school-age child, and a young adolescent. Injuries affecting unossified bones or growth centers are invisible radiographically.

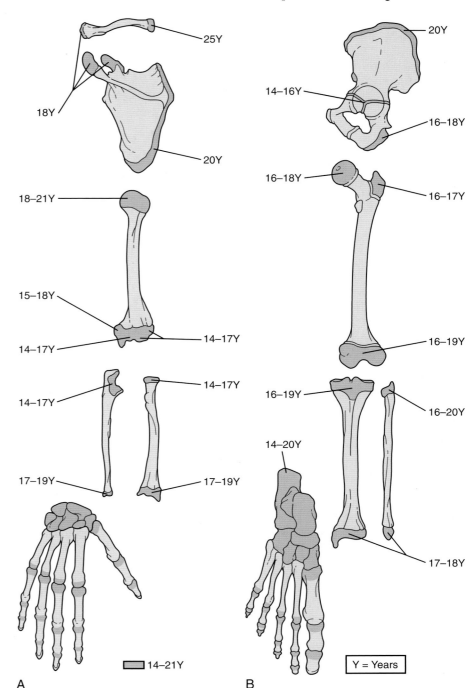

Figure 21-3. Ages at physeal closure.

25Y

18Y

20Y

18–21Y

15–18Y

14–17Y

14–17Y

14–17Y

14–17Y

17–19Y

17–19Y

14–21Y

20Y

14–16Y

16–18Y

16–18Y

16–17Y

16–19Y

16–19Y

16–20Y

14–20Y

17–18Y

Y = Years

A   B

bones heal more rapidly and have a remarkable capacity for remodeling.

Finally, numerous genetic, metabolic, endocrine, renal, and inflammatory processes can affect not only growth and ultimate height but also skeletal maturation—in some cases delaying it and in others accelerating it. Comparison of the patient's actual bone age, as determined by the number of radiographically visible ossification centers, with his or her chronologic age can help in the diagnosis of these underlying disorders.

Physical Assessment

History

Key historical points in the evaluation of problems not resulting from trauma include the following:

1. Age at onset of symptoms
2. Mode of onset
3. Clinical course including the manner and rate of progression and associated signs and symptoms
4. Past medical history with an emphasis on the prenatal and perinatal history in the infant or young child
5. Family history, especially of genetic, metabolic, and musculoskeletal problems

This information helps considerably in narrowing the list of differential diagnostic possibilities.

When the patient's problem is the result of trauma, it is important to obtain the following historical points:

1. The time and place of the accident and whether it was witnessed
2. The mechanism of injury including the degree of force applied and the direction of force, if known (e.g., if a fall, from what height, onto what surface? Was the child running or walking (momentum)? In what posi-

tion did the child land? Was there any head injury or loss of consciousness?)
3. The child's behavior since the time of injury (e.g., decreased movement, guarding, refusal to walk or limping, any altered level of consciousness)
4. Complaint of pain (if so, how severe, and can it be localized?)
5. Prior treatment or first aid
6. Past medical history of serious illness and prior injuries
7. Family history of musculoskeletal problems

This information helps localize the site or sites of injury and potential injury severity, points to the risk of possible associated injuries, gives clues to the possible existence of underlying disorders that may predispose to injury, and may occasionally raise a suspicion of abuse.

Physical Examination

The orthopedic examination involves a systematic assessment of posture, stance, and gait; the symmetry or asymmetry of paired musculoskeletal structures and their motion; muscle strength and tone; and neurovascular status. In pediatrics, the patient's developmental level is a major consideration, not only in terms of the interpretation of findings, but also in terms of the manner in which the examination is conducted. Patience and often some degree of creativity are required on the part of the examiner if the patient is very young. Often, much information can be gleaned from an initial period of observation of the child's demeanor and spontaneous activity. This can be assisted by providing age-appropriate toys for him or her to play with while the history is being taken and by engaging the patient in play (if circumstances permit) before starting the more formal physical examination. This also helps to alleviate anxiety and gain the child's trust, enhancing his or her cooperation. As in all examinations of infants and children, taking time to establish the child's trust in the examiner is helpful. After spontaneous activity is observed, the relevant parts of the orthopedic examination are typically done by region.

A complete orthopedic examination that assesses each bone, muscle, joint, tendon, and ligament is lengthy, detailed, and rarely indicated. Even in multiple-trauma victims and patients whose symptoms point toward an underlying systemic disorder, each region is screened and a full assessment done only of those regions where local musculoskeletal abnormalities are found. Similarly, in patients with focal injuries or deformities, the examination can generally be focused on the region involved, with the clinician bearing in mind referral patterns for pain and the maxim that all extremities "begin at the back." Finally, in performing routine physical examinations on healthy children, after a general screening examination of spontaneous movement, posture, gait, station, and stance, the assessment of the musculoskeletal system is focused on areas at risk for the child's age (e.g., the hip for dislocation in the neonate, the spine for scoliosis in the preadolescent and adolescent).

Regional Musculoskeletal Examination

In the regional examination the area of concern is inspected visually for spontaneous movement, guarding, size, swelling, deformity, and the appearance of overlying skin, and the findings are compared with those for its paired structure. After this, the normal side and then the affected side are gently palpated for warmth, induration, and tenderness. Muscle mass, tone, and reflexes on the affected side are compared with those on the normal side, and the presence or absence of spasm is noted. If asymmetry in muscle mass is detected, the circumference is measured bilaterally at a point equidistant from a fixed bony landmark. The child is then asked to move the extremity or handed objects to get him or her to do so, and active motion is observed. If this appears limited, passive range of motion is tested first on the normal and then on the affected side, taking care not to cause severe pain. Strength is tested against gravity and then against resistance (Table 21-1), being careful to stay within the limits of pain. Then sensation and vascular status are also evaluated.

Joints are further inspected to determine whether there is erythema, obliteration of landmarks that may indicate presence of effusion, evidence of deformity, and position of comfort. Further evaluation to detect joint effusion is done by pressing on one side of a visible joint while feeling for the protrusion of fluid on the other. The joints are palpated to check for evidence of heat and tenderness, range of motion is assessed, and evidence of pain on motion is determined.

Assessment of ligamentous stability around joints is discussed under specific sections of the regional examination. However, it is important to remember that in cases of acute trauma, especially when deformity or hemarthrosis is evident on initial assessment, tests of ligamentous stability should be deferred, the extremity splinted, and radiographs obtained to check for possible underlying fracture.

Axial Skeleton and Upper Extremity Examination

Trunk and Neck. With the examiner in front and the patient standing, the sternocleidomastoid muscles, the bony prominences of the clavicles, and the respective heights of the acromioclavicular joints, nipples, and anterior iliac crests and sides of the chest wall are inspected for symmetry. The patient is then turned and viewed from behind, and the shoulder and scapular height, the muscle bulk of the trapezius muscles, and the height of the posterior iliac crests and of the depressions over the sacroiliac joints are checked for symmetry. Trapezius strength is determined by having the patient shrug his or her shoulders, first against gravity and then against resistance, as the examiner presses down on the shoulders. The muscles supplying the scapula are tested by having the patient press his or her outstretched arms against a wall. Winging of the scapula during this maneuver is suggestive of weakness of the serratus anterior muscle. The line of the spinous processes of the vertebrae is observed for straightness, and the position of the head over the trunk is noted. Normally the head is aligned over the midline of the sacrum.

Next, the sternocleidomastoid and paraspinous muscles of the neck are palpated to assess for bulk, tone, tenderness, and spasm, and the spinous processes of the cervical

Table 21-1 Grading of Muscle Strength

GRADE	PHYSICAL FINDING
0/5	No movement seen
1/5	Muscle can move joint with gravity eliminated
2/5	Muscle can move joint against gravity but not against added resistance
3/5	Muscle can move joint against slight resistance
4/5	Muscle can move joint against moderate added resistance
5/5	Normal strength

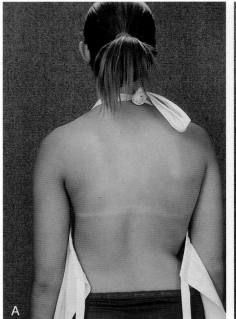
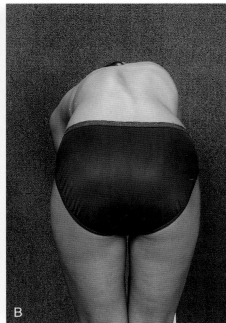
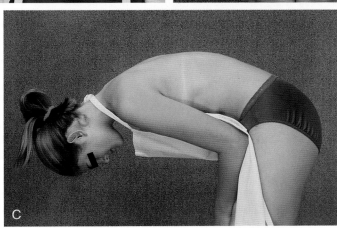

Figure 21-4. Adams Forward Bend test. **A,** Scoliosis can be difficult to detect on observation of the standing patient. **B,** With the child bending forward and observed from behind, it is much easier to appreciate the asymmetrical trunk rotation seen in scoliosis. **C,** Viewing the patient from the side, one can more easily see even subtle degrees of kyphosis and note lack of reversal of normal lordosis.

vertebrae are palpated to assess for tenderness and step-off. In the immobilized trauma patient these observations are made largely with the patient supine on a backboard and then log-rolled onto his or her side. Importantly, in checking for neck injury, the cervical spine can be cleared clinically if the patient is awake and alert and has no complaint of neck pain, no evidence of tenderness or paraspinous muscle spasm, and no extremely painful injury elsewhere. If the patient's level of consciousness is not normal or there is a major distracting injury, the cervical spine cannot be cleared, even if radiographic findings are normal, because spinal cord injury can be present in the absence of bony abnormalities.

Range of neck motion is assessed by having the patient move his or her head. A normal child can touch his or her chin to the chest, extend the neck to look directly above, and bend laterally to 45 degrees. He or she is also capable of symmetrical lateral rotation when turning the head from side to side. Strength is tested by applying pressure to the forehead while the patient flexes his or her neck and to the occiput as the patient extends, and by applying resistance to the opposite side of the head as the patient bends and rotates laterally.

Thoracolumbar Spine. Viewed from the side, the normal child has a lordotic curve in the cervical area with a bony prominence at C7, a mild thoracic kyphosis, a lumbar lordosis, and a sacral kyphosis. Each patient is checked for the presence, absence, or accentuation of these curves. The midline of the back is inspected for evidence of abnormal pigmentation and the presence of hemangiomas, nevi, hairy tufts, dimples, masses, or defects, which may be associated with underlying bony or neural anomalies (see Chapter 15).

Flexion, extension, rotation, and lateral bending of the thoracolumbar spine are primarily motions of the thoracolumbar junction and the lumbar area. Most children can bend forward to touch their toes, bend laterally 20 to 30 degrees (with the pelvis held stable by the examiner's hands on the iliac crests), and rotate 20 to 30 degrees in either direction.

Examination of the back for spinal deformity is assisted by the use of the Adams Forward Bend test (Fig. 21-4). For this, the examiner stands behind the patient, who is then asked to bend forward with arms extended and the palms of the hands together. The surface of the back in the lumbar and thoracic regions is examined for asymmetrical elevation of the paravertebral spinous area, thus indicating a structural rotation of the spine and the possibility of scoliosis (see Fig. 21-4B). The examiner should also note any evidence of missing spinous processes (stepoff) or their deviation from the midline and palpate the paravertebral muscles for spasm and tenderness. Increased kyphosis, especially in the thoracic region, may be detected when viewing the patient from the side (see Fig. 21-4C),

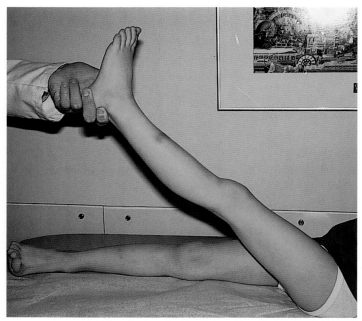

Figure 21-5. Straight leg raising test. With the patient supine, the limb to be tested is grasped behind the ankle and elevated into hip flexion with the knee in full extension. If pain is produced well before 90 degrees of flexion is achieved, the test is positive, indicating irritation of a sciatic nerve root.

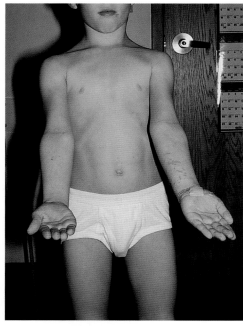

Figure 21-6. Carrying angle. The normal relationship of the extended supinated forearm to the upper arm is not a straight line but involves 5 to 10 degrees of lateral or valgus angulation.

as can lack of reversal of the lumbar lordosis, which may indicate muscle spasm or abnormality of the lumbar spine. Leg length inequality may be evaluated during the upright standing portion of this test (see "Lower Extremity Examination" later) and, if present, should be corrected with appropriate lifts under the short side in order not to cause a false Forward Bend test.

Any examination of the spine must include a neurologic assessment of strength, tone, reflexes, and sensation. The straight leg raising test (Fig. 21-5) can be helpful in demonstrating nerve root pathology in patients with slipped disks, spinal or paraspinal masses, or inflammatory processes. The test is performed with the patient lying supine on the examining table. The limb to be tested is grasped behind the ankle and elevated passively into hip flexion with the knee fully extended. This maneuver stretches the sciatic nerve as it passes behind the hip joint, and if one of its several roots has been irritated by a protruded disk, mass, or inflammatory process, pain will be felt with only 15 to 30 degrees of hip flexion. Normally the straight leg can be brought to 90 degrees of hip flexion without difficulty.

Shoulder. When examining the shoulder, first the position of the upper limbs is observed, at the same time noting whether there is any swelling, asymmetry of height, or visible landmarks and looking for any difference in spontaneous movement. Prominent landmarks that are easily palpable include the acromion process lying laterally and subcutaneously, the clavicle, the spine of the scapula, the coracoid process, and the bicipital groove. Any displacement or tenderness of these structures should be noted. Swelling of the glenohumeral joint capsule and atrophy of the shoulder muscles are best appreciated by viewing from above with the patient seated and by comparison with the normal side.

Assessing range of motion is important because many shoulder problems are manifested by a loss of normal motion. The shoulder is a ball-and-socket joint with six components of movement. Abduction, a function of the

deltoid muscle, is tested by having the patient raise the extended, supinated arm up so that the hand is directly above the shoulder (180-degree abduction). To test adduction, the patient is asked to flex his or her shoulder to 20 to 30 degrees and then draw the upper arm diagonally across his or her body (75 degrees is normal). Flexion is assessed by having him or her raise the extended pronated arm up and forward until it is parallel to the floor; extension is tested by having him or her return the arm to the neutral position and then lift the arm up and backward (45 to 60 degrees is normal). To check rotation, the upper arm is held to the side with the elbow flexed to 90 degrees and the child is asked to turn the forearm toward the body (medial) and then out to the side (lateral) (60 to 90 degrees is normal).

Elbow. In the normal relationship of the extended, supinated forearm to the upper arm, there is 5 to 10 degrees of lateral (valgus) angulation, termed the *carrying angle* (Fig. 21-6). When this angle is greater than 10 degrees, the deformity is termed *cubitus valgus* and, when less or reversed, *cubitus varus (gunstock deformity)*. The range of motion of the hinge joint of the elbow has four components: extension, a function of the triceps (normally to 0 degrees of flexion); flexion, a function of the biceps (normally to 145 degrees); supination (normally to 90 degrees); and pronation (80 to 90 degrees). The latter two components are tested by having the patient turn the palm up and down respectively, with the elbow flexed.

Because of the proximity of the brachial artery and the median, radial, and ulnar nerves to the elbow joint, injuries of the elbow necessitate a careful neurovascular examination.

Wrist and Hand. During examination of the wrist and hand, one should observe skin color, check capillary refill, and palpate the radial and ulnar pulses to assess circulation. Any swelling or edema should be noted, as well as any abnormal posture or position. The presence of intra-articular fluid in the wrist is manifested by swelling and tenderness, especially evident dorsally, and by restriction of wrist motion. Wrist motion has four components: flexion with the hand held down (normally 70 to

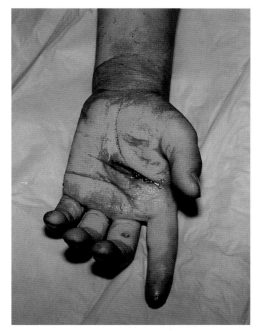

Figure 21-7. Extensor tendon overpull. This boy's palm laceration involved the flexor tendons to his index finger. With his hand at rest, his index finger lies in extension, in contrast to his other fingers, which are partially flexed. (Courtesy Robert Hickey, MD, Children's Hospital of Pittsburgh.)

Table 21-2	Signs of Neural Dysfunction with Injury of the Upper Extremity

NERVE	SIGN
Radial	↓ Strength of wrist and finger extensors ↓ Sensation in web space between thumb and index finger, dorsum of hand to proximal interphalangeal joints, and radial aspect of ring finger
Ulnar	↓ Strength of wrist flexion and adduction ↓ Strength of finger spread ↓ Sensation over ulnar aspect of palm and dorsum of hand, little finger, and ulnar aspect of ring finger
Median	↓ Strength of wrist flexion and abduction ↓ Strength of flexion of proximal interphalangeal joints ↓ Strength of opposition of thumb to base of little finger ↓ Sensation over radial aspect of palm, thumb, index, and long fingers
Anterior interosseous	↓ Strength of flexion of the distal interphalangeal joints of the index finger and thumb

80 degrees); extension with the hand held up (normally 70 degrees); and ulnar and radial deviation (normally 25 degrees and 15 to 20 degrees, respectively).

Examination of hand function can be particularly challenging in young children because of lack of cooperation and developmental limitations. Observation of the position at rest (normally a loose fist with all the fingers pointing in the same direction and with the same degree of flexion) and of use during play is often helpful. Having the parent perform various hand and finger motions while trying to get the child to imitate these can be helpful in some cases. Handing the child a small object such as a key or a thin piece of paper such as a dollar bill may suffice for assessing opposition of thumb to fingers, which in the older child is tested by having him or her touch the tip of the thumb to the tip of the little finger. Normal ranges of motion in the hand are 90 degrees of flexion and 45 degrees of extension for the metacarpophalangeal joints, full extension and 100 degrees of flexion for the proximal interphalangeal (PIP) joints, and full extension and 90 degrees of flexion for the distal interphalangeal joints.

Because the bones of the hand are subcutaneous, displaced fractures and dislocations are readily evident on inspection. Laceration or rupture of the tendons is common because of their superficial location. Those involving flexor tendons result in extensor tendon overpull (Fig. 21-7), with the affected digit lying in greater extension than its neighbors at rest. Conversely, extensor tendon lacerations result in flexor muscle overpull, with the opposite result.

Functional testing of the tendons and intrinsic muscles of the hand is generally possible in older children. They can be asked to extend the fingers at the metacarpophalangeal joints and each interphalangeal joint. Function of the flexor digitorum profundus muscle is tested by holding the PIP joint extended while the patient flexes the tip of the finger. To test the superficialis flexor tendon, adjacent distal interphalangeal joints are held in extension and the patient is asked to flex the finger being tested at the PIP joint. The intrinsic muscles of the hand are

evaluated by having the child adduct and abduct the fingers toward and away from the middle finger. Sensation is best tested using two-point discrimination and pinprick in older children and by touch in very young children.

Muscle strength in the upper extremity is largely tested during assessment of range of motion of the joints, with and without resistance. Signs of neural dysfunction with injury of the upper extremity are listed in Table 21-2.

Lower Extremity Examination

Hip. Examination of the hip begins by assessing gait (see later discussion) and stance, checking the latter to see if the anterior superior and posterior superior iliac spines and the greater trochanters are level. If not, a leg length discrepancy should be suspected and leg length measured. Total length is measured from the bottom of the anterior superior iliac spine to the medial malleolus of the ankle with the patient supine. If inequality is found, the knees are flexed to 90 degrees with the feet flat on the examination table. If, as the examiner looks from the foot of the examination table, one knee appears higher than the other, the tibias are unequal in length; if one knee is anterior to the other when viewed from the side, the discrepancy involves the femurs. If total leg lengths are equal, the inequality apparent when the patient is standing may be due to pelvic obliquity or flexion contracture of the hip. The latter may also be associated with a compensatory accentuation of lumbar lordosis.

The thighs are checked next for symmetry and signs of atrophy. If atrophy is found, circumference should be measured and compared at a fixed point below the greater trochanters.

Because the hip lies deep and is surrounded by muscles, direct inspection is impossible and palpation is of limited value (though the femoral triangle, greater trochanter, and posterior aspect should be palpated to check for tenderness). As a result, assessment of the position of comfort (abduction and external rotation are seen with effusion, hemarthrosis, and fracture [see Figs. 21-15C and 21-91B]), weight bearing, range of motion, and pain on motion are particularly important (for hip examination in the neonate, see "Developmental Dislocation of the Hip" later).

In evaluating range of motion of the hip, care must be taken to distinguish true hip motion from that occurring in combination with pelvic rotation or trunk flexion. The

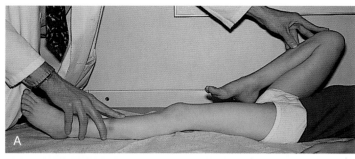

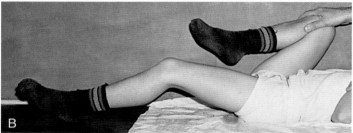

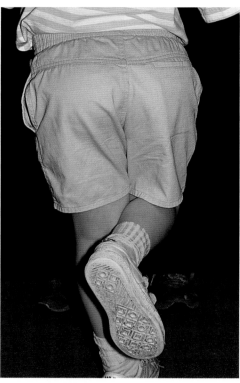

Figure 21-8. Thomas test. This test of range of hip extension is performed by flexing both hips, then holding one in flexion while the patient is asked to extend the other leg. **A,** Normally, full extension is achieved. **B,** Inability to fully extend the hip, seen in this boy with Legg-Calvé-Perthes disease, indicates the presence of a flexion contracture of the hip and constitutes a positive Thomas test.

Figure 21-9. Trendelenburg test. This test is performed to check for weakness of the hip abductors. While lifting his right foot, this patient's left abductor muscles stabilize his pelvis with a slight rise of the pelvis on the right. If left hip abductor weakness were present, the right pelvis would tilt downward when the right leg was lifted.

range of hip flexion is normally about 120 degrees. It is tested with the child lying supine. The hip to be tested is passively flexed while the contralateral hip and pelvis are observed or stabilized by one hand. The limit of flexion is reached when movement of the contralateral pelvis is noted. Alternatively, both hips can be flexed simultaneously to stabilize the pelvis and eliminate truncal flexion. The Thomas test is performed by flexing both hips so that the thighs touch the abdomen. Then one is held in place, thereby eliminating lumbar lordosis and movement of the lumbosacral joint, and the patient is asked to extend the hip to be tested. Normally he or she should be able to extend the hip to 0 degrees of flexion (Fig. 21-8A). Failure to do this indicates the presence of a hip flexion contracture, which is a positive result on the Thomas test (Fig. 21-8B). Next, the knee and thigh are held with the hip and knee flexed to 90 degrees and internal and external rotation are tested and recorded in degrees. Abduction and adduction are also checked with the hip flexed to 90 degrees. While the examiner places the thumb and index finger of one hand over the patient's pelvis, attempting to span the distance between the anterior superior iliac spines, the hip to be tested is abducted and then adducted. The limit is determined by the point at which the pelvis begins to move (normally 45 degrees of abduction and 30 degrees of adduction). Extension is tested with the patient prone by having him or her lift the leg up from the table (normal, 20 to 30 degrees). Internal and external rotation are also tested with the patient prone and the hip and leg in extension.

When hip abductor weakness is suspected on the basis of the finding of a gait abnormality, the Trendelenburg test (Fig. 21-9) is performed. This involves having the child stand and asking him or her to lift one leg up. Normally the pelvis should rise slightly on the side of the leg that is lifted. If instead it drops, abductor weakness is present on the opposite side, and the Trendelenburg test is positive.

Knee. Importantly, knee pain is a common reason for seeking orthopedic care and it is often referred from the

hip; thus any patient presenting with knee pain should always be examined for possible limitation of hip motion or pain on motion of the hip.

The knee examination begins with the examiner viewing the joint from the front, side, and back, looking for differences in contour, swelling or masses, and changes in overlying skin. From the front, the knee is inspected for valgus (lower leg points away from the midline) or varus (lower leg deviates toward the midline) deformity and for evidence of effusion, manifested by obliteration of the normal depressions around the patella or by generalized swelling. In viewing the knee from its lateral aspect, the examiner looks for incomplete extension resulting from flexion contracture or excess hyperextension (recurvatum deformity), as well as for symmetry of the tibial tuberosities. From the rear, the popliteal fossae are checked for symmetry and evidence of swelling. The thighs are also observed for comparative size and contour.

The knees are palpated to assess warmth and check for tenderness along the medial and lateral joint lines, the medial and collateral ligaments, the patella and its supporting ligaments, the femoral and tibial condyles, and the tibial tubercles. Palpation is easier with the knee flexed because the skeletal landmarks are more readily seen and felt, and the muscles, tendons, and ligaments are relaxed in this position.

When there is evidence of a marked effusion, landmarks are obscured and the patella is readily ballotable. This is seen with intra-articular hemorrhage, arthritis, and synovitis, and range of motion is usually significantly limited. If landmarks are only mildly obscured (suggestive of a mild joint effusion or fluid collection in the bursae), pressure should be applied over the suprapatellar pouch with the thumb and index finger of one hand milking down any fluid present while simultaneously pushing the patella

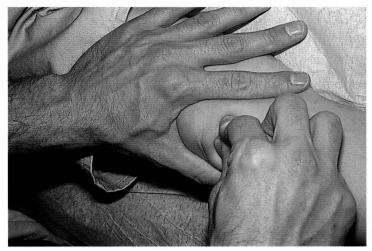

Figure 21-10. Test for small knee joint effusions. Moderate pressure is applied over the suprapatellar pouch with the thumb and index finger of one hand, milking any fluid present downward. The other hand simultaneously pushes the patella up toward the femur. When an effusion is present, the patella becomes ballotable and a palpable click is felt as the patella strikes the front of the distal femur.

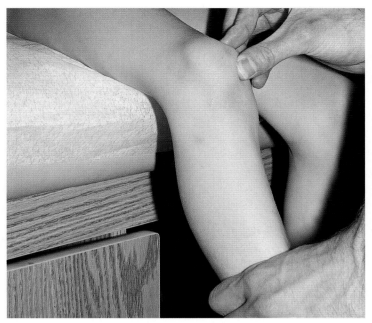

Figure 21-11. Apprehension test for a subluxating or dislocating patella. With the patient sitting and the knee supported in 30 degrees of flexion, the patella is gently pushed laterally. Any abnormal amount of lateral displacement, pain, or apprehension constitutes a positive test.

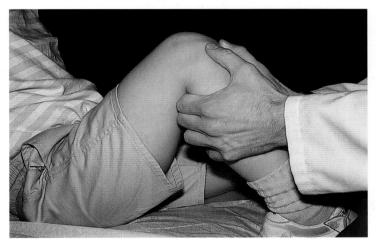

Figure 21-12. Anterior and posterior drawer tests for cruciate ligament stability. With the patient supine, the hips flexed to 45 degrees, and the knees flexed to 90 degrees, the examiner grasps the proximal tibia with his or her fingers behind the knee and thumbs on the anterior joint line and makes a gentle pull-push motion. Forward movement of more than 0.5 to 1 cm indicates anterior cruciate instability, representing a positive anterior drawer test. Similar posterior motion on pushing indicates posterior cruciate instability, representing a positive posterior drawer test.

up toward the femoral condyles with the other hand (Fig. 21-10). If fluid is present, the patella is ballotable and a palpable click is noted as the patella strikes the front of the femur.

The knee is primarily a hinge joint and is normally capable of 130 to 140 degrees of flexion and 5 degrees of hyperextension. However, it can also rotate approximately 10 degrees internally and externally, and this involves rotation of the tibia on the femur. Flexion is tested with the patient either sitting or lying prone. To test extension, the examiner can either have the patient sit and try to straighten the leg to 0 degrees of flexion or try to lift the straightened leg from the examination table while lying supine. Rotation is assessed by turning the foot medially and then laterally with the knee flexed.

With the knees flexed to 80 to 90 degrees, the patellas should face forward when viewed from the front and be located squarely at the ends of the femurs when seen from the side. The apprehension test (Fig. 21-11) is performed to check for a subluxating or dislocating patella. With the patient sitting, the examiner supports the lower leg and holds the knee flexed to 30 degrees. The patella is then gently pushed laterally. Any abnormal amount of lateral displacement, pain, or apprehension in response to this maneuver indicates a positive test.

Ligamentous stability of the knee should be assessed in the mediolateral and anteroposterior planes. In patients with acute injuries, especially those involving significant pain and swelling, this should be deferred until radiographs have been obtained to check for associated fractures.

The abduction/adduction stress test is used to determine the degree of stability of the medial and lateral collateral ligaments. With the supine patient's thigh moved to the side of the examination table and the knee flexed to 30 degrees, the examiner holds the distal thigh in one hand while grasping the inside of the lower leg with the other. To test the medial collaterals, the examiner applies valgus stress by pressing medially against the distal thigh with the upper hand while gently abducting the lower leg. To check the lateral collaterals, the examiner applies varus stress by pressing laterally on the inside of the distal thigh while gently adducting the lower leg. Normally the joint line should open no more than 1 cm on either side.

Anteroposterior ligamentous stability is provided by the anterior and posterior cruciate ligaments of the knee. They are tested by the anterior and posterior drawer and Lachman tests. The former are performed with the patient supine; the hip and knee flexed to 45 and 90 degrees, respectively; and the foot planted on the examining table, stabilized by the examiner's thigh or buttock. The examiner then grasps the proximal tibia with his or her fingers behind the knee and the thumbs over the anterior joint line and gently pulls and pushes (Fig. 21-12). In a positive anterior drawer test, the tibia moves forward more than 0.5 to 1 cm, indicating instability of the anterior cruciate ligament. Movement backward more than 0.5 to 1 cm indicates instability of the posterior cruciate ligament. In the Lachman test (Fig. 21-13) for anterior cruciate tears,

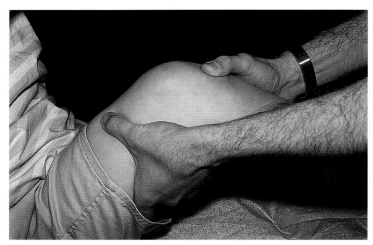

Figure 21-13. Lachman test for anterior cruciate ligament tear. With the knee flexed to 15 degrees, the distal femur is grasped with one hand and the proximal tibia with the other, with the thumb on the joint line. The tibia is moved forward while the femur is pushed backward. Any abnormal displacement of the tibia on the femur indicates anterior cruciate instability and represents a positive test.

the knee is flexed to 15 degrees. The examiner grasps the distal femur with one hand and the proximal tibia with the other. The thumb of the lower hand is placed on the joint line, and the femur is pushed backward as the tibia is pulled forward. Abnormal anterior displacement of the tibia on the femur can be seen and felt if instability is present. The amount of excursion is estimated in millimeters, and the end point is recorded as soft or firm.

Ankle. Examination of the ankle begins with inspection for evidence of deformity, swelling, change in color of overlying skin, and abnormal position (especially with weight bearing). Palpation is performed to detect warmth and localize tenderness. In the neutral position the long axis of the foot should be at 90 degrees to the long axis of the tibia. Normally a child can dorsiflex 20 degrees and plantar flex 30 to 50 degrees from the neutral position, as well as invert and evert approximately 5 degrees. Dorsiflexion and plantar flexion can be checked by observing passive and active motion (with and without resistance) but are perhaps most easily tested by having the ambulating child walk on his or her heels and toes, respectively. Similarly, inversion is tested by having him or her walk on the outside of the feet and eversion by having him or her walk on the medial sides.

Tests for ligamentous instability can be important following severe ankle sprains. The anterior drawer test is used to assess the stability of the anterior talofibular ligament. With the patient's legs dangling over the side of the examination table and the foot in a few degrees of plantar flexion, the examiner grasps the anterior aspect of the distal tibia with one hand while holding the calcaneus cupped in the palm of the other. The calcaneus is then drawn anteriorly while the tibia is pushed posteriorly. Normally there should be no movement, but with instability of the anterior talofibular ligament, the talus slides anteriorly. Lateral instability is seen only with major tears of the anterior talofibular and calcaneofibular ligaments, occasionally accompanied by tears of the posterior talofibular ligament, and is tested by inverting the calcaneus with one hand while grasping the distal tibia with the other. When instability is present, the talus gaps and rocks in the ankle mortise. Medial instability is exceptionally rare because of the strength of the fan-shaped deltoid ligament. To test for medial instability, the tibia and calcaneus

are held in the same manner as they are in testing lateral instability, but the foot is everted instead. Gross gaping of the ankle mortise is felt when there is a major tear.

Gait and Gait Disturbances

Between the onset of walking and 3 years of age, children tend to have a wide-based gait and toddlers often hold their arms out to the side to assist balance. By 3 years of age, children achieve a normal smooth and rhythmical heel-to-toe gait, consisting of two main phases: stance and swing. The stance phase begins when the heel strikes the ground, bears all the weight, and progresses to foot flat, midstance, and push-off as weight is transferred from the heel to the metatarsal heads. The swing phase starts with acceleration after push-off and progresses through midswing to deceleration just before heel strike. During the swing phase, as the leg moves forward, so does the opposite arm. Because stance occupies 60% of the time and weight is borne in this phase, most gait disorders are more evident during the stance phase than during the swing phase. Normally the distance between the two heels (width of the base) is between 5 and 10 cm, the pelvis and trunk shift laterally about 2.5 cm from stance to stance, the center of gravity rises and falls no more than 5 cm, and the pelvis rotates forward about 40 degrees during swing.

Gait is best observed by having the patient walk back and forth in a hall or in a room with a mirror at one end. As the patient walks, the examiner focuses first on overall movement and then on the motion of the pelvis, hips, thighs, knees, lower legs, ankles, and feet in succession, both coming and going. In doing so, he or she looks for the pattern of heel-to-toe motion, for shortening of the stance phase, for evidence of limitation of joint motion or weakness, and for positional changes of the extremities. Checking the patient's shoes for signs of abnormal wear is also helpful.

Most acute and many chronic disturbances of gait in childhood are caused by pain. Others stem from weakness or spasticity caused by neurologic or muscular disorders, from leg length inequality, or from deformity. Important historical points are the time of onset of the abnormal gait and the circumstances surrounding it; the duration; whether the abnormal gait is constant or intermittent and, if intermittent, the time of day it is most apparent (AM, juvenile rheumatoid arthritis; PM, neuromuscular disorders—symptoms becoming more apparent with fatigue); and its relation to activity or exercise including its effect on running or climbing stairs. The examiner should note any associated pain and its location, bearing in mind referral patterns (low back to buttocks and lateral thigh; hip to groin, medial thigh, knee, and sometimes buttock) and attempting to determine whether the pain is constant (suggestive of tumor or infection) or intermittent.

Gait Disturbances Stemming from Pain, Limb Length Inequality, or Stiffness. An antalgic gait is a limp caused by pain on weight bearing that results in shortening of the stance phase on the affected side. It can be due to pain referred from the back or pain anywhere in the lower extremity. Causes include trauma, pathologic fracture, infection, inflammatory disorders and other sources of arthritis, malignancy, tight shoes, foreign body in the shoe, and a lesion on the sole of the foot. Careful physical examination combined with a complete history usually enables localization of the problem.

Patients with leg length inequality manifest depression of the trunk and pelvis during the stance phase on the shorter leg and circumduction of the longer leg during swing. Some children try to compensate for the leg length inequality by toe-walking on the shorter extremity.

Patients with limited hip motion compensate by thrusting the pelvis and trunk forward in the swing phase. When knee flexion is limited, children tend to hike up the pelvis on the involved side during the swing phase and circumduct the leg to clear the foot from the floor. A circumduction gait can also be related to a painful condition involving the ankle or a limitation of ankle motion. By circumducting the leg laterally during swing phase, the patient reduces the need for ankle motion.

Gait Disturbances Resulting from Weakness or Spasticity. Patients with weakness of the hip abductors (gluteus medius muscle) have a Trendelenburg gait. Because they are unable to maintain a level pelvis and linear progression of their center of gravity, their pelvis tilts toward the unsupported side and their shoulder lurches toward the weak side during stance phase to maintain their center of gravity over the foot. Patients with weakness of the gluteus maximus (seen most commonly in children with Duchenne muscular dystrophy) have to hyperextend their trunk and pelvis to maintain their center of gravity posterior to the hip joint (see Fig. 15-58). Proximal muscle weakness may also be demonstrated by observing a child getting up from the floor unassisted. A Gower sign indicates weak hip extensors and abductors, necessitating that the patient use his arms to assist in standing by placing his hands on his anterior thighs and pushing up, progressively moving his hands upward along the thighs until erect posture is achieved (see Fig. 15-57). Children with weakness of the quadriceps femoris muscle may have a relatively normal gait on level ground but difficulty climbing stairs. Weakness of the dorsiflexors of the foot results in footdrop and a steppage gait. Because the foot hangs down during swing phase, the patient must lift the knee higher than usual to help the foot clear the floor and the forefoot tends to slap the floor on impact because smooth deceleration of the foot cannot be controlled. When the plantar flexors are weak, the patient is unable to push off at the end of the stance phase and so the heel and forefoot come off the floor at the same time.

An equine gait, characterized by toe-walking or a toe-to-heel sequence during the stance phase, is seen in children with heel cord contracture and limited dorsiflexion. It is usually indicative of an underlying neurologic problem with spasticity. Patients with spastic cerebral palsy who are able to ambulate often manifest a stiff-legged scissors gait, in which one foot crosses over the other during the swing phase. Vestibular or cerebellar dysfunction or generalized weakness tends to result in a wide-based ataxic gait because of abnormal balance. Absence of the normal arm swing with walking is seen in patients with paresis or cerebellar disease.

Intoeing and Out-toeing. The angular difference between the long axis of the foot and the forward line of progression during walking is called the *foot progression angle*. A minus value is assigned to intoeing, a plus value to out-toeing. The normal range varies from 5 to 10 degrees to 10 to 20 degrees, respectively. The remaining rotational profile of the lower extremities can be examined with the patient in the prone position (Fig. 21-14). The foot axis can be determined by a line marked from the middle of the heel on the plantar surface to the lateral side of the second toe (Fig. 21-14A). The hip excursion is the difference between the angular measure of the maximum prone internal rotation (Fig. 21-14B) and that for external rotation (Fig. 21-14C), and in the young child is usually negative, representing more internal rotation than external rotation. In the adolescent and adult, usually there is more external rotation, or a positive hip excursion angle. Finally, the axis of the tibia and fibula can be determined by looking down the lower extremity in the prone knee-flexed position and comparing the axis of the plane of motion of the knee (Fig. 21-14D) with the transmalleolar axis (Fig. 21-14E) estimated by palpating the malleoli. The normal axis is 15 to 25 degrees externally rotated.

Femoral anteversion, internal tibial torsion, and metatarsus adductus are common causes of excessive intoeing, or pigeon toe, and femoral eversion and external tibial torsion are common causes of out-toeing, or slew foot (see "Disorders of the Lower Extremity" later).

Musculoskeletal Trauma

The normal impulsiveness and inquisitiveness of children combined with their lack of caution and love of energetic activities place them at a relatively high risk for accidental injury. The incidence of trauma is further increased by the prevalence of child abuse (see Chapter 6). In fact, beyond infancy, trauma is the leading cause of death in children and adolescents and is a source of significant morbidity. Musculoskeletal injuries are common, whether seen in isolation or as part of multisystem trauma. Although the management of life-threatening injuries to the airway, circulation, and central nervous system (CNS) must take precedence over treatment of accompanying musculoskeletal injuries in cases of multiple trauma, it must be kept in mind that fractures can result in significant blood loss. This is particularly true of pelvic and femoral fractures. Furthermore, prompt attention must be given to assessment of the status of neurovascular structures distal to obvious fractures because failure to recognize compromise may result in permanent loss of function. Finally, traumatic hip dislocations must be reduced within 6 to 12 hours if the risk of aseptic necrosis and long-term morbidity is to be minimized.

Fractures

Diagnosis

One of the many variables that complicate the diagnosis of the skeletally injured child is that the child, already in pain, is frightened by his or her recent experience and by the strangeness of the hospital or emergency department setting. Many children are too young to give a firsthand history, and the cooperation of toddlers is often limited. The parents are likely to be anxious as well. A calm, empathetic manner is necessary to allay their fears. Taking a thorough history before making any attempt to perform a physical assessment helps the examiner establish rapport with the patient and the family. This should include questions concerning the type and direction of the injuring force, the position of the involved extremity at the time of the accident, and the events immediately following the injury such as measures taken at the scene of the accident. The presence of underlying disorders and the possibility of contamination of an open wound should be determined as well. Physicians also should be alert to signs suggestive of inflicted injury or child abuse. These include a history in which the mechanism of injury does not fit the type and/or severity of the fracture found, an unusual delay in presentation, and/or radiographic evidence of old healing fractures for which no medical attention was ever sought.

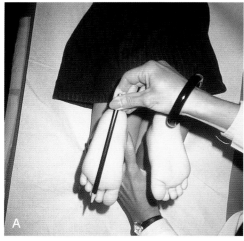

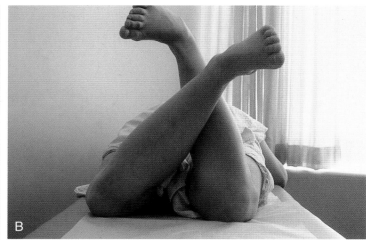

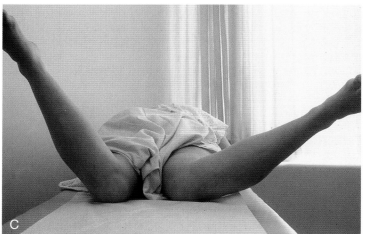

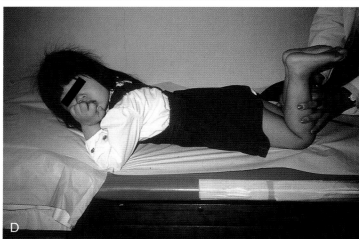

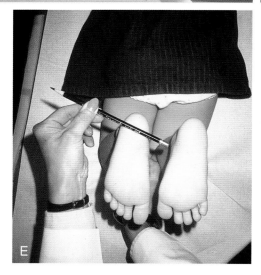

Figure 21-14. Evaluation of the rotational profile of the lower extremities. **A,** The foot axis is determined by a line marked from midheel to the lateral aspect of the second toe. Hip excursion is the difference between the angular measure of maximum prone internal rotation **(B)** and maximum prone external rotation **(C).** The tibia-fibula axis is determined by comparing the axis of the plane of motion of the knee with the patient prone and knees flexed **(D)** to the transmalleolar axis **(E).**

In cases of suspected fracture, splinting, elevation, and topical application of ice may help reduce discomfort and local swelling. Splinting is particularly important for displaced and unstable fractures because it prevents further soft tissue injuries and reduces the risk of fat embolization. When pain is moderate to severe and there are no cardiovascular or CNS contraindications, analgesia should be administered promptly. Contrary to the opinion of many physicians, this does not obscure physical findings. Tenderness is not reduced significantly, swelling remains, and patient cooperation during the examination may be considerably greater.

Before beginning the physical examination, it is wise for the examiner to talk with the child to further gain his or her trust. Older infants and toddlers are often more comfortable when allowed to sit on a parent's lap, and use of puppets or toys can reduce fear and help gain their cooperation. Because comparison of paired extremities is an integral part of orthopedic assessment, it is best to begin by examining the uninjured side and it is wise to defer palpation of the most likely site of the injury on the affected side until last. If young children are highly anxious, it can be useful to instruct the parent in how to perform passive range of motion and palpation.

The first step in the physical examination is visual inspection of the injured area. The gross position of the extremity should be noted, and attention given to the presence or absence of deformity, distortion or abnormal

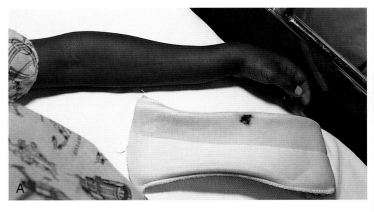

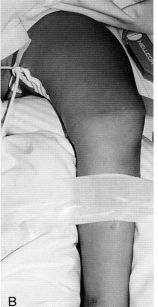

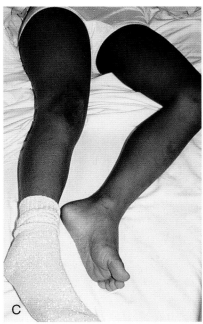

Figure 21-15. Visible abnormalities seen on inspection in children with fractures. **A,** Distortion and angulation of the distal forearm in a child with fractures of the radius and ulna. **B,** Swelling and angulation of the proximal thigh resulting from a femur fracture. **C,** Longitudinal shortening of the thigh in a child with a proximal femur fracture. Note the characteristic externally rotated position of the injured leg. The child was struck by a car, sustaining a fracture of the femoral neck.

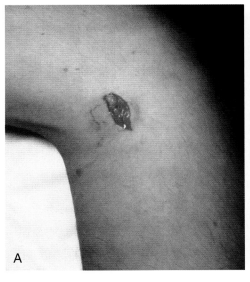

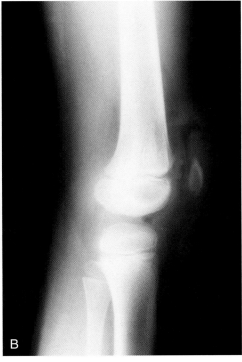

Figure 21-16. **A,** Penetrating injury of the knee. This child was struck by a stone propelled by the blades of a power lawn mower. Though the laceration appeared to be minor, serosanguineous fluid flowed from it on movement of the knee, suggesting penetration of the joint capsule. This was confirmed on exploration in the operating room. **B,** Air is seen within the knee joint and in the overlying soft tissues in a child who sustained a deep laceration that penetrated the joint capsule. (**A,** Courtesy Bruce Watson, MD.)

angulation, and longitudinal shortening (Fig. 21-15). The overlying skin and soft tissues are examined for evidence of swelling, ecchymoses, abrasions, punctures, and lacerations. Comparison with the opposite extremity and measurement of circumference can be helpful when findings are subtle.

The location of open wounds is important in ascertaining whether an underlying fracture is open or closed and in assessing the risk of joint penetration. Small puncture wounds or lacerations overlying bony structures from which a bloody, fatty exudate is oozing usually reflect communication with the medullary cavity of a fractured bone. Similarly, punctures or tears over joints that weep serous or serosanguineous fluid, especially when drainage is increased on moving the joint, must be assumed to communicate with the joint capsule (Fig. 21-16A). In

patients with penetrating joint injuries, radiographs may demonstrate air in the joint, but absence of this does not rule out capsular penetration (see Fig. 21-16B). Probing of open wounds that are highly likely to communicate with a fracture or joint is contraindicated. The wound should be cleaned and covered with a sterile dressing until its extent can be determined under sterile conditions in the operating room.

After inspection of the most obviously injured area, palpation and assessment of active and passive motion can be performed. It is crucial to remember that in examining an injured limb the entire extremity must be evaluated in order to detect less obvious associated injuries. Localized swelling and tenderness on palpation are significant findings and should alert the examiner to the high likelihood of an underlying fracture. Pain on motion

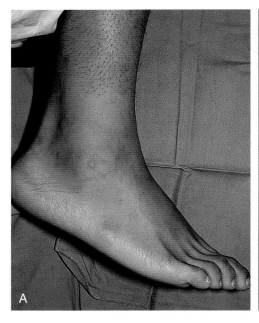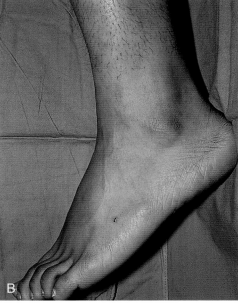

Figure 21-17. Salter-Harris type I fracture of the distal fibula. **A,** Slight swelling is present over the lateral malleolus. The degree of swelling can be truly appreciated only by comparing the injured ankle with its normal counterpart, shown in **B.** The patient had point tenderness over the affected malleolus. The findings differ from those seen in an ankle sprain, in which tenderness and swelling are greatest over the ligaments inferior to the malleolus (see Fig. 21-65).

and limitation of motion signal the need for careful scrutiny as well. Assessment of motion involves observation of spontaneous movement, attempts to get the patient to voluntarily move the involved part through its expected range, and passive movement. Particular attention should be paid to the adjacent proximal and distal joints to avoid missing associated injuries. It can be difficult, however, to determine whether motion is limited because of pain, an associated injury, or fear and lack of cooperation.

Clinical findings vary depending on the nature of the fracture. Undisplaced growth plate fractures typically present with mild, localized swelling and point tenderness at the level of the epiphysis (Fig. 21-17). Because ligamentous injury is relatively uncommon in a child, the finding of point tenderness should suffice to prompt treating the injury as a fracture until proven otherwise. Often initial radiographs appear normal and the fracture is confirmed only on follow-up when repeat radiographs disclose evidence of healing. Swelling is typically mild and occasionally imperceptible in cases of torus or buckle fractures and of undisplaced transverse and spiral fractures. Careful palpation should disclose focal tenderness, however. Usually, the patient also experiences some degree of discomfort on motion in some planes or on weight bearing, but it must be remembered that limitation of movement or function can be minimal in patients with such incomplete fractures. In contrast, fractures that completely disrupt the bone and displaced fractures are accompanied by more prominent swelling; more diffuse tenderness; and severe pain, which is markedly increased on motion (Fig. 21-18; see also Fig. 21-15A and B). Crepitus may also be evident on gentle palpation. In examining children with these findings, manipulation must be kept to a minimum to prevent further injury.

Assessment of neurovascular function distal to the injury is essential in evaluating any child with a potential fracture. This includes checking the integrity of pulses and speed of capillary refill, as well as testing sensory and motor function. Strength and sensation should be compared with those of the contralateral extremity. Assessment of two-point discrimination is probably the best test of sensory function. Evidence of neurovascular compromise necessitates urgent, often operative, orthopedic treatment. In addition, this assessment is crucial before and after reduction of displaced fractures to determine if the procedure itself has impaired function in any way. Persis-

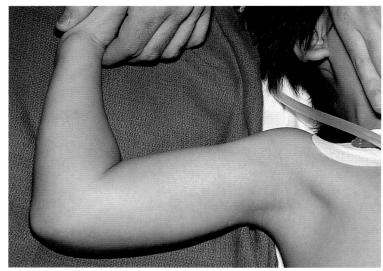

Figure 21-18. Fracture with overlying soft tissue swelling. This child has a displaced supracondylar fracture of the distal humerus with moderate soft tissue swelling. The degree of swelling becomes evident if the size of the elbow area is compared with the size of the patient's wrist.

tence of intense pain following fracture reduction should provoke suspicion of ischemia.

Supracondylar fractures of the humerus, fractures of the distal femoral shaft and proximal tibia, fracture-dislocations of the elbow and knee, and severely displaced ankle fractures are particularly likely to be associated with neurovascular injury.

Even relatively minor fractures of the tibia, forearm bones, metatarsals, and femur can result in compartment syndrome, in which bleeding and edema collection within a closed fascial compartment produce increased pressure that causes neurovascular compromise and muscle ischemia. This should be strongly suspected in patients who complain of intense pain that is aggravated by passive stretching of the muscles. On palpation the area is noted to be swollen and tense, at times even hard. The patient may complain of paresthesias and show pallor and decreased pulses. However, it is important to also be aware of the fact that vascular compromise can be present in a patient who has normal distal pulses and good peripheral perfusion (see "Compartment Syndromes" later).

In all cases of suspected extremity fractures the injured part should be properly splinted and elevated, an ice pack applied, and analgesia administered while the patient awaits transport to the radiography suite. However, to obtain high-quality radiographs, obstructing splints must be removed temporarily. This presents no major problem in patients with partial or nondisplaced fractures but can create difficulties in patients with severe displaced fractures. To ensure that manipulation is minimal in these patients, splint removal, positioning for radiographs, and splint reapplication should be supervised by a physician and not done merely at the discretion of the x-ray technician.

At a minimum, two radiographs taken at 90-degree angles are obtained, anteroposterior (AP) and lateral views being the most common. Oblique views are helpful in fully disclosing the nature and extent of many fracture patterns, especially when the injury involves the ankle, elbow, hand, or foot. They can also prove useful in detecting subtle spiral fractures and in cases in which the AP and lateral views are normal, yet a fracture is strongly suspected. Radiographs should include the joints immediately proximal and distal to a fractured long bone, because there may be associated bony or soft tissue injuries in these areas as well. Such associated injuries easily can be missed on clinical examination when assessment of motion is limited by pain or when patient cooperation is limited. It is necessary to obtain comparison views of the opposite side, especially when evaluating patients with suspected physeal injuries who may have very subtle radiographic abnormalities. These views can also prove invaluable in detecting cortical disruptions. In some cases of displaced or angulated fractures, potentially complex intra-articular fractures, and vertebral and pelvic fractures, a CT scan can be useful. A bone scan may be necessary to detect subtle stress fractures.

Particular care should be taken in interpreting pediatric radiographs because of the high incidence of subtle or even normal findings in patients with fractures. If the clinical picture strongly suggests a fracture, appropriate treatment should be initiated, even if the radiograph appears normal. Reassessment in 1 to 2 weeks can then clarify the exact nature of the injury.

Fracture Patterns

Fractures should be described in terms of anatomic location, direction of the fracture line, type of fracture, and degree of angulation and of displacement. When the growth plate is involved, use of the Salter-Harris classification system is recommended.

Any specific mechanism of injury results in a readily definable pattern of force application, which tends to produce a typical fracture pattern. Because of this, it is often possible to infer the likely mechanism of injury once the fracture pattern is documented radiographically. If the vector of the direct force is perpendicular to the bone, a transverse fracture is most likely to result, whereas direct force applied at any angle to the bone produces an oblique fracture pattern. Examples of situations resulting in transverse and short oblique fractures include falls in which an extremity strikes the edge of a table, counter, or chair; direct blows with an object such as a stick; and karate chops. These fractures are commonly seen as a result of accidents or fights and in the battered child syndrome. Comminuted fractures generally result from high-velocity, direct forces such as those characteristic of vehicular accidents, falls from heights, or gunshot wounds. Impacted fractures are produced by forces oriented in a direction parallel to the long axis of the bone. Application of indirect force commonly results in spiral, greenstick, or torus fractures in children.

A common example of a nondisplaced spiral fracture is the toddler's fracture (see Fig. 21-43), which results from a fall with a twist. Typically, the child was either running, turned, and then fell; jumped and fell with a twist; or got his or her foot caught and fell while twisting to extricate himself or herself. If a child's arm or leg is forcibly pulled and twisted, a similar fracture pattern may be seen. Greenstick and torus fractures of the radius or ulna are incurred usually when the child falls on an outstretched arm with the wrist dorsiflexed. Vigorous repetitive shaking while holding a child by the hands, feet, or chest results in small metaphyseal chip or bucket-handle fractures, a major feature of the shaken-baby syndrome (see Chapter 6 and Figs. 6-27 and 6-28). Table 21-3 summarizes the major features of these various fracture patterns, which are illustrated in Figures 21-19 through 21-27.

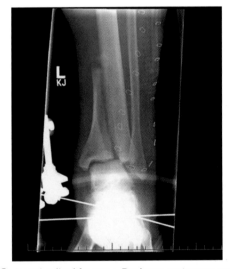

Figure 21-19. Longitudinal fracture. During a motocross competition this teenager missed a jump and was thrown 20 feet in the air, then fell to the pavement below, landing directly on his foot. The force of the impact was transmitted upward through his ankle, resulting in this vertical tibia fracture.

Table 21-3	Patterns of Fractures	
FRACTURE PATTERN	**MAJOR FEATURE**	**RADIOGRAPHIC APPEARANCE**
Longitudinal	Fracture line is parallel to the axis of a long bone	Fig. 21-19
Transverse	Fracture line is perpendicular to the axis of a long bone	Fig. 21-20 and see Fig. 21-28
Oblique	Fracture line is at an angle relative to the axis of a bone	Fig. 21-21
Spiral	Fracture line takes a curvilinear course around the axis of a bone	Fig. 21-22 and see Fig. 21-43
Impacted	Bone ends are crushed together, producing an indistinct fracture line	Fig. 21-23
Comminuted	Fracturing forces produce more than two separate fragments	Fig. 21-24
Bowing	Bone bends to the point of plastic deformation without fracturing	Fig. 21-25
Greenstick	Fracture is complete except for a portion of the cortex on the compression side of the fracture, which is only plastically deformed	Fig. 21-26 and see Fig. 21-25B
Torus	Bone buckles and bends rather than breaks	Fig. 21-27 and see Fig. 21-29

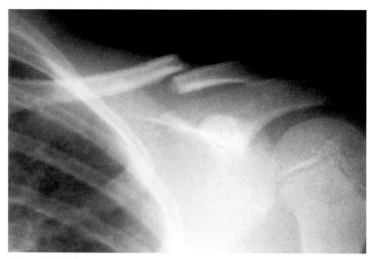

Figure 21-20. Transverse fracture of the midportion of the clavicle. The fracture line is perpendicular to the long axis of the bone.

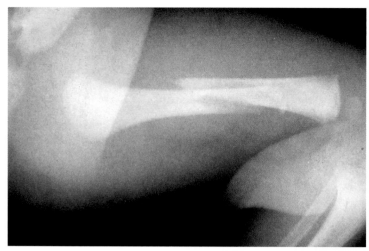

Figure 21-21. Oblique fracture of the midportion of the femur. The fracture line is angled relative to the axis of the bone.

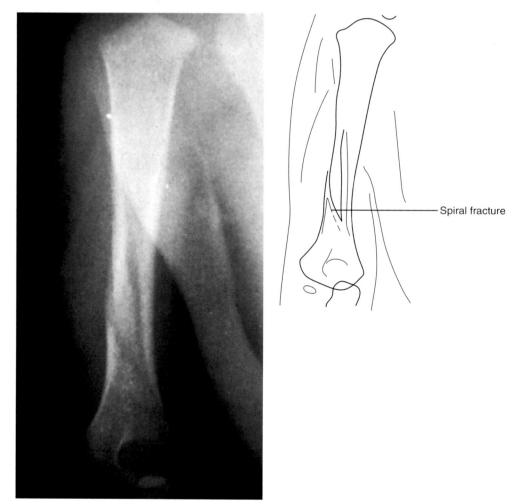

Figure 21-22. Spiral fracture of the humerus. The fracture line takes a curvilinear course around the axis of the bone.

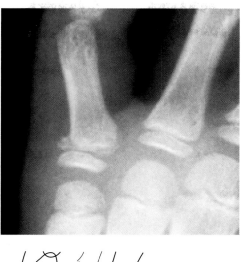

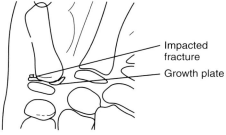

Figure 21-23. Impacted fracture of the base of the proximal phalanx resulting from axial loading. The fracture line is indistinct, and the fragments appear to be crushed together. The fracture does not actually involve the growth plate but is located just distal to it in the proximal metaphysis.

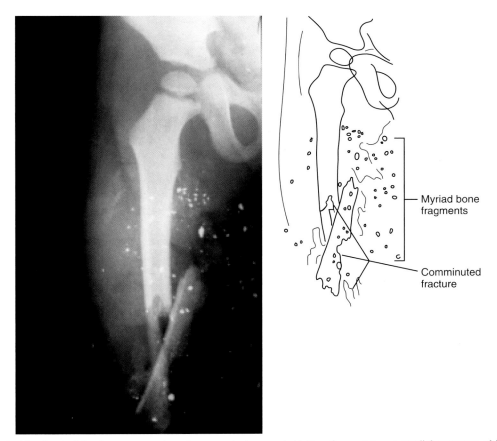

Figure 21-24. Comminuted fracture of the femur secondary to a gunshot wound. Notice the numerous small fragments of bone in the adjacent soft tissues.

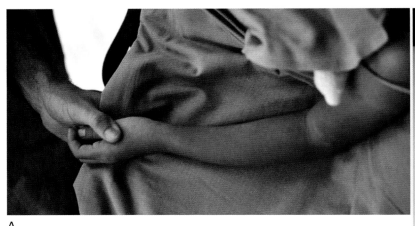

A

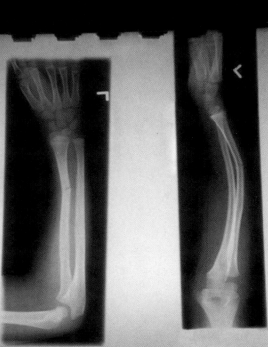

B

Figure 21-25. Plastic deformation. **A,** While playing soccer, this school-age child fell onto his outstretched arm. On impact another player who fell with him landed on the arm, resulting in this bowing deformity of the forearm. **B,** On x-ray plastic deformation of both the ulna and radius are seen, along with a greenstick fracture of the radius. This necessitated manipulation under anesthesia to straighten the arm before casting.

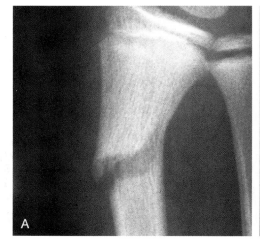

A

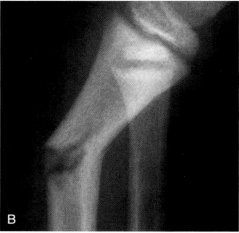

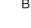

B

Figure 21-26. Greenstick fracture of the distal radius. **A,** In this anteroposterior view of the distal radius, a fracture line is seen that is complete except for a portion of the cortex on the compression side of the fracture. **B,** The lateral radiograph demonstrates more clearly the disrupted and compressed cortices. This resulted from a fall on the outstretched arm with the wrist in dorsiflexion.

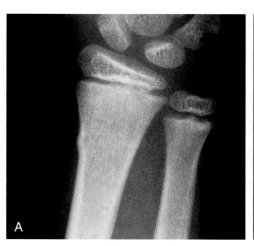

A

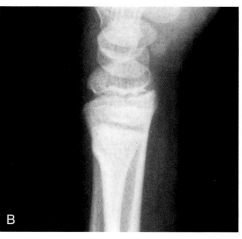

B

Figure 21-27. Torus fracture of the distal radius resulting from a fall on an outstretched arm. **A,** An anteroposterior radiograph of the wrist shows a minor torus or buckle fracture of the radius. **B,** The lateral radiograph shows the dorsal location of the deformity. This injury can be expected to completely remodel.

The anatomic location of the fracture line simply refers to that portion of the bone to which the injury force was applied. Table 21-4 presents types of fractures classified by anatomic location. These fractures are illustrated in Figures 21-28 through 21-36. There is some degree of overlap in this method of categorization, however.

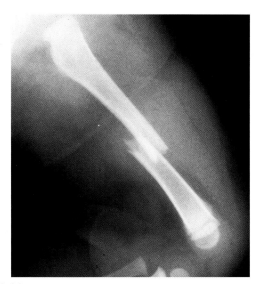

Figure 21-28. Diaphyseal fracture. A transverse fracture line crosses the diaphyseal region of the femur. A moderate amount of overlap exists at the fracture site.

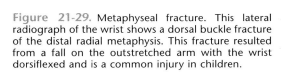

Figure 21-29. Metaphyseal fracture. This lateral radiograph of the wrist shows a dorsal buckle fracture of the distal radial metaphysis. This fracture resulted from a fall on the outstretched arm with the wrist dorsiflexed and is a common injury in children.

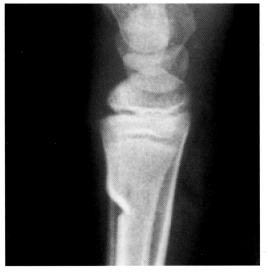
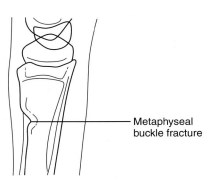

Metaphyseal buckle fracture

Physeal Fractures

An estimated 15% of all fractures in children involve the physis. Because the adjacent epiphyseal plate is not ossified in the young child and therefore is invisible on a radiograph, the fracture may be mistaken for a minor sprain or missed altogether, only to manifest itself at a later date in the appearance of slowed or failed longitudinal limb growth or in the development of an angular deformity. Even if diagnosed and properly treated, physeal injuries may still result in longitudinal or angular abnormalities. This risk is especially high in children with physeal fractures involving the distal femur, proximal tibia, or radial head and neck. Most physeal disruptions occur through the zone of cartilage cell hypertrophy within the physeal plate and thus do not result in permanent damage to the plate. However, a small proportion of disruptions involve the resting or germinal layer of the physis and may disrupt the cells permanently, resulting in eventual deformity despite adequate reduction of the fracture fragments.

Because of the potential for long-term morbidity in patients with physeal fractures, great attention has been focused on the classification, diagnosis, treatment, and prognosis of physeal fractures. The Salter-Harris classification scheme is the system most commonly used in North America to classify physeal injuries (Fig. 21-37).

Salter-Harris Type I. This injury consists of a fracture running horizontally through the physis itself, resulting in a variable degree of separation of the epiphysis from

Table 21-4   Classification of Fractures by Anatomic Location

TYPE	SITE	RADIOGRAPHIC APPEARANCE
Diaphyseal	Fracture involves the central shaft of a long bone.	Fig. 21-28 and see Figs. 21-21, 21-22, and 21-25
Metaphyseal	Fracture involves the widened end of a long bone.	Fig. 21-29 and see Fig. 21-26 and Figs. 6-27 and 6-28
Epiphyseal	Fracture involves the chondro-osseous end of a long bone. Such fractures can also be classified as Salter-Harris fractures.	Fig. 21-30
Articular	Fracture involves the cartilaginous joint surface.	Fig. 21-31 (see also Figs. 21-40 and 21-41)
Intercondylar	Fracture is located between the condyles of a joint. This is one variant of articular fracture and could also be subclassified as a Salter-Harris fracture.	Fig. 21-31A
Physeal	Fracture involves the growth center of long bone. These are subclassified according to the Salter-Harris system.	Fig. 21-32
Condylar	Fracture traverses the condyle of a joint.	Fig. 21-33
Supracondylar	Fracture line is located just proximal to the condyles of a joint.	Fig. 21-34
Epicondylar	Fracture involves an area juxtaposed to the condylar surface of a joint.	Fig. 21-35
Subcapital	Fracture is located just below the epiphyseal head of certain bones.	Fig. 21-36

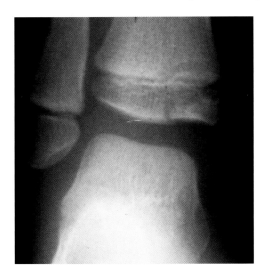

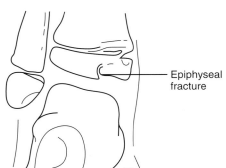

Epiphyseal fracture

Figure 21-30. Epiphyseal fracture. A fracture involving the medial aspect of the epiphysis of the distal tibia is seen in this anteroposterior radiograph of the ankle in a 4-year-old girl. A slight stepoff is present at the articular surface. This could also be classified as a Salter-Harris type III fracture.

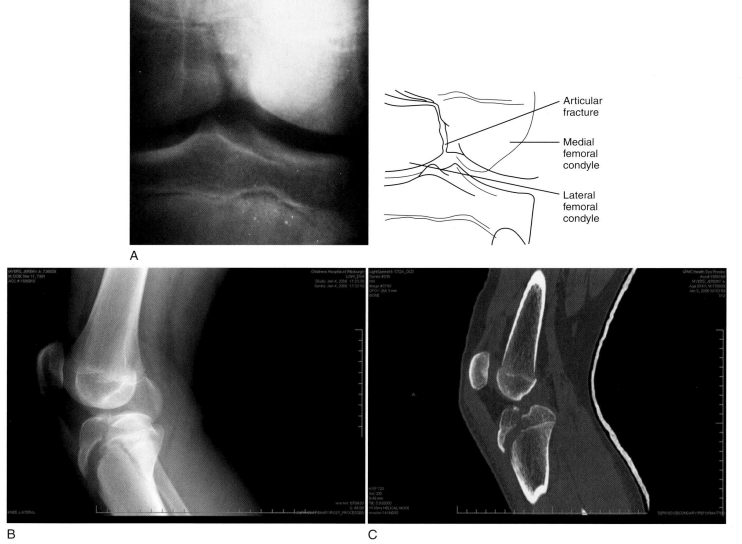

Articular fracture

Medial femoral condyle

Lateral femoral condyle

A

B   C

Figure 21-31. Articular fractures. **A,** This anteroposterior view of the knee demonstrates intra-articular extension of a fracture line that exits at the junction of the medial and lateral femoral condyles. The condyles are separated by only a few millimeters. This can also be termed an *intercondylar fracture.* **B,** On coming down from a rebound, a 14-year-old basketball player landed with a twist with his knee in extension. The lateral radiograph demonstrates intra-articular extension of a fracture line that starts at the tibial tubercle and exits in the middle of the knee joint. **C,** On computed tomography scan the degree of intra-articular displacement of the fracture is better appreciated.

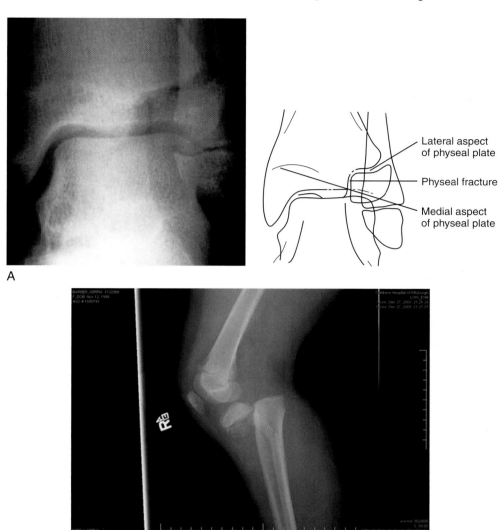

Figure 21-32. Physeal fractures. **A,** A fracture of the lateral aspect of the tibial epiphysis through the lateral aspect of the physeal plate is seen in this anteroposterior view of the ankle of a 13-year-old boy. Also called a Tillaux fracture, this pattern is seen in adolescents in whom the medial aspect of the distal tibial physis has closed but not the lateral aspect. It can also be classified as a Salter-Harris type III fracture. **B,** A 7-year-old restrained backseat passenger involved in a head-on collision motor vehicle accident suffered a direct impact to the front of his lower leg due to violent displacement of the front seat. This resulted in shearing of the proximal tibial epiphysis from the metaphysis. The lateral view of the knee demonstrates complete separation of the epiphysis from most of the metaphysis. This degree of posterior displacement of the metaphysis can be associated with compression of the popliteal artery. This can also be classified as a Salter-Harris type II fracture because a small metaphyseal fragment remains attached to the epiphysis.

A

B

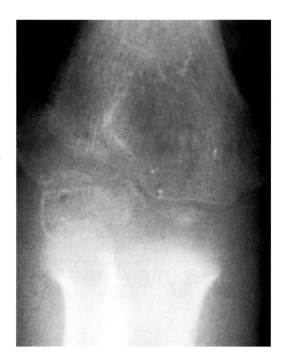

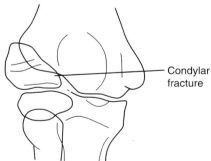

Figure 21-33. Condylar fractures. This anteroposterior radiograph of the elbow shows a fracture of the lateral condyle of the distal humerus. The condyle is displaced proximally and radially. The fragment is always larger than it appears on a radiograph because of the large amount of unossified cartilage present in the distal humerus.

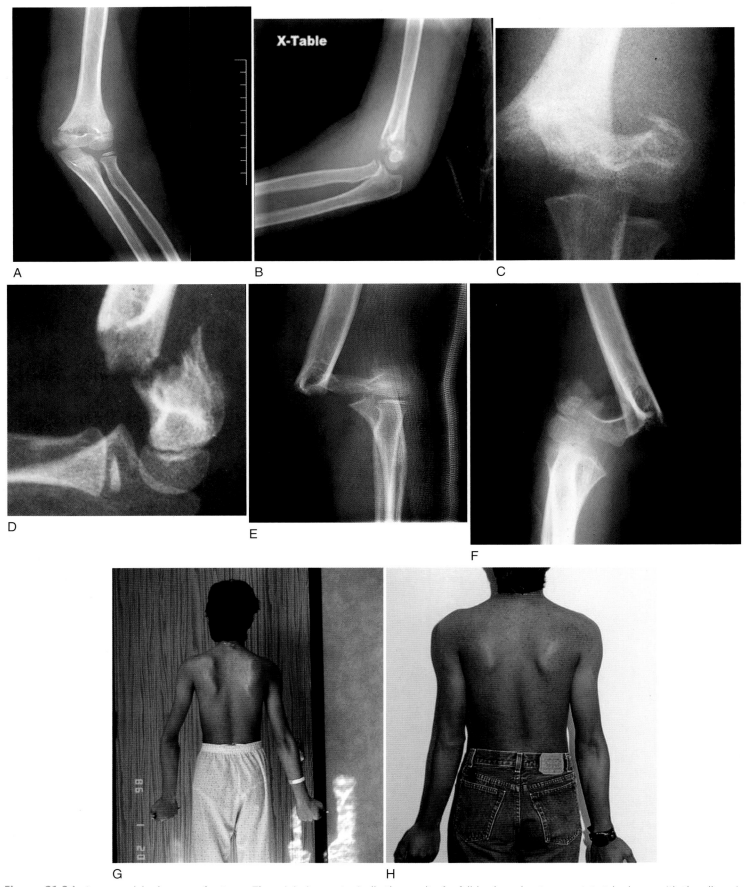

Figure 21-34. Supracondylar humerus fractures. These injuries are typically the result of a fall backward onto an outstretched arm with the elbow in hyperextension. This transmits the force of the impact to the distal humerus, driving the distal fragment posteriorly. Most require surgery to realign, reduce, and stabilize the fracture. **A,** This 8-year-old fell backward off a swing, landing on his hand with his elbow extended. The anteroposterior radiograph shows the fracture line crossing through the olecranon fossa in the supracondylar region of the distal humerus. While there is marked soft tissue swelling, degree of displacement appears mild. **B,** In the lateral view moderate posterior displacement of the distal fragment is evident. There is also a positive fat pad sign. **C,** In another boy, following a more severe backward fall, the AP radiograph shows the distal fragment displaced radially, and **D,** in the lateral view, significant posterior displacement is evident. **E** and **F,** In this case an 8-year-old fell backward from a barn window onto his extended arm. This resulted in a severely displaced (type III) supracondylar fracture with associated injury to the brachial artery and vascular insufficiency of the forearm and hand, manifest by a cool hand and absent pulses. The distal fragment is displaced posterolaterally. In such cases the brachial artery may be placed on "stretch" over the proximal fragment or may be entrapped between fragments. This is a true surgical emergency requiring immediate surgery to reduce the fracture and restore distal blood flow. **G,** This boy has cubitus valgus deformity of his left elbow as a result of incorrect healing of a supracondylar fracture. **H,** This was corrected by a distal humerus osteotomy, restoring normal contour to the elbow.

the metaphysis. The amount of separation depends on the degree of periosteal disruption. Radiographs are often normal; hence the diagnosis frequently must be made clinically on the basis of the findings of point tenderness and mild soft tissue swelling over the site of an epiphysis (Fig. 21-38; see also Fig. 21-17). This injury usually results from a shearing force. Prognosis is usually favorable.

Salter-Harris Type II. Also produced by shearing forces, this injury consists of a fracture line running a variable distance through the physis and exiting through the metaphysis on the side opposite the site of fracture initiation. A fragment consisting of the entire epiphysis with an attached metaphyseal fragment is thus produced (Fig. 21-39). Prognosis is generally favorable with adequate reduction.

Salter-Harris Type III. Intra-articular shearing forces can produce a fracture line running from the articular surface through the epiphysis and then exiting through a portion of the physis. This creates a separate epiphyseal fragment with no connection to the metaphysis (Fig. 21-40; see also Figs. 21-30 and 21-32A). Prognosis may be quite poor. Accurate anatomic reduction is required to achieve the best possible outcome.

Salter-Harris Type IV. In this fracture the fracture line starts at the articular surface, runs through the epiphysis across the physis, and exits the metaphysis. A single fragment consisting of both the epiphysis and attached metaphysis is thus created (Fig. 21-41). Like the Salter-Harris type III fracture, the injury results from the application of a shearing force. Prognosis may be poor despite seemingly good anatomic restoration of the fracture fragments. Open reduction and internal fixation is virtually always necessary. Salter-Harris type III and type IV fractures also can be classified as intra-articular fractures.

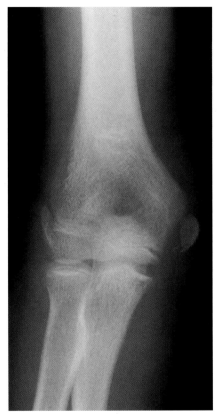

Figure 21-35. Epicondylar fracture. This 10-year-old tripped while playing soccer and fell onto his arm with a valgus strain on the elbow. The anteroposterior radiograph shows a moderately displaced medial epicondylar fracture. These injuries are sometimes associated with dislocation of the elbow, in which case there is marked swelling of the entire elbow.

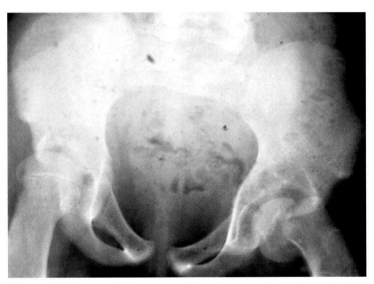

Figure 21-36. Subcapital fracture. This anteroposterior radiograph of the pelvis shows a displaced subcapital fracture of the left femur. This particular injury may be seen acutely as the result of significant trauma or may develop slowly as a result of gradual slipping at the physeal level.

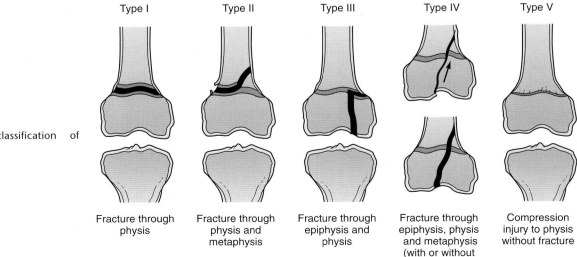

Figure 21-37. Salter-Harris classification of physeal injuries.

Type I	Type II	Type III	Type IV	Type V
Fracture through physis	Fracture through physis and metaphysis	Fracture through epiphysis and physis	Fracture through epiphysis, physis and metaphysis (with or without displacement)	Compression injury to physis without fracture

▢ Physis   ▪ Fracture line

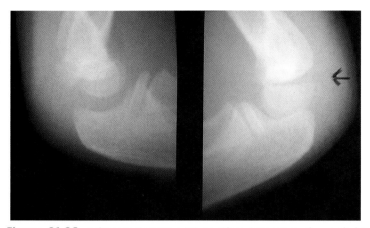

Figure 21-38. Salter-Harris type I injury. Close inspection shows slight widening of the distal humeral epiphysis *(right, arrow)*. Clinically, the patient had pain, tenderness, and decreased range of motion of the elbow. (Courtesy Jocelyn Ledesma Medina, MD.)

Salter-Harris Type V. This type of fracture is the product of a crushing injury to the physis without physeal fracture or displacement. Radiographic diagnosis is virtually impossible to make at the time of injury; hence this fracture must be diagnosed on clinical grounds. Distinction between a Salter-Harris type I and a Salter-Harris type V fracture is often possible only when a subsequent growth abnormality has been appreciated. Prognosis is quite poor for normal growth (Fig. 21-42).

Fracture Treatment Principles

The healing and remodeling capacity of the growing bones of a child is considerably greater than that of an

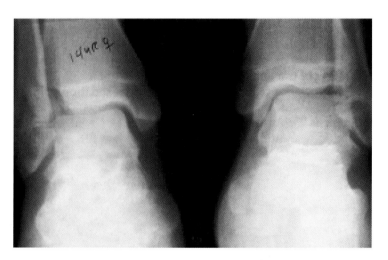

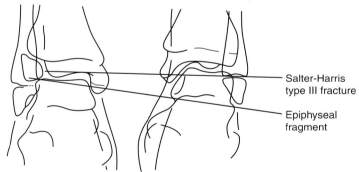

Figure 21-40. Salter-Harris type III injury. Comparison view of both ankles reveals a fracture involving the lateral aspect of the right distal tibial epiphysis. This configuration creates a separate fragment without any connection to the metaphysis.

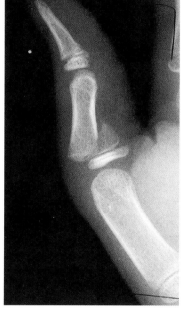

Figure 21-39. Salter-Harris type II injury. On this lateral radiograph of the thumb, the fracture is seen to involve the proximal phalanx. The fracture line runs through the physis and exits through the metaphysis on the side opposite the site of fracture initiation. A fragment consisting of the entire epiphysis with the attached metaphyseal fragment is produced.

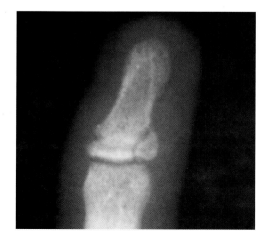

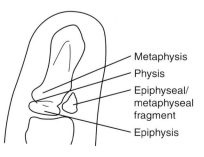

Figure 21-41. Salter-Harris type IV injury. This patient incurred a fracture of the distal phalanx of the index finger. The fracture line starts at the articular surface, runs through the epiphysis across the physis, and exits through the metaphysis. A single fragment consisting of the epiphysis and the attached metaphysis is thus created.

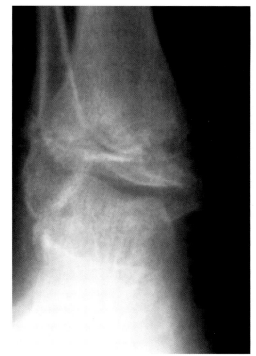

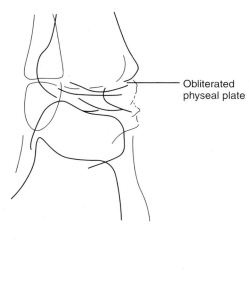

Obliterated physeal plate

Figure 21-42. Salter-Harris type V injury. This anteroposterior radiograph of the ankle taken several weeks after a crush injury sustained in an automobile accident reveals obliteration of the distal tibial physeal plate. As is often the case, original radiographs taken at the time of injury looked normal. This fracture must be suspected on clinical grounds, and the patient treated and followed accordingly.

adult; the younger the child and the closer the fracture to the epiphysis, the greater is this capacity for regeneration. As a result, healing is rapid, necessitating a shorter period of immobilization; nonunion is rare. Furthermore, in planning fracture reductions, the remodeling capability and the likely addition to bone length as a result of overgrowth must be considered. For example, in managing a toddler with a femur fracture that is displaced in the plane of motion of the adjacent joint, the bone ends must overlap to account for overgrowth and a degree of angulation can be accepted because this will ultimately be corrected by remodeling. The amount of angulation and the degree of overlap of fracture fragments that can be accepted are difficult to state in numeric terms. Acceptable position is determined in part by the child's age, the nature and position of the fracture, the bone involved, the appearance and condition of the adjacent soft tissues, and the presence or absence of other systemic injuries. Remodeling has its limitations, however. Rotational deformities and angular deformities that are not in the axis of adjacent joint motion are not effectively remodeled. Thus these must be corrected at the time of initial fracture reduction.

Nondisplaced fractures are simply casted or splinted. Because of the relative rarity of ligamentous injuries before epiphyseal closure, patients with an appropriate clinical history and point tenderness over an epiphysis are presumed to have a fracture and should be treated accordingly, even if radiographs are normal. Most displaced fractures not involving the physis can be treated by closed reduction and casting. As a general rule, open reduction and internal fixation are usually reserved for the management of Salter-Harris type III and type IV fractures that have any degree of displacement; for certain open fractures; and for fractures associated with continued neurovascular compromise. Depending on the time of presentation, degree of displacement, and severity of soft tissue swelling, reduction or casting may have to be deferred pending application of traction and subsidence of edema.

The importance of adequate analgesia and sedation before the performance of closed-reduction procedures warrants emphasis. Too often reduction is performed without the benefit of appropriate analgesia and justified by the rationale that "it will only hurt for a minute." This reasoning is callous because that excruciating "minute" may seem an eternity to the child. After reduction and/or immobilization in a cast or splint, pain should be markedly alleviated, although some analgesia is likely to be necessary for a day or two. Persistence or recurrence of considerable discomfort signifies a complication and warrants prompt reevaluation.

Care must be taken in describing the nature of the injury and its prognosis and in explaining the rationale for proposed treatment measures to the parents. A simpler explanation in terms geared to his or her developmental level should be given to the child. Written instructions regarding home care measures, necessary parent observations, and worrisome signs that signal the need for prompt reevaluation are invaluable.

Special Cases
Clavicular Fractures. Fractures of the clavicle are common. They are caused by lateral compression forces (as can occur in the process of delivery of the newborn or in falls onto the shoulder), by transmission of forces through the glenohumeral joint in a fall to the side on an outstretched arm, or occasionally by a direct blow or impact on the clavicle itself. Most involve the midshaft or distal clavicle. Greenstick fractures are more common in infants and toddlers, whereas through-and-through fractures are more typical of older children and adolescents (see Fig. 21-20). Severe displacement and angulation are usually prevented by the thick periosteum that envelops the clavicle. Clinically, the child complains of pain in the shoulder, is noted to avoid moving the arm on the involved side, and often splints it by holding the arm close against the chest. Tenderness and mild swelling are evident on palpation of the fracture site. Complications are rare, and treatment consists of the application of a padded figure-of-eight splint for 2 to 3 weeks for purposes of immobilization and to prevent foreshortening of the clavicle on healing. Older children may be more comfortable with the addition of a sling for the first few days. Slings are not advisable for toddlers because they need to be able to hold

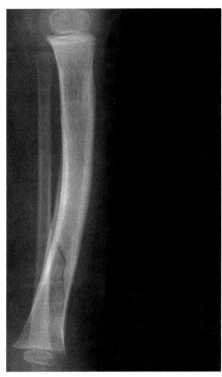

Figure 21-43. Toddler's fracture. This spiral fracture of the distal tibia was the result of a fall with a twist. The fracture was invisible when the child was seen initially but is evident along with subperiosteal new bone formation on this follow-up film taken 2 weeks later.

both arms out when walking in order to maintain balance. Forewarning parents that a hard bump will appear as the fracture heals and that this is due to callus formation is advisable because the clavicle's superficial location makes the site of callus formation prominent.

Medial clavicular fractures are rare and are caused by high-impact forces and often are associated with injuries of mediastinal structures. Thus, they warrant meticulous evaluation including chest CT and often angiography.

Fractures involving the distal tip of the clavicle in infants (beyond the neonatal period) and toddlers are likely to be the result of abuse (see Fig. 6-36).

Toddler's Fracture. One of the most common orthopedic injuries seen in children between the ages of 1 and 5 years is the toddler's fracture. The child usually has a sudden onset of refusal to bear weight on one leg or of an antalgic limp. Typically this develops after a fall with a twist, to which the unsteady toddler is unusually prone. The child may have gotten his or her foot caught and fallen while trying to extricate himself or herself, may have fallen while running and making a sudden change of direction, or fallen with a twist on jumping. Not uncommonly the actual fall is unwitnessed, and the parents are unsure about the nature of the accident. The injury results in a spiral or short oblique fracture of the distal tibia or the junction of the mid and distal tibia (Fig. 21-43). Because the thick periosteum tends to be only partially disrupted, soft tissue swelling is often minimal and tenderness may be subtle. Furthermore, many of these fractures are radiographically invisible or so subtle as to be difficult to detect, although some degree of soft tissue swelling may be evident on the film. In some cases an oblique view may be revealing. Without radiographic evidence of a fracture, the physician must rely on the examination findings to make a clinical diagnosis.

It is generally best to allow the child to remain seated in the parent's lap during the examination. This helps calm the child and ensures a more subdued response to palpation of the uninvolved areas. Attention should first be turned to the normal extremity. The ankle, knee, and hip should be placed through their range of motion. Next, the entire foot, tibia, fibula, and femur should be palpated. The child will cry if upset, but nothing about the examination should otherwise exacerbate the child's baseline irritability. Attention is then directed to the involved extremity, and a similar examination is performed. Palpation over the fracture site usually will be revealed either by a withdrawal reaction or, more commonly, by an increase from baseline irritability, usually manifested by a change in the child's facial expression and in the pattern of crying. In suspected cases in which it is difficult to determine if tenderness is present, a gentle passive twist applied to the tibia may elicit pain. Localized bone tenderness or pain on passive twisting in this setting is clinical proof of a fracture, even if radiographs are normal. In attempting to assess frightened and highly uncooperative toddlers, it is best to give them time to calm down and then either have the parent perform palpation or introduce puppets and palpate using the puppet's hands.

Treatment consists of either long- or short-leg casting for approximately 4 weeks. Infection must be included in the differential diagnosis of the limping child in this 1- to 5-year age group but usually can be ruled out by lack of fever, absence of local erythema, and normal blood values. If there is no clear history of a fall, only a mild limp, no evidence of localized tenderness, and radiographs are normal, it may be best to defer treatment and observe the child closely.

Fractures Involving the Elbow. Supracondylar, condylar, intercondylar, and epicondylar humerus fractures and proximal radius and ulna fractures all involve the elbow, and the major mechanism is a fall onto the arm with the elbow in hyperextension. In a young infant, a fracture through the cartilaginous portion of the distal humerus at the level of the condyles is known as a transcondylar fracture. Because of the lack of ossification, these are difficult to diagnose on routine x-rays. This may necessitate an MRI study or arthrogram to confirm the diagnosis in an infant with a swollen elbow. Given the force necessary to cause these fractures, when they are seen in an infant who is not yet standing and walking, inflicted trauma must be suspected (Fig. 21-44).

Supracondylar fractures account for about 50% of elbow injuries and usually result from a fall backward onto an outstretched hyperextended arm, which typically results in some degree of posterior displacement of the distal humeral fragment (see Fig. 21-34). A grading system, developed by Gartland and useful in describing severity of injury, includes: Type 1—nondisplaced, Type 2—partial displacement with intact posterior cortex, and Type 3—displaced with complete disruption of the posterior cortex. When due to abuse, the mechanism is usually a grab and yank into hyperextension (see Fig. 6-38). More rarely, a direct blow to the posterior aspect of the distal humerus is the cause, in which case the distal fragment is angulated anteriorly. Pain, swelling, and tenderness are most prominent over the posterior aspect of the distal humerus. A significant risk of associated neurovascular injury exists in patients with such fractures.

Lateral condylar fractures are in part interarticular (see Fig. 21-33). Typically they result from a fall onto an extended and abducted arm. Swelling and tenderness are prominent over the lateral aspect of the elbow. These fractures are generally unstable and often require pinning to ensure optimal reduction.

Medial epicondylar fractures stem from falls in which the elbow is hyperextended and abducted from the body,

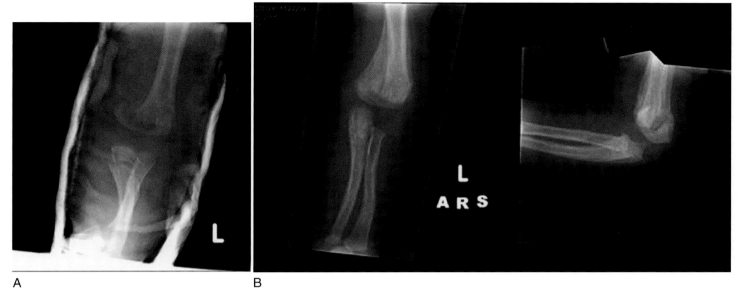

Figure 21-44. Inflicted elbow fractures. This 10-month-old was brought in with a history of a minor fall and decreased use of his arm. **A,** However, radiographs revealed displaced transverse fractures of both the distal humerus and proximal ulna along with marked soft tissue swelling. These findings were incompatible with the reported mechanism of injury and instead were the result of grabbing the arm and yanking the elbow into hyperextension with severe force. **B,** Follow-up films 1 month later show prolific subperiosteal new bone formation.

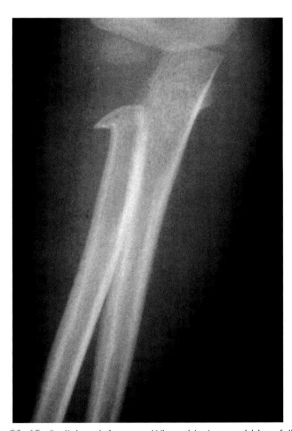

Figure 21-45. Radial neck fracture. When this 4-year-old boy fell off his bike, the position of his arm on impact resulted in transmission of a valgus force across the elbow joint, resulting in this impaction fracture of the radial neck. Radial neck fractures may require reduction to restore normal supination and pronation of the forearm.

subjecting it to a valgus stress (see Fig. 21-35). They are also commonly seen in association with elbow disloca-tions. These children have swelling and tenderness cen-tered over the medial aspect of the elbow.

Radial head and neck fractures are usually the result of a fall onto an outstretched, supinated arm (Fig. 21-45). Local swelling and tenderness are centered over the proxi-mal radius, although pain is often referred to the wrist. Because they often are accompanied by other fractures, care should be taken to search for associated injuries.

Radiographic findings in patients with fractures about the elbow can be subtle, and oblique and comparison views may be necessary to reveal them. Key signs sugges-tive of a fracture in the absence of fracture lines are the posterior fat pad sign and displacement of the anterior humeral line. The fat pad sign consists of the upward and outward displacement of the posterior fat pad of the distal humerus (Fig. 21-46A and B and see Fig. 21-34B), which is normally invisible. The finding of a fat pad indicates the presence of a hemarthrosis, and it can be seen in patients with fractures involving the distal humerus, proximal radius, or proximal ulna. The anterior humeral line is a line drawn through the anterior cortex of the humerus and normally intersects the middle third of the capitel-lum. As just noted, hyperextension injuries of the distal humerus resulting in fractures typically displace the distal humeral fragment posteriorly. As a result, the anterior humeral line intersects the anterior third of the capitellum if displacement is slight or misses it entirely if displace-ment or angulation is marked (Fig. 21-46B).

Hand and Finger Fractures. Although a complete dis-cussion of the examination of the hand and hand injuries is beyond the scope of this chapter, several key points bear emphasis, as appropriate assessment and management are essential if long-term dysfunction is to be prevented (see Figs. 21-87 and 21-88).

Phalangeal Fractures. The most common mechanism of injury producing phalangeal fractures in young chil-dren is a crush injury caused by getting their fingers caught in a door or by the weight of a heavy object falling on them. Crush injuries continue to be common in older children and adolescents, but contact sports and fistfights assume an increasing causative role in this age group.

Meticulous attention must be paid to the assessment of neurovascular and tendon function to detect subtle abnor-malities that may reflect significant injury with the poten-tial for long-term complications. This can be difficult in young children. However, much information can be gained from observing the position of the hands at rest

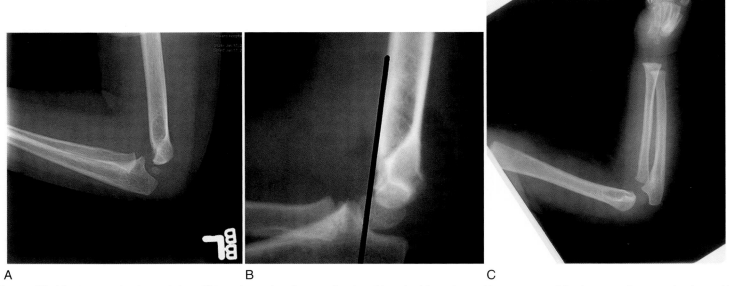

A   B   C

Figure 21-46. A, Posterior fat pad sign. Although no clear fracture line is evident in this patient with a supracondylar fracture, the posterior fat pad is readily visible, being displaced upward and outward from the posterior aspect of the distal humerus. The finding indicates presence of a joint effusion, which following trauma is blood, and in about 70% of cases with no visible fracture line, an occult fracture is present. **B,** Anterior humeral line. A line drawn through the anterior cortex of the humerus in another patient with a positive fat pad intersects the anterior third of the capitulum, indicating posterior displacement of the distal humeral fragment. **C,** Normal elbow for comparison. (**B,** Courtesy Richard B. Towbin, MD, Children's Hospital of Philadelphia.)

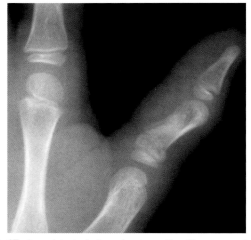

Figure 21-47. Angulated phalanx fracture. Significant angular deformity is seen in this impaction fracture of the proximal phalanx of the thumb. Such fractures require careful reduction to prevent permanent disability.

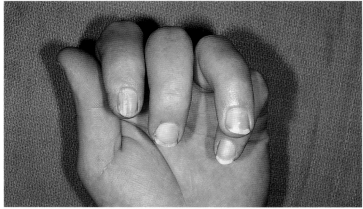

Figure 21-48. Rotational deformity resulting from a hand injury. With rotational deformity the plane of the nail of the involved finger is seen to deviate from its normal orientation. (Courtesy Neil Jones, MD, University of California, Los Angeles.)

and during spontaneous movement, as well as by watching motion as the parents hand objects to the child.

Complete phalangeal fractures typically angulate as a result of the action of the intrinsic muscles of the hand. Any fracture associated with shortening, significant angulation (Fig. 21-47), or rotational deformity and any intra-articular fracture must be appropriately reduced. Shortening and rotation are best detected by comparison of the injured hand with its normal opposite. Comparison of the planes of the fingernails of both hands with the forearms supinated and the fingers partially flexed is particularly useful in detecting rotational abnormalities (Fig. 21-48).

Determination of the degree of angulation and identification of intra-articular fractures are best done radiographically. X-ray findings can be subtle, necessitating careful comparison with radiographs of the normal hand. Obtaining oblique, as well as AP and lateral views, is also important.

Chip fractures at the base of the middle or distal phalanges may be associated with avulsion of the flexor or

extensor tendons, which may necessitate surgical repair. Clinically, an extensor tendon injury may be manifested by flexor tendon overpull (Fig. 21-49), and conversely, flexor tendon injuries may result in extensor overpull (see Fig. 21-7).

Crush injuries of the distal phalanges associated with partial or complete nail avulsions often result in open fractures with laceration of the nail bed (Fig. 21-50). These require careful cleansing, débridement, nail bed repair, and antibiotic prophylaxis.

The volar plate is a cartilaginous plate located at the base of the middle phalanx of each finger. Intra-articular fractures involving the PIP joint may fracture or tear this structure as well. The typical mechanism of injury is usually a blow to the end of the finger in hyperextension. Often a chip of bone avulsed from the middle phalanx is seen radiographically. Clinically, pain and swelling are especially marked over the volar aspect of the PIP joint. A hyperextension deformity of the involved PIP joint may be seen when the fingers are extended, or pain or locking may be noted on attempted flexion. Pain is exacerbated on passive hyperextension and reduced on passive flexion.

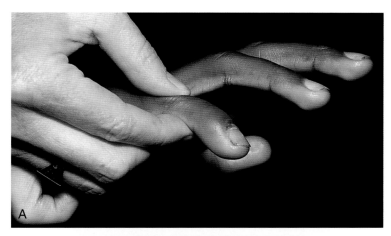

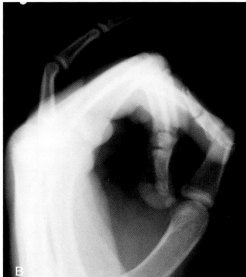

Figure 21-49. Distal phalanx fracture with extensor tendon injury. **A,** Another player's shoulder landed on this boy's finger. The finger was swollen and painful and maximally tender at the base of the distal phalanx, and the patient was unable to extend the distal interphalangeal joint. **B,** Radiograph revealed separation of the epiphysis at the base of the distal phalanx.

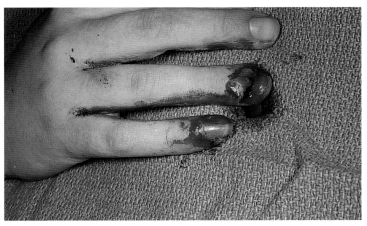

Figure 21-50. Crush injury of the distal phalanx. This child's finger was slammed in a car door. He incurred a crush fracture of the distal phalanx, partial avulsion of the nail, and a nail bed laceration. By definition, this is an open fracture. (Courtesy Neil Jones, MD, University of California, Los Angeles.)

Volar plate injuries may also accompany dislocation of the PIP joint (see "Ligamentous Injuries" later).

Metacarpal Fractures. The boxer's fracture, an impacted fracture of the neck of the fifth and often the fourth metacarpal, is among the most common of these injuries (Fig. 21-51). It occurs as a result of direct impact with a

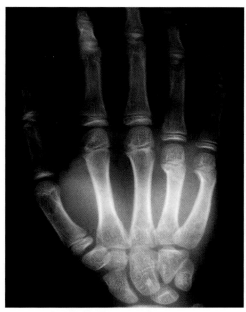

Figure 21-51. Boxer's fracture. This adolescent presented with pain and swelling of the lateral aspect of his right hand after punching a wall in a fit of temper. Radiographically he has typical boxer's fractures of the necks of the fourth and fifth metacarpals with volar displacement of the distal fragments.

partially clenched fist (typically resulting from punching another person or a wall) and is most commonly seen in aggressive adolescents. It can also result from a fall onto a clenched fist. Clinically, depression of the involved knuckle or knuckles may be noted, along with more proximal swelling and discoloration. The involved metacarpals may also appear shortened. An associated rotational deformity, if present, is manifested by rotation of the nails of the corresponding fingers (see Fig. 21-48). If the injury stems from punching another person in the mouth, care must be taken to check for overlying breaks in the skin caused by the opponent's teeth. These are infection-prone wounds and may communicate with metacarpophalangeal joints. Radiographically, volar angulation of the distal segment is typically found. If this exceeds 15 to 20 degrees or a rotational deformity is present, the patient should be referred to an orthopedist or hand surgeon for reduction. Nondisplaced, minimally angulated fractures can be treated with an ulnar gutter splint.

Metatarsal Fractures. Most metatarsal fractures are the result of a heavy object dropping onto the foot and thus are crush injuries. Falls in which the patient twists the forefoot or in which the forefoot is caught in plantar flexion can produce transverse fractures (Fig. 21-52), and injuries of the foot with the ankle inverted and the foot in plantar flexion can avulse the tuberosity from the base of the fifth metatarsal. Mild, localized swelling and point tenderness are noted over the site of a metatarsal fracture; weight bearing is painful, if not impossible. A short-leg cast provides maximal relief. This must be distinguished from the normal finding of a secondary ossification center, termed the *os vesalianum,* at the base of the fifth metatarsal. The edges of the latter are smooth, rounded, and sclerotic (Fig. 21-53).

Adolescents involved in long-distance running or walking may incur stress fractures of the shafts of the second and third metatarsals, which are the site of maximal stress and weight application during the push-off phase of walking and running. Pain often increases insidiously and tends to be poorly localized. Swelling may be imperceptible. These are often microfractures and may be radiographically invisible until healing becomes detect-

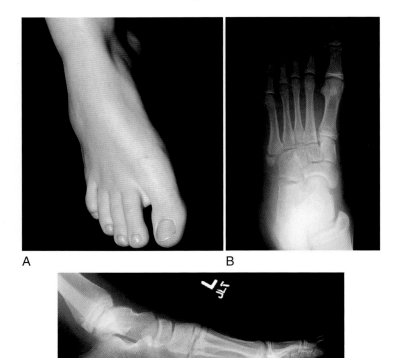

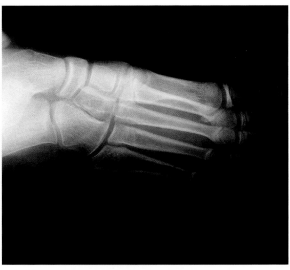

Figure 21-53. Os vesalianum. Many children have a secondary ossification center at the base of the fifth metatarsal. This can be distinguished from a fracture by the fact that its edges are smooth, rounded, and sclerotic. (Courtesy Jocelyn Ledesma Medina, MD.)

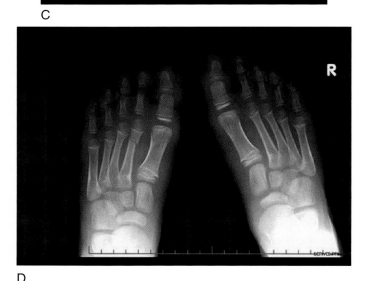

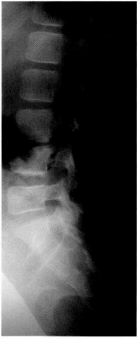

Figure 21-54. Lap belt fracture. This flexion/distraction injury occurred through the body of the L4 vertebra when the child's body hyperflexed over a lap belt in a head-on automobile collision.

Figure 21-52. Transverse metatarsal fractures. **A,** This adolescent fell forward with her forefoot twisted under her. Swelling over the proximal portion of the fifth metatarsal was prominent. **B** and **C,** AP and lateral radiographs show a transverse fracture of the proximal fifth metatarsal. **D,** This boy caught his left foot on steps and fell with his forefoot in plantar flexion, thereby incurring a transverse fracture of the distal portion of his second metatarsal.

able 3 to 4 weeks after onset. Earlier detection is possible with bone scans.

Lap Belt Fractures. Increased awareness of the importance of using seat belts to prevent serious multiple trauma in auto accidents and adherence to recommendations to place children in the back seat of the car have resulted in an increase in the incidence of lap belt fractures in children. In a head-on collision, the head and torso of a child wearing only a lap belt are thrown forward, resulting in hyperflexion of the lumbar spine over the fulcrum of the lap belt and often causing a flexion/distraction injury. This may produce a compression fracture of a lumbar vertebra

or, more likely, a shear fracture through the body of the vertebra, as well as the pedicle and spinous process. This is best seen on a lateral radiograph of the lumbar spine (Fig. 21-54). An AP view of the spine may show lateral displacement of a portion of the involved vertebral body. Because the fulcrum of the injury is anterior where the lap belt contacts the anterior abdominal wall, this injury produces a characteristic rectangular bruise and abrasion over the lower abdomen. Associated intra-abdominal injury, especially a ruptured viscus, is common, and the resultant abdominal pain may overshadow that of the vertebral injury. Hence whenever a lap belt bruise is seen during the physical examination, great care should be taken in palpating the back for localized tenderness or spasm, and immobilization of the torso and lower back should be maintained until CT scan of the lumbar spine is obtained to confirm the presence or absence of fracture and determine whether or not a fracture, when present, is stable or unstable. Fortunately, increased use of three-point belts in back seats is reducing the frequency of this injury.

Pelvic Avulsion Fractures. Pelvic avulsion fractures are a phenomenon unique to adolescents, with a peak occurrence between 13 and 14 years of age in girls and 15 and 17 years of age in boys. This stems from the fact that the secondary centers of ossification in these young people have not yet fused to the pelvis. These fractures are typically seen in adolescents who are in top physical condition and involved in competitive sports, especially track and field (e.g., sprinting and jumping), soccer, and football. The incidence of these fractures is increasing with the rising participation of adolescents in competitive sports. Most result from a sudden, violent muscular contraction while the ipsilateral extremity is held in a static position or when a muscle is suddenly lengthened during isometric contraction. As the muscle power exceeds the strength of the tendinous unit, it is torn from the apophysis or secondary ossification center. Avulsion fractures of the ischial tuberosity are the most common. They tend to occur during sprinting and are due to the sudden, powerful contraction of the hamstring muscles when the hip is flexed and the knee extended (Fig. 21-55A). Avulsions of the anterior inferior and anterior superior iliac spines (see Fig. 21-55B and C) are caused by strong contractions of the rectus femoris and sartorius muscles, respectively. These, too, tend to happen during running, often during an abrupt directional change. Some cases of anterior inferior/superior iliac spine avulsions occur with kicking. At the time of injury, the patient experiences sudden pain at the site and difficulty walking. On examination, point tenderness and swelling are noted over the involved apophysis and weakness on active hip motion is seen secondary to pain.

In viewing radiographs, it is important to compare the involved side with the normal side to detect displacement of the avulsed fragment and to avoid mistaking a normal apophysis for a fracture.

Treatment is conservative and consists of a few days of bed rest until the pain subsides, followed by 2 to 6 weeks of crutch-walking, with a gradual increase in weight bearing as pain allows. Thereafter, careful reconditioning facilitates a safe return to full activity, usually within 6 to 10 weeks.

Pathologic Fractures. Children with severe osteopenia or osteoporosis, whether stemming from an inherited disorder or disuse secondary to neurologic or neuromuscular disease, are at considerably increased risk of incurring fractures as the result of minor falls or even during routine physical therapy exercises. Localized bone lesions including those caused by osteomyelitis, tumors, or cysts, can cause localized cortical thinning as they expand. Impact on the involved bone can then also result in a pathologic fracture. Examples of some of these conditions and representative fractures are presented in Chapter 6 (see Figs. 6-75 and 6-76).

Compartment Syndromes. A compartment syndrome arises whenever the interstitial tissue fluid pressure exceeds the capillary perfusion pressure within a muscle compartment. In clinical practice the interstitial pressure elevation must reach approximately 35 to 45 mm Hg for this to occur. Because the enclosed fascial boundary of the involved muscle compartment is unyielding, hemorrhage or edema within it can cause interstitial pressure to rise to such levels, resulting in muscle ischemia and neurovascular compromise. Compartment syndromes are not rare in childhood and can be seen after open or closed fractures, crush injuries, or prolonged pressure on an extrem-

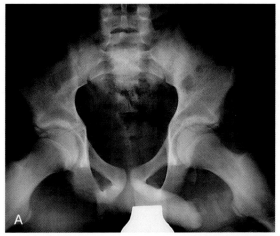

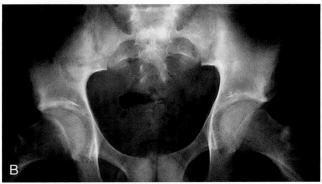

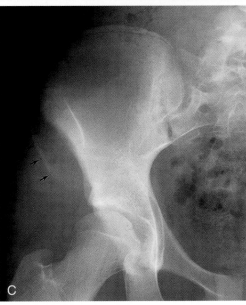

Figure 21-55. Pelvic avulsion fractures. **A,** Ischial tuberosity avulsion fracture. This 14-year-old football player sprinting for a touchdown fell on his stomach and experienced sharp left hip pain. He could not bear weight after the incident and was found to have tenderness over the left buttock and pain with abduction and flexion of the left hip. The avulsed fragment is best seen on this frog-leg view. **B,** Anterior inferior iliac spine avulsion fracture. While running in gym class, this 15-year-old boy experienced the sudden onset of left hip pain and difficulty walking. He had point tenderness over the anterior inferior iliac spine and full range of hip motion but experienced pain on flexion and internal rotation. If compared with the right, the avulsed apophysis is evident. **C,** Another 15-year-old boy, who developed sudden onset of right hip pain and inability to bear weight while kicking a soccer ball, has a large avulsion fracture of the anterior superior iliac spine *(arrows)*. (**A** and **B,** Courtesy Janet Kinnane, MD, Children's Hospital of Pittsburgh.)

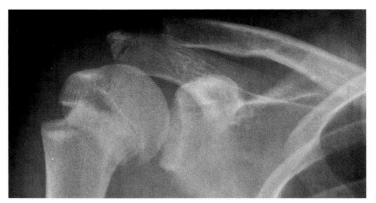

Figure 21-56. Epiphyseal separation. Because of the elasticity and relatively greater strength of the ligaments, forces that would have resulted in dislocation in an older adolescent have instead caused epiphyseal separation and displacement of the proximal humeral epiphysis in this prepubescent child. (Courtesy Department of Pediatric Radiology, Children's Hospital of Pittsburgh.)

ity, which can occur in a comatose child who has been lying on an extremity for several hours. A displaced fracture of the proximal tibial metaphysis is the fracture most likely to be complicated by a compartment syndrome. Other fractures that are well documented to predispose to the development of this problem include supracondylar humerus fractures and displaced forearm fractures.

Prompt and accurate diagnosis of a compartment syndrome is essential because, if definitive treatment is not implemented within 4 to 6 hours of onset, permanent neuromuscular damage will result. The clinical findings in compartment syndrome are quite classic. The involved extremity is swollen and tense to palpation. The patient complains of severe pain that is unrelieved by elevation, immobilization, and routine doses of narcotics. Passive movement of the terminal digits (fingers or toes) exacerbates the pain, and active motion is avoided. In view of the fact that pulses may never be diminished or absent despite a full-blown, florid compartment syndrome, the diagnosis or decision to treat should never be based solely on the presence or absence of the peripheral pulses. Because clinical diagnosis can be difficult, especially in the uncooperative or comatose child, intracompartmental needle pressure readings are recommended.

Emergent surgical decompression of the fascial covering of all involved compartments is necessary to prevent irreversible muscle and nerve damage. Following fascial decompression, relief of pain and return of active muscle power are immediate.

Ligamentous Injuries

Dislocations

The ligaments of a child have great elasticity and are relatively strong compared with bony structures, especially the physis (Fig. 21-56). Consequently, joint dislocations and ligamentous disruptions are rather unusual in childhood; when seen, they are usually the result of severe trauma and are commonly associated with fractures. In some instances the dislocation is obvious and the fracture subtle or even invisible radiographically (Fig. 21-57), but often the fracture is the prominent clinical finding and the dislocation less apparent. Hence the emphasis in pediatric orthopedics is on examining the entire extremity and on including the joints proximal and distal to a suspected fracture site in the radiographic examination. Failure to diagnose the full extent of injury can result in permanent morbidity. It must also be remembered that in

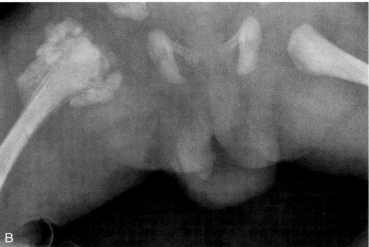

Figure 21-57. Fracture-dislocation, right hip. This young infant presented following a serious automobile accident with what appeared to be a traumatic hip dislocation without an associated fracture. **A,** The right femoral head is displaced laterally and superiorly. **B,** The follow-up film taken 2 weeks later reveals vigorous callus formation around the proximal femur and periosteal new bone formation both proximally and distally, thus confirming the existence of associated femoral fractures. (Courtesy Department of Pediatric Radiology, Children's Hospital of Pittsburgh.)

infants epiphyseal separations before ossification can simulate dislocations. For example, separation of the distal humeral epiphysis in infancy presents a radiographic picture suggestive of posterior displacement of the olecranon. The most frequent sites of dislocation in children are the hip, patellofemoral joint, and interphalangeal joints.

Hip dislocations in the young are usually the result of falls. In children younger than 5 years of age, the softness of the acetabulum and relative ligamentous laxity enable dislocation without the application of extreme force, and thus there may be no associated fractures. In older children, violent force is required and dislocation is commonly accompanied by fractures of the femur and acetabulum. In most instances the femoral head dislocates posteriorly. The child presents in severe pain with the involved leg held in adduction, internally rotated and flexed (Fig. 21-58). A position of extension, external rotation, and abduction is adopted by patients with the less common anterior dislocation. When the child also has an impressive femoral fracture, his or her pain may be attributed to that and the positional findings missed, unless the clinician specifically looks for them. Even in patients without an obvious associated fracture, epiphyseal separation or avulsion of an acetabular fragment may have occurred. Prompt reduction is important, both to relieve pain and to reduce the risk of secondary avascular necrosis of the femoral head. Postreduction films are important because these are more likely to disclose the fact that an epiphyseal separation has occurred and tend to show incomplete reduction if a radiolucent intra-articular fragment is present.

In patellofemoral dislocations the patella usually dislocates laterally (Fig. 21-59). This may occur as the result of laterally directed shearing forces or of a hyperextension injury. Patients with ligamentous laxity appear particularly susceptible. In most instances the patella has relocated by the time the patient is seen. If not, it is seen as a bulge lateral to its usual anterior location and the patient is in severe pain. In such cases x-rays should be deferred, the leg should be extended immediately, and the patella pushed back into place. This maneuver promptly alleviates pain. Other findings on examination include prominent swelling and hemarthrosis, tenderness along the medial patellar border, a positive apprehension test (see "Knee" and Fig. 21-11), and increased lateral mobility of the patella. Avulsion fractures of the lateral femoral condyle or medial patella are common associated injuries. Application of ice, rest, and use of a knee immobilizer for 3 weeks are recommended. Currently there is disagreement on whether surgical intervention should be considered after the first episode or deferred until a recurrence.

True shoulder dislocations are seen only in adolescents after epiphyseal fusion. On examination of the shoulder, a loss of the rounded contours lateral and anterior to the acromion is found. When the humeral head dislocates anteriorly, it is displaced medially beneath the coracoid process, where it can be palpated (Fig. 21-60). These patients usually support the affected arm with the opposite hand, with the shoulder in moderate internal rotation. Patients with posterior shoulder dislocations have evidence

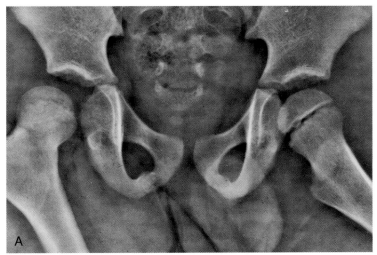

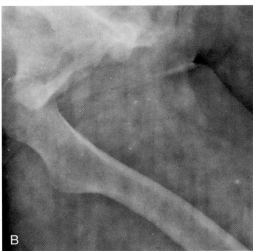

Figure 21-58. Traumatic posterior hip dislocation. This child suffered an impaction injury in an automobile accident. **A,** In the AP view the right femoral head appears to be displaced laterally and superiorly. The femur is also adducted and internally rotated. **B,** The frog-leg view discloses the severity of displacement posteriorly.

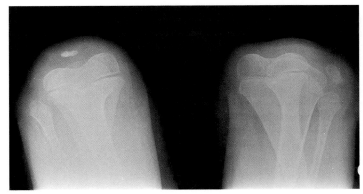

Figure 21-59. Patellar dislocation. In this flexion view obtained before relocation, the left patella is displaced laterally and there is marked swelling. (Courtesy Department of Pediatric Radiology, Children's Hospital of Pittsburgh.)

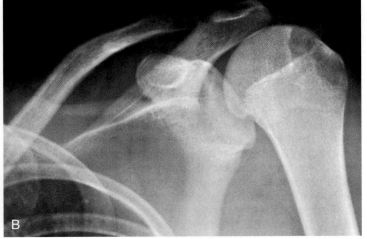

Figure 21-60. **A,** Anterior dislocation of the right shoulder. The humeral head is not in the glenoid fossa but is displaced anteriorly. **B,** The normal relationship is seen in this comparison view of the left shoulder. The injury occurred when the patient was taking a back swing for a hockey shot. The patient felt a pop with the immediate onset of severe pain. Note that his epiphyses have fused. (Courtesy Department of Pediatric Radiology, Children's Hospital of Pittsburgh.)

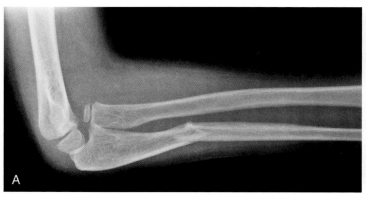
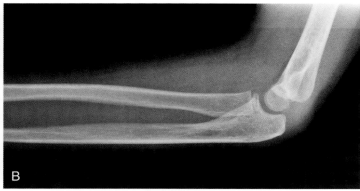

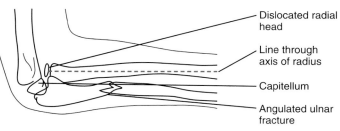

- Dislocated radial head
- Line through axis of radius
- Capitellum
- Angulated ulnar fracture

Figure 21-61. Monteggia fracture. **A,** A displaced fracture of the proximal right ulna is accompanied by dislocation of the radial head. A line drawn through the long axis of the radius would intersect the distal humerus above the level of the capitellum. **B,** The comparison view of the left arm shows the normal position of the radial head. (Courtesy Department of Pediatric Radiology, Children's Hospital of Pittsburgh.)

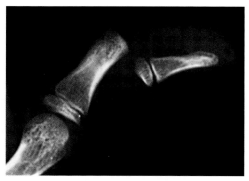

Figure 21-62. Interphalangeal joint dislocation. The distal phalanx of the thumb is dislocated dorsally. (Courtesy Department of Pediatric Radiology, Children's Hospital of Pittsburgh.)

of a fullness posterior to the glenoid cavity and are unable to externally rotate the involved upper extremity.

Separation of the proximal humeral epiphysis or major fracture-dislocations are seen in younger children subjected to forces that would cause shoulder dislocation after puberty (see Fig. 21-56).

Elbow dislocations are rare in the absence of an associated fracture. The fracture may be as subtle as a nonossified fragment avulsed from the medial epicondyle or as prominent as a displaced fracture of the ulna or radius. An example of the latter is the *Monteggia fracture,* which results from a fall onto the hand with the elbow extended and the forearm rotated radially, producing a varus stress. In this situation a displaced fracture of the proximal ulna is accompanied by dislocation of the radial head. A radial dislocation should be suspected if a line drawn through the long axis of the radius fails to pass through the capitellum on any view (Fig. 21-61). Less frequently, fractures of the radius are associated with dislocation of the radioulnar joint, and fractures of the olecranon may be accompanied by dislocation of the radius. A fall onto an extended or partially flexed arm with the forearm supinated can result in posterior dislocation of both the radius and ulna with tearing of the anterior portion of the joint capsule and of the medial collateral ligaments. This injury may be associated with fracture of the medial epicondyle (see Fig. 21-35), the coronoid process, the olecranon, or the proximal radius. Clinically the forearm is

shortened and there is an obvious deformity and marked swelling of the posterior aspect of the elbow. A high risk of neurovascular compromise and compartment syndrome exists in patients with this injury.

Dislocation of an interphalangeal joint results in an obvious deformity and is an intensely painful injury (Fig. 21-62). Avulsion fractures, volar plate fractures, and tendinous or capsular injury may be associated with it and difficult to detect radiographically. These must be suspected if range of motion is incomplete following relocation. In some cases the associated injury makes closed reduction impossible.

Sprains

A sprain is a ligamentous injury in which some degree of tearing occurs, often as a result of excessive stretching or twisting. As noted in the section on fractures, sprains are less common in children with open epiphyses than they are in older adolescents whose epiphyses have fused. When sprains do occur in these younger patients, they tend to be milder and may be associated with Salter-Harris fractures. This stems from the fact that the growth plate, being weaker than the ligaments, tends to give before significant ligamentous tearing can occur. Thus in children, physeal fractures tend to result from forces that would produce a sprain in older adolescents or adults.

In many other instances a suspected sprain is actually a small avulsion fracture. If the portion avulsed is ossified, the small fragment may be detectable radiographically, but if the fragment is cartilaginous, it will be radiographically invisible. A particular example of this is the gamekeeper's thumb, which is often associated with a small avulsion fracture of the proximal phalanx (Fig. 21-63). In it, an injury causing forceful abduction of the thumb results in rupture of the ulnar collateral ligament at the base of the thumb. Adequate examination necessitates stress testing of the radial and ulnar collateral ligaments by applying varus and valgus stress, respectively, with the thumb in extension. However, this is often impossible until pain has been reduced by a digital nerve block. If more than 20 degrees of instability is found on stressing the ulnar collaterals, the patient should be referred to an orthopedist or hand surgeon for possible surgical repair.

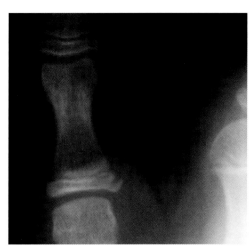

Figure 21-63. Gamekeeper's thumb. A small avulsion fracture of the epiphysis at the base of the proximal phalanx is associated with rupture of the ulnar collateral ligament. The injury occurred when the patient fell while skiing and the strap of his ski pole forcefully abducted his thumb on impact.

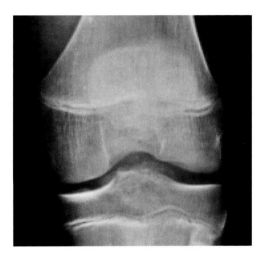

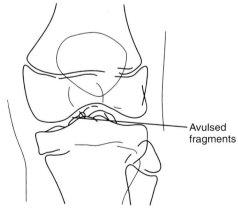

Avulsed fragments

Figure 21-64. Avulsion fracture of the left tibial spine as the result of a soccer injury (anteroposterior view). Also present were a tear in the cruciate ligament and a lipohemarthrosis. (Courtesy Department of Pediatric Radiology, Children's Hospital of Pittsburgh.)

Failure to correct the problem results in a loss of resistance to abduction and a weak pinch.

Before epiphyseal closure, Salter-Harris fractures and avulsion fractures of the distal fibula or tibia should be strongly suspected in children with "sprainlike" injuries of the ankle. Similarly, injuries that rupture the cruciate ligaments of the knee in adults usually avulse the tibial spine in children (Fig. 21-64). These are the result of a

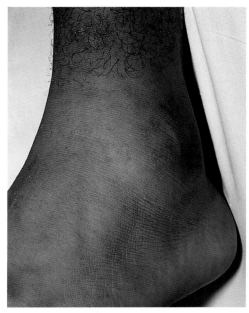

Figure 21-65. Ankle sprain. Marked tenderness and swelling were maximal inferior to the malleolus of this 17-year-old youth. The anterior talofibular, calcaneofibular, and posterior talofibular ligaments were all tender. This is in contrast to the findings seen with a Salter-Harris type I fracture of the distal tibia (see Fig. 21-17).

Table 21-5	Classification of Sprains	
GRADE OF SPRAIN	**DEGREE OF TEARING**	**CLINICAL FINDINGS**
I	A small percentage of ligamentous fibers is disrupted	Pain on motion Local tenderness Mild swelling
II	A moderate percentage of fibers is torn	Pain on motion More diffuse tenderness Moderate swelling, may have joint effusion Mild instability
III	The ligament is completely disrupted	Severe pain on motion Marked swelling, usually with joint effusion Marked tenderness Joint instability

blow to the knee, forcing it into hyperextension along with a valgus or varus stress. Following physeal closure in adolescence, sprains are seen with some frequency.

Sprains are classified in three grades according to severity (Table 21-5). In contrast to physeal fractures, swelling and tenderness are more likely to be prominent and occur early. They are most evident over the involved ligament or ligaments, not over the epiphysis. Pain on motion is often more marked in patients with sprains than in patients with physeal fractures.

Ankle Sprains. An ankle sprain in an adolescent patient is typically caused by a severe inversion stress injury, and the presenting findings are diffuse pain and tenderness along with swelling centered below the lateral malleolus, although the superior margin of swelling may cover the malleolus (Fig. 21-65). Areas of maximal tenderness may be found over the anterior talofibular ligament alone or over both it and the calcaneofibular ligament. Rarely the posterior talofibular ligament is also torn in patients with particularly severe sprains, and tenderness and swelling are noted over its course as well. Little pain occurs on dorsiflexion or plantar flexion, but marked pain occurs on passive inversion. Tests for ligamentous stability are described earlier (see "Ankle").

Knee Sprains. Patients with major knee sprains present with marked pain, refusal to bear weight, and swelling resulting from hemarthrosis. Tears of the medial or lateral collateral ligaments of the knee are seen in adolescents and are usually the result of a direct blow that applies valgus or varus stress, respectively. A football tackle and being hit by a car from the side are common reported mechanisms. Tenderness is prominent over the involved ligaments. Major tears result in ligamentous instability detected by the adduction/abduction stress test (see "Knee"). Tibial spine avulsion fractures (see Fig. 21-64) and anterior cruciate ligament tears stem from falls in which the knee is hyperflexed, often a fall from a bicycle or a fall while skiing. Tenderness is marked anteriorly, and instability is demonstrated by the anterior drawer and Lachman tests (see "Knee" and Figs. 21-12 and 21-13).

Because of the frequency of associated fractures in children and adolescents, patients with apparent sprains and hemarthroses should not undergo tests of ligamentous stability until radiographs have been obtained and the possibility of an unstable fracture has been ruled out.

Shoulder Separation. A shoulder separation involves a ligamentous tear at the acromioclavicular joint, usually resulting from a fall onto an outstretched, adducted arm. Clinically the lateral aspect of the clavicle appears to ride higher on the injured side than on the normal side, and with application of pressure it may be forced back into its normal position. If it can also be moved forward and backward, the coracoclavicular ligaments have been torn as well.

Evaluation and Management. In evaluating patients with possible sprains, careful attention must be given not only to assessment of swelling, tenderness, and joint stability, but also to evaluation of adjacent bony structures and to musculotendinous function (see "Physical Examination" earlier). Complete evaluation may be impossible if initial presentation has been delayed for several hours and secondary effusion, soft tissue swelling, and muscle spasm are pronounced. In such instances it may be necessary to immobilize the affected joint with a splint and have the patient return for reevaluation in 24 to 72 hours when the swelling has abated.

Rest, the application of ice, use of analgesic anti-inflammatory agents such as ibuprofen, and perhaps use of an Ace wrap or taping, suffice for grade I sprains. Subjective improvement occurs in a few days. Grade II and grade III sprains require a longer period of immobilization. Splinting or casting for a few to several weeks is generally necessary. Grade III sprains may require surgical intervention.

Subluxation of the Radial Head (Nursemaid's Elbow)

Subluxation of the radial head is the most common elbow injury in childhood and one of the most common ligamentous injuries. The mechanism is one of sudden traction applied to the extended arm. The injury is seen predominantly in children between the ages of 1 and 4 years. The typical history is one of a parent's suddenly pulling the child up by the arm to prevent a fall; of the child, in a fit of temper, attempting to pull away from the parent; or of a child being swung by an arm. However, in a number of cases the injury is due to the child's grabbing onto some object in an effort to avoid falling. This type of injury can also occur in an infant who is rolled over with

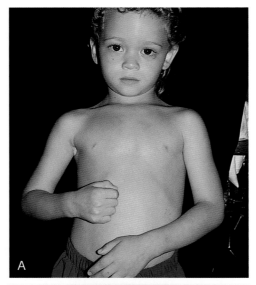

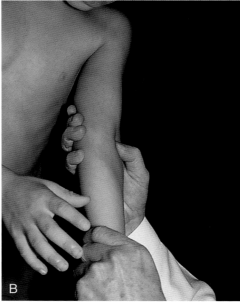

Figure 21-66. Nursemaid's elbow. **A,** The affected arm is held close to the body with the elbow flexed and the forearm pronated. **B,** The reduction maneuver consists of supinating the forearm while pressing down on the radial head.

an extended arm trapped beneath his or her trunk. After a brief initial period of crying, the child calms down but is unable to use the affected arm, which is held close to the body with the elbow flexed and forearm pronated (Fig. 21-66A). If old enough to talk, the child may complain of elbow, forearm, or even wrist pain. Physical examination reveals no bony tenderness and no evidence of swelling, but on assessment of passive motion, the child resists any attempt at supination and cries in pain. Mild limitation of elbow flexion and extension may also be noted.

Pathologically, when the radial head is subluxated by the sudden pull on the arm, the annular ligament is torn at the site of its attachment to the radius and the radial head slips through the tear. When the traction is released and the radial head recoils, the proximal portion of the annular ligament becomes trapped between the radial head and the capitellum (Fig. 21-67). This limits motion and produces the child's pain. Radiographs are normal because the radial head is not truly subluxated. When a patient presents with a typical history, is found to have no evidence of tenderness, and resists supination, x-ray

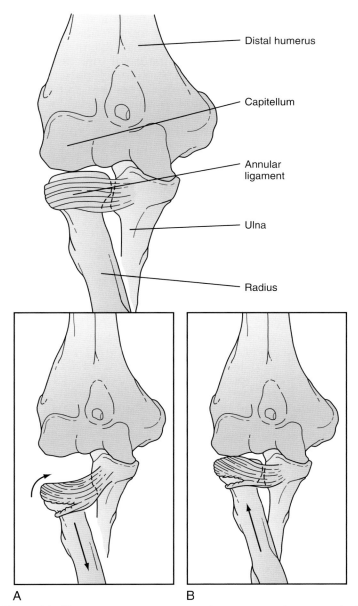

- Distal humerus
- Capitellum
- Annular ligament
- Ulna
- Radius

A   B

Figure 21-67. Nursemaid's elbow. **A,** Sudden traction on the outstretched arm pulls the radius distally, causing it to slip partially through the annular ligament and tearing it in the process. **B,** When traction is released, the radial head recoils, trapping the proximal portion of the ligament between it and the capitellum.

studies are unnecessary. Reduction, as described later, should be attempted.

Treatment consists of supinating the child's forearm with the elbow in a flexed position while applying pressure over the radial head (see Fig. 21-66B). A click can be perceived as the annular ligament is freed from the joint. Occasionally this maneuver fails, in which case the forearm should be supinated and extended with traction applied distally while pressing down on the radial head. If this fails as well, pronation with the elbow in extension may be attempted. On reduction, pain relief is immediate and return of function is evident within 10 to 15 minutes. Clinicians often recommend that the child wear a sling for 10 days to reduce use and to allow the annular ligament to heal; compliance is difficult to ensure, however.

If presentation has been delayed for several hours, there may be a longer delay between reduction and resumption of normal use and it may be necessary to administer acetaminophen for 12 to 14 hours to relieve residual aching. Parents should be cautioned to avoid maneuvers that cause excessive traction on the arm because there is a significant risk of recurrence.

Extremity Pain with Ligamentous Laxity

Children with significant and generalized ligamentous laxity have hypermobile joints and are vulnerable to excessive stretching or stress on ligamentous and musculotendinous structures. They are also somewhat more susceptible to joint dislocations. The phenomenon is seen in up to 18% of girls and 6% of boys. After periods of vigorous physical activity, these children often complain of arthralgias, shin or muscular pain, and occasionally have evidence of joint swelling. Episodes tend to occur in the evening or at night; are self-limited, lasting 1 to several hours; and respond to rest and acetaminophen or ibuprofen. Many of these children have been accused of attention-getting behavior and hypochondriasis. Others have been dismissed as having "growing pains," and some have undergone extensive testing for rheumatic disorders. A history of greater than average activity on the preceding day and of recurrent short-lived pain usually without objective swelling, combined with findings of ligamentous laxity on examination (Fig. 21-68), should point to this diagnosis. The rarity of joint swelling and the absence of fever and other systemic symptoms help to rule out rheumatic and collagen vascular disorders.

Once the problem is correctly diagnosed, patients can minimize discomfort by avoiding sudden increases in level of activity, when possible, and by taking a mild anal-

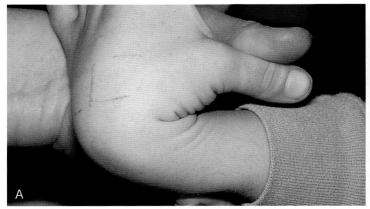
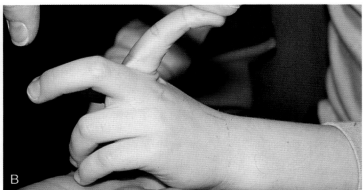

A   B

Figure 21-68. Ligamentous laxity. This child shows findings typical of the joint hypermobility seen with ligamentous laxity. **A,** He is able to hyperflex the wrist on the forearm. **B,** He can also hyperextend the distal interphalangeal joint and the metacarpophalangeal joint.

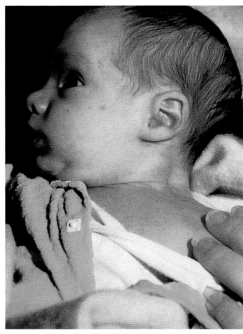

Figure 21-69. Congenital torticollis. The "tumor" of congenital torticollis is seen as a swelling in the midportion of the sternocleidomastoid muscle. It is firm on palpation, and the muscle itself is shortened. The head tilts toward the affected side, and the chin rotates in the opposite direction. (Courtesy James Reilly, MD, A. I. duPont Hospital for Children.)

gesic prophylactically before going to bed after a day of unusually vigorous activity. Graduated strengthening exercises may also be helpful. This is particularly true for children who want to participate in gymnastics or competitive sports.

Disorders of the Neck and Spine

Children with disorders of the axial skeleton most commonly present with some type of deformity. Pain or dysfunction of the associated spinal cord and nerve roots may also prompt evaluation. Because these conditions often progress with growth, awareness and early recognition are important to assist early institution of appropriate treatment and to minimize resultant morbidity.

Congenital Torticollis

Congenital torticollis, or "wryneck," is a positional abnormality of the neck produced by fibrosis and shortening of the sternocleidomastoid muscle. It is thought to be secondary to abnormal intrauterine positioning or to birth trauma resulting in the formation of a hematoma within the muscle belly. Usually the condition is recognized at or shortly after birth. A palpable swelling or "tumor" is often noted within the muscle. With subsequent fibrosis, the characteristic deformity of torticollis develops, consisting of head tilt toward the affected side with rotation of the chin to the opposite side (Fig. 21-69). Passive rotation is diminished toward the side of the torticollis, and lateral side bending is limited toward the side away from the torticollis. Although the mass usually disappears in the first several weeks of life, contracture of the muscle persists and, if untreated, may result in craniofacial disfigurement with flattening of the face on the affected side. Gentle passive stretching exercises and positioning the child's crib so that external stimuli will cause him or her to turn the head and neck away from the side of deformity

may be beneficial. If these measures fail, surgical release of the contracted muscle may be indicated.

Considerations in the differential diagnosis include Klippel-Feil syndrome; inflammatory or infectious conditions of the head, neck, or nasopharynx; posterior fossa or brainstem neoplasm; traumatic cervical spine injury; and atlantoaxial rotary subluxation. However, with the exception of the Klippel-Feil anomaly, the other conditions tend to occur considerably later in childhood. In addition, a hip examination should be performed and an AP pelvis radiograph obtained for each infant with torticollis because hip instability or dysplasia is present in approximately 20% of these children.

Klippel-Feil Syndrome

Patients with Klippel-Feil syndrome have a congenital malformation of the neck that results from a failure of segmentation in the developing cervical spine. The condition varies greatly in severity, depending on the number of vertebrae that are fused (Fig. 21-70A and B). More severely affected individuals exhibit a short, broad neck with the appearance of "webbing," a low hairline, and gross restriction of motion (Fig. 21-70C and D). The condition may be associated with other congenital malformations such as a Sprengel deformity (see Fig. 21-81); rib deformities; scoliosis; CNS defects; and cardiac, pulmonary, and renal anomalies. Secondary neurologic problems are rare, but accelerated degenerative changes may occur at mobile spinal segments adjacent to the involved vertebrae.

On occasion, range-of-motion exercises or bracing may be tried to improve mobility or correct the deformity. Surgery, except for cosmesis or the treatment of neurologic dysfunction, is rarely indicated. Mild forms of the malformation may be diagnosed only as a result of radiographs taken for other reasons.

Scoliosis

Scoliosis is a condition in which there is curvature of the spine occurring in the lateral plane. It occurs in structural forms, characterized by a fixed curve, and "functional" forms, characterized by a flexible or correctable curve. By anatomic necessity, this lateral deviation is associated with vertebral rotation, such that when this deformity occurs in the thoracic spine, a chest wall deformity, or "rib hump," develops (Fig. 21-71). When it occurs in the lumbar spine, a prominence of the flank may be noted (Fig. 21-72). Often there is a primary structural curve with an adjacent secondary compensatory curve. Most cases of structural scoliosis are idiopathic and have their onset in early adolescence. A familial predisposition has been documented, but inheritance appears to be multifactorial. Females are affected more often than males, and their curvature is more likely to worsen. Infantile (0 to 3 years) and juvenile (3 to 10 years) forms of idiopathic scoliosis are seen, though much less commonly. Those with onset in infancy rapidly develop plagiocephaly with flattening of the head on the concave side of the curve and a corresponding prominence on the opposite side of the head. Affected infants also have an increased incidence of associated hip dysplasia, congenital heart disease, inguinal hernia, and mental retardation. Structural scoliosis can also occur in conjunction with neuromuscular conditions such as cerebral palsy (Fig. 21-73), myelomeningocele, spinocerebellar degeneration, polio, and spinal cord tumors; myopathic disorders including arthrogryposis or muscu-

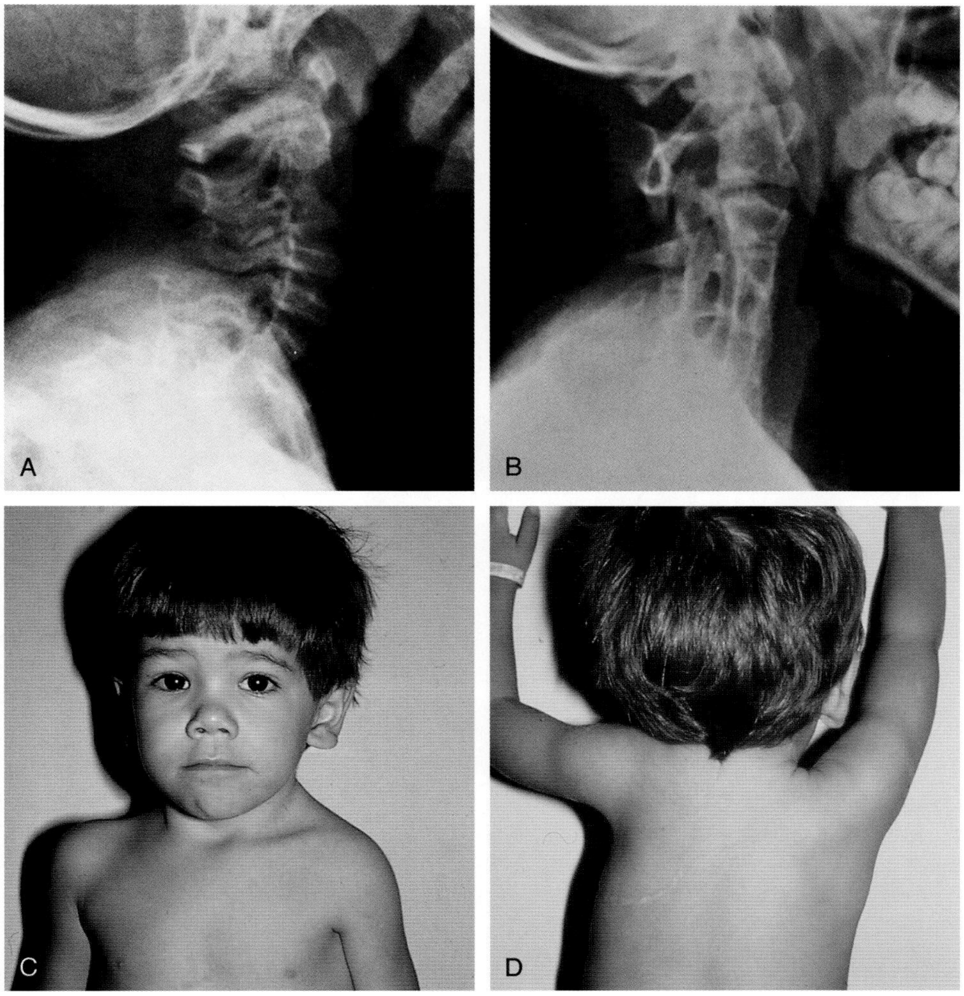

Figure 21-70. Klippel-Feil syndrome. **A,** This radiograph shows mild osseous involvement with fusion of the upper cervical segments. **B,** Another patient shown in this radiograph has severe osseous involvement in which C3-C7 are fused and hypoplastic. **C,** Clinically the neck appears short and broad in the anterior view of this young child. **D,** In this posterior view the hairline is low and an associated Sprengel deformity is present, the left scapula being hypoplastic and high riding. As a result, the patient is unable to fully raise his left arm. Typical webbing of the neck is not appreciable in this child.

Table 21-6	Causes of Scoliosis

Structural Scoliosis
Idiopathic
Congenital
Neuromuscular
Other conditions that may result in scoliosis
   Myopathic disorders
   Neurofibromatosis
   Mesenchymal disorders
   Osteochondrodystrophies
   Metabolic disorders
   Trauma, surgery, irradiation, burns

Functional Scoliosis
Herniated lumbar disks
Postural derangements
Limb length inequality
Irritative or inflammatory disorders
Hysteria

lar dystrophy; congenital spinal anomalies (Fig. 21-74A and B) such as hemivertebrae, trapezoidal vertebrae, unsegmented vertebrae; neurofibromatosis (Fig. 21-75) and mesenchymal disorders; and a variety of other conditions (Table 21-6). These neuromuscular and congenital forms of scoliosis tend to have more rapid progression of curvature than is true of idiopathic scoliosis, and infants with congenital spinal anomalies have a high incidence of associated genitourinary anomalies.

Apparent nonstructural, flexible, or "functional" scoliosis may be seen in association with poor posture; limb length inequality; or flexion contracture of a hip or knee, in which case the curve disappears when the child is seated. It can also be seen with paraspinous muscle spasm after a

back injury; as the result of splinting because of pain in cases of pyelonephritis, appendicitis, or pneumonia; or in patients with a herniated intervertebral disk and secondary nerve root pain (see Fig. 21-80A; see also Table 21-6). These forms resolve with treatment of the primary disorder.

Except in curvatures resulting from inflammatory or neoplastic processes and from herniation of an intervertebral disk, pain is rarely a complaint in children and adolescents with scoliosis. In fact, patients with pain, signs of nerve root compression, or evidence of new-onset peripheral neurologic deficits should undergo thorough evaluation for a treatable underlying cause.

The clinical signs found during examination in a patient with scoliosis can be separated into true pathognomonic findings and associated stigmata, which may also occur in otherwise normal, nonscoliotic children. The only true pathognomonic sign of scoliosis is the presence of a curve noted on forward bending, which constitutes a positive Adams Forward Bend test (see "Thoracolumbar Spine" earlier). An associated convex posterior chest wall prominence (termed *rib hump*) or paralumbar prominence may also be noted on forward bending (see Fig. 21-71B). The rib hump and paralumbar prominence are manifestations of the vertebral rotational deformity seen in scoliosis.

Frequently a diagnosis of scoliosis is based not on a positive forward bend test, but rather on the presence of so-called stigmata signs. These signs include shoulder asymmetry, unilateral scapular prominence, waist asymmetry, and small chest or paralumbar humps (see Figs. 21-71A, 21-72, and 21-75A). Any or all of these stigmata signs may be present in a child with true scoliosis, but the mere presence of these stigmata does not always imply the

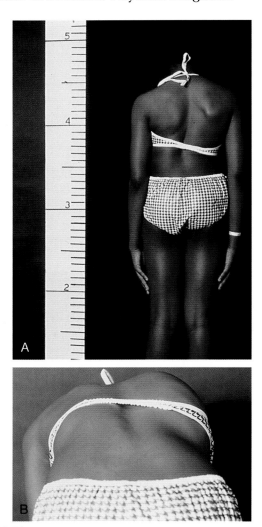

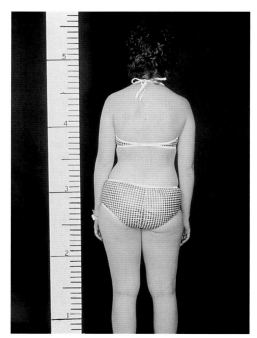

Figure 21-71. Moderate idiopathic thoracic scoliosis in an adolescent. **A,** Scapular asymmetry is easily discernible in the upright position. This results from rotation of the spine and attached rib cage. **B,** Forward flexion reveals a rib hump deformity.

Figure 21-72. Lumbar scoliosis. Pelvic obliquity is present, with prominence of the left flank.

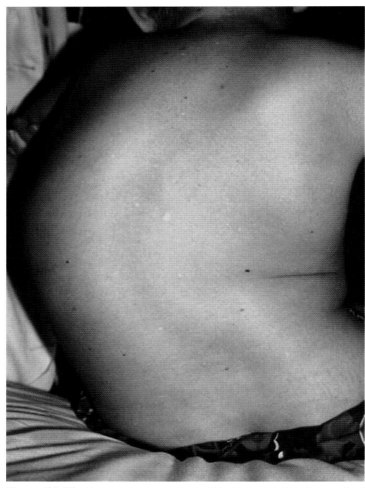

Figure 21-73. Neuromuscular scoliosis. This 12-year-old boy has cerebral palsy and scoliosis. Note that his sitting balance is affected by the curve of his spine, which extends from the upper thorax to his pelvis, resulting in pelvic obliquity and inability to sit independently. This is typical of spinal deformity in patients with neuromuscular disorders.

presence of scoliosis. Body asymmetry is a frequent occurrence in the normal nonscoliotic child. A carefully performed Adams Forward Bend test always determines whether the stigmata signs are associated with true scoliosis or simply evidence of body asymmetry.

Because screening studies have shown that up to 5% of school-age children and adolescents have lateral curvatures, routine screening by primary care physicians is important. Hence the forward bend test should be part of all examinations in children from age 6 to 7 years until the end of puberty (see "Thoracolumbar Spine" earlier). When true clinical scoliosis is found, the patient should be referred for orthopedic evaluation no matter how small the curve is felt to be. It is probably safer and more cost-effective for the primary care physician to make the referral without obtaining prior radiographs, because typical office radiographs done for scoliosis screening are usually not of high quality. Standing, full-torso x-rays taken on 36-inch (90-cm)-long cassette films with special grids are much more helpful and more readily available in the orthopedic clinic or office. Once a diagnosis of scoliosis has been made, follow-up x-rays are routinely obtained no more frequently than at 6- to 9-month intervals. The goal of close follow-up is to detect progression of curvature early and implement treatment to prevent or reduce it when needed. Idiopathic curves of 25 to 30 degrees or more and lesser curves showing rapid progression are

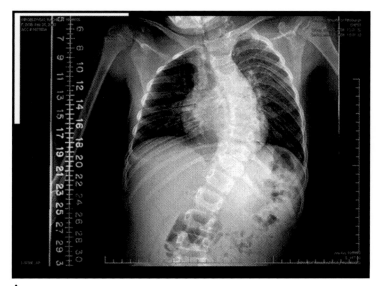

A

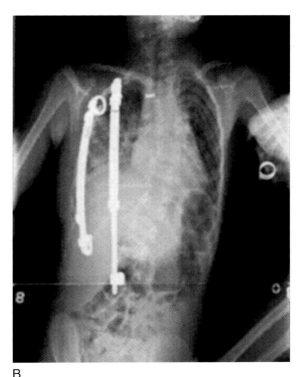

B

Figure 21-74. Congenital scoliosis. **A,** This 7-year-old was born with fusion of ribs 5 to 10 on her right side. She also has congenital failure of segmentation of several vertebrae. Both of these anomalies contributed to her progressive scoliotic deformity. **B,** She was treated with an opening thoracostomy (separation of the ribs) and insertion of a Vertical Expandable Prosthetic Titanium Rib (VEPTR, Synthes). This device allows for spinal growth and expansion of the chest cavity by repeated surgical expansions at 6-month intervals.

treated with spinal bracing and an exercise program. Children with curves exceeding 45 to 50 degrees or those with curves that progress rapidly despite bracing require operative intervention.

Patients with untreated curvatures exceeding 75 to 80 degrees inevitably suffer significant secondary cardiopulmonary problems including decreased vital capacity, shunting, decreased oxygen saturation, and cor pulmonale.

Newborns and infants should be screened for congenital and infantile forms of scoliosis. This is often best done by holding the infant prone on the examiner's hand and can be done while assessing for parachute reflex.

Kyphosis

Kyphosis is a condition in which there is curvature of the spine in the sagittal plane. The thoracic spine normally has a kyphotic curvature of 25 to 50 degrees, with a similar amount of lordosis in the lumbar spine in the sagittal plane. Excessive kyphosis may be purely postural in nature or may be associated with a number of pathologic conditions. The latter include congenital vertebral anomalies, spinal growth disturbance known as Scheuermann disease (Fig. 21-76), neuromuscular afflictions, skeletal dysplasias, and metabolic diseases (Fig. 21-77). Kyphosis can also develop after spinal trauma or surgery. Patients with a structural deformity may complain of backache aggravated by motion. The deformity is best viewed from the lateral position on forward bending. Evaluation of the effects of posture and of application of pressure over the apex of the curve assists diagnosis and decisions regarding treatment.

Postural kyphosis is usually seen in preadolescents and consists of a flexible thoracic kyphosis that is correctable on hyperextension. Most affected children have a compensatory increase in lumbar lordosis. Radiographic findings are normal. Treatment consists of an exercise program designed to strengthen trunk and abdominal muscles, which are usually weak in these patients.

Scheuermann disease, a disorder of unknown etiology, is the most common cause of fixed kyphotic deformity. It can be distinguished clinically from postural kyphosis by its inherent stiffness and the greater magnitude of the deformity. The deformity fails to correct or is only partially correctable on hyperextension or on the application of pressure over the apex of the curve. Lateral radiographs reveal anterior wedging of three or more consecutive vertebral bodies that are located at the apex of the curve. Radiographic evidence of end-plate erosion of the involved vertebrae often exists, and Schmorl nodules are a common associated finding (see Fig. 21-76).

Exercises and bracing are quite effective in treating mild structural kyphosis in the growing spine. However, when the deformity is severe and fixed, surgical correction and stabilization may be indicated.

Spondylolisthesis

Spondylolisthesis is a condition characterized by the translation or forward displacement of one vertebral body over another and is seen most commonly at the lumbosacral articulation. The problem may develop as a result of insufficiency or fatigue fractures of the pars interarticularis (isthmic), congenital dysplasia of the posterior spinal elements (dysplastic), or degenerative changes in the disk and facets (degenerative), or it may occur secondary to pathologic lesions within the vertebra and its elements (pathologic). Isthmic spondylolisthesis (spondylolysis) is by far the most common type (Fig. 21-78). Patients with a congenital predisposition may show alarming degrees of slippage. The condition is often associated with low back pain that increases with strenuous activities and abates with rest. Some patients have symptoms of nerve root irritation. This necessitates differentiation from inflammatory and neoplastic processes and from disk herniation.

Examination often reveals loss of normal lumbar lordosis, tenderness of the involved posterior elements, paravertebral muscle spasm, and secondary tightness of the hamstring muscles. A stepoff deformity may be evident on palpation of the spinous processes. Range of motion is

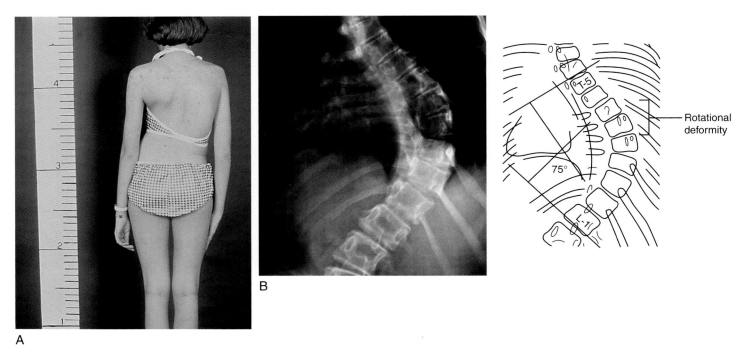

Figure 21-75. Severe thoracic scoliosis secondary to neurofibromatosis. **A,** Note the chest wall deformity and that the patient's head is not centered over the pelvis. **B,** The severe curvature is more apparent on this radiograph. The angle of measurement (here, 75 degrees) is determined by the intersection of lines drawn perpendicular to the vertebrae at the ends of the curve (Cobb method).

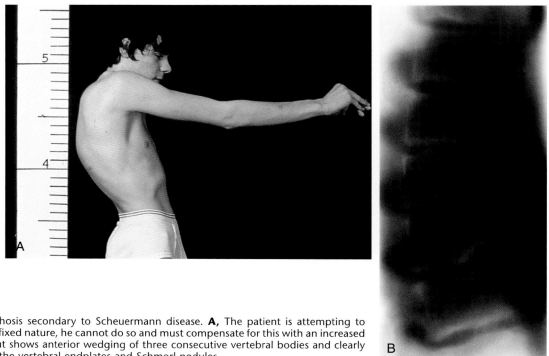

Figure 21-76. Moderate thoracic kyphosis secondary to Scheuermann disease. **A,** The patient is attempting to correct the deformity, but because of its fixed nature, he cannot do so and must compensate for this with an increased lumbar lordosis. **B,** This tomographic cut shows anterior wedging of three consecutive vertebral bodies and clearly demonstrates the associated erosion of the vertebral endplates and Schmorl nodules.

often limited in extension because of pain. Nerve root signs may be present. In its most severe form, spondyloptosis, the L5 vertebral body may completely translate off the sacrum, and the patient characteristically exhibits a waddling gait, a transverse abdominal crease, flattened buttocks, and flexion deformities of the hips and knees, as well as foreshortening of the torso (Fig. 21-79A and B). Characterization and grading of the process are accomplished with radiographs. The oblique view may reveal a spondylolysis and the lateral view the degree of spondylolisthesis (Fig. 21-79C; see also Fig. 21-78).

In mild to moderate cases, treatment consists of appropriate exercises and bracing. Patients with progressive slippage require surgical fusion, and those with neural involvement may also require nerve root decompression. In cases of severe spondylolisthesis with cosmetic deformity, functional impairment, and neurologic dysfunction, surgical reduction of the deformity may be attempted but is not easy, nor is it without risk to the adjacent neural structures.

Herniated Intervertebral Disk

Although relatively common in adults, herniated disks occur only rarely in children and infrequently in adoles-

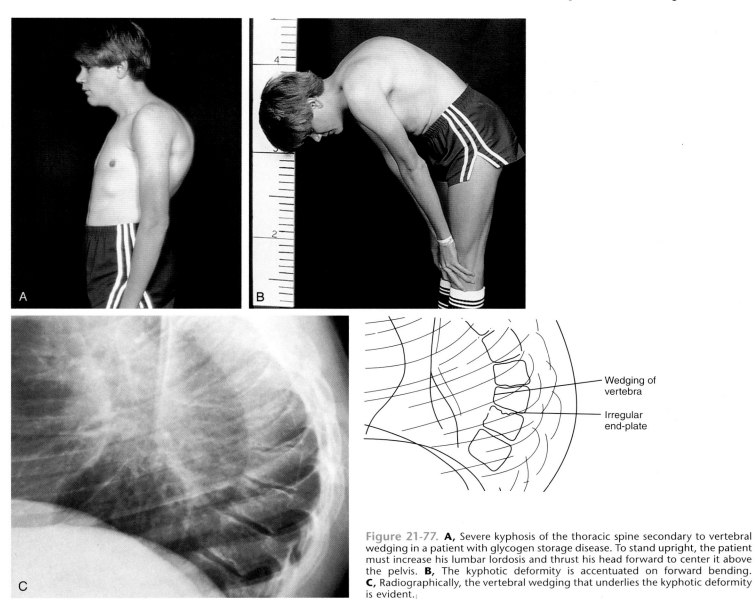

Figure 21-77. **A,** Severe kyphosis of the thoracic spine secondary to vertebral wedging in a patient with glycogen storage disease. To stand upright, the patient must increase his lumbar lordosis and thrust his head forward to center it above the pelvis. **B,** The kyphotic deformity is accentuated on forward bending. **C,** Radiographically, the vertebral wedging that underlies the kyphotic deformity is evident.

Figure 21-78. Radiograph of a moderate isthmic spondylolisthesis in a 14-year-old boy. The forward slippage of L5 on the sacrum was the result of a fatigue fracture of the pars interarticularis.

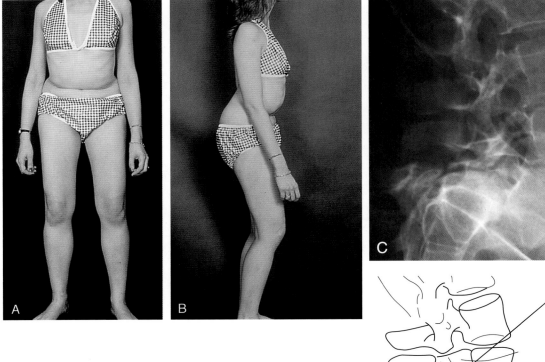

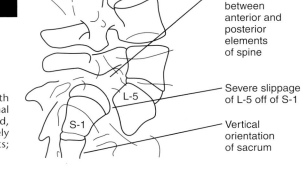

No visible
continuity
between
anterior and
posterior
elements
of spine

Severe slippage
of L-5 off of S-1

Vertical
orientation
of sacrum

L-5

S-1

Figure 21-79. Spondyloptosis in a 16-year-old girl. **A,** A cosmetic deformity is common with this magnitude of spondylolisthesis. The torso is foreshortened, and a transverse abdominal crease is present. **B,** In the lateral view the torso is thrust forward, the buttocks are flattened, and there are flexion deformities of the hips and knees. **C,** The L5 vertebra has completely translocated off the sacrum as the result of a congenital insufficiency of the posterior elements; the lumbar spine has essentially migrated anteriorly and into the pelvis.

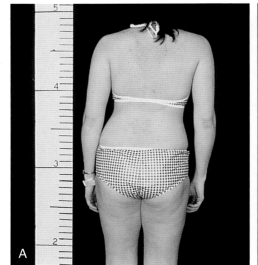

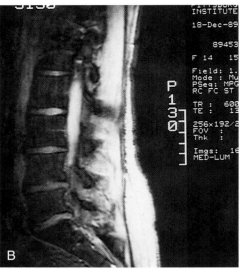

Figure 21-80. Herniated intervertebral disk. **A,** Diskogenic scoliosis is evident in a 16-year-old girl with a herniated disk at L4-L5. The trunk is shifted away from the affected side. The normal lumbar lordosis is absent, and spinal motion is severely limited. **B,** On sagittal MRI, the L4-L5 disk bulges posteriorly, compressing the cauda equina. (**B,** Courtesy Department of Pediatric Radiology, Children's Hospital of Pittsburgh.)

cents. They are almost always limited to the lower two segments of the lumbar spine. A history of antecedent trauma is not uncommon. Lower extremity radicular symptoms predominate. Patients often describe a peculiar "pulling" sensation in a lower extremity or liken their pain to a "toothache" in the distribution of the L5 or S1 nerve roots (see Fig. 15-1). They also may complain of numbness or weakness in the involved limb. Forward flexion, sitting, coughing, and straining aggravate the neurologic symptoms.

On examination, an antalgic scoliosis of the lumbar spine may be apparent, which the patient is unable to reduce (Fig. 21-80A). Inability to reverse the normal lumbar lordosis is noted, and symptoms may be aggravated by attempts at flexion. The straight leg raising test is often positive (radicular symptoms being reproduced when the limb is raised by the examiner [see "Thoracolumbar Spine" and Fig. 21-5]), and neurologic abnormalities may be found on sensory, motor, and reflex testing, although these may be subtle. Plain radiographs usually show no abnormality, other than a possible diskogenic scoliosis, but the diagnosis may be verified by myelography, CT, or MRI (Fig. 21-80B). The differential diagnosis may include hematogenous disk space infection or vertebral osteomy-

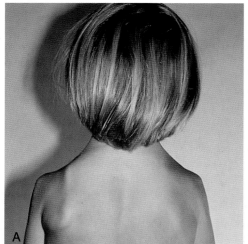
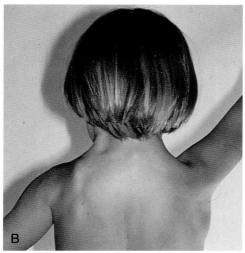

Figure 21-81. Sprengel deformity. **A,** The left scapula is high riding and hypoplastic, and its vertebral border is prominent. **B,** Shoulder motion is severely limited, particularly in abduction. (Courtesy Dana Mears, MD.)

elitis, spinal cord or neural element tumor, and spondylolisthesis with nerve root irritation.

Nonsurgical treatment consisting of rest and anti-inflammatory agents may be successful, but if a profound neurologic deficit is present or if incapacitating symptoms persist, surgical disk excision may be indicated. Intradiskal chemonucleolysis, as employed for adults, is contraindicated for children, and conservative treatment of radiographically proven disk herniation is not as effective in adolescents as it is in adults.

Disorders of the Upper Extremity

Because of the importance of prehensile function, disorders affecting any area of the upper limb can result in significant impairment of motor development during childhood. Knowledge of the normal anatomy and actions of the shoulder, arm, elbow, forearm, wrist, and hand is vital for assessment of abnormalities and institution of appropriate treatment.

Sprengel Deformity

A Sprengel deformity is a congenital malformation characterized by an abnormally small, high-riding scapula. In most cases it is unilateral. The etiology is unknown, but there appears to be a familial predisposition and the condition may be associated with a variety of other congenital anomalies including Klippel-Feil syndrome (see Fig. 21-70) and rib and vertebral malformations. Scoliosis and torticollis may be associated abnormalities. Cosmetic deformity and limited shoulder motion on the affected side are the usual complaints.

On examination, the scapula is noted to be hypoplastic and high riding in association with asymmetry of the base of the neck and shoulders (Fig. 21-81A). Shoulder motion is usually severely limited, particularly in abduction (Fig. 21-81B). This is due to limited scapular motion because the scapula is often tethered to the cervical spine by a fibrous omovertebral band, which is frequently ossified. Radiography confirms the abnormal size and position of the scapula.

Nonsurgical treatment consisting of stretching and range-of-motion exercises may be instituted but is rarely successful. Surgery may be undertaken on occasion for

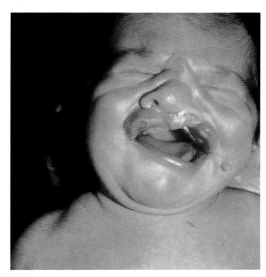

Figure 21-82. Congenital pseudarthrosis of the clavicle. There is a bulbous, nontender swelling in the region of the midclavicle. The medial aspect of the clavicle is prominent. This patient has associated anomalies. Radiographic appearance is shown in Figure 6-73.

cosmetic and functional reasons and may consist of excision of the prominent superior aspect of the scapula or of release and reduction of the scapula accomplished by positioning it inferiorly on the chest wall. Although care must be taken during the procedure to prevent brachial plexus injury, surgery performed before adolescence usually improves appearance and restores some function.

Congenital Pseudarthrosis of the Clavicle

Congenital pseudarthrosis of the clavicle is a rare congenital disorder usually manifested by a painless, nontender bulbous deformity in the region of the midclavicle. It is thought to result from a failure of maturation of the ossification center of the clavicle. It generally involves the right side and on occasion may be associated with other congenital anomalies and can be seen in patients with neurofibromatosis 1. In cleidocranial dysostosis the entire clavicle may be absent or may have an appearance similar to that of congenital pseudarthrosis.

On examination, the clavicle appears foreshortened with a prominence evident in its midportion (Fig. 21-82;

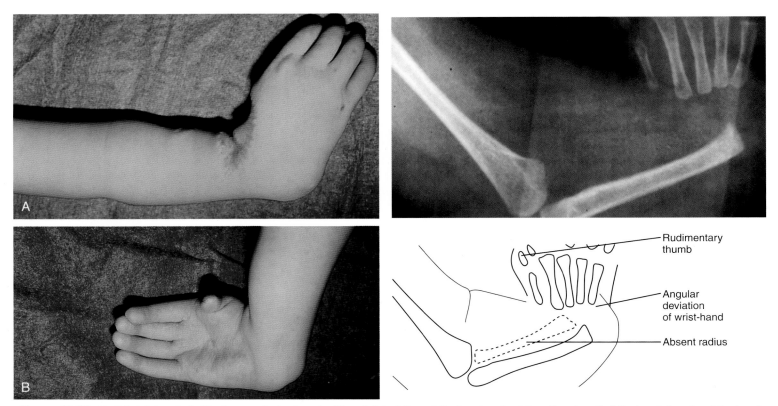

Figure 21-83. Radial club hand. **A,** The forearm is shortened with radial deviation of the hand and wrist on the ulna. **B,** A flexion deformity of the hand and wrist on the forearm and a hypoplastic thumb are present. **C,** Radiograph shows absence of the radius, dislocation of the carpus, and a rudimentary thumb, all characteristic of radial club hand. (Clinical photographs courtesy Joseph Imbriglia, MD, Allegheny General Hospital, Pittsburgh.)

see Fig. 6-77 for radiographic appearance). Palpation reveals hypermobility of the two ends of the clavicle and crepitance. Generally, range of motion of the shoulder is normal. This condition characteristically involves no functional impairment and requires no treatment. Although clavicular fracture as a result of birth trauma may present a similar appearance, it is easily distinguished because of tenderness over the region of deformity.

Radial Club Hand

Radial club hand is the result of congenital absence or hypoplasia of the radial structures of the forearm and hand. Associated muscular structures and the radial nerve are hypoplastic or absent. The anomaly is rare and affects more male than female subjects. Its characteristic clinical presentation is one of a small, short, bowed forearm and aplasia or hypoplasia of the thumb, and the residual hand is deviated radially (Fig. 21-83A and B). Radiographs show absence of bones in the affected area (Fig. 21-83C).

Treatment is best instituted early with passive stretching exercises and corrective casting. Surgical treatment consists of centralization of the hand on the "one-bone forearm" to maximize function.

Ganglion of the Wrist

A ganglion is a benign cystic mass consisting of an accumulation of synovial fluid or gelatin in an outpouching of a tendon sheath or joint capsule. The exact etiology is unknown, but it is thought to be related to a herniation of synovial tissue with a ball-valve effect. Antecedent

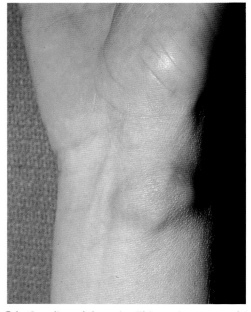

Figure 21-84. Ganglion of the wrist. This cystic mass overlying the wrist joint and flexor tendons was asymptomatic and nontender.

trauma may be reported. These masses may be present over the dorsal or volar aspects of the wrist and are generally located toward the radial side (Fig. 21-84). Occasionally they are seen on the dorsum of the foot or adjacent to one of the malleoli of the ankle (see Fig. 21-108). Their size may fluctuate with time and activity. On examination they may be either firm or fluctuant, and they can be transilluminated. Although most are asymptomatic, an occasional patient may complain of pain and tenderness.

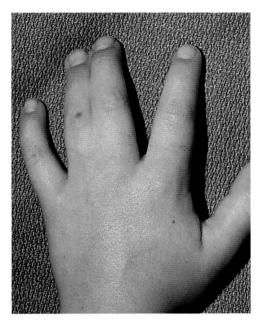

Figure 21-85. Syndactyly. This child has mild syndactyly involving soft tissues of the middle and ring fingers without bony involvement. (Courtesy Joseph Imbriglia, MD, Allegheny General Hospital, Pittsburgh.)

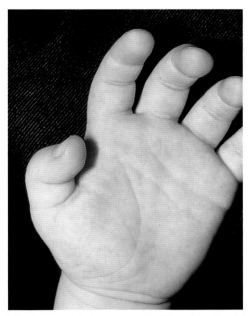

Figure 21-86. Congenital trigger thumb. There is a fixed flexion deformity at the interphalangeal joint of the thumb resulting from tightness of the tendon sheath of the flexor pollicis longus. The remainder of the hand appears normal.

Treatment is generally unnecessary for patients who are asymptomatic, and surgery is not routinely advised because the recurrence rate may be as high as 20%. Occasionally, patients desire removal for cosmetic or psychological reasons. Aspiration, injection, or rupture of these cysts does not eradicate them. Surgical excision with obliteration of the base of the ganglion is the most successful treatment for the occasional patient in whom treatment is indicated.

Syndactyly

Syndactyly is a relatively common congenital anomaly involving failure of the digits of the hands or feet to separate. It is both more common and more disabling in the upper extremity. Bilateral involvement is usual, and a positive family history is not uncommon. It may be associated with other congenital anomalies, particularly Apert syndrome and Streeter dysplasia. Great variation in the degree of fusion exists. In mild cases, only the skin is joined, making reconstructive surgery simple (Fig. 21-85). In more severe cases the nails, deeper structures, and bones may be conjoined, contributing to deformity and growth abnormalities and making reconstructive treatment more difficult.

Congenital Trigger Thumb

A congenital trigger thumb is characterized by a fixed or intermittent flexion deformity of the interphalangeal joint of the thumb that may be present at birth or may develop shortly thereafter (Fig. 21-86). It is thought to result from tightness of the tendon sheath of the flexor pollicis longus in the region of the metacarpophalangeal joint. The flexion deformity generally cannot be reduced, although in milder cases it may be passively correctable, with a snapping sensation felt as the tendon passes through the stenosed pulley mechanism. If passively correctable,

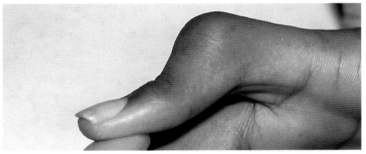

Figure 21-87. Boutonnière deformity of the finger. A fixed flexion contracture of the proximal interphalangeal joint exists, along with hyperextension of the distal joint secondary to volar migration of the lateral bands of the extensor mechanism. This is the result of an unrecognized or inadequately treated injury to the extensor tendon at its insertion on the middle phalanx.

splinting in extension occasionally results in correction; otherwise, surgery is required.

Boutonnière (Buttonhole) Deformity

A boutonnière deformity of a finger is the end result of a traumatic avulsion of the central portion of the extensor tendon at its insertion on the middle phalanx that went unrecognized at the time of initial injury. The mechanism of injury is usually a blow to the tip of the finger that drives it into forced flexion against resistance, although a laceration over the dorsum of the finger involving the extensor tendon may produce a similar deformity if tendon involvement is not recognized and repaired at the time. Initially, there may be local tenderness over the dorsal aspect of the PIP joint without deformity. With time, however, the lateral bands of the extensor mechanism migrate volarly, producing a flexion deformity of the PIP joint with a secondary extension deformity of the distal joint (Fig. 21-87). If the injury is recognized early, healing may occur with splinting of the PIP joint in extension. Later, open surgical repair may be necessary to improve function.

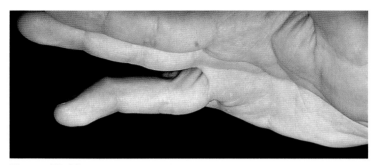

Figure 21-88. Mallet finger with secondary swan-neck deformity. This is the result of avulsion of the extensor tendon from its insertion at the base of the distal phalanx, which was not recognized at the time of injury. The patient shows a flexion deformity of the distal interphalangeal joint and secondary hyperextension of the proximal interphalangeal joint.

Mallet Finger/Swan-Neck Deformity

A mallet finger is the result of avulsion of the extensor tendon from its insertion at the base of the distal phalanx of a finger. It occurs as a result of a blow to the extended finger against resistance. The tendon alone, or a portion of the distal phalanx into which it inserts, may be involved. The clinical appearance is that of a "dropped finger" or flexion deformity of the distal interphalangeal joint with inability to actively extend the joint (see Fig. 21-49). If not recognized and treated at the time of the initial injury, the condition becomes chronic and contracture of the extensor mechanism may occur, with a secondary hyperextension deformity of the PIP joint producing a swan-neck deformity (Fig. 21-88). Treatment consists of splinting the distal joint in an extended position, open reduction if a large fragment of bone is involved, or surgical repair in chronic cases.

Disorders of the Lower Extremity

Normally developed and functional lower extremities permit locomotion with ease and a minimal amount of energy expenditure. A disability resulting from a deformed, shortened, or painful lower limb can be considerable (see "Gait and Gait Disturbances" earlier).

Many problems of the lower extremities occurring in childhood are congenital and, if they remain unrecognized or are unsuccessfully treated, can result in lifelong disability. Knowledge of the normal anatomy and function of the hip, knee, ankle, and foot is necessary to accurately recognize and treat abnormalities in this region (see "Lower Extremity Examination" earlier).

Developmental Dislocation of the Hip

Developmental dislocation of the hip, formerly referred to as *congenital dislocation of the hip,* consists of displacement of the femoral head from its normal relationship with the acetabulum. It is a relatively frequent problem, with an incidence of 1 to 2 per 1000 births. It is generally detectable at birth or shortly thereafter. Female infants are affected significantly more frequently than male infants, and unilateral dislocation is twice as frequent as bilateral. Developmental dislocation may be divided into idiopathic and teratogenic types. Idiopathic dislocation is more frequent, and patients often have a positive family history

for the defect. Its severity varies from subluxated, to dislocated and reducible, to dislocated and irreducible. This type of developmental dislocation may be related to abnormal intrauterine positioning or restriction of fetal movement in utero, which impedes adequate development and stability of the hip joint complex. The relaxing effect of hormones on soft tissue during pregnancy may also contribute, with affected infants perhaps being more sensitive to the pelvic relaxation effects of maternal estrogen. A history of breech presentation is not uncommon, and these patients often exhibit generalized ligamentous laxity. Teratogenic dislocations of the hip represent a more severe form of the disorder and are probably the result of a germ plasm defect. They occur early in fetal development and result in malformation of both the femoral head and the acetabular socket. Associated congenital anomalies are common in infants whose dislocations are teratogenic including clubfoot deformity, congenital torticollis, metatarsus adductus, and infantile scoliosis.

The importance of careful hip evaluation in the newborn and at early infant visits cannot be overemphasized. Early diagnosis enables prompt institution of treatment and results in a better outcome. A knowledge of the clinical signs and skill in techniques of examination are necessary.

Typically, the infant with a dislocated hip has no noticeable difference in the position in which the leg is held, although some affected infants may hold the leg in a position of adduction and external rotation. If the dislocation is unilateral, the skinfolds of the thighs and buttocks are often asymmetrical and the involved lower extremity appears shorter than the opposite side (Fig. 21-89A). This foreshortening is accentuated by holding the hips and knees in 90 degrees of flexion (Galeazzi sign). In patients with bilateral dislocations, this asymmetry is not present. In a truly dislocated hip, the most consistent physical finding is that of limited abduction (see Fig. 21-89B). Additional diagnostic maneuvers may assist in establishing the diagnosis. In patients with reducible dislocations, the Ortolani sign is positive when a palpable clunk is felt on abduction and internal rotation (relocation) of the hip. The Barlow test is positive if, with the knees flexed and hips flexed to 90 degrees, the hips are gently adducted with pressure applied on the lesser trochanter by the thumb. A palpable clunk indicating posterior dislocation is appreciated if the hip is unstable or dislocated. When the hip is dislocated and irreducible, only limitation of abduction is apparent.

The radiographic findings of a developmental hip dislocation are characteristic. The femoral head is generally located lateral and superior to its normal position, and the acetabulum may be shallow, with lateral deficiency and a characteristic high acetabular index or slope (Fig. 21-89C and D). Reduction of the dislocated hip is apparent if, on abduction of the hip to 45 degrees, a line drawn through the axis of the metaphysis of the neck crosses the triradiate cartilage (Fig. 21-89 diagram). Since ossification is not evident radiographically until 3 to 6 months of age, ultrasound evaluation of the hip is often helpful in determining the acetabular/femoral head relationships. Furthermore, in developmental dislocation, ossification may be delayed even longer, because normal articulation forces are absent.

In teratogenic hip dislocation, there may be hypoplasia of both the acetabular and femoral sides with noncongruent development of one or both of these structures. The early radiographic findings, however, are similar to those already mentioned.

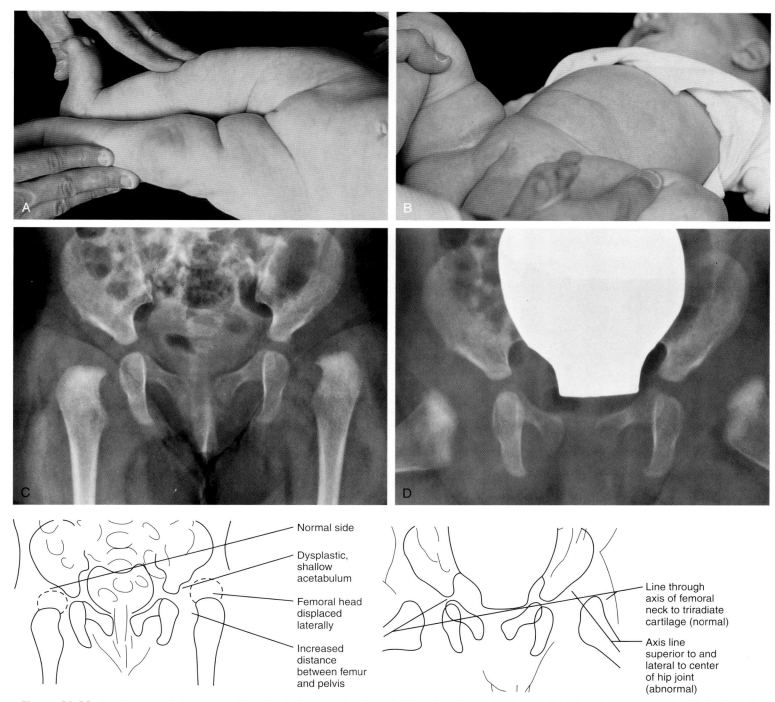

Figure 21-89. Developmental dislocation of the hip. **A,** In cases of unilateral dislocation, the involved extremity is foreshortened and the thigh and groin creases are asymmetric. **B,** Limited abduction of the involved hip is seen. This is a consistent finding in infants with a dislocated and irreducible hip. **C,** In this anteroposterior radiograph obtained in a 3-month-old child, the proximal left femur is displaced upward and laterally, and the acetabulum is shallow. The femoral head is not visible on the radiograph because of the delayed ossification associated with developmental hip dislocation. **D,** In the frog-leg view, the long axis of the affected left femur is directed toward a point superior and lateral to the triradiate cartilage, in contrast with that of the right, which points directly toward this structure.

Successful correction of congenital hip dislocation depends on early diagnosis and institution of appropriate treatment. In the first 6 months of life, use of a Pavlik harness, which permits gentle motion of the hip in a flexed and abducted position, may achieve and maintain a satisfactory reduction. Between 6 and 18 months of age, gentle closed reduction and immobilization in a spica cast with or without surgical release of the contracted iliopsoas and adductor muscles is indicated. After the age of 18 months, reduction by manipulative measures is difficult owing to contractures of the associated soft tissues. In such instances open reduction is usually indicated. In cases of teratogenic dislocation, underlying maldevelopment makes the outcome less satisfactory, even with optimal management.

With early recognition and appropriate treatment, a relatively normal hip with satisfactory function can be anticipated in cases of idiopathic hip dislocation. Failure of concentric reduction or complications such as avascular necrosis of the femoral head, resulting from overzealous attempts at closed reduction in long-standing cases, may result in a lifelong disability characterized by pain and stiffness in the hip; an antalgic, lurching gait; and shortening of the involved limb.

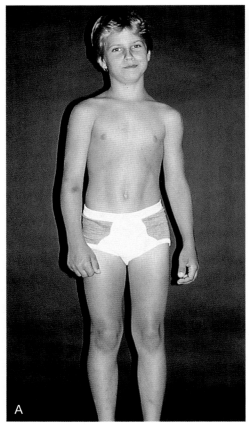

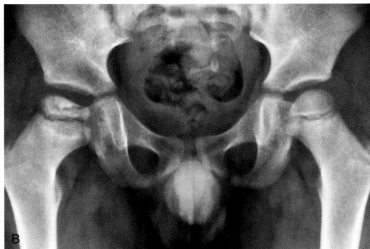

Figure 21-90. Legg-Calvé-Perthes disease. **A,** This 7-year-old boy is small for his chronologic age. He is bearing less weight on the involved right leg (note the slightly flexed right knee). On examination a hip flexion contracture, detected by a positive Thomas test (see Fig. 21-8B), and an abductor lurch gait were found. **B,** In this anteroposterior radiograph, the right femoral epiphysis is flattened and fragmented. The proximal femur is also displaced inferiorly and laterally.

Legg-Calvé-Perthes Disease

In Legg-Calvé-Perthes disease (coxa plana), impairment of the blood supply to the developing femoral head results in avascular necrosis. The etiology is unknown. Current theories implicate traumatic disruption of the blood supply and recurrent episodes of synovitis, during which increased intra-articular pressure compromises blood flow to the developing ossific nucleus, as causative. The disorder generally becomes manifest between the ages of 4 and 11 years, with a higher incidence in boys. Affected children often exhibit delayed skeletal maturation and are small for their age. Unilateral involvement is the rule, and if a bilateral case is suspected, some form of epiphyseal dysplasia must be ruled out. The severity of the disease varies greatly, depending on the extent to which the femoral head is affected. Younger children generally have milder involvement, as a larger portion of the femoral head is still cartilaginous and less dependent on vascular supply.

Typically onset is insidious. The child may present with symptoms characteristic of toxic synovitis without radiographic findings. Many children present with a painless limp, and others complain of thigh or knee pain, fatigue on walking, or hip stiffness. Generally, the patient bears less weight on the involved leg when standing and there is a flexion contracture of the involved hip (Fig. 21-90A; see also Fig. 21-8B), with the lower extremity held in a slightly externally rotated position. Pain and limitation of motion are encountered on attempts at internal rotation and abduction. The Trendelenburg sign (failure to maintain a level pelvis when standing on the involved limb) is positive.

Early radiographic findings may include failure of progressive development of the femoral ossific nucleus, a subchondral radiolucent fracture line (Caffey sign), and evidence of slight subluxation. However, in early cases, radiographs may be completely normal, though a nuclear bone scan may be useful in verification of impairment of the blood supply to this region. Later, fragmentation of the femoral ossification center may be evident with flattening of the femoral head, extrusion, and frank subluxation (Fig. 21-90B).

The disease is self-limited, typically lasting for 1 to 2 years. Although revascularization and reconstitution of the femoral head always occur, loss of mechanical integrity of the head with flattening and fragmentation of its surface may result in an irreversible predisposition to degenerative change. Most treatments are based on the principle of "containment" and the maintenance of a normal relationship of the femoral head within the acetabulum so as to minimize permanent joint incongruity. In young children with minimal symptoms and radiographic findings, decreased activity and close observation may be all that is necessary. Anti-inflammatory agents and traction are used during episodes of synovitis. In more severe cases, abduction casting, bracing, or surgical treatment with femoral or acetabular osteotomy to reposition the femoral head deeper within the acetabulum may be employed. In patients whose disease is recognized late or who fail to respond to appropriate measures, permanent degenerative change is common and salvage-type surgery may be necessary.

Slipped Capital Femoral Epiphysis

Slipped capital femoral epiphysis, a disorder seen early in puberty, involves displacement of the femoral head from the femoral neck through the epiphyseal plate. It is seen more frequently in males and occurs bilaterally in approximately 25% of cases. Most commonly, it occurs at the onset of puberty in obese children with delayed sexual maturation. Although the etiology is unclear, it is generally thought that hormonal changes at the time of puberty may result in loss of mechanical integrity of the growth

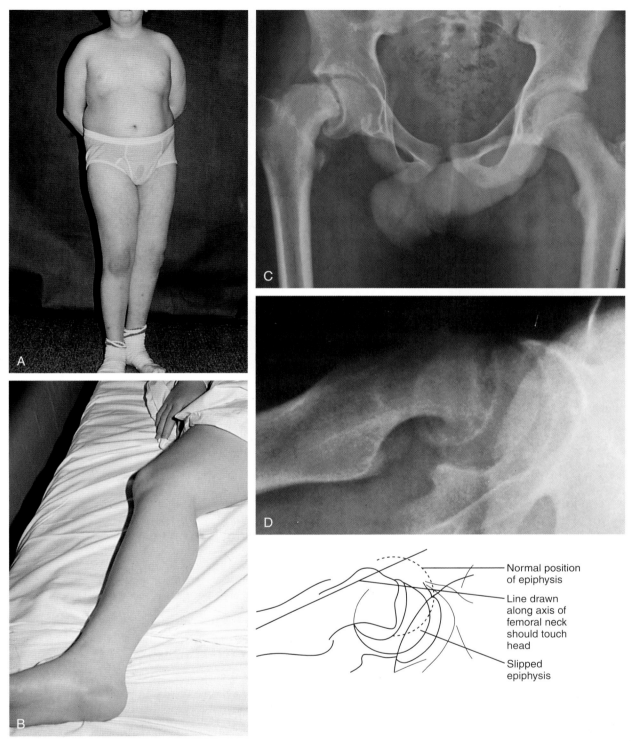

Figure 21-91. Slipped capital femoral epiphysis. **A,** This obese boy presented with a painful limp during early puberty. Note his reluctance to bear weight on the involved right leg. **B,** When he lies supine, the affected leg is positioned in external rotation because this minimizes discomfort. Attempts at motion produce pain in the acutely slipped epiphysis. **C,** In the anteroposterior radiograph the right femoral head is displaced medially in relation to the femoral neck as a result of epiphyseal separation. **D,** In the lateral view the femoral head is seen to be displaced posteriorly in relation to the femoral neck. A line drawn along the axis of the femoral neck should normally touch the head.

plate, and that if the epiphysis is then subjected to excessive shear stress, slippage through this area may occur. This condition differs from traumatic epiphyseal fractures because the translational displacement occurs through a different portion of the growth plate. In some cases an underlying connective tissue disorder such as Marfan syndrome or an endocrinologic problem such as hypothyroidism can be identified.

The clinical presentation is quite characteristic, although the duration of symptoms varies. The patient presents with a painful limp and may or may not have a history of recent trauma, which is usually minor, or pain may have developed after jumping. This injury may have precipitated a slip in the previously weakened epiphysis or may have increased the degree of displacement of a slip that was already in progress. The pain may be perceived as being in the hip or in the thigh or knee. The lower extremity is held in an externally rotated position secondary to deformity at the site of physeal displacement (Fig. 21-91A and B). An antalgic and abductor lurch gait is

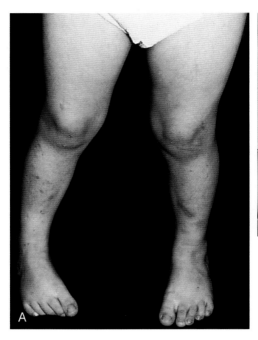

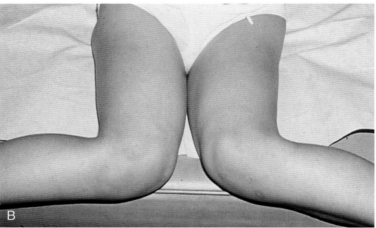

Figure 21-92. Femoral anteversion. **A,** The condition occurs bilaterally, and in the standing view, both legs appear to turn inward from the hip down. **B,** On assessment of range of motion, the degree of internal rotation of the hips is found to be greater than normal. (Courtesy Michael Sherlock, MD, Lutherville, Md.)

usually apparent. A flexion contracture may be noted, and range of hip motion tends to be diminished in all planes, particularly internal rotation. Slight shortening of the involved lower extremity is observed in some patients.

Radiographic findings vary from a widened and radiolucent physis (preslip) to a frank deformity with displacement of the femoral head on the proximal femur posteriorly and inferiorly in relation to its normal counterpart (Fig. 21-91C and D). The degree of slippage and deformity correlates with the extent of incongruity of the hip joint and the later development of degenerative change and painful symptoms. Prompt intervention to prevent further displacement is an important factor in preventing lifelong problems, and awareness of the condition, a high index of suspicion, and early recognition are key factors in improving prognosis.

In patients with minimally or moderately displaced slips, stabilization of the slip with in situ pin fixation is indicated. In severe slips, especially those that have slipped acutely, pinning may be the treatment of choice initially, but development of avascular changes secondary to disruption of the blood supply to the femoral head may occur and complicate the outcome. When the disease is recognized late and deformity is severe, proximal femoral osteotomy may be necessary. Children with unilateral slipped epiphyses must be monitored closely for signs of involvement of the opposite limb.

Femoral Anteversion

Femoral anteversion may be viewed as a normal variation of lower extremity positioning in the developing child. In utero and at birth, the femoral neck sits in an anteverted position relative to that of the adult. During childhood it remodels to a position of slight anteversion and normal alignment of the lower extremities. In certain children, however, delayed rotational correction may result in persistent intoeing. An unsightly gait, kicking of the heels, and tripping on walking or running are frequent related complaints. There may be a history of sitting on the floor with knees bent and the lower legs turned outward in a reversed tailor position. Generally the condi-

tion is bilateral and is not associated with other musculoskeletal problems.

On examination, the child is noted to stand with the thighs, knees, and feet all turned inward. An increase in internal rotation over external rotation is apparent on assessment of range of motion of the hip (Fig. 21-92). Radiographic findings are normal. No treatment is indicated, other than reassurance that the condition will correct with growth and instructions to avoid sitting in the predisposing position.

Genu Varum (Physiologic Bowleg)

Genu varum, or bowleg, is usually a normal variation of lower extremity configuration, seen in the 1- to 3-year-old age group. It is generally recognized shortly after ambulation begins and may be associated with laxity of other joints and internal tibial torsion. Examination reveals diffuse bowing of the lower extremities with an increased distance between the knees that is accentuated on standing (Fig. 21-93). Varus positioning of the heel with pronation of the feet may be noted on weight bearing. The child may walk with a waddling gait and kick the heels on running to clear the feet from the ground and avoid hitting the contralateral limb. Laxity of joint capsular structures may be noted with application of a reduction force.

Radiographs of children with physiologic bowing show normal osseous and physeal development and may reveal a gentle symmetrical bowing of the femur and tibia. Although there may be slight beaking of the medial metaphyses of the femur and tibia adjacent to the knee joint, there is no fragmentation of the epiphyses or irregularity of the growth plate, as is seen in *Blount disease* (see Fig. 21-96).

Treatment is rarely indicated, as this condition resolves with growth; in fact, a valgus deformity of the knees may be noted later, at approximately 4 to 5 years of age. Casting, bracing, and corrective shoes are unnecessary, and there is no indication for surgery.

Less commonly, genu varum is of pathologic origin. Conditions such as rickets (see Fig. 6-78) or other metabolic abnormalities, epiphyseal dysplasia, various forms of dwarfism, and pathologic growth disturbances such as

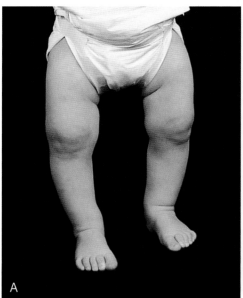

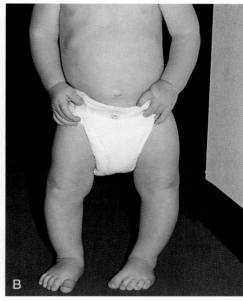

Figure 21-93. Physiologic genu varum. **A,** The mild symmetrical bowing seen in this 1-year-old boy represents a normal variation of lower extremity configuration that occurs in toddlers; correction occurs with growth and remodeling. The bowing is diffuse and involves the upper and lower portions of the legs. **B,** This child has more severe physiologic bowing, which resulted in frequent tripping and a waddling gait. He also had associated ligamentous laxity and intoeing on the left.

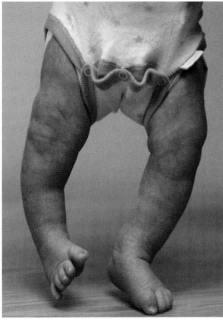

A

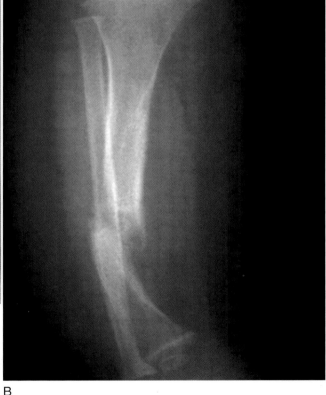

B

Figure 21-94. Pathologic genu varum. **A,** This 11-month-old child has a unilateral, right-sided bow leg deformity. When unilateral, genu varum is not a result of intrauterine positioning and necessitates radiographs to determine the cause of the deformity. **B,** In this case the bowing was caused by a congenital pseudarthrosis of the tibia, a condition frequently associated with neurofibromatosis 1 (see Chapter 15).

Blount disease may be causative and can be diagnosed on the basis of radiographic findings if the diagnosis is not obvious clinically. Unilateral bowing is not a result of intrauterine positioning and should prompt investigation for an underlying disorder (Fig. 21-94).

Genu Valgum (Physiologic Knock-Knee)

Genu valgum, or knock-knee, is a normal variation of lower extremity configuration, generally noted in children between 3 and 5 years of age. The phenomenon is part of the normal process of remodeling of the lower extremities during growth and development. It is more frequently seen in females and may be associated with ligamentous laxity. While standing, the child is noted to have an increased distance between the feet when the medial aspects of the knees touch one another (Fig. 21-95). Not uncommonly, the child will place one knee behind the other in an attempt to get the feet together. In some cases, valgus alignment of the feet and a pes planus deformity may be noted. Radiographs reveal no osseous or physeal abnormalities, but accentuation of the angular deformity of the knee secondary to ligamentous laxity is seen on weight-bearing views. One must rule out the possibility of an underlying metabolic condition such as rickets or renal disease. Treatment is generally not indicated, as the condition gradually corrects with time.

Blount Disease

Blount disease is an isolated growth disturbance of the medial tibial epiphysis manifested as an angular varus deformity of the proximal tibia with apparent progressive genu varum. Unilateral and bilateral involvement are seen with nearly equal frequency. The etiology of this condition is unknown, although it appears to be more common in African Americans. It may represent a compression injury to the medial growth plate of the proximal tibia.

On careful examination, a localized angular deformity of the proximal tibia is apparent (Fig. 21-96A and B), in contrast to the diffuse bowing of the lower extremities seen in patients with physiologic bowleg. Generally there is no evidence of the ligamentous laxity commonly associated with physiologic bowing. Radiographs reveal fragmentation of the medial epiphysis of the tibia associated with beaking and loss of height in this region, as well as the characteristic angular deformity (see Fig. 21-96C). A satisfactory response to treatment depends on accurate diagnosis and early recognition, as bracing or surgical osteotomy with realignment of the leg may prevent further progression.

Osgood-Schlatter Disease

Osgood-Schlatter disease is a traction apophysitis of the tibial tubercle that tends to develop during the adolescent growth spurt. It occurs somewhat more frequently in males than in females. It is thought that differential rates of growth in the osseous and soft tissue structures and stress on the apophyses produced by vigorous physical activity are contributing factors. Bilateral involvement is usual. Patients have a history of gradually increasing pain and swelling in the region of the tibial tubercle. Discomfort is accentuated by vigorous physical activity, kneeling, or crawling and is relieved by rest.

On examination, a localized tender swelling is noted in the region of the tibial tubercle and patellar tendon (Fig. 21-97A). The knee joint is otherwise normal on examination, with the exception that some patients show limitation of knee flexion with reproduction of their pain. Radiographs may reveal only soft tissue swelling in the region of the proximal tibial apophysis or irregularity of ossification of this structure (see Fig. 21-97B). In long-standing cases, frank fragmentation of the apophysis may be seen.

The problem, although self-limited, typically persists for 6 to 24 months. If the condition is only occasionally bothersome and does not limit activities, treatment is unnecessary. Use of ibuprofen, as needed, for relieving pain and curtailing activities that produce pain are suffi-

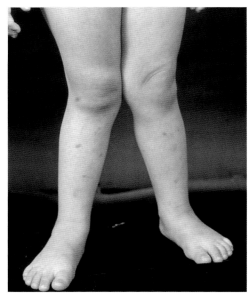

Figure 21-95. Genu valgum. This 3½-year-old girl shows moderate knock-knee. Ligamentous laxity and mild pes planus are associated problems.

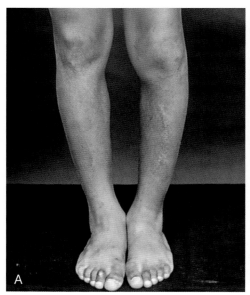
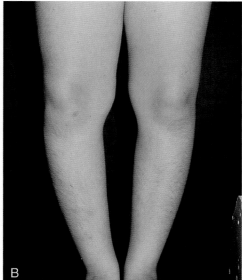
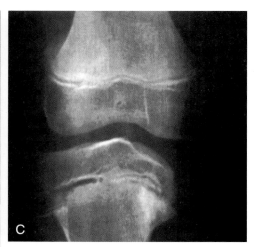
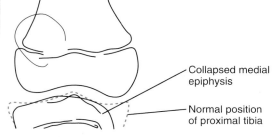

Figure 21-96. Blount disease. **A,** This patient has a unilateral angular deformity of the proximal left tibia that gives the appearance of genu varum. **B,** Both proximal tibias are bowed in another patient as a result of fragmentation and loss of height of the medial epiphyses. In contrast with physiologic bowing, the thighs are straight. **C,** This radiograph shows the typical fragmentation, loss of height, and angular deformity or beaking of the medial portion of the proximal tibia.

Collapsed medial epiphysis

Normal position of proximal tibia

Figure 21-97. Osgood-Schlatter disease. **A,** Localized swelling is evident in the region of the tibial tubercle. This is generally tender on palpation. The knee is otherwise normal on examination, with the possible exception of mild limitation of flexion. **B,** Irregularity and fragmentation of the tibial tubercle are seen in this radiograph. In less severe cases of shorter duration, soft tissue swelling or irregularity of ossification may be the only finding.

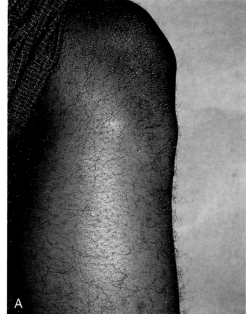
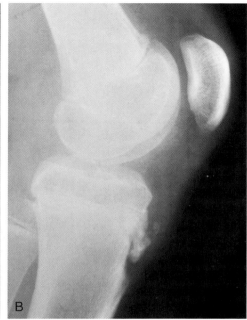

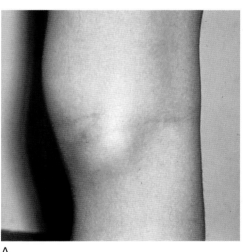
A

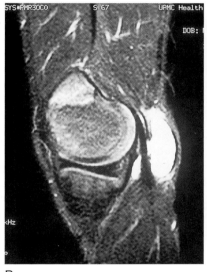
B

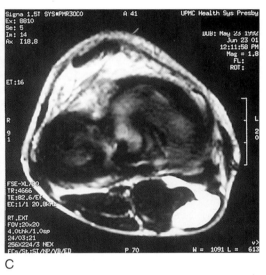
C

Figure 21-98. Popliteal (Baker) cyst. **A,** A localized swelling appears in the region of the semimembranosus tendon. This may arise from the synovial lining of the semimembranosus bursa. **B,** Sagittal plane MRI from another child with a Baker cyst shows the posterior location. **C,** A transverse plane MRI demonstrates the posterior and medial position of cyst and its close relation to the gastrocnemius muscle.

cient treatment for most patients. If severe pain and a limp are present, a short period of immobilization in a splint or cast may be beneficial. Steroid injection is contraindicated because this may cause deterioration of the tendon and provides little in the way of long-term relief.

Popliteal (Baker) Cyst

Popliteal cysts occurring in childhood are encountered most commonly in children between 5 and 10 years of age and occur significantly more frequently in boys than in girls. They are located in the posteromedial aspect of the knee joint in the region of the semimembranosus tendon and medial gastrocnemius muscle belly. Pathologically a fibrous tissue or synovial cyst filled with synovia-like fluid is seen. In contrast to those seen in adults, popliteal cysts in childhood generally do not communicate with the joint capsule but originate instead beneath

the semimembranosus tendon, presumably as a result of chronic irritation. Occasionally, vague pain is noted but evaluation is usually sought because of a recently noted painless mass.

On examination, a soft, nontender, cystic mass is found in the described location (Fig. 21-98A). Range of motion of the joint is normal unless the cyst is particularly large, limiting flexion. The knee is otherwise normal, and radiographs show no osseous abnormality. An MRI clearly delineates the cyst and its position in relation to nearby structures (Fig. 21-98B and C). Popliteal cysts are benign and may resolve over time, although surgical excision is reasonable if desired.

Anterior Patellar Disorders

Pain located in or around the patella is a frequent complaint, especially in the adolescent. Once thought to

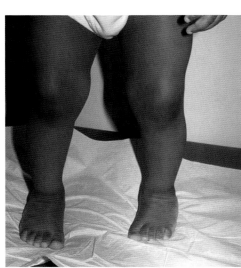

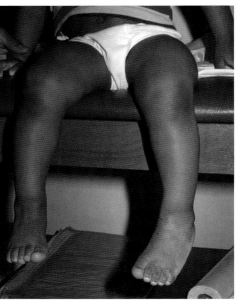

Figure 21-99. Internal tibial torsion. **A,** On weight bearing the hip, thigh, and knee are normally oriented and the patella faces anteriorly, but the lower leg and foot turn inward. The deformity results in prominent intoeing on walking, which may cause the child to trip frequently. **B,** In this view of the child while sitting, it is easy to appreciate that the lateral malleolus is positioned anteriorly to the medial malleolus. This shifts the ankle mortise and foot to a medially oriented position.

A   B

involve irregular changes in the articular cartilage of the patella and termed *chondromalacia,* the true sources of pain in this region are still not completely understood. Two primary causes for this group of symptoms have been identified, however. One is mechanical malalignment of the patellofemoral mechanism, either congenital or acquired. In such cases the patella does not track congruously in the femoral groove, and subsequent alignment problems or quadriceps atrophy can lead to increased stress on the tissues producing pain. The second cause may relate to overuse of the patellofemoral joint leading to chronic fatigue of the tissues, intrasubstance failure, and a painful inflammatory response.

Onset of symptoms may be insidious or may abruptly follow trauma. The patient complains of diffuse aching behind the patella that is exacerbated by climbing stairs, pedaling a bicycle, or prolonged sitting. On examination the patella is found to be tender, and application of pressure over the patella with the knee slightly flexed elicits pain. In the case of mechanical malalignment, tenderness may be greatest on palpation of the lateral or medial edge of the patella near the facets. In overuse problems, tenderness may be noted either at the quadriceps attachment proximally or at the inferior pole where the infrapatellar tendon attaches. In either case, when the examiner holds a hand over the patella as the patient flexes and extends the knee, a grating sensation may be felt.

Treatment is aimed at the underlying cause. If malalignment is the primary source of the problem, quadriceps strengthening exercises and avoidance of high mechanical loads such as deep knee bends and weight lifting may suffice. Occasionally, surgical release of the retinaculum on the lateral side may be necessary. When overuse is causative, a reduction of activities to assist initiation of healing and oral administration of anti-inflammatory agents followed by a stepwise return to normal activities is effective. Evaluation of training schedule and techniques and modifications where indicated may prevent recurrence.

Internal Tibial Torsion

Internal tibial torsion is a nonpathologic variation in the normal development of the lower leg in children

younger than the age of 5 years. It is a rotational deformity that is thought to result from internal molding of the foot and leg in utero. The child is usually brought for evaluation because of concern about prominent intoeing on walking and frequent tripping.

On examination, the hips and knees are found to be normally aligned, with the patellas facing anteriorly, but the lower legs and feet are rotated inward. The lateral malleolus, which is normally positioned slightly posterior to the medial malleolus, may be in alignment with it or even anteriorly displaced, thus causing the ankle mortise to shift to a medially directed orientation, resulting in intoeing (Fig. 21-99). The rotational deformity can be detected by having the patient lie prone on the examining table with the knees flexed (see Fig. 21-14E). Radiographs reveal no osseous abnormalities. Treatment is seldom indicated; remodeling gradually corrects the condition as the child grows and develops. Children who have a habit of sitting on their feet on the floor may inhibit the normal remodeling process and should be discouraged from doing so. Bracing and special shoes have little effect and are not recommended.

Congenital Clubfoot

Congenital clubfoot (talipes equinovarus) is a teratogenic deformity of the foot that is readily apparent at birth. It is seen more frequently in male infants than female infants and has an incidence of 1 in 1000 live births. Etiology is probably multifactorial. Findings from familial incidence studies point toward an underlying genetic predisposition. Abnormal intrauterine positioning and pressure at a critical point in development may contribute as well. Neural, muscular, and osseous abnormalities are other proposed predisposing conditions. A near equal frequency of unilateral and bilateral involvement exists. The deformity is characterized by three primary components: (1) the entire foot is positioned in plantar flexion (equinus); (2) the hindfoot is maintained in a position of fixed inversion (varus); and (3) the forefoot exhibits an adductus deformity, often combined with supination (Fig. 21-100A to C). In the newborn period the deformity may be passively correctable to some extent. With time, however, deformities become more fixed as a result of contracture of soft tissue structures.

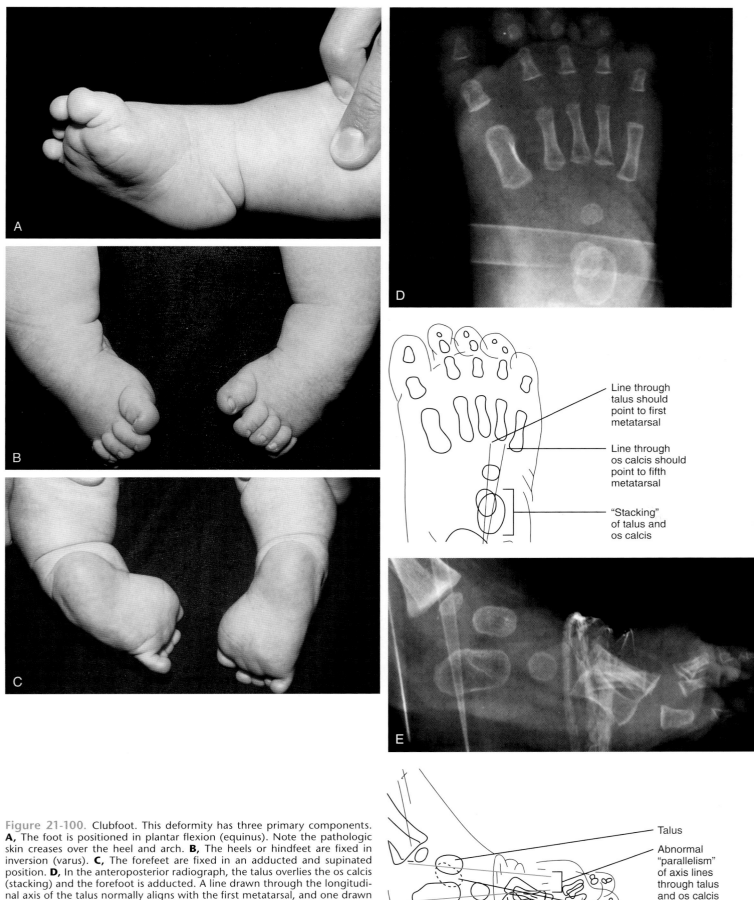

Figure 21-100. Clubfoot. This deformity has three primary components. **A,** The foot is positioned in plantar flexion (equinus). Note the pathologic skin creases over the heel and arch. **B,** The heels or hindfeet are fixed in inversion (varus). **C,** The forefeet are fixed in an adducted and supinated position. **D,** In the anteroposterior radiograph, the talus overlies the os calcis (stacking) and the forefoot is adducted. A line drawn through the longitudinal axis of the talus normally aligns with the first metatarsal, and one drawn through the axis of the os calcis normally aligns with the fifth metatarsal. **E,** This lateral radiograph shows that the foot is in equinus and the axes of the talus and os calcis are nearly parallel. They normally intersect at an approximately 45-degree angle. (Compare with normal shown in Fig. 21-101.)

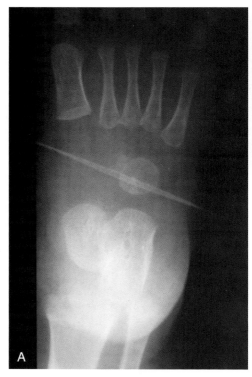

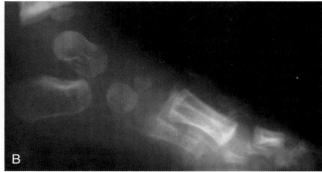

Figure 21-101. Normal foot. Anteroposterior **(A)** and lateral **(B)** views of the foot of a slightly older child show the normal orientation of the tarsal bones, as compared with the findings in congenital clubfoot (shown in Fig. 21-100D and E).

The primary pathologic finding is that of a rotational deformity of the subtalar joint with the os calcis internally rotated beneath the talus, producing the characteristic varus deformity of the heel and mechanically creating a block to dorsiflexion of the foot. The navicular bone is in a medially displaced position on the head or neck of the talus, producing the characteristic adductus deformity of the forefoot (Fig. 21-100D and E). Contractures of the Achilles and posterior tibial tendons and of the medial ankle and subtalar joint capsules appear to be secondary factors that contribute to the difficulty in obtaining anatomic reduction. Congenital absence of certain tendinous structures may be found in rare instances. A small atrophic-appearing calf is frequently noted without pathologic change in its osseous or soft tissue structures. The typical congenital clubfoot deformity must be differentiated from similar foot deformities secondary to neurologic imbalance resulting from myelodysplasia, spinal cord tethering, or degenerative neurologic conditions. Occasionally, tibial hemimelia with deficiency of this bone may present a similar clinical picture. The condition should not be confused with the nonteratogenic occurrence of isolated metatarsus adductus. Its association with arthrogryposis and congenital dislocation of the hips should also be kept in mind.

The roentgenographic difference between a clubfoot and a normal foot can be appreciated by comparing Figure 21-100D and E with Figure 21-101A and B.

Early treatment consists of attempts at manipulation and serial casting or cast wedging with progressive correction. When the child is seen late or closed treatment is unsuccessful, open reduction and surgical release of the contracted soft tissues is indicated. Generally these measures should be undertaken before the age at which walking is expected in order to prevent the deformity from impeding the child's motor and social development.

Metatarsus Adductus

Metatarsus adductus (metatarsus varus) is a deformity of the forefoot in which the metatarsals are deviated medi-

ally. The condition is probably the result of intrauterine molding and is usually bilateral. Other than the deviation, there are no pathologic changes in the structures of the foot. There is a wide spectrum of severity and resultant intoeing, but otherwise patients are asymptomatic. Clinically it should be distinguished from the more severe and complex deformity of congenital clubfoot, as it carries a more benign prognosis.

Examination is best performed with the foot braced against a flat surface or with the patient standing. With the hindfoot and midfoot positioned straight, the affected forefoot assumes a medially deviated or varus position (Fig. 21-102A and B). A skin crease may be located over the medial aspect of the longitudinal arch. When mild, the deviation may be passively correctable by the physician or actively correctable by the patient. Active correction may be demonstrated by gentle stroking of the foot, stimulating the peroneal muscles to contract. In more severe cases, the deviation may be only partially corrected by these maneuvers. Some patients have an associated internal tibial torsion deformity, but their calf muscle is normal in size. Radiographs demonstrate the abnormal deviation of the metatarsals medially without other osseous abnormalities (Fig. 21-102C).

Treatment depends on the severity of the condition. In mild cases, passive manipulation of the deformity by the mother several times a day may suffice. In moderate cases, a combination of manipulative stretching and reverse or straight-last shoes may be indicated. More severe cases, which are not passively correctable and which exhibit a prominent deformity and skin crease, necessitate serial manipulation and casting for 6 to 8 weeks. If the deformity persists despite these measures, surgical intervention may be required. Treatment should be undertaken before anticipated ambulation so as to prevent impairment of the patient's motor and social development.

Metatarsus Primus Varus (Adductus)

Metatarsus primus varus is a congenital and often hereditary foot deformity characterized by a broad fore-

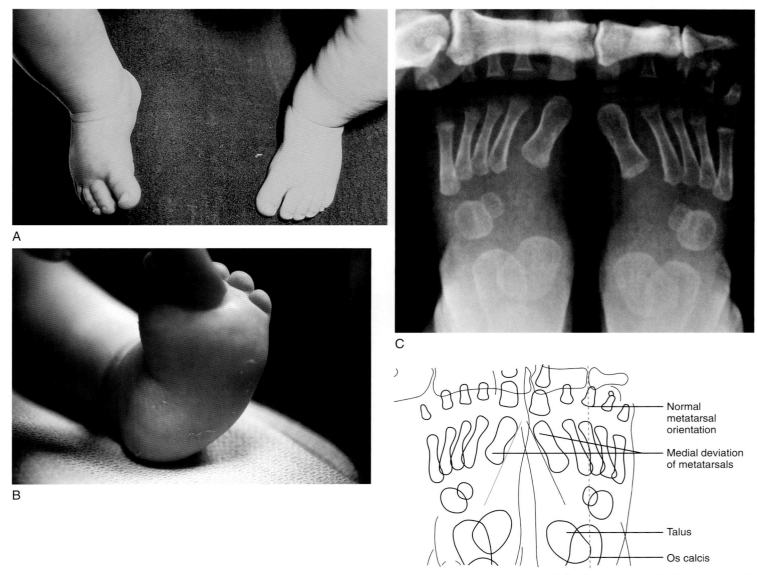

Figure 21-102. Metatarsus adductus. **A,** In this view from above, the forefeet are seen to be deviated medially, but otherwise the feet are normal. **B,** When the feet are viewed from the plantar aspect, rounding of the lateral border can be appreciated, along with a crease on the medial side. **C,** In the AP radiograph, all five metatarsals can be seen to be deviated medially with respect to the remainder of the foot; otherwise, the bony structures are normal. The relationship of the talus and os calcis is normal, unlike the relationship in clubfoot.

foot with medial deviation of the first metatarsal. It is significantly more frequent in females than in males. Examination reveals a wide forefoot with medial deviation of the first metatarsal and normal orientation of the second through fifth metatarsals. Often an associated varus deviation of the great toe exists (Fig. 21-103A). Over time, a secondary hallux valgus deformity and bunion may be produced by the abnormal forces exerted on the great toe with weight bearing and ambulation (see Fig. 21-103B). The heel may seem narrow, but this is more apparent than real. Pronation of the forefoot may be present as well. Radiographs confirm the diagnosis by revealing an increased space between the first and second metatarsals and a large first intermetatarsal angle. The first ray through the tarsometatarsal joint may be medially oriented, forming the basis for the deformity.

In mild cases no treatment may be necessary. In moderate or severe cases, foot strain symptoms, bunion pain, and shoe-fitting problems may necessitate treatment. Surgical osteotomy of the medial cuneiform or first metatarsal in conjunction with bunion correction can satisfactorily eliminate the deformity.

Congenital Vertical Talus

Congenital vertical talus is a teratogenic anomaly of the foot noted at birth and characterized by a severe flatfoot deformity. The underlying pathology is a malorientation of the talus, which assumes a more vertical position than normal. The adjacent navicular is dorsally displaced, articulating with the superior aspect of the neck of the talus and causing the forefoot to assume a dorsiflexed and valgus orientation. In effect, these deformities are the opposite of those seen in congenital clubfoot. The etiology of this condition is unknown, although it may be associated with other musculoskeletal or organ system anomalies. Pathologic analysis reveals normal development of the bones but an abnormal relationship. As in clubfoot, associated soft tissue contractures may occur, particularly of the Achilles tendon, toe extensors, and anterior tibial tendon.

Clinically the deformity is recognizable as a calcaneovalgus foot with loss of the arch or, on some occasions, a rocker-bottom-type foot with a prominent heel (Fig. 21-104A and B). The head of the talus is often palpable on the medial plantar aspect of the midfoot. The deformity is usually fixed, but passive correction may be obtainable

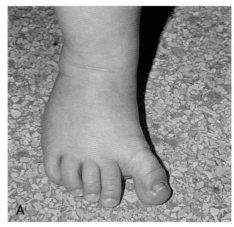
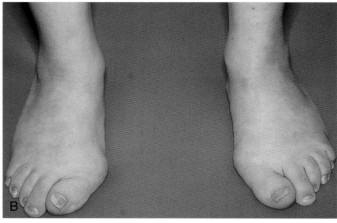

Figure 21-103. Metatarsus primus varus. **A,** The first metatarsal and great toe are deviated medially, and the forefoot is broad. The other metatarsals are normally oriented. **B,** Bilateral metatarsus primus varus with hallux valgus. The forefeet are broad, and the great toes deviate laterally. (**A,** Courtesy Michael Sherlock, MD, Lutherville, Md.)

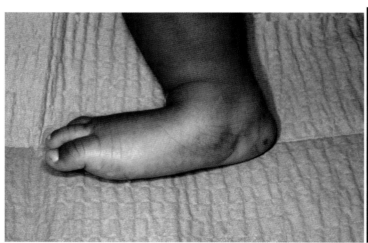
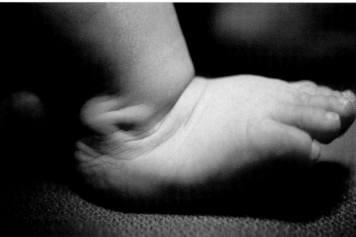

A

B

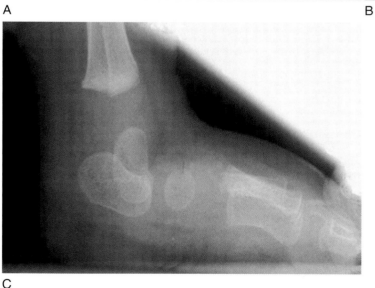

C

Figure 21-104. Congenital vertical talus. **A,** The normal longitudinal arch of the foot is absent; a rocker-bottom type deformity is present; and the forefoot is fixed in dorsiflexion, which is even more evident in **B. C,** On this radiograph the talus is oriented vertically, and its position does not change with flexion or extension of the ankle. The calcaneus is also fixed in equinus position, resulting in a rigid flat foot deformity (see Fig. 21-101B for comparison.)

in some instances, particularly if the talus is oriented in a less severe oblique position. Radiographs mirror the clinical appearance, showing a vertical orientation of the talus, a calcaneus deformity of the os calcis, and valgus orientation of the forefoot (see Fig. 21-104C; see also Fig. 21-101B for a normal comparison).

Initially, attempts at manipulation and serial casting are indicated. However, if this is unsuccessful, as is often the case, surgery may be necessary.

Calcaneovalgus Foot Deformity

Physiologic calcaneovalgus is another deformity of the foot thought to result from intrauterine molding. It is normally a supple deformity that is passively correctable, in contrast with the rigid foot characteristic of congenital vertical talus. The condition is evident at birth and at times is associated with a contralateral metatarsus adductus. No underlying pathologic changes occur in the foot, and no osseous deformities other than the positional one exist. On examination, the foot is noted to be held in a dorsiflexed and everted position with some loss of the normal longitudinal arch (Fig. 21-105). Tightness of the anterior tibial tendon and laxity of the Achilles tendon may be noted in association with the positional deformity. Radiographs reveal no pathologic bony changes. Nonoperative treatment is usually successful and consists of serial casting to eliminate the deformity. Later, wearing shoes with inner heel wedges and longitudinal arch supports may help prevent recurrence and improve ambulation.

Pes Planus (Flatfoot)

Pes planus, or physiologic flatfoot, is an extremely common condition to which there is a familial predisposition. It is characterized by laxity of the soft tissues of the foot resulting in loss of the normal longitudinal arch, with pronation or eversion of the forefoot and valgus or lateral orientation of the heel (Fig. 21-106). Secondary tightness of the Achilles tendon may exist. Generally the condition is asymptomatic in children, and evaluation is sought primarily because of parental concern about the appearance of the foot and the possibility of future problems. Occasionally, affected patients report discomfort after long walks or running.

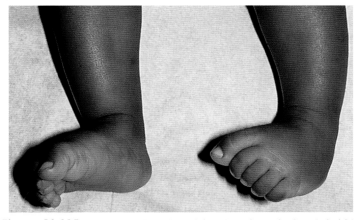

Figure 21-105. Calcaneovalgus foot deformity. The right foot is held in a position of eversion and dorsiflexion. This deformity is supple and thus is passively correctable. The contralateral foot exhibits a metatarsus adductus deformity, giving the feet a "windswept" appearance.

On examination the characteristic appearance is easy to recognize, and laxity of other joints, particularly the thumb, elbow, and knee, may be noted. Weight-bearing radiographs reveal loss of the normal longitudinal arch without osseous abnormality. Treatment is unnecessary if the condition is asymptomatic. Corrective shoes with arch supports are of no use unless symptoms of foot strain are present.

Accessory Tarsal Navicular

An accessory tarsal navicular results from formation of a separate ossification center on the medial aspect of the developing tarsal navicular at the insertion site of the posterior tibial tendon. The condition is not uncommon and is usually associated with a pes planus deformity. Clinically, patients exhibit a bony prominence on the medial aspect of the foot that tends to rub on the shoe, thus producing a painful bursa (Fig. 21-107A). Radiographs reveal either a separate ossification center or bone medial to the parent navicular, or a medial projection of the navicular when fusion has occurred (Fig. 21-107B and C). Cast immobilization may be helpful in acutely painful cases. Long-term improvement can be obtained by wearing soft, supportive shoes with longitudinal arches and a medial heel wedge. Recalcitrant symptoms warrant surgical intervention.

Ganglion of the Foot

A ganglion, or synovial cyst, may develop on the foot. These benign masses are similar to those more commonly seen on the wrist. They originate from outpouchings of a joint capsule or tendon sheath. Trauma may be a predisposing factor in their formation. They are most commonly found on the dorsal or medial aspect of the foot. The mass is soft and nontender and transilluminates. It does not produce symptoms, other than difficulty in fitting shoes (Fig. 21-108). If this occurs, surgical excision may be indicated.

Cavus Feet and Claw Toes

Cavus feet and claw toes are deformities produced by a muscular imbalance within the foot. Although they may occur for unknown reasons, often they are manifestations

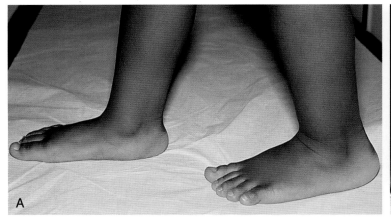
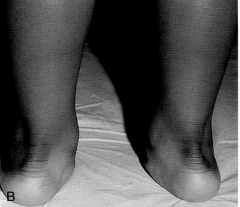

Figure 21-106. Pes planus (flatfoot). **A,** Laxity of the soft tissue structures of the foot results in a loss of the normal longitudinal arch and pronation or eversion of the forefoot. **B,** Viewed from behind, the characteristic eversion of the heels is appreciated more readily.

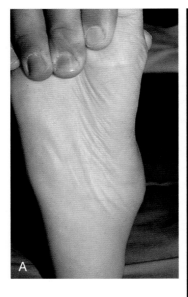

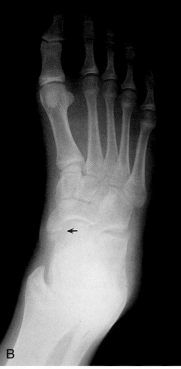

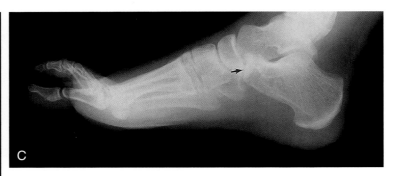

Figure 21-107. Accessory tarsal navicular. **A,** A bony prominence produced by the formation of a separate ossification center of the tarsal navicular is present over the medial aspect of the midfoot. It is covered by a painful bursa, produced by chronic rubbing of the prominence against the medial side of the patient's shoe. Patients with this problem usually have a pes planus deformity as well. **B** and **C,** AP and lateral radiographs of the foot demonstrate the accessory navicular. The posterior tibialis tendon attaches to the small accessory bone and may contribute to continued irritability and tenderness in this area. Similar extra ossicles are often present asymptomatically on the opposite foot.

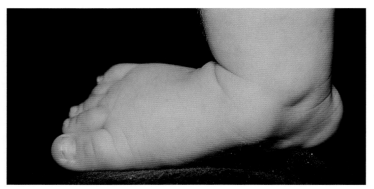

Figure 21-108. Ganglion of the foot. A prominent soft tissue mass is present over the medial aspect of the midfoot. This represents a ganglion of the posterior tibial tendon sheath.

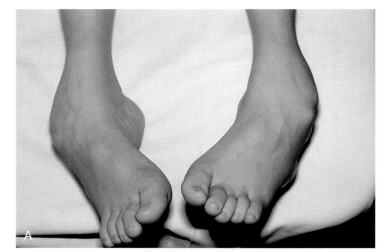

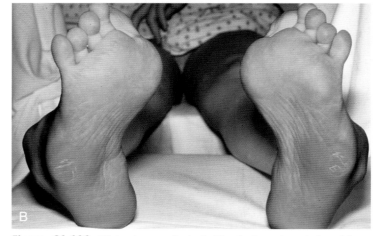

of an underlying neurologic disorder such as Charcot-Marie-Tooth disease (see Chapter 15 and Fig. 15-62), Friedreich ataxia, or spinal cord tethering (see Fig. 15-37). These conditions should be considered in evaluating each patient presenting with these deformities, particularly if the problem is unilateral. Cavus feet exhibit a high arch with a varus or inversion deformity of the heel. Usually the metatarsal heads appear prominent on the plantar aspect of the foot (Fig. 21-109). This phenomenon is accentuated by overlying callosities that develop as a result of abnormal weight bearing. With claw toes, the metatarsophalangeal joints are held in extension with the PIP joints in flexion and the distal joint in the neutral or slightly flexed position (Fig. 21-110). Calluses tend to develop over the PIP joints as the result of rubbing against shoes. Neurologic examination may reveal motor weakness, most often involving the anterior tibial, toe extensor, and peroneal muscles.

Logical treatment necessitates identifying and treating the underlying pathologic condition when possible. Nonsurgical measures for managing the deformities and ameliorating the symptoms consist of the wearing of customized shoes and use of a metatarsal bar to relieve

Figure 21-109. Bilateral cavus feet. **A,** The feet are inverted and have high arches. The deformity is often a feature of neuromuscular disorders, as in this case where it is the result of Charcot-Marie-Tooth disease. **B,** In addition to the high arches and varus (inverted) heels seen in the view of the plantar surface, the prominence of the metatarsal head region is apparent. Callosities have developed over the lateral borders of the feet as a result of abnormal weight bearing.

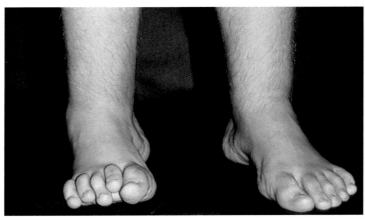

Figure 21-110. Unilateral claw toes. This child with a tethered spinal cord has unilateral claw toe deformities. The metatarsophalangeal joints are held in extension while the proximal interphalangeal joints are fixed in flexion.

pressure on the metatarsal heads and to correct the extension deformities at the base of the toes. However, surgical correction is often necessary.

Generalized Musculoskeletal Disorders

Numerous systemic disorders have significant musculoskeletal manifestations. Those relating to genetic, endocrine, collagen vascular, neurologic, and hematologic problems are discussed in their respective chapters. Four conditions with major musculoskeletal manifestations—cerebral palsy, spina bifida, osteogenesis imperfecta, and arthrogryposis—are discussed in this section.

Cerebral Palsy

Cerebral palsy refers to a group of fixed, nonprogressive neurologic syndromes resulting from static lesions of the developing CNS. Depending on the timing of injury, signs may be present at birth or they may become evident in infancy or early childhood. The primary cerebral insult may be intrauterine or perinatal infection; a prenatal or perinatal vascular accident; anoxia due to placental insufficiency, difficult delivery, or neonatal pulmonary disease; hyperbilirubinemia resulting in kernicterus; or neonatal hypoglycemia. After the newborn period, CNS infections, trauma, and vascular accidents may, when severe, produce the disorder. Abnormal motor function is the most obvious result and may take the form of a spastic neuromuscular disorder (65% of cases), athetosis (25%), or rigidity and/or ataxic neuromuscular dysfunction (10%). Sensory deficits and intellectual impairment are common, and there is a significant incidence of associated seizure disorders.

Because of the number and variety of possible insulting factors, each of which has its own spectrum of severity, there is a broad range in the location and extent of neural damage, and thus in the degree of functional impairment. Patients with severe afflictions generally have early evidence of gross neuromuscular dysfunction. Those with milder involvement may have subtler abnormalities and may be diagnosed only after they fail to achieve normal developmental and motor milestones. Patterns of the affliction include involvement of one or two limbs (monoplegia or hemiplegia), of both lower extremities (diplegia),

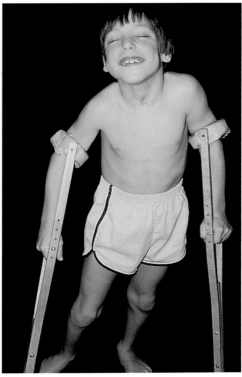

Figure 21-111. Cerebral palsy. Typical patient with spastic quadriplegia. Note the secondary muscle atrophy especially evident in the lower extremities. He requires crutches to ambulate, seizure medication, and a specialized educational program. His neuromuscular abnormalities are the result of a one-time central nervous system insult and are not progressive.

of all four extremities (quadriplegia) (Fig. 21-111), or of all limbs with poor trunk and head control (pentaplegia). Those patients with a spastic disorder exhibit flexion contractures of the involved limbs, hyperreflexia, and spasticity; those with athetosis exhibit the characteristic movement disorder. Mixed involvement is apparent in some patients. Neurologic examination often reveals the persistence of primitive reflexes. Patients with severe involvement that inhibits sitting and ambulation suffer disuse atrophy of involved muscles and skeletal demineralization that increases their risk of pathologic fractures (see Figs. 6-75 and 6-76).

Another complication seen in children with severe spasticity, especially with quadriplegia, is hip dislocation (Fig. 21-112). This and associated arthritic changes are the result of significant and prolonged imbalance of muscle pull about the hip. In 50% of these cases associated pain is problematic, necessitating hip replacement. Administration of medications that reduce muscle spasm and carefully timed and selected surgical procedures described later are helpful in preventing dislocation. Oral Baclofen can also be helpful in reducing spasticity, ameliorating the pain due to associated muscle spasm, and in prevention of contractures and bone and joint deformity. In cases in which the maximum oral dosage is not sufficient to control spasticity or produces unwanted side effects, consideration should be given to intrathecal Baclofen administration using a Baclofen pump, as delivery of the drug directly to the spinal cord/CNS does not produce the systemic effects seen with the oral route.

In evaluating patients with apparent cerebral palsy, one must be careful to rule out a progressive neurologic disorder such as intracranial or spinal cord neoplasms, degenerative neurologic conditions, and tethering of the spinal cord.

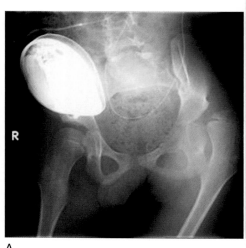

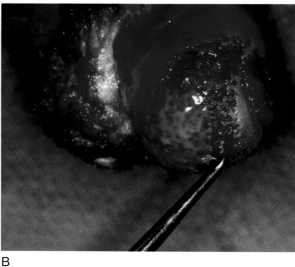

A   B

Figure 21-112. Hip dislocation in cerebral palsy (CP). **A,** This 9-year-old with quadriplegic CP has a dislocated left hip as a result of spasticity and unbalanced muscle pull. This is a source of significant pain in about 50% of cases whether or not the child is ambulatory, and surgical treatment is indicated. Note the Baclofen pump on the right. **B,** This is the proximal femur removed from another child with severe spasticity and a painful dislocated hip. Note the erosion of the articular cartilage. This and disuse osteoporosis make it easy for a metal probe to perforate the femoral head.

Optimal treatment necessitates a team approach. In addition to general pediatric, neurologic/neurosurgical, and orthopedic care, these patients often need the services of a urologist and physical, occupational, and speech therapists, and they may need to be enrolled in individualized educational programs. Family counseling is a necessity. From an orthopedic standpoint, emphasis is placed on optimizing neuromuscular function by attempting to assist the achievement of progressive motor milestones including the ability to sit, stand, walk, and perform activities of daily living. Exercises, bracing, and surgical procedures all have a role, and the institution of specific measures must be timed to fit the pace of growth and development of the individual child. Encouragement and cautious optimism are important. Surgical treatment usually takes the form of soft tissue release to relieve flexion deformities, tendon transfer to optimize functional use of the extremities, osteotomy to correct deformities, and occasionally selective neurectomy to inhibit overactive muscle units.

Pharmacologically, intramuscular injection of botulinum toxin may provide temporary reduction in spasticity and thus may assist physical therapy.

Spina Bifida Cystica (Myelomeningocele)

The myelodysplasias are a group of congenital deformities that result from defective closure of the caudal portion of the neural tube during embryonic development. When the failure of closure involves only the posterior vertebral elements, it is termed a *meningocele;* when it involves neural and vertebral elements, a *myelomeningocele.* In patients with myelomeningocele, the loss of neurologic function that results from abnormal cord and spinal root development has dire consequences for the developing musculoskeletal system. Affected children often require neurosurgical closure of the defect at birth to allow healing and prevent infection, and most need a ventriculoperitoneal shunt to prevent or control hydrocephalus. Because of lack of bladder innervation and control, careful urologic follow-up is necessary as well.

The skeletal manifestations seen in spina bifida are the result of imbalances in muscle function of the trunk and extremities. The neurologic loss roughly corresponds to the level of the spine at which the defect lies. In those patients with thoracic myelomeningocele, complete lack

of sensation and motor function is seen in the lower extremities, and ambulating and functional capacity is limited. On the other hand, in those individuals whose defect is at a low lumbar or sacral level, the weakness and subsequent deformity may be limited to the foot, or hip extensors and abductors, and to bladder dysfunction.

As with cerebral palsy, treatment by a multidisciplinary team of physicians, nurses, and therapists is helpful in reducing complications and maximizing function. Physical therapy (PT) is important in helping to maintain motion and maximize strength of those muscles that are working. Bracing, in addition to PT, helps prevent secondary joint contractures, which can significantly impair function. Surgical intervention may be necessary to help rebalance unequal muscle forces and to release contractures if they occur. A kyphotic deformity (Fig. 21-113A to C) of the spine can make bracing, sitting, and lying uncomfortable and may necessitate surgical correction with spinal rods and fusion.

Osteogenesis Imperfecta

Osteogenesis imperfecta (OI) is a family of inherited disorders characterized most notably by brittle bones. Nearly 90% of cases have been determined to be the result of mutations in either the COL1A1 or COL1A2 genes, which code for production of the proα 1 and 2 polypeptide chains, which are then assembled into a triple helix composed of 2 proα 1 chains and 1 proα 2 to form type I collagen—the major structural protein of bone and other connective tissues. Thus far, hundreds of different mutations of these genes have been identified as causative of varying phenotypes of OI. Nearly all are autosomal dominant. Some of these mutations are characterized by production of structurally abnormal collagen. In other cases, the mutant allele is not expressed, resulting in secretion of about 50% of expected levels of structurally normal type I collagen (see also Chapter 1). Histologically, bone mass is decreased and trabeculae are reduced in both number and thickness. Ossification is decreased, and when structurally abnormal collagen is produced, osteoid is poorly organized. The end result is a significant increase in susceptibility to fractures.

The most widely accepted system of classification of these disorders, developed by Silence in the 1970s, uses a combination of clinical features and course, radiographic

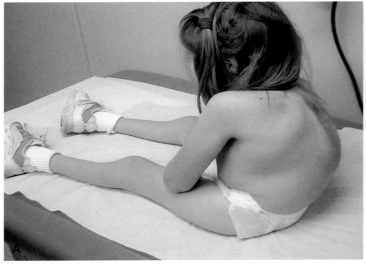

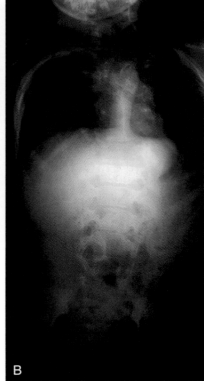

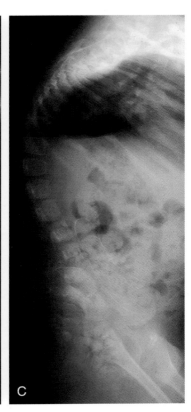

Figure 21-113. Spina bifida. **A,** This child with thoracic-level spina bifida has an obvious kyphotic deformity. The scars on her back are from surgical closure of her myelomeningocele. **B** and **C,** Anteroposterior and lateral radiographs of the spine demonstrate that kyphosis is secondary to incomplete posterior osseous support.

findings, and genetic factors to divide cases into four main types. In type I, nearly all cases are characterized by reduced production of structurally normal collagen, whereas in types II to IV some proportion of the type I collagen produced is structurally abnormal. Phenotypically, patients with types I and IV have mild to moderate (less often moderately severe) fragility, and those with types II and III have severe disease. Patients with the two milder forms typically experience a distinct decrease in fracture frequency with the onset of puberty, which then reverses in the fifth or sixth decade, or after menopause in women.

Considerable phenotypic variation exists between and within types, due predominantly to the large number of possible sites for mutations to occur on the COL1 genes. Some cases of intrafamilial variability are the result of genetic mosaicism within a parent.

Although the causative mutations affect all connective tissues in the body, their primary clinical manifestations involve the skeleton because of the greater structural demands placed on bones. Estimates of incidence of cases of type I range from 1 in 15,000 to 30,000 live births, and from 1 in 20,000 to 60,000 of type II. Type III occurs in approximately 1 in 70,000. Cases of type IV are thought to be much less common, but the exact incidence of type IV is unknown because it is likely that many patients with milder disease are never diagnosed, and there is evidence that a number of other cases have been misclassified as having type I in the past. The same is probably true of patients with milder forms of type I whose sclerae are not noticeably blue.

Osteogenesis Imperfecta Type I

OI type I is the most common form and is usually the mildest clinically. Two subtypes exist: A (the great majority) in which teeth are normal and B (unusual) in which dentinogenesis imperfecta is a feature (see Fig. 20-35). All have blue or grayish-blue sclerae at birth (Fig.

21-114A), although the degree varies and tends to lessen with age.

Bony fragility ranges from mild to moderate (up to 10% have no fractures). Although an occasional patient incurs a fracture during delivery, most experience their first after they begin to cruise or walk. The most common sites are the long bones of the arms and legs. Healing is normal with good callus formation and occurs without deformity.

Radiographically, bones appear normal in infancy, save for the presence of wormian bones within the sutures of the calvarium (Fig. 21-114B and see Fig. 15-28); however, over time, some degree of osteopenia becomes evident along with thinning of the cortices (Fig. 21-114C). In some patients vertebral flattening is noted in later childhood and adolescence.

Growth is normal with ultimate stature within the expected range or at its lower limits. Kyphoscoliosis is seen only occasionally. Other common clinical features include mild femoral bowing at birth and generalized ligamentous laxity with joint hypermobility. Easy bruisability and slight thinning of the skin are present in some patients. Approximately 50% of individuals with OI type I develop progressive hearing loss beginning in the late teens or twenties. The loss has both sensorineural and conductive components, the latter stemming from fractures and/or fusion of the ossicles of the middle ear.

Osteogenesis Imperfecta Type II

OI type II is the severest form and is usually lethal in the perinatal period. Most cases are the result of new mutations, although parental germline mosaicism is occasionally causative. Intrauterine growth is severely retarded, and affected infants are born prematurely with innumerable poorly healed fractures and prominent deformities due to extreme bony fragility. The sclerae are a dark blue-black; the facies is triangular with micrognathia and a small beaked nose; and the calvarium is large in relation

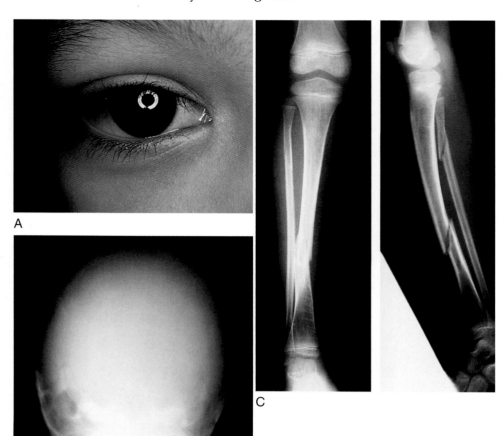

Figure 21-114. Osteogenesis imperfecta (OI) type I. **A,** Blue sclera. **B,** Wormian bones. Multiple wormy, irregular lucencies are seen over the occipitoparietal area. This finding is characteristic of all children with OI types I, II, and III and is seen in more than 50% of patients with OI type IV. **C,** Cortical thinning is evident, especially distal to the oblique fracture of the tibia in this child with OI type I who incurred his fractures jumping off a chair. (**A** and **C,** Courtesy Thomas Daley, MD, St. Joseph's Hospital, Paterson, NJ.)

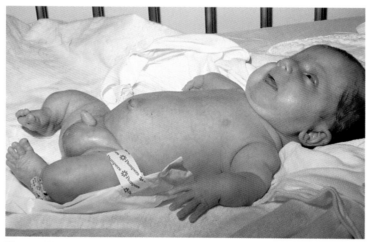

Figure 21-115. Osteogenesis imperfecta type II. This infant was born with multiple fractures and limb deformities. The thighs are fixed in abduction and external rotation. His sclerae are a dark bluish-gray. He died of respiratory insufficiency in the first month of life as the result of his small thorax.

to the face and remarkably soft. Other clinical features include marked shortening of the extremities and severe bowing of the legs with hips flexed and thighs fixed in abduction and external rotation (Fig. 21-115). The combination of a short trunk (due to vertebral flattening) and a small chest cage predisposes to severe/progressive pulmonary insufficiency and congestive heart failure.

Radiographs reveal extreme undermineralization of the entire skeleton; prominent vertebral flattening; very thin hypoplastic beaded ribs; and long bones (especially the femurs) that are broad and telescoped, resembling a concertina in appearance.

Death usually supervenes within a few days to weeks of delivery due to cardiopulmonary complications.

Osteogenesis Imperfecta Type III

Like type II, this form is usually the result of new mutations, less commonly of parental germline mosaicism. The majority are born with multiple fractures and deformities due to fractures in utero. Those who are not incur multiple fractures within the first 1 to 2 years. Birth weights are usually low, and length is short. The extremities are foreshortened, and tibial bowing is prominent (Fig. 21-116A). Sclerae are blue to pale blue and gradually lighten with age. The calvarium is relatively large in comparison with the face, which is triangular with a small chin and frontotemporal bossing (Fig. 21-116B). Dentinogenesis imperfecta is seen in more than half of cases. Bony fragility is moderately severe to severe, and fractures occur with minimal trauma. Healing is impaired and often associated with hyperplastic callus and angulation. Repeated fractures of long bones over time result in progressive limb shortening and deformity.

Radiographically severe diffuse osteopenia and thin cortices are evident, and this tends to worsen with age (Fig. 21-116C). The calvarium is markedly undermineralized with wormian bones seen within sutures (see Fig. 21-114B). The ribs are thin and hypodense. In some patients cystic changes develop in the metaphyses of long bones between 2 and 5 years of age. These are a manifestation of severe disorganization of growth plate structure, which significantly impairs linear growth, and combined with vertebral flattening results in markedly reduced stature. Rapidly progressive kyphoscoliosis is a feature in many older patients and predisposes to cardiopulmonary complications. Other clinical features include ligamentous laxity (seen in 50%) and early-onset hearing loss.

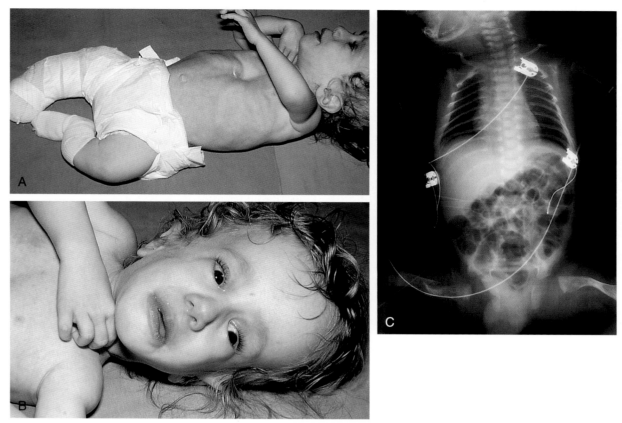

Figure 21-116. Osteogenesis imperfecta type III. **A,** Note the extremely small stature of this 5-year-old child and the deformities of the rib cage and lower extremities. A recent fracture has been splinted. **B,** In this close-up, the characteristic craniofacial features are seen, consisting of a triangular facies, a broad nose, and frontal and temporal bossing. The sclerae may be normal in color, as in this child, or light blue or gray. **C,** Radiograph of an affected infant shows dwarfed, deformed femurs with a new fracture in the midshaft of the right femur. Note also the thin, peculiarly shaped ribs.

About 25% experience easy bruisability, and a number of affected children also report heat intolerance and excessive sweating.

Osteogenesis Imperfecta Type IV

OI type IV, generally considered the least common of the four major types of OI, is divided into two major subsets, A (a minority) with normal dentition and B (the majority) with dentinogenesis imperfects (see Fig. 20-35). Sclerae are normal in color or slightly gray. Degree of bony fragility ranges widely from mild to moderately severe. Birth weight and length are normal, and mild femoral bowing is seen in most affected newborns. Occasionally fractures occur in utero or at delivery, but most do not experience their first break until after the perinatal period, usually after they begin to walk. Although most fractures heal without deformity, in some instances mild angulation and long bone shortening may occur.

Radiographically, bones may appear normal early on, but with age cortical thinning and osteopenia become increasingly evident. Linear growth tends to be mildly impaired, and by age 2 to 3 years most affected children are at or below the third percentile. Generalized ligamentous laxity with joint hypermobility and bowing of the lower extremities and/or valgus knees are not uncommon. Up to a third develop scoliosis in late childhood/early adolescence. Hearing loss is unusual.

Other Types of Osteogenesis Imperfecta

Since the Sillence classification was formulated in the 1970s, major advances in testing for defects in type I col-

lagen have enabled more accurate classification of cases into the four major types of OI. In addition, three other clinical types have been identified more recently (V-VII), none of which has any detectable deficit in type I collagen. Types V and VI are autosomal dominant, and type VII is autosomal recessive. All are rare.

Osteogenesis Imperfecta Type V. Affected children have normal sclerae and teeth but moderate to severe fragility of long bones and vertebrae, as well as ligamentous laxity. Callus produced in the course of fracture healing is distinctly hyperplastic. Radiographically a radiodense band is seen in all affected patients who were still growing in the metaphyses of long bones near the epiphyses. Another feature unique to this type is calcification of the interosseous membrane between the ulna and radius, which limits supination and pronation of the forearm.

Osteogenesis Imperfecta Type VI. Patients with type VI have normal to slightly blue sclerae and normal teeth. Mild to moderate osseous fragility is seen (often to a greater degree than in type IV), with onset of fractures occurring in the first 6 to 18 months. Vertebral compression fractures are especially common. Histologically there is evidence of defective mineralization of the bony matrix with accumulation of osteoid.

Osteogenesis Imperfecta Type VII. In these children sclerae are blue but teeth are apparently normal. Osteopenia is significant, and bony fragility moderate to severe. Fractures are often present at the time of delivery and those involving long bones of the lower extremities often result in deformity. Both coxa vara, a downward curvature of the femoral neck causing adduction of the thigh, and rhizomelia (shortening of the proximal extremities) have been described.

Diagnosis

With close attention to clinical findings and course, as well as radiographic features and family history, the diagnosis of OI types II and III is relatively obvious and of types I and IV is usually straightforward. The major exception involves the very small minority of cases of type IV A—with normal teeth and sclerae—and of type IA, whose sclerae are not noticeably blue. Routine laboratory studies that reflect bone and mineral metabolism are normal and thus unhelpful. Thus far determination of standards for the normal range of bone density in growing children is in its infancy. Further, while measurements in children with mild forms of OI reveal that densities are usually somewhat low, many are still within what is currently considered the normal range.

When a clinical diagnosis cannot be made with any degree of assurance and when an exact diagnosis is necessary, analysis of collagen synthesis by fibroblasts obtained via skin biopsy can be performed. However, the process takes 3 to 4 months. It must also be remembered that the results will be normal in children with types VI to VII.

Prenatal diagnosis is possible for families who have had a child with type II or III OI (whose genetic defect has been identified) using DNA analysis of chorionic villous sampling. Ultrasound is also of use for these types between 15 and 18 weeks' gestation. Routine specific genetic testing is as yet unfeasible.

Differential Diagnosis

Generally there is no confusion in the diagnosis of type III OI. The same is true of most type II cases, although occasionally they must be distinguished from thanatophoric dysplasia, achondrogenesis, and autosomal recessive hypophosphatasia.

The major differential diagnostic considerations in cases of types I and IV are child abuse and idiopathic juvenile osteoporosis.

Distinction from abuse (see Chapter 6) is usually possible clinically because infants and children with previously undiagnosed mild OI and an acute fracture are brought in for care promptly, by parents who are appropriately concerned and give a history of a mechanism of injury that fits the fracture pattern found, although the amount of force reported is somewhat less than usually required to cause a fracture. Further, most of these fractures involve the diaphyses of the long bones of the extremities. The metaphyseal fractures seen commonly in abuse victims are exceptionally rare in children with OI, and typically one does not find multiple fractures of varying ages for which no prior care has been sought. Finally, skull fractures are rare in OI and retinal hemorrhages, subdural hematomas, and visceral injuries are not seen, with the rare exception of the infant or child with OI who is also a victim of abuse.

The major source of potential confusion is the infant with mild OI and normal sclerae who has incurred one or more nondisplaced fractures in utero or during delivery that were not diagnosed in the newborn period. If he or she then presents with a first symptomatic fracture within the ensuing few months, old healing fractures will be found. Again, timing of presentation, parental demeanor, consistency with mechanism, and family history and psychosocial history should all be scrutinized carefully in making the distinction. Consultation with a specialist in abuse and neglect can be very helpful.

Idiopathic juvenile osteoporosis is an exceptionally rare disorder of unknown etiology. In affected children osteopenia and fractures are most evident in the vertebrae, less so in the long bones, and measurements of bone density are well below normal. This condition improves dramatically in adolescence. Family history is negative for unusually frequent fractures.

Treatment

Patients with OI types I and IV usually require only routine orthopedic care for their fractures and counseling regarding accident prevention and safety. Palliative supportive care and minimal handling are the only measures available for infants with OI type II. Treatment of infants and children with OI type III is geared toward minimizing the frequency of fractures and preventing deformities. In infancy this may mean limited handling of the child and use of a padded carrying device. Later, bracing and surgical treatment in the form of osteotomies and internal stabilization of long bones with intermedullary rod fixation may be necessary. Maintenance of activity and the avoidance of repeated prolonged periods of immobilization help prevent disuse atrophy.

Early investigational trials of intravenous pamidronate in patients with severe fragility have shown some promise in reducing fracture frequency. However, only preliminary results on small numbers of patients are available, and data on long-term side effects exist. Growth hormone, which stimulates bone and collagen metabolism, has shown some promise in children with more severe forms of OI type I. It is, however, contraindicated in patients with kyphoscoliosis because it increases the rate of progression of deformity, and also in children with types II to IV because its stimulant effect on collagen metabolism only serves to increase secretion of abnormal collagen.

Arthrogryposis

Arthrogryposis is a nonprogressive muscular disorder of unknown etiology that appears to be related to either failure of development of or degeneration of muscular structures. Neural factors have been implicated in its pathogenesis because in some instances the spinal cord has been found to be reduced in size, with a decreased number of anterior horn cells. Generally all limbs are involved. On occasion the disease may be confined to one or a few limbs only. Primary manifestations consist of joint contractures with secondary deformities and limited motion. Deformities include clubfoot; dislocated hips; and contractures of the knees, elbows, wrists, and hands (Fig. 21-117). Motion of the involved joints is severely limited, but patients can generally compensate for this functional limitation. Radiographs show relatively normal-appearing bones and joints, but fat density is noted in the areas where muscles are normally seen. On pathologic analysis, there is a striking absence of muscle tissue with strands of fat permeating the area.

Orthopedic treatment is aimed at providing optimal motor function. Range-of-motion exercises may maintain what motion is present but rarely result in an increase. Surgery rarely results in improved range of motion but is indicated to restore functional position in those patients with clubfoot and/or hip dislocation. Gradual recurrence of the deformity after surgery is not uncommon, however.

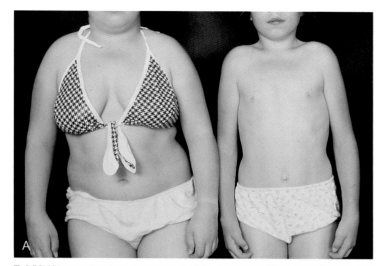

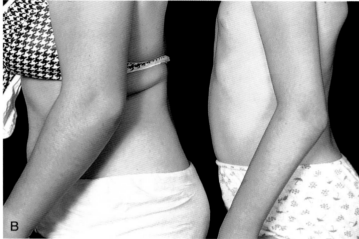

Figure 21-117. Arthrogryposis. **A,** Two sisters with the generalized form of the disorder. Note the stiff posture and tubular appearance of the limbs. Motion of all joints is limited as a result of failure in the development of or the degeneration of muscular structures. Their stature is short. **B,** The lateral view highlights the flexion contractures of the elbows.

Sports Medicine

The benefits of physical activity and sports have been touted not only by the health care professions but also by school officials, sports enthusiasts, the media, and insurers. They include improved physical fitness and flexibility; an increased sense of physical well-being; and reduction of stress, tension, and anxiety at all ages. Further, a well-selected activity can be a source of considerable physical pleasure and enjoyment. In childhood and adolescence, physical activity and sports can increase self-confidence and self-esteem, especially when the child is able to achieve mastery of skills and, thereby, a sense of competence and accomplishment. Participation in team sports can also assist development of interactive social skills including cooperation, conflict resolution, and discipline and give a child a sense of "fitting in." Furthermore, when physical activity is and remains a source of fun and enjoyment from an early age, it can set the stage for a lifelong pattern or habit of being active with the attendant long-term benefits of cardiovascular health, good weight control, optimal bone density, and reduction of risk of developing type 2 diabetes.

In the first half of the 20th century, sports in childhood consisted primarily of free play and "pick-up games" in yards, on streets, in alleys, and on empty lots with little or no adult supervision. Spontaneity, flexibility, and in many cases greater inclusiveness (kids of differing ages and skill levels) were typical, and although competition was a feature, it tended to be less prominent than is true of organized sports. In contrast, today greater danger in many urban neighborhoods; limited numbers of children in others; lack of access to playgrounds or other sports facilities; and competing demands of television, computers, and homework have reduced the opportunity for unstructured free play. Furthermore, with many children entering day care at an early age and progressing through preschool to elementary school and beyond, constant adult supervision of play is often the norm. These factors have contributed to the strong trend over the past few decades toward increasing organization of sports. As a result, participation of children in either formally or informally organized sports activities is nearly universal and has become part of normal childhood experience. Physical education may begin as early as age 4 and extend through adolescence and is now nearly equal for boys and girls.

This trend toward increasing organization has had its pluses and minuses. It can be positive when there is good coaching and supervision that takes developmental levels and readiness into consideration, has reasonable goals for participation, and good methods for achieving them. Elements of such programs include emphasis on learning basic skills while gradually increasing level and intensity of activity; on developing the social skills necessary for good teamwork; on good sportsmanship and having fun more than winning; and use of praise, encouragement, and enthusiasm to motivate progress. Other good practices include fair processes in team selection; matching competitors by size and skill level; teaching the rules and the reasons for them; placing emphasis on safety and setting strict limits on dangerous practices; and teaching safe practice techniques with reasonable time limits on practices and games to reduce risk of overuse and other injuries. An added benefit has been a trend toward construction of better facilities and development and use of improved equipment. Conversely, when coaches and parents place unrealistic demands and expectations on children that exceed their developmental abilities and readiness to participate, when competitiveness and winning become the goals and only the best players get praise and the opportunity to play, and when criticism and demeaning remarks are used as "motivators," then spontaneity and enjoyment are lost and sports become a source of stress. In such situations, many children lose interest and motivation and come away with a sense of frustration and failure. In fact, greater emphasis on competition from peers, coaches, and parents and higher expectations for increased performance in ever-younger children now account for a significant rise in the incidence of adult-type injuries appearing in children. This is in addition to the injury patterns that are unique to childhood. It also may be partially responsible for a significant drop-off in sports participation during the middle school teen years.

Development of Athletic Skills

Having a basic understanding of child development is integral to optimal parental encouragement of physical activity and to safe and effective coaching of sports programs. Acquisition of motor milestones during infancy and childhood follows a relatively orderly and predictable course, albeit with a wide range of normal variation in rate.

This development in concert with advances in cognitive and social ability is dependent on physical growth and on myelination and neural maturation with corresponding increases in sensory/motor integration, as well as on each child's own curiosity and desire to master new movements and activities. Although it has been demonstrated that having freedom and encouragement to explore and experiment at their own pace (without undue restriction or criticism) fosters developmental advances, there is no evidence that participation in early training programs either hastens this process or improves later performance in sports.

In the early school years, further maturation assists acquisition of additional basic motor skills, development of mature patterns of sport-related skills (Table 21-7), and then trying out these skills in varying combinations (*transitional skills*). There is evidence that instruction and practice can help refine motor skills in children in this age range. Cognitively and socially, young school-age children do not have the wherewithal to make true teamwork or team play realistic, however. During later childhood and early puberty, ongoing maturation enhances the ability to further refine skills and enables understanding of strategy and practice of true teamwork. Throughout the elementary and middle school years, there is a gradual increase in cardiopulmonary endurance in both sexes, and this, coupled with the fact that strength is relatively comparable in boys and girls, makes coed participation and competition feasible and safe.

With puberty, the growth spurt results in major increases in muscle mass and strength, as well as in exercise capacity or cardiopulmonary endurance. Girls tend to mature earlier and more gradually, while boys often enter puberty somewhat later but at a more rapid rate, ultimately ending up much larger and stronger than most of their female counterparts. This makes coed participation, especially in contact sports, less safe for girls. During the pubertal growth spurt, bones grow relatively faster than surrounding soft tissues, resulting in a temporary period of decreased flexibility or tightness, especially of the hamstring muscles and ankle dorsiflexors. This phenomenon can predispose to injury, and preparticipation stretching exercises are advisable as a preventive measure (see Fig. 21-123). Throughout childhood and well into puberty, the open epiphyses of growing bones are vulnerable to injury when subjected to shearing stresses and heavy weight loads. This necessitates care in strength training and avoidance of weightlifting and related sports until skeletal maturity is achieved.

The wide range of normal variation of onset and pace of puberty results in significant differences in size and maturation of individuals of the same age and sex. This has led to the practice of matching children and teams by weight or size to reduce risk to smaller children in contact sports. Use of maturation indexing, matching by Tanner stage or maturity level, is gaining interest, and although there are no hard data yet regarding effectiveness, it does have an inherent logic and may be preferable, given the fact that a pubertal child of the same size as a prepubertal child is likely to be much stronger. To date, however, this practice has not gained wide acceptance.

Table 21-8 presents in summary form the developmental progression of motor and cognitive development along with corresponding recommendations for athletic education and training. Importantly, no data currently exist regarding optimal age for beginning participation in the various organized sports.

The Preparticipation Sports Physical Examination

Recognition of the rise in injury incidence and of new types of injury in children, especially when participating in programs that do not adequately factor in neuromus-

Table 21-7	Average Age at Acquisition of Mature Patterns of Sports-Related Motor Skills	
SKILL	**BOYS (YR)**	**GIRLS (YR)**
Throwing	6	8
Kicking	7	8
Hopping and catching	7-8	7-8
Hitting balls and shooting baskets	10-14	10-14

Table 21-8	Developmental Skills for Sports and Sports Recommendations during Childhood	
EARLY CHILDHOOD (2 TO 5 YR)	**MIDDLE CHILDHOOD (6 TO 9 YR)**	**LATE CHILDHOOD (10 TO 12 YR)**
Motor Skills • Limited fundamental skills • Limited balance skills **Learning** • Extremely short attention span • Poor selective attention • Egocentric learning—trial and error • Visual and auditory cues are important **Vision** • Not fully mature before ages 6 to 7 (farsighted) • Difficulty tracking and judging velocity of moving objects **Sports Recommendations** • Emphasize fundamental skills with minimal variation and limited instruction • Emphasize fun, playfulness, exploration, and experimentation rather than competition • *Activities:* Running, swimming, tumbling, throwing, catching	**Motor Skills** • Continued improvement in fundamental skills • Posture and balance become more automatic • Improved reaction times • Beginning transitional skills **Learning** • Short attention span • Limited development of memory and rapid decision making **Vision** • Improved tracking • Limited directionality **Sports Recommendations** • Emphasize fundamental skills and beginning transitional skills • Flexible rules of sports • Allow free time in practices • Short instruction time • Minimal competition • *Activities:* Entry-level soccer and baseball	**Motor Skills** • Improved transitional skills • Ability to master complex motor skills • Temporary decline in balance control at puberty **Learning** • Selective attention • Able to use memory strategies for sports such as football and basketball **Vision** • Adult patterns **Sports Recommendations** • Emphasis on skill development • Increasing emphasis on tactics and strategy • Emphasize factors promoting continued participation • *Activities:* Entry level for complex skill sports (football, basketball)

Modified from Nelson MA: Developmental skills and children's sports. Physician Sportsmed 19:67-79, 1991.

cular and cognitive development, has led to increased interest in more formal medical monitoring of child and adolescent athletes.

In an effort to foster safer participation, a task force was formed composed of representatives from the American Academy of Family Practice, the American Academy of Pediatrics, the American Medical Society for Sports Medicine, the American Orthopaedic Society for Sports Medicine, and the American Osteopathic Association for Sports Medicine. Their charge was to develop recommendations and standards for the format of the preparticipation evaluation (PPE) of youngsters before entry into competitive sports programs. Initial recommendations were published in 1992 and were subsequently refined and updated in 1997.

The primary goals of the PPE are as follows:
1. Detection of underlying medical problems or conditions that are characterized by the following:
   - May predispose to injury (e.g., patellofemoral malalignment)
   - Are potentially disabling (e.g., prior injury)
   - Are potentially life threatening (e.g., hypertrophic cardiomyopathy)

Such conditions may warrant further evaluation and testing, a rehabilitation or preconditioning program, or selection of an alternative sport.
2. Assessment of the following:
   - General health
   - Physical maturation
   - Fitness level and proficiency for a particular sport (including strength, flexibility, and joint stability)

This helps in determining whether a preconditioning program may be indicated or whether selection of an alternative sport may be advisable.
3. Compliance with insurance and legal requirements
4. Counseling regarding health-related issues
   - Nutrition and healthy diet
   - Avoidance of high-risk or unhealthy behaviors (e.g., drugs, alcohol, fighting, promiscuity)
   - Importance of safe training and play techniques and safety equipment
   - What sports are safe for the individual
5. Ideally, assessment of cognitive and social readiness; interest level, goals, and motivation; psychosocial supports at home and at school; and current life stresses are included.

The person performing the examination may be the primary care physician or, in some instances, a sports medicine physician or a physician with a specific interest in this area. It is generally recommended that an examination be done at least every 2 years, more frequently if there is a change in the physical condition of the child or a change in the sports level. However, most states and school systems require yearly examinations. The assessment is best performed at least 6 to 8 weeks before beginning participation to allow for time to correct any deficiencies that may need rehabilitation or warrant a preconditioning program.

Three major formats/sites of examination may be used:
- Locker room examination: Students line up and are seen one at a time by a team physician who usually has an interest in or expertise in sports medicine.
- Station method: The examination is divided into components, each with a station that may be staffed by a nurse, physician, trainer, or coach. Stations include weight/height, vision, vital signs, and general examination. Dental and nutrition stations are optional.
- Office method: The child is examined by his own primary care physician.

Both the locker room and station methods tend to be performed in a noisy milieu (making auscultation difficult). They afford limited privacy and have the disadvantage of the physician's not knowing or having an established relationship with the child or adolescent. They do, however, have the advantage of having physicians who tend to be more well versed in sports medicine, are reputed to be more efficient, and are less costly. The office method affords privacy, a quiet environment, and greater opportunity for individual attention and counseling. When there has been long-standing continuity of care, the physician knows the child's past medical, surgical, injury, growth, developmental, family, and psychosocial histories. Furthermore, the established physician-patient relationship assists assessment of maturity, readiness, motivation, and psychosocial stressors that may affect performance, and it can enhance efficacy of counseling and compliance with recommendations. It may have the disadvantage of the physician's having limited knowledge of the sport and its requirements.

The forms designed by the PPE task force for the history, physical examination, and clearance to participate (Figs. 21-118 to 21-120) are well crafted for meeting the goals of the PPE. They are regarded by experts as the best available, and we encourage their use (especially the history form), although states and school systems often have their own less inclusive forms.

Ideally, the history form is given to the prospective athlete in advance of the examination date, with instructions to complete it together with his or her parents. (Requiring a parental signature may be advisable to ensure that the parent's input is included.) Athletes may need to be reassured that the primary goal of the PPE is to identify potential problems that can be remedied, whenever possible, not to exclude them from play. This form is then reviewed with the athlete at the time of the examination. Questions are designed to screen for conditions most likely to result in problems or to be associated with significant risk for injury, reinjury, disability, or sudden death. Positive responses also help to highlight areas that need special attention in performing the physical examination. Particular areas of emphasis include exercise- or postexercise-related cardiopulmonary, neurologic, and musculoskeletal symptoms; family history of early and sudden cardiac deaths; past medical, surgical, injury, and heat illness histories; and identification of chronic or recent illnesses (especially the possibility of myocarditis and mononucleosis) that may be sources of increased risk or necessitate limits on participation.

The cardiovascular, pulmonary, and musculoskeletal portions of the physical examination have the highest yield in identifying potential problems. Attention is also paid to identifying visual problems that warrant protective eyewear (i.e., being functionally one-eyed), the abdominal examination for detection of visceromegaly, and genital examination (when having a single testicle warrants extra protection during contact sports).

In addition to screening for hypertension, the cardiac examination should focus on findings that may suggest a previously undetected disorder that may place the athlete at risk when playing sports of high aerobic intensity. These include hypertrophic cardiomyopathy, aortic stenosis, coarctation, other cardiomyopathies, myocarditis, and certain arrhythmias. Attention is paid to pulse quality and regularity; amplitude of pulses in upper and lower extremities; precordial activity; and auscultation in supine, as well as squatting and standing, positions because in some (though not all) cases of hypertrophic cardiomyopathy

PREPARTICIPATION PHYSICAL EVALUATION

HISTORY

DATE OF EXAM_____

Name_____ Sex_____ Age_____ Date of birth_____

Grade_____ School_____ Sport(s)_____

Address_____ Phone_____

Personal physician_____

In case of emergency, contact

Name_____ Relationship_____ Phone (H)_____ (W)_____

Explain "Yes" answers below.
Circle questions you don't know the answers to.

Yes No

1. Have you had a medical illness or injury since your last check up or sports physical? ☐ ☐
   Do you have an ongoing or chronic illness? ☐ ☐
2. Have you ever been hospitalized overnight? ☐ ☐
   Have you ever had surgery? ☐ ☐
3. Are you currently taking any prescription or nonprescription (over-the-counter) medications or pills or using an inhaler? ☐ ☐
   Have you ever taken any supplements or vitamins to help you gain or lose weight or improve your performance? ☐ ☐
4. Do you have any allergies (for example, to pollen, medicine, food, or stinging insects)? ☐ ☐
   Have you ever had a rash or hives develop during or after exercise? ☐ ☐
5. Have you ever passed out during or after exercise? ☐ ☐
   Have you ever been dizzy during or after exercise? ☐ ☐
   Have you ever had chest pain during or after exercise? ☐ ☐
   Do you get tired more quickly than your friends do during exercise? ☐ ☐
   Have you ever had racing of your heart or skipped heartbeats? ☐ ☐
   Have you had high blood pressure or high cholesterol? ☐ ☐
   Have you ever been told you have a heart murmur? ☐ ☐
   Has any family member or relative died of heart problems or of sudden death before age 50? ☐ ☐
   Have you had a severe viral infection (for example, myocarditis or mononucleosis) within the last month? ☐ ☐
   Has a physician ever denied or restricted your participation in sports for any heart problems? ☐ ☐
6. Do you have any current skin problems (for example, itching, rashes, acne, warts, fungus, or blisters)? ☐ ☐
7. Have you ever had a head injury or concussion? ☐ ☐
   Have you ever been knocked out, become unconscious, or lost your memory? ☐ ☐
   Have you ever had a seizure? ☐ ☐
   Do you have frequent or severe headaches? ☐ ☐
   Have you ever had numbness or tingling in your arms, hands, legs or feet? ☐ ☐
   Have you ever had a stinger, burner, or pinched nerve? ☐ ☐
8. Have you ever become ill from exercising in the heat? ☐ ☐
9. Do you cough, wheeze, or have trouble breathing during or after activity? ☐ ☐
   Do you have asthma? ☐ ☐
   Do you have seasonal allergies that require medical treatment? ☐ ☐

Yes No

10. Do you use any special protective or corrective equipment or devices that aren't usually used for your sport or position (for example, knee brace, special neck roll, foot orthotics, retainer on your teeth, hearing aid)? ☐ ☐
11. Have you had any problems with your eyes or vision? ☐ ☐
    Do you wear glasses, contacts, or protective eyewear? ☐ ☐
12. Have you ever had a sprain, strain, or swelling after injury? ☐ ☐
    Have you broken or fractured any bones or dislocated any joints? ☐ ☐
    Have you had any other problems with pain or swelling in muscles, tendons, bones or joints? ☐ ☐
    If yes, check appropriate box and explain below.
    ☐ Head ☐ Elbow ☐ Hip
    ☐ Neck ☐ Forearm ☐ Thigh
    ☐ Back ☐ Wrist ☐ Knee
    ☐ Chest ☐ Hand ☐ Shin/calf
    ☐ Shoulder ☐ Finger ☐ Ankle
    ☐ Upper arm ☐ Foot
13. Do you want to weigh more or less than you do now? ☐ ☐
    Do you lose weight regularly to meet weight requirements for your sport? ☐ ☐
14. Do you feel stressed out? ☐ ☐
15. Record the dates for your most recent immunizations (shots) for:
    Tetanus_____ Measles_____
    Hepatitis B_____ Chickenpox_____

FEMALES ONLY

16. When was your first menstrual period?_____
    When was your most recent menstrual period?_____
    How much time do you usually have from the start of one period to the start of another?_____
    How many periods have you had in the last year?_____
    What was the longest time between periods in the last year?____

Explain "Yes" answers here:_____
_____
_____
_____
_____
_____
_____
_____
_____
_____

I hereby state that, to the best of my knowledge, my answers to the above questions are complete and correct.

Signature of athlete_____ Signature of parent/guardian_____ Date_____

Figure 21-118. Preparticipation history form. (From Smith DM [ed]: American Academy of Family Physicians, American Academy of Pediatrics, American Medical Society for Sports Medicine, American Orthopaedic Society for Sports Medicine, American Osteopathic Association for Sports Medicine: Preparticipation Physical Evaluation Monograph, ed 2. Minneapolis, 1997, pp 1-49.)

PREPARTICIPATION PHYSICAL EVALUATION

PHYSICAL EXAMINATION

Name_____ Date of birth_____

Height_____Weight_____% Body fat (optional)_____Pulse_____BP___/___(___/___,___/___)

Vision R 20/ _____ L 20/ _____   Corrected: Y   N   Pupils: Equal _____   Unequal _____

	NORMAL	ABNORMAL FINDINGS	INITIALS*
MEDICAL			
Appearance			
Eyes/ears/nose/throat			
Lymph nodes			
Heart			
Pulses			
Lungs			
Abdomen			
Genitalia (males only)			
Skin			
MUSCULOSKELETAL			
Neck			
Back			
Shoulder/arm			
Elbow/forearm			
Wrist/hand			
Hip/thigh			
Knee			
Leg/ankle			
Foot			

*Station-based examination only

Figure 21-119. Preparticipation physical examination form. (From Smith DM [ed]: American Academy of Family Physicians, American Academy of Pediatrics, American Medical Society for Sports Medicine, American Orthopaedic Society for Sports Medicine, American Osteopathic Association for Sports Medicine: Preparticipation Physical Evaluation Monograph, ed 2. Minneapolis, 1997, pp 1-49.)

PREPARTICIPATION PHYSICAL EVALUATION
CLEARANCE FORM

☐ **Cleared**

☐ **Cleared after completing evaluation/rehabilitation for:**_____
_____
_____
_____

☐ **Not cleared for:**_____**Reason:**_____

Recommendations:_____
_____
_____
_____

Name of physician (print/type)_____**Date**_____

Address _____**Phone**_____

Signature of physician_____, **MD or DO**

Figure 21-120. Clearance to play form. (From Smith DM [ed]: American Academy of Family Physicians, American Academy of Pediatrics, American Medical Society for Sports Medicine, American Orthopaedic Society for Sports Medicine, American Osteopathic Association for Sports Medicine: Preparticipation Physical Evaluation Monograph, ed 2. Minneapolis, 1997, pp 1-49.)

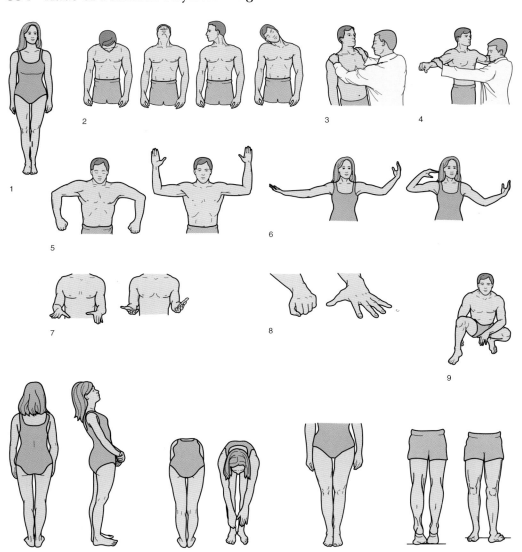

Figure 21-121. Two-minute musculoskeletal screening examination. (From Smith DM [ed]: American Academy of Family Physicians, American Academy of Pediatrics, American Medical Society for Sports Medicine, American Orthopaedic Society for Sports Medicine, American Osteopathic Association for Sports Medicine: Preparticipation Physical Evaluation Monograph, ed 2. Minneapolis, 1997, pp 1-49.)

1. Inspection, athlete standing, facing toward examiner (symmetry of trunk, upper extremities).
2. Forward flexion, extension, rotation, lateral flexion of neck (range of motion, cervical spine).
3. Resisted shoulder shrug (strength, trapezius).
4. Resisted shoulder abduction (strength, deltoid).
5. Internal and external rotation of shoulder (range of motion, glenohumeral joint).
6. Extension and flexion of elbow (range of motion, elbow).
7. Pronation and supination of elbow (range of motion, elbow and wrist).
8. Clench fist, then spread fingers (range of motion, hand and fingers).
9. "Duck walk" four steps (motion of hip, knee, and ankle; strength; balance).
10. Inspection, athlete facing away from examiner (symmetry of trunk, upper extremities).
11. Back extension, knees straight (spondylolysis/spondylolisthesis).
12. Back flexion with knees straight, facing toward and away from examiner (range of motion, thoracic and lumbosacral spine; spine curvature; hamstring flexibility).
13. Inspection of lower extremities, contraction of quadriceps muscles (alignment, symmetry).
14. Standing on toes, then on heels (symmetry, calf; strength; balance).

and other sources of left ventricular outlet obstruction, a systolic murmur that increases on rising from squatting is noted. This is in contrast to the flow murmur heard in well-conditioned athletes that decreases on standing.

Murmurs that increase on standing from a squat position, diastolic murmurs and those grade III or greater, pulse irregularities other than physiologic changes with respiration, unequal pulses in upper and lower extremities, and decreased pulse amplitude all warrant further evaluation by a cardiologist, as do any positive responses to cardiovascular questions on history.

Exercise-induced asthma, the most common pulmonary problem affected by exercise, can often be identified by history of cough, shortness of breath, or chest tightness with exercise. Nevertheless, in many cases the condition remains unrecognized. Although peak flow readings before and after exercise challenge done in the office (running up and down stairs or jumping rope for 3 to 5

minutes) may detect additional cases, research suggests that the best method is field testing of pulmonary function before and after a 1-mile run. Unfortunately, the latter is often impractical.

The contours, symmetry, range of motion, and stability of the neck, back, shoulders, elbows, wrists, hands, hips, knees, ankles, and feet can be assessed quickly and efficiently using the 2-minute musculoskeletal screening examination (Fig. 21-121). When this is combined with additional attention to areas highlighted by the history, the vast majority of musculoskeletal abnormalities that may benefit from preconditioning programs or rehabilitation are identified, with concomitant reduction of risk of injury and disability.

Use of routine laboratory tests has been found unnecessary. Furthermore, studies of mass electrocardiographic and echocardiographic screenings have proved to have

Table 21-9	Classification of Sports by Contact/Collision Risk	
CONTACT OR COLLISION	**LIMITED CONTACT**	**NONCONTACT**
Basketball	Baseball	Archery
Boxing*	Bicycling	Badminton
Diving	Cheerleading	Body building
Field hockey	Canoeing or kayaking	Bowling
Football (tackle)	(white water)	Canoeing or kayaking
Ice hockey[†]	Fencing	(flat water)
Lacrosse	Field events	Crew or rowing
Martial arts	High jump	Curling
Rodeo	Pole vault	Dancing[‡]
Rugby	Floor hockey	Ballet
Ski jumping	Football (flag)	Modern
Soccer	Gymnastics	Jazz
Team handball	Handball	Field events
Water polo	Horseback riding	Discus
Wrestling	Racquetball	Javelin
	Skating	Shot put
	Ice	Golf
	In-line	Orienteering[§]
	Roller	Power lifting
	Skiing	Race walking
	Cross-country	Riflery
	Downhill	Rope jumping
	Water	Running
	Skateboarding	Sailing
	Snowboarding[¶]	Scuba diving
	Softball	Swimming
	Squash	Table tennis
	Ultimate Frisbee	Tennis
	Volleyball	Track
	Windsurfing or surfing	Weight lifting

*Participation not recommended by the American Academy of Pediatrics.
[†]The American Academy of Pediatrics recommends limiting the body checking allowed for hockey players 15 years and younger to reduce injuries.
[‡]Dancing has been further classified into ballet, modern, and jazz since previous statement was published.
[§]A race (contest) in which competitors use a map and compass to find their way through unfamiliar territory.
[¶]Snowboarding has been added since previous statement was published.
From American Academy of Pediatrics, Committee on Sports Medicine and Fitness 2000-2001: Medical conditions affecting sports participation. Pediatrics 107:1205-1209, 2001.

Table 21-10	Classification of Sport by Level of Aerobic Intensity and by Degree of Static and Dynamic Demands		
HIGH TO MODERATE INTENSITY			
High to Moderate Dynamic and Static Demands	*High to Moderate Dynamic and Low Static Demands*	*High to Moderate Static and Low Dynamic Demands*	
Boxing*	Badminton	Archery	
Crew or rowing	Baseball	Auto racing	
Cross-country skiing	Basketball	Diving	
Cycling	Field hockey	Horseback riding	
Downhill skiing	Lacrosse	(jumping)	
Fencing	Orienteering	Field events	
Football	Race walking	(throwing)	
Ice hockey	Racquetball	Gymnastics	
Rugby	Soccer	Karate or judo	
Running (sprint)	Squash	Motorcycling	
Speed skating	Swimming	Rodeo	
Water polo	Table tennis	Sailing	
Wrestling	Tennis	Ski jumping	
	Volleyball	Water skiing	
		Weight lifting	
LOW INTENSITY			
Low Dynamic and Low Static Demands			
Bowling			
Cricket			
Curling			
Golf			
Riflery			

*Participation not recommended by the American Academy of Pediatrics.
From American Academy of Pediatrics, Committee on Sports Medicine and Fitness, 2000-2001: Medical conditions affecting sports participation. Pediatrics 107:1205-1209, 2001.

high cost and low yield in detecting potentially life-threatening cardiac abnormalities (probably because of their low incidence). Hence these studies should be reserved for cases in which results of history and physical examination indicate the need for further cardiac assessment. Although the rare case of an asymptomatic child with no findings on examination may escape detection, use of a thorough screening assessment as just described will identify the vast majority of children at risk.

As noted earlier, though maturation indexing has generated interest it has not gained wide acceptance. Nevertheless, Tanner staging may have a role in selecting lower-risk activities and providing advice with regard to intensity of training. For example, a girl at Tanner stage 2 is entering a period of maximum growth velocity during which female athletes may have limited joint flexibility and may be particularly predisposed to overuse syndromes.

Strength and endurance may be other factors that are potentially helpful in the preparticipation evaluation. These include body composition (skinfolds); endurance (12-minute or 1.5-mile run); flexibility (stretch, reach); agility (Illinois agility test); power (vertical jump); and balance (single-leg stance), although exact standards for many of these have yet to be defined.

In addition, participation clearance for a particular level of sport must be matched with the safety of the sport. The American Academy of Pediatrics has classified sports into risk categories (Tables 21-9 and 21-10) on the basis of

contact/collision risk, degree of aerobic intensity required, and static and dynamic demands placed on the body during play. Although the categorizations are quite helpful, it is important to recognize that they do not factor in the competitiveness of a given sports program or its intensity of training, and they do not include factors that predispose to overuse injuries.

Clearance for participation in organized youth sports is generally divided into three categories: (1) full, unrestricted participation is allowed; (2) approval of coach, trainer, or team physician is required, and the athlete may have defined limits on participation or require rehabilitation; and (3) clearance is deferred because of underlying disease process or the need to evaluate further for such a process before giving clearance.

Risk of Injury

In early and middle childhood, risk of sports-related injury is relatively low. Being smaller and having less muscle strength than adolescents, children achieve less velocity and thus encounter less force in falls and collisions. In this age range, injuries are more likely to be incurred during recreational play and in the process of learning a new sport. With puberty, gains in size, strength, and speed combine with increased competitiveness and intensity of play to substantially increase both the incidence and severity of injuries. Even so, the majority of injuries incurred during organized sport are minor in nature; less than 10% are serious; and catastrophic spinal and head injuries and sudden cardiac, pulmonary, and heat-related deaths are rare events. Injuries are more likely to occur during practice sessions because practices outnumber formal competitions or games, although incidence of injuries per unit of time played is greater during the latter.

The incidence of overuse injuries, in particular, has risen in parallel with the trend toward increasing organization of sports. Children are especially prone to overuse injuries during periods of rapid growth, when the rate of bone growth exceeds that of surrounding soft tissues, resulting in decreased flexibility. Intensive training for a particular sport, especially when initiated at a low level of fitness; abrupt increases in level of activity; lack of preconditioning; and participation in multiple sports during the course of a year are other predisposing factors, as are training practices that fail to teach children proper athletic techniques and to monitor and limit repetitive motions.

Youths with ligamentous laxity (up to 7% of school-aged children) and joint malalignment (such as patellofemoral tracking disorder) may be injury prone without special preconditioning. Children and adolescents who resume competitive participation following a musculoskeletal injury, without full rehabilitation (return of normal strength, flexibility, and range of motion), have a significant risk for reinjury.

In female athletes, especially gymnasts, dancers, and long-distance runners, undue calorie restrictions to maintain "ideal weight," in combination with intensive training regimens, result in amenorrhea; decreased estrogen levels; and loss of bone density, which has been demonstrated to predispose to early hip and vertebral fractures.

Environmental factors can also be sources of significant risk. These include weather conditions such as high heat and humidity (with attendant risk of dehydration and heat illness) and extreme cold or swimming in cold water (frostbite, hypothermia). Children are particularly prone to hyperthermia and hypothermia because of their larger surface area–to-volume ratio. They also have a decreased rate and delay in onset of sweating, compared with adults, making it more difficult for them to dissipate heat. Finally, they have to be encouraged to drink adequate fluids, as their own thirst levels tend not to be adequate to ensure replacement of losses. Finally, uneven or unsafe field conditions or playing surfaces; improper, poorly designed, or ill-fitting equipment (including shoes); and lack of or failure to use appropriate safety gear are other significant factors.

Participation in some types of organized sports carries an inherently greater risk and thus higher rates and degrees of severity of injury. This is by virtue of their requiring higher levels of aerobic intensity, their placing high static and/or dynamic stresses on the body, or because high-velocity contacts or collisions are part of the activity. Among these, competitive wrestling, football, and gymnastics are the top three, followed by cross-country skiing, soccer, basketball, track, volleyball, softball, and baseball in approximate order of frequency (see classification system of sport activities based on contact-collision risk [Table 21-9], as well as on aerobic intensity required and on static and dynamic demands encountered [Table 21-10]). Such sports may present especially high risks to children with underlying chronic health conditions (see section Sport Selection and Participation for Children with Underlying Problems or Chronic Conditions).

Two areas of sport are specifically not recommended by the AAP: boxing because of high risk of eye and head injury; and weight lifting, power lifting, maximal lifts, and body building because of concerns regarding epiphy-seal injuries (especially of the wrist) and apophyseal separations of the vertebrae in children and adolescents who have not reached skeletal maturity.

Nonorganized recreational sports are not without their own hazards, in part because of less supervision and inconsistent compliance with recommended safety measures. Those in which high-speed or angular momentum is attained carry particularly high risks for significant trauma. These include bike riding, skateboarding, in-line skating, trampoline jumping, and riding motor bikes and all-terrain vehicles.

Risk Reduction and Injury Prevention

One of the first steps in prevention is identification of children at potential risk for injury using the PPE and referral for further evaluation, if indicated, to a preconditioning exercise program to increase strength, aerobic fitness and/or flexibility, or for preseason sport-specific training, as indicated. In cases in which children are found to have conditions that make certain activities potentially harmful, counseling by physicians and coaches regarding safe and enjoyable alternative sports that are of interest to the child can be most helpful.

Coaches who are well trained in teaching and coaching their sport, as well as in health and safety issues, and who place their players' interests first are crucial figures in promoting safety. Best practices include the following:

1. Meeting with prospective players before the preseason to do these things:
   - Emphasize the importance and purpose of the PPE and of honesty in completing the history form
   - Outline expected skill and fitness levels for preseason tryouts
   - Suggest or oversee safe, well-supervised preparticipation conditioning or sport-specific training programs
2. During the preseason and season
   - Implementing graduated training regimens in which youths can improve skills at a reasonable pace. Such regimens also emphasize the following:
   - Warm-up and cool-down periods
   - Learning proper skill techniques (e.g., throwing, kicking)
   - Limiting the number of repetitions of a single activity (such as throws for a pitcher)
   - Placing appropriate limits on practice duration and time in play
   - Having flexibility to modify the regimens to meet individual athletic needs
   - Familiarizing athletes with the rules of the game and their basis in consideration for safety, along with promotion of strict officiating
   - Promoting, even insisting on, safe playing facilities and conditions
   - Ensuring appropriate use of proper equipment of good design and good fit
   - Insisting on use of recommended safety gear (Table 21-11)
   - Fostering gradual acclimatization to hot/humid weather conditions, ensuring frequent rest periods, encouraging drinking fluids, and limiting time for practice
   - Insisting on prompt evaluation of injuries or worrisome symptoms, as well as complete rehabilitation before return to play

In Table 21-12 common injuries seen in athletes participating in a number of specific sports are enumerated along

Table 21-11	Safety Gear and Field Safety Modifications

RECOMMENDED/REQUIRED DEVICES	SPECIFIC SPORT(S)
Helmets	Bike riding, skating, baseball (batting), football, hockey
Elbow/wrist/knee guards	Skating, skateboarding
Shin guards	Soccer
Chest protectors	Baseball catcher
Mouthguards	Contact sports
Protective eyewear*	Racquet sports, water sports, contact sports (unless incorporated into helmet)
Groin cups	Football, hockey

FIELD MODIFICATIONS	SPORT
Breakaway bases	Baseball
Stationary goal cages	Soccer

*Mandatory for all functionally one-eyed individuals and those who have had eye surgery or prior eye trauma per American Academy of Pediatrics, Committee on Sports Medicine and Fitness.
From American Academy of Pediatrics, Committee on Sports Medicine and Fitness, 1995-96: Protective eyewear for young athletes. Pediatrics 98:311-313, 1996.

with prevention strategies recommended by the American Academy of Orthopaedic Surgeons and the American Academy of Pediatrics.

Conditioning and Training

The rise in participation of youth in sports activities and the ever-increasing desire to improve performance have led to new concern for understanding the physiologic responses of the growing child to regular and increasingly demanding exercise regimens. The most general of these measures is the maximum oxygen uptake (VO_2 max). Studies of VO_2 max, which includes cardiovascular, pulmonary, and musculoskeletal function, have shown that there is relatively little difference between children and adults, and only slightly less function in girls versus boys. It is of note, however, that training does not improve VO_2 max in children. The biggest increase seems to occur with the pubertal growth spurt. In contrast with aerobic function, children do not do as well anaerobically (as measured by the anaerobic threshold), apparently because they cannot utilize glycogen as efficiently as adults. These factors are important in considerations of the two major types of sports training programs, endurance and strength training.

Endurance training consists of a long-term specific exercise program designed to increase exercise capability during prolonged sports participation; in many instances its purpose is to increase the athlete's fatigue resistance. This is done by specifically increasing the amounts of "overload" on a graduated basis and may be sport specific, for example, running. Basic to endurance training is aerobic conditioning, which requires sustained rhythmic movement of large muscle groups at a level of intensity that results in increases in heart rate and respiratory rate. The recommended frequency is 3 to 5 times per week for approximately 15 minutes. In monitoring the training program of the pediatric athlete, it is essential to avoid overload situations that can cause tissue damage and lower performance. All programs need to take into account duration, frequency, and intensity. In young children, conditioning is often best approached through play activi-

ties that are more attractive to them with their shorter attention spans. Importantly, those devising training programs should take into consideration that children are not miniature adults.

Strength training involves the use of progressive resistance exercises to increase the ability to exert force or resist force. It is designed to enhance ability to perform a sport and to assist in injury prevention by increasing strength. This is to be distinguished from weight lifting, which is considered a sport, is not a conditioning program, and is not recommended for the immature skeleton. Experts generally agree that a carefully controlled and closely supervised progressive program in the prepubescent athlete may be effective in increasing strength, although it does not increase muscle mass before puberty. Rather, it appears to increase firing of motor neurons and synchronization of motor units. Close supervision by a knowledgeable adult, who monitors technique and the intensity and duration of sessions, is essential to ensure optimum benefit and prevent injury. Training begins with no added load until the child has developed consistently good technique. Then low weight or resistance can be added. When the child is comfortably able to do between 8 and 15 repetitions, then weight or resistance can be added in small increments. The American Orthopaedic Society for Sports Medicine (AOSSM) Workshop on Strength Training recommends two to three sessions per week of 20 to 30 minutes each including a warm-up and cool-down period. When improved general fitness is also a goal, strength training should be combined with a tailored aerobic conditioning program. Specific strengthening exercises and their target muscle groups are presented in Table 21-13, and exercises designed to strengthen the muscles of the shoulder girdle are shown as an example in Figure 21-122A to E.

Strength training can be especially beneficial in preconditioning athletes with ligamentous laxity and in those with patellofemoral malalignment. By strengthening muscles around the involved joints, most commonly the shoulder and knee, joint stability may be improved and the risk of glenohumeral and patellar subluxations and of other injuries may be reduced. Finally, carefully supervised and graduated strength training is an important part of postinjury rehabilitation.

Stretching exercises can prove valuable as part of a preconditioning program, in warm-ups before sport participation, and in rehabilitation. They are designed to enhance flexibility or ease of movement of a joint through its normal range of motion. A stretching program is particularly important for children and adolescents during growth spurts, when bone growth outstrips that of the soft tissues surrounding adjacent joints, thereby decreasing flexibility. Examples of stretching exercises are presented in Fig. 21-123A to G. Children should be supervised closely, at least initially, to ensure that their movements are slow and smooth, progressing to the point at which resistance is felt, whereupon they should hold still without bouncing for a count of 10.

Sport Selection and Participation for Children with Underlying Problems or Chronic Conditions

The prevalence of children and adolescents with chronic health problems has significantly increased over the past few decades, largely due to advances in medical and

Table 21-12	Sport-Specific Injury Prevention Strategies*

BALLET/DANCE

Common Injuries

Repetitive hyperextension of the spine

Sprains, tendinitis, stress fractures of the lower extremity

Talar impingement

Snapping hip (iliopsoas tendinitis, trochanteric bursitis)

Prevention Strategies

Initiate a program of strengthening and stabilization exercises for the trunk.

Initiate a stretching and strengthening program for tight hip flexors and weak abductors/external rotators; work the hip within available range of motion.

Treat precursor conditions (shin splints, metatarsalgia).

Initiate a program of strengthening and proprioception exercises for the ankle and calf; encourage low-impact training (Pilates method, pool workouts).

Avoid pointe work until strength and skill permit; ensure that pointe shoes are fitted professionally.

Limit pointe work and pliés if the ankle is swollen or if there is any restricted joint motion.

Ensure calcium intake is adequate.

BASEBALL/SOFTBALL

Common Injuries

Throat injuries (to catchers)

Head and eye injuries

Rotator cuff impingement/tendinitis

Medial epicondylitis

Ankle injuries

Prevention Strategies

Use proper protective equipment (helmets, throat guards for catchers, breakaway bases).

Limit the number of throws and teach proper throwing technique.

Initiate a program of strengthening for the shoulder and a graduated preseason training program.

BASKETBALL

Common Injuries

Patellar tendinitis

Ankle injuries

Prevention Strategies

Initiate a program of stretching, strengthening, and overall conditioning exercises.

Use braces and taping for ankles.

FIELD HOCKEY

Common Injuries

Ankle sprains

Knee sprains

Back pain (often discogenic or vertebral end plate)

Prevention Strategies

Use proper protective equipment (lace-up ankle braces and/or tape).

Initiate a program of strengthening exercises for the quadriceps and hamstrings.

Initiate a program of exercises to maintain overall flexibility and neutral spine posture.

FOOTBALL

Common Injuries

Concussions

Neck injuries

Stingers and burners

Low back stress fractures

Pelvic contusions

Dehydration

Heat-related illnesses

Prevention Strategies

Teach proper tackling techniques.

Use proper protective equipment (helmets, face masks, mouth guards).

Ensure frequent water breaks are scheduled in high temperature/high humidity conditions.

Remove helmet frequently.

Ensure proper hydration during practice and competition.

GYMNASTICS

Common Injuries

Repetitive flexion, hyperextension, and compression stresses at the thoracolumbar junction and on the lumbar vertebrae

Capsulitis and dorsal impingement at the wrist

Radial epiphysitis

Osteochondritis dissecans at the elbow

Ulnar collateral sprains of the elbow

Shoulder instability

Tendinitis of the biceps and supraspinatus muscles

Prevention Strategies

Initiate a program of strengthening exercises for the abdomen and trunk and exercises to maintain the spine in a neutral position.

Use tape or braces to protect the wrist.

Limit weight bearing and impact on the upper extremities to protect the elbow and wrist.

Limit extreme or repetitive abduction and external rotation of the shoulder.

Initiate a program of strengthening exercises for the rotator cuff and scapular stabilizers.

ICE HOCKEY

Common Injuries

Concussions

Lacerations about the head and face

Acromioclavicular sprains

Glenohumeral subluxations/dislocations

Ligament sprains in the knee

Contusions of the quadriceps

Prevention Strategies

Use proper protective equipment (mouthguard, well-padded full-cage helmet with good strap *around* the chin) (Note: Many helmets are equipped with only a strap that goes under the chin).

Initiate a program of strengthening exercises for the upper body, especially the rotator cuff and scapular stabilizers, and the quadriceps and hamstrings.

Ensure that the net can slide out of the holes in the ice when athletes strike the pipes.

Increase padding in the thigh guard by using football thigh pads because these are larger and thicker.

SOCCER

Common Injuries

Concussion

Contusions about the head

Tibial shaft fractures

Prevention Strategies

Teach proper "heading" techniques and avoid excessive heading.

Avoid heading a water-soaked ball.

Use shin guards.

SWIMMING

Common Injuries

Rotator cuff impingement/tendinitis

Medial patellofemoral pain (from breaststroke)

Spondylolysis

Prevention Strategies

Initiate program of strengthening, stretching, and flexibility exercises for the shoulder, rotator cuff, upper back, and scapular stabilizers.

Limit use of hand paddles or devices that create added resistance in the water.

Use fins to provide greater leg drive and reduce demands on the shoulder.

TENNIS

Common Injuries

Rotator cuff impingement/tendinitis

Medial epicondylitis

Lateral epicondylitis

Spondylolysis

Prevention Strategies

Initiate a program of strengthening and flexibility exercises for the back, shoulder, and abdominal muscles, especially strengthening the rotator cuff and scapular stabilizers and improving flexibility in the hamstrings and hip flexors.

Use proper mechanics and equipment to prevent elbow injuries.

| Table 21-12 | Sport-Specific Injury Prevention Strategies*—cont'd |

TRACK AND FIELD

Common Injuries	*Prevention Strategies*
Stress fractures of the lower extremity	Ensure proper diet and conditioning, gradually increasing speed and intensity.
	Initiate a cross-training program.
Sesamoiditis	Ensure good shoe fit.
Shin splints	Avoid downhill running and sudden stops.
Iliotibial band syndrome	

WRESTLING

Common Injuries	*Prevention Strategies*
Glenohumeral subluxation/dislocation	Initiate a preseason program of strengthening exercises for the rotator cuff, scapular
Acromioclavicular and sternoclavicular sprains	stabilizers, quadriceps mechanism, and hamstrings.
Meniscal tears	Avoid quick stops in dangerous positions during practice and competition.
Skin infections (herpes virus, bacteria [impetigo], tinea corporis)	Ensure that mats are cleaned daily with commercial antiseptic solution.
	Teach athletes to seek medical attention for rapid treatment of any questionable skin lesions to prevent spread of infection.
	Conduct skin checks before tournaments.
Auricular hematomas (with resultant cartilage deformity [cauliflower ear])	Use proper protective equipment (snug-fitting head gear with ear protectors).
	Drain any blood in the auricle promptly to prevent cartilage deformity.

*Injuries and prevention strategies are not listed in any particular sequence. Both lists provide general examples and are not intended to represent each injury or prevention strategy.
From Barfield WR, Gross RH: Injury prevention. In Sullivan JA, Anderson SJ (eds): Care of the Young Athlete. Elk Grove Village, Ill, American Academy of Orthopaedic Surgeons, American Academy of Pediatrics, 2000.

| Table 21-13 | Preconditioning Strengthening Exercises |

EXERCISE	TARGET MUSCLE(S)
The empty can	Supraspinatus
Prone horizontal abduction	Deltoid, infraspinatus, teres minor
90-degree/90-degree external rotation	Teres minor
Side-lying external rotation	Infraspinatus, teres minor
Superman	Lower trapezius
Abdominal curls	Rectus abdominis
Quad set	Quadriceps
Straight leg raise	Quadriceps: May perform progressive resistance exercises with more weight on ankle
Knee curls	Hamstrings: progressive resistance exercises with more weight on ankle
Toe raises/toe-walking	Gastrocnemius/soleus
Heel walking	Anterior tibialis

Modified from Goldberg B, Pappas AM, Cummings NM: Considerations for sports selection and preparatory training. In Goldberg B (ed): Sports and Exercise for Children with Chronic Health Conditions: Guidelines for Participation by Leading Pediatric Authorities. Champaign, Ill, Human Kinetics Publishers, 1995.

| Table 21-14 | Disease-Specific Benefits of Exercise |

DISEASE	BENEFITS
Cardiac disorders	Improved cardiac function and aerobic capacity
Asthma	Possible reduced severity of EIB
Cystic fibrosis	Improved respiratory muscle endurance
	Improved clearance of airway mucus
Insulin-dependent diabetes mellitus	Increased insulin sensitivity
	Increased glucose utilization
	Prevention of obesity
	Reduction in associated CAD risk factors
Muscular dystrophy	Maintain muscle strength and endurance
	Prevention of disuse atrophy
	Maintain ambulation
Cerebral palsy	Prevent joint contractures
	Improve ambulation and other motor function
	Improved aerobic capacity
Arthritis	Preserve range of motion
	Decreased joint stiffness
	Prevent disuse muscle atrophy and osteopenia
	Possible decreased rate of progression of joint disease
Renal disease	Improved blood pressure
	Improved lipoprotein profiles
	Improved glucose tolerance

CAD, coronary artery disease; EIB, exercise-induced bronchospasm.
From Nelson MA, Harris SS: The benefits and risks of sports and exercise for children with chronic health conditions. In Goldberg B (ed): Sports and Exercise for Children with Chronic Health Conditions: Guidelines for Participation by Leading Pediatric Authorities. Champaign, Ill, Human Kinetics Publishers, 1995.

surgical treatment modalities that have substantially increased life span and quality of life. With improved general health has come greater interest in participation in sports on the part of these children. This has been bolstered by increased recognition of the importance of avoiding the natural tendency to overprotect "vulnerable" children by concerned parents and subspecialists and by programs like the Special Olympics. The latter has greatly expanded opportunities for handicapped children in sports and clearly demonstrated the benefits of sport and the enjoyment that can be derived. Indeed, research and experience has shown that the majority of children with chronic health conditions can reap many of the same benefits as those noted in normal children and that the benefits well outweigh the risks when careful attention is given to safe sport selection and preconditioning. Furthermore, many such children are actually able to significantly improve their physical health and reduce risk for obesity as a result (Table 21-14). Psychosocial benefits may be even greater in terms of reducing the sense of isolation many such children feel, increasing their level of enjoyment in life and even helping them to forget their disease, for at least a time.

The preparticipation evaluation of these youngsters, though similar to that for children in good general health, must focus additional attention on the following:

1. The exact nature of and current status of the child's disease
2. The effect of the disorder on stamina and skill acquisition
3. The child's current fitness and skill levels
4. Whether specific sports pose undue risk for injury or complications
5. Whether special considerations are necessary in terms of the following:
   - Therapeutic intervention
   - Preconditioning and training

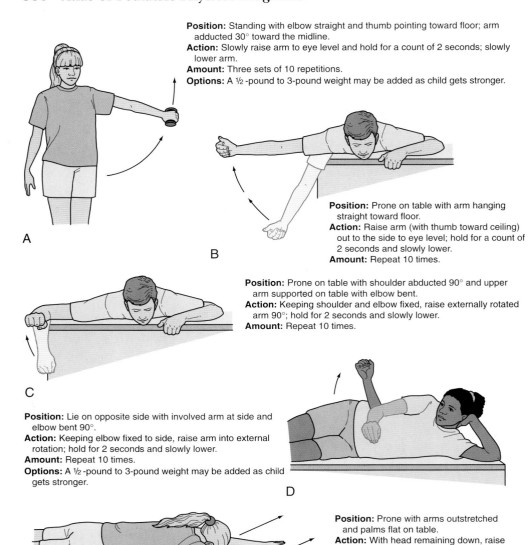

Position: Standing with elbow straight and thumb pointing toward floor; arm adducted 30° toward the midline.
Action: Slowly raise arm to eye level and hold for a count of 2 seconds; slowly lower arm.
Amount: Three sets of 10 repetitions.
Options: A ½-pound to 3-pound weight may be added as child gets stronger.

A

Position: Prone on table with arm hanging straight toward floor.
Action: Raise arm (with thumb toward ceiling) out to the side to eye level; hold for a count of 2 seconds and slowly lower.
Amount: Repeat 10 times.

B

Position: Prone on table with shoulder abducted 90° and upper arm supported on table with elbow bent.
Action: Keeping shoulder and elbow fixed, raise externally rotated arm 90°; hold for 2 seconds and slowly lower.
Amount: Repeat 10 times.

C

Position: Lie on opposite side with involved arm at side and elbow bent 90°.
Action: Keeping elbow fixed to side, raise arm into external rotation; hold for 2 seconds and slowly lower.
Amount: Repeat 10 times.
Options: A ½-pound to 3-pound weight may be added as child gets stronger.

D

Position: Prone with arms outstretched and palms flat on table.
Action: With head remaining down, raise arms as high as possible overhead; hold for a count of 3.
Amount: Repeat 10 times.

E

Figure 21-122. Shoulder-strengthening exercises. **A,** Empty can. **B,** Prone horizontal abduction. **C,** 90-degree/90-degree external rotation. **D,** Side-lying external rotation. **E,** Superman. (From Goldberg B, Pappas AM, Cummings NM: Consideration for sports selection and preparatory training. In Goldberg B [ed]: Sports and Exercise for Children with Chronic Health Conditions. Guidelines for Participation from Leading Pediatric Authorities. Champaign, Ill, Human Kinetics Publishers, 1995.)

- Special protective devices
- Modifications in training techniques, rules, duration of play periods, rest periods, etc.

Children with PPE findings suggestive of high-risk cardiac abnormalities and children with moderate to severe pulmonary disease need referral to a subspecialist for complete evaluation including exercise stress testing.

Following the PPE and any necessary subspecialty or physical therapy assessment, level of clearance for participation can be determined, and the child and his or her parents can be informed of necessary limits. Suggestions can be made regarding activities that are not only safe but at which the child has a realistic chance of success.

To facilitate decision making, the American Academy of Pediatrics, through the Committee of Sports Medicine, has recommended specific participation levels for competitive sports for children and adolescents with either chronic disease or underlying physical defects on the basis of risk (Table 21-15). This classification system has a number of "Qualified Yes" recommendations that indicate the need for consultation with relevant subspecialists regarding the individual child's needs. This is necessitated by the fact that there are often significant differences in level of severity of a disorder and degree of disability, and therefore in ability to participate.

Specific examples of clearance decisions might include the following:
1. No restrictions: Small ventricular septal defect or atrial septal defect
2. Clearance with recommendations:
   - Child with exercise-induced asthma—cleared but must take bronchodilator 15 to 20 minutes before exercise; must be allowed to stop and rest if becoming short of breath or otherwise symptomatic
   - Girl with patellofemoral malalignment—cleared following preparticipation strengthening program
3. Qualified clearance:
   - Down syndrome child who wants to participate in contact sport—cleared pending cervical spine x-rays to rule out atlantoaxial instability.
4. Not cleared:
   - For swimming—child with poorly controlled seizure disorder
   - For contact sport—child with osteogenesis imperfecta, cardiac pacemaker, hemophilia
5. No competitive sports:
   - Child with hypertrophic cardiomyopathy
   - Child who has undergone open heart surgery within past 6 months
   - Symptomatic mitral valve prolapse

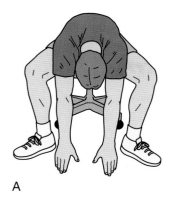
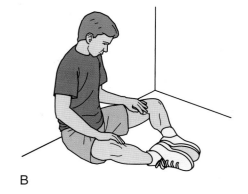

A

Position: Sitting on a stool with hips extended and externally rotated.
Action: Gradually bend forward toward floor until a gentle stretch is felt in the lower back; hold for 10 seconds.
Amount: Repeat 10 times.

B

Position: Sitting with back against a wall and soles of feet together.
Action: Gently push down on the inside of thighs; hold for count of 30 and then relax.
Amount: Repeat 10 times.

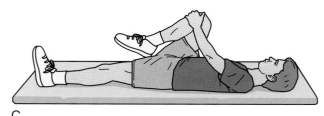

C

Position: Supine on table.
Action: Bring one knee toward chest while keeping opposite leg straight; gently pull on knee and hold for a count of 30.
Amount: Repeat 10 times each side.

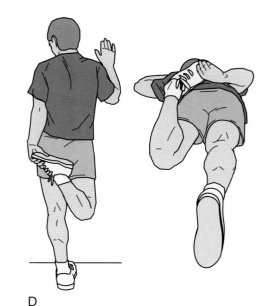

D

Position: Either standing with ipsilateral arm against wall for support or in prone position.
Action: Grab right foot with left hand and gently pull foot toward buttock. Hold for a count of 10.
Amount: Repeat 20 times, alternating legs.

E

Position: Supine with one leg bent to chest and hands locked behind knee.
Action: Slowly straighten knee until gentle stretch is felt; hold for count of 10.
Amount: Three sets of 10 repetitions on each side.

Figure 21-123. Stretching exercises to enhance flexibility. **A,** Lumbar stretch. **B,** Hip adductor stretch. **C,** Hip flexor stretch. **D,** Quadriceps stretch. **E,** Hamstring stretch.

The classification and clearance process is often further defined by specific organizations for the disability. For example, the National Association of Sports for Cerebral Palsy, the National Wheelchair Athletic Association, and the International Sports Organization for the Disabled are responsible for deciding which disabled athletes will compete in the Special Olympics, as well as in what category. The need for adaptive equipment is controlled and classified by the organizing agencies and can include such devices as wheelchairs, custom seating devices for boats, and outrigger ski poles.

In helping these children with sport selection, the physician must try to achieve a balance between necessary limits and encouraging activity. This is aided by clear knowledge of the nature of the child's problem and of the demands and risks of specific sports, as well as information on the level of competitiveness and training demands of the proposed sports program. Although children with chronic conditions may not be able to participate in some sports, there is still a wide array of safe alternative sports available to them (see Tables 21-9 and 21-10 and Goldberg in the Bibliography). In conferring with the child and family, it is generally possible to find one or more activities that are of interest to the child, that are safe for him or her, and at which the athlete has a reasonable chance to improve and succeed. Teaching the child to recognize

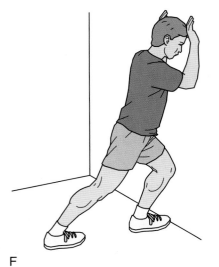

Position: Stand a little distance from wall, resting forearms and forehead against wall.
Action: Bend one knee while keeping opposite leg straight and foot flat on the floor until a gentle stretch is felt in calf of straight leg. Hold for a count of 10.
Amount: Three sets of 10 repetitions on each side.

F

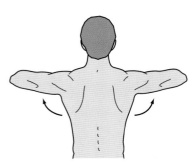

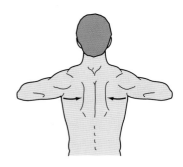

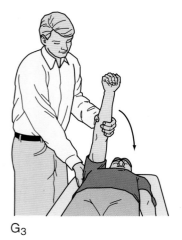

G₂

Position: Supine on table; assistant must stabilize scapula on the thoracic wall.
Action: Slowly push arm across chest; hold for a count of 5.
Amount: Repeat 10 times.

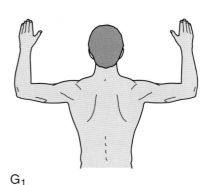

G₁

G₃

Position: Sitting with elbows bent 90°.
Action: Raise (abduct) arm to shoulder level; pinch shoulder blades together; rotate arms toward ceiling, hold for a count of 5, then slowly reverse movements.
Amount: 25 sets of 5 repetitions.

Position: Supine with assistant stabilizing scapula on thoracic wall and arm in neutral rotation.
Action: Slowly bring arm up overhead toward table; hold for a count of 5.
Amount: Repeat 10 times.

Figure 21-123 cont'd. F, Gastrocnemius/soleus stretch. **G,** Shoulder stretches: G1, standing abduction/external rotation; G2, glenohumeral adduction stretch; G3, glenohumeral forward elevation stretch. Note: Stretching slowly until resistance is felt and then holding still in that position for 10 seconds are important. (From Goldberg B, Pappas AM, Cummings NM: Consideration for sports selection and preparatory training. In Goldberg B [ed]: Sports and Exercise for Children with Chronic Health Conditions. Guidelines for Participation from Leading Pediatric Authorities. Champaign, Ill, Human Kinetics Publishers, 1995.)

Table 21-15	Sport Participation Recommendations for Children with Underlying and Chronic Health Conditions*

CONDITION	MAY PARTICIPATE
Atlantoaxial instability (instability of the joint between cervical vertebrae 1 and 2) *Explanation:* Athlete needs evaluation to assess risk of spinal cord injury during sports participation.	Qualified yes
Bleeding disorder *Explanation:* Athlete needs evaluation.	Qualified yes
Cardiovascular disease	
Carditis (inflammation of the heart) *Explanation:* Carditis may result in sudden death with exertion.	No
Hypertension (high blood pressure) *Explanation:* Those with significant essential (unexplained) hypertension should avoid weight and power lifting, body building, and strength training. Those with secondary hypertension (hypertension caused by a previously identified disease) or severe essential hypertension need evaluation. The National High Blood Pressure Education Working Group defined significant and severe hypertension.	Qualified yes
Congenital heart disease (structural heart defects present at birth) *Explanation:* Those with mild forms may participate fully; those with moderate or severe forms or who have undergone surgery need evaluation. The 26th Bethesda Conference defined mild, moderate, and severe disease for common cardiac lesions.	Qualified yes
Dysrhythmia (irregular heart rhythm) *Explanation:* Those with symptoms (chest pain, syncope, dizziness, shortness of breath, or other symptoms of possible dysrhythmia) or evidence of mitral regurgitation (leaking) on physical examination need evaluation. All others may participate fully.	Qualified yes
Heart murmur *Explanation:* If the murmur is innocent (does not indicate heart disease), full participation is permitted. Otherwise, the athlete needs evaluation (see congenital heart disease and mitral valve prolapse).	Qualified yes
Cerebral palsy *Explanation:* Athlete needs evaluation.	Qualified yes
Diabetes mellitus *Explanation:* All sports can be played with proper attention to diet, blood glucose concentration, hydration, and insulin therapy. Blood glucose concentration should be monitored every 30 minutes during continuous exercise and 15 minutes after completion of exercise.	Yes
Diarrhea *Explanation:* Unless disease is mild, no participation is permitted because diarrhea may increase the risk of dehydration and heat illness. See Fever.	Qualified no
Eating disorders Anorexia nervosa Bulimia nervosa *Explanation:* Patients with these disorders need medical and psychiatric assessment before participation.	Qualified yes
Eyes Functionally one-eyed athlete Loss of an eye Detached retina Previous eye surgery or serious eye injury *Explanation:* A functionally one-eyed athlete has a best-corrected visual acuity of less than 20/40 in the eye with worse acuity. These athletes would suffer significant disability if the better eye were seriously injured, as would those with loss of an eye. Some athletes who previously have undergone eye surgery or had a serious eye injury may have an increased risk of injury because of weakened eye tissue. Availability of eye guards approved by the American Society for Testing and Materials and other protective equipment may allow participation in most sports, but this must be judged on an individual basis.	Qualified yes
Fever *Explanation:* Fever can increase cardiopulmonary effort, reduce maximum exercise capacity, make heat illness more likely, and increase orthostatic hypertension during exercise. Fever may rarely accompany myocarditis or other infections that may make exercise dangerous.	No
Heat illness, history of *Explanation:* Because of the increased likelihood of recurrence, the athlete needs individual assessment to determine the presence of predisposing conditions and to arrange a prevention strategy.	Qualified yes
Hepatitis *Explanation:* Because of the apparent minimal risk to others, all sports may be played that the athlete's state of health allows. In all athletes, skin lesions should be covered properly, and athletic personnel should use universal precautions when handling blood or body fluids with visible blood.	Yes
Human immunodeficiency virus infection *Explanation:* Because of the apparent minimal risk to others, all sports may be played that the athlete's state of allows. All athletes should cover their skin lesions properly, and athletic personnel should use universal health precautions when handling blood or body fluids with visible blood.	Yes
Kidney, absence of one *Explanation:* Athlete needs individual assessment for contact, collision, and limited-contact sports.	Qualified yes
Liver, enlarged *Explanation:* If the liver is acutely enlarged, participation should be avoided because of risk of rupture. If the liver is chronically enlarged, individual assessment is necessary before collision, contact, or limited-contact sports are played.	Qualified yes
Malignant neoplasm *Explanation:* Athlete needs individual assessment.	Qualified yes
Musculoskeletal disorders *Explanation:* Athlete needs individual assessment.	Qualified yes
Neurologic disorders	
History of serious head or spine trauma, severe or repeated concussions, or craniotomy. *Explanation:* Athlete needs individual assessment for collision, contact, or limited-contact sports and also for noncontact sports if deficits in judgment or cognition are present. Research supports a conservative approach to management of concussion.	Qualified yes

Continued

Table 21-15 Sport Participation Recommendations for Children with Underlying and Chronic Health Conditions*—cont'd	
CONDITION	**MAY PARTICIPATE**
Seizure disorder, well-controlled	Yes
Explanation: Risk of seizure during participation is minimal	
Seizure disorder, poorly controlled	Qualified yes
Explanation: Athlete needs individual assessment for collision, contact, or limited-contact sports. The following noncontact sports should be avoided: archery, riflery, swimming, weight or power lifting, strength training, and sports involving heights. In these sports, occurrence of a seizure may pose a risk to self or others.	
Obesity	Qualified yes
Explanation: Because of the risk of heat illness, obese persons need careful acclimatization and hydration.	
Organ transplant recipient	Qualified yes
Explanation: Athlete needs individual assessment.	
Ovary, absence of one	Yes
Explanation: Risk of severe injury to the remaining ovary is minimal.	
Respiratory conditions	
Pulmonary compromise including cystic fibrosis	Qualified yes
Explanation: Athlete needs individual assessment, but generally, all sports may be played if oxygenation remains satisfactory during a graded exercise test. Patients with cystic fibrosis need acclimatization and good hydration to reduce the risk of heat illness.	
Asthma	Yes
Explanation: With proper medication and education, only athletes with the most severe asthma will need to modify their participation.	
Acute upper respiratory infection	Qualified yes
Explanation: Upper respiratory obstruction may affect pulmonary function. Athlete needs individual assessment for all but mild disease. See Fever.	
Sickle cell disease	Qualified yes
Explanation: Athlete needs individual assessment. In general, if status of the illness permits, all but high exertion, collision, and contact sports may be played. Overheating, dehydration, and chilling must be avoided.	
Sickle cell trait	Yes
Explanation: It is unlikely that persons with sickle cell trait have an increased risk of sudden death or other medical problems during athletic participation, except under the most extreme conditions of heat, humidity, and possibly increased altitude. These persons, like all athletes, should be carefully conditioned, acclimatized, and hydrated to reduce any possible risk.	
Skin disorders (boils, herpes simplex, impetigo, scabies, molluscum contagiosum)	Qualified yes
Explanation: While the patient is contagious, participation in gymnastics with mats, martial arts, wrestling, or other collision, contact, or limited-contact sports is not allowed.	
Spleen, enlarged	Qualified yes
Explanation: A patient with an acutely enlarged spleen should avoid all sports because of risk of rupture. A patient with a chronically enlarged spleen needs individual assessment before playing collision, contact, or limited-contact sports.	
Testicle, undescended or absence of one	Yes
Explanation: Certain sports may require a protective cup.	

*This table is designed for use by medical and nonmedical personnel. "Needs evaluation" means that a physician with appropriate knowledge and experience should assess the safety of a given sport for an athlete with the listed medical condition. Unless otherwise noted, this is because of variability of the severity of the disease, the risk of injury for the specific sport, or both.
From American Academy of Pediatrics, Committee on Sports Medicine and Fitness, 2000-2001: Medical conditions affecting sports participation. Pediatrics 107:1205-1209, 2001.

when to stop and rest (e.g., starting to get short of breath or to tire) is also important. For further details on evaluation of risks, clearance considerations, and sport selection for individual disorders, see Goldberg (1995).

Having helped with sport selection, the physician can also encourage and help assist an individualized and graduated preparticipation conditioning or training program, which can often incorporate rehabilitative physical therapy. He or she can also help to identify sport programs that allow participation with flexibility and modifications. Monitoring the child's progress over time is also advisable.

Rehabilitation and Return to Play

Rehabilitation of the pediatric athlete following injury involves restoring the individual to normal activity so that he or she may return to sports as quickly as possible. Decisions regarding timing of return to play must be made with the athlete's best interest and safety foremost. This necessitates monitoring of progress, assessment of readiness, and determination (in consultation with coaches) of

the usefulness of additional protective equipment and/or of the need for changes in skill technique or training regimen (especially important for children with overuse injuries).

Return to Play Following Musculoskeletal Injury

Rehabilitation of musculoskeletal injury encompasses the reparative and healing process and assists return to prior level of activity through the use of physical modalities and therapeutic exercises. Inflammation and repair are important phases that have different interventions. In the inflammatory stages of an acute injury, tissue swelling and the inflammatory response require rest or splinting to prevent further injury and protect the injured part during the early phase of the healing process, along with application of ice packs or ice massage and judicious use of oral anti-inflammatory agents. Once the acute phase of injury has passed, then protected mobility and the use of heat to mobilize the repair process are appropriate. Use of ultrasound, a high-energy source that when applied to the body can produce deep heat and is selectively absorbed by muscle and connective tissue (because of their high water content), can be quite helpful.

Therapeutic exercises are effective after initial healing is well under way, although well-moderated early exercises may be used on occasion. These are applied in a graduated manner to bring back strength and flexibility. They fall into the categories of passive, active-assisted, active, active-resistive, isometric, and strengthening exercises. These therapeutic exercises may be viewed as a transition between the acute injury and conditioning exercises. Programs must be specific to the area of injury, goal oriented, appropriately paced, and well supervised by physical therapists or knowledgeable trainers. *Return to play is safe when the athlete is symptom free with normal strength, flexibility, and range of motion.*

Return to Play Following Concussion

The issue of timing of return to play of the athlete who has incurred a concussion is one of particular importance, the reason being that suffering a second concussion while the athlete is still symptomatic from a first can result in the catastrophic phenomenon known as *second impact syndrome.* This is characterized by relentless cerebrovascular congestion and edema with loss of autoregulation of cerebral blood flow, usually culminating in herniation and death.

Concussion is defined as a condition characterized by temporary impairment of neurologic function following a head injury. Important to remember is that loss of consciousness and amnesia, though common, are not always seen. Other acute symptoms may include dizziness, headache, drowsiness, confusion, disorientation, delayed response times, difficulty concentrating, emotional lability or inappropriateness, visual changes, and impaired coordination. These may be seen singly or in any combination.

In the acute situation, obviously any athlete with prolonged loss of consciousness, abnormal neurologic findings, persistently altered mental status, or progression of acute symptoms merits prompt transfer to the hospital for further evaluation and imaging. In milder cases of head injury, a sideline assessment of mental status (orientation, ability to concentrate, and short-term memory) and of neurologic status (strength, sensation, coordination) is indicated to determine if any signs and symptoms of concussion are present. If these are negative, provocative exertional tests that increase intracranial pressure (push-ups, sit-ups, sprints, or Valsalva maneuver) are performed. If any concussive symptoms are present on mental status or neurologic screening or are provoked by exertional tests, further participation is contraindicated. If symptoms are mild and duration is brief (<15 minutes), some authorities believe the youth may return to play, while others advocate deferring return for a day or so. When symptoms persist, it is generally agreed that the athlete should not compete until he or she has been asymptomatic both at rest and on exertion for at least a week. Most recommend neurosurgical evaluation and/or neuroimaging when symptoms persist beyond a week. Athletes who have a prior history of concussion may warrant a longer period of inaction (2 to 4 weeks or more).

Return to Play Following Exacerbation of Underlying Disorder

For recommendations regarding return to play of athletes who incur other injuries or exacerbation of symptoms of chronic diseases, see Goldberg (1995), Sullivan and Anderson (2000), and Garrett and coworkers (2001) in the Bibliography.

Bibliography

Ablin DS, Greenspan A, Reinhart M, Grix A: Differentiation of child abuse from osteogenesis imperfecta. Am J Radiol 154:1035-1046, 1990.

Aegerter E, Kirkpatrick JA Jr: Orthopedic Diseases: Physiology, Pathology, Radiology, 4th ed. Philadelphia, WB Saunders, 1975.

American Academy of Neurology, Quality Standards Subcommittee: Practice parameter: The management of concussion in sports (summary statement). Neurology 48:581-585, 1997.

American Academy of Pediatrics, Committee on Sports Medicine: Participation in competitive sports. Pediatrics 81:737-739, 1988.

American Academy of Pediatrics, Committee on Sports Medicine and Fitness: Strength training by children and adolescents. Pediatrics 107:1470-1472, 2001.

American Academy of Pediatrics, Committee on Sports Medicine and Fitness and Committee on School Health: Organized sports for children and preadolescents. Pediatrics 107:1459-1461, 2001.

American Orthopaedic Association: Manual of Orthopaedic Surgery, 6th ed. Philadelphia, The Association, 1985.

American Society for Surgery of the Hand: The Hand: Examination and Diagnosis. Edinburgh, Churchill Livingstone, 1983.

American Society for Surgery of the Hand: The Hand: Primary Care of Common Problems. Aurora, Colo, Churchill Livingstone, 1985.

Bachman D, Santora S: Orthopedic trauma. In Fleisher GR, Ludwig S (eds): Textbook of Pediatric Emergency Medicine, 4th ed. Philadelphia, Lippincott Williams & Wilkins, 2000.

Canale GT: Campbell's Operative Orthopaedics, 9th ed. St Louis, Mosby, 1999.

Chang FM: The disabled athlete. In Stanitski CL, DeLee JC, Drez D (eds): Pediatric and Adolescent Sports Medicine, vol 3. Philadelphia, WB Saunders, 1994.

Ferguson AB Jr: Orthopedic Surgery in Infancy and Childhood, 5th ed. Baltimore, Williams & Wilkins, 1981.

Garrett WE, Kirkendall DT, Squire DL (eds): Principles and Practice of Primary Care Sports Medicine. Philadelphia, Lippincott Williams & Wilkins, 2001.

Garrick JG: Sports medicine. Pediatr Clin North Am 24:737-747, 1977.

Goldberg B (ed): Sports and Exercise for Children with Chronic Health Conditions: Guidelines for Participation from Leading Pediatric Authorities. Champaign, Ill, Human Kinetics Publishers, 1995.

Herring JA: Tachdjian's Pediatric Orthopedics, 3rd ed. Philadelphia, WB Saunders, 2002.

Hoppenfeld S: Physical Examination of the Spine and Extremities. New York, Appleton-Century-Crofts, 1976.

Kelly JP, Rosenberg JH: Diagnosis and management of concussion in sports. Neurology 48:575-580, 1997.

Lombardo JA: Preparticipation physical evaluation. Primary Care 11: 3-21, 1982.

Lonstein JE: Moe's Textbook of Scoliosis and Other Spinal Deformities, 3rd ed. Philadelphia, WB Saunders, 1995.

Lovell WW, Winter RB: Pediatric Orthopedics, 4th ed. Philadelphia, JB Lippincott, 1996.

Ogden JA: Skeletal Injury in the Child, 3rd ed. New York, Springer, 2000.

Rang M: Children's Fractures, 2nd ed. Philadelphia, JB Lippincott, 1983.

Rockwood CA Jr, Wilkins KE, King RE: Fractures in Children, vol 3, 3rd ed. Philadelphia, JB Lippincott, 1991.

Salter RB: Textbook of Disorders and Injuries of the Musculoskeletal System, 3rd ed. Baltimore, Williams & Wilkins, 1999.

Scoles PV: Pediatric Orthopedics in Clinical Practice, 2nd ed. Chicago, Year Book, 1988.

Simon RR, Koenigsknecht SJ: Orthopedics in Emergency Medicine: The Extremities. New York, Appleton, 1982.

Smith DM (ed): American Academy of Family Physicians, American Academy of Pediatrics, American Medical Society for Sports Medicine, American Orthopaedic Society for Sports Medicine, American Osteopathic Association for Sports Medicine: Preparticipation Physical Evaluation Monograph, ed 2. Minneapolis, 1997, pp 1-49.

Staheli LT: Fundamentals of Pediatric Orthopedics, 2nd ed. Wickford, RI, Lippincott-Raven, 1998.

Stanitski CL, DeLee JC, Drez D (eds): Pediatric and Adolescent Sports Medicine, vol 3. Philadelphia, WB Saunders, 1994.

Sullivan JA, Anderson SJ (eds): Care of the Young Athlete. Elk Grove Village, Ill, American Academy of Orthopaedic Surgeons, American Academy of Pediatrics, 2000.

Sullivan JA, Grana WA (eds): The Pediatric Athlete. Parkridge, Ill, American Academy of Orthopaedic Surgery, 1989.

CHAPTER 22

Craniofacial Anomalies

A. Corde Mason, Joseph E. Losee, and Michael L. Bentz

Even when identified prenatally, the birth of an infant with a congenital anomaly is disheartening and anxiety-laden for the parents. Infants with anomalies that involve the craniofacial domain are met with additional apprehensions, as the face is so central to human uniqueness and recognition, significantly affecting integration and socialization. Negotiating the hours and days after such a birth is often punctuated with a loss of words to explain findings on examination and their implications. Parents are concerned and interested in the extent of the anomalies and their short- and long-term effects on the welfare of their new child. They are interested in treatment options and strategies and are also experiencing a cascade of emotions that may range from guilt to fear.

The pediatrician, neonatologist, and reconstructive surgeon are often closely involved in the initial evaluation and care of these infants and their families. Although craniofacial anomalies may occur as isolated events, they frequently occur with other anomalies that suggest a syndromic etiology, unifying the presentation. Many such syndromes are rare, and diagnosis can be challenging, with the physician trying to jar a memory that has not been tapped since residency. Complicating recall is a nomenclature that is not intuitive even to those facile with Latin. As such, communication of findings among health care providers may prove difficult, as words are often lacking to effectively document the initial findings of their examinations. These data, however, are vitally important to the ultimate diagnosis and often become clear only after a genetic evaluation places the findings into familiar, though infrequently used, medical terms. Once an eponym has been assigned, the natural history of these syndromes may not be completely familiar to the practitioner. Thereafter, workups for evaluation of associated occult pathology are required.

The intent of this chapter is to acquaint the clinician with a lexicon of terms that will enable him or her to describe findings on examination, to review facial clefting, and to describe several of the more commonly encountered craniofacial syndromes, detailing their presentations and natural histories. As with many clinical queries, a reacquaintance with embryology and anatomy significantly assists understanding.

Embryology and Anatomy

The formation of the structures that constitute the skull and face proceeds along a series of developmental pathways that occur between 4 and 7 weeks after conception. By the fourth week of gestation, the fetus exhibits distinguishable caudal and cephalic ends. In addition, three distinct cellular reserves are identifiable. Endoderm, mesoderm, and ectoderm each are evident, and their migration and differentiation lead to the formation of various end organs and tissues. The skeletal system including the bones of the skull and face evolves from cells originating from the neural crest and from mesoderm that segregates to form the paraxial and lateral plates. On either side of the neural tube, paraxial mesoderm further divides into segmented tissue blocks that are known as somitomeres in the cephalic region and somites from the occiput caudally. These mesenchymal cells give rise to fibroblasts, chondroblasts, and osteoblasts, which further migrate within the cephalic domain to participate in the formation of the bones of the *neurocranium,* the protective vault that encases the brain. At the same time, the mesenchymal differentiation of neural crest cells in the head region participates in the formation of the *viscerocranium,* the facial skeleton. The foundation is thus laid for the development of what is postnatally identified as the craniofacial domain.

The substrata of the neurocranium continue to develop, forming various plates that mature toward the recognized eight bones of the skull (Fig. 22-1). The frontal, occipital, sphenoid, ethmoid, and paired temporal and parietal bones, which encase and protect the developing brain, remain segregated prenatally, assisting ultimate parturition. The spaces between these bones are as important as the bones themselves and represent the fontanelles and sutures of the cranium.

The fontanelles represent intersections of the various cranial sutures. They are found at the angles of the parietal bones, as these bones are located most centrally within the skull construct. The anterior fontanelle, the largest, lies at the corners of the two parietal and frontal bones, and the posterior fontanelle lies at the intersection of the two parietal and occipital bones. The posterior fontanelle closes within the first 6 months of life, and the anterior fontanelle closes between 12 and 18 months of age.

The sutures represent the articulating surfaces between two adjacent bones of the cranium. There are two sets of sutures, the coronal and lambdoid, as well as the sagittal and metopic (Fig. 22-2). The metopic suture is positioned between the two portions of the frontal bone and is usually fused in the term infant at delivery. The sagittal (interparietal) suture lies between the two parietal bones and extends from the midpoint of the frontal bone backward to the uppermost angle of the occipital bone. The coronal (frontoparietal) and lambdoid (occipitoparietal) sutures lie transversely; the coronal sutures connect the frontal bone with the parietal bones, while the lambdoid sutures connect the occipital bone to the parietal bones. In the case of normal prenatal and postnatal development, the sutures remain open or unfused for several months after the birth of the infant. This assists birth, by allowing for molding of the infant's head as it passes through the vaginal canal, and allows for the rapid increase in the infant's brain volume, which doubles in the first 6 months of life and again by 2 years of age. The sagittal and coronal sutures are usually the first to close, or ossify, and do so in a posterior to anterolateral direction. Prenatal or postnatal premature fusion of the sutures results in craniosynostosis and deformation of the bony skull. Depending on the number, position, and timing of suture closure, several ramifications may evolve that affect the midface and lower face of the developing infant.

The facial skeleton, or viscerocranium, is supported on a scaffold of 14 bones—the vomer and mandible and the paired nasal, maxilla, lacrimal, zygoma, palatal, and inferior nasal concha (Fig. 22-3). By the end of the fourth gestational week, the neural crest–derived mesenchyme differentiates to form three facial prominences: the maxillary, mandibular, and frontonasal. Over the course of the

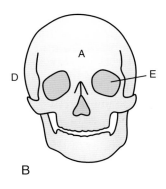

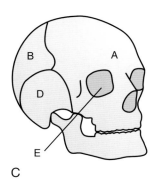

Figure 22-1. Bones of the human skull in lateral **(A)**, anteroposterior **(B)**, and oblique **(C)** presentation. A, Frontal. B, Parietal. C, Occipital. D, Temporal. E, Ethmoid.

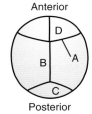

Figure 22-2. Cranial sutures as viewed from the vertex of the skull. A, Coronal. B, Sagittal. C, Lambdoidal. D, Metopic.

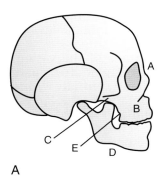

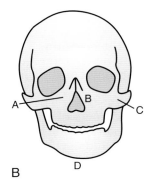

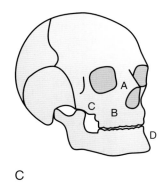

Figure 22-3. Bones of the human face in lateral **(A)**, anteroposterior **(B)**, and oblique **(C)** presentation. A, Nasal. B, Maxilla. C, Zygoma. D, Mandible. E, Palatal.

Table 22-1	Clefting Characteristics	
	CLEFT LIP ± PALATE	**ISOLATED CLEFT PALATE**
Cleft Incidence	60% 1 in 700	40% 1 in 1000
Sex	M > F (2:1)	M = F
Race	Asian > white > African American (3:2:1)	No difference

next 2 weeks, migration and fusion result in the sculpture of the facial features supported by the underlying bony face. The frontal-nasal prominence gives rise to the forehead, bridge of the nose, and medial and lateral nasal prominences that further define the lower nose. The maxillary prominence evolves into the cheeks and lateral aspect of the upper lip, and the mandibular prominence develops into the lower lip. Abnormal migration, fusion, or disruption of established events during this cascade results in anomalies.

Cleft Lip and Palate

Cleft lip and palate are the most common craniofacial congenital anomalies encountered (Table 22-1). Affecting approximately 1 in 700 individuals in the United States or about 15,000 live births per year, it is probable that practicing pediatricians will care for at least one affected child in a career. Although the cleft may be a component of an identifiable syndrome, it more commonly occurs as a solitary defect. Children with clefting present multiple

challenges and are optimally cared for in a multidisciplinary care setting. Infants may have difficulty with feeding and weight gain, may have significant middle ear disease and hearing deficits, and may exhibit speech and other developmental delays. During infancy and childhood various procedures are performed to restore esthetic and functional integrity to the lip and/or palate. Not surprisingly, these children often need support in adjusting psychologically to the societal implications of their deformity and to time spent in the hospital for operative interventions. An understanding of the basics of lip and palate clefting is therefore useful.

Facial clefting is frequently categorized into the cleft lip, with or without cleft palate (CLP) and the isolated cleft palate (CP). Epidemiologically, a distinction is notable between the two with respect to incidence, race, and sex. Approximately 1 in 600 live births are affected with a CLP, occurring twice as often in males. Asians constitute the largest population of affected infants, followed by whites, then African Americans. CP is less frequently encountered, with an incidence of 1 in 1000 live births. Although females are affected slightly more often than males, no race predilection has been identified.

The etiology of lip and palatal clefting is not fully understood, but it is believed to be multifactorial with both genetic and environmental components contributing. During the end of the fifth week of gestation, lip and palatal development begins with the formation of the maxillary prominences and the lateral and medial nasal prominences around the nasal pits. As the maxillary prominences grow medially, the medial nasal prominences are displaced toward the midline and fuse, forming the intermaxillary segment. This segment contains three domains, which are destined to become the philtrum of the upper lip, the portion of the upper jaw carrying the incisors, and the triangular primary palate. During the same period of gestation, the maxillary prominences develop outgrowths called the palatine shelves, which are intended to lie in a horizontal orientation above the tongue for ultimate fusion in the midline, forming the secondary palate. They fuse anteriorly with the primary palate, completing the division between the nasal canals and the oropharynx. Failure of fusion of the palatine shelves results in secondary palatal clefting, whereas partial or complete lack of fusion of the maxillary prominence with the medial nasal prominence on one or both sides results in lip clefting with or without clefting of the primary and secondary palates (Fig. 22-4). This developmental cascade is complete by the 12th week of gestation. During this vulnerable period anatomic interference (malposition of the tongue due to mandibular hypoplasia as in the Pierre Robin sequence), miscues in cell differentiation and migration, or teratogens (phenytoin, retinoids, steroids, lithium, and maternal smoking) may lead to clefting in the developing fetus.

Lip and palatal clefts are typically identified at the time of the newborn's first physical examination. Multiple care providers are typically recruited for the optimal care of these infants. Initial focus by the pediatrician should be a thorough examination to exclude other obvious or occult anomalies suggesting that the cleft is a component of a syndrome. Multiple syndromes are associated with clefting; however, a syndromic etiology comprises the minority of patients in whom clefting occurs. The majority of newborns have isolated cleft anomalies; as such, they are usually otherwise healthy infants and the primary concern is one of feeding. Initial difficulties develop from the inability of the infant to create an airtight seal to suckle effectively. Nasal regurgitation is frequent. Not surprisingly, newborns with large palatal clefts or clefts involving both the lip and palate are more severely impeded, while babies with an isolated cleft lip tend to have fewer difficulties. Upright positioning and adaptive nipples can assist with preventing regurgitation and achieving effective closure around the nipple to obtain a seal. Breastfeeding is possible for infants with clefting; in fact, because the breast is more compliant, the infant may fare better in creating a seal around the breast, yielding greater feeding success, particularly in infants with narrower clefts. For those in whom breastfeeding is not successful, maternal breast milk may be bottle-fed using adaptive nipples. The benefits of feeding breast milk should not be discounted in this population of children, who are more prone to middle ear disease. As with any newborn, infant weight and growth should be monitored closely; however, in this patient population it is not unusual for poor weight gain to be noted in the first 2 to

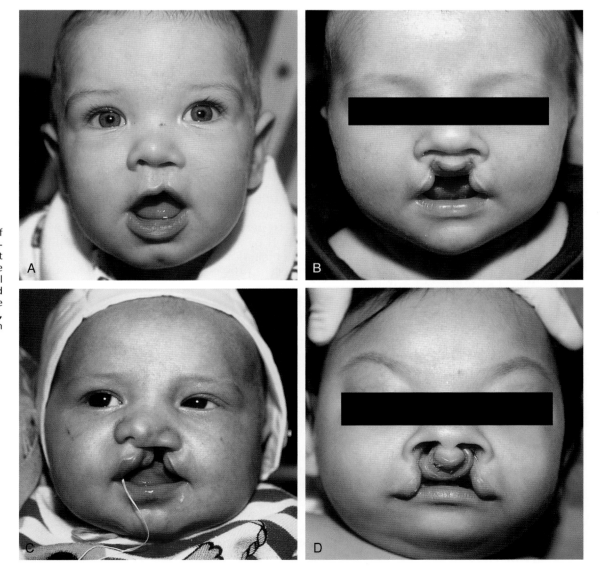

Figure 22-4. The spectrum of lip clefting. **A,** Left-sided unilateral cleft lip with minimal soft tissue involvement or "forme fruste." **B,** Incomplete bilateral cleft lip. **C,** Complete left-sided unilateral cleft lip. Note the associated nasal deformity. **D,** Complete bilateral cleft lip with associated palatal clefting.

3 months of life. Thereafter, infants typically progress well and are able to make up weight.

Eustachian tube ventilatory impairment secondary to disruption of the muscular sling of the soft palate in infants with posterior palatal clefting leads to frequent bouts of otitis media. Although early cleft closure has been shown to reduce this incidence, many children continue to be affected with significant middle ear pathology. Careful monitoring of the ears for both purulent and nonpurulent middle ear effusions is therefore important, and early otolaryngologic involvement is warranted for placement of tympanostomy tubes for middle ear ventilation. Persistent effusions, particularly in infancy, may result in conductive hearing loss with subsequent delays in speech and language development. Additionally, sensorineural hearing loss may be identified in up to a third of children with palatal clefting, underscoring the importance of continued surveillance through adulthood.

Surgical reconstruction of facial clefts is a multistep endeavor, the particulars of which depend on the specific deformity. In general, however, interventions are targeted toward esthetic improvement, maintenance of normal maxillofacial growth, and restoration of palatal function in an effort to assist normal phonation. Reparative strategies continue to evolve, and controversy exists as to optimal timing and optimal procedure. Typically the cleft lip/nasal deformity repair is scheduled at 2 to 3 months of age. Some centers preoperatively manipulate the cleft defect using orthodontics. Orthodontics involves the use of customized intraoral mouthpieces that promote realignment of the cleft segments. In some centers palate repair may be combined with the initial lip repair, but in most the palate repair is performed several months later. Optimal hearing and speech acquisition evolve when palatal integrity is restored before the second birthday. As such, palate closure is typically performed before 2 years of age despite concerns that early surgical interventions involving the midface may have a negative impact on maxillofacial growth and result in midface retrusion. Studies continue to try to define intervals when interventions can be performed with a minimum of untoward effects.

Unique errors of speech articulation are common to patients with cleft palate and are more likely to develop in children who undergo delayed palatal repair. Hypernasal speech may occur in patients in whom the soft palate is foreshortened and allows air to escape into the posterior nasal vestibule. For these patients a pharyngeal flap procedure may be performed whereby a peninsula of the posterior pharynx is attached to the soft palate. This recruited tissue serves to lengthen the palate and substantially alleviates hypernasal speech.

Between ages 7 and 10, during mixed dentition an alveolar bone graft is usually recommended to permit normal eruption of the canine on the affected side(s). As the child develops an awareness of self, the lip scar resulting from earlier repair often becomes an issue and revision can be performed to improve the upper lip's appearance. The end of adolescence marks the completion of the child's facial skeletal growth. At this time residual nasal deformities, which usually involve a broad and inferiorly displaced nasal ala, may be targeted. Malalignment of the upper and lower jaws may additionally exist due to deficient maxillary growth. Once mandibular growth is complete, surgical correction involving advancement of the midface can be performed to restore normal occlusion. Further procedures may involve the grafting of bone to residual bony defects in the upper alveolar ridge, as well as repair of any

identified palatal fistulas that affect speech or impede eating or drinking. As this brief discussion outlines, the family of a newborn with a facial cleft can anticipate numerous procedures spanning the entire childhood of their infant before reaching the end of the restorative journey. The impact of these interventions on the child is certainly profound.

Deformational Plagiocephaly

The term plagiocephaly, derived from the Greek words *plagio* (oblique, twisted, or slanted) and *kephale* (head), describes an asymmetric cranium and has multiple origins. Asymmetry may develop in utero due to genetic abnormalities that permit early sutural synostosis as in several recognized syndromic synostoses. In addition, mechanical forces exerted on the fetal skull due to multiple gestations, reduced maternal pelvic volume, or fetal neurologic abnormalities may lead to a misshapen, uneven skull. Ex utero, the neonatal cranium is recognized to be quite malleable, and persistent mechanical forces on it can lead to a molding effect that may or may not be desired.

Deformational plagiocephaly describes occipital flattening, with resulting changes to the craniofacial skeleton, occurring in the perinatal period and presenting as a unilateral or bilateral deformity. It is the most common type of plagiocephaly, with an incidence ranging from 5% to 48% of healthy newborns. Though likely not a new entity, recognition and diagnosis of deformational plagiocephaly have certainly increased since the early 1990s with the American Academy of Pediatrics' (AAP) recommendation to place newborns supine at sleep. This practice guideline has had impressive effects on reducing the incidence of sudden infant deaths from 40% to 9%. Compliance with the recommendation, however, has resulted in an estimated 51% of infants spending a majority of time on their backs. As such, the infant skull generally comes to rest on one side of the occiput, and a persistent sleep position develops. This leads to sustained forces on the developing malleable infant skull.

Early evidence of these pressures results in localized occipital alopecia. If allowed to continue, abnormal molding or flattening of the underlying cranium occurs, resulting in plagiocephaly. Studies characterizing the demographics of this condition reveal a male predominance and right-sided unilateral predilection. Paralleling follow-up studies showing compliance with the "Back to Sleep" campaign greatest among Caucasian populations, an increased incidence in deformational plagiocephaly among Caucasian children has been noted (95% Caucasian, 2% African American, 2% Hispanic). Finally, multiparity is an identified risk factor and torticollis is present in association with the deformity in up to 20% of infants affected.

Classically, deformational plagiocephaly is a postnatal acquired condition. However, it is important to recognize that a condition of congenital deformational plagiocephaly has been found to occur up to 10% of the time. Acquired deformational plagiocephaly is believed to occur when infants are placed supine and assume a position of comfort that most likely corresponds to their previous intra-uterine lie. Newborns are typically unable to lift and midline their heads until 3 months of life, when neuromotor control has matured. When the infant is allowed to develop a persistent sleep position, this adopted behavior is subsequently difficult or impossible to change. This persistent sleep position, usually with the head turned to the right, results in constant compressive forces exerted against the expanding infant skull. These forces result in a unilateral occipital flattening and resulting anterior displacement of the ipsilateral craniofacial features.

A careful history and an attentive examination diagnose deformational plagiocephaly. Typically, infants with deformational plagiocephaly have relatively normal symmetric heads at birth but asymmetry evolves over subsequent weeks to months. On examination, the infant's face and skull should be observed from anterior, posterior, and vertex positions. Initially, the infant is placed in the parental lap facing forward and the examiner evaluates the anterior craniofacial skeleton for symmetry (Fig. 22-5). In this view, head tilt, as well as the forehead, orbits, midface, and mandible, are critically assessed. In up to 80% of infants with typical unilateral deformational plagiocephaly, the ipsilateral forehead will be displaced anteriorly, creating the illusion of asymmetrical enlargement. The ipsilateral palpebral fissure is often vertically elongated, and the ipsilateral cheek is displaced anteriorly, again creating the illusion of asymmetrical enlargement. The mandibular midline can be displaced to the affected side, a result of contralateral head tilt and ipsilateral head twist due to associated torticollis. The infant is then turned facing the parent as the examiner evaluates the posterior head. Careful attention is given to the mastoid skull. In typical deformational plagiocephaly, the mastoid skull base is symmetric. The infant is then placed supine with the head in the examiner's lap and feet in the parent's lap for vertex perspective. In typical deformational plagiocephaly, an occipital flatness is associated with ipsilateral ear, forehead, and cheek anterior displacement, resulting in the characteristic parallelogram skull shape (Fig. 22-6).

As noted earlier, associated muscular torticollis is frequently seen in children with deformational plagiocephaly. In the anterior view, particular attention is paid to head tilt and twist. Infants with deformational plagiocephaly, both acquired and congenital, routinely have contralateral sternocleidomastoid (SCM) muscle "stiffness" rather than true muscle atrophy and fibrosis. This is due to persistent intrauterine or postnatal positioning. The normal SCM muscle functions in tilting the head ipsilaterally and twisting the head contralaterally. In typical deformational plagiocephaly, the contralateral SCM muscle is affected and foreshortened, resisting full extension. This results in a contralateral head tilt and ipsilateral head twist. With the child's head in the examiner's lap, palpation of the contralateral SCM demonstrates a slight tightness and tenderness. Attempts at contralateral head twist are met with resistance and agitation.

Treatment strategies begin with prevention. Primary care providers for newborns are instrumental in educating

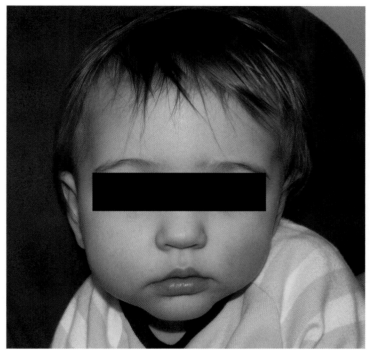

Figure 22-5. Infant with right-sided deformational plagiocephaly demonstrating anterior craniofacial changes: an advanced forehead, ear, and cheek.

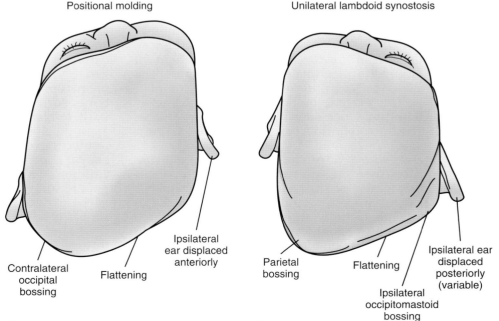

Positional molding

Unilateral lambdoid synostosis

Figure 22-6. Vertex views. **A,** Right-sided deformational plagiocephaly exhibiting a parallelogram head shape. **B,** Right-sided lambdoid craniosynostosis exhibiting a trapezoid-like head shape.

Contralateral occipital bossing

Flattening

Ipsilateral ear displaced anteriorly

Parietal bossing

Flattening

Ipsilateral ear displaced posteriorly (variable)

Ipsilateral occipitomastoid bossing

A

B

new parents about methods of reducing the risk of deformational plagiocephaly. Although supine position should be stressed during unattended sleep periods, as it has significantly reduced the incidence of sudden infant deaths, a significant amount of prone positioning or "tummy time" for the awake, observed infant is recommended to prevent the evolution of a persistent sleep pattern and to promote shoulder girdle strengthening affording infant mobility. Additionally, the infant's head resting position during sleep should be alternated from left to right sides. The infant should spend minimal time in car seats or other seating that maintains supine positioning.

With increasing awareness of deformational plagiocephaly, parents seek professional advice for this condition at an earlier age. This allows for the institution of behavioral modification that has a greater likelihood of success. The two factors that affect the treatment plan and ultimate outcome are (1) age at presentation and (2) severity of the deformity. No universal treatment plan has been agreed on; however, there is a general consensus on the approach to the child with deformational plagiocephaly. For the infant who presents with deformational plagiocephaly younger than 5 to 6 months of age, behavioral modifications are implemented. These include an attempt at repositioning the infant's head during sleep. This can be attempted with the placement of a rolled-up receiving blanket so that the rounded side of the head is placed dependent against the mattress, off-loading the affected side of the occiput. Parents are advised to alter the infant's position in the crib to encourage less time spent on the affected side. Because sleeping space is frequently against a room wall, the crib should be positioned so that the infant is forced to lie on the unaffected side to receive auditory and visual stimuli from toys, mobiles, and activity in the room. During feeding, parents are encouraged to position the child so that arm cradling removes pressure from the affected side of the skull. When awake, observed prone placement in the form of "tummy time" is recommended. On initial evaluation of the infant, care is taken to note any evidence of head tilt or twist that would indicate muscular torticollis. If torticollis is diagnosed, neck exercises should be taught to the parents as part of the management. Neck exercises have been recommended with each diaper change. These exercises include gently rotating the child's head so that the chin touches the shoulder and is held for 10 seconds. This is performed for three repetitions bilaterally, stretching the SCM muscle. The head is then tilted so that the ear touches the ipsilateral shoulder, again for three repetitions and held for 10 seconds and performed bilaterally, stretching the trapezius muscle. Finally, chin-to-chest stretches complete the program. This exercise program takes approximately 2 additional minutes per diaper change. These infants are monitored on a monthly basis until 5 to 6 months of age.

Those infants who at 5 to 6 months of life (1) fail conservative management, (2) present with initial moderate to severe deformities, or (3) have concomitant anterior craniofacial deformities are candidates for external cranioplasty with an orthotic device. These custom-fitted molding-helmets assist skull reshaping. The soft helmet is constructed after either obtaining a custom plaster mold of the infant's head, or the generation of a CT scan. An outer layer of polyethylene copolymer with an inner layer of polyethylene foam is fashioned such that the device is tight where the head is prominent yet permits growth where the head is flat. Children with deformational plagiocephaly typically present to the craniofacial surgeon at

approximately 6 months of age, having failed conservative therapy. Helmet therapy is optimally started as soon as indicated in an attempt to capitalize on the yet malleable cranial bones. Best results occur when therapy is initiated between 6 and 8 months of age; when started after age 12 months remolding has been less successful in the experience of most clinicians. A compliant, dedicated caretaker is required for success as older infants may not eagerly embrace the helmet at first. Initially, children go through a short "warm-up" period and then are encouraged to spend 23 hours a day in the helmet. With consistency, infants quickly adapt with typical alacrity and have been reported to experience separation angst once therapy is discontinued. Children are serially seen at 2- to 3-month intervals and receive a developmental/neurological examination, as well as an assessment of the progress of contour remodeling.

In summary, although the "Back to Sleep" campaign has decreased the incidence of SIDS dramatically, an unfortunate sequel of deformational plagiocephaly has reached epidemic proportions today. In the past decade, the diagnosis of deformational plagiocephaly has been codified. Primary care providers must be aware of this condition and, in turn, educate parents in its prevention. Should preventative measures fail, deformational plagiocephaly can be successfully treated with behavior modification and/or cranial molding helmet therapy.

Craniofacial Anomalies

Multiple craniofacial anomalies have been characterized in the literature. The majority are quite rare. Due to developmental origins, these syndromes may be segregated anatomically into the regions of the head in which the majority of findings are identified. This allows for an analysis of syndromes that primarily affect the skull, midface, and lower face or mandible. The following discussion reviews several of the more common syndromes of interest from each of these facial domains.

The Skull

Craniofacial anomalies that affect the skull are often identified when the head of a newborn or growing infant appears to be abnormally shaped. Anomalous sutural closure is frequently the etiology of these misshapen calvariae. Craniosynostosis, or craniostenosis, is defined as premature closing of the sutures between the cranial bones during development, resulting in deformities of the skull. *Primary* craniosynostosis originates from pathology at an involved suture, whereas *secondary* craniosynostosis results from dysgenesis of the underlying brain that directs cranial expansion. This distinction is noteworthy because children with secondary synostosis generally do not require surgical intervention.

The classification of craniosynostosis is separated into simple or complex depending on whether one or more than one suture is involved (Table 22-2). The compensatory forces exerted on the developing skull result in various recognized patterns or shapes. Generally, the skull will grow in a direction parallel to the prematurely fused suture. A *brachycephalic* skull is shortened in the anteroposterior dimension due to bilateral coronal suture synostosis. *Acrocephaly*—literally, "tower skull"—describes a skull in which the height of the anterior cranium is greater

Table 22-2	Skull Shape Nomenclature	
NAME	**SUTURE(S) INVOLVED**	**SHAPE**
Acrocephaly	Bilateral coronal	Skull height greater anteriorly, slanting downward posteriorly
Brachycephaly	Bilateral coronal	Wide, taller skull shortened in anteroposterior dimension
Oxycephaly	Bilateral coronal	Taller skull, shortened in both width and anteroposterior dimension
Turricephaly	Bilateral coronal	Tall skull
Plagiocephaly	Unilateral coronal or unilateral lambdoidal	Asymmetrical skull
Scaphocephaly	Sagittal	Anteroposterior elongation with bitemporal narrowing
Trigonocephaly	Metopic	Narrow, triangular, ridged forehead
Kleeblattschädel	Bilateral coronal, lambdoidal, and metopic	Cloverleaf deformity

than that of the posterior cranium, resulting in a skull that slants from front to back. As a result, the skull grows to a greater extent in both width and height. When bicoronal fusion occurs later in development, the width, as well as the anteroposterior dimension, is reduced and the skull is taller, resulting in *oxycephaly*. If the upward growth of the skull is augmented due to premature bicoronal closure, *turricephaly* results. *Plagiocephaly* describes an asymmetrical cranium. Skull development that occurs during unilateral coronal or unilateral lambdoidal synostosis may lead to this conformation. Importantly, not all cases of plagiocephaly are attributable to sutural synostosis, as deformational mechanisms may lead to cranial asymmetry as well (see previous section). Infants with *scaphocephaly* usually have sagittal suture synostosis evidenced by temporal narrowing and compensatory elongation of the skull in the anteroposterior dimension. When the metopic suture alone is fused, the forehead is noted to be narrow and triangular with a prominent ridge. *Trigonocephaly* describes the shape of this skull. The most severe skull dysmorphology and intracranial compromise result from fusion of the coronal and lambdoid sutures bilaterally and of the anterior metopic suture. Compensatory bulging at the remaining open sagittal suture leads to a trifoliate appearance described as the cloverleaf deformity, or *kleeblattschädel*.

The incidence of craniosynostosis varies from 1:1500 to 1:1900 live births. The frequency appears equal in all ethnic populations but varies between genders depending on which suture is involved. Its etiology is likely quite heterogeneous and perhaps, in some instances, multifactorial. Genetics certainly does play a role in some cases. Recent investigations have identified mutations in the genome and downstream protein products that result in the patterns of suture fusion and systemic anomalies associated with more than 100 described syndromic craniosynostoses. The origin of simple craniosynostosis, however, remains elusive. Some indirect evidence suggests that mechanical compression may contribute to suture closure in humans because twins and infants delivered from a breech position have an increased incidence of craniosynostosis. Some theorize that skull compression leads to ischemia and/or fibrosis at the suture line and thereby contributes to early fusion.

Nonsyndromic, Simple Craniosynostoses

Up to 70% of simple, isolated craniosynostoses (those involving only a single cranial suture) occur sporadically. Autosomal dominant and recessive familial patterns have been identified in 8% of cases. Estimating risk for subsequent pregnancies is difficult, but if one parent and child are affected, subsequent pregnancies have a quoted 50% risk of recurrence. Simple sagittal synostosis, more frequently identified in males with a male-to-female ratio of 4:1, is the most commonly encountered simple craniosyn-

ostosis, representing 57% of cases. Simple coronal synostosis occurs less often, with even fewer reported cases of isolated metopic synostosis. True lambdoidal synostosis is extremely rare.

Sagittal Synostosis. Sagittal synostosis results from premature fusion of the sagittal suture, resulting in a scaphocephalic skull shape with an increased anteroposterior length and a reduction in the width of the skull (Fig. 22-7). Isolated nonsyndromic sagittal synostosis is the most common form of craniosynostosis. Typically sporadic in occurrence, only about 2% of patients demonstrate a genetic etiology. A 4:1 male predominance is recognized with no race predilection. In general, the majority of infants with sagittal synostosis are at low risk for intracranial hypertension and minimal risk for abnormal brain development, as the remaining cranial sutures are patent, allowing for compensatory expansion of the neurocranium and normal brain growth.

The involved sagittal suture may be variably affected, ranging from predominantly anterior fusion, to predominantly posterior fusion, to complete fusion. Reflective of these variances, the skull shape may be differentially misshapen. Patients with isolated anterior sagittal suture fusion will manifest frontal bossing, whereas those with isolated posterior suture fusion will exhibit occipital bossing. Bossing of both the frontal and occipital domains with associated biparietal narrowing results from complete fusion of the suture.

Diagnosis is made via observation of these findings on physical examination. In addition, a midline ridge may be palpable. CT in axial, coronal, and three-dimensional constructs confirms the diagnosis and is instrumental in planning operative strategies.

Surgical intervention strives to reshape the calvarium, targeting the anterior and posterior prominences while widening the biparietal dimension. Various techniques are used and depend on the age of the infant at operation. Infants younger than 1 year of age are candidates for strip sagittal suturectomy (excision of the affected suture)—with or without further cranial vault remodeling. In centers where only suturectomy is performed, either via an open or endoscopic approach, ultimate skull shape remodeling is assisted by the use of molding helmets. These orthotic devices exploit the recognized continued growth of the brain and its effects on the overlying skull. Worn 23 hours daily for several months, they redirect skull growth toward a symmetric, normal shape. Some centers, however, target the abnormal anterior and posterior prominences at the time of surgery. In these instances, in addition to removal of the affected suture, the occiput and frontal bones are concomitantly reshaped. A helmet is then employed to complete the process of remolding the skull by facilitating widening in the biparietal dimension. The skulls in infants over the age of a year are relatively less malleable and therefore must be targeted with

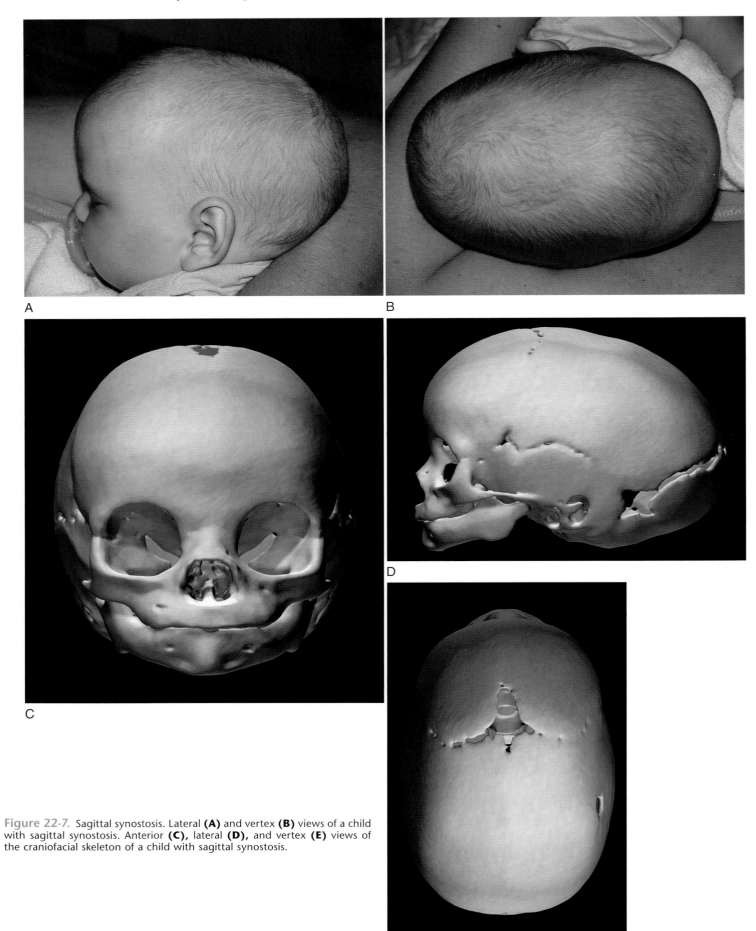

A

B

C

D

E

Figure 22-7. Sagittal synostosis. Lateral **(A)** and vertex **(B)** views of a child with sagittal synostosis. Anterior **(C)**, lateral **(D)**, and vertex **(E)** views of the craniofacial skeleton of a child with sagittal synostosis.

cranial vault remodeling, in which the various bones are reshaped and secured with plates or wire fixation.

Coronal Synostosis. The coronal sutures may be affected either unilaterally or more infrequently bilaterally, resulting in anterior plagiocephaly and anterior brachycephaly, respectively. Bicoronal synostosis is more often syndromically associated. Nonsyndromic unilateral coronal synostosis has an estimated incidence of 1:2500 and accounts for 15% to 30% of cases of craniosynostosis. Its etiology is unknown, but proposed causes include fetal head constraint, thyrotoxicosis, and certain vitamin deficiencies.

Synostosis of a single coronal suture results in a widened ipsilateral palpebral fissure, an elevated and anteriorly positioned ipsilateral ear, a nasal root deviation toward the affected suture, chin deviation away from the affected suture, and a superiorly and posteriorly displaced supraorbital rim and eyebrow known as the "harlequin eye" deformity. These findings (Fig. 22-8) on physical examination are consistent with the diagnosis, and sutural obliteration is then documented by CT. Most children do not exhibit findings of intracranial hypertension but should have a neurosurgical and ophthalmologic evaluation. Providing no evidence of intracranial hypertension exists, surgical remodeling of the skull is usually planned between 10 and 12 months. This is achieved by targeting the anterior cranial vault (frontal and parietal bones) and the supraorbital bar. Postoperatively, children are frequently assessed to assure that aesthetic outcomes are optimal. Forehead and orbital changes will be readily apparent postoperatively; facial changes like nasal root position and ear position are noted to correct more slowly as the child ages.

Metopic Synostosis. The metopic suture is the first cranial suture to fuse, typically beginning before age 2. It is unique in that it is the only suture that disappears and is indiscernible in the adult skull. Premature fusion leads to a "keel"-shaped trigonocephalic head (Fig. 22-9). Trigonocephaly is a relatively uncommon entity with an incidence of between 1:2500 and 1:15,000 births and accounting for 10% to 20% of isolated craniosynostoses. Males are affected more often than females with an identified sex ratio of 3:1. Examination of the skull and face in affected patients may reveal hypotelorism, upward slanting of the eyelids laterally, and a triangular shape to the forehead and supraorbital ridge. A bony ridge may be palpable over the metopic suture. Though typically an isolated condition, 8% to 15% of children affected with trigonocephaly will have associated anomalies involving the extremities or the central nervous, cardiac, or genitourinary systems. Evaluation is completed with a CT scan to confirm sutural synostosis.

An ophthalmologic evaluation is warranted because these children are at increased risk for the development of astigmatism and strabismus. Further, though its incidence in this population is less than 4%, the presence of intracranial hypertension must be excluded. Although literature exists suggesting no developmental delay in these children, other studies have shown an increased incidence of cognitive delay, not attributable to sequelae of intracranial hypertension. Therefore it is recommended that development in these infants be closely monitored.

The severity of the deformity determines whether surgical intervention is indicated. In those with sutural synostosis lacking significant skull deformity, no treatment is indicated. Those with obvious forehead deformity are candidates for anterior cranial vault remodeling. In these infants surgical intervention is planned for within the first year of life and involves remodeling of the frontal bones and the supraorbital rim to achieve improved contour.

Lambdoid Synostosis. Lambdoid synostosis may involve one or both of the lambdoid sutures and is the rarest of the craniosynostoses. A raised ridge may be palpable over the involved suture on examination, and there is often a mastoid bulge of the affected side of the occiput with contralateral occipital parietal bossing (Fig. 22-10).

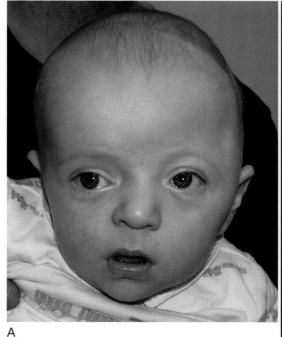

A

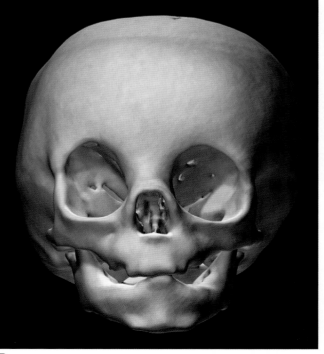

B

Figure 22-8. Unilateral coronal synostosis. **A,** Photograph of a child with left-sided unilateral coronal synostosis. **B,** Anterior view of the craniofacial skeleton of a child with right-sided unilateral coronal synostosis.

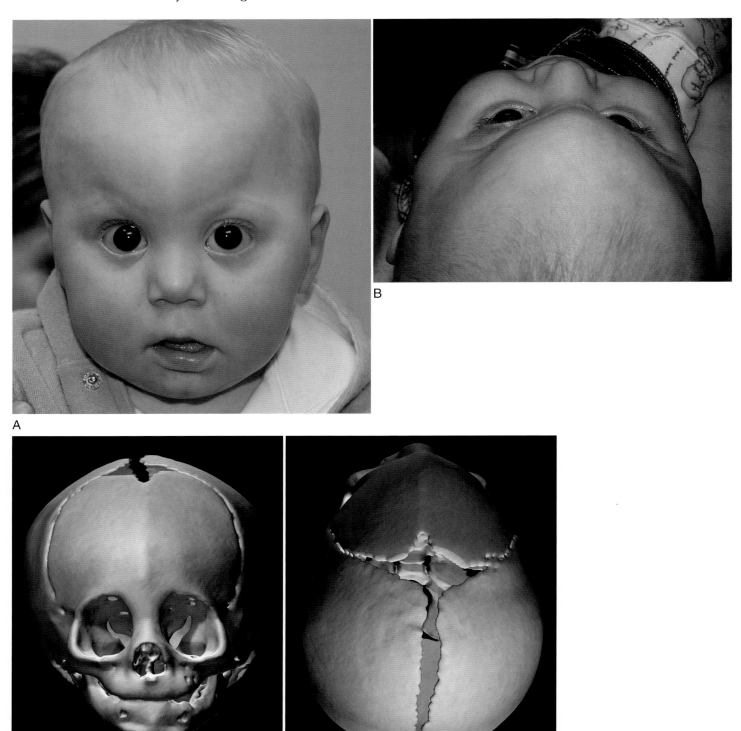

Figure 22-9. Metopic synostosis. Anterior **(A)** and vertex **(B)** views of a child with metopic synostosis. Anterior **(C)** and vertex **(D)** views of the craniofacial skeleton of a child with metopic synostosis.

From the vertex view (see Fig. 22-6), a trapezoid head-shape is seen, with contralateral frontal bossing, posterior displacement of the ipsilateral ear, and ipsilateral occipitomastoid bossing. This view best distinguishes true lambdoid suture synostosis from far more prevalent deformational plagiocephaly, which does not involve sutural fusion. CT confirms sutural fusion and assists planning for any indicated reconstructive surgery. Those with significant or progressive deformity undergo surgery between 6 and 12 months of age with surgical plans designed to reshape the entire occiput.

Syndromic, Complex Craniosynostoses

Craniosynostoses involving more than one suture are more rarely encountered and often adhere to an autosomal dominant inheritance pattern. These include the Apert, Crouzon, Pfeiffer, and Jackson-Weiss syndromes, which involve multiple sutures in addition to systemic

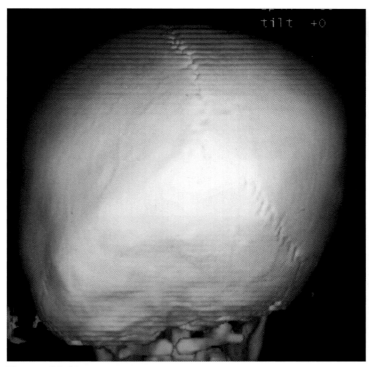

Figure 22-10. Lambdoid synostosis. Posterior view of the craniofacial skeleton of a child with left-sided lambdoid synostosis.

Table 22-3	Gene Mutations Associated with Craniofacial Syndromes	
GENE/PROTEIN	**SYNDROME**	**CHROMOSOME**
FGFR1	Pfeiffer	8
FGFR2	Apert	10
	Crouzon	
	Pfeiffer	
	Jackson-Weiss	
	Beare-Stevenson	
FGFR3	Muenke	4
	Crouzon with AN	
TWIST	Saethre-Chotzen	7
Treacle	Treacher Collins	5

AN, acanthosis nigricans.

anomalies. In the 1990s, a glimpse into the etiology of these four phenotypic clinical entities was made possible because of advances and resultant findings at the molecular-genomic level. Central to this new knowledge is the fibroblast growth factor receptor (FGFR) and the role of various mutations in its gene that are associated with a number of craniosynostotic syndromes.

The FGFRs are a family of four tyrosine kinase transmembrane receptors expressed in high levels in bone that bind extracellular fibroblast growth factors (FGFs). FGFs are structurally similar proteins that command a significant role in the growth and differentiation of various cells of mesenchymal and neuroectodermal origin. They are also involved with chemotaxis, angiogenesis, apoptosis, and spatial patterning within developing tissues. Structurally similar, the 17 known FGFs lack affinity toward specific FGFRs and consequently any FGF may stimulate any FGFR. Three domains have been identified on the FGFR molecule: a cytoplasmic domain, a transmembrane domain, and an extracellular domain consisting of three immunoglobulin-like regions. The binding of an FGF to the FGFR occurs at two of these immunoglobulin-like regions and leads to dimerization of two FGFRs. These events then stimulate the third immunoglobulin-like region, which mediates a complex cascade of intracellular activity. These intracellular signals orchestrate various developmental pathways including those present in the developing fetal cranial sutures and neurocranium. FGFRs are responsible for restraining growth. Thus mutations that decrease their activity would likely result in augmented growth and are described as "hypermorphic" mutations. Early fusion of a cranial suture is a hypermorphic event.

Various point mutations have been discovered in the FGFRs (Table 22-3). Three of the FGFRs—FGFR1, FGFR2, and FGFR3—are associated with craniosynostotic syndromes when mutations occur. The *FGFR1* gene maps to chromosome 8. Mutations of this gene are associated with one form of Pfeiffer syndrome. The *FGFR2* gene resides on

chromosome 10. The phenotypic syndromes that may result from the greater than 43 amino acid substitutions identified vary. Indeed, mutations of this receptor are associated with the Apert, Crouzon, Pfeiffer, or Jackson-Weiss phenotype depending on the location and type of substitution that occurs. The *FGFR3* gene is found on human chromosome 4, and nucleotide changes within this gene are associated with Muenke syndrome and a phenotype of Crouzon syndrome that manifests with acanthosis nigricans.

Although the association between the FGFRs and the various craniosynostotic syndromes shapes our understanding of the origins of the respective anomalies, much remains to be learned before that understanding is complete. As is evident, the syndromes are genomically related yet phenotypically distinct. Not surprisingly, the clinical diagnosis, management, and prognosis for each of these syndromes, as well as for each individual afflicted with a syndrome, vary. Accordingly, the following sections examine each syndrome in more specific detail.

Apert Syndrome. Apert syndrome is an autosomal dominant disorder with incomplete penetrance and a birth prevalence of 5.5 to 16 per 1 million live births. The majority of cases are sporadic. The defect has been localized to chromosome 10q. More than 98% of cases of Apert syndrome have identifiable mutations in the *FGFR2* gene. The etiology involves nucleotide changes, leading to missense amino acid substitutions that result in phenotypic changes. Apert syndrome accounts for 4.5% of all craniosynostoses.

Clinical features may be divided into craniofacial, extremity, and visceral anomalies (Fig. 22-11). The two hallmarks of the disorder are craniosynostosis and symmetrical extremity syndactyly. Infants typically have a misshapen skull. This is the result of coronal suture synostosis resulting in brachycephaly and the appearance of a disproportionately high cranium. Mean lengths and weights of these newborns are frequently above the 50th percentile. Eyes are often wide set, or hyperteloric, resulting from an underlying widened metopic and sagittal suture that closes between 2 and 4 years of age. As a result of hypoplasia, the midface may appear retruded, with a downturned mouth. As a result of midface deficiency, the posterior choanae may be hypoplastic, leading to obstruction of the nasopharyngeal airway. Although choanal stenosis is common, atresia is rare. A cleft palate may be present, and stylohyoid calcification is evident in 38% to 88% of patients.

Because orbital depth is foreshortened, children with Apert syndrome are at risk for significant eye injury. Owing to shallow orbits, the globes of the eyes may be proptotic

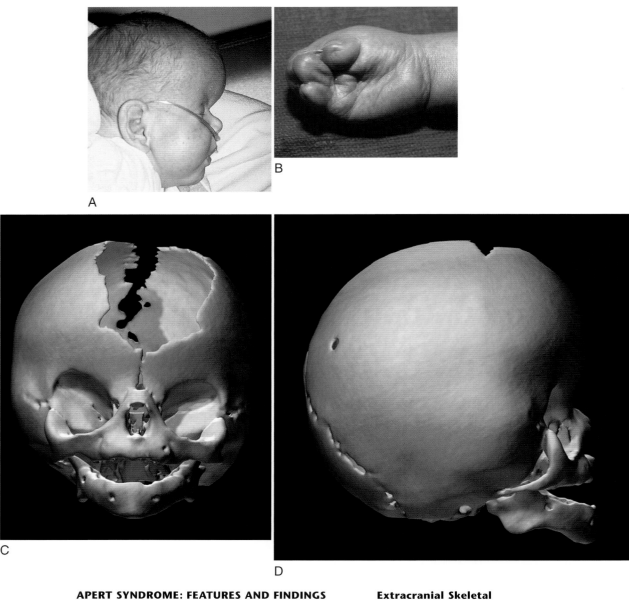

APERT SYNDROME: FEATURES AND FINDINGS

Craniofacial	**Extracranial Skeletal**
Brachycephaly due to coronal suture synostosis	Symmetrical syndactyly of the hands
Hypertelorism	Cervical spine fusion
Proptosis	Shortened humeri
V-pattern exotropia	**Other**
Midface hypoplasia	Cardiovascular anomalies
Choanal stenosis	Hydronephrosis
Cleft palate	Cryptorchidism
Stylohyoid calcification	Tracheal anomalies
Conductive hearing deficits	Obstructive sleep apnea
	Diffuse acne

Figure 22-11. Apert syndrome. **A,** Lateral view of a child with Apert syndrome. **B,** Syndactyly of the hand. Anterior **(C)** and lateral **(D)** views of the craniofacial skeleton of a child with Apert syndrome. Note the expansive anterior fontanelle in the anteroposterior view.

and exotropic. Corneal abrasions and exposure keratosis may occur. Attention to infant crib positioning and toddler surveillance during acquisition of walking skills is important to prevent abrasions and traumatic injuries. In addition, the application of lubricating ointment during sleep and instillation of artificial tears during the day should be practiced for corneal protection. Strabismus, a common finding, exhibits a V pattern with exotropic upward gaze divergence and an esotropic downward gaze. Patients frequently develop visual acuity abnormalities that include myopia, hyperopia, and/or associated astigmatism.

Children with Apert syndrome are more likely to encounter middle ear infections than their peers. Otitis media is common and likely related to eustachian tube dysfunction, which may be associated with midface anomalies or an associated cleft palate. Attention to bouts of otitis media and early otolaryngologic evaluation and placement of myringotomy tubes are essential to ensure proper hearing and language development. Neurosensory hearing loss is uncommon in these children. However, conductive hearing deficiencies are frequently encountered, largely due to effusions and other sequelae of chronic or recurrent otitis media.

Intracranially, various anomalies have been described including megalocephaly, hypoplastic white matter, heterotopic gray matter, frontal encephalocele, and agenesis of the corpus callosum. Although ventriculomegaly may be identified on head imaging, significant hydrocephalus with intracranial hypertension is not common in these children, though progressive hydrocephaly may evolve on occasion. In evaluation, an early baseline MRI scan may be obtained to define specific brain anomalies. All infants should have a baseline CT scan and serial examinations to monitor for possible evolving intracranial hypertension.

The impact of the craniocerebral anomalies on infant intelligence is an appropriate parental concern. Not surprisingly, cognitive function may be impaired in the presence of intracranial anomalies. Because 72% of children with Apert syndrome are noted to have brain anomalies, they are more likely to have developmental delays and cognitive deficits. Although a family setting that includes a nurturing environment has been shown to significantly improve cognitive development, proper timing of release of the synostotic coronal sutures may also alter some of the previously noted deficits. Because age at operation has been shown to affect intelligence, children who are operated on before their first birthday but after 3 months of age are more likely to have intelligence quotients (IQs) greater than 80. Unfortunately, children who had similar procedures before 3 months of age trended toward lower IQs and required further operations.

Infants with Apert syndrome also exhibit extracranial findings. Although the axial skeletal system is always involved, the central skeleton may be affected as well. Cervical spine fusion occurs in 70% of patients, with increasing frequency as the child ages. Levels C3-C4 and C5-C6 are commonly affected. Patients should have cervical radiographs to assess for vertebral abnormalities, particularly before anesthesia for surgery. The extremities are always involved to some degree, specifically bilateral fusion of the digits of the hands and feet, which identify patients with the syndrome. Symmetrical syndactyly of the second, third, and fourth digits is common, resulting in a "mitten hand" appearance (see Fig. 22-11B). The first and fifth digits can present separately from the central hand mass. Staged reconstruction can usually be performed to separate the digits, allowing for opposition and a more functional hand. In addition, the more proximal upper extremity may exhibit limitations in range of motion, particularly at the shoulder and elbow. The humerus may be shortened.

Visceral anomalies may also be present. Cardiovascular and genitourinary anomalies have been noted to occur in 10% of patients. Cardiac anomalies may include atrial or ventricular septal defect, coarctation of the aorta, patent ductus arteriosus, pulmonic stenosis, or more complex lesions. Hydronephrosis and cryptorchidism in males are encountered. Infants may require echocardiography and renal ultrasonography early to examine for occult findings. Less frequently, anomalies of the respiratory system (1%) and gastrointestinal system (1%) may occur. Infants may develop respiratory insufficiency secondary to airway compromise resulting from tracheal abnormalities that prevent adequate distention of the trachea. Obstructive sleep apnea, which can evolve into cor pulmonale, may be present due to the distorted and malpositioned facial bones contributing to upper airway obstruction. Indeed, patients who snore and/or are disproportionately somnolent should be evaluated appropriately with an overnight oximetry sleep study to document desaturations. Patients identified with obstructive sleep apnea do benefit from nasal continuous positive airway pressure.

Finally, the skin of patients with Apert syndrome may display excessive sweating. Patients have been shown to have an increased number of sweat glands and prominent sebaceous glands. During adolescence the skin becomes oily, and in 70% of patients acne erupts on the face, chest, and back.

Crouzon Syndrome. Crouzon syndrome is a craniosynostosis syndrome that may be inherited via an autosomal dominant pattern with incomplete penetrance or may present as a sporadic new case. First identified in 1912, up to 60% of cases are new mutations, many of which are associated with advanced paternal age older than 35 years. Representing approximately 5% of craniosynostoses, Crouzon syndrome has a birth prevalence of 15 to 16 per 1 million live births and is associated with the *FGFR2* gene located on chromosome 10. The syndrome is genetically heterogeneous, explaining its variability of expression. Up to 25 nucleotide alterations have been identified that lead to amino acid substitutions at the site of the *FGFR2* gene on chromosome 10, resulting in the classic Crouzon syndrome phenotype.

Craniofacial findings include brachycephalic craniosynostosis due to bilateral coronal suture fusion (Fig. 22-12). Significant hypertelorism is usually present with shallow orbits that create ocular exophthalmos and proptosis. Midface involvement includes maxillary hypoplasia, a short and beaked nose, and bifid uvula with or without cleft palate. Maxillary hypoplasia juxtaposed with normal mandibular growth yields an appearance of mandibular prognathism. Intracranial anomalies often exist including anomalous venous drainage and hydrocephalus. Hydrocephalus is present with greater frequency in patients with Crouzon syndrome than in patients with Apert syndrome. Chiari I malformations are present in 71% of cases, with associated hindbrain herniation in a similar percentage of patients. This is likely related to early closure of the lambdoid sutures, which commonly occurs in these children. Early MRI is therefore recommended to evaluate for hydrocephalus and provide a baseline for follow-up. Another unusual craniofacial finding noted in 50% of Crouzon patients is calcification of the stylohyoid ligament.

Otopathology is frequently encountered in the patient with Crouzon syndrome. Externally the ears are usually normal in appearance, although approximately 50% are set low on the face. Patients often suffer conductive hearing loss due to middle ear effusions and inner ear pathology, which is present due to midface anomalies. Eustachian tube function is impeded due to these anomalous anatomic arrangements, predisposing to multiple bouts of otitis media. In addition, patients with Crouzon syndrome may suffer neurosensory hearing deficits, as well as mixed losses. Therefore infants should be carefully evaluated for hearing deficits and serially monitored throughout development. Early referral to otolaryngology colleagues for treatment of identified conductive and neurosensory hearing losses can optimize auditory outcomes for the individual in many instances.

Extracranially, approximately one quarter of patients have radiographic abnormalities of the cervical spine. Cervical vertebral fusion at the C2-C3 and C5-C6 levels may be identified either in childhood or in adulthood. In addition, patients may exhibit butterfly vertebrae, which may fuse later in life. Cervical spine flexion-extension radiographs should be considered before anesthesia and should be updated due to the progressive character of the cervical vertebral fusion witnessed in these patients.

Pfeiffer Syndrome. First described in 1964, Pfeiffer syndrome (PS) (Fig. 22-13) is a less commonly encountered syndromic craniosynostosis that is also associated with mutation of the fibroblast growth factor receptor. Mutations in the *FGFR1* and *FGFR2* genes on chromosomes 8

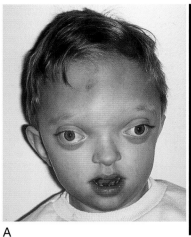
A

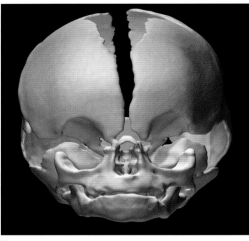
B

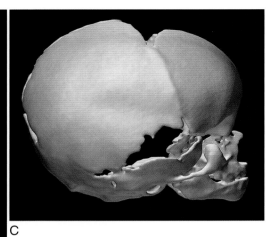
C

CROUZON SYNDROME: FEATURES AND FINDINGS
Craniofacial
Brachycephaly due to coronal suture synostosis
Hydrocephaly with Chiari I malformation
Hypertelorism
Proptosis
Midface hypoplasia
"Beaked" nose

Cleft palate
Stylohyoid calcification
Conductive and/or neurosensory hearing deficit
Extracranial Skeletal
Cervical spine fusion
Other
Acanthosis nigricans

Figure 22-12. Crouzon syndrome. **A,** Photograph of a child with Crouzon syndrome. Anterior **(B)** and lateral **(C)** views of the craniofacial skeleton of a child with Crouzon syndrome.

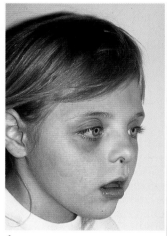
A

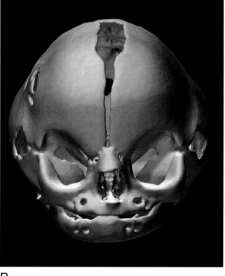
B

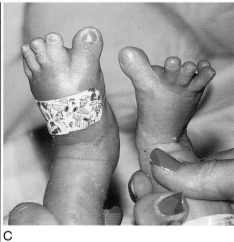
C

PFEIFFER SYNDROME: FEATURES AND FINDINGS

	Type I	Type II	Type III
Craniofacial			
Acrocephaly, or turribrachycephaly (oxycephaly,) due to coronal suture synostosis	+		+
Kleeblattschädel sutural deformity		+	
Hydrocephaly		+	
Midface hypoplasia	+	++	++
"Beaked" nose	+	+	+
Hypertelorism	+	+	+
Proptosis	+	++	+
Blindness		+	
Choanal atresia		+	+
Mental retardation		+	+
Extracranial Skeletal			
Broad, radially deviated thumbs	+	+	+
Broad, medially deviated great toes	+	+	+
Soft-tissue syndactyly	+	+	+
Elbow ankylosis		+	+

Figure 22-13. Pfeiffer syndrome. **A,** Photograph of a child with Pfeiffer syndrome. **B,** Anterior view of the craniofacial skeleton of a child with Pfeiffer syndrome. **C,** Characteristic medially deviated, broad great toes seen in Pfeiffer syndrome.

and 10, respectively, lead to one of three recognized clinical subtypes. Classic PS, or type I, is associated with normal intelligence and good prognosis. About 95% of patients with type I have mutations in *FGFR2,* whereas 5% have mutations in *FGFR1.* This subtype trends toward a more autosomal dominant inheritance pattern, whereas types II and III PS are more sporadic in occurrence. Both types II and III are associated with mutations in *FGFR2* and are uncommon. They are associated with mental retardation and have a poor prognosis. Infants with severe multisutural synostosis, the kleeblattschädel anomaly, characteristic hands and feet, and ankylosis of the elbows represent type II PS. Patients with type III PS resemble those with type II but lack the cloverleaf skull.

Infants with PS have some degree of craniofacial dysmorphism. Type I PS may exhibit acrobrachycephaly or turribrachycephaly due to symmetrical or asymmetrical coronal suture synostosis. In addition, maxillary hypoplasia with a depressed midface and small beaked nose is evident. Hypertelorism, proptosis, and strabismus are common ocular findings. Type II PS patients, due to presumed early sutural fusion, have impressive cranial anomalies, with characteristic temporal bulging identified as the kleeblattschädel deformity (cloverleaf skull), often associated with hydrocephalus. The midface is more severely affected, exhibiting orbital stenosis, extreme proptosis, and blindness. Severe midface hypoplasia may include choanal atresia that contributes to upper airway obstruction.

Extracranially, all types of PS display broad, symmetric thumbs that deviate radially, as well as medially deviated great toes. The distal phalanx of the thumb is broad, and the proximal phalanx is triangular in shape and may even be absent. The middle phalanges may be absent as well. Soft tissue syndactyly is noted between digits 2 and 3 (and sometimes 3 and 4) of both the hands and feet. Also, the thumbs and great toes may be shortened, and types II and III PS may exhibit elbow ankylosis.

Not surprisingly, infants with PS experience frequent bouts with otitis media. These episodes, in combination with underlying midface anomalies, contribute to a significant incidence of conductive hearing loss. In addition, infants may lack external auditory canals. Thus infants should have otologic evaluation early and be monitored closely. Visceral gastrointestinal manifestations of PS occur with less frequency and include pyloric stenosis and malpositioned anus.

Crouzon Syndrome with Acanthosis Nigricans. A unique group of patients sharing a specific Ala391Glu mutation on *FGFR3* has recently been identified. These patients exhibit craniofacial features similar to those of Crouzon syndrome but also have an associated cutaneous finding. Besides the characteristic facies, their skin is affected with acanthosis nigricans, a verrucous hyperplasia and hypertrophy of the skin with associated hyperpigmentation and accentuated skin markings. It is distributed in the axillae, neck, chest, abdomen, breasts, perioral and periorbital regions, and nasolabial folds. Multiple melanocytic nevi are also frequently noted over the face, trunk, and extremities.

Muenke Syndrome. Muenke syndrome is a recently described FGFR-associated craniosynostosis that results from a Pro250Arg substitution in the *FGFR3* gene. Patients with Muenke syndrome are characterized by coronal craniosynostosis, the severity of which may be quite variable. In addition, sensorineural hearing deficits and skeletal anomalies of the hands and feet have been described. Variable cognitive deficits and developmental delays have also been identified in the 61 individuals reported to date.

Jackson-Weiss Syndrome. Jackson-Weiss syndrome is an autosomal dominant craniosynostotic and acrosyndactylic syndrome first described in a single, large Amish pedigree in 1976. Although often incomplete and variably expressed, penetrance is high within pedigrees. This allows for a spectrum of phenotypic findings, which etiologically are associated with mutations in the *FGFR2* gene on chromosome 10.

Clinical findings in affected infants include craniosynostosis with varying degrees of severity, midface hypoplasia, and structural abnormalities of the feet. Although a few individuals have no clinical or radiographic evidence of face or skull dysmorphology, the majority exhibit some degree of coronal suture craniosynostosis. Most individuals present with facial asymmetry and a broad forehead and turricephaly. Midface hypoplasia, cleft palate, hypertelorism, nasal beaking, mandibular prognathism, and strabismus are also described. Significant hearing deficits are common and may be conductive, neurosensory, or mixed in nature. Individuals may develop with normal intelligence or be challenged with moderate to mild mental retardation.

All affected patients display some degree of feet anomalies. Although one instance of third and fourth finger syndactyly has been reported, generally the hand is not involved. Short, broad metatarsals; calcaneocuboid bony fusion; and anomalous tarsal bone shape are present minimally. Medial deviation of the great toe and partial cutaneous syndactyly of the second and third toes may exist. Other individuals have been reported with partial duplications of the distal phalanges of the great toe. Clearly, radiographic evaluation of the hands and feet is necessary to fully characterize the extent of skeletal anomalies that exist.

Beare-Stevenson Syndrome. Beare-Stevenson syndrome is a recognized rare craniosynostotic syndrome related to mutation in the FGFR2 and is remarkable for its cutaneous manifestations. Affected patients exhibit mild craniosynostosis and some degree of mental retardation. Although cutis gyrata or redundant skin folds and acanthosis nigricans help to identify the syndrome, patients may also have findings including pyloric stenosis, an anteriorly displaced anus, and genitourinary anomalies.

Saethre-Chotzen Syndrome. First described in the early 1930s but more clearly defined in 1975, Saethre-Chotzen syndrome exhibits considerable clinical variability. Expressed as an autosomal dominant pattern of inheritance with incomplete penetrance, a deletion on chromosome 7 has been identified as the origin of this phenotype. Missense mutations in the *TWIST* gene that resides in this region are associated with this syndrome. The TWIST protein is a transcription factor that regulates gene expression by interacting with DNA. Although no mutations in the *FGFR* genes have been identified as yet, Saethre-Chotzen syndrome shares several phenotypic similarities with syndromes related to FGFR mutations.

The craniofacial domain is frequently affected. Although craniosynostosis may be absent, when it is present, patients may exhibit variable and often asymmetrical skull dysmorphisms. Coronal synostosis leading to brachycephaly, metopic stenosis with resultant trigonocephaly, and lambdoidal fusion causing occipital flattening may occur. In addition, infants are noted to have a straight nasal bridge, flattened forehead, hypertelorism, ptosis, and facial asymmetry. Midface involvement includes palatal clefting, hearing loss, and external ear anomalies. Children are usually of normal intelligence, although mild to moderate mental retardation has been reported.

Extracranially, vertebral abnormalities involving the cervical and lumbar spine may exist, as well as syndactyly of the second and third toes. The most common hand anomaly noted is a mild syndactyly between the second and third fingers. Fifth finger clinodactyly; a single flexion crease; a short fourth metacarpal; and a short, angulated thumb have all been reported as well.

The Midface

Although debate exists as to the etiology of most of the midface craniofacial syndromes, anomalous development in substrata originating from the branchial arches is a common element. These syndromes can be quite complex because they affect many facial structures including the eyes, ears, soft tissues, and skeleton of the midface. Accordingly, the defects are among the most challenging to reconstruct, with patients requiring multiple procedures and interventions. These syndromes are often also associated with mandibular anomalies, which place this population of infants at significant risk for early respiratory compromise, due to ineffective ventilation from upper airway obstruction. In severe cases, early tracheotomy is required to provide a secure airway.

Mandibulofacial Dysostosis (Treacher Collins Syndrome)

The Treacher Collins syndrome (TCS) is defined by a constellation of findings that affect the midface and mandible (Fig. 22-14). Since 1900, when TCS was first described,

300 to 400 cases have been reported with a suspected incidence of 1 in 50,000 live births. Inheritance can follow a variably expressed autosomal dominant pattern within pedigrees, although 50% of cases are thought to represent de novo mutations. The gene has been mapped to chromosome 5 situated between the colony stimulating factor receptor *(CSFR)* gene and the osteorectin *(SPARC)* gene. It encodes treacle, a protein product generously expressed in various fetal and adult tissues whose specific function remains unclear but may be related to signal transduction between the cytoplasm and nucleus. The genetic miscue results in anomalies of structures originating from the first and second branchial arches and the nasal placode in the developing fetus.

The hallmarks of the syndrome include midface and mandibular dysmorphology and tend to be bilateral with involvement of the ear, eye, malar region (cheek), and mandible. Intelligence is usually average to above average. The malar region, a second branchial arch derivative, is variably hypoplastic with both bony and soft tissue involvement. Hypoplasia of the zygoma, which lends central support to the cheek, may be quite severe, manifesting as an obvious lateral facial cleft. The lateral aspects of the orbits can similarly be deficient, leading to temporal concavity, reduced bitemporal distance, and reduced cephalic length. Thus the neurocranium may appear misshapen, although craniosynostosis is not a feature of the syndrome. In addition, midline structures such as the nasal choanae are often atretic, and a cleft palate or a cleft lip may be present.

The overlying soft tissues reflect the underlying bony deficiencies in the region and include anomalies of the eyelid and its adnexal structures, preauricular-cheek skin, the temporal fossa, and the external ears. The eyelids

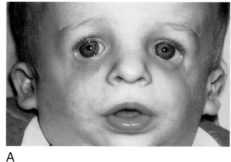

A

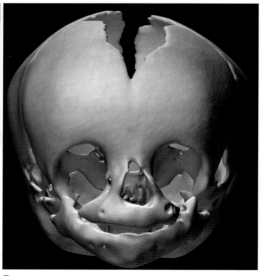

B

MANDIBULOFACIAL DYSOSTOSIS (TREACHER COLLINS SYNDROME): FEATURES AND FINDINGS

Craniofacial (Usually Bilateral Findings)	
Bilateral zygoma hypoplasia	Absent lower eyelashes
Bony deficiency of lateral orbits	Preauricular hair
Maxillary hypoplasia	Bilateral external ear deformities
Choanal stenosis	Bilateral external auditory canal stenosis or atresia
Cleft palate with or without cleft lip	Auditory ossicle hypoplasia or ankylosis
Downward-slanting palpebral fissure	Conductive hearing deficits
Colobomas	Retrognathia due to mandibular hypoplasia
Lower eyelid hypoplasia	Bite malocclusion
	Temporomandibular joint dysfunction

Figure 22-14. Mandibulofacial dysostosis. **A,** Photograph of a child with mandibulofacial dysostosis. **B,** Anterior view of the craniofacial skeleton of a child with mandibulofacial dysostosis.

appear antimongoloid with a downward slant of the palpebral fissure that results from colobomas and hypoplasia of the lower lids and the lateral canthi. The eyelid cilia (eyelashes) are often absent. Preauricularly, a tongue-shaped extension of hair may be present. The ears typically exhibit symmetrical, bilateral outer and middle ear malformations. The external ears, or pinnae, may be absent, malformed, or malpositioned. Symmetrical external auditory canal stenosis or atresia is identified in most patients in association with middle ear hypoplasia or atresia, the severity of which usually parallels that of the involved external ear. Although the auditory ossicles may be absent, more frequently they are hypoplastic, ankylosed to the wall of the middle ear's tympanic recess. As such, most patients suffer a conductive hearing loss that is often mirrored in its severity by the extent of external ear malformation. Fortunately, many of these children can significantly benefit from the use of hearing aids because the inner ear is usually spared and normal. Hearing should therefore be assessed early to allow for early fitting of hearing aids to promote language acquisition.

A derivative of the third branchial arch, the mandible is usually hypoplastic, resulting in retrognathia and malocclusion. Because both the maxilla and mandible are involved, the temporomandibular joint (TMJ) is often dysfunctional, with errant muscles of mastication. An anterior open bite of varying severity exists, depending on the degree of mandibular hypoplasia, which is segregated into subtypes to assist with the timing and planning for subsequent reconstructive efforts. Type I TMJ-mandibular deficiency describes a retrognathic mandible with a minor anterior open bite and minimal hypoplasia of the glenoid fossa. The TMJ therefore functions normally. Moderate glenoid fossa hypoplasia is found in type IIA, but TMJ function remains good. In contrast, type IIB TMJ-mandibular deficiency describes severe mandibular retrognathia and anterior open bite with more severe glenoid fossa hypoplasia. Although the TMJ is more anteriorly and medially located, it functions with an acceptable degree of rotation. A type III mandible is free-floating with no lower jaw articulation against the cranial base. Retrognathia is severe. A tracheostomy is generally required postnatally due to the precarious airway.

The airway is a significant concern for newborns affected with TCS and, depending on the extent of malformation, may place the infant at impending risk of respiratory embarrassment. Maxillary hypoplasia tends to constrict the nasal passages, leading to some degree of choanal stenosis or atresia, compromising airflow through the upper airway in the nasal-dependent newborn. Mandibular micrognathia and lingual retroposition further impinge on the upper airway, obstructing the oropharynx and hypopharyngeal spaces. In less severely affected newborns, special infant positioning and monitoring may be necessary early in life. However, a tracheostomy may be necessary for severely affected infants to provide a secure airway.

The midface anomalies may have a significant impact on the early care of the infant with TCS. The infant's ability to successfully feed may be impaired, particularly if comfortable respiration is impeded. In these instances, gavage feeding can be used to ensure acquisition of adequate nutrition. More definitive interventions, like tracheostomy or gastrostomy tube placement, may be necessary in the long term, depending on the severity and origin of respiratory insufficiency with feeding activities. Early care must also target the infant's sight and hearing, as well as

initiating reconstructive planning. A full head CT with special sections through the petrous portions of the temporal bones should be performed early during the first 6 months of life to document the extent of craniofacial involvement including external, middle, and inner ear pathology. A complete ophthalmologic examination to evaluate the function of the extraocular muscles, rule out corneal exposure, and examine visual acuity complements the initial workup.

Facial reconstruction is challenging because it targets the zygomatic/orbital region, maxillomandibular region, nasal region, soft tissues, external ears, and auditory canals and middle ears. For this reason, reconstructive efforts span several years and involve multiple procedures. Unless corneal exposure is an issue prompting earlier intervention, reconstruction is typically performed when the child is 5 to 7 years of age and generally yields good long-term results. The time for mandibular reconstruction depends on the type of mandibular deformity present. Types I, IIA, and IIB do not benefit from reconstruction of the TMJ and thus involve lengthening only of the mandible. Reconstruction involves osteotomies through the mandibular rami, preserving the native TMJ. Distraction osteogenesis then corrects deficiencies of the anteroposterior and height dimensions, as new bone growth (osteogenesis) is stimulated behind the serially lengthened severed mandible. The most favorable results are achieved when the patient is at early skeletal maturity, ages 13 to 15 in females and ages 15 to 16 in males. The type III deformity requires glenoid fossa construction, which is performed as part of the zygomatic and orbital reconstruction. First-stage reconstruction is usually initiated at 6 to 10 years of age. Mandibular lengthening may proceed as previously described. Most patients benefit from reconstructive rhinoplasty to correct the nasal mid-dorsal hump and mild to moderately wide nasal bridge. Postponing rhinoplasty until after orthognathic reconstruction is complete is preferable. The soft tissue deficits of the eyelid-adnexal region are esthetically and functionally challenging to reconstruct. Eyelid skin-muscle flaps and full-thickness skin grafts are used, but often with limited cosmetic outcomes.

The hollow temporal fossa may be rebuilt with vascularized tissue from a remote anatomic region, as a local source of tissue for augmentation is usually lacking. The external ear can be reconstructed through a staged approach that involves the sculpture of autologous rib cartilage into a scaffold that is placed in a posterior auricular skin envelope and allowed to mature before elevation and positioning with tragus reconstruction. Ear reconstruction is optimally performed around 6 to 7 years of age when the ribs have matured to a degree that allows for an adequate volume for harvest. The external ear canals and middle ear can then be targeted, with significant resultant gains in hearing. The external and internal ear reconstructions should be closely coordinated between the plastic surgeon and the otologist, with the external reconstruction performed first.

Acrofacial Dysostosis (Nager Syndrome)

Nager and deReynier, in 1948, characterized the first of a series of infants with anomalies that involved branchial arch deformations similar to those observed in the Treacher Collins syndrome, but additionally were associated with upper extremity anomalies. Although an autosomal dominant inheritance pattern is presumed, the majority of the less than 40 reported cases are sporadic in occurrence, and little is understood about the etiology of this craniofacial syndrome. Males are affected almost twice as often as females. Nager syndrome manifests with mandibulofacial dysostosis, and patients present with hypoplasia of the zygoma, downward slant of the palpebral fissures, colobomas of the lower eyelid, and maxillary hypoplasia (Fig. 22-15). Although these findings are generally less severe than those found in TCS, the associated mandibular hypoplasia tends to be of greater consequence in the Nager patient. As such, respiratory decompensation is frequent and up to 40% of patients require tracheostomy during the first year of life. Ear involvement includes preauricular skin tags, bilateral external ear anomalies, and stenosis or atresia of the external auditory canal, with resultant conductive hearing deficits. The majority of children have identified palatal anomalies; clefting is present in one third.

Discriminatingly, the radial aspect of the forearms and hand are abnormal in all children with Nager syndrome. Proximal fusion of the two forearm bones, or radioulnar synostosis, is observed in one third of children, and all cases exhibit either hypoplasia or aplasia of the thumbs. The toes may be involved. Although less often a component of the syndrome, visceral findings affecting the kidneys, spine, and genitalia have been identified. Developmentally, children progress, provided that hearing deficits are appropriately targeted, thereby optimizing conductive hearing losses.

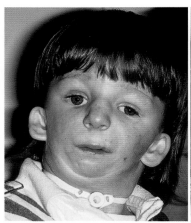 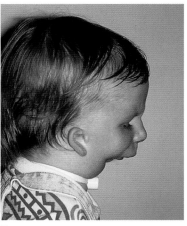

A   B

ACROFACIAL DYSOSTOSIS (NAGER SYNDROME): FEATURES AND FINDINGS
Craniofacial (Usually Bilateral Findings)
Bilateral zygoma hypoplasia
Bony deficiency of lateral orbits
Maxillary hypoplasia
Choanal stenosis
Cleft palate with or without cleft lip
Downward-slanting palpebral fissure
Colobomas
Lower eyelid hypoplasia
Absent lower eyelashes
Preauricular hair
Bilateral external ear deformities
Bilateral external auditory canal stenosis or atresia
Auditory ossicle hypoplasia or ankylosis
Conductive hearing deficits
Severe mandibular hypoplasia
Bite malocclusion
Temporomandibular joint dysfunction
Extracranial Skeletal
Radioulnar synostosis
Thumb hypoplasia or aplasia

Figure 22-15. Acrofacial dysostosis. **A** and **B,** Photographs of children with acrofacial dysostosis.

Oculo-Auriculo-Vertebral Spectrum (Goldenhar Syndrome and Hemifacial Microsomia)

The oculo-auriculo-vertebral syndrome, or spectrum, is a collection of facial anomalies that are believed by many experts to represent a spectrum of phenotypes exhibited secondary to a heterogeneous developmental field defect (Fig. 22-16). It includes several named entities including the Goldenhar syndrome, craniofacial microsomia, and hemifacial microsomia. Classically, hemifacial microsomia defined a condition that primarily affected ear, oral, and mandibular development; Goldenhar syndrome additionally included vertebral anomalies and epibulbar dermoids. Due to significant overlap noted between the two conditions, a segregation of the two into separate syndromes has been called into question; instead, each is proposed as a possible phenotypic variant of a common underlying developmental aberration. To date, the debate is not settled.

Over the past decades, several etiologic theories have been advanced implicating chromosomes, teratogens, vascular accidents, and adhesion molecules. A number of chromosomal anomalies have been associated, including deletions of 5p, 6q, 18q, and 22q; trisomies of chromosomes 7, 9, and 18; and sex chromosome aneuploidy, including 49,XXXXY, 47,XXY, 47,XXX, and 49,XXXXX. Direct causality of these has not been established, and indeed their observation may be coincidental. Several teratogenic factors have been associated, including maternal diabetes, thalidomide exposure, primidone, and retinoic acid. Vascular disruption has been suggested as a nidus for development of these features. This view postulates that stapedial arterial development is precluded or halted secondary to hematoma formation, leading to sequelae within its branchial arch watershed. Intrauterine compression of the area resulting in compromise has also been offered as a reason for the evolution of hemifacial microsomia. Disturbed chondrogenesis of the occipital bones and of the vertebral bodies, in which defective mineralization and resorption of cartilage is observed, has provided tissue evidence for a yet undefined primary defect in mesenchymal development. Ectodermal nondisjunction of the otic pit from surrounding tissue postulates that adhesion molecules may be responsible for the inability of the developing otic vesicle to separate from the surface ectoderm as it sinks into the mesenchymal substrata during the fourth week of gestation. The result is a tethering of the surrounding tissue, which exerts forces that affect the developing inner and middle ear and cervical spine, as well as resulting in regional growth restrictions. Partial separation allows for mesenchymal tissue influx, leading to dermoid and coloboma development. Although many theories exist, no one theory convincingly reconciles all identified phenotypes. Therefore it is suggested that more than one etiologic factor may exist, leading to the spectrum of findings that are observed.

Consistent with its associated ambiguity, characterization and therefore discussion often vary depending on the source. For the purposes of this discussion, the findings witnessed in the Goldenhar syndrome and hemifacial microsomia are referred to as the oculo-auriculo-vertebral spectrum (OAVS). As such, OAVS's incidence varies from 1 in 3500 to 1 in 19,500 live births, depending on the data source. A male-to-female ratio of 3:2 is observed, with a similar ratio of lateralization favoring the right side of the body. Most cases are sporadic, although familial patterns have been identified.

Affected infants exhibit anomalies in facial structures of first and second branchial arch derivation, although

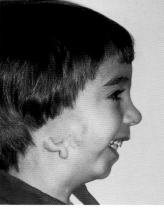

OCULO-AURICULO-VERTEBRAL SPECTRUM: FEATURES AND FINDINGS

Craniofacial
Facial asymmetry
Unilateral maxillary, temporal, and zygomatic hypoplasia
Epibulbar dermoids with fine hairs
Unilateral colobomas of upper eyelids
Esotropia or exotropia
Preauricular appendages
Pretragal fistula
External ear deformities
External auditory canal stenosis or atresia
Conductive hearing deficits
Macrostomia due to mandibular dysgenesis
Lateral facial cleft
Cleft lip with or without cleft palate
Central Nervous System
Seventh cranial nerve palsy
Microcephaly
Hydrocephaly
Encephaloceles
Extracranial Skeletal
Cervical vertebral fusion
Spina bifida
Hemivertebrae
Butterfly, fused, or hypoplastic vertebrae
Scoliosis
Rib anomalies
Cardiovascular
Ventricular septal defect
Tetralogy of Fallot
Transposition of the great vessels
Coarctation of the aorta
Pulmonic stenosis
Dextrocardia
Other
Pulmonary dysplasia
Tracheoesophageal fistula
Renal anomalies
Imperforate anus

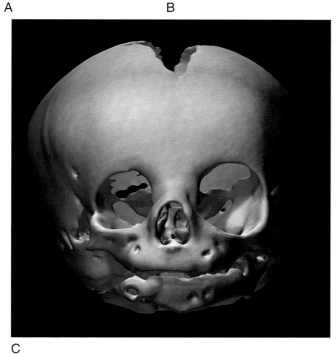

Figure 22-16. Oculo-auriculo-vertebral spectrum. **A** and **B,** Photographs of a child with oculo-auriculo-vertebral spectrum. **C,** Anterior view of the craniofacial skeleton of a child with right-sided OAV spectrum anomalies (hemifacial microsomia).

approximately half have additional anomalies other than those classically described. Findings may be divided into those affecting the craniofacial domain, the central nervous system, the skeleton, cardiovascular anomalies, and other systemic findings. The majority of cases have some degree of facial asymmetry that may become apparent only as the child grows. The maxillary, temporal, and malar bones are hypoplastic and flattened on the affected side. The mandible may be either aplastic or hypoplastic. Up to one third may have bilateral involvement, although one side is generally more affected than the other. As noted earlier, right-sided involvement is seen with greater frequency. Smooth epibulbar dermoids often with fine hairs are common unilateral findings inferotemporally at the limbus of the eye. Unilateral colobomas of the upper eyelids and oculomotor disorders including esotropia and exotropia are other ocular findings. The region of the ear is always involved to some degree and may exhibit preauricular appendages and pretragal blind-ended fistulae. The pinna may be missing or hypoplastic and malpositioned anteriorly and inferiorly. Occasionally both ears are involved, but more commonly only one ear is affected. The external auditory canal may be atretic or stenotic, leading to conductive hearing impairment, which is far more common than neurosensory losses in this cohort of

patients. The mandible is affected in one third of cases, with noted agenesis of the ramus and associated macrostomia or lateral facial cleft. The affected mandible is almost always on the same side as the anomalous ear. The palatal and tongue muscles may be hypoplastic and paralyzed, affecting feeding success. Further, a unilateral or bilateral cleft lip and/or palate occurs in up to 15% of infants.

The central nervous system may be involved and, not surprisingly, the degree of involvement is predictive of the child's intellectual capabilities. Involvement of nearly all cranial nerves has been reported, with lower facial weakness a frequent observation. Brain anomalies including microcephaly, encephaloceles, hydrocephaly, lissencephaly, holoprosencephaly, corpus callosum hypoplasia, and the Arnold-Chiari malformation have been described. Fusion of cervical vertebrae and fusion of the atlas to the occiput may occur in up to one third of cases. More caudally, the spine may exhibit spina bifida; hemivertebrae; butterfly, fused, or hypoplastic vertebrae; scoliosis; and rib anomalies. Congenital heart disease is reported with structural defects including ventricular septal defects, tetralogy of Fallot, transposition of the great vessels, aortic coarctation, pulmonic stenosis, and dextrocardia. External carotid artery hypoplasia is an interesting vascular anomaly found in some patients, perhaps reflective of more cephalic developmental defects. Other less frequently encountered systemic anomalies have been identified that include pulmonary parenchymal dysplasia, tracheoesophageal fistula, renal abnormalities, and imperforate anus.

The Mandible

Isolated mandibular malformations are more rare, with the exception of the Pierre Robin sequence (PRS). PRS is not a syndrome; rather, it is a sequence defined as a constellation of findings that result from a single gestational misfortune that leads to subsequent developmental sequelae. It may appear as an entity alone or in association with other syndromes.

Pierre Robin Sequence

The tendency of the tongue to fall back into the upper airway of newborns causing respiratory distress and cyanosis was termed *glossoptosis* by Pierre Robin in a cohort of infants in 1923. Since then, an appreciation and understanding of what is now accepted as the Pierre Robin sequence have evolved (Fig. 22-17). Recognized as a triad of micrognathia, glossoptosis, and palatal clefting, PRS is a developmental anomaly that may significantly threaten the newborn. Prolonged hypoxia, respiratory failure, feeding problems, aspiration pneumonia, failure to thrive, and death may all result if appropriate, expedient interventions are not executed.

The Pierre Robin sequence evolves due to abnormally hypoplastic development of the mandible between weeks 7 to 11 of gestation. As a result, the tongue is positioned high within the nasopharynx resting against the cranial base, unable to drop lower due to mandibular position. As the palatal shelves initiate medial growth, the malpositioned tongue physically obstructing their union impedes midline fusion. A U-shaped palatal cleft results. At birth the newborn as an obligate nose breather frequently suffers upper airway obstruction from a tongue that, though of normal size, easily falls back into the nasopharynx, especially when the infant is positioned supine.

The origin of mandibular hypoplasia in these infants is felt to be heterogeneous. Intrauterine positional deformation in which the head is flexed with the chin resting on the chest preventing appropriate growth is one hypothe-

sis. A second hypothesis is that mandibular hypoplasia occurs intrinsic to a coexisting malformation syndrome, such as Stickler syndrome. Neuromuscular anomalies have also been proposed as reasons preventing normal intrauterine mandibular movement in the developing fetus and thereby initiating the sequence. Unifying all of these events is the resultant abnormally small mandible, setting the stage for the evolution of findings identified as PRS. For this reason, PRS is not regarded as a specific disease entity. Although more commonly an isolated, nonsyndromically associated sequence, PRS is diagnosed in association with recognizable syndromes in 25% to 40% of cases.

Pierre Robin sequence may occur as frequently as 1 in 2000 live births, with reported mortalities ranging from 19% to 65%. Most mortality is attributed to respiratory failure secondary to upper airway obstruction. As such, the pediatrician who evaluates the infant at delivery must be prepared for all eventualities. It is prudent to advise the parents of potential respiratory difficulties that the infant may experience in the ensuing weeks. Because PRS may be a component of a yet undefined syndrome, it is best to avoid premature labeling at the time of delivery. Identification of the newborn as experiencing respiratory distress is crucial for timely management. As an obligate nose breather, the infant will have little tolerance for obstruction of the upper airway. Micrognathia narrows the nasopharynx, leading to an increase in airway resistance for which the infant attempts to compensate by recruiting accessory muscles of respiration. Substernal and intercostal retractions become evident as a component of the respiratory pattern. As more negative pressure is generated, the tongue may be further pulled into the pharynx, exacerbating the airway obstruction. Noisy breathing and stridor are audible evidence of the at-risk airway. Infants observed to be in distress might improve with prone positioning. Although prone positioning is rarely a definitive measure, it should be tried because it may make the infant more comfortable by allowing the tongue to drop anteriorly, at least partially relieving the obstruction. Pulse oximetry, blood gas monitoring, and polysomnographic studies are recommended in the early phases of management to assess efficiency of respiration. If the infant continues to exhibit signs of respiratory distress or presents with frank apnea, intubation is indicated to ensure a secure airway. Should anatomy preclude successful endo-

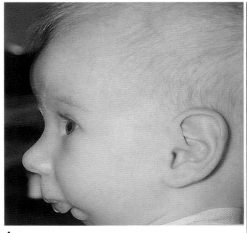

A

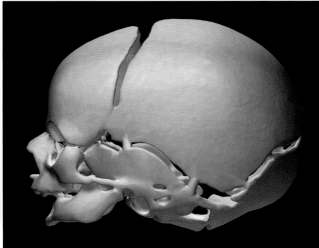

B

Figure 22-17. Pierre Robin sequence. **A,** Lateral view of a child with Pierre Robin sequence, characterized by severe micrognathia and cleft palate. **B,** Lateral view of the craniofacial skeleton of a child with Pierre Robin sequence. Note the small, retruded mandible. (**A,** Courtesy Wolfgang Losken, MD.)

tracheal intubation, an emergent tracheostomy should be performed. This, however, is rarely necessary.

Protection of airway patency is obviously of great concern. Several techniques have been used to ensure adequate ventilation and oxygenation, some of which have fallen in and out of favor. The tongue lip adhesion (TLA) or glossopexy, in which the tongue is sutured to the lower lip, displacing it out of the nasopharynx, has been abandoned by many due to dehiscence and frequent need for reoperation at the time of last publication of this atlas. Since then, however, it has gained favor in several institutions with refinements in technique that involve a dual musculomucosal adhesion. With this innovation, dehiscence rates have dropped convincingly, making it an appealing alternative to tracheostomy if conservative methods have failed in airway management. Further, graduation from nasogastric tube feedings to oral feedings in infants with TLA occurred in up to 75% of infants requiring the procedure. At the time of palatal repair, usually around 9 to 12 months of age, the adhesion is taken down. This coincides nicely with the amount of time necessary for infant mandibular growth to overcome its contribution to airway compromise. Should a TLA fail to alleviate airway obstruction, either distraction of the mandible or a tracheostomy is indicated. Distraction of the mandible involves making bilateral osteotomies in the infant mandible and gradually pulling it to length as new bone is laid down in the intervening space. It can be performed fairly rapidly, and some centers report good success. Tracheostomy bypasses the obstructed nasopharynx and should be the procedure of last resort. The frequency with which tracheostomy is currently performed varies among centers. As the morbidity and complications associated with tracheostomy are not insignificant in the first year of life, its indications deserve careful consideration.

Due to respiratory insufficiency, up to 55% of infants with PRS may experience feeding difficulties. Those with significant hypoxemia with feedings or inadequate caloric intake require gavage feeding. Gastrostomy tube placement is rarely necessary, usually only in cases associated with syndromic central nervous system involvement.

Outcomes for children with PRS vary. Advances in monitoring have led to improved outcomes, and generally children do well. Strategies for initial and long-term management continue to evolve, though. As such, care plans that foster optimal outcomes for these children should be individually developed.

Summary

Clefting and craniofacial syndromes represent a number of interesting and at times challenging medical and surgical entities that fortunately afflict a relatively small number of newborns. Medical science has only recently begun to delineate why these developmental anomalies occur and unfortunately may have little to offer in the way of intervention owing to the early occurrence of the developmental miscues. The impact on those affected and their families can be devastating. Encouragingly, early thorough evaluations and appropriate interventions can significantly benefit the lives of these children. Many health care providers are pivotal to the success of these endeavors. Indeed, multidisciplinary teams consisting of pediatric specialists, otologists, reconstructive surgeons, dietitians, and therapists convincingly optimize the outcomes for these children and should be enlisted where available.

Bibliography

Ades LC, Mulley JC, Senga LP, et al: Jackson-Weiss syndrome: Clinical and radiographical findings in a large kindred and exclusion of the gene from 7p21 and 5qter. Am J Med Genet 51:121-130, 1994.

Aleck K: Craniosynostosis syndromes in the genomic era. Semin Pediatr Neurol 11:256-261, 2004.

Cohen MM, Kreiborg S: An updated pediatric perspective on the Apert syndrome. Am J Dis Child 147:989-993, 1993.

Cohen MM Jr, Rollnick BR, Kaye CI: Oculoauriculovertebral spectrum: An updated critique. Cleft Palate J 26:276-286, 1989.

Danziger I, Brodsky L, Perry R, et al: Nager's acrofacial dysostosis: Case report and review of the literature. Int J Pediatr Otorhinolaryngol 20:225-240, 1990.

Gorlin RJ: Fibroblast growth factors, their receptors and receptor disorders. J Cranio-Maxillofac Surg 25:69-79, 1997.

Keating RF: Craniosynostosis: Diagnosis and management in the new millennium. Pediatr Ann 26:600-620, 1997.

Losee JE, Mason AC: Deformational plagiocephaly: Diagnosis, prevention, and treatment. Clin Plastic Surg 32:53-64, 2005.

Ocampo RV, Persing JA: Sagittal synostosis. Clin Plastic Surg 21:563-574, 1994.

Posnick JC: Treacher Collins syndrome: Perspectives in evaluation and treatment. J Oral Maxillofac Surg 55:1120-1133, 1997.

Posnick JC: Unilateral coronal synostosis (anterior plagiocephaly): Current clinical perspectives. Ann Plast Surg 36:430-447, 1996.

Prevel CD, Eppley BL, McCarty M: Acrocephalosyndactyly syndromes: A review. J Craniofac Surg 8:279-285, 1997.

Singer L, Sidoti EJ: Pediatric management of Robin sequence. Cleft Palate Craniofac J 29:220-223, 1992.

Wilkie AOM, Wall SA: Craniosynostosis: Novel insights into pathogenesis and treatment. Curr Opin Neurol 9:146-152, 1996.

CHAPTER 23

Otolaryngology

Robert F. Yellon, Timothy P. McBride, and Holly W. Davis

The importance of pediatricians and family physicians having an understanding of and experience with otolaryngologic problems and being skilled in techniques of examination of the head and neck region cannot be overemphasized. One study revealed that more than one third of all visits to pediatricians' offices were prompted by ear symptoms. When nasal and oral symptoms are included, ear, nose, and throat pathology accounts for more than 50% of all visits. With patience and proper equipment, pediatricians can complete a thorough examination on almost all children. If a disorder fails to respond to therapy or becomes chronic or recurrent, or if an unusual problem is encountered, then consultation with a pediatric otolaryngologist should be sought.

Successful examination of the ears, nose, and oropharynx of a young child can present some challenges, especially with older infants and toddlers, who fail to appreciate the need for (and thus often vigorously resist) examination. This can be a particular problem in children who have had previous bad experiences. Patience, warmth, humor, and careful explanation on the part of the examiner help reduce fear and enhance cooperation.

Whenever possible, the child should be allowed to sit on the parent's lap. Pacifiers, puppets and other toys, and tongue blades with faces drawn on them can all serve to reduce anxiety, enlist the child's trust, and distract attention. Gradual introduction of the equipment can also be helpful, especially if done in a playful way. The child can be asked to blow out the otoscope light while the examiner turns it off, urged to catch the light spot as the examiner moves it around, and even allowed to look in the parent's or examiner's ears (Fig. 23-1A to D). Parents can also help demonstrate maneuvers for opening the mouth, panting to depress the tongue, and holding the head back. Although this may take a little additional time at the outset, it often saves considerable time in the long run and makes future follow-up examinations far easier.

Ear Disorders

Ear pain (otalgia), discharge from the ear (otorrhea), and suspected hearing loss are three of the more common and specific otic symptoms for which parents seek medical attention for their children. Less specific symptoms such as pulling or tugging at the ears, fussiness, and fever are also frequently encountered, particularly in children younger than 2 years of age.

History should center on the nature and duration of symptoms, character of the clinical course, and possible antecedent treatment. Because many infections of the ear are recurrent and/or chronic, the parent should be asked about previous medical or surgical therapy (e.g., antibiotics, myringotomy, tube insertion).

A brief review of the anatomy of the ear is helpful in developing a logical approach to any clinical abnormalities that may be encountered. The ear is conveniently divided into the following three regions (Fig. 23-2):

1. The ***external ear*** includes the pinna, or auricle, and the external auditory canal, up to and including the tympanic membrane.
2. The ***middle ear*** is made up of the middle ear space, the inner surface of the eardrum, the ossicles, and the mastoid.
3. The ***inner ear*** comprises the cochlea (hearing), the labyrinth and semicircular canals (balance), and the main nerve trunks of the seventh and eighth cranial nerves.

The examination should include inspection of the auricle, periauricular tissues, and external auditory canal and visualization of the entire tympanic membrane including assessment of its mobility in response to positive and negative pressure. This often necessitates clearing the canal of cerumen or discharge by using a curette, cotton wick, lavage, or suction (Fig. 23-3A and B). Use of a surgical otoscope head or an examining microscope assists visualization during the cleaning process. These procedures should be performed carefully and gently and attempted only after the child has been carefully immobilized to avoid trauma (Fig. 23-4). It is extraordinarily easy to injure the canal during the process of cleaning the external ear. Hence great care must be taken; otherwise bleeding from the ensuing trauma obscures the examination and upsets the patient and parent. Both the patient and parent should be given a clear explanation of the procedure beforehand. Allowing older children to handle and look through the equipment before cleaning the ear reduces anxiety and enhances cooperation (see Fig. 23-3C).

Because the external auditory canal is often angulated in infants and young children, gentle lateral traction on the pinna is frequently necessary to assist visualization of the eardrum itself (Fig. 23-5). In infancy the tympanic membrane tends to be oriented at a greater angle (Fig. 23-6A and B); the landmarks are less prominent; and the skin that lines the canal, being loosely attached, moves readily on insufflation of air, simulating a normally mobile eardrum. To avoid confusion, the canal should be inspected as the speculum is inserted to ensure that the transition between canal wall and tympanic membrane is visualized.

The pneumatic otoscope is the most valuable diagnostic tool when signs or symptoms of otitis media are present. Pediatricians, family practitioners, and otolaryngologists who treat children should be skilled in its use. Practical advice on the use of this instrument is as follows:

1. Use adequate light. A bright halogen lamp is better than an ordinary light bulb. Replace bulbs routinely every 4 to 6 months, and provide for routine battery charging.
2. Choose a speculum of sufficient size to allow adequate penetration (10 to 15 mm) into the external canal for good eardrum visualization.
3. Restrain the patient (on the parent's lap or on the examining table).
4. Brace the hand holding the otoscope on the child's head to avoid ear canal trauma.

When otoscopic findings are unclear or it is difficult to obtain a good air seal for pneumatic otoscopy, tympanometry can be highly useful in evaluating patients older than 8 months of age (Fig. 23-7). The procedure is not of value in young infants because the abundance of loose connective tissue lining the ear canal and the laxity of the cartilage at the entrance increase canal wall compliance and invalidate the results.

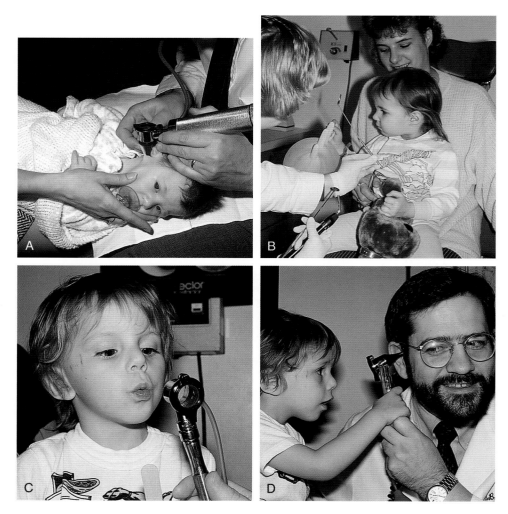

Figure 23-1. Techniques to assist examination of a child's ears, nose, and oropharynx. **A,** Young infants often can be examined on their mother's lap, with gentle immobilization provided by the parent and the examiner's hand. **B,** Having a toddler or preschooler sit on the mother's lap and using puppets, other toys, and tongue blades with faces drawn on them while gradually introducing the examining instruments reduce anxiety and enlist cooperation. **C** and **D,** Making a game of blowing out the otoscope light and allowing the patient to check the examiner first convey that otoscopy does not have to hurt.

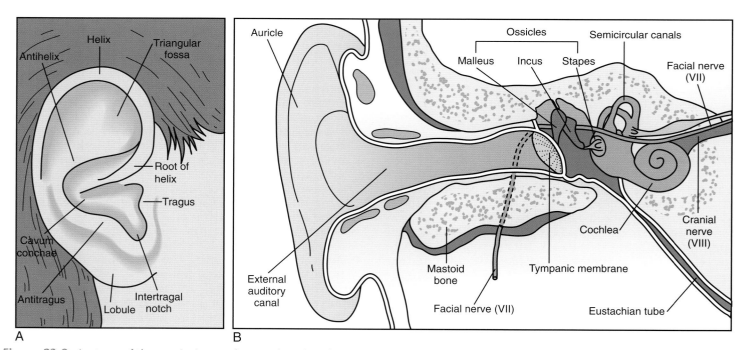

Figure 23-2. Anatomy of the ear. **A,** A normal external ear (auricle or pinna) is shown, with its various landmarks labeled. It is helpful to refer to such a diagram in assessing congenital anomalies. **B,** This coronal section shows the various structures of the hearing and vestibular apparatus. The three main regions are the external ear, middle ear, and inner ear. The eustachian tube connects the middle ear and the nasopharynx and serves to drain and ventilate the middle ear.

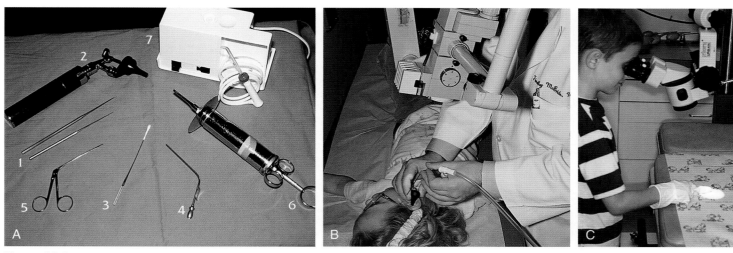

Figure 23-3. **A,** Equipment for cleaning the external auditory canal. The curette *(1)* is the implement most commonly used to remove cerumen. Use of a surgical otoscope head *(2)* makes the process considerably easier. Additional implements include cotton wicks *(3)* and a suction tip *(4)* for removal of discharge or moist wax, alligator forceps *(5)* for removing foreign bodies, and an ear syringe *(6)* and motorized irrigation apparatus *(7)* for removing firm objects or impacted cerumen. Lavage is contraindicated when there is a possible perforation of the tympanic membrane. If the motorized apparatus is used for irrigation, it must be kept on the lowest power setting to avoid traumatizing the eardrum. **B,** Use of suction is often necessary when there is copious exudate. **C,** Allowing the child to look through the examining microscope may help him or her cooperate with the examination.

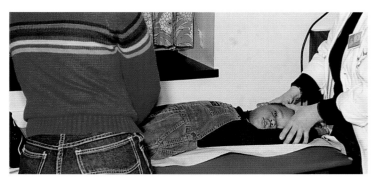

Figure 23-4. Method of immobilization for cleaning. An assistant holds the child's arms and simultaneously immobilizes the child's head with the thumbs. The parent firmly holds the hips and thighs. This prevents motion by the child during cleaning of the ear canal and is also useful for otoscopy in young children.

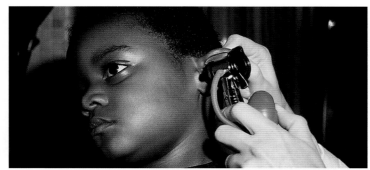

Figure 23-5. Because the external auditory canal usually is angulated in children, lateral traction on the pinna is often required to straighten the canal and improve visualization of the tympanic membrane.

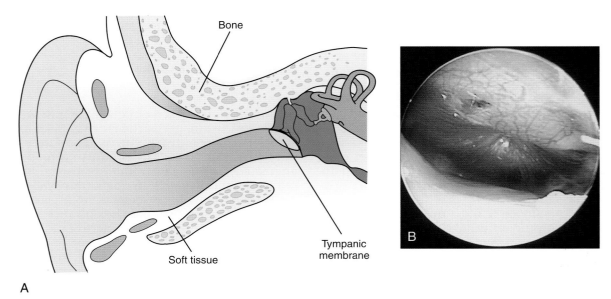

Bone

Soft tissue

Tympanic membrane

A

Figure 23-6. Angulation of the tympanic membrane in infancy. **A,** The relationship between the ear canal and eardrum is different in the infant, with the drum being tilted at an angle of 130 degrees. **B,** Greater care is required in examining an infant's eardrum because of this angulation and because the landmarks are less prominent.

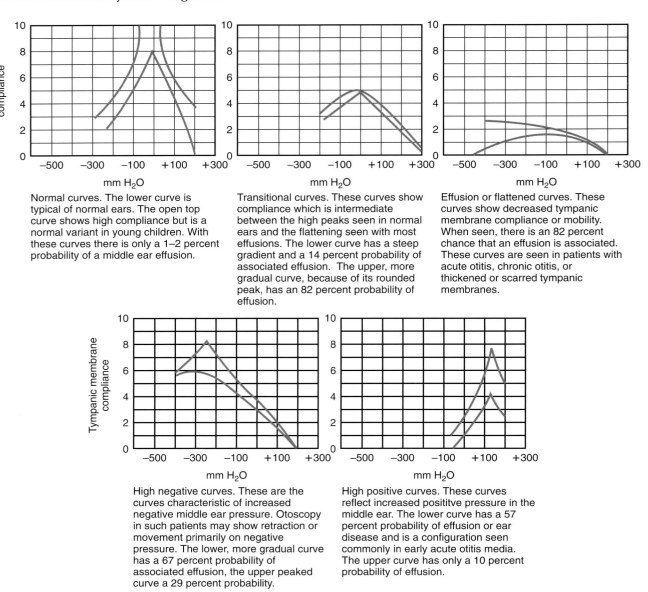

Normal curves. The lower curve is typical of normal ears. The open top curve shows high compliance but is a normal variant in young children. With these curves there is only a 1–2 percent probability of a middle ear effusion.

Transitional curves. These curves show compliance which is intermediate between the high peaks seen in normal ears and the flattening seen with most effusions. The lower curve has a steep gradient and a 14 percent probability of associated effusion. The upper, more gradual curve, because of its rounded peak, has an 82 percent probability of effusion.

Effusion or flattened curves. These curves show decreased tympanic membrane compliance or mobility. When seen, there is an 82 percent chance that an effusion is associated. These curves are seen in patients with acute otitis, chronic otitis, or thickened or scarred tympanic membranes.

High negative curves. These are the curves characteristic of increased negative middle ear pressure. Otoscopy in such patients may show retraction or movement primarily on negative pressure. The lower, more gradual curve has a 67 percent probability of associated effusion, the upper peaked curve a 29 percent probability.

High positive curves. These curves reflect increased positive pressure in the middle ear. The lower curve has a 57 percent probability of effusion or ear disease and is a configuration seen commonly in early acute otitis media. The upper curve has only a 10 percent probability of effusion.

Figure 23-7. Tympanometric patterns of various conditions of the middle ear. (Courtesy Mrs. Ruth Bachman, Pittsburgh, Pa.)

Because otitis media can be a reflection of both immunologic and anatomic abnormalities, the practitioner should be suspicious of possible underlying immune or temporal bone defects when seeing patients with chronic or frequently recurrent otitis media. The temporal bone is the bony housing for the auditory and vestibular systems. In addition, it provides bony protection for the facial nerve as it crosses from the brainstem to the facial muscles. The growth and development of this bone are affected in syndromes such as Treacher Collins that are characterized by altered midface growth (Fig. 23-8). The soft tissues attached to the temporal bone, such as the muscles controlling eustachian tube function, can be abnormal in children with cleft palates (see section "Palatal Disorders"). As a result, children with these disorders tend to have an increased incidence of otitis media.

Children with chronic effusions who complain of hearing loss, those whose parents complain that they do not listen, those with speech delays, or those with suspected congenital malformations must have their hearing evaluated by audiometry, evoked otoacoustic emissions, or brainstem evoked potentials. Patients with vertigo and/or problems of balance and those with facial weakness or asymmetry warrant testing of both hearing *and* vestibular

function. These children, and those suffering from malformations, may require CT, MRI, or genetic studies in select cases to clarify the nature of the problem.

Disorders of the External Ear

The Four "D"s

Examination of each child's ear begins with inspection of the auricle and periauricular tissues for four important signs—discharge, displacement, discoloration, and deformity (the four "D"s). The canal is normally smooth and angulated slightly in an anterior direction. Cerumen is often present; it varies in color from yellowish-white to tan to dark brown. It is secreted from glands interspersed among the hair follicles at the entrance to the ear canal, and it may have some bacteriostatic activity. When cerumen obstructs the view, it must be removed to allow adequate visualization of the canal and tympanic membrane. When soft and moist, cerumen is easily removed with a curette. Removal may be more difficult if the cerumen is dry and flaky and may require removal with alligator forceps or, at times, instillation of drops. In some children, cerumen solidifies or has been packed in with

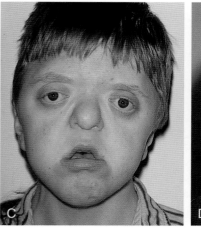
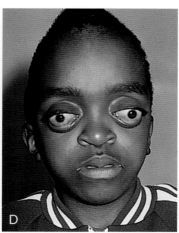
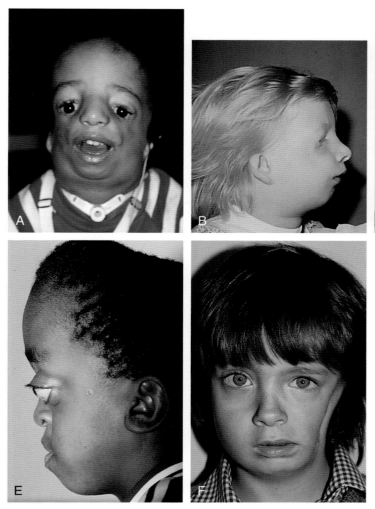

Figure 23-8. Syndromes affecting the growth of the temporal bone and midface that predispose patients to recurrent or chronic otitis media and chronic recurrent sinus infections. **A** and **B,** Treacher Collins syndrome. Note the maxillary hypoplasia, micrognathia, and auricular deformity. **C,** Apert syndrome. **D** and **E,** Crouzon syndrome. Both are characterized by severe maxillary and midfacial hypoplasia. **F,** Hemifacial microsomia with unilateral hypoplasia. (**B** to **F,** Courtesy Wolfgang Loskin, MD, University of North Carolina, Chapel Hill.)

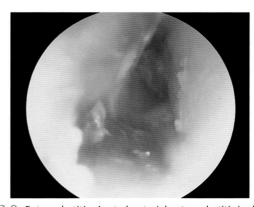

Figure 23-9. External otitis. Acute bacterial external otitis is characterized by intense pain that is worsened by traction on the pinna, along with purulent exudate and intense canal wall inflammation.

cotton-tipped applicators, forming a firm plug that impedes sound conduction and requires softening for removal. Irrigation is contraindicated if there is any possibility that the eardrum may not be intact.

Discharge. Discharge is a common complaint with a number of possible causes. When there is thick, white discharge and erythema of the canal wall, the physician should gently pull on the pinna. If this maneuver elicits pain and the canal wall is edematous, primary otitis externa is the likely diagnosis (Fig. 23-9), although prolonged drainage from untreated otitis media with perforation may present a similar picture (see "Disorders of the Middle Ear" later). When the middle ear is the source of

otic discharge, the tympanic membrane is abnormal and should show evidence of perforation (see Fig. 23-27). The major predisposing condition to primary otitis externa is prolonged presence of excessive moisture in the ear canal, which promotes bacterial or fungal overgrowth. Thus this is a common problem in swimmers. Another major source is the presence of a foreign body in the ear canal (see Fig. 23-19), which stimulates an intense inflammatory response and production of a foul-smelling purulent discharge. Thus when otic drainage is encountered, the discharge must be gently removed under appropriate magnification to assess the condition of the tympanic membrane and rule out the presence of foreign objects. This can be accomplished either by gentle siphoning and wiping with cotton wicks or by careful suctioning (see Fig. 23-3).

If the history indicates that the drainage is persistent or recurrent despite therapy, a culture should be obtained to determine both the causative organism and its sensitivity to antimicrobial agents. Treatment consists primarily of topical otic antimicrobial/steroid preparations. Systemic antibiotics should be given when pain is severe; when there is evidence of otitis media; or when, despite attempts at cleaning, there is still uncertainty about an infection of the middle ear. Parenteral antibiotics may be required when the process has extended, producing cellulitis of the periauricular soft tissues.

Displacement. Displacement of the pinna away from the skull is a worrisome sign. The most severe condition causing displacement is mastoiditis, resulting from extension of a middle ear infection through the mastoid air cells and out to the periosteum of the skull. In addition

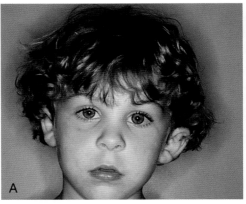
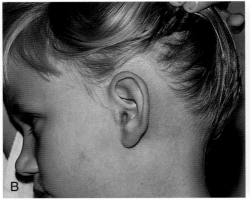
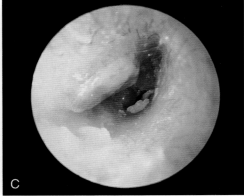

Figure 23-10. Mastoiditis. **A,** This frontal photograph clearly shows the left auricle displaced anteriorly and inferiorly. **B,** In another patient, viewed from the side, erythema can be appreciated over the mastoid process. **C,** On otoscopy, erythema and edema of the canal wall are evident and the postero-superior portion of the canal wall sags inferiorly. (**C,** Courtesy Michael Hawke, MD.)

to displacement, important clinical signs of mastoiditis include erythema and edema of the pinna and the skin overlying the mastoid, exquisite tenderness on palpation of the mastoid process, a sagging ear canal, purulent otorrhea, fever, and usually toxicity (Fig. 23-10). This condition is now considered unusual and is seen mainly in patients with long-standing, untreated, or inadequately treated otitis media. Recognition, prompt institution of parenteral antibiotic therapy, and myringotomy are crucial because there is significant risk of central nervous system (CNS) extension. Radiographs show haziness of the mastoid air cells; a CT scan helps delineate the extent of involvement and assists the surgical approach (Fig. 23-11). Mastoidectomy is indicated in cases complicated by bone erosion, or CNS extension, and in those in which intravenous (IV) antibiotics and myringotomy fail to produce complete resolution.

Other conditions characterized by displacement of the pinna away from the head include parotitis, primary cellulitis of periauricular tissues, and edema secondary to insect bites or contact dermatitis. Parotitis is differentiated by finding prominent induration and enlargement of the parotid gland anterior and inferior to the external ear, together with blunting of the angle of the mandible on palpation (see Figs. 12-25 and 12-26). Primary cellulitis is characterized by erythema and tenderness but can often be distinguished clinically from mastoiditis by the presence of associated skin lesions that antecede the inflammation (Fig. 23-12). In cases secondary to untreated external otitis or otitis media with perforation, the picture may be clinically similar. Localized contact dermatitis and angioedema may be erythematous, but they are also pruritic and nontender. The former condition is characterized by microvesicular skin changes (Fig. 23-13), whereas in the latter condition, a precipitating insect bite can often be identified on inspection (Fig. 23-14).

Discoloration. Discoloration is another important sign and is commonly a feature of conditions producing displacement. Erythema of the pinna is common when there is inflammation, with or without infection (see Figs. 23-10B and 23-12 to 23-14). Ecchymotic discoloration may be encountered with trauma. When this overlies the mastoid tip, the area immediately posterior to the pinna, it is termed a *Battle sign* (Fig. 23-15A) and usually reflects a basilar skull fracture. In such cases the canal wall should be checked for tears and the tympanic membrane for perforation or a hemotympanum (blood behind the tympanic membrane) (see Fig. 23-15B). These findings are generally more helpful in making the diagnosis than

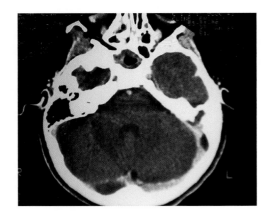

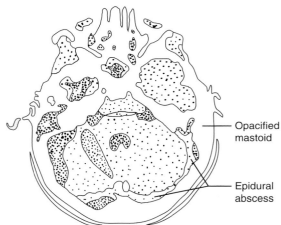

Figure 23-11. Mastoiditis. The CT image shows acute left-sided mastoiditis with the complication of an associated epidural abscess delineated in the diagram.

routine skull x-rays, which are often inconclusive. CT can usually confirm the diagnosis of a basilar skull fracture. Recognition that bruising of the pinna and/or postauricular area can be a manifestation of child abuse is most important (see Chapter 6).

Deformity. When the external ear is grossly misshapen or microtic, associated anomalies of middle ear and inner ear structures are common and hearing loss may be significant (Fig. 23-16). Severe deformities stem from developmental anomalies of the branchial arches, which contribute to both external ear and middle ear structures. Such abnormalities warrant a thorough evaluation in infancy to ensure early recognition and treatment of hearing loss. Deformity of the pinna can be the result of

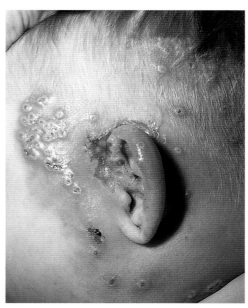

Figure 23-12. Periauricular and auricular cellulitis. This infant had mild postauricular seborrhea and developed varicella. The vesicular varicella lesions that clustered at sites of prior skin irritation became secondarily infected with group A β-streptococci, resulting in cellulitis with intense erythema, edema, and tenderness of the auricle and periauricular tissues. In this case the external canal was normal. (Courtesy Ronald Chludzinski, MD.)

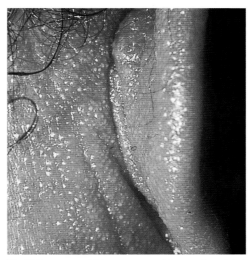

Figure 23-13. This young girl became sensitive to the nickel posts of her earrings and developed periauricular contact dermatitis. The auricle and periauricular skin are erythematous and covered by a weeping, pruritic microvesicular eruption. (Courtesy Michael Sherlock, MD, Lutherville, Md.)

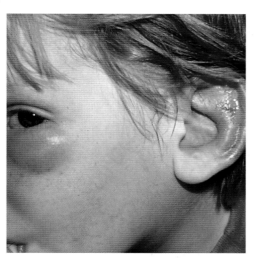

Figure 23-14. Angioedema. This youngster had pruritic, nonpainful, non-tender erythema and swelling of his ear and infraorbital region. Close examination of the latter revealed the punctum of an insect bite. Another punctum on his ear was obscured by crusting following scratching. (Courtesy Michael Sherlock, MD, Lutherville, Md.)

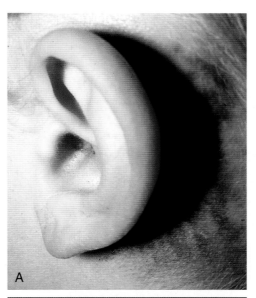

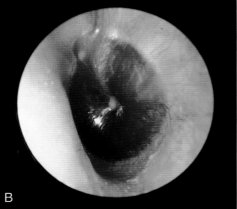

Figure 23-15. Basilar skull fracture. **A,** The presence of a basilar skull fracture involving the temporal bone is often signaled by postauricular ecchymotic discoloration, termed the *Battle sign.* **B,** The force of the blow may also cause tearing of the ear canal or, as shown here, middle ear hemorrhage with hemotympanum. Depending on timing of examination, this may appear red or blue. (**B,** Courtesy Michael Hawke, MD.)

hereditary factors or exposure to teratogens, but at times it is simply produced by unusual intrauterine positioning. Most deformities are minor. In some instances they may be part of a picture of multiple congenital anomalies (Fig. 23-17A to C; see also Fig. 23-8 and Chapter 1), but in most cases they represent isolated, minor malformations that are of little significance other than cosmetic (Fig. 23-17D).

Preauricular sinuses and cysts constitute two of the more common congenital abnormalities. These are congenital remnants located anterior to the pinna with an overlying surface dimple (Fig. 23-18A). These cysts are vulnerable to infection and abscess formation (Fig. 23-18B), which necessitates incision and drainage in conjunction with antistaphylococcal antibiotics. Once infection has occurred, recurrence is common unless the entire cyst is completely excised. This procedure should be undertaken once inflammation has subsided.

Foreign Objects and Secondary Trauma

It is not unusual for children to put paper, beads, and other foreign objects into their ear canals (Fig. 23-19A). Small insects also on occasion may become trapped in the external ear (see Fig. 23-19B). In some cases small objects may be embedded in cerumen and missed on inspection.

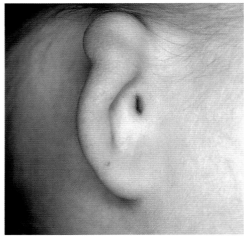

Figure 23-16. Microtia and atresia of the right external ear. In this otherwise normal child, the pinna failed to develop properly and the external canal was atretic. Audiometric testing revealed a 60-dB hearing loss. Such isolated deformities stem from abnormal development of the first and second branchial arches.

As noted earlier, if present for more than a few days, the foreign material stimulates an inflammatory response and production of a purulent discharge that is often foul-smelling and may obscure the presence of the inciting foreign body. Removal of some objects can be accomplished by use of alligator forceps or by irrigation of the ear canal; others—particularly spherical objects—require use of a Day (right angle) hook or suction (Fig. 23-19C; see also Fig. 23-3). Foreign objects may also be the source of painful abrasions or lacerations of the external auditory canal or even perforation of the tympanic membrane. Insertion of pencils or sticks into the ear canal by the child and parental attempts to clean the canal with a cotton swab are the most common modes of such injury.

Exposure to concussive forces such as a direct blow (which may be accidental or inflicted) or an explosion can also result in perforation (Fig. 23-20A and B). Patients with traumatic perforations must be carefully assessed for signs of injury to deeper structures. If tympanic membrane perforation occurs as a result of penetration by a foreign object or of concussive forces, the physician must be particularly aware of the possibility of middle ear or inner ear damage. Evidence of hearing loss, vertigo, nystagmus, facial nerve injury, or cerebrospinal fluid leak should prompt urgent otolaryngologic consultation because an emergent surgical exploration may be indicated.

Disorders of the Middle Ear

The normal tympanic membrane is thin, translucent, neutrally positioned, and mobile. The ossicles, particu-

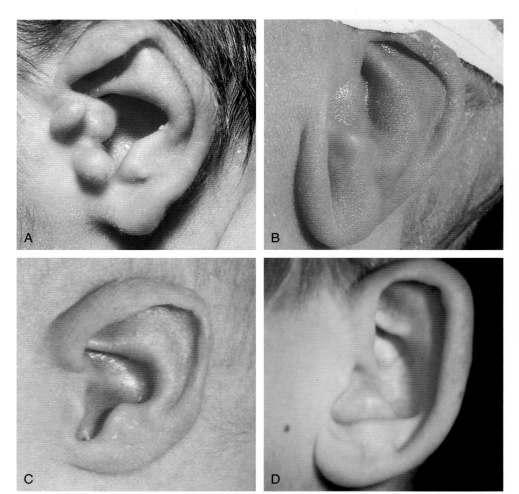

Figure 23-17. Minor congenital auricular deformities. **A,** In this infant the superior portion of the helix is folded over, obscuring the triangular fossa; the antihelix is sharply angulated; and there are three preauricular skin tags. **B,** This neonate with orofaciodigital and Turner syndromes has a simple helix and a redundant folded lobule. The ear is low set and posteriorly rotated, and the antitragus is anteriorly displaced. **C,** This infant with Rubinstein-Taybi syndrome has an exaggerated elongated intertragal notch. **D,** Lop ear in an otherwise normal child. The auricular cartilage is abnormally contoured, making the ear protrude forward. (**C,** Courtesy Michael Sherlock, MD, Lutherville, Md.)

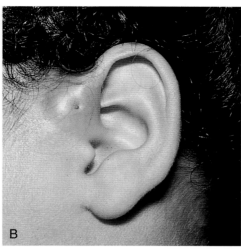

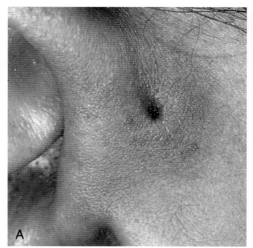

Figure 23-18. Preauricular sinuses. **A,** These branchial cleft remnants are located anterior to the pinna and have an overlying surface dimple. **B,** In this child the sinus has become infected, forming an abscess. (**A,** Courtesy Michael Hawke, MD.)

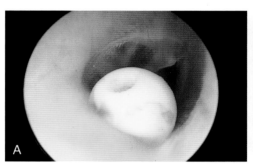

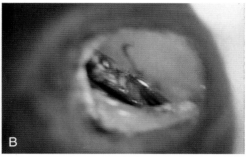

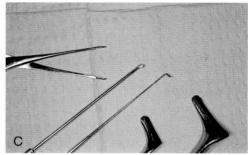

Figure 23-19. Otic foreign bodies. **A,** This child inserted a bead into her ear. The object must be removed carefully to prevent further trauma. **B,** This patient experienced a period of intense buzzing, pain, and itching in the ear that abated after a few hours. If the tympanic membrane is intact, olive or mineral oil may be used to drown the insect. **C,** A blunt-tipped, right-angled Day hook, small wire loop curette, Hartmann forceps, and an alligator forceps (and see Fig. 23-3A) are useful instruments for removing foreign bodies from the external auditory canal.

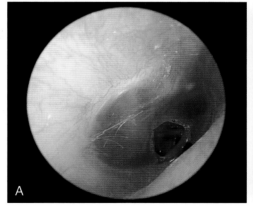

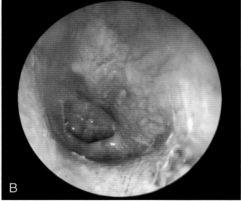

Figure 23-20. Traumatic perforations of the tympanic membrane. **A,** This 8-year-old boy's tympanic membrane was perforated by a forceful slap on the ear. **B,** Even more severe damage with thickening and hemorrhage is seen in this victim of a blast injury caused by an explosion. (**A,** Courtesy Michael Hawke, MD.)

larly the malleus, are generally visible through the membrane (Fig. 23-21). Adequate assessment of the tympanic membrane requires that the examiner note four major characteristics: (1) thickness, (2) degree of translucence, (3) position relative to neutral, and (4) mobility. Application of gentle positive and negative pressure using a properly sealed pneumatic otoscope (Fig. 23-22) produces brisk movement of the eardrum when the ear is free of disease and abnormal movement when fluid is present, when the drum is thickened or scarred, or when there is an increase in either positive or negative pressure (Fig. 23-23). An abnormality in any one of the four major characteristics suggests middle ear pathology.

Acute Otitis Media

Acute otitis media is the term used to describe acute infection and inflammation of the middle ear. Associated inflammation and edema of the eustachian tube mucosa appear to play key roles in the pathogenesis by impeding drainage of the middle ear fluid. In some children, anatomic or chronic physiologic abnormalities of the eustachian tube predispose to infection. The problem is commonly seen in conjunction with an acute upper respiratory tract infection, and its onset is often heralded by a secondary temperature spike one to several days after the onset of respiratory symptoms. The major offending organisms are bacterial respiratory pathogens. The most commonly isolated organisms and their relative frequency are shown in Figure 23-24A. Figure 23-24B demonstrates the rise of penicillin-resistant *Streptococcus pneumoniae*. A small proportion of cases constitute an exception to these percentages, that is, those in which otitis is accompanied by conjunctivitis. Nontypable *Haemophilus influenzae* is found to be causative in 70% to 75% of these cases. Increas-

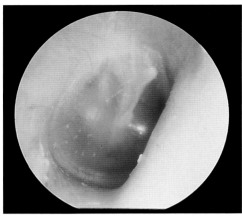

Figure 23-21. A normal tympanic membrane. The drum is thin and translucent, and the ossicles are readily visualized. It is neutrally positioned with no evidence of bulging or retraction. (Courtesy Sylvan Stool, MD.)

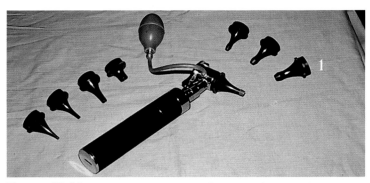

Figure 23-22. Pneumatic otoscopy. This procedure requires proper equipment including a pneumatic otoscope head and an appropriately sized speculum to achieve a good air seal. When a seal is difficult to obtain despite proper speculum size, the head and tubing should be checked for air leaks. If none is found, application of a piece of rubber tubing to the end of the speculum (shown attached to the otoscope) or use of a soft speculum (1) may solve the problem.

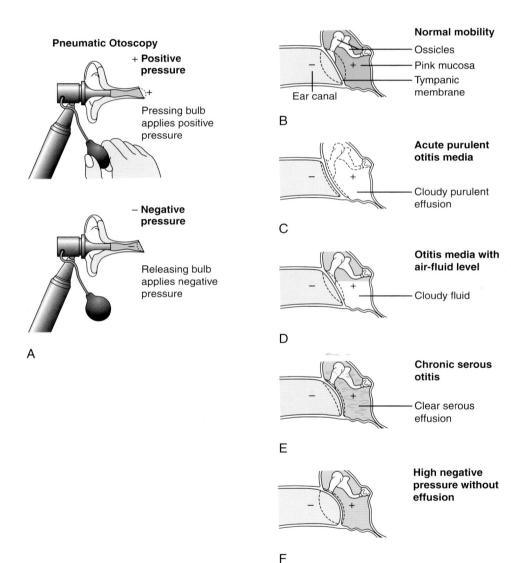

Pneumatic Otoscopy

+ Positive pressure

Pressing bulb applies positive pressure

− Negative pressure

Releasing bulb applies negative pressure

A

Normal mobility

— Ossicles
— Pink mucosa
— Tympanic membrane

Ear canal

B

Acute purulent otitis media

— Cloudy purulent effusion

C

Otitis media with air-fluid level

— Cloudy fluid

D

Chronic serous otitis

— Clear serous effusion

E

High negative pressure without effusion

F

Figure 23-23. Technique and findings in pneumatic otoscopy. **A,** The speculum is inserted into the ear canal to form a tight seal. The bulb is then gently and slowly pressed and released while the mobility of the drum is assessed. Pressing on the bulb applies positive pressure; letting up applies negative pressure. **B,** A normal drum moves inward and then back. **C,** In cases of acute otitis media in which the middle ear is filled with purulent material, the drum bulges toward the examiner and moves minimally. **D,** In cases of acute otitis media with an air-fluid level, mobility may be nearly normal. In some patients, however, the drum may be retracted, indicating increased negative pressure. If this is the case, mobility on positive pressure may be reduced while movement on negative pressure is nearly normal or only mildly decreased. **E,** This is the same pattern as that seen commonly in children with chronic serous otitis. **F,** In cases of high negative pressure and no effusion, application of positive pressure produces little or no movement, but on negative pressure the drum billows back toward the examiner.

ing rates of β-lactamase positivity in these organisms, as well as the rising incidence of penicillin-resistant *S. pneumoniae,* has necessitated use of high-dose amoxicillin and/ or greater use of β-lactamase-resistant antibiotic regimens whenever this syndrome is seen.

In acute otitis media the classic findings on inspection of the tympanic membrane are erythema and injection; bulging that obscures the malleus; thickening, often with a grayish-white or yellow hue, reflecting a purulent effusion; and reduced mobility (Fig. 23-25A). However, crying rapidly produces erythema of the eardrum, and thus erythema in a crying child is of little diagnostic value. The patient is usually febrile and, if old enough, typically complains of otalgia. However, in many cases this "text-

BACTERIOLOGY OF ACUTE
OTITIS MEDIA (AOM)

PENICILLIN-RESISTANT *S. PNEUMONIAE*
United States (1979–1998)

Figure 23-24. Bacterial pathogens in otitis media. **A,** Distribution of pathogens cultured in acute otitis media. **B,** Increasing percentage of isolates of penicillin-resistant *Streptococcus pneumoniae* in otitis media. (**A,** Courtesy Charles Bluestone, MD, Children's Hospital of Pittsburgh; **B,** from Doern GV: Trends in antimicrobial susceptibility of bacterial pathogens of the respiratory tract. Am J Med 99(Suppl):3S-7S, 1995; Jacobs N, Bajaksouzian S, Zilles A, et al: Susceptibility of *Streptococcus pneumoniae* and *Haemophilis influenzae* to ten oral antimicrobial agents based on pharmocodynamic parameters: 1997, US Surveillance Study. Antimicrob Agents Chemother 43:1901-1908, 1999.)

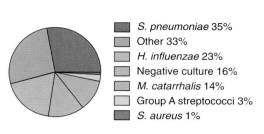
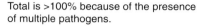

S. pneumoniae 35%
Other 33%
H. influenzae 23%
Negative culture 16%
M. catarrhalis 14%
Group A streptococci 3%
S. aureus 1%

Total is >100% because of the presence of multiple pathogens.

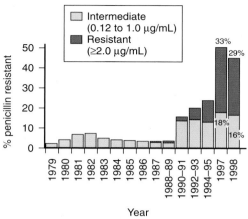

A

B

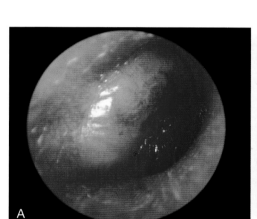
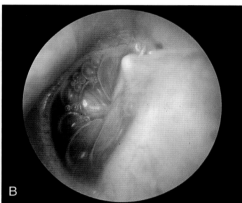
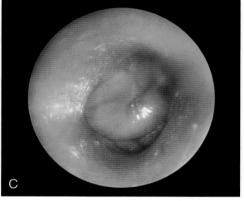

Figure 23-25. Acute otitis media. **A,** This is the textbook picture: an erythematous, opaque, bulging tympanic membrane. The light reflex is reduced, and the landmarks are partially obscured. Mobility is markedly reduced. **B,** In this acutely febrile child who complained of otalgia, the presence of both air and fluid formed bubbles separated by grayish-yellow menisci. Even though the drum was not injected, this finding, combined with fever and otalgia, is consistent with acute infection. **C,** In this child the tympanic membrane was injected at the periphery, and a yellow purulent effusion caused the inferior portion to bulge outward. Mobility was markedly reduced. (**A,** Courtesy Michael Hawke, MD.)

book picture" is not seen. This is probably due in part to time of presentation, the virulence of the particular pathogen, and host factors.

Accuracy in diagnosis necessitates meticulous care during otoscopy and knowledge of the various modes of presentation. Children may have fever of a few hours' duration and otalgia (or if very young, fever and irritability) yet have no abnormality on otoscopy. If reexamined the following day, many of these patients have clear evidence of acute otitis media. Some have erythema and bubbles or air-fluid or air-pus levels (a result of venting by the eustachian tube) without bulging and with nearly normal mobility of the eardrum (see Fig. 23-25B). In still other cases the drum may be full and poorly mobile with cloudy fluid behind it but with minimal erythema (see Fig. 23-25C). In some patients the drum is retracted, moves primarily or only in response to negative pressure, and shows signs of inflammation and/or a cloudy effusion.

Occasionally the signs and symptoms of otitis media may be accompanied by formation of a bullous lesion on the surface of the tympanic membrane, a condition termed *bullous myringitis* (Fig. 23-26). These children usually complain of intense pain. Whereas this phenomenon is most commonly associated with mycoplasmas in adults, any of the usual pediatric pathogens (see Fig. 23-24) can be causative in children. Finally, acute otitis media may, by virtue

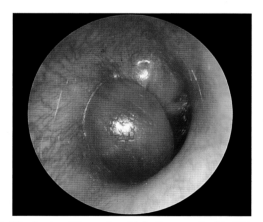

Figure 23-26. Acute otitis media with bullous myringitis. This patient was febrile and extremely uncomfortable. On otoscopy an erythematous bullous lesion is seen obscuring much of the tympanic membrane. This phenomenon, called *bullous myringitis,* is caused by the usual pathogens of otitis media in childhood. The bullous lesion commonly ruptures spontaneously, providing immediate relief of pain.

of increasing middle ear pressure, result in acute perforation of the tympanic membrane. On presentation the canal may be filled with purulent material; however, tugging on the pinna usually does not elicit pain, and erythema and edema of the canal wall are minimal or

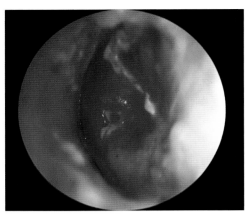

Figure 23-27. Acute otitis media with perforation. In this child, increased middle ear pressure with acute otitis resulted in perforation of the tympanic membrane. The drum is thickened, and the perforation is seen at the 3 o'clock position.

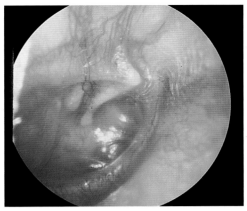

Figure 23-28. Serous otitis media. This patient has a chronic serous middle ear effusion. The tympanic membrane is retracted, thickened, and shiny. Behind it is a clear yellow effusion. Mobility was decreased and primarily evident on negative pressure. The child was not acutely ill but did have decreased hearing. (Courtesy Sylvan Stool, MD.)

absent. Cleansing with a cotton wick or suction usually reveals an inflamed drum with a barely visible perforation (Fig. 23-27).

Just as clinical findings of acute otitis media vary, so do symptoms. Although some patients have severe otalgia, others may complain of sore throat, mild ear discomfort, ear popping, or decreased hearing yet have floridly inflamed eardrums. Fever may be absent.

Radiographic studies are generally of little value in the diagnosis of acute otitis media. When a temporal bone CT scan is obtained in a patient with acute otitis media and fluid in the middle ear, fluid will also be present in the mastoid cavity. This will be interpreted by a radiologist as clouding of the mastoid because it may be difficult to distinguish between the CT findings of acute otitis media and those of acute mastoiditis. In such instances it is important that the physician look at the patient's clinical signs rather than rely on radiographic findings to make the diagnosis.

In addition to treating patients with an appropriate antimicrobial agent and analgesics when necessary, follow-up examination is important. This is best done 2 to 3 weeks after diagnosis, when complete resolution can be expected in more than 50% of children. The purpose of reevaluation is to identify those patients who have persistent serous effusions and require ongoing surveillance. Selected patients with mild, uncomplicated acute otitis media may be observed without antimicrobial therapy, but follow-up examination is still necessary.

Otitis Media with Effusion ("Serous Otitis Media")

Serous effusion in the middle ear may result from an upper respiratory tract infection, or it may be the residual of treated acute otitis. In many instances this effusion is not spontaneously cleared but instead remains in the middle ear for weeks or months, resulting in a persistent clear gray or yellow effusion behind the eardrum (Fig. 23-28). Persistence appears to result in part from eustachian tube dysfunction with poor drainage and ventilation. Pneumatic otoscopy often reveals poor mobility of the tympanic membrane, and mobility is noted primarily on negative pressure. The latter is thought to develop as a result of absorption of middle ear gases by mucosal cells, creating a vacuum that persists with the fluid because of failure of ventilation by the eustachian tube. Such long-standing effusions impair hearing and may be subject to bacterial invasion and thus predispose to recurrent middle ear infection. Persistence of bilateral serous effusions for

more than 3 to 4 months with hearing loss is an indication for myringotomy and insertion of tubes (see Fig. 23-30A and B) to improve hearing and reduce risk of recurrent infection.

Chronic-Recurrent Otitis Media

Chronic or chronic-recurrent otitis media with effusion (COME) is common in young children. Patients subject to this condition appear to have significant and prolonged eustachian tube dysfunction. This "otitis-prone" state may be a seemingly isolated phenomenon, or it can be a feature of a number of syndromes characterized by palatal dysfunction or malformation or by facial hypoplasia or deformity. These conditions include cleft palate, Crouzon syndrome, Down syndrome, the mucopolysaccharidoses and mucolipidoses (see Fig. 23-8, and section "Palatal Disorders"). Chronic obstructive adenoidal hypertrophy may also be a predisposing condition. Less commonly, immunodeficiency and the immotile cilia syndrome are identified as underlying etiologic conditions.

Chronic otitis media is associated with significant morbidity in terms of intermittent or chronic hearing impairment, intermittent discomfort, and the ill effects of recurrent infection. Over months or years, the process produces permanent myringosclerotic changes in which the tympanic membrane becomes whitened, thickened, and scarred (Fig. 23-29A). Chronic perforations are common (Fig. 23-29B). Patients with persistent middle ear infections despite medical therapy, those with frequent recurrences, and children with chronic severe tympanic membrane retraction (Fig. 23-29C) appear to benefit from surgical drainage and insertion of tympanostomy tubes that vent the middle ear (Fig. 23-30). Persistence of a serous effusion for longer than 3 to 4 months with significant hearing loss is also an indication for myringotomy and insertion of tubes. Once placed, tubes should be checked at intervals for presence and patency. Spontaneous extrusion generally occurs 6 to 24 months after insertion. When tubes have been inserted, it is wise to prevent contamination of the middle ear with water. The need for earplugs in children with tubes or a perforation is the subject of some controversy, but in general their use is still recommended.

Protection of the Exposed Middle Ear with Earplugs or Ear Defenders

Earplugs, or ear defenders, come in all shapes and sizes. They vary in cost from inexpensive, premolded earplugs

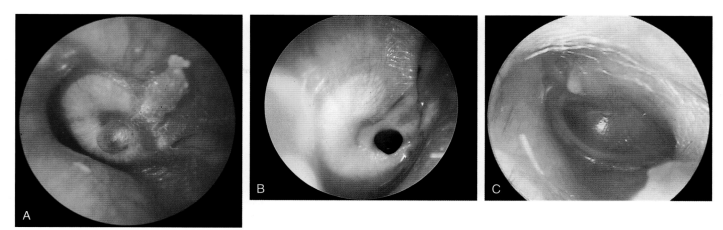

Figure 23-29. Sequelae of chronic otitis media. **A,** Much of this child's tympanic membrane is scarred and thickened, and a thinned dimeric area balloons out of the inferior central portion. **B,** The eardrum is markedly thickened, scarred in an arc from 12 to 5 o'clock, and has a large chronic perforation. **C,** Severe retraction of the tympanic membrane is seen in this patient. The membrane adheres to the malleus. (**A** and **B,** Courtesy Sylvan Stool, MD; **C,** courtesy Alejandro Hoberman, MD, Children's Hospital of Pittsburgh.)

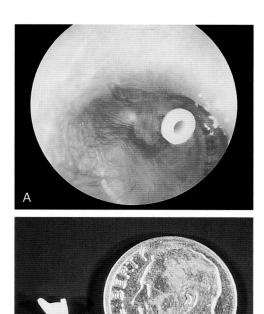

Figure 23-30. A, Tympanic membrane of patient with a history of chronic otitis media, with tympanostomy tube in place. The tube serves to vent the middle ear, improve hearing, and reduce the frequency of infection. **B,** The tympanic membrane is slightly smaller than the size of a dime. A typical tube takes up approximately 15% of the tympanic membrane's surface area. There are many different types in a variety of shapes, materials, sizes, and colors. Selection is based on specific pathology and surgeon preference. (**A,** Courtesy Sylvan Stool, MD.)

to expensive, custom-molded devices. The general purpose of an earplug is to prevent water from entering the external ear canal and contaminating the middle ear space. "Wax" earplugs act like a putty that can be molded into the particular shape that comfortably blocks the individual's ear canals. A preformed ear defender is held in place by the conchal bowl and provides reasonable protection for children. The ear defenders vary in shape, and a child needs to be fitted for an age-appropriate size. Although custom-made ear plugs are not of critical importance, they do provide a better fit and are more comfortable, and compliance with their use tends to be greater. Children have a propensity to lose or misplace these devices, and it

is best to focus on obtaining functional earplugs that are easily replaceable at minimal cost.

Other Middle Ear Disorders

Though considerably less common than otitis media and serous otitis media, a number of other disorders involving the tympanic membrane are important because of potential severity.

Mass Lesions Involving the Tympanic Membrane. The most common and one of the most serious mass lesions of the eardrum is a **cholesteatoma.** It can present as a defect in the tympanic membrane through which persistent drainage occurs, or it can appear as a white cystic mass behind or involving the eardrum. It consists of trapped epithelial tissue that grows beneath the surface of the membrane (Fig. 23-31). Although a few are congenital, the majority are sequelae of untreated or chronic-recurrent otitis media. If a cholesteatoma is not removed surgically, it continues to enlarge; becomes locally destructive; and can erode the mastoid bone, destroy the ossicles, and even invade the inner ear structures or cranium. A progressive hearing impairment is usually a feature of this condition.

Granulomas or *polyps* of the tympanic membrane (Fig. 23-32) can also develop in children with chronic middle ear infections. The most common cause of aural polyps in children is an old, retained tympanostomy tube. Cholesteatoma is another predisposing condition. These tissues often bleed easily, which can frighten the patient, the parent, and the physician. Left untreated, polyps can enlarge to fill the canal and by expansion can progressively damage the drum and the ossicles. Therefore prompt surgical removal is indicated if therapy with topical and oral antimicrobials is unsuccessful.

Distortions of the Tympanic Membrane. Thin, dimeric portions of the eardrum may be observed in patients with chronic middle ear disease, or they may develop after extrusion of a tympanostomy tube (Fig. 23-33; see also Fig. 23-29A). These thinned areas are the result of abnormal healing of perforations and are hypermobile on pneumatic otoscopy. The important points to note on examination are whether the pocket is fully visible or partly hidden, its location with respect to the ossicles, and whether or not it is dry. If the ear canal and drum are not dry, an active infection and/or cholesteatoma is present. In cases of severe deformity, aggressive therapy

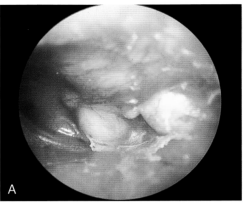
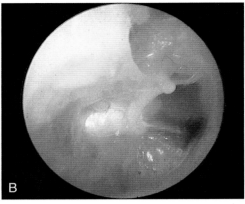
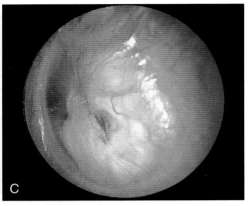

Figure 23-31. Cholesteatomas. **A,** Congenital cholesteatoma noted in a young child with spontaneous ear drainage. No previous history of ear infections existed. **B** and **C,** Acquired cholesteatomas, which generally present after a long history of chronic middle ear disease.

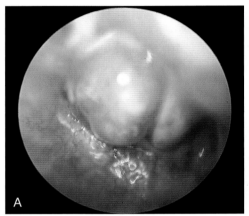
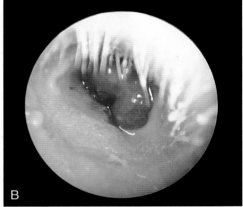

Figure 23-32. Granulomas and polyps of the tympanic membrane. **A,** Growth of this polypoid granuloma was stimulated by the inflammatory process of chronic middle ear infection. **B,** These polyps, which protrude through a tympanic membrane perforation, have enlarged to entirely fill the external ear canal. Because of the possible attachment of the polyp to the facial nerve or the ossicles of the middle ear, removal of polyps requires extreme caution. (**A,** Courtesy Sylvan Stool, MD.)

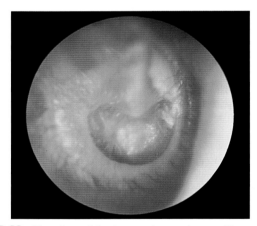

Figure 23-33. Dimerism of the tympanic membrane. Otoscopy demonstrates a severely retracted atrophic segment of the eardrum that also has multiple white scars (tympanosclerosis). The thinned portions are the result of abnormal healing of perforations and tend to be hypermobile on otoscopy. (Courtesy Sylvan Stool, MD.)

including ventilation of the middle ear and excision of the pocket may be necessary.

Nasal Disorders

A child's nose is examined most commonly for disturbances in external appearance, excessive drainage, or blockage of airflow and interference with breathing. Epistaxis is also frequently encountered.

Nasal Examination

The nasal examination can be difficult in younger children. It is best done with the child sitting on a parent's lap or in a chair. The child's head is held in a neutral position, not tilted up.

An otoscope with a wide speculum (≥4 mm) is the most practical instrument. The examiner should gently brace his or her free hand on the child's upper lip to prevent sudden head movement from pushing the speculum tip into the nose, which could lead to nasal trauma, and should try to look toward the back of the nose rather than up into the nose. If the child is old enough to comply, he or she is asked to breathe through his or her mouth so as not to fog up the lens on the otoscope. If a nasal spreader-type speculum is used, a headlight is desirable. The septum, the anterior edges of the middle and inferior turbinates, and the nasal floor are inspected, and the quality of nasal secretions is noted. With practice and when there is minimal congestion, adenoidal size can be assessed.

A more thorough examination is possible using a nasal endoscope; this enables full visualization of internal nasal structures. Before starting, the nose is sprayed with a decongestant to shrink the nasal mucosa and with a topical anesthetic. With patience, older children can be coaxed through the insertion and examination. Allowing them to hold and inspect the device, test the light, look at themselves on the monitor, and even insert the tip into their nose assists cooperation (Fig. 23-34A to C). Most children younger than 5 years of age require immobilization in a papoose board. If suctioning is necessary, having the patient take a deep breath and hold it before applying

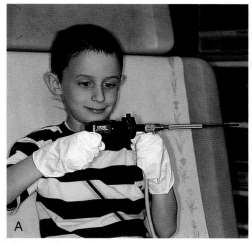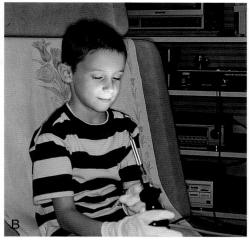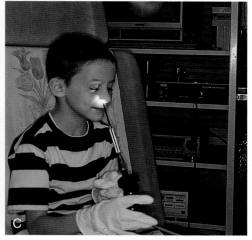

Figure 23-34. Nasal endoscopic examination. **A,** A child holding and feeling the endoscope. **B,** When he shines the light on himself, the endoscope shows his face on the monitor. **C,** By holding it at the entrance to his nose, he sees that the instrument is neither hot nor painful.

suction reduces discomfort. The nasal endoscope is a useful tool, and this type of examination can be done readily in the otolaryngologist's office.

Nasal Congestion and Obstruction

Upper Respiratory Infections in Early Infancy

In infancy and early childhood the nasal passages are small and easily obstructed by processes that produce mucosal edema and coryza, whether infectious, "allergic," or traumatic. In the first 1 to 3 months, infants are obligate nose breathers and therefore can have significant respiratory distress from nasal congestion alone. Young infants with upper respiratory tract infections may, in addition to nasal discharge, have tachypnea and mild retractions and often have to interrupt feeding to breathe, which can result in the swallowing of significant amounts of air, leading to a secondary increase in spitting up after feeding and to intestinal gas pain. These secondary problems can be minimized by instructing parents to hold these infants up on their shoulders and burp them for 10 to 15 minutes after feedings. Instillation of saline nose drops to loosen secretions, followed by nasal suctioning before meals and naps, also provides a measure of relief. Oral decongestants are ineffective and often produce marked irritability when given to infants in the first year of life. Fortunately, these upper respiratory tract infections are generally brief and clear within a few days.

On occasion, infants with upper respiratory tract infection go on to have persistent, purulent, or serosanguineous nasal discharge. Culture of discharges persisting longer than 10 to 14 days may disclose heavy growth of a single pathogen. Preliminary studies of empirical antimicrobial therapy in such infants suggest that this produces rapid and effective resolution of symptoms when compared with a placebo. Thus this picture of prolonged nasal discharge probably represents a *bacterial ethmoiditis,* the infant equivalent of sinusitis.

Nasopharyngitis Secondary to Gastroesophageal Reflux (Reflux Rhinitis)

Infants with gastroesophageal reflux disease (GERD) may develop persistent nasal congestion and rhinorrhea with varying degrees of mucosal inflammation and edema in response to exposure to gastric juices. Snoring and/or coughing during sleep are common associated symptoms. Although vomiting or frequent spitting, sometimes with passage of regurgitated material through the nose, may be reported, often such symptoms are absent. The GERD section at the end of this chapter details the spectrum of signs and symptoms that may assist in diagnosis of GERD-related nasal disorders.

Congenital Causes of Nasal Obstruction

Congenital causes of nasal obstruction include choanal atresia, choanal stenosis, and mass lesions such as tumors, cysts, and polyps.

Choanal Atresia and Stenosis. Choanal atresia may be bony (90%) or membranous (10%), bilateral or unilateral. Newborns with bilateral choanal atresia manifest severe respiratory distress at delivery, with cyanosis that is relieved by crying and returns with rest (paradoxical cyanosis). The true nature of the problem can elude detection if the physician relies solely on passing soft feeding catheters through the nose to determine patency because these can buckle or curl within the nose. The correct diagnosis is best made by using a van Buren urethral sound or a firm plastic suction catheter (both No. 8 French). This is passed gently along the floor of the nose, close to the septum. If bony resistance is encountered, the diagnosis of choanal atresia is suspected (Fig. 23-35A) and can be confirmed by obtaining a CT scan of the nose and nasopharynx with fine overlapping cuts (see Fig. 23-35B).

Immediate relief of respiratory distress may be accomplished by insertion of an oral airway (or a firm nipple from which the tip has been cut away) into the mouth. Definitive studies can then be performed to aid in planning surgical correction. Infants with unilateral choanal atresia (Fig. 23-36) are usually asymptomatic at birth; however, with time they develop a persistent unilateral nasal discharge.

Choanal stenosis or anterior nasal (piriform aperture) stenosis is also generally asymptomatic in the newborn period, but acquisition of an upper respiratory tract infection can result in significant respiratory compromise. When either lesion is suspected, nasal endoscopy or probing with a urethral sound is indicated. If the sound meets resistance, further evaluation is required. In most cases symptomatic therapy using saline nose drops and nasal suctioning is sufficient to help the infant through the upper respiratory tract infection. With growth, the problem usually abates, but in some cases surgery may be required.

Congenital Mass Lesions. Congenital mass lesions are another source of nasal obstruction. These are particularly likely to become apparent during the first 2 years of life. The modes of presentation vary; some lesions are manifest primarily by symptoms of obstruction and are detected by diagnostic radiography; others become visually evident within a nostril or as a subcutaneous mass located near the root of the nose. Occasionally these patients have recurrent nasal infections and/or epistaxis. All such masses merit thorough clinical and radiographic evaluation because many have intracranial connections.

An *encephalocele* is an outpouching of brain tissue through a congenital bony defect in the midline of the skull. Some patients have craniofacial deformities and a rounded subcutaneous swelling between the eyes or adjacent to the nose. Overlying skin may be somewhat hairy. In other instances the neural tissue prolapses into the nasopharynx, resulting in signs and symptoms of nasal obstruction without obvious external anomalies (Fig. 23-37A). Occasionally a grapelike mass may be seen (via direct nasopharyngoscopy) within the nares or protruding into the pharynx. The mass is usually identified by diagnostic radiography. CT (Fig. 23-37B) is particularly helpful in delineating the extent of the mass and the underlying bony defect. Repair requires a collaborative effort by specialists in otolaryngology, neurosurgery, and in some cases plastic surgery.

Nasal dermoids are embryonic cysts containing ectodermal and mesodermal tissue. They present as round, firm subcutaneous masses located on the dorsum of the

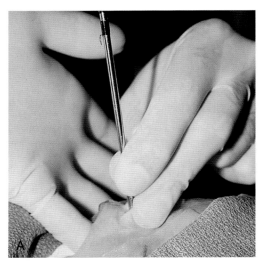

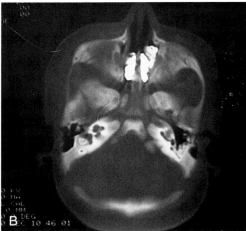

Figure 23-35. Choanal atresia. **A,** This infant manifested severe respiratory distress at delivery, with paradoxical cyanosis. Attempts to pass a urethral sound suggested bony obstruction of the choanae bilaterally. **B,** A CT scan done after instillation of radiopaque dye reveals pooling of the dye within the nose anterior to the choanae, confirming complete obstruction.

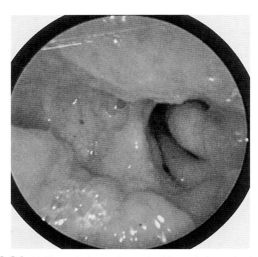

Figure 23-36. Unilateral choanal atresia. Viewed through the nasopharyngoscope, the left choana is clearly patent, whereas the right is atretic. The child had a history of unilateral nasal discharge.

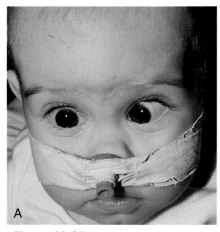
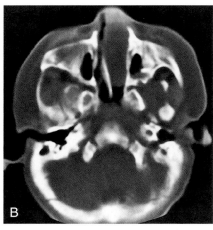
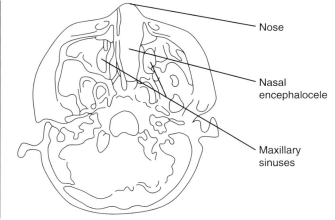

Figure 23-37. Nasal encephalocele. **A,** This normal-appearing infant had signs of severe nasal obstruction, necessitating insertion of a nasopharyngeal airway to relieve distress. **B,** A CT scan shows a large nasal mass lesion that fills one nostril and pushes the nasal septum into the other. This lesion proved to be an encephalocele extruding through a bony defect in the skull base (extrusion seen on another CT cut).

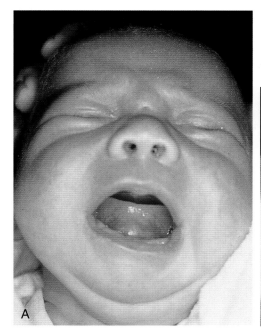
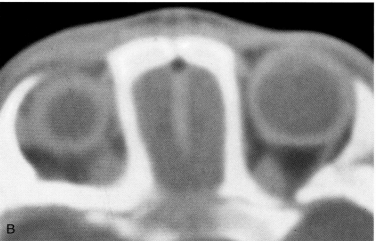

Figure 23-38. Nasal dermoid. **A,** A firm, round mass with a central dimple is seen over the bridge of this infant's nose. **B,** CT scan demonstrates a bony dehiscence of the nasal bridge with a nasal dermoid extending into the anterior cranial vault in the area of the foramen cecum.

nose, close to the midline (Fig. 23-38A). Examination of the overlying skin frequently reveals a small dimple, at times with extruding hair. Some of these cysts have deep extensions down to the nasal septum or through the cribriform plate into the cranium. Thorough evaluation using axial and coronal CT scans (see Fig. 23-38B) and MRI is necessary to determine extent and plan repair. If such cysts are not removed, secondary infection is common and often results in fistula formation.

Small skin tags are frequently seen around the nasal vestibule and should be removed to improve appearance.

Papillomas (Fig. 23-39) are similar growths that occur on the distal nasal mucosa near the mucocutaneous junction. These growths should be excised to improve appearance and confirm diagnosis; they do not cause obstruction.

Acquired Forms of Nasal Obstruction
Adenoidal and Tonsillar Hypertrophy. The lymphoid tissue that constitutes the tonsils and adenoids is relatively small in infancy, gradually enlarges until 8 to 10 years of age, and then usually begins to shrink in size. In most instances this normal process of hypertrophy results in mild to moderate enlargement of these structures and does not constitute a problem. A small percentage of children, however, develop marked adenoidal and tonsillar hypertrophy, with attendant symptoms of nasal obstruction and rhinorrhea. A few even have difficulty swallowing solid foods. Recurrent infection appears to be the most common inciting factor, although atopy may play a role in some cases. Occasionally, mononucleosis is the initiating event, resulting in rapid enlargement of adenoidal and tonsillar tissues that is then slow to resolve (see "Tonsillitis/Pharyngitis" later and see Chapter 12). In most children, progressive adenoidal enlargement appears to be the cumulative result of a series of upper respiratory tract infections. The consequent obstruction to normal flow of secretions then starts a vicious circle, making the child more vulnerable to recurrent infections of the ears, sinuses, and nasopharynx, which in turn further exacerbate the adenoidal and tonsillar hypertrophy.

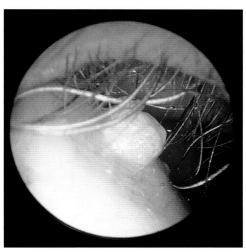

Figure 23-39. Nasal papillomas present as warty growths at the mucocutaneous junction of the nares. (Courtesy Michael Hawke, MD.)

Regardless of mode of origin, when adenoidal hypertrophy is marked, blockage of the nasal airway becomes severe and results in mouth breathing, chronic rhinorrhea, inability to blow the nose, and snoring during sleep (Fig. 23-40A). Speech becomes hyponasal and muffled. The child holds his or her mouth open and has little or no airflow through the nares, and his or her tonsils may also meet in the midline (see Fig. 23-40B). A cephalometric lateral neck x-ray examination reveals a large adenoidal shadow impinging on the nasal airway (see Fig. 23-40C). For many patients these features are noted primarily in the course of acute illness; however, a number of children have symptoms even when free of acute infection. In a minority of cases obstruction is so severe as to produce sleep disturbance. This is characterized by restlessness and retractions when recumbent, snoring, and possibly prolonged sleep apnea with frequent waking. Some patients begin to sleep sitting up, and many manifest daytime fatigue. Symptoms are worse during sleep because relaxation of the pharyngeal muscles further increases the degree of upper airway obstruction. In severe cases this

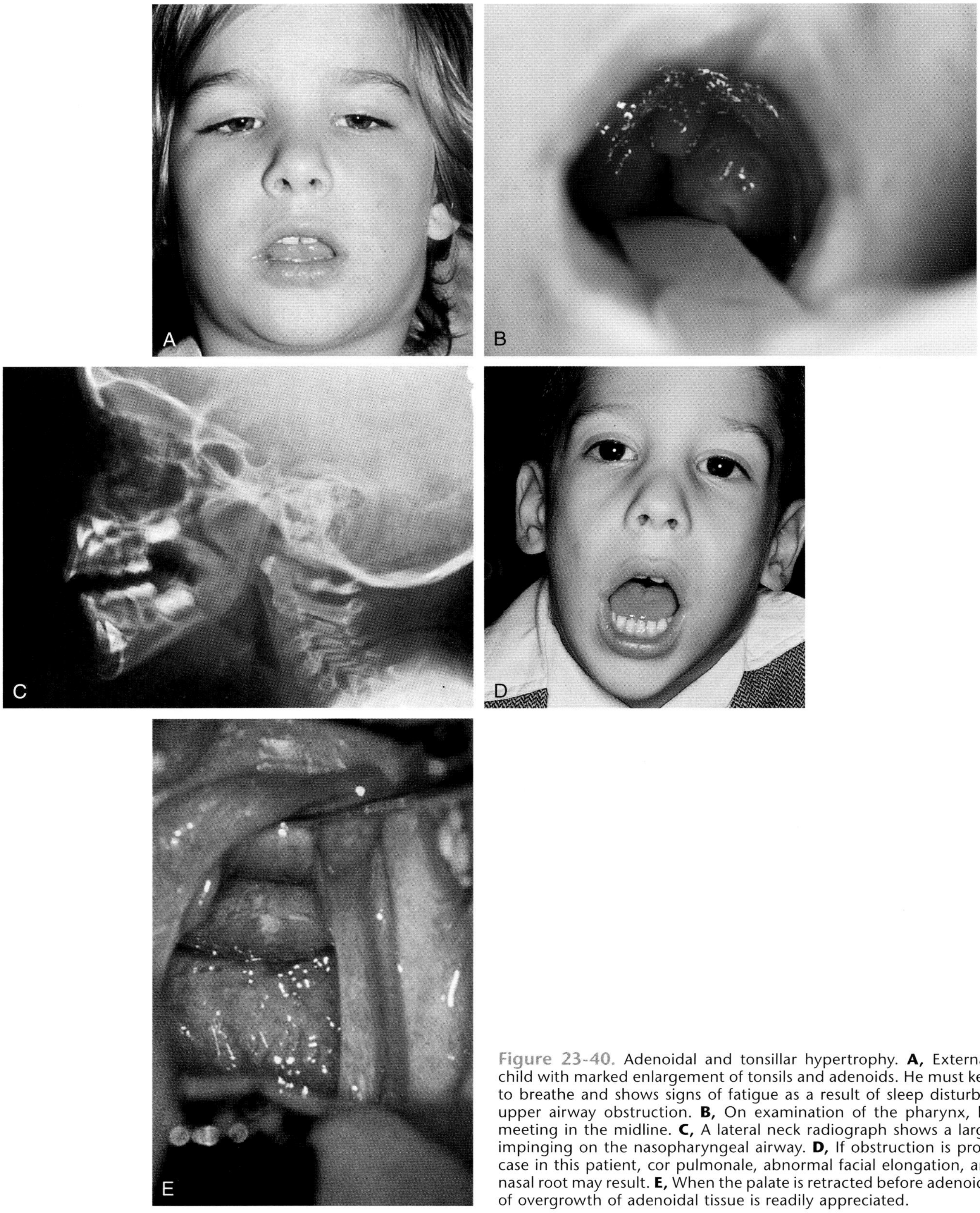

Figure 23-40. Adenoidal and tonsillar hypertrophy. **A,** External appearance of a child with marked enlargement of tonsils and adenoids. He must keep his mouth open to breathe and shows signs of fatigue as a result of sleep disturbance caused by his upper airway obstruction. **B,** On examination of the pharynx, his tonsils are seen meeting in the midline. **C,** A lateral neck radiograph shows a large adenoid shadow impinging on the nasopharyngeal airway. **D,** If obstruction is prolonged, as was the case in this patient, cor pulmonale, abnormal facial elongation, and widening of the nasal root may result. **E,** When the palate is retracted before adenoidectomy, the extent of overgrowth of adenoidal tissue is readily appreciated.

results in periods of hypoxia and hypercarbia, leading to intermittent apnea and waking. Because a patient may look relatively healthy when awake (with the exception of having to breathe through the mouth), it is important to observe for retractions and to assess the pattern of breathing after the child has been recumbent for a period of time or, better still, during a nap. Use of continuous pulse oximetry during this period of observation enables documentation of presence or absence of oxygen desaturation.

If obstruction persists for a prolonged period of time, cor pulmonale (with signs of right ventricular hypertrophy on electrocardiogram and chest radiograph) and abnormal facial growth may result (see Fig. 23-40D).

Management of patients with adenoidal hypertrophy depends in part on the severity and the duration of the obstruction. In milder cases of short duration or in patients with intermittent symptoms, careful monitoring; treatment of atopy, when present; and institution of a 2- to 4-

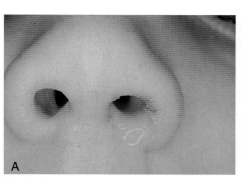

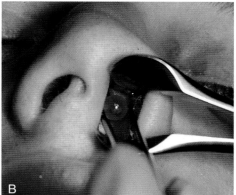

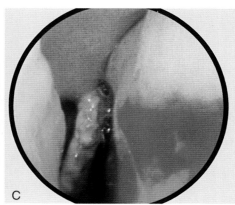

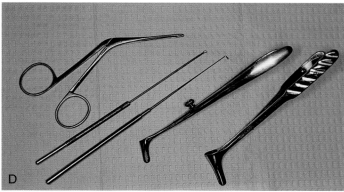

Figure 23-41. Nasal foreign body. **A,** This child had a unilateral, foul-smelling nasal discharge. **B,** Aspiration of the discharge in this patient revealed a red bead that was removed with a Day hook. **C,** A piece of cardboard is seen in this child's nostril. Note the mucosal abrasion from a prior attempt at removal. **D,** Hartmann forceps, a small wire loop curette, and a right-angle Day hook are the instruments used most commonly for removal of nasal foreign bodies. Nasal spreaders assist visualization and create a wider space for inserting the desired instrument. Note that bleeding or aspiration of the nasal foreign body may occur, especially with uncooperative toddlers. Thus consideration should be given for removal of nasal foreign bodies in the operating room with general anesthesia and a controlled airway. (**A,** Courtesy Michael Hawke, MD; **C,** from Becker W: Atlas of Ear, Nose, and Throat Diseases, 2nd ed. Stuttgart, Germany and New York, Thieme, 1983.)

week course of antimicrobial therapy with a β-lactam-stable agent may result in significant shrinkage of hypertrophied tonsillar and adenoidal tissues. Children with persistent symptoms despite therapy and those with sleep disturbance or cor pulmonale should undergo adenoidectomy, during which the extent of adenoidal overgrowth can be fully appreciated (see Fig. 23-40E). Children with major orthodontic abnormalities and nasal obstruction also should be considered for adenoidectomy before orthodontic correction.

Nasal Foreign Bodies. As with the external ear, it is not unusual for small children to put beads, paper, pieces of sponge, plastic toys, or other foreign material into their noses. Such foreign objects are irritating to the nasal mucosa and soon incite an intense inflammatory reaction with production of a thick, purulent, foul-smelling discharge that helps to hide their presence. Intermittent epistaxis may accompany the discharge. Because most children younger than 5 years of age are unable to blow their noses and are afraid or unable to tell their parents what they have done, the object is not expelled and the problem often goes unrecognized until symptoms develop and medical attention is sought. A unilateral nasal discharge and/or a foul smell are the typical chief complaints and should lead the clinician to suspect a foreign body immediately (Fig. 23-41A).

Speculum examination may readily disclose the object (Fig. 23-41B and C), but often the purulent discharge obscures the view, necessitating removal with an absorbent swab or via gentle suction. Even when visualization is accomplished, removal can be difficult because children are easily frightened at the prospect of instrumentation, and their struggling can result in mucosal injury during attempts at removal (see Fig. 23-41C). To minimize problems, topical anesthetic spray and a topical vasoconstrictor can be applied, and the child can be restrained with a papoose board. Older patients or calm young children may do well sitting in a parent's lap, if the examiner is

patient, reassuring, and willing to explain each step carefully. The discharge may then be removed by swab or suction. If the object is anterior to the turbinates, removal can be attempted using suction; a small wire loop curette; a right-angled Day hook for spherical objects; or alligator, or Hartmann, forceps for material that can be grasped (Fig. 23-41D). Consultation with an otolaryngologist should be sought for removal of objects located more posteriorly or those not readily removed on initial attempts. A major concern is that in the attempted removal, a deeply situated foreign body may be dislodged into the nasopharynx, leading to aspiration or, worse, laryngeal obstruction. In such cases the best course of action is to remove the object after the airway has been secured with an endotracheal tube in the operating room, with the patient under general anesthesia. Significant bleeding may occur during attempted removal of an intranasal foreign body, and this is another reason to strongly consider general anesthesia with an endotracheal tube to secure the airway.

Nasal Polyps. Polyps are thought to be the end result of recurrent infection and/or inflammation, although in a portion of cases, atopy may play a contributing role. Polyps originate in the ethmoid or, less commonly, the maxillary sinuses and protrude through the sinus ostia into the nasal cavity. The phenomenon is unusual in children younger than 10 years of age, with the exception of patients with cystic fibrosis, 25% of whom develop polyps, some as early as infancy. Symptoms consist of those of progressive nasal obstruction, frequently with associated discharge. Recurrent sinusitis is a common complication as a result of impaired sinus drainage. In some cases chronic sinusitis may be the cause of polyp formation. Affected patients with acute infections may also have intermittent epistaxis. Involvement may be unilateral or bilateral. On examination, moist, glistening pedunculated growths that may have a smooth or a grape-like appearance are seen (Fig. 23-42). Bilateral opacification of the ethmoid and maxillary sinuses is commonly found on radiography. Polyps must be distinguished from a nasal glioma or encephalocele, which may have a similar appearance and can produce identical symptoms. These neural mass lesions are more common in infancy but may present in older children. Therefore, CT of the sinuses and skull base should be considered for children with polypoid nasal lesions who do not have cystic fibrosis.

Surgical removal of the polyps is indicated to relieve nasal obstruction, reduce the risk of secondary sinusitis, and diminish the possibility of altered facial growth. Another problem seen in children with chronic polyps (most frequently those with cystic fibrosis) consists of widening of the nasal root and prominence of the malar areas of the face (Fig. 23-43).

Nasal Trauma

Blunt nasal trauma is frequently encountered in pediatrics. In the majority of instances it results only in minor swelling and mild epistaxis, which is readily controlled by application of pressure over the nares (see Chapter 2 for nasal trauma incurred during delivery). However, more severe injuries do occur and have a significant potential for long-term morbidity and deformity if not identified and treated appropriately. These injuries include displaced nasal fractures (Fig. 23-44A and B), which, if not reduced, result in permanent deformity; septal deviation or dislocation, with or without an associated fracture (Fig. 23-45), which produces unilateral impairment of airflow; and septal hematomas (Fig. 23-46A), which, if not drained promptly, may lead to abscesses (see Fig. 6-25) and cause destruction of nasal cartilage resulting in a saddle-nose deformity (Fig. 23-46B). Finally, profuse bleeding that is difficult to stop or recurs readily suggests trauma to deeper structures of the face or frontal bones and warrants prompt stabilization and meticulous clinical and radiographic assessment (see Chapter 20).

In evaluating patients with nasal trauma, the nasal bridge should be inspected for swelling or deformity (the latter may not be apparent if swelling is marked) and the septum palpated for tenderness, crepitus, or excessive

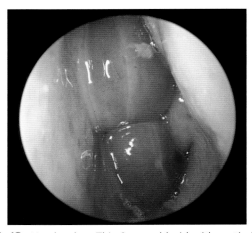

Figure 23-42. Nasal polyp. This 2-year-old girl with cystic fibrosis was referred because of nasal obstruction and nocturnal snoring of a few months' duration. A large grayish polyp was found in the left nostril. Any child presenting with a nasal polyp should be tested for cystic fibrosis.

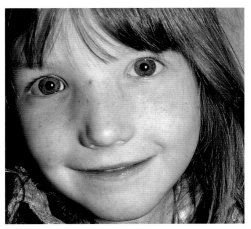

Figure 23-43. Sequelae of chronic nasal polyps. This 7-year-old girl with cystic fibrosis and recurrent nasal polyps shows secondary alteration in facial growth consisting of a broadened nasal root and prominence of the malar areas. This occurred despite several resections.

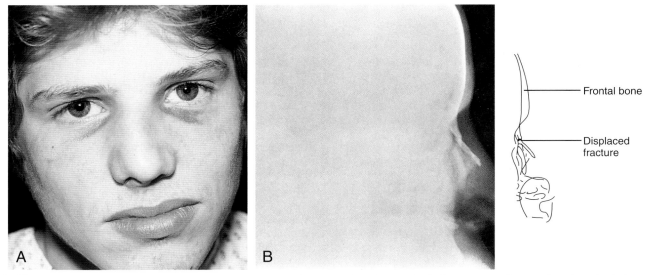

Figure 23-44. Displaced nasal fracture. **A,** This teenager was hit on the nose while playing football. On external inspection there is obvious deformity, and there are ecchymoses under both eyes. Crepitus was evident on palpation. **B,** A lateral radiograph of another patient shows a displaced fracture of the proximal portion of the nasal bone, delineated on the diagram.

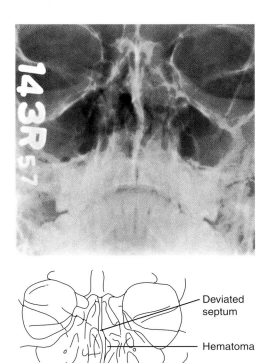

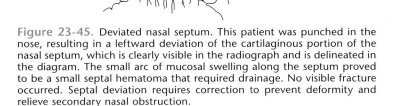

Figure 23-45. Deviated nasal septum. This patient was punched in the nose, resulting in a leftward deviation of the cartilaginous portion of the nasal septum, which is clearly visible in the radiograph and is delineated in the diagram. The small arc of mucosal swelling along the septum proved to be a small septal hematoma that required drainage. No visible fracture occurred. Septal deviation requires correction to prevent deformity and relieve secondary nasal obstruction.

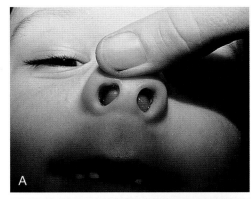

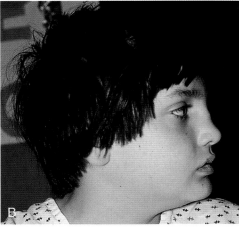

Figure 23-46. Septal hematoma. This patient incurred facial trauma **(A)** resulting in multiple fractures of the nasal and orbital bones and submucosal bleeding along the nasal septum. Such septal hematomas must be drained promptly to reduce the risk of abscess formation and to prevent cartilage necrosis, which ultimately results in a saddle-nose deformity **(B).** (**A,** Courtesy Robert Hickey, MD, Children's Hospital of Pittsburgh, Pa.)

mobility. The nares should be cleared of clots, and the septum assessed for position and presence of swelling, which would suggest a hematoma. A hematoma is soft on palpation of the septum with a cotton-tipped applicator. Examination of the oropharynx is also helpful in determining if blood is flowing posteriorly. When marked swelling, severe tenderness, deformity, crepitus, or septal deviation is found, radiography is indicated. However, radiographs should be interpreted with caution because a large portion of the nasal skeleton in children is composed of cartilage rather than bone and serious nasal injuries can be present despite a seemingly normal x-ray film. Septal hematomas, displaced fractures, and bleeding that fails to cease readily with direct pressure necessitate prompt consultation with an otolaryngologist.

Epistaxis

Although often due to direct trauma, nasal bleeding in childhood has a number of other causes including infection, mucosal irritation, bleeding disorders, vascular anomalies, and hypertension. Patients with these conditions may have apparently spontaneous bleeding or epistaxis triggered by minor external trauma or by forceful sneezing and blowing. Profuse bleeding that is difficult to stop is most characteristic of acute thrombocytopenia, vascular anomalies, and severe hypertension. Mild bleeding that is readily controlled by application of pressure suggests mucosal infection or irritation that promotes bleeding from small superficial veins located on the ante-

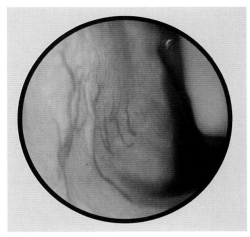

Figure 23-47. Dilated septal vessels of Kiesselbach plexus, which tend to bleed in response to mucosal infection or irritation. (From Becker W: Atlas of Ear, Nose, and Throat Diseases, 2nd ed. Stuttgart and New York, Thieme, 1983.)

rior nasal septum (Fig. 23-47). In all cases the problem should be taken seriously and investigated carefully to correctly diagnose and appropriately treat the primary source of the problem.

In approaching patients with epistaxis, the following historical points should be addressed:
1. Is the problem acute or recurrent?
2. Was external trauma, sneezing, or blowing a triggering event?

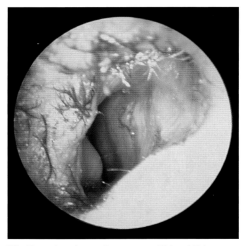

Figure 23-48. Excoriated nasal septum. This child presented with an upper respiratory tract infection and a history of intermittent epistaxis with nasal blowing and nocturnal epistaxis with blood noted on his pillow in the mornings. He had a purulent nasal discharge *(lower right)* and a diffusely excoriated erythematous septum. Cultures of nose and throat specimens grew group A β-streptococci.

3. What is the duration of the current bleed and the approximate volume of blood loss (handkerchiefs soaked, hemodynamic status, etc.)?
4. Is the bleeding unilateral or bilateral?
5. Has the patient been having symptoms suggestive of an upper respiratory tract infection or nasal allergy?
6. Has the child manifested other signs and symptoms of an underlying coagulopathy or of hypertension?
7. Has the patient been taking medication, especially aspirin, ibuprofen, or other nonsteroidal anti-inflammatory agents?

Physical assessment must address the patient's general well-being in addition to careful examination of the nose. Hemodynamic status is of particular importance when hemorrhage has been profuse.

After observation of the external appearance of the nares, the nose is cleared of clots and discharge, if present. Then the septum and mucosa are inspected for possible points of hemorrhage, signs of obstruction, mass lesions, and foreign objects. The oropharynx should also be examined for posterior flow of blood, especially in cases in which no point of bleeding is evident on inspection of the nasal mucosa. Otolaryngologic consultation should be sought in cases involving profuse bleeding that does not readily cease on application of pressure and may require nasal packing or other surgical treatment.

Epistaxis Caused by Infection and Mucosal Irritation

In many patients with nontraumatic epistaxis, examination reveals unilateral or bilateral septal erythema and friability or excoriation (Fig. 23-48). The history given is one of intermittent bleeding, especially with sneezing, blowing the nose, or during sleep (the child's pillow is found spotted with blood). The phenomenon is commonly attributed to digital manipulation of the nose in response to itching. However, in view of the sensitivity of the mucosa to painful stimuli, picking to the point of excoriation is rather unlikely. In many instances erythematous friable areas are impetiginous or represent the combined effects of inflammation (the result of nasopharyngitis, sinusitis, or allergic rhinitis) and trauma caused by forceful sneezing and blowing. When infection is suspected, culturing of the friable area for a predominant bacterial

pathogen (especially group A β-hemolytic streptococci or coagulase-positive staphylococci) may prove rewarding. In patients with no history of or no findings consistent with upper respiratory tract infection, mucosal drying may be responsible. This occurs most commonly in winter as a result of drying of the air by central heating systems. Although application of topical antibiotic ointment, water-based lubricants, humidification, and antihistamines (for atopic patients) may provide some relief, when bacterial pathogens are found, oral antimicrobial therapy is more likely to be successful.

Patients with nasal polyps who have an intercurrent infection and children with nasal foreign bodies with secondary infection and inflammation are also highly prone to intermittent epistaxis and blood-tinged nasal discharge.

Epistaxis Caused by Bleeding Disorders

Despite application of pressure, epistaxis in patients with coagulopathies is more likely to be prolonged and carries a greater risk of significant blood loss. Although many such patients have known bleeding disorders, a few may present with prolonged or recurrent nosebleeds as one of the initial manifestations of their problem. This is most typical of idiopathic thrombocytopenia, aplastic anemia, and acute leukemia. When epistaxis arises in the context of a bleeding disorder, the personal history, family history, and/or other physical findings should point to the diagnosis (see Chapter 11), which can then be confirmed by hematologic studies (complete blood count and differential, platelet count, prothrombin time and partial thromboplastin time, and coagulation profile).

Acute management depends in part on the source of the coagulopathy (e.g., factor replacement or platelet transfusion) and in part on severity of bleeding. Topical application of a vasoconstrictor such as epinephrine and insertion of absorbable synthetic material that aids coagulation (Gelfoam or Surgicel) can be helpful in patients with thrombocytopenia and an anterior point of bleeding. The risks of secondary infection with packing must be given careful consideration in patients undergoing immunosuppressive therapy. Prophylactic antimicrobials should be administered to patients requiring packing to avoid secondary infections.

Epistaxis Caused by Vascular Abnormalities

In a minority of children with recurrent epistaxis, the history reveals significant bleeding that typically drains from one side of the nose. This suggests a localized vascular abnormality. The most commonly encountered problem is that of a dilated septal vessel or plexus, which may be a sequela of prior inflammation (see Fig. 23-47). This may be visible anteriorly but also can be located high on the septum, requiring nasal endoscopy for identification. Cauterization is generally curative. In children older than 7 years of age, anterior septal lesions can be cauterized in the office with silver nitrate after application of a topical anesthetic and vasoconstrictor. Younger children and many patients with posterior lesions may need general anesthesia for cauterization.

Two relatively rare vascular anomalies also may be the source of recurrent nasal bleeding: telangiectasias and angiofibromas. Patients with **hereditary hemorrhagic telangiectasia** (Osler-Weber-Rendu disease) have an autosomal dominant disorder characterized by formation of cutaneous and mucosal telangiectatic lesions that begin to develop in childhood and gradually increase in number with age. These lesions appear as bright red, slightly raised, star-shaped plexuses of dilated small vessels that blanch on pressure (Fig. 23-49). Mucosal telangiectasias may bleed spontaneously or in response to minor trauma. Recurrent epistaxis is a common mode of presentation in childhood. Multiple telangiectasias are evident on close examination. Hematuria and/or gastrointestinal bleeding may be seen separately or in combination with epistaxis.

Juvenile nasopharyngeal angiofibroma is a rare vascular tumor seen predominantly in adolescent boys. Although benign, it is locally invasive and destructive and may involve the maxillary sinuses, palate, sphenoid sinus, and portions of the skull base. The most common mode of presentation is one of profuse, often recurrent epistaxis. Some patients also have symptoms of nasal obstruction with secondary rhinorrhea, and a small percentage may have visual, auditory, or other cranial nerve disturbances. On examination, a purplish soft tissue mass may be seen through the nares or on nasopharyngoscopy. In addition to standard radiographs, CT, MRI, and angiography may be necessary to assess the extent of the tumor (Fig. 23-50). Carefully planned excision is then the treatment of choice.

Epistaxis Caused by Hypertension
In contrast to the adult population, hypertension is an unusual source of epistaxis in childhood. However, it should be considered, especially in patients with antecedent headache and spontaneous, profuse bleeding that is difficult to stop. Patients with such a history may have previously undiagnosed coarctation of the aorta or chronic renal disease with severe secondary hypertension, and they should be examined with these possibilities in mind. It must be remembered that after significant blood loss, blood pressure may drop to normal levels.

Disorders of the Paranasal Sinuses and Adjacent Structures

The paranasal sinuses are air-filled, bony cavities that lie within the facial bones of the skull, adjacent to the nasal passages. They develop through a gradual enlargement of pneumatized cells that evaginate from the nasal cavity. This process occurs over the course of childhood and adolescence; there is a wide normal range in the duration of this process and in the ultimate size of the sinuses and their ostia (Fig. 23-51). In infancy the ethmoid and maxillary sinuses are partially pneumatized, but they are small and not readily demonstrable on radiographs (although they can be readily seen on a CT scan). Therefore radiographs are of little diagnostic value until after the first 2 years of life. The sphenoid sinus is not evident until about 5 to 6 years, and the frontal sinuses are not well developed until after 7 to 8 years of age (Fig. 23-52).

The sinuses are lined by ciliated respiratory epithelium, which produces and transports mucous secretions. They drain into the nasal cavity through various small openings, which are located under the middle turbinate. Several points of clinical importance warrant emphasis. First, the ostia of the sinuses are small and thus easily obstructed by mucosal edema. Further, there are many important structures adjacent to the sinuses that are vulnerable to involvement if a disease process spreads beyond a sinus. These include the orbit, the brain, and the cavernous sinus. The roots of the maxillary teeth lie in the floor of the maxillary sinuses. Therefore dental infections may drain into the maxillary sinuses, resulting in recurrent or chronic sinusitis. Hence the dentition should be thoroughly inspected in evaluating any child with suspected sinus infection (see Chapter 20).

Sinusitis

During the first several years of life, infection of the maxillary and/or ethmoid sinuses is more common than is generally appreciated. Frontal sinusitis becomes important after about 10 years of age. The probable pathogenesis is mucosal swelling (whether the result of upper respira-

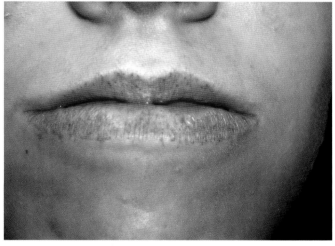

Figure 23-49. Hereditary hemorrhagic telangiectasia. Numerous telangiectasias dot the lips and palatal mucosa of this boy who had problems with recurrent epistaxis. (Courtesy Bernard Cohen, MD, Johns Hopkins Hospital.)

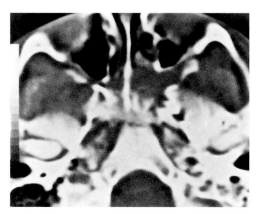

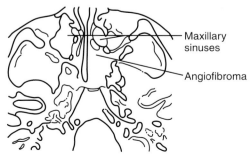

Figure 23-50. Juvenile nasopharyngeal angiofibroma. CT scan is helpful in assessing the extent of this locally invasive vascular tumor. In this cut, an enhancing mass (an angiofibroma, as delineated in the diagram) is seen occupying the posterior portion of the left nostril, deviating the septum and compressing the ipsilateral maxillary sinus.

Maxillary sinuses

Angiofibroma

THE PARANASAL SINUSES

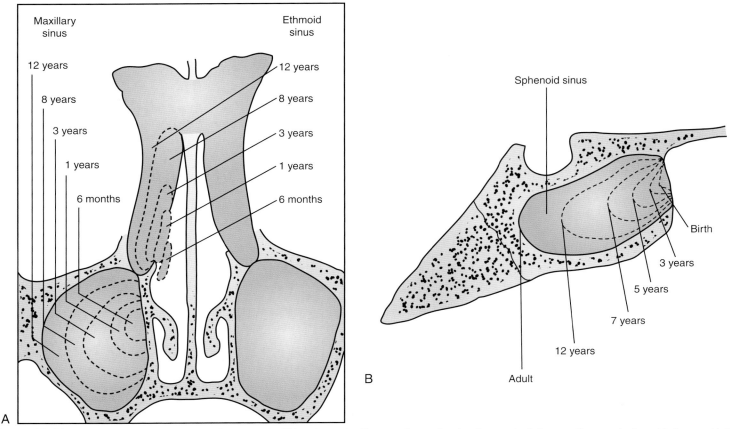

Figure 23-51. Development of the paranasal sinuses. **A,** This schematic diagram shows the development of the maxillary and ethmoid sinuses. Note that development occurs throughout childhood and may not be complete until 12 years of age. **B,** The sphenoid sinus, which sits under the pituitary fossa, develops slowly and may not even be well aerated for the first 5 to 6 years of life.

tory tract infection, allergic rhinitis, or chemical irritation), resulting in obstruction of the sinus ostia. This impedes drainage of secretions; promotes mucous plugging; and, if prolonged, sets the stage for proliferation of bacterial pathogens with resultant infection. Both bacterial and viral pathogens have been isolated from pediatric patients. The most commonly identified bacteria are *S. pneumoniae,* nontypable *H. influenzae,* and *Moraxella catarrhalis.* The viral agents include adenoviruses and parainfluenza viruses. As in adults, no good correlation exists between results of nasopharyngeal and sinus aspirate cultures. There is, however, an approximately 80% correlation between middle meatus and sinus cultures.

As with otitis media, a number of conditions predispose children to sinus infections by virtue of alterations in anatomy and/or physiology. These conditions include midfacial anomalies or deformities, particularly when maxillary hypoplasia is part of the picture (see Fig. 23-8); cleft palate (see "Palatal Disorders" later); nasal deformity and/or septal deviation, whether congenital or acquired; mass lesions including hypertrophied adenoids, nasal foreign bodies, polyps, and tumors; abnormalities of mucus production and/or ciliary action such as cystic fibrosis and ciliary dyskinesia; immunodeficiency; atopy; dental infection; and barotrauma.

Clinical Presentations

In young children, sinusitis is primarily a disorder of the ethmoid and maxillary sinuses, and the clinical picture differs considerably from that seen in adolescents and adults. The most common picture is one of a prolonged upper respiratory tract infection that has shown no sign of amelioration after 7 to 10 days. Cough and/or persistent nasal discharge (of any character—thin, thick; clear, cloudy; white, yellow, or green) are the major complaints. The cough is usually loose or wet; it is prominent during the day but may be worse on waking in the morning and/or on first going to bed at night. Patients tend to clear their throats and sniff or snort frequently, especially after sleep. Halitosis or "fetor oris" is commonly noted by parents. In a minority of children, periorbital swelling, most noticeable on awakening, may be reported (Fig. 23-53). A small percentage of patients have a low-grade fever, and a few may complain of headache, facial discomfort, sore throat, or abdominal pain (thought to be due to gastric irritation from swallowing the infected postnasal discharge).

Often, physical examination alone is of little help in distinguishing sinusitis from an upper respiratory tract infection. Findings may include purulent nasal and postnasal discharge with erythema of the nasal mucosa and pharynx, but, as noted previously, this is not uniformly seen. Halitosis may be pronounced and strongly suggests sinusitis in the absence of evidence of dental infection, severe pharyngitis, or nasal foreign body. Sinusitis is also probable when features of the aforementioned picture are accompanied by signs of a maxillary dental abscess (see Chapter 20). Tenderness to percussion over the sinuses suggests sinusitis but is not seen in the majority of patients with the "prolonged upper respiratory tract infection" picture. The clinical spectrum is wide; any combination of the aforementioned symptoms and signs may be present, and sinusitis should be suspected, even if the course is relatively brief, whenever clinical findings are strongly suggestive.

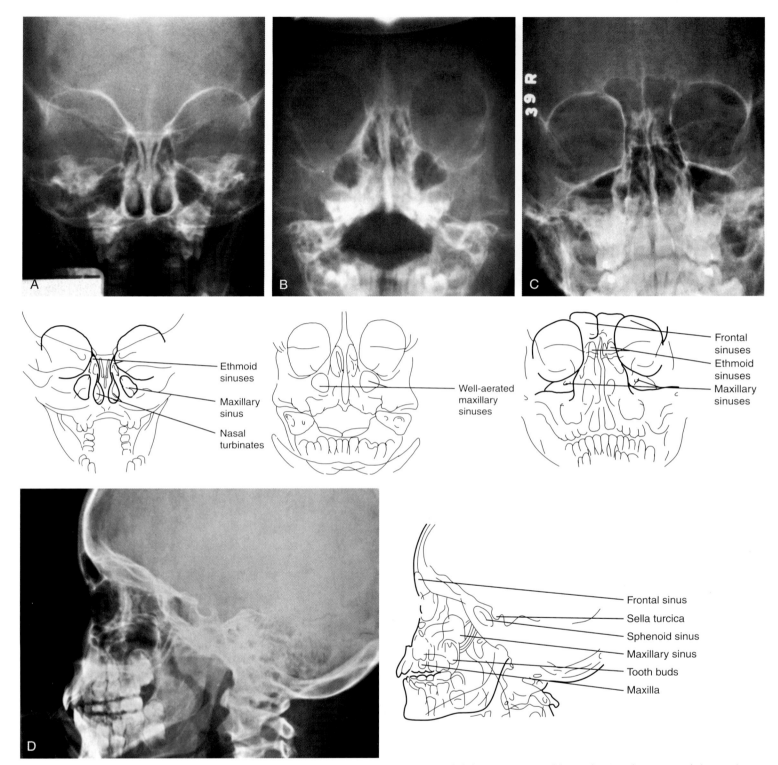

Figure 23-52. Normal radiography of the sinuses. Radiography is currently the most helpful noninvasive tool for evaluating the paranasal sinuses. Interpretation requires appreciation of the normal pattern of development and the findings in health and with disease. **A,** Anteroposterior, or Caldwell, view shows clear ethmoid sinuses in an 18-month-old child. The bony margins are sharp, and the sinus cavities are dark. **B,** The Waters view of the same child shows normal maxillary sinuses with sharply defined bony margins. The cavities appear black. **C,** After age 6 or 7, the Caldwell view is taken posteroanteriorly. In this 8-year-old boy, the bony margins of both the ethmoid and frontal sinuses are sharply defined. Because the calvaria is superimposed, it can be difficult to appreciate frontal sinus clouding on this view alone, particularly with bilateral disease. Therefore evaluation of the frontal sinuses requires close scrutiny of both Caldwell and lateral views. **D,** Lateral view of an 8-year-old child shows pneumatization of the frontal and sphenoid sinuses. Bony margins are sharply defined. The frontal sinuses appear black, but the sphenoid is somewhat gray because there are more overlying structures. Note that the roots of the maxillary teeth are embedded in the floor of the maxillary sinus. Note that plain sinus radiographs are quite inaccurate when compared with sinus CT.

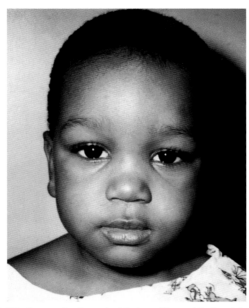

Figure 23-53. Sympathetic periorbital swelling with sinusitis. This 2-year-old boy was seen late in the afternoon with fever, wet cough, decreased activity, and mild infraorbital puffiness. The swelling was neither red, indurated, nor tender and reportedly had been more marked on awakening in the morning. He also had a scant cloudy nasal discharge. His chest radiograph was normal, but sinus films showed opacification of the maxillary sinuses.

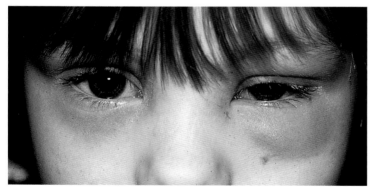

Figure 23-54. This child with sinusitis had prominent erythematous periorbital edema and signs of purulent conjunctivitis. The redness raised concerns of periorbital cellulitis, but the area was nontender and not indurated. Presence of periorbital swelling is a helpful clue in diagnosing sinusitis in children with other suggestive signs and symptoms. (Courtesy Ellen Wald, MD, Children's Hospital of Pittsburgh.)

A less frequent mode of presentation in young children is that of an acute upper respiratory tract infection that is unusually severe, which is characterized by high fever and copious purulent nasal discharge. Facial discomfort and periorbital swelling (nontender, nonindurated, and most marked on waking) are common with this picture. The edematous area may be normal in color or mildly erythematous (Fig. 23-54) and is thought to result from impairment of venous blood flow caused by increased pressure within the infected sinuses. Some of these patients also have conjunctival erythema and discharge. If periorbital erythema is intense or the area is indurated or tender, periorbital cellulitis should be suspected. Occasionally a child with sinusitis has the typical findings of sympathetic edema but without high fever or the prolonged upper respiratory tract infection picture.

Older children and adolescents with acute maxillary and/or ethmoid sinusitis may have either of the previously described symptom pictures but are more likely to complain specifically of headache and/or facial pain. The headache may be perceived as frontal, temporal, or even retroauricular. Facial discomfort can be described as malar pain or a sense of pressure or fullness. Occasionally, patients complain that their teeth hurt (in the absence of dental pathology). When the frontal sinuses are involved, frontal or supraorbital headache is prominent, often perceived as dull or pulsating. The sphenoid sinus is rarely a site of isolated sinus infection, but it is often involved in pansinusitis, in which case occipital and postauricular pain may be reported in addition to discomfort in other sites. Frequently the headache is intermittent. When constant, it varies in severity. This variability appears to be related to degree of drainage. Patients reporting copious "postnasal drip" tend to have less pain. Discomfort and congestion are often most marked on waking, probably as a result of recumbency and lack of gravity-promoted drainage. Some patients also report aggravation of pain with head movement, particularly on bending down and then straightening up. Swallowed discharge often produces significant abdominal discomfort as well. Coughing is often a feature but tends to be less prominent than in younger children. Physical findings include purulent (often blood-streaked) nasal and postnasal discharge, erythema of the nasal mucosa, and halitosis. Tenderness on sinus percussion is common. As with younger children, the clinical spectrum is wide and highly variable.

Ancillary Diagnostic Methods

When patients have most of the signs and symptoms of sinusitis, the diagnosis can be made on clinical grounds and treatment started empirically. This is particularly true for the younger child with the prolonged upper respiratory tract infection picture. Amoxicillin remains the drug of first choice for patients who are not allergic to penicillin. If there is no clear clinical improvement in 3 to 4 days, switching to amoxicillin/clavulanate or a comparable antimicrobial is indicated. If this also fails to produce clinical improvement in 3 to 4 days, resistant pneumococci may be the likely culprits, and high-dose amoxicillin/clavulanate (80 to 90 mg/kg/day), clindamycin, or an agent to which the organism is likely to be sensitive is indicated. In less clear-cut cases, ancillary tools and tests are often necessary. The usefulness of the various diagnostic methods in evaluating suspected sinusitis is still under study. Radiography appears to be the most helpful noninvasive tool in children older than 2 years of age. Radiographs are most useful in patients in whom the clinical picture is not distinct enough to distinguish between sinusitis and allergic rhinitis and in patients who fail to respond to antimicrobial therapy as noted earlier. Findings of complete opacification, mucosal thickening greater than 4 mm, or an air-fluid level on standard radiography (Fig. 23-55) are strongly associated with positive findings on sinus aspiration. However, the wide range of variability in development and configuration of the sinuses can make interpretation difficult. Plain radiographs of the sinuses have been shown to both overestimate and underestimate the degree of sinusitis when compared with CT of the sinuses. The CT scan (Fig. 23-56) is the most sensitive modality for diagnosis and is considered the gold standard, but it can be falsely positive in patients with viral upper respiratory tract infections, is expensive, and requires sedation of the younger patient for an adequate examination. Thus it should be reserved for patients with possible complications of sinusitis, underlying anatomic abnormalities, or suspected chronic sinusitis who fail to respond to a prolonged course of antimicrobial therapy.

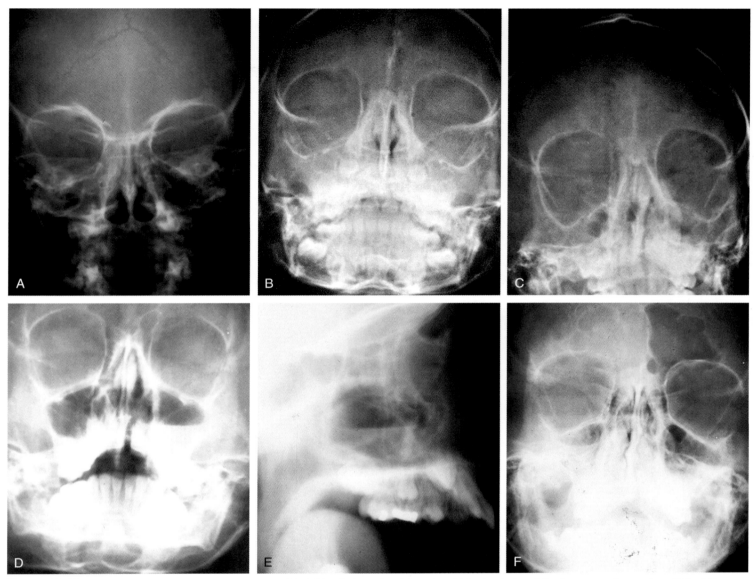

Figure 23-55. Radiographic findings in sinusitis. **A,** In this Caldwell view, the right ethmoid is clouded and the bony margins are less distinct than on the left. **B,** In this Waters view, complete opacification of both maxillary sinuses is evident. The bony margins are visible but faint. **C,** This child has significant mucosal thickening of the maxillary sinuses. Thickening of greater than 4 mm has a strong association with positive culture on sinus aspirate. **D** and **E,** In another patient an air-fluid level can be seen in the left maxillary sinus on both Waters and lateral views. **F,** Differential opacification of the right frontal sinus is evident in this child who had fever and headache. (**D** and **E,** Courtesy J. Ledesma-Medina, MD; **F,** courtesy CD Bluestone, MD, Children's Hospital of Pittsburgh.)

Needle aspiration of the sinuses is conclusive but invasive and not without risk. It is, however, justified in patients with severe symptoms, patients with CNS or orbital extension, those not responding to treatment, and those who are immunocompromised or immunosuppressed.

At minimum, therapy consists of a 10- to 14-day course (or until the patient is symptom free for 7 days) of an antimicrobial agent suitable to the likely spectrum of organisms (see preceding paragraph). It is not unusual for a 3- to 4-week course of therapy with a β-lactam-stable agent to be required. Analgesia is given as needed for discomfort and perhaps an oral antihistamine or topical intranasal steroid spray in patients known to have allergic rhinitis. Some children with intense headaches or facial pain experience symptomatic relief by using topical nasal vasoconstrictors and warm compresses during the first 1 or 2 days of therapy. Patients with sinusitis should be instructed to avoid swimming underwater or diving until completion of therapy because the resultant barotrauma aggravates symptoms and may promote intracranial spread of infection.

Complications of Sinusitis

Infectious sinusitis is important not only because of the discomfort it causes, but also because there is a significant risk of extension of infection and secondary complications. This risk stems from several anatomic factors. First, the sinuses surround the orbits superiorly, medially, and inferiorly. The bony plates that make up the sinus walls are thin and porous, and their suture lines are open in childhood. This is especially true of the lamina papyracea, which separates the ethmoid air cells from the orbits (Fig. 23-57). Increased sinus pressure occurring as a result of ostial blockage and fluid collection can cause separation of portions of these bony septa and can compromise their blood supply. The resultant necrosis promotes extension of infection. Facial vascular anatomy also contributes to the spread of infection. The veins of the face, nose, and sinuses drain in part into the orbit and then into the ophthalmic venous system, which is in direct continuity with the cavernous sinus. The ophthalmic veins have no valves and thus may provide less defense against spread of infection. The orbit is also devoid of lymphatics, which

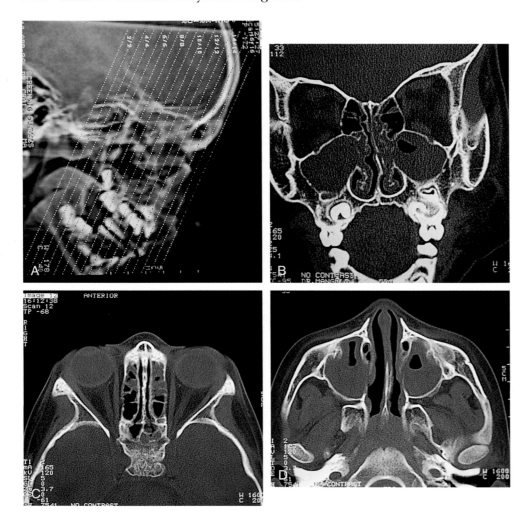

Figure 23-56. CT findings in acute sinusitis. **A,** In the topographic view the examiner can identify the position of each slice and also has an excellent view of the adenoid bed. **B,** The coronal view shows the maxillary-ethmoidal relationship in conjunction with the orbit. Note that the ethmoids are clear but the right maxillary sinus is completely opacified, and the left maxillary sinus is nearly so with only a small air pocket visible. **C,** This axial view shows patchy ethmoidal clouding. **D,** Marked mucosal thickening of both maxillary sinuses is shown in this axial view.

helps explain the ease of periorbital edema formation when there is increased sinus pressure. The relative looseness of the subcutaneous tissues of the face also assists edema collection and may aid in spread of infection. As a result of these factors, direct extension of infection can occur: (1) into the periorbital soft tissues, producing periorbital cellulitis; (2) through the bony walls into the orbits, resulting in orbital cellulitis or a subperiosteal abscess within the bony orbit; (3) via erosion outward through the frontal bone, producing a Pott puffy tumor; or (4) via erosion inward through the frontal bone, resulting in an epidural abscess. On rare occasions, hematogenous seeding of bacteria may occur.

Fortunately, improved recognition of sinus infection and early use of antimicrobial therapy, whether before or early in the course of recognized extension, have reduced the frequency, severity, and morbidity of these disorders.

Pott puffy tumor and epidural abscess, being direct complications of frontal sinusitis, are discussed next. Periorbital and orbital cellulitis, stemming at times from sinusitis and at times from other predisposing conditions, are covered in the subsequent section.

Pott Puffy Tumor. Frontal sinusitis assumes importance after 8 to 10 years of age (once the frontal sinuses have begun to form) and has the potential for serious complications, particularly when neglected or inadequately treated. Erosion occurring anteriorly through the frontal bone results in formation of a subperiosteal abscess, classically known as a *Pott puffy tumor*. This is seen as an erythematous frontal swelling that has a doughy consistency and is exquisitely tender (Fig. 23-58). Affected patients tend to be toxic, febrile, and extremely uncomfortable. Prompt surgical drainage is of utmost importance. A CT scan should be obtained before surgical drainage to evaluate the extent of the abscess and identify other sites of spread. Osteomyelitis of the frontal bone is present, and long-term IV antimicrobials are required for Pott puffy tumor.

Epidural Abscess. Another potential complication of frontal sinusitis is the formation of an epidural abscess as the result of erosion through the posterior wall of the frontal bone. This should be suspected in patients with frontal sinusitis who have unusually high temperature, unusually severe headache, signs of toxicity, or altered sensorium. Diagnosis is best confirmed by CT scan (Fig. 23-59) and MRI. Although IV antimicrobial therapy and careful monitoring may suffice in management of small lesions, larger abscesses necessitate neurosurgical consultation and surgical intervention. Brain abscesses are also possible (see Fig. 15-48).

Periorbital and Orbital Infections

Periorbital Cellulitis Caused by Spread from Adjacent Sinusitis

Periorbital cellulitis is the mildest of the complications of infectious sinusitis. The cellulitis is confined to tissues outside the orbit, with spread blocked in part by the orbital septum (see Fig. 23-57). When sinusitis is the underlying condition, the ethmoid or maxillary sinuses are the structures primarily affected. Typically, patients are younger

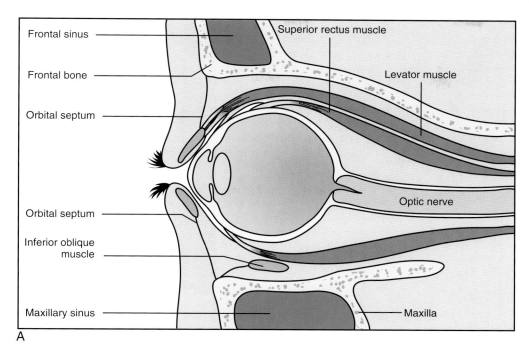

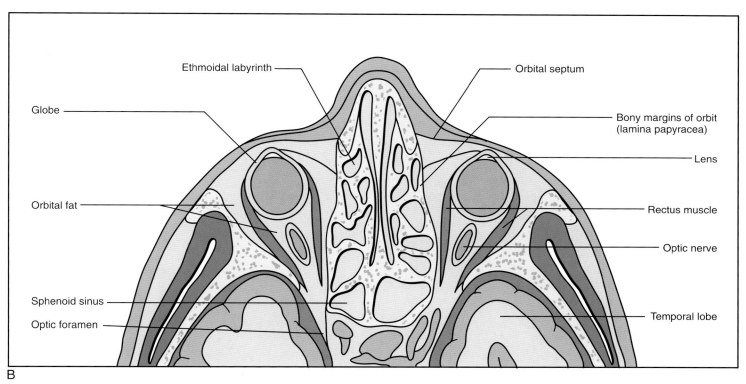

Figure 23-57. The anatomy of the orbit. **A,** Sagittal section shows the relationship of the orbit to the maxillary and frontal sinuses and the position of the orbital septum within the eyelid. The latter structure appears to serve as an anatomic barrier, helping to prevent the spread of infection from periorbital tissues into the orbit. **B,** In this horizontal section the close relationship of the orbit to the ethmoid sinuses is apparent.

than 4 or 5 years of age and have an antecedent history of upper respiratory tract infection with or without conjunctivitis, otitis, or sinusitis. This is superseded by the sudden appearance of lid and periorbital swelling. In contrast to the uncomplicated sympathetic edema seen in some patients with sinusitis, the swelling in children with periorbital cellulitis is usually unilateral and is erythematous, indurated, and tender (Fig. 23-60). Conjunctival injection and discharge may also be seen. In many patients a secondary increase in temperature accompanies the onset of swelling, but although most patients appear uncomfortable, toxicity is unusual. The course of periorbital cellulitis resulting from extension of sinus infection is milder and characterized by much slower progression than is true of cases resulting from hematogenous spread.

Periorbital Cellulitis Caused by Hematogenous Spread

When periorbital cellulitis is the result of hematogenous seeding, the organisms tend to be more virulent, the onset more explosive, and the course more fulminant. Typically the patient experiences sudden onset of high fever (often after a mild upper respiratory tract infection) accompanied by the appearance of erythematous, indurated, and tender periorbital swelling, which progresses rapidly and

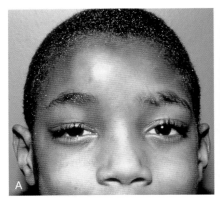
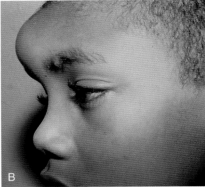
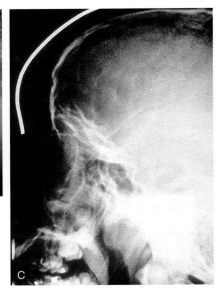

Figure 23-58. Pott puffy tumor. **A** and **B,** This patient had fever, headache, and an erythematous swelling over the forehead that was exquisitely tender and had a doughy consistency. **C,** A lateral radiograph shows frontal sinus clouding, irregularity of the frontal bone, and marked soft tissue swelling that is highlighted by a wire placed over the forehead and scalp. (**C,** Courtesy Kenneth Grundfast, MD, Boston Medical Center.)

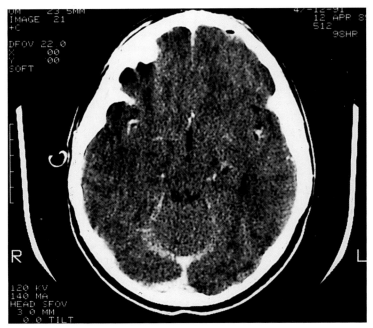

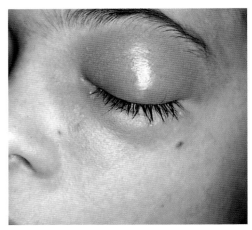

Figure 23-60. Periorbital cellulitis. Intense erythema and edema of the lids are evident. The swollen tissues were indurated and tender on palpation. Ocular motion was normal. Underlying ethmoid sinusitis was confirmed by CT scan.

Figure 23-59. Epidural abscess. This patient had lethargy, high fever, left eye pain, and periorbital swelling after 1 week of severe nasal congestion. A CT scan, obtained to rule out orbital involvement, revealed a small epidural abscess behind the left frontal bone. Note the small central air pocket.

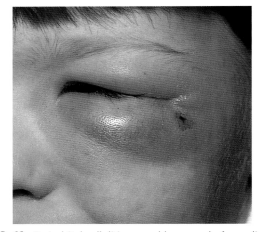

Figure 23-61. Periorbital cellulitis caused by spread of an adjacent facial infection. This child developed fever and erythematous, tender periorbital swelling a few days after incurring an abrasion as a result of a fall.

is accompanied by signs of systemic toxicity. The majority of these patients are younger than 1 year of age or only slightly older, and bacteremia with *S. pneumoniae* or *H. influenzae* type B is usual. Widespread use of the *H. influenzae* type B vaccine has dramatically reduced the incidence of *H. influenzae* B–induced cellulitis.

Periorbital Cellulitis Caused by Spread from Adjacent Facial Infection

More than 50% of children with periorbital cellulitis have neither sinusitis nor bacteremia as a predisposing condition. Rather, the patients appear to suffer from extension of nearby facial infection to periorbital tissues. They may have a history of antecedent trauma to the orbit or nearby facial structures often with a break in the skin (Fig. 23-61) or one of a primary skin infection (impetigo, a pustule, a chalazion, infected dermatitis, or insect bite).

They subsequently experience a temperature spike and evolution of periorbital and eyelid edema. This group tends to be somewhat older, generally older than 5 years of age. *Staphylococcus aureus* and group A β-hemolytic streptococci are the predominant offending organisms.

Diagnostic Studies

A number of cultures are often obtained in an attempt to isolate the causative pathogen in cases of periorbital cellulitis. Needle aspiration of the leading edge of the cellulitis has perhaps the highest yield but requires caution. It is perhaps best avoided when the inflamed area does not extend well beyond the orbital rim because of the risk of eye injury if the patient moves suddenly, despite efforts to immobilize his or her head. Cultures of adjacent skin wounds, when present, are also commonly positive. Nasopharyngeal and conjunctival drainage reveals the offending organism in about one half to two thirds of cases, respectively. Blood cultures are positive in about one third of patients overall, with the highest incidence found in cases caused by hematogenous spread. Sinus radiographs show opacification in more than two thirds of patients without antecedent trauma or skin lesions and in about 40% to 50% of patients with such a history. Ethmoid opacification is the predominant finding. Middle meatus culture, but not nasal culture, may be useful for detection of the sinus pathogen. Radiographic interpretation can be difficult, however, because overlying edema may give a false impression of clouding. In addition, standard radiographs are relatively useless in most cases of hematogenous origin because the patients are typically younger than 1 year of age. CT, however, is an excellent tool for assessing the extent of infection and the presence or absence of sinus opacification, as well as for detecting evidence of early orbital involvement.

Because of the severity and the potential for further extension and hematogenous spread, aggressive IV antimicrobial therapy is urgently required. This necessitates empirical selection of agents to cover likely pathogens, pending culture results. Patients also require close monitoring for signs of complications.

Orbital Cellulitis

In orbital cellulitis, infection extends into the orbit itself. It may take the form of undifferentiated cellulitis, or it may later evolve into a subperiosteal or orbital abscess. Patients tend to have a history similar to that of patients with periorbital cellulitis but are generally more ill, toxic, and lethargic. The most common source of spread is an adjacent, infected ethmoid sinus, although extension from a nearby facial infection occasionally occurs. Causative organisms are the same as those in periorbital cellulitis. Patients old enough to be articulate describe intense, deep retro-orbital pain aggravated by ocular movement. Edema and erythema of the lid and periorbital tissues are often so marked that it is impossible to open the eye without use of lid retractors (Fig. 23-62A and B). Tenderness is exquisite. If the lid can be retracted, the clinician may find proptosis, conjunctival inflammation with chemosis and purulent discharge, decreased extraocular motion, and some loss of visual acuity. Ophthalmologic consultation is required.

Aggressive IV antimicrobial therapy and close monitoring for evolution and CNS complications are vital in the management of orbital cellulitis. CT is proving exceptionally useful for determining the presence or absence of abscesses (see Fig. 23-62C). When a subperiosteal abscess is present or the clinical ocular examination shows deterioration, surgical drainage combined with an ethmoidectomy is indicated. It is now possible to perform the ethmoidectomy and abscess drainage endoscopically in selected patients. Optimal management necessitates a team approach involving pediatrics, otolaryngology, ophthalmology, and at times neurosurgery.

Local complications of orbital cellulitis include abscess formation, optic neuritis, retinal vein thrombosis, and panophthalmitis. CNS complications may result from direct extension or spread of septic thrombophlebitis. Meningitis, epidural and subdural abscesses, and cavernous sinus thrombosis have been described. All are characterized by marked toxicity and alteration in level of consciousness. Cavernous sinus thrombosis is heralded by sudden, bilateral, pulsating proptosis and chemosis in association with increased toxicity and obtundation.

Atopic Disorders

Allergic Rhinitis with Postnasal Discharge

Patients with allergic rhinitis appear to be more susceptible to infectious sinusitis than nonatopic individuals, probably as a result of mucosal swelling in response to allergen exposure and alterations in ciliary action. They can also have symptoms mimicking sinusitis in the absence of infection, and this can be a source of confusion. Two major clinical pictures are seen. In the first, nasal congestion, nighttime cough, and morning throat clearing are prominent. Some patients may complain of morning nausea, and a few may have morning emesis with vomitus containing large amounts of clear mucus.

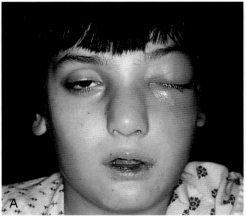
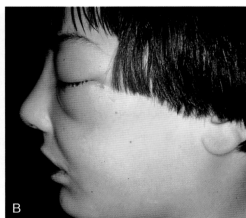
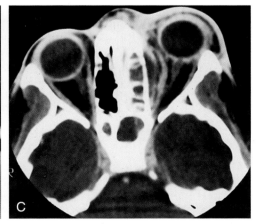

Figure 23-62. Orbital cellulitis. **A** and **B,** This child had a fever, severe toxicity, and marked lethargy. He experienced intense orbital and retro-orbital pain and showed a limited range of ocular motion with associated exacerbation of pain. **C,** This CT scan shows preseptal swelling, proptosis, and lateral displacement of the globe and orbital contents by a subperiosteal abscess.

Fever is absent, and in contrast with infectious sinusitis, nasal discharge is never purulent, there is no halitosis, and daytime cough is not prominent. Patients may complain of itching of the nose and eyes, and some have frequent sneezing. On examination, the nasal mucosa is edematous but does not appear inflamed. Discharge, if present, is clear. Patients also tend to have the typical allergic facies (see Chapter 4) with Dennie lines, allergic shiners, and cobblestoning of the conjunctivae. Environmental control and antihistamines provide symptomatic relief for most of these children.

Vacuum Headache

The second potentially confusing clinical picture is that of the allergic sinus headache, or vacuum headache. In this condition, older atopic individuals complain of intense facial or frontal headache, without fever or other evidence of infection. This occurs during periods in which patients are having exacerbation of allergic symptoms, after swimming in chlorinated pools, or while flying on an airplane. The phenomenon appears to be caused by acute blockage of sinus ostia by mucosal edema, with subsequent creation of a vacuum within the sinus as a result of oxygen consumption by mucosal cells. The resultant negative pressure pulls the mucosa away from the walls of the sinus, producing the pain. In these patients the nasal mucosa tends to be pale and swollen but without discharge. Sinuses may be tender to percussion but are clear radiographically. Symptoms respond promptly to application of a topical vasoconstrictor and warm compresses over the face. Improvement is maintained by antihistamines and decongestants.

Oropharyngeal Disorders

Oropharyngeal Examination

Adequate examination of the pharynx is important in pediatrics because of the frequency of pharyngeal infections. However, the procedure can be challenging at times. The small size of the mouth and difficulty of depressing the tongue in infancy, lack of cooperativeness in toddlers, and fear of gagging with use of tongue blades in older children can impede efforts. These problems can be minimized with a few simple techniques. Infants and young children, when placed supine with the head hyperextended on the neck, tend to open their mouths spontaneously, enabling visualization of the anterior oral cavity and assisting insertion of a tongue blade to depress the tongue and inspect the posterior palate and pharynx. When examining older children, asking them to open their mouths as wide as possible and pant "like a puppy dog" or say "ha ha" usually results in lowering of the posterior portion of the tongue, revealing the posterior palatal and pharyngeal structures. Because conditions involving the lips, mucosa, and dentition are presented in Chapter 20, this section concentrates on palatal and pharyngeal disorders.

Palatal Disorders

Palatal malformations range widely in severity and can significantly affect feeding, swallowing, and speech. In addition, by altering normal nasal and oropharyngeal physiology, they place affected patients at increased risk for chronic recurrent ear and sinus infections.

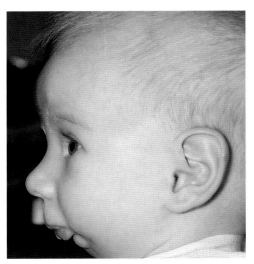

Figure 23-63. Pierre Robin syndrome, characterized by severe retromicrognathia and cleft palate. In this infant the micrognathia produced posterior displacement of the tongue, resulting in airway obstruction that necessitated a tracheotomy. (Courtesy Wolfgang Loskin, MD, University of North Carolina, Chapel Hill.)

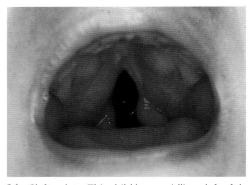

Figure 23-64. Cleft palate. This child has a midline cleft of the soft palate. The hard palate, alveolar ridge, and lip are spared. (Courtesy Ms. Barbara Elster, Cleft Palate Center, Pittsburgh.)

Cleft Palate

Palatal clefts are among the most severe abnormalities encountered. They stem from a failure of fusion during the second month of gestation and have an incidence of about 1 in every 2000 to 2500 births. They are usually but not always associated with a cleft lip. The defect is often isolated in an otherwise normal child. In many cases there is a positive family history for the anomaly. A number of teratogens have also been linked to the malformation. In a small percentage of cases the cleft palate is one of multiple congenital anomalies in the context of a major genetic syndrome such as the Pierre Robin anomaly (Fig. 23-63) and trisomies 13 and 18 (see Chapter 1).

The extent of the cleft varies: Some involve only the soft palate (Fig. 23-64); others extend through the hard palate but spare the alveolar ridge (Fig. 23-65A). Still others are complete (Fig. 23-65B and C). The defect may be unilateral or bilateral. The four major types of congenital cleft palate follow:

Type I Soft palate only (see Fig. 23-64)
Type II Unilateral cleft of soft and hard palate (see Fig. 23-65A)
Type III Unilateral cleft of soft and hard palate extending through the alveolar ridge (see Fig. 23-65B)
Type IV Bilateral cleft of soft and hard palate extending through the alveolar ridge (see Fig. 23-65C)

These anomalies create a number of problems beyond the obvious cosmetic deformity. In infancy, a cleft palate pre-

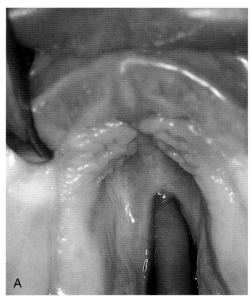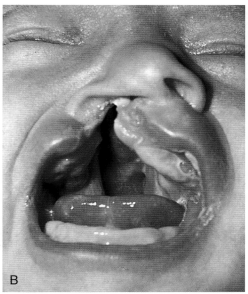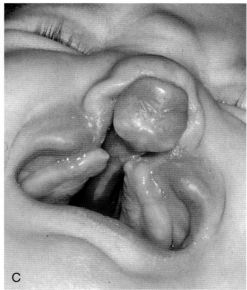

Figure 23-65. Cleft palate. **A,** Cleft of the hard and soft palate, sparing the alveolar ridge. Complete clefts of the palate, alveolar ridge, and lip may be unilateral **(B)** or bilateral **(C)**. (**A** and **C,** Courtesy William Garrett, MD; **B,** courtesy Michael Sherlock, MD, Lutherville, Md.)

vents the child from creating an effective seal when nursing and hampers feeding. In addition, formula tends to reflux into the nasopharynx with resultant choking. This necessitates patience during feeding, use of palatal obturators or specially designed nipples or feeding devices, and careful training of parents in feeding techniques that facilitate nursing and prevent failure to thrive. Eustachian tube function is uniformly abnormal, and before repair, all patients have chronic middle ear effusions that are frequently infected. Even after repair, recurrent middle ear disease (characterized by negative pressure and effusions, and possibly cholesteatomas) remains a problem. Hearing loss, with its potential for hampering language acquisition, ultimately occurs in more than 50% of patients. Despite corrective surgery, palatal function is never totally normal, and many patients continue to have hypernasal speech and difficulties in articulation, necessitating long-term speech therapy. Secondary dental and orthodontic problems are routine as well.

The multitude of problems and the need for frequent medical visits and multiple operations, in combination with the often-associated cosmetic deformity, can have a significant psychological impact on the child and family. Optimal management necessitates a multidisciplinary team, preferably coordinated by a primary care physician who is aware of the patient's individual needs and those of his or her family. Timing of corrective surgery remains somewhat controversial. Cleft lips are repaired at about 3 months, but scheduling of palatal repair must be individualized depending on the size and extent of the cleft. Defects of the soft palate are generally repaired at about 8 months, and the hard palate is closed either surgically or by use of a prosthetic plate. Most patients also require early myringotomy with insertion of tubes at the time of lip repair to help manage the chronic middle ear disease. Adenoidectomy is contraindicated because of adverse effects on palatal function, unless airway obstruction is severe and resistant to antimicrobial therapy. Upper (partial) adenoidectomy may be required in selected patients with severe airway obstruction.

Another disorder of clinical importance, **submucous cleft of the palate,** is often overlooked in infancy. The condition is characterized by a bony U-shaped notch, pal-pable in the midline, at the juncture of the hard and soft portions of the palate (Fig. 23-66A). There also may be palpable midline thinning of the soft palate. The anomaly results from a failure of the tensor veli palatini muscle to insert properly in the midline. Some children have an associated double or notched (bifid) uvula that, when present, serves as a clue to the existence of the palatal abnormality (see Fig. 23-66A and B). The bifid uvula may be an isolated anomaly, however. Although not subject to the feeding difficulties seen in children with overt clefts, children with submucous clefts have similar problems with eustachian tube dysfunction and recurrent middle ear disease. Speech is often mildly hypernasal. Recognition is particularly important when considering tonsillectomy and adenoidectomy for recurrent tonsillitis and otitis because surgical removal of the adenoids in these children can result in severe speech and swallowing dysfunction; hence these procedures may be contraindicated. In selected cases of severe adenoidal hypertrophy, upper (partial) adenoidectomy may be an option.

High-Arched Palate

High-arched palate, a minor anomaly, is a common clinical finding (Fig. 23-67). Although usually an isolated variant of palatal configuration, it occasionally occurs in association with congenital syndromes. Long-term orotracheal intubation of premature infants creates an iatrogenic form of the problem. Although generally clinically insignificant, the high arch can be associated with increased frequency of ear and sinus infections and hyponasal speech in severe cases.

Tonsillar and Peritonsillar Disorders

Tonsillitis/Pharyngitis

As noted earlier, the tonsils and adenoids are quite small in infancy, gradually enlarge over the first 8 to 10 years of life, and then start to regress in size. When evaluating the tonsils, particularly during the course of an acute infection, or when monitoring patients for chronic enlargement, it is helpful to use a standardized size-grading

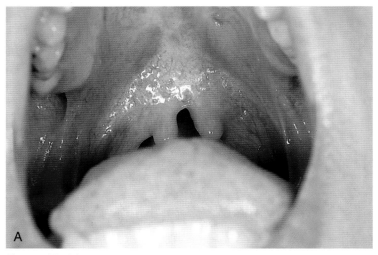

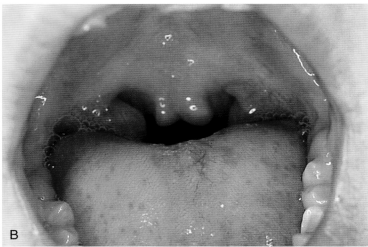

Figure 23-66. Submucous cleft of the palate. **A,** This girl shows failure of normal midline fusion of the palatal muscles, resulting in midline thinning of the soft palate. Palpation confirms the area of weakness. A U-shaped notch can also be felt in the midline at the junction of the hard and soft palate. She also has a bifid uvula. **B,** This child was found to have a notched uvula on pharyngeal examination. This may serve as a clue to the presence of a submucous palatal cleft, or it may be an isolated anomaly.

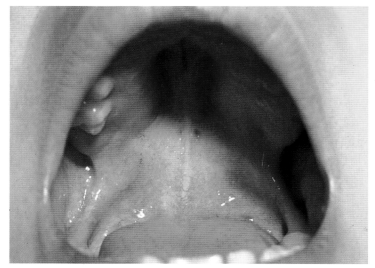

Figure 23-67. High-arched palate. This is a common minor anomaly, usually isolated, but occasionally associated with genetic syndromes.

system, as shown in Figure 23-68. Inspection of the palate is also important in assessing patients with tonsillopharyngitis because lesions characteristic of particular pathogens are often present on the soft palate and tonsillar pillars (see Chapter 12).

The tonsils appear to serve as a first line of immunologic defense against respiratory pathogens and are frequently infected by viral and bacterial agents. The most commonly identified organisms are group A β-hemolytic streptococci, adenoviruses, coxsackieviruses, and the Epstein-Barr (EB) virus. There is a wide range of severity in symptoms and signs, regardless of the pathogenic organism. Sore throat is the major symptom, and it may be mild, moderate, or severe. When severe, it is typically associated with dysphagia. Erythema is the most common physical finding and varies from slightly to intensely red (Fig. 23-69). Additional findings may include acute tonsillar enlargement, formation of exudates over the tonsillar surfaces, and cervical adenopathy. In a small percentage of cases the findings suggest a given pathogen. Patients with fever, headache, bright red and enlarged tonsils (with or without exudate), palatal petechiae (Fig. 23-69B), tender and enlarged anterior cervical nodes, and perhaps abdom-

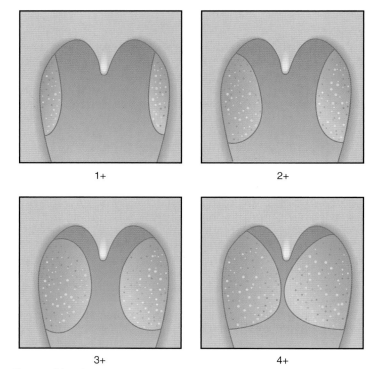

Figure 23-68. Grading of tonsillar size for children with acute tonsillopharyngitis and those with chronic tonsillar enlargement. This grading system is particularly useful in serial examinations of a given patient. (Modified from Feinstein AR, Levitt M: Role of tonsils. N Engl J Med 282: 285-291, 1970. Copyright © 1970 Massachusetts Medical Society. All rights reserved.)

inal pain are likely to have streptococcal infection. Patients with marked malaise, fever, exudative tonsillitis, generalized adenopathy, and splenomegaly are probably suffering from EB virus mononucleosis (Fig. 23-69C, and see Chapter 12). Those with conjunctivitis, nonexudative tonsillar inflammation, and cervical adenopathy may have adenovirus. Yellow ulcerations with red halos on the tonsillar pillars strongly suggest coxsackievirus infection, whether or not other oral, palmar, or plantar lesions are present (see Chapter 12). Unfortunately, the majority of patients with tonsillopharyngitis do not have such clear-cut clinical syndromes. Patients with streptococcal infection may have only minimal erythema; in its early stages, mono-

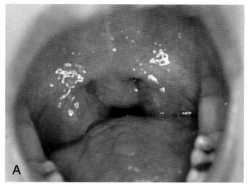

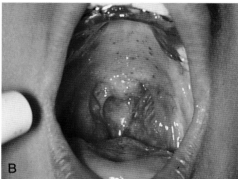

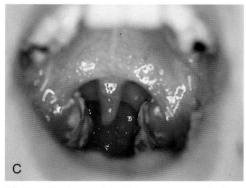

Figure 23-69. Tonsillopharyngitis. This common entity has a number of causative pathogens and a wide spectrum of severity. **A,** The diffuse tonsillar and pharyngeal erythema seen here is a nonspecific finding that can be produced by a variety of pathogens. **B,** This intense erythema, seen in association with acute tonsillar enlargement and palatal petechiae, is highly suggestive of group A β-streptococcal infection, though other pathogens can produce these findings. **C,** This picture of exudative tonsillitis is most commonly seen with either group A streptococcal or Epstein-Barr virus infection. (**B,** Courtesy Michael Sherlock, MD, Lutherville, Md.)

nucleosis may consist of fever, malaise, and nonexudative pharyngitis without other signs; and although streptococci and EB virus are the most common sources of exudative tonsillitis and palatal petechiae, other pathogens produce these findings as well.

Because of the variability in the clinical picture and the importance of identifying and treating group A β-hemolytic streptococcal infection to prevent both pyogenic (e.g., cervical adenitis, peritonsillar, retropharyngeal and parapharyngeal abscesses) and nonpyogenic (e.g., rheumatic fever) complications, a screening throat culture is advisable for patients with even mild signs or symptoms of tonsillopharyngitis. In obtaining this culture, the clinician swabs both tonsils and the posterior pharyngeal wall to maximize the chance of obtaining the organism. In the first 3 years of life, when streptococcal infection is suspected (because of history of exposure, signs of pharyngitis, or scarlatiniform rash), it is helpful to obtain a nasopharyngeal culture as well. For reasons as yet unclear,

the nasopharyngeal culture is often positive when the throat culture is negative in this age group.

Treatment is symptomatic for all forms of tonsillopharyngitis except that caused by group A β-hemolytic streptococci, which requires a 10-day course of penicillin, amoxicillin, or erythromycin. As the secondary attack rate of group A β-hemolytic streptococci within families is 50%, parents should be instructed to notify the physician if other family members develop symptoms of upper respiratory or pharyngeal infection within the ensuing few weeks. If so, they can then be examined and specimens obtained for culture, or they can be treated empirically. Follow-up is also important. As noted earlier, the tonsillitis of mononucleosis may appear mild early in the course of the illness, yet tonsillar inflammation and enlargement may progress over a few to several days to produce severe dysphagia and even airway obstruction. Thus parents should be instructed to notify the physician if such signs develop. Follow-up is also important in monitoring for other complications and for frequent recurrences.

Recurrent Tonsillitis

Frequent recurrences of tonsillitis, despite antibiotic therapy when indicated, must be handled on an individual basis. In some cases frequent recurrences of streptococcal infection can be traced to other family members. When they are treated along with the patient, the cycle of recurrences often ends. In other instances frequent recurrent tonsillar infections have no traceable source within the family, and they are significantly debilitating. In children with six or more episodes in any 1 year, five episodes a year for 2 consecutive years, or three episodes per year for 3 consecutive years, tonsillectomy has a favorable outcome in reducing both frequency and severity of sore throats.

Uvulitis

Uvulitis is characterized by inflammation and edema of the uvula. In addition to throat pain and dysphagia, affected patients commonly complain of a sense of having "something in their throat" or a gagging sensation. The phenomenon has been reported in association with pharyngitis caused by group A β-hemolytic streptococci, in which cases the uvula is bright red and often hemorrhagic (Fig. 23-70A). The condition has also been noted in association with mononucleosis, both in the presence and the absence of exudative tonsillitis (Fig. 23-70B), and with other viral agents as well (Fig. 23-70C). Uvulitis has also been reported in a patient with concurrent epiglottitis. In this case the child was anxious, toxic, febrile, and drooling, with a more severe clinical picture than that seen with streptococcal or EB virus infection. Culture of the uvular surface grew *H. influenzae* type B.

Peritonsillar Abscess or Cellulitis

A peritonsillar abscess is one that forms between the tonsil and constrictor muscle and extends into the soft palate. Patients are usually school age or older, and they typically have a history of having developed an antecedent sore throat a week or two earlier, which was not cultured or treated, or for which the child was given an incomplete course of antimicrobial therapy. The patient may experience initial improvement but then has a sudden onset of high fever and severe throat pain, which is worse on one side. The pain usually radiates to the ipsilateral ear and is associated with marked dysphagia, such that the patient spits out saliva to avoid swallowing. On examination, the child often appears toxic and has obvious enlarge-

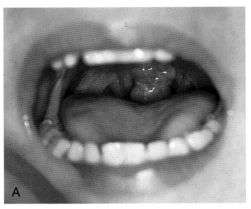
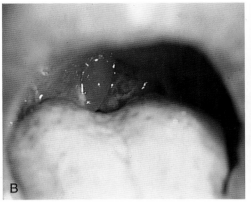
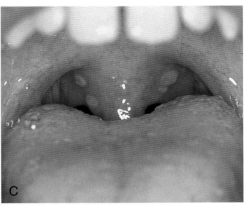

Figure 23-70. Uvulitis. **A,** The uvula appears markedly erythematous and edematous, with pinpoint hemorrhages, in this case caused by β-streptococci. **B,** In this child with mononucleosis the tonsils are enlarged and covered with a gray membrane, and the uvula is edematous and erythematous. The patient had respiratory compromise because of the severity of his tonsillar and adenoidal hypertrophy. **C,** The vesicular lesions on the swollen, painful uvula of this patient suggest a viral etiology, probably involving an enterovirus.

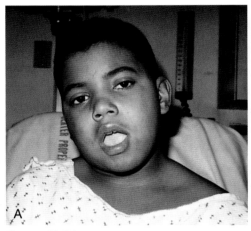
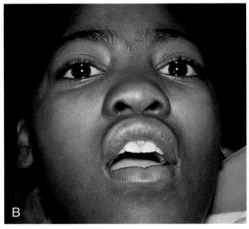
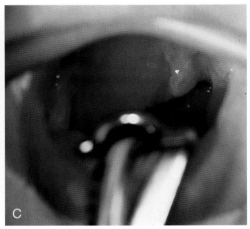

Figure 23-71. Peritonsillar abscess. **A,** This patient demonstrates the torticollis often seen with a peritonsillar abscess in an effort to minimize pressure on the adjacent inflamed tonsillar node. **B,** Sympathetic inflammation of the pterygoid muscles causes trismus, limiting the patient's ability to open the mouth. **C,** This photograph, taken in the operating room, shows an intensely inflamed soft palatal mass that obscures the tonsil and bulges forward and toward the midline, deviating the uvula.

ment of the ipsilateral tonsillar node, which is exquisitely tender. Many patients have torticollis, tilting the head toward the involved side to minimize pressure of the sternocleidomastoid muscle on the adjacent tonsillar lymph node (Fig. 23-71A). Speech is thick and muffled because of splinting of the tongue and pharyngeal muscles. Trismus, or limitation of mouth opening, is often noted as a result of inflammation of the adjacent pterygoid muscles (Fig. 23-71B). If visualization of the pharynx is possible (despite the trismus), a bright red, smooth mass is seen in the supratonsillar area projecting forward and medially, obscuring the tonsil, and deviating the uvula to the opposite side (Fig. 23-71C). Group A β-hemolytic streptococci and *S. aureus* are the most common pathogens. Mixed infections with gram-positive and gram-negative aerobic, as well as anaerobic pathogens, are common. Patients with mononucleosis, concurrently infected with group A streptococci and treated with steroids, are reportedly at risk for developing a rapidly evolving peritonsillar abscess.

If fluctuance is evident on palpation, operative drainage is necessary in addition to antibiotic therapy to prevent spontaneous rupture with secondary aspiration or other complications such as airway obstruction or spread of infection to adjacent areas. When fluctuance is not present, the patient is in a cellulitic stage and management consists of IV antimicrobial therapy and serial reexamination.

Because of the risks of rupture, prompt otolaryngologic consultation is suggested from the outset.

Tonsillar Lymphoma

The majority of children, whether well or acutely ill with tonsillitis, have tonsils that are symmetrical in size. When a child has an asymmetrically enlarged tonsil without evidence of infection, the possibility of a lymphoma should be considered (Fig. 23-72). Thorough history of recent health status and meticulous regional and general examination are in order. Particular attention should be paid to cervical and other nodes and to the size and consistency of abdominal viscera. Hematologic studies may also be helpful. In the absence of other evidence, a brief period of observation may be justified. If other findings are suggestive or enlargement continues during observation, excisional biopsy is indicated.

Penetrating Oropharyngeal Trauma

Penetrating oral injuries are fairly common in childhood and are usually the result of falling with a stick, pencil, straw, or lollipop in the mouth. Gunshot wounds and external stab wounds are unusual occurrences in the pediatric population, but their incidence begins to increase in adolescents. Prophylactic antimicrobial therapy is indi-

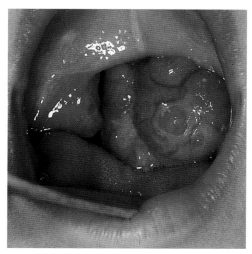

Figure 23-72. Tonsillar lymphoma. This adolescent had painless dysphagia. Examination revealed marked unilateral tonsillar enlargement. The asymmetry and degree of enlargement prompted tonsillectomy. Pathologic examination confirmed a tonsillar lymphoma.

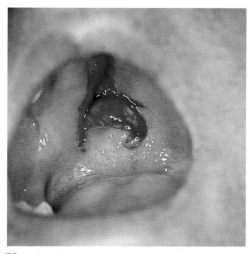

Figure 23-73. Palatal laceration. This large, complex laceration occurred when this boy fell with a piece of metal tubing in his mouth. A flap of palatal tissue has retracted away from the tear, warranting surgical approximation.

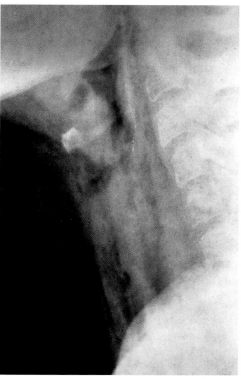

Figure 23-74. Retropharyngeal air dissection. This lateral neck radiograph of a child with a puncture wound of the posterior pharyngeal wall reveals extensive air dissection through the retropharyngeal soft tissues. Subcutaneous air has tracked anteriorly as well.

cated for all penetrating injuries because of the high risk of secondary infection.

The majority of intraoral injuries involve the palate and consist of simple lacerations. Many of these injuries heal spontaneously and require no repair. Large lacerations producing excessive bleeding or mucosal flaps must be sutured (Fig. 23-73).

Penetration of the posterior pharyngeal wall may result in a number of complications. These patients merit careful clinical evaluation of the oropharynx and neck; neck radiographs should also be obtained. Whenever an object penetrates the pharyngeal wall, it introduces oral flora into the retropharyngeal soft tissues, setting the stage for development of infection and abscess formation (see "Retropharyngeal Abscess" later and Fig. 23-76). This complication is seen predominantly in patients who fail to seek care immediately after the injury. However, it can develop even in treated patients. Symptoms generally begin a few to several days after the initial trauma. Fever, pain, dysphagia, and signs of airway compromise predominate.

In a number of patients with posterior pharyngeal tears, penetration results in dissection of air through the retro-pharyngeal soft tissues (Fig. 23-74). Such children may complain of throat and neck pain. Subcutaneous emphysema may be noted clinically. Occasionally, signs of airway compromise develop with this complication. Therefore hospitalization for observation is advisable when this sequela is encountered.

When penetration involves posterolateral structures (e.g., the tear is located near the tonsil or tonsillar pillar), the possibility of vascular injury must be considered. Deep penetration in this area can puncture or nick the internal carotid artery or nearby vessels, resulting in hemorrhage or, more commonly, gradual hematoma formation. Clues to vascular injury are lateral pharyngeal or peritonsillar swelling and fullness or tenderness on palpation of the neck on the side of the wound. Radiographs should confirm soft tissue swelling. Patients with peritonsillar tears should be admitted for observation even in the absence of these signs. Findings that suggest vascular involvement warrant magnetic resonance or CT angiography or, more rarely, formal angiography. Neck exploration for vessel repair may be required.

Upper Airway Obstruction

Acute Upper Airway Obstruction

Few conditions in pediatrics are as emergent and potentially life-threatening as those causing acute upper airway obstruction. In these conditions, expeditious assessment and appropriate stabilization are often life saving. In contrast, underestimation of severity of distress, overzealous attempts at examination or invasive procedures, and efforts by the unskilled to intervene may have catastrophic results.

The major causes are severe tonsillitis with adenoidal enlargement (see "Tonsillar and Peritonsillar Disorders" earlier and Fig. 23-70B), retropharyngeal abscess, epiglottitis, croup or laryngotracheobronchitis, foreign body aspiration, and angioedema (see Chapter 4). All are characterized by stridor, retractions that are primarily suprasternal and subcostal (unless distress becomes severe and retractions generalize), and mild to moderate increases in heart and respiratory rates. For purposes of assessment, it is helpful to classify the disorders into two categories—supraglottic and subglottic—on the basis of major signs and symptoms listed in Table 23-1.

The key to appropriate management is a brief history detailing the course and associated symptoms, followed by rapid assessment of clinical signs to determine the approximate level of airway involvement and the degree of respiratory distress (Table 23-2). This can be done for the most part through visual inspection, without ever touching the patient. It is particularly important to avoid upsetting a child with upper airway obstruction who shows signs of fatigue or cyanosis or meets any of the other criteria for severe respiratory distress. Such disturbances can serve only to worsen distress and may precipitate complete obstruction. Therefore when a child has signs of moderately severe or severe obstruction, his or her parents should be allowed to remain with him or her; any positional preference (if manifested) should be honored; and oral examination, venipuncture, IV line placement, and radiographs should be deferred until the airway is secure. Once the initial assessment is done, the most skilled personnel available are assembled to stabilize the airway. This procedure is best accomplished under controlled conditions in the operating room.

Supraglottic Disorders
See also "Tonsillar and Peritonsillar Disorders" earlier.

Retropharyngeal Abscess. A retropharyngeal abscess usually involves one of the retropharyngeal lymph nodes that run in chains through the retropharyngeal tissues on either side of the midline. Because these nodes tend to atrophy after 4 years of age, the disorder is seen primarily in children younger than 3 or 4 years old. The major causative organisms are group A β-hemolytic streptococci, although *S. aureus* is found in some cases. Mixed infections with gram-positive and gram-negative aerobes, as well as anaerobes, are common as well.

The child with a retropharyngeal abscess generally has a history of an acute, febrile upper respiratory tract infection or pharyngitis beginning several days earlier, which may have improved transiently. Suddenly, the child's condition worsens with development of a high spiking fever, toxicity, anorexia, drooling, and dyspnea. On examination, the patient is restless and irritable and tends to lie with his or her head hyperextended, simulating opisthotonos. Quiet gurgling stridor is heard. If respiratory distress is not severe, the pharynx can be examined, and a fiery red asymmetrical swelling of the posterior pharyngeal wall may be observed pushing the uvula and ipsilateral tonsil forward (Fig. 23-75A). Even with direct examination, this swelling can be difficult to appreciate at times. A portable lateral neck radiograph taken on inspiration and with the neck in extension (with a physician in attendance) shows marked widening of the prevertebral soft tissues (Fig. 23-75B), which are normally no wider than a vertebral body.

It should be noted that false-positive radiographic findings of prevertebral soft tissue swelling, in the absence of retropharyngeal pathologic findings, are common when lateral neck radiographs are not taken on inspiration and with the neck extended. When a retropharyngeal abscess is diagnosed, prompt otolaryngologic consultation should be sought to determine if the mass is fluctuant, necessitating surgical drainage, or if it is in an early cellulitic phase, requiring serial re-examination. A CT scan can be helpful in this regard (Fig. 23-75C). High-dose IV antimicrobial therapy is necessary whether or not drainage is required.

As noted earlier, a retropharyngeal abscess may occasionally form in an older child after a puncture wound of the posterior pharyngeal wall (Fig. 23-76). Signs of infection develop acutely a few days later. In these cases oral flora are found on culture.

Parapharyngeal Abscess. Lateral neck space abscesses can also occur in infants and young children. Most patients are toxic with high spiking fevers. The history and clinical picture are nearly identical to those of children with retropharyngeal abscess. However, these patients have torticollis, bending toward the affected side, and examination of the neck reveals diffuse anterolateral swelling that is exquisitely tender (Fig. 23-77A). Oral inspection may reveal medial displacement of the tonsil

Table 23-1	Clinical Features of Acute Upper Airway Disorders	
CLINICAL FINDING	**SUPRAGLOTTIC DISORDERS**	**SUBGLOTTIC DISORDERS**
Stridor	Quiet and wet	Loud
Voice alteration	Muffled	Hoarse
Dysphagia	+	−
Postural preference*	+	−
Barky cough	−	+ Especially with croup
Fever	+	+ Usually with croup
Toxicity	+	−
Trismus	+ Usually with peritonsillar abscess	−
Facial edema	−	+ Usually with angioedema

Epiglottitis—patient characteristically sits bolt upright, with neck extended and head held forward; *retropharyngeal abscess*—child often adopts opisthotonic posture; *peritonsillar abscess*—patient may tilt head toward affected side.
From Davis HW, Gartner JC, Galvis AG, et al: Acute upper airway obstruction: Croup and epiglottitis. Pediatr Clin North Am 28:859-880, 1981.

Table 23-2	Estimation of Severity of Respiratory Distress		
CLINICAL FINDING	**MILD**	**MODERATE**	**SEVERE**
Color	Normal	Normal	Pale, dusky, or cyanotic
Retractions	Absent to mild	Moderate	Severe and generalized with use of accessory muscles
Air entry	Mild ↓	Moderate ↓	Severe ↓
Level of consciousness	Normal or restless when disturbed	Anxious, restless when undisturbed	Lethargic, depressed

From Davis HW, Gartner JC, Galvis AG, et al: Acute upper airway obstruction: Croup and epiglottitis. Pediatr Clin North Am 28:859-880, 1981.

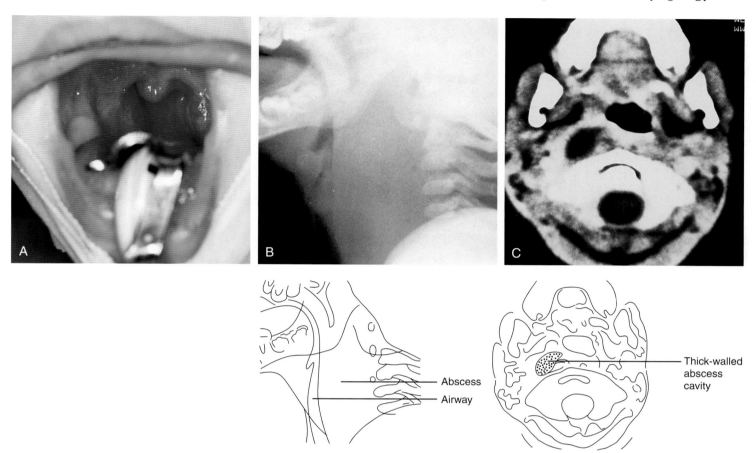

Figure 23-75. Retropharyngeal abscess. A young child presented with high fever, drooling, quiet stridor, and an opisthotonic postural preference. **A,** Pharyngeal examination in the operating room revealed an intensely erythematous, unilateral swelling of the posterior pharyngeal wall. **B,** A lateral neck radiograph shows prominent prevertebral soft tissue swelling that displaces the trachea forward. **C,** On CT scan, a thick-walled abscess cavity is evident in the retropharyngeal space. The highly vascular wall enhanced with contrast injection.

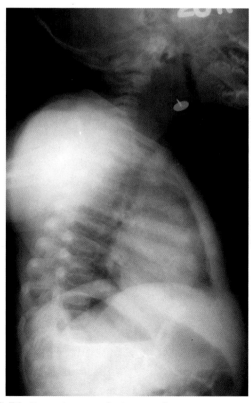

Figure 23-76. Retropharyngeal abscess after a puncture wound. This child tried to swallow a tack that punctured and became lodged in the posterior pharyngeal wall. The incident was unwitnessed, and he came to medical attention only when he developed fever and began drooling. (Courtesy Robert Gochman, MD, Schneider Children's Hospital, Long Island Jewish Medical Center.)

or lateral pharyngeal wall. A CT scan is essential to confirm the diagnosis (Fig. 23-77B). Parapharyngeal cellulitis is treated with IV antimicrobials. Abscesses are treated with prompt drainage to prevent rupture with aspiration of purulent material, erosion into vascular structures, and extension to adjacent sites or into the mediastinum.

Epiglottitis (Supraglottitis). Epiglottitis, perhaps the most acutely emergent form of acute upper airway obstruction, is an infection caused by *H. influenzae* type B. Its incidence has dropped precipitously since introduction of the *H. influenzae* B vaccine. Hence many younger practitioners have never seen a case, increasing the risk of delayed diagnosis. Epiglottitis is characterized by marked inflammation and edema of the pharynx, epiglottis, aryepiglottic folds, and ventricular bands. The peak age range is 1 to 7 years, but infants and older children may be affected. Onset is sudden and progression rapid; most patients are brought to medical attention within 12 hours of the first appearance of symptoms. Generally the child is entirely well until several hours before presentation, when he or she abruptly spikes a high fever. This is rapidly followed by progressive quiet stridor, severe throat pain with dysphagia and drooling, and soon thereafter by dyspnea and anxiety.

On examination, the child is usually toxic, anxious, and remarkably still, sitting bolt upright with neck extended and head held forward (unless obstruction is mild or fatigue has supervened) (Fig. 23-78A to C). Quiet gurgling stridor and drooling are evident, along with dyspnea and retractions. If the child will talk, which is unusual, the voice is muffled. This clinical picture is so typical that, when seen, the best course of action after initial assess-

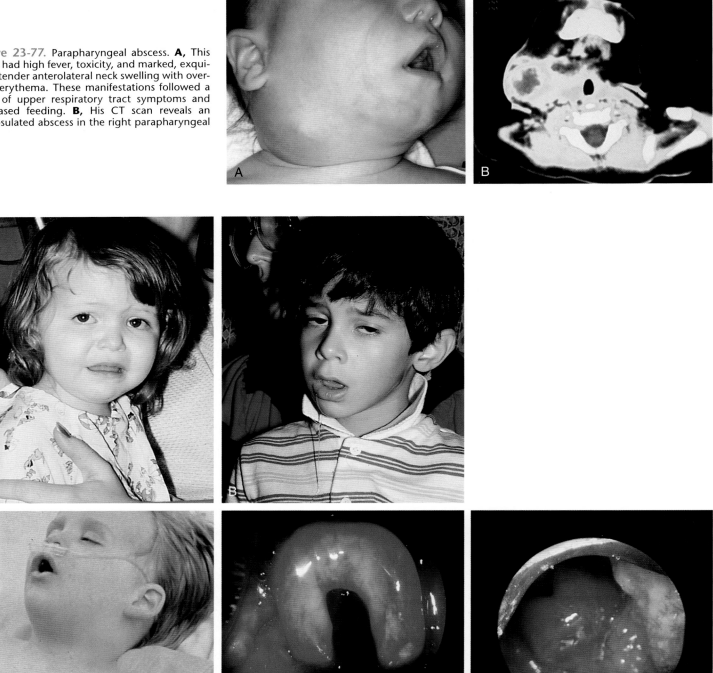

Figure 23-77. Parapharyngeal abscess. **A,** This infant had high fever, toxicity, and marked, exquisitely tender anterolateral neck swelling with overlying erythema. These manifestations followed a week of upper respiratory tract symptoms and decreased feeding. **B,** His CT scan reveals an encapsulated abscess in the right parapharyngeal area.

Figure 23-78. Epiglottitis. **A to C,** These three patients with acute epiglottitis demonstrate the varying degrees of distress that may be seen, depending on age and time of presentation. **A,** This 3-year-old seen a few hours after onset of symptoms was anxious and still but had no positional preference or drooling. **B,** This 5-year-old, who had been symptomatic for several hours, holds his neck extended with head held forward, is mouth breathing and drooling, and shows signs of tiring. **C,** This 2-year-old was in severe distress and was too exhausted to hold his head up. **D and E,** In the operating room the epiglottis can be visualized and appears intensely red and swollen. It may retain its omega shape or resemble a cherry.

ment is prompt airway stabilization, usually intubation under controlled conditions by experienced personnel in the operating room. At this time the epiglottis/supraglottis is found to be markedly swollen and erythematous (Fig. 23-78D and E). After airway stabilization, cultures can be obtained and IV antimicrobial therapy initiated. Obtaining a radiograph before transfer to the operating room is contraindicated; it adds nothing and may precipitate decompensation.

On occasion, children present with a similar history but milder symptoms and signs. In these cases, presentation is early or the child is older than average. Respiratory distress is minimal, and visualization of the pharynx can be attempted (without use of a tongue blade) if the child will voluntarily open his or her mouth. In some instances a swollen epiglottis is seen projecting above the tongue. When the history suggests epiglottitis/supraglottitis but clinical findings are mild and the diagnosis is not con-

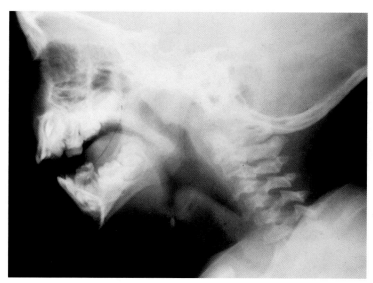

Figure 23-79. Mild epiglottitis or supraglottitis. This lateral neck radiograph demonstrates mild epiglottic swelling and thickening of the aryepiglottic folds.

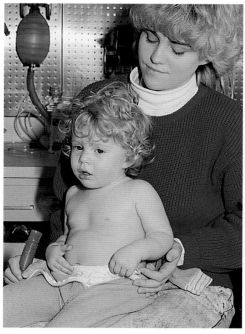

Figure 23-80. Croup. This toddler with moderate upper airway obstruction caused by croup had suprasternal and subcostal retractions. Her anxious expression was the result of mild hypoxia confirmed by pulse oximetry.

firmed by attempted noninvasive visualization, a portable lateral neck x-ray examination (done in the emergency department with a physician in attendance) can be useful. It may reveal mild epiglottic enlargement ("thumb-print sign"; Fig. 23-79) or merely swelling of the aryepiglottic folds and ventricular bands. If either is found, the diagnosis is confirmed. Hypopharyngeal dilatation may also be seen. Intubation is generally advisable in the former instance despite mild symptoms, but close observation on IV antibiotic therapy (covering for *H. influenzae* type B) may suffice when mild supraglottitis is the only finding.

Subglottic Disorders

Croup or Laryngotracheobronchitis. Croup, an acute respiratory illness, is characterized by inflammation and edema of the pharynx and upper airways, with maximal narrowing in the immediate subglottic region. There is probably a component of laryngospasm as well. The majority of cases are caused by viral pathogens, with parainfluenza, respiratory syncytial virus, adenoviruses, influenza viruses, and echoviruses being the agents most commonly identified. The peak season is between October and April in the Northern Hemisphere. The disorder primarily affects children between the ages of 6 months and 3 years. This is probably because their airways are narrower, and the mucosa is both more vascular and more loosely attached than in older children, enabling greater ease of edema collection. Older children can be affected, however.

Typically the child has had symptoms of a mild upper respiratory tract infection with rhinorrhea, cough, low-grade fever, and perhaps a sore throat for 1 to 5 days before developing symptoms of croup. The change is generally sudden and usually occurs at night or during a nap. The child awakens with fever, loud inspiratory stridor, a loud "barky" or "seal-like" cough, and hoarseness. The severity of symptoms and the course vary widely and are highly unpredictable. Duration averages 3 days but can be as brief as 1 day or as long as a week. Most patients have a waxing and waning course, with symptoms more severe at night, but it is impossible to predict which night will be the worst. Some patients remain relatively mildly affected throughout the course, while others progress either slowly or rapidly to severe distress. Airway drying, probably in part as a

result of mouth breathing necessitated by nasal congestion (especially while sleeping), appears to aggravate the cough and possibly the element of laryngospasm.

Physical findings are highly variable, depending on degree of distress at the time of presentation. Most affected children are moderately febrile but not toxic and have a loud barky cough and loud inspiratory stridor, with suprasternal and subcostal retractions (Fig. 23-80) and a mild decrease in air entry. A small percentage of patients with more extensive airway inflammation may have wheezing on auscultation. Distinguishing the stridor of croup from the wheezing of asthma is most important. Many patients improve substantially as a result of exposure to cool night air during the trip to the emergency department. Some have restlessness or agitation reflecting hypoxia, and a few have severe distress. In these more severely affected patients, stridor may be both inspiratory and expiratory, with generalized retractions. If impairment of airflow is extreme, fatigue supervenes, stridor abates, and retractions diminish. *This must not be mistaken for clinical improvement.* A clinical scoring system that helps in grading severity of distress is presented in Table 23-3. In mild to moderate cases the pharynx can be visualized and reveals only mild erythema. *Oral examination should be deferred in severe cases until the airway is secure.* Radiography can be helpful in demonstrating subglottic narrowing—the "steeple sign" (Fig. 23-81A). However, this is not necessary for patients with mild disease, and it is contraindicated for those with severe distress.

Management depends largely on severity of distress when the child is seen and on clinical response to mist therapy. Most patients have mild disease, improve considerably on mist alone, and can be managed at home with humidification. Parents must, however, be instructed to watch for signs of increasing distress, which would warrant return to the hospital. Aerosolized racemic epinephrine is effective in reducing airway obstruction caused by croup. It is particularly useful for children with moderate obstruction who do not show marked improvement on mist alone, and it can provide significant relief for children with

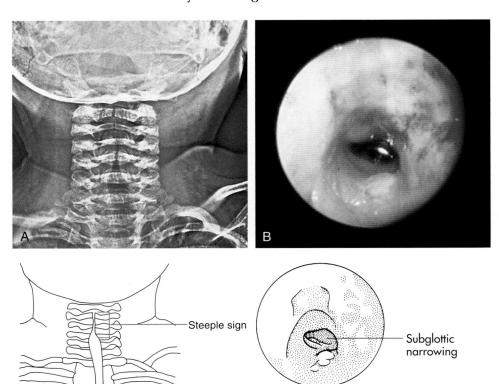

Figure 23-81. Croup. **A,** This radiograph reveals a long area of narrowing extending well below the normally narrowed area at the level of the vocal cords. The finding is often termed the *steeple sign.* **B,** In this patient, direct visualization revealed subglottic narrowing so severe that only tracheotomy would enable establishment of an adequate airway. (**A,** Courtesy Sylvan Stool, MD.)

Table 23-3	Croup Scoring System			
CLINICAL FINDING	**0**	**1**	**2**	**3**
Stridor	None	Mild	Moderate inspiratory at rest	Severe, on inspiration and expiration, or none with markedly decreased air entry
Retractions	None	Mild	Moderate	Severe, marked use of accessory muscles
Air entry	Normal	Mild decrease	Moderate decrease	Marked decrease
Color	Normal	Normal (0 score)	Normal (0 score)	Dusky or cyanotic
Level of consciousness	Normal	Restless when disturbed	Anxious, agitated when undisturbed	Lethargic, depressed

Modified from Taussig LM, Castro O, Beaudry PH, et al: Treatment of laryngotracheobronchitis (croup): Use of intermittent positive-pressure breathing and racemic epinephrine. Am J Dis Child 129:790-793, 1975.

severe distress. This agent, though effective, is short acting, and rebound tends to occur. Thus patients requiring racemic epinephrine should generally be admitted for further observation. Administration of intramuscular dexamethasone (sometimes followed by a 2- to 3-day course of oral prednisone) appears to reduce the severity of symptoms and thus the need for hospitalization.

Patients in severe distress who do not improve dramatically after treatment with racemic epinephrine, as well as those who steadily worsen in the hospital despite mist and aerosol treatments, merit airway endoscopy and stabilization, via intubation or tracheotomy under controlled conditions in the operating room. The choice of procedure remains controversial and is perhaps best made in accordance with the skills of the personnel and facilities available at the individual institution. In some instances, subglottic narrowing is so severe as to necessitate tracheotomy (see Fig. 23-81B). Attempts at emergency tracheotomy in the emergency department are fraught with hazard and should be avoided at all costs.

Bacterial Tracheitis. In a small percentage of cases, children with a crouplike picture are atypically toxic, markedly febrile, and have rapidly progressive airway obstruction necessitating urgent intubation and occasion-ally tracheotomy. Bronchoscopy before airway stabilization reveals severe inflammation; edema; and a copious, purulent subglottic exudate that contains large numbers of bacteria. Most of these patients appear to have a history of viral croup with sudden worsening. It is thus thought that the disorder may represent secondary bacterial infection. However, there is still some speculation that this disorder may represent an unusually virulent form of viral laryngotracheobronchitis.

Foreign Body Aspiration. Foreign body aspiration is seen for the most part in older infants and toddlers. The story is usually one of a sudden choking episode while the child was eating material that the immature dentition is ill equipped to chew. Such foods include nuts, seeds, popcorn, raw vegetables such as carrots and celery, and hot dogs. Occasionally the episode occurs when the child is chewing on a small object, a toy, or a detachable portion of a toy. If the object lodges in the larynx, asphyxiation results unless the Heimlich maneuver or back blows are performed promptly. In the majority of cases the foreign material clears the larynx and lodges in the trachea or a bronchus (more commonly, the right mainstem). After the choking spell, there is a silent period usually lasting up to several hours (occasionally days or weeks), after which the

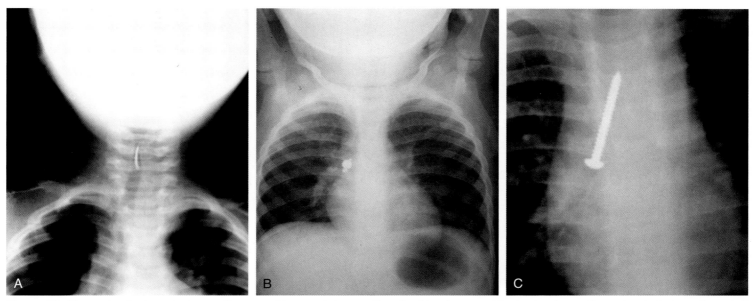

Figure 23-82. Foreign body aspiration. Radiopaque objects and those well outlined by air are readily visualized on radiographs. **A,** A piece of eggshell is seen in the subglottic portion of the trachea, clearly outlined by the air column. **B,** An earring lies in the entrance of the right mainstem bronchus. **C,** A screw is seen lodged in the right mainstem bronchus and projecting into the trachea. (**A,** Courtesy Mananda Bhende, MD, Children's Hospital of Pittsburgh; **B** and **C,** courtesy Robert Gochman, MD, Schneider Children's Hospital, Long Island Jewish Medical Center.)

child develops cough, stridor (if the object is lodged in the trachea) or wheezing (if it is lodged in a bronchus), and respiratory distress. In this acute phase, when the object is situated in a bronchus, wheezing may be unilateral and associated with decreased breath sounds. Later, diffuse wheezing may be heard, simulating asthma or bronchiolitis.

Lateral neck and chest radiographs may reveal aspirated objects that are radiopaque or outlined by the air column (Fig. 23-82A to C), enabling localization before endoscopy. However, most cases involve materials not visible on radiographs, although other radiographic clues may be present. Partial obstruction of a bronchus creates a ball-valve effect, allowing air in during inspiration but preventing its egress on expiration. This produces hyperinflation of one or more lobes of the lung on the same side as the foreign body (Fig. 23-83), which may be evident on the plain chest film. In subtler cases, chest fluoroscopy may highlight the differential inflation and deflation, showing mediastinal shift away from the side of the foreign body on exhalation (Fig. 23-84). These findings are particularly likely if the patient is seen fairly soon after the aspiration episode.

When there is a delay in seeking medical attention (usually because the aspiration episode was unwitnessed and onset of symptoms insidious), the patient may have cough and fever. In these instances, atelectasis and a mediastinal shift toward the side of the foreign body may be found on the chest radiograph (Fig. 23-85). This finding also may be seen acutely when the bronchus is totally obstructed. Many patients presenting acutely have no detectable radiographic abnormality after foreign body aspiration. Hence when clinical suspicion is high, given the history and physical findings, rigid endoscopic examination (with forceps for foreign body removal available) is indicated despite normal plain films. Conversely, when physical findings and x-ray films are normal and the history is questionable, a period of close observation may be indicated.

Unfortunately, in up to 50% of cases, the aspiration episode is not reported because the parent does not relate it to the child's symptoms or did not witness the choking

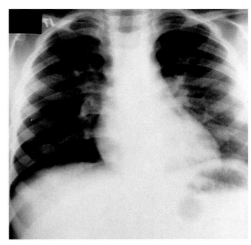

Figure 23-83. Foreign body aspiration with ipsilateral hyperinflation. This 18-month-old child was eating popcorn when he suddenly began choking. Within a few hours, he developed significant respiratory distress and his chest radiograph revealed massive hyperinflation of the right lung caused by the ball-valve effect of a piece of popcorn lodged in the right mainstem bronchus. (Courtesy Department of Radiology, Uniontown Hospital, Uniontown, Pa.)

spell. For this reason, this diagnosis should be considered and specific questions asked regarding possible aspiration whenever a young child has acute onset of cough and stridor or experiences a first episode of wheezing.

Chronic Upper Airway Obstruction

Laryngeal Examination

In children with a subacute or chronic airway disorder, a laryngeal examination is necessary to arrive at a definitive diagnosis. If a child is in distress or has acutely decompensated, this examination should be done in an operating room where rigid ventilating bronchoscopes and an anesthesiologist are available as backup. When the child is not in significant distress and the airway has been stable, laryngoscopy can be performed by an otolaryngologist in

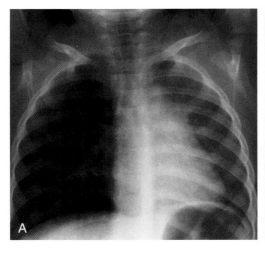

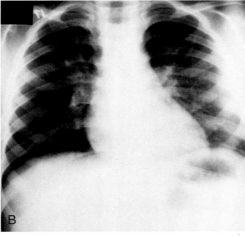

Figure 23-84. Foreign body aspiration, inspiratory and expiratory radiographs. **A,** This inspiratory film taken during fluoroscopy suggests hyperinflation of the right lower and middle lobes. **B,** This becomes much more evident on exhalation, when the hyperinflation persists and the mediastinum shifts to the opposite side. (Courtesy Robert Gochman, MD, Schneider Children's Hospital, Long Island Jewish Medical Center.)

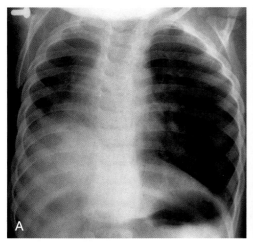

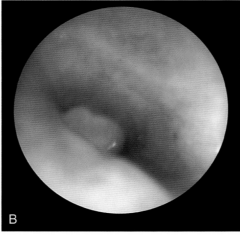

Figure 23-85. Foreign body aspiration—delayed presentation. **A,** With delay in presentation of partial obstruction or with complete obstruction of a bronchus, radiographic findings consist of atelectasis and a mediastinal shift *toward* the side of the foreign body. **B,** In this case a peanut was found completely obstructing the bronchus. (Courtesy Robert Gochman, MD, Schneider Children's Hospital, Long Island Jewish Medical Center.)

the office or emergency department using a flexible fiberoptic nasopharyngolaryngoscope (Fig. 23-86A). These are now available in a range of diameters suitable for pediatric patients. Letting the older child handle the scope (with close supervision) and look through the lens assists cooperation. The child is then prepared by spraying the nasal mucosa with a decongestant and topical lidocaine. With careful preparation, most patients can be examined in the parent's lap or an examination chair, but the toddler usually requires immobilization in a papoose board. The fiberoptic tube is then gently inserted into the nose and guided through past the palate (see Fig. 23-86B). If the child is exclusively mouth breathing, the soft palate may be apposed to the posterior pharyngeal wall. Asking the child to try to breathe through the nose a few times moves the palate forward, assisting passage. Anatomic abnormalities and dynamic motion of the supraglottic and glottic structures are easily seen with this device. Asking the child to phonate by saying the letter *e* enables observation of cord movement. In infants, cord movement is generally observed with crying. Although less well seen, the subglottic space can generally be viewed as well.

Subglottic Stenosis

Subglottic stenosis is a disorder in which the subglottic region of the trachea is unusually narrow in the absence of infection. In some instances the stenosis is the result of abnormal cricoid development and is therefore congenital. In other cases narrowing is the long-term result of injury and scarring from prior intubation. Regardless of the source, these children tend to develop stridor and

respiratory distress with each upper respiratory tract infection. A few are identified by virtue of having an atypically prolonged episode of croup. Some also have stridor with crying, even when well. Neck x-rays may present a similar appearance to that seen with croup (steeple sign [see Fig. 23-81A]).

The problem generally improves with growth, but up to 40% of these children develop such severe distress with colds that tracheotomy and reconstruction are required. Figure 23-87A shows laryngeal findings resulting from endotracheal tube trauma with formation of obstructing granulation tissue that later developed into severe glottic and subglottic stenosis requiring tracheotomy (Fig. 23-87B). Figure 23-88 shows the endoscopic view of a child with a laryngeal laceration and fracture due to blunt neck trauma who required tracheotomy and later developed subglottic stenosis.

Laryngomalacia

Laryngomalacia, a congenital condition, accounts for greater than 70% of cases of persistent stridor in infants. The problem is the result of unusual flaccidity of the laryngeal structures, especially the epiglottis and the arytenoid cartilages. The etiology is uncertain, but it is thought to be caused by lack of neural coordination of the laryngeal muscles, with the result that supraglottic structures hang over the airway entrance like a set of loose sails over a sailboat (Fig. 23-89).

Clinically these infants tend to have mild inspiratory stridor that is worse when they are lying supine and tends to improve when they are placed in the prone position or their necks are slightly hyperextended. The condition is usually benign and rarely interferes with feeding or respiration. The diagnosis can be confirmed only by direct visualization of the larynx during active respiration. This is important in that it is necessary to document that the stridor is not the result of a more dangerous condition.

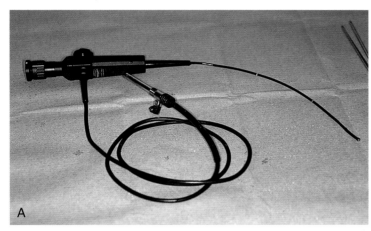

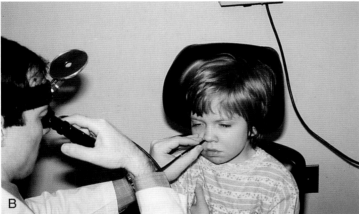

Figure 23-86. Fiberoptic laryngoscopy. **A,** The flexible fiberoptic laryngoscope. **B,** With careful preparation the patient can tolerate insertion of the flexible fiberoptic tubing and the examination.

Once the examination has been completed, the parents can be reassured that the condition is usually benign and that with growth the stridor typically abates by the end of the first year and a half of life. Management consists of observation, with particularly close monitoring during upper respiratory tract infections. GERD often occurs concomitantly with laryngomalacia, and empirical treatment of GERD often results in reduction of stridor. The occasional infant with unusually severe obstruction must be managed surgically.

Even though a child has the classic presentation of laryngomalacia, other significant airway problems may mimic this disorder, and thus endoscopy to confirm the diagnosis is always required. For example, Figure 23-90A shows an endoscopic view of a vallecular cyst that displaced the epiglottis in a posterior direction, creating airway obstruction that mimicked laryngomalacia. Cyst excision was curative (Fig. 23-90B).

Vocal Cord Paralysis

Paralysis of the vocal cords may be present at birth, or it may develop in the first 2 months of life. It may be bilateral or unilateral. The underlying problem is generally located somewhere along the vagus nerve and may be found in the central nervous system or in the periphery. Even though many cases are idiopathic, a thorough evaluation must be done in an effort to locate the lesion and identify its source. Ten percent of chronic stridor cases in neonates are thought to be due to this condition.

Infants with unilateral cord paralysis have stridor, hoarseness, and a weakened voice or cry. The airway diameter is generally adequate for respiration, and unless a secondary lesion is present, it is rarely necessary to perform a tracheotomy. This problem is most often caused by a cardiac abnormality because the recurrent laryngeal nerve is looped around these structures as it passes through the chest.

In contrast, bilateral vocal cord paralysis is a life-threatening condition that presents with stridor and cyanosis because the vocal cords are unable to abduct on inspiration with consequent severe narrowing of the aperture between the cords (Fig. 23-91). As the problem is usually associated with a depressed laryngeal cough reflex,

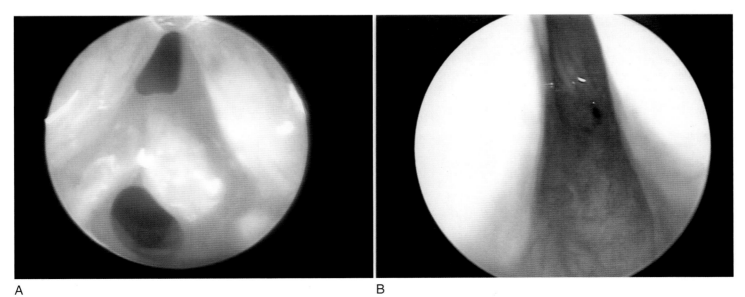

A
B
Figure 23-87. **A,** Glottic granulation tissue from prolonged intubation. **B,** Severe posterior glottic and subglottic stenosis. The granulation tissue and mucosal injury in **B** organized into a severe scar with a pinhole airway necessitating chronic tracheotomy.

aspiration is common. A tracheotomy is essential to secure the airway. Hydrocephalus or an Arnold-Chiari malformation is often the underlying problem because each causes compression of the vagus nerve as it leaves the brainstem. Neurosurgical intervention may correct the problem and allow eventual decannulation.

Juvenile Laryngeal Papillomatosis

Juvenile laryngeal papillomatosis is a condition in which multiple benign papillomas develop and grow on the vocal cords. In a few patients they may extend to involve the pharyngeal walls or tracheal mucosa. They are of viral origin, and there is some evidence of transmission during delivery to children born to mothers with condylomata acuminata. The main symptom is hoarseness, but stridor may develop in children with large lesions or tracheal extension. Radiographs are usually normal. The diagnosis should be considered in patients with chronic hoarseness and in those with atypically prolonged croup. On laryngoscopy, irregular warty masses are seen (Fig. 23-92). Biopsy is required to confirm the diagnosis. Excision can be performed using forceps, a laser, or a powered microdebrider, but it is often followed by regrowth. Tracheotomy should be avoided if at all possible because this may promote seeding farther down the tracheobronchial tree.

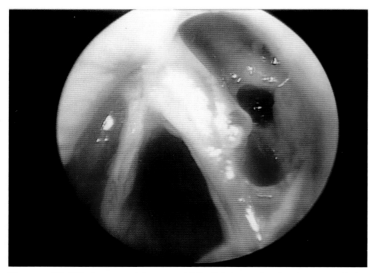

Figure 23-88. Laryngeal trauma. This child sustained a fracture of the thyroid cartilage from blunt neck trauma. This is the endoscopic view of the laceration to the right side of the right true vocal cord. This child required open repair and tracheotomy for airway stabilization.

Vascular Compression of the Trachea

Persistent expiratory wheezing or stridor that is unresponsive to bronchodilators may result from vascular compression of the trachea (Fig. 23-93) or tracheobronchomalacia. Symptoms are exacerbated by infections with increased respiratory requirements and increased secretions. Importantly, vascular compression of the trachea and tracheomalacia produce *expiratory* stridor. This is in contrast to laryngomalacia, which produces *inspiratory* stridor.

Esophageal Foreign Bodies

Ingestion of foreign objects is relatively common in older infants and toddlers, who are prone to putting almost anything they can pick up into their mouths. Coins, small toys, and pieces of toys are the objects most frequently found. Most traverse the esophagus, stomach, and intestines without incident and are of little concern. A small percentage of swallowed foreign bodies, being too large to pass through to the stomach, become lodged in the esophagus (usually at the level of the cricopharyngeus [C6] and less commonly at the level of the aorta [T4] or the diaphragmatic inlet [T11-12]). With mild obstruction, the child may refuse solid foods (although 17% of patients are asymptomatic); with moderate obstruction, liquids often are refused as well, or the child may appear to choke with drinking. When obstruction is nearly complete, the child may begin drooling. If the object is particularly large, it may compress the trachea as well, producing signs of upper airway obstruction. Older patients may complain of neck or substernal pain or discomfort, especially with swallowing.

Patients who have significant symptoms of esophageal or respiratory obstruction and those who have ingested sharp, potentially toxic, or caustic objects should undergo prompt endoscopic removal. Those who have ingested smooth objects and have mild symptoms can be observed for 12 hours and then have a repeat x-ray examination. If the object has passed into the stomach, endoscopy can be avoided. Otherwise, endoscopic removal is indicated.

Although in many cases there is a clear history of ingestion, in a significant percentage the ingestion was not witnessed. A high level of suspicion is often required to make the diagnosis, and the possibility of an esophageal foreign body should be considered in evaluating any young child for a sudden change in eating pattern. Plain radiographs detect metallic and other radiopaque objects (Fig. 23-94). Most ingested objects are plastic, however,

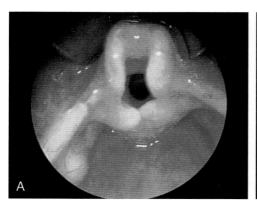
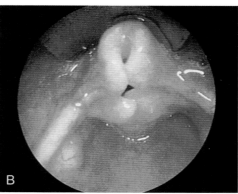

Figure 23-89. Laryngomalacia. **A,** Note the omegoid shape of the epiglottis and the elongation of the arytenoid cartilages. **B,** This is the larynx during inspiration. Note that the forces of the inspired air lead to collapse of the laryngeal inlet. Infolding of the epiglottic surfaces and the arytenoid cartilages causes partial airway obstruction.

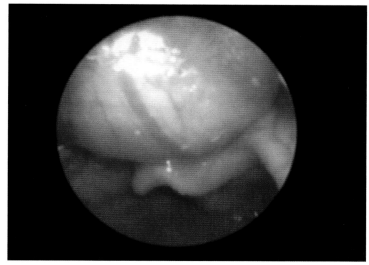

A

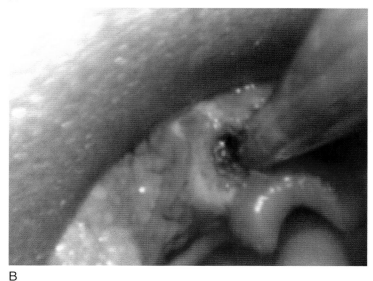

B

Figure 23-90. **A,** Vallecular cyst. Large mucous retention cyst in the vallecula displacing the epiglottis in a posterior direction leading to severe airway obstruction and stridor that mimicked laryngomalacia. **B,** Endoscopic excision of the superior cyst wall was curative.

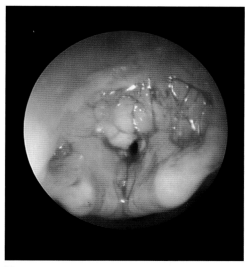

Figure 23-92. Laryngeal papillomas. Multiple smooth, warty growths are seen nearly occluding the larynx in this child who had a history of chronic hoarseness.

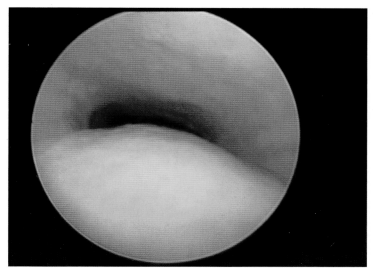

Figure 23-93. Vascular compression of the trachea. Anomalous innominate artery compression of the distal anterior tracheal wall. The presentation of this child was that of intractable wheezing during expiration that did not respond to bronchodilators. The child improved following thoracotomy for lifting (pexy) of the innominate artery off the trachea by sewing it to the inner surface of the sternum.

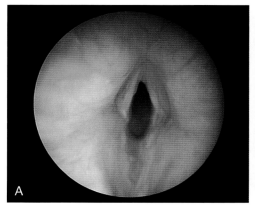

A

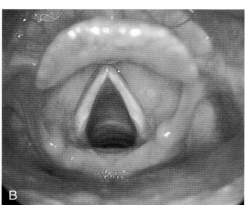

B

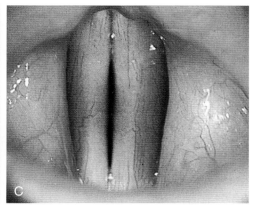

C

Figure 23-91. Bilateral vocal cord paralysis. **A,** The marked narrowing of the aperture between the cords stems from loss of ability to abduct on inspiration. The voice may be normal in some cases because the vocal cords can adduct. This is in contrast to normal opening and closing on inspiration and expiration as seen in **B** and **C.**

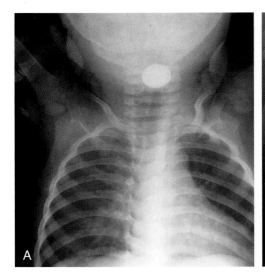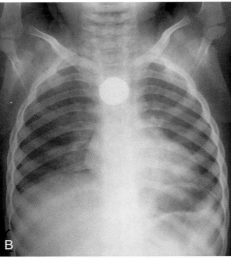

Figure 23-94. Esophageal foreign bodies. **A,** This youngster accidentally swallowed a coin. He complained of throat pain and refused oral intake. When initially seen, the coin was lodged high in the esophagus. **B,** After observation overnight, repeat radiography revealed that the coin had moved down but was still lodged in the esophagus. The patient underwent endoscopic removal. Note that asymmetrical objects in the esophagus are oriented in the coronal plane, whereas in the trachea, they lie in the sagittal plane (see Fig. 23-82A). (Courtesy Robert Gochman, MD, Schneider Children's Hospital, Long Island Jewish Medical Center.)

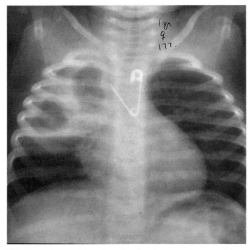

Figure 23-95. Esophageal foreign body. An unwitnessed ingestion of this safety pin led to a period of anorexia followed by fever and respiratory distress. The point of the pin had perforated the esophageal wall and pleura, causing a secondary right upper lobe pneumonia. (Courtesy Robert Gochman, MD, Schneider Children's Hospital, Long Island Jewish Medical Center.)

and require barium swallow or in some cases endoscopy for detection. Delays in diagnosis can result in stricture formation or, more rarely, esophageal perforation with secondary pneumomediastinum, mediastinitis, pneumonia (Fig. 23-95), and/or large vessel hemorrhage.

Otolaryngologic Manifestations of Gastroesophageal Reflux Disease

Over the past 2 decades, increased recognition and study of gastroesophageal reflux disease (GERD) have led to greater understanding of the disorder and its protean manifestations. As noted earlier, infants with GERD may develop nasopharyngeal congestion with varying degrees of mucosal inflammation, edema, and rhinorrhea. This is the result of exposure of mucosal surfaces to gastric juices. Affected infants who are still obligate nose breathers may have respiratory distress with feeding (sucking) and are often reported to snore during sleep. Some, but by no means all, have a history of vomiting and/or frequent

spitting up, and parents may report that at times some of the regurgitated material comes out the nose.

Reflux has also been associated with cough and wheezing, especially during sleep. In most cases this reflects a reflex bronchospastic response to esophageal mucosal irritation, whereas in others, more severe reflux into the posterior pharynx with aspiration may be causative. In the latter, severe bouts of coughing and bronchospasm with patchy infiltrates on chest radiograph may be seen. Infants who aspirate repeatedly may be noted on bronchoscopy to have cobblestoning of the posterior tracheal mucosa (Fig. 23-96A) and may also have prominent edema and inflammation of glottic structures (Fig. 23-96B). Chronic or intermittent hoarseness can be an associated feature. GERD has also been found to be causative in cases of recurrent croup. In still other infants, reflux of even a minute amount of gastric contents onto the vocal cords can precipitate intense laryngospasm with attendant apnea. This tends to occur when the baby is laid down shortly after a feeding. If the apnea is unwitnessed and laryngospasm is prolonged, this can prove fatal. As noted earlier, subclinical GERD is common in infants with laryngomalacia and it is also present in the majority of infants with acquired subglottic stenosis.

In addition to vomiting or spitting up, infants with GERD may have a range of symptoms of esophagitis. These may include crying after every few swallows with feeding (as reflux is induced by swallowing); refusal to feed; and arching and writhing movements of the neck and back, which constitute Sandifer syndrome. It is important to recognize that Sandifer movements; other symptoms of esophagitis; and snoring, cough, and bronchospasm that are worse during sleep can all occur in isolation or in any combination, and that they are often seen in the absence of overt vomiting and spitting. Hence when infants have these symptoms persistently, evaluation for GERD and/or empirical therapy should be instituted.

Neck Disorders

Neck disorders including adenitis, congenital cysts, and vascular and lymphatic masses and tumors are commonly managed by otolaryngologists. Limitations of space have required us to be selective in presenting disorders in this chapter. The reader is referred to Chapter 12 for a discus-

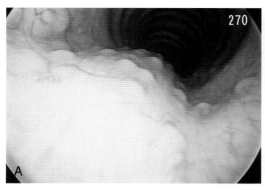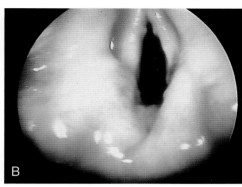

Figure 23-96. Airway manifestations of gastroesophageal reflux. **A,** This cobblestoned appearance of the posterior tracheal mucosa is the result of chronic inflammation in an infant with severe gastroesophageal reflux and recurrent aspiration. **B,** In this infant there is so much edema of the arytenoid mucosa that the arytenoids obscure the view of the posterior portion of the vocal cords. (**A,** Courtesy Anil Gungor, MD, Anadolu Foundation Healthcare System, Cayirova Mevkii, Gebze, Turkey.)

sion of cervical adenitis and to Chapter 17 for a description of mass lesions.

Acknowledgments

The authors would like to acknowledge and thank Children's Hospital of Pittsburgh, Department of Radiology, and University of Pittsburgh School of Medicine, Department of Neuroradiology, for providing many of the radiographs and CT scans in this chapter.

Bibliography

Bluestone CD, Stool SE (eds): Pediatric Otolaryngology, 4th ed. Philadelphia, WB Saunders, 2002.
Bluestone CD, Wald ER, Shapiro GC: The diagnosis and management of sinusitis in children: Proceedings of a closed conference. Pediatr Infect Dis J 4:549-555, 1985.
Bowen AD, Ledesma-Medina J, Fujioka M, et al: Radiologic imaging in otorhinolaryngology. Pediatr Clin North Am 28:905-939, 1981.
Davis HW, Gartner JC, Galvis AG, et al: Acute upper airway obstruction: Croup and epiglottitis. Pediatr Clin North Am 28:859-880, 1981.
Gellady AM, Shulman ST, Ayoub EM: Periorbital and orbital cellulitis in children. Pediatrics 61:272-277, 1978.
Gwaltney JM Jr, Phillips CD, Miller RD, Riker DK: Computed tomographic study of the common cold. N Engl J Med 330:25-30, 1994.
McAlister WH, Lusk R, Muntz HR: Comparison of plain radiographs and coronal CT scans in infants and children with recurrent sinusitis. Am J Roentgenol 153:1259-1264, 1989.
McGuirt WF (ed): Pediatric Otolaryngology Case Studies. Garden City, NY, Medical Examination, 1980.
Rosenfeld R, Bluestone CD (eds): Evidence-Based Otitis Media. Hamilton, Ontario, BC Decker, 1999.
Ungkanont K, Yellon R, Weissman J, et al: Head and neck space infections in infants and children. Otolaryngol Head Neck Surg 112:375-382, 1995.
Wald ER: Acute sinusitis in children. Pediatr Infect Dis J 2:61-68, 1983.
Wald ER, Milmoe GI, Bowen A'D, et al: Acute maxillary sinusitis in children. N Engl J Med 304:749-754, 1981.
Weber AL, Baker AS, Montgomery WW: Inflammatory lesions of the neck, including fascial spaces—evaluation by computed tomography and magnetic resonance imaging. Isr J Med Sci 28:241-249, 1992.

Index

Note: Page numbers followed by *f* or *t* indicate figures and tables, respectively.

A

Abdomen
distention of, bilious vomiting with, 637-639, 638f-640f
injury to, 198-200, 199f, 200f, 213
scaphoid, 625, 627f
Abdominal mass, 436-437, 436f-437f, 649-655
causes of, 650t
imaging of, 649
inflammatory, 655, 657f
location of, 649, 649f
in neonates, 649-651, 650f-652f
in older children and adolescents, 655, 657f
in toddlers and young children, 651, 652f-657f, 653-654
Abdominal pain, 382-385
causes of, 645-648, 647f-649f
functional disorders causing, 382-383
recurrent, 383, 383t
right-sided or lower, differential diagnosis of, 709, 709t, 710t-711t
Abdominal wall
congenital defects of, 665-667, 666f, 667f
hernias involving, 667-668, 667f, 668f
Abdominoscrotal hydrocele, 556
Abducens nerve (CN VI) palsy
esotropia in, 719-720
increased intracranial pressure and, 581, 582f
Abetalipoproteinemia, hemolytic anemia in, 413
Abrasions
in child abuse, 173, 175f, 176f
corneal, 752-753, 753f
genital, 688, 688f
orofacial, 771
Abruptio placentae, 40, 40f
Abscess
anorectal, 673-674, 673f
apocrine gland, 468-469, 469f
Bartholin gland, 702-703, 706f
brain, 583, 584f
breast, 60, 60f, 469, 469f, 665
cold, in skeletal tuberculosis, 493f, 494
dental, 769, 769f, 770f
epidural, 916, 918f
parapharyngeal, 926-927, 928f
pelvic appendiceal, 694-695, 694f
perifollicular, 468, 468f
peritonsillar, 923-924, 924f
periungual (paronychia), 468, 468f
retropharyngeal, 926, 927f
scalp, 469-470, 470f
skin and soft tissue, 467-470, 468f-470f
urachus, 538, 539f
Absence seizure, 593-594, 593f
Abuse. See Child abuse; Sexual abuse.
Acanthocytic anemia, 413, 414f
Acanthosis nigricans, 336, 337f
in Beare-Stevenson syndrome, 881
Crouzon syndrome with, 881
in insulin resistance, 372, 373f
Acceleration/deceleration forces, head injuries caused by, 191-192
Accessory tarsal navicular, 841, 842f
Acetabular index or slope, in developmental hip dislocation, 828, 829f
Achalasia, 390, 390f
Achilles reflex, 563, 566f

Acidosis
lactic, in mitochondrial diseases, 31
renal tubular, 516, 518f
Acne, 312-313, 313f
neonatal. See Cephalic pustulosis, neonatal.
Acoustic neurofibromatosis, bilateral, 568-569, 569t
Acquired immunodeficiency syndrome. See HIV/AIDS.
Acrobrachycephaly, 879
Acrocephaly, 872-873, 873t
Acrodermatitis, papular, 453-454, 455f
Acrofacial dysostosis, 883-884, 884f
Acromegaly, 354
Acromioclavicular joint, 243
Acropustulosis, infantile, 301-302, 302f
Actinomycotic adenitis, 478t
Activated protein C (APC) resistance, thrombosis in, 428
Adams forward bend test, 785, 785f, 819, 820f
Addison disease, 337, 362, 364f
Adenitis. See Lymphadenitis.
Adenohypophysis, 352-355, 353f-355f
Adenoidal hypertrophy, 905-907, 906f
Adenoma sebaceum, in tuberous sclerosis, 569, 570f
Adenomatous polyps, 645, 646f
Adenopathy. See Lymphadenopathy.
Adenosine deaminase deficiency, in severe combined immunodeficiency, 121-122
Adenovirus infection, 446, 447f, 476t
vulvovaginitis from, 698
ADHD (attention-deficit hyperactivity disorder), 89-91, 90t
Adhesions
intestinal obstruction from, 641
labial. See Labial adhesions.
preputial, after circumcision, 549-550, 550f
Adnexal measurements, normal, 727f
Adrenal cortex, 361-363
Adrenal glands, 361-364
Adrenal hemorrhage, 200, 200f
Adrenal hyperplasia, congenital, 363, 365f, 369, 560f
Adrenal insufficiency, 236, 362-363, 364f, 365f
Adrenal mass, 651
Adrenal medulla, 363-364
Adrenal neuroblastoma, 651, 652f-654f, 653
Adrenocortical carcinoma, 438, 438f
Adrenocorticotropic hormone (ACTH)
deficiency of, isolated, 363, 365f
regulation of, 354, 355f
Aerobic intensity, classification of sport by, 855t
Agammaglobulinemia, congenital, 117, 117f
Age
body mass index for, 348f, 349t
gestational. See Gestational age.
hemoglobin levels by, 404t
maternal
Down syndrome and, 10, 10t
Klinefelter syndrome and, 14-15
ossification centers and, 781, 782f, 783f
physeal closures by, 783f
stature percentiles by, 348f
AIDS. See HIV/AIDS.
Airway emergency, EXIT procedure for, 623, 625f

Airway obstruction
stridor in, 606-608
upper
acute, 925-931, 926t, 927f-932f
chronic, 931-934, 933f-936f
respiratory distress, estimation of severity, 623, 624f, 625f
wheezing in, 608-610
Airway remodeling, in asthma, 107, 107f
Alagille syndrome, 399, 400f, 529-530, 530f
Albinism, 335, 741-742, 742f
ocular, 742, 742f
partial, 335-336, 336f
Albinoidism, 742
Albright hereditary osteodystrophy, 359, 360f
Alcohol use, maternal, fetal alcohol syndrome from, 30, 30f
Alder-Reilly bodies, 422, 423f
Aldosterone, synthesis of, 365f
Alleles, 1
Allen object recognition cards, 714, 715f
Allergen immunotherapy, for hymenoptera sensitivity, 95-96
Allergic alveolitis, extrinsic, 111-112
Allergic bronchopulmonary aspergillosis, 112, 113f, 609, 609f, 632f
Allergic cobblestoning, 113, 113f
Allergic conjunctivitis, 112-113, 113f, 114f, 733
Allergic contact dermatitis, 287-288, 290f, 291f
Allergic rhinitis, 98-102, 99f-101f, 101t
with postnasal discharge, 919-920
Allergic salute, 100, 100f
Allergic shiner, 99, 99f
Allergic sinus headache, 920
Allergic vulvitis, 694
Allergy. See also Hypersensitivity disorders.
to drugs, 98, 99f
to food, 97-98, 97f, 98t
to hymenoptera venom, 94-97, 97f
ocular, 112-113, 113f, 114f
respiratory disease and, 102-112
Allergy tests, 93, 95f, 95t
Alopecia
friction, 339-340, 340f
scarring, 340
from systemic insult, 337, 339f
in systemic lupus erythematosus, 255, 256f
traction, 340, 340f
in trichorrhexis nodosa, 339, 340f
in trichotillosis (trichotillomania), 340, 341f
Alopecia areata, 337-338, 339f
Scotch-plaid nail pitting in, 337, 345f
Alport syndrome, 527, 527f, 528f
ALTE (apparently life-threatening event), 616
Alveolitis, extrinsic allergic, 111-112
Amblyopia, 724-725, 726f
ametropic, 717, 725, 726f
anisometropic, 717, 724-725, 726f
deprivation, 724, 726f
strabismic, 725, 726f
treatment of, 725
Amelogenesis imperfecta, 764, 764f, 765f
Ametropic amblyopia, 717, 725, 726f
Amnion nodosum, 41, 41f
Amniotic bands, 47, 48f
Amniotic fluid, meconium staining of, 43, 43f
Amoxicillin, for sinusitis, 914
Amplatzer Duct Occluder, 158, 158f
Amplatzer Septal Occluder, 157, 157f
Anagen effluvium, 337

Anal abnormalities, in sexual abuse, 223, 223f
Anal fissure, 642, 643f, 674
Anal sphincter, spontaneous relaxation of, 231-232
Anal variants, normal, 231-232, 232f
Analgesia, for fracture pain, 792, 805
Anaphylactoid reaction, 94
　drug-induced, 98
Anaphylaxis, 93-98, 94f, 95f, 96f
　causes of, 96f
　from hymenoptera sting, 95-97
　symptoms of, 96f
Androgen, synthesis of, 365f
Androgen insensitivity, 365, 369, 535, 536f
Anemia
　acanthocytic, 413, 414f
　aplastic, 202, 203f, 428, 429f
　congenital dyserythropoietic, 410, 412f
　Cooley, 408, 408f, 532
　from decreased red cell production, 405-410
　definition of, 403
　Diamond-Blackfan, 410
　Fanconi, 428, 428f
　hemolytic. See Hemolytic anemia.
　hypochromic microcytic, 405-409
　　chronic inflammatory states and, 408-409
　　iron deficiency and, 405-406, 405f, 406f
　　lead poisoning and, 406-408, 407f
　　sideroblastic, 409, 409f
　　thalassemia and, 408, 408f
　from increased red cell destruction, 410-418
　iron deficiency, 405-406, 405f, 406f
　　lead poisoning and, 407
　macrocytic
　　with megaloblastic body movements, 409-410, 409f-412f
　　without megaloblastic body movements, 410
　normocytic normochromic, 410
　　with elevated reticulocyte count, 411-414
　sideroblastic, 409, 409f
　spur cell, 413, 414f
　symptoms of, 404, 405f
Anesthetics, topical
　dermatitis from, 287, 291f
　in gynecologic examination of prepubertal patient, 680
Aneuploidy, 2-3, 3f
Aneurysm, coronary artery, in Kawasaki syndrome, 270, 270f
Angelman syndrome, 18, 19-20, 19f
Angioedema, 114, 115f
　versus cellulitis, 473
　of ear, 894, 895f
　hereditary, 114-115
　in urticaria, 303
Angiofibroma
　juvenile nasopharyngeal, epistaxis in, 911, 911f
　in tuberous sclerosis, 569, 570f
Angiokeratoma corporis diffusum, 529, 529f
Angioma, tufted, 327, 327f
Angiomatosis, leptomeningeal, in Sturge-Weber syndrome, 573
Angiomyolipoma, renal, 521, 521f, 570
Angioneurotic edema, 607
Angle kappa, 721, 722f
Angular scoliosis, in neurofibromatosis 1, 566, 568f
Aniridia, 432-433, 433f, 736-737, 737f
Aniseikonia, 717
Anisocoria, 748-749
Anisometropic amblyopia, 717, 724-725, 726f
Ankle
　examination of, 247, 247f, 790
　sprains of, 815-816, 815f
Ankyloblepharon, 728
Ankyloglossia, 659, 761, 761f
Anogenital warts, 313-314
Anomaly. See Congenital anomalies.
Anorectal abscess, 673-674, 673f
Anorectal anomalies, 670-674
Anterior chamber, 735-736, 735f, 736f

Anterior drawer test, 789, 789f, 790
Anterior fontanelle, 867, 868f
Anthropometric measurements, 378, 379f, 379t, 380f, 380t
Antibiotics
　for acne, 313
　for breast abscess, 665
　for epidermolytic hyperkeratosis, 280
　for gonorrhea, 706
　for staphylococcal diaper dermatitis, 296
　for streptococcal scarlet fever, 457
Antidiuretic hormone (ADH), 356
Anti–double stranded DNA antibodies, in systemic lupus erythematosus, 258
Antifungal agents
　for candidal vulvovaginitis, 699
　for diaper dermatitis, 296, 297
　for tinea capitis, 342
　for tinea diaper dermatitis, 297
　topical
　　for seborrheic dermatitis, 285
　　for tinea, 292, 294
Antigravity muscular control, 66-67, 68f, 69f
Antihistamines, for urticaria, 304
Antihypertensive agents, hirsutism from, 531
Antinuclear antibodies (ANAs), in systemic lupus erythematosus, 258, 258f
Antiphospholipid antibody syndrome, systemic lupus erythematosus and, 255, 256
Antipruritics
　for atopic dermatitis, 283-284
　for scabies, 310
Antiretroviral therapy, 506
Anti-RNP antibodies
　in mixed connective tissue disease, 262
　in systemic lupus erythematosus, 258
Antithrombin III deficiency, thrombosis in, 428
α_1-Antitrypsin deficiency, versus asthma, 111
Antituberculous drugs, 496
Anus, imperforate, 8f, 521, 522f, 670-671, 671f-673f, 673
　ambiguous genitalia and, 559, 560f
Aorta, coarctation of
　balloon angioplasty for, 155-156, 156f
　echocardiography in, 146, 148f
　radiographic appearance of, 137, 137f
　rib notching in, 138, 140f
Aortic arch
　double, 137-138, 138f
　right, 137, 137f
Aortic stenosis
　cardiac catheterization for, 154
　radiographic appearance of, 136-137, 137f
　Ross procedure for, 151, 152f
　with small annulus, Konno procedure for, 151, 152f, 153
APECED syndrome, 359
Apert syndrome, 877-879, 878f, 893f
Aphthous stomatitis
　in Behçet's disease, 271, 769
　in PFAPA syndrome, 272, 768-769
Aphthous ulcers, recurrent, 768-769, 768f
Apical bullous lung disease, 631, 632f
Aplasia cutis congenita, 11f, 341, 342f
Aplastic anemia, 202, 203f, 428, 429f
Apnea, 616-617
　central, 617
　mixed, 617
　sleep, 616, 879
Apocrine gland abscess, 468-469, 469f
Apparent life-threatening event (ALTE), 616
Appendages, testicular, 552
　torsion of, 553, 554f, 669-670, 670f
Appendicitis, 647, 711t
　acute, 645-647, 647f
　differential diagnosis for, 647-648
　with pelvic appendiceal abscess, 694-695, 694f
Appendicovesicostomy, 541, 543f
Apprehension test, 789, 789f
Appropriate for gestational age (AGA), 37, 39f

Apt-Downey test, 642
Arachnodactyly
　Beals congenital contractural, 21, 22f
　in Marfan syndrome, 21, 22f
Arginine vasopressin (AVP), 356
Arrhythmias, 140-144, 141f-144f
Arterial blood gases, 622, 622t
Arterial switch procedure, for transposition of the great arteries, 151, 151f
Arterial thrombosis, 427
Arteriohepatic dysplasia, 399, 400f, 529-530, 530f
Arthralgia, 241
Arthritis
　in hemophilia, 426, 426f, 427f
　in Henoch-Schönlein purpura, 266, 267f
　idiopathic, juvenile, 253
　infectious, 253-254
　Lyme, 253, 254f, 462
　psoriatic, 253, 253f
　pyogenic, 253
　in rheumatic disease, 241
　rheumatoid. See Rheumatoid arthritis, juvenile.
　in rubella, 443
　septic, 488-491, 489t, 490f
　in systemic lupus erythematosus, 241, 257
　viral, 253-254
Arthrocentesis, in septic arthritis, 490
Arthrogryposis, 848, 849f
Arthropathy. See also Osteoarthropathy; Spondyloarthropathy.
　Jaccoud, 257
Aryepiglottic folds, edema of, 618, 619
Ash-leaf spots, 334, 336f, 569, 571f
Asperger syndrome, 87
Aspergillosis, allergic bronchopulmonary, 112, 113f, 609, 609f, 632f
Aspiration
　evaluation of, 617-618, 617f-619f
　of foreign body, 111, 111f, 930-931, 931f, 932f
　of meconium, 52, 52f
　needle, 661
Association(s), 7
　CHARGE, 27-28, 27f
　VATER/VACTERL, 28, 28f
Asthma, 102-111
　airway remodeling in, 107, 107f
　versus bronchiolitis, 108-109, 109t
　clinical index of, 110t
　cough in, 602
　cough-variant, 606
　definition of, 102
　diagnosis of, 102-107, 103f, 104t-106t
　differential diagnosis of, 108-111, 109f, 109t, 110t, 111f
　exacerbations of, severity of, 104, 105t
　versus foreign body aspiration, 111, 111f
　incidence of, 102, 102f
　mortality in, 102, 103f
　pathogenesis of, 104f
　peak expiratory flow rate in, 102, 103f, 104
　persistent, factors predictive of, 110, 110t
　physical examination in, 105-107, 108, 109f
　pulmonary function tests in, 104-105, 105f
　pulsus paradoxus in, 106, 106t
　radiography in, 107-108, 108f
　versus respiratory infection, 110-111
　seasonality of, 102, 103f
　steroid-dependent, 108, 109f
　triggers of, 102
　wheezing in, 609
Astigmatism, 716f, 717
Astrocytoma, 440
　cerebral, increased intracranial pressure in, 583, 583f
　subependymal, in tuberous sclerosis, 570, 572f
Asymmetrical tonic neck reflex (ATNR), 65-66, 66f, 83-84
Ataxia-telangiectasia, 122, 573-574, 573f

Atelectasis, in systemic lupus erythematosus, 256, 256f
Athetoid or ataxic cerebral palsy, 84
Athlete's foot, 292, 294f
Athletics. *See* Sports.
Atopic dermatitis, 280-284
    differential diagnosis of, 283
    herpes simplex infection with, 284, 452, 453f
    IgE level in, 122-123
    keratosis pilaris in, 281, 283f
    lichenification in, 282f
    phases of, 281, 281f-282f
    pityriasis alba in, 283, 283f
    treatment of, 283-284
Atopic disorders, sinusitis versus, 919-920
Atopic keratoconjunctivitis, 113, 113f
Atrial contractions, premature, 140, 142f
Atrial isomerism, 134, 135f
Atrial pacemaker, wandering, 140, 142f
Atrial septal defect
    closure of, 157, 157f
    echocardiography in, 144, 145f
    heart size in, 135-136, 136f
Atrial septoplasty, 156, 156f
Atrial septostomy, balloon, 156
Atrioventricular block, third-degree, 144, 144f
Atrioventricular septal defect
    electrocardiography in, 138, 141f
    partial form of, 144, 145f
Attachment, development of, 79
Attention-deficit hyperactivity disorder, 89-91, 90t
Audiogram, 88, 88f
Aural fistula, 46, 46f
Auricular cellulitis, 894, 895f
Auspitz sign, in psoriasis, 279, 279f
Autism, 87-88
Autistic spectrum disorder, 87
Autoimmune hepatitis, 400
Autosomes, 1
    abnormalities of, 9-13
Avulsion fracture
    pelvic, 811, 811f
    of tibial spine, 815, 815f, 816
Avulsion injury
    dental, 775, 775f
    orofacial, 772, 772f
Axillary freckling, in neurofibromatosis 1, 566, 567f
Axillary lesions, 664-665
Axillary lymph nodes, 477, 481f
Axonal shearing, diffuse, in shaken baby syndrome, 195, 197f

B
B cell(s), development of, 116, 116f
B cell disorders, 117-118, 117f, 118f
    with T cell disorders
        partial, 122-123, 122f, 123f
        severe, 119-122, 120t, 121f
Babble, 77
Babinski reflex, 563, 566f
Baby bottle caries, 235f, 236-237, 767, 767f
Back, physical examination of, 785-786, 785f, 786f
Baclofen, in cerebral palsy, 843
Bacteremia, periorbital cellulitis from, 917-918
Bacteria, intracellular, 422, 423f
Bacterial conjunctivitis, 732, 733f
Bacterial cystitis, 519-520, 520f, 520t
Bacterial endocarditis
    retinopathy in, 745-746, 745f, 746f
    signs of, 132-133, 133f
Bacterial infection
    of bone and joint, 482-491, 483f-490f
    exanthematous, 454-463, 456f-463f
    in meningitis, 459, 459f, 585, 585f
    of oral cavity, 769-770, 769f-771f
    of skin and soft tissue, 298, 299f, 464-475, 465f-474f

Bacterial tracheitis, 930
Bacterial vaginosis, 692t, 704-705, 705f
Baker cyst, 245, 247, 247f, 835, 835f
Balanitis, 551
Ballard assessment of gestational age, 33, 35f
Ballet, injury prevention in, 858t
Band keratopathy, in juvenile rheumatoid arthritis, 252, 252f
Barium enema, in gastrointestinal obstruction, 634, 634f
Barium esophagram, 634, 635f
    in double aortic arch, 137-138, 138f
Barlow test, in developmental hip dislocation, 828
Bartholin gland abscess, 702-703, 706f
Bartonella henselae, 481
Basal cell carcinoma, 431, 432f
Baseball, injury prevention in, 858t
Basilar skull fracture, 894, 895f
Basophilic stippling, 407, 407f
Basophils, normal values for, 419t
Batten disease, 422
Battle sign, 894, 895f
Beals congenital contractural arachnodactyly, 21, 22f
Beare-Stevenson syndrome, 881
Beau lines, in Kawasaki syndrome, 268, 269f
Becker muscular dystrophy, 588, 588t
Beckwith-Wiedemann syndrome, 40, 372, 372f, 433, 623, 624f
Behçet's disease, 270-272, 272f
Bell phenomenon, in third nerve palsy, 722, 722f
Benign extra-axial fluid collections (BEAFCs), 212-213
Benzoyl peroxide, for acne, 313
Berger disease, 266
Bicycle ergometry, 621
Biliary atresia, extrahepatic, 398-399, 399f
Biliary tract disease, 648
Bilirubin, elevated. *See* Hyperbilirubinemia.
Bimanual (vaginal-abdominal) examination, 685
Bimanual rectal examination, 751
Biopsy
    esophageal mucosal, 634
    muscle, in juvenile dermatomyositis, 265
    rectal, suction, in Hirschsprung disease, 639, 640f
    transbronchial, 622
Biotin deficiency, with parenteral nutrition, 381, 382f
Bird-breeder's lung, 111
Birth trauma, 42-44, 42f-45f
    bruising and petechiae in, 43, 43f
    caput succedaneum and, 42, 42f
    clavicle fracture and, 42-43
    fat necrosis in, 43, 43f
    meconium staining and, 43, 43f
    nasal deformities in, 43-44, 44f
    peripheral nerve damage and, 44, 44f, 45f
Bite marks, in child abuse, 173, 177f
Bites. *See* Insect bites and stings.
Black eyes, after forehead contusion, 202, 202f
Bladder
    exstrophy of, 541, 544f
    neurogenic, 546, 547f
        non-neurogenic, 547, 547f
    rhabdomyosarcoma of, 546f
Blade septoplasty, 156, 156f
Blalock-Taussig shunt, 149, 149f
Blaschkoid distribution
    in incontinentia pigmenti, 322, 323f
    in pigmentary mosaicism, 333-334, 335f
Blast cells, 418, 420f
Blastoma. *See also* Neuroblastoma; Retinoblastoma.
    pulmonary, 629, 630f
Bleeding. *See also* Hematoma; Hemorrhage.
    gastrointestinal. *See* Gastrointestinal bleeding.
    nasal, 424, 909-911, 909f-911f
    variceal, 645

Bleeding disorders, 422-427. *See also* Coagulation disorders; Thrombosis.
Bleeding time (BT), 424, 425
Blepharitis, 728
Blepharophimosis, 725, 727f
Blepharoptosis, 725-726, 727f
Blistering
    in epidermolysis bullosa, 320-322, 321f, 322f
    in incontinentia pigmenti, 322, 323f
Blistering distal dactylitis, 206, 298, 299f
Blood
    maternal versus fetal, Apt-Downey test for, 642
    in urine, 509, 514-515, 516f
Blood pressure
    elevated. *See* Hypertension.
    examination of, 127
Blood smear, 403, 404f
Blount disease, 834, 834f
Blue diaper syndrome, 510
Blue dot sign, 553, 554f, 669-670, 670f
Blue nevus, 332, 332f
Blueberry muffin rash, in congenital rubella, 498, 498f
Bobble-head doll syndrome, 595
Bochdalek hernia, 625
Body lice, 310-311, 312f
Body mass index, 347, 348f, 349t
Bohn nodules, 760, 760f
Boil, 468, 468f
Bone. *See also* Skeletal *entries.*
    brittle, temporary, 209
    demineralization of, from disuse, 209, 209f
    lytic lesions of, in cancer, 438, 439f
Bone age, radiography of, 347
Bone cyst, fracture in, 209, 210f
Bone demineralization, 209, 209f
Bone infection, 482-488, 483f-489f. *See also* Osteomyelitis.
Bone pain, in osteomyelitis, 483
Bone scan
    in acute osteomyelitis, 484, 486f
    in child abuse, 184, 185f, 189, 190f
Bone tumors, 439, 441f
"Boot-shaped" heart, 135, 135f
Bordetella pertussis, 600-601, 600f
Borrelia burgdorferi, 461
Borrelia vincentii, 770
Boutonnière deformity, 827, 827f
Bowleg
    physiologic, 832-833, 833f
    in rickets, 359, 361f
Boxer's fracture, 809, 809f
Brachial plexus trauma, in newborn, 44, 45f
Brachycephaly, 872-873, 873t, 875, 877, 879
Brain. *See also* Central nervous system.
    abscess of, 583, 584f
    atrophy of, in AIDS, 503, 505f
    injury to. *See* Head trauma.
    tumors of, 431-432, 432f, 440-441
Brainstem glioma, 440-441, 583, 584f
Branchial arch anomalies, 662, 663f
Branchial cleft anomalies, 662, 663f
Branchial cleft cyst, 478t, 661, 661f
Branding injuries, inflicted, 178, 179f
Breast
    abscess of, 60, 60f, 469, 469f, 665
    development of
        female, 350f, 351, 352f
        premature, 368, 368f
    lesions of, 665, 665f
    nipple discharge from, 665
Breast milk, bioactive substances in, 54, 377t
Breastfeeding, 54-63
    benefits of, 54, 375, 376t
    breast examination in, 55-56, 55f, 56f
    breast size and, 55
    cup feeding and, 62f, 63
    double-pumping and, 61, 62f
    drug therapy during, 55
    engorgement in, 59
    evaluation of, 55-57, 55f-57f

Breastfeeding (Continued)
finger feeding and, 62f, 63
holding positions in, 57-59, 58f
impetigo and, 60, 60f
latch in, 56-57, 56f, 57f
mastitis and, 60, 60f
maternal history and, 54-55, 54f
milk transfer assessment in, 60-61, 61t
nipple trauma in, 57, 57f, 59, 59f
of premature infants, 61-63, 61f, 62f
problems in, 59-61
rusty pipe syndrome in, 61, 61f
stools in, 53, 53f
supplemental nursing system in, 62-63, 62f
yeast infection and, 59-60, 60f
Breath sounds, 598, 598f
Breech presentations, bruising and petechiae in, 43, 43f
Bronchial foreign body, 633f
Bronchiectasis, 602-603, 604f
hypogammaglobulinemia and, 117, 117f
Bronchiolitis
versus asthma, 108-109, 109t
obliterative, 610, 612f
Bronchogenic cyst, 601, 608, 608f, 633f
Bronchopulmonary aspergillosis, allergic, 112, 113f, 609, 609f, 632f
Bronchopulmonary dysplasia, 50, 52f, 610
Bronchopulmonary foregut malformations, 627-630, 629f, 630f
Bronchoscopy
flexible fiberoptic, 621-622, 621f
rigid, of inhaled foreign body, 602, 603f
Brown syndrome, vertical eye deviation in, 723, 723f
Brucellosis, 476t
Bruises
accidental, 201-202, 202f
in cancer, 430
differential diagnosis of, 201-205, 202f-205f
genital, 688, 688f
inflicted, 167-173, 168f-175f
documentation of, 171, 173
oral, 179, 181f
myoglobinuria and, 171, 175f
in newborn, 43, 43f
orofacial, 772
from subcultural healing practices, 202, 203f
Wood lamp examination of, 171, 175f
Bruit, 129t
Brush spots, 738
Bruxism, craniomandibular dysfunction and, 779
Bubonic plague, 481-482
Buccal cellulitis, 473, 473f
"Bucket handle" deformity, 670, 671f
Buffalo hump, in Cushing syndrome, 361, 362f
Bulbocavernosus reflex, 535
Bullous impetigo, 465, 466f
Buphthalmos, in Sturge-Weber syndrome, 573, 573f
Burkitt lymphoma, 433, 434f
Burns
in child abuse, 173, 175, 178-179, 178f-180f, 178t
differential diagnosis of, 45f-47f
cigarette
accidental, 207
inflicted, 178-179, 180f
lesions mistaken for, 207, 207f
contact, 178, 179f
curling iron, 179f, 206, 206f
differential diagnosis of, 205-207, 205f-207f
immersion, 175, 178, 178f, 178t
iron, 179f, 206, 206f
oral, 772, 773f
space heater, 179f, 206
Butane lighter, inflicted burns with, 179, 180f
Buttonhole deformity, 827, 827f

C
C1 esterase inhibitor, absence of, in hereditary angioedema, 114-115
Café-au-lait spots, 336-337, 338f
conditions associated with, 566, 567t
in McCune-Albright syndrome, 367, 368f
in neurofibromatosis 1, 566, 567f
Caffey's disease, 211, 212f
Calcaneovalgus foot, 840-841, 841f
Calcification
cortical, in congenital toxoplasmosis, 497, 497f
intracranial
in Sturge-Weber syndrome, 573
in tuberous sclerosis, 570, 571f
Calcinosis
in CREST syndrome, 259, 261f
in juvenile dermatomyositis, 263, 263f, 264
in scleroderma, 261-262
Calcium, imbalance of, 359-360, 360f, 361f, 361f
Calculi, renal, 515-516
Callus formation, in fracture healing, 181, 182f, 184, 185f
Camptomelic dwarfism, 364
Cancer, 429-441. See also Tumor(s).
abdominal findings in, 436-437, 436f-437f
in ataxia-telangiectasia, 574
chest findings in, 434, 435f-436f, 436
head and neck findings in, 431-434, 432f-435f
liver, 437
musculoskeletal system in, 438-440, 439f-441f
neurologic symptoms in, 440-441
ocular findings in, 432-433, 432f-434f
orofacial findings in, 433-434, 434f-435f
predisposing diseases and, 430, 430t
signs and symptoms of, 429-430, 430t
skin lesions in, 430-431, 430f-432f
testicular, 556, 556f
thyroid, 356, 434, 478t
urogenital tract in, 437-438, 438f
Candidal diaper dermatitis, 295, 296f
in AIDS, 505f
versus streptococcal impetigo, 466
Candidiasis
chronic mucocutaneous, 119
oral, 770, 771f
vaginal discharge in, 692t
vulvovaginitis in, 699, 700f
Canker sores, 768-769, 768f
Capillary and capillary/venous malformations, 328-329, 329f
Capital femoral epiphysis, slipped, 830-832, 831f
Caput succedaneum, 42, 42f
Carbohydrate malabsorption, 388
Carbuncle, 468
Carcinoma. See Cancer; Tumor(s).
Cardiac. See also Heart.
Cardiac anomalies, in Apert syndrome, 879
Cardiac apex and situs discordance, in congenital heart disease, 134, 134f, 135f
Cardiac catheterization, interventional
for closure of defects, 157-158, 157f-158f
in congenital heart disease, 153-158, 154f-158f
for creation or enlargement of defects, 156, 156f
for valvular obstruction, 153-154, 154f
for vascular stenosis, 155-156, 155f-156f
Cardiac examination, 127-133, 128f-133f, 129t, 130t, 132t. See also Cardiovascular assessment.
Cardiac involvement
in juvenile rheumatoid arthritis, 253
in scleroderma, 262
in systemic lupus erythematosus, 255-256
Cardiac rhabdomyosarcoma, in tuberous sclerosis, 570
Cardiac surgery, for congenital heart disease, 146, 149-153, 149f-153f

Cardiomyopathy, in AIDS, 503, 506f
CardioSEAL device, 157, 157f
Cardiothoracic ratio, 598
Cardiovascular assessment
cardiac examination in, 127-133, 128f-133f, 129t, 130t, 132t
chest radiography in, 133-138, 134f-140f
echocardiography in, 144-146, 145f, 148f
electrocardiography in, 138-144, 141f-144f
laboratory aids in, 133-146
in sports preparticipation examination, 851, 854
Cardiovascular disease. See Heart disease.
Caries, dental, 235f, 236-237, 766-767, 767f
Carotid bruit, 129t
Carrying angle, 786, 786f
CASR gene mutation, 359
Cataract, 738-740, 738f-740f, 738t, 739t
differential diagnosis of, 738, 738t
in galactosemia, 739, 739f
lamellar, 739, 739f
polar, 739, 739f
in rubella, 739, 739f
syndromes associated with, 738, 739t
Catheterization, cardiac. See Cardiac catheterization, interventional.
Cat's eye reflex. See Leukocoria.
Cat-scratch disease, 481, 481f, 661-662, 662f
Causalgia, 272
Caustic ingestion, esophageal stricture after, 390-391, 391f
Cavus foot, 841-843, 842f
CD18 deficiency, in leukocyte adhesion deficiency, 123
CD154 (CD40 ligand) deficiency, in hyper IgM syndrome, 122
Celiac disease, 236, 389-390, 389f, 390f
Cellulitis, 471-474
auricular and periauricular, 894, 895f
buccal, 473, 473f
from extension of infection, 474
facial, 474, 769, 770f
hematogenous, 473, 473f, 916-919, 918f
necrotizing, 474-475, 474f
orbital, 919, 919f
periorbital, 916-919, 918f
peritonsillar, 923-924, 924f
wound-related, 471-473, 472f
Central nervous system
abnormalities of, hypopituitarism and, 351-352, 353f
injuries to, in child abuse, 190-196, 192f-198f
malformations of, 575-581, 576f-581f
in systemic lupus erythematosus, 257, 257f
tumors of, 431-432, 432f, 440-441
hypopituitarism in, 352
in neurofibromatosis, 567, 569
Central shunt, 149, 149f
Cephalhematoma, in newborn, 42, 42f
Cephalic pustulosis (neonatal acne), 318-319, 320f
Cerebellar tumors, 583, 584f
Cerebral artery dysplasia, in neurofibromatosis 1, 568
Cerebral atrophy, in shaken baby syndrome, 195, 197f
Cerebral contusions, in child abuse, 195, 196f
Cerebral edema
increased intracranial pressure in, 582, 582f
in shaken baby syndrome, 195, 197f
Cerebral gigantism, 39, 85
Cerebral palsy, 81-84, 82f-84f, 82t, 843-844
abnormalities in primitive reflexes and equilibrium responses in, 83-84
abnormalities of tone in, 82, 82f, 83f
athetoid or ataxic, 84
diagnostic criteria for, 82t
findings associated with, 84
hemiplegic, 83, 83f
hip dislocation in, 843, 844f
hypotonic, 84
physical examination in, 81-84, 82f, 82t, 83f

Cerebral palsy (*Continued*)
  prognosis in, 84
  scoliosis in, 818, 820f
  spastic diplegia and quadriplegia in, 83-84, 84f, 843, 843f
Cerebrospinal fluid, in congenital syphilis, 501
Cervical lymph nodes, 475, 476f, 477
Cervical lymphadenopathy, 475, 476f, 477, 477f
  benign reactive, 661, 661f, 662f
  differential diagnosis of, 478t, 661-662, 662f
  infectious causes of, 475, 476t
  in mononucleosis, 450
Cervical mass, 623, 625f
Cervical spine
  congenital atrophy of, 591, 591f
  fusion of, 879
Cervical teratoma, respiratory distress in, 623, 625f
Cervicothoracic neuroblastoma, 432, 433f
Cervix
  nulliparous, normal, 684, 684f
  strawberry, in *Trichomonas vaginalis*, 704, 705f
CFTR gene, 610, 612
Chadwick sign, 711
Chalazion, 728, 729f, 730f
Chancre, syphilitic, 702, 702f
Charcot-Marie-Tooth disease, 590-591, 590f, 841-843, 842f, 843f
CHARGE association, 27-28, 27f
Chédiak-Higashi syndrome, 422, 423f
Cherry red spot, 746, 746f, 747, 747f
Chest
  auscultation of, 598, 598f
  inspection of, 597
  palpation of, 597-598
  percussion of, 598
Chest disease. *See* Pulmonary disorders.
Chest wall
  deformities of, 663-664, 664f
  masses of, 434, 435f
Chickenpox. *See* Varicella.
Child abuse, 161-239. *See also* Neglect; Sexual abuse.
  abdominal injuries in, 198-200, 199f, 200f
    differential diagnosis of, 213
  abrasions in, 173, 175f, 176f
  bite marks in, 173, 177f
  bone scan in, 184, 185f, 189, 190f
  bruises, welts, and scars in, 167-173, 168f-175f
    differential diagnosis of, 201-205, 202f-205f
    documentation of, 171, 173
    myoglobinuria and, 171, 175f
    oral, 179, 181f
    Wood lamp examination of, 171, 175f
  burns in, 173, 175-178, 178-179, 178f-180f, 178t
    cigarette or cigarette lighter, 178-179, 180f
    contact, 178, 179f
    differential diagnosis of, 205-207, 205f-207f
    immersion, 175, 178, 178f, 178t
  central nervous system injuries in, 190-196, 192f-198f
  deaths due to, 161
  definition of, 163
  emotional, 238
  epidemiology of, 161-163, 162t-164t
  fractures in, 180-188, 182f-190f
    clavicular, 187, 189f
    compression/distraction (three-point bending), 187, 188f
    diagnostic imaging of, 188-190, 190f
    diaphyseal, 186-187, 186f-189f
    differential diagnosis of, 207-211, 209f-212f
    hand, 188, 190f
    head injury and, 184
    healing of, 181-182, 182f, 184, 185f
    long bone, 184, 186-187, 186f-189f
    metaphyseal, 182-183, 182f, 183f

Child abuse (*Continued*)
    multiple, bone scan in, 184, 185f
    oblique, 186-187, 187f
    rib, 183-184, 184f, 185f, 200, 201f
    skull, 194, 194f, 195f
    spiral, 186, 186f
    supracondylar, 187, 189f
    torus (buckle), 187, 187f
    transverse, 187, 187f
    vertebral, 188, 190f
  head trauma in, 190-196, 192f-198f
    clinical picture of, 194-195, 194f-197f
    differential diagnosis of, 211-213, 214f
    morbidity and mortality associated with, 190-191
    neuroimaging of, 195-197, 198f
    pathophysiology and biomechanics of, 191-192
    pathophysiology of shaking and, 192-194, 192f, 193f
  injury patterns in, 167-200
  intrathoracic injuries in, 200, 201f
    differential diagnosis of, 213
  lacerations in, 173, 175f, 176f, 179-180, 181f
  methods used in, 164t
  misleading or deceptive history in, 164, 164t
  nasal injuries in, 180, 181f
  oral injuries in, 179-180, 181f
    differential diagnosis of, 213
  versus osteogenesis imperfecta, 848
  passive, 232-237, 234f-235f, 238t. *See also* Neglect.
  physical, 163-213
    presenting signs and symptoms in, 164, 165t
    red flags for, 165-167, 167t
    restraint injury in, 173, 177f
    risk factors for, 162-163, 162t-164t
    skeletal injuries in
      diagnostic imaging of, 188-190, 190f
      types of, 180-188, 182f-190f
    slashing and stab wounds in, 173, 176f
    strangulation injury in, 173, 177f
    subgaleal hematoma in, 167, 170f
    suffocation in, 161
    surface marks in, 167-179, 168f-180f
      differential diagnosis of, 201, 202f-207f, 207
    suspected
      history and physical examination in, 164-165, 166t
    tourniquet injury in, 173, 177f
      differential diagnosis of, 207, 207f
    triggers of, 164
    weapons used in, 164t, 169, 174f
  reporting of, 238-239
Chin, laceration of, 772, 773f
Chlamydia trachomatis
  culture for, 680
  pneumonia in, 599-600, 600f
  sexually transmitted, 692t, 697t, 706-708
Choanal atresia, 903, 904f
  in CHARGE association, 27, 27f
Choanal stenosis, 903-904
Choledochal cyst, 399, 399f, 648, 654, 656f
Cholesteatoma, 901, 902f
Chondrodystrophy, 347, 349
Chondromalacia patellae, 247, 836
Chordee, 547-548, 549f
Chorea, 257, 595
Choreoathetosis, 595
Chorioamnionitis, 41, 41f
Chorioretinitis, in congenital toxoplasmosis, 497
Choroid plexus papilloma
  hydrocephalus in, 576
  increased intracranial pressure in, 583, 583f
Choroid rupture, 754, 754f
Choroiditis, 744. *See also* Retinochoroiditis.
"Christmas tree" deformity, in jejunoileal atresia, 638, 638f

Chromosome(s)
  abnormalities of, 2-4, 3f, 4t, 10f
  analysis of, 1-2
  autosomal, abnormalities of, 9-13
  morphology and nature of, 1-2, 1f, 2f
  sex, abnormalities of, 13-15
Chromosome 15, imprinting disorders and, 18, 18f
Chronic obstructive pulmonary disease (COPD), 111
Churg-Strauss vasculitis, 265
Cigarette burns, in child abuse, 178-179, 180f
Ciliary dyskinesia, 603
Cimetidine, for recurrent aphthous ulcers, 769
Circumcision
  buried penis after, 548, 549f
  meatal bridges after, 549, 550f
  meatal stenosis after, 549, 549f
  preputial adhesions and skin bridges after, 549-550, 550f
Circumvallate placenta, 40, 40f
Classic cradle, in breastfeeding, 58f, 59
Clavicle
  congenital pseudarthrosis of, 209-210, 210f, 825-826, 825f
  fracture of, 187, 189f, 796f, 805-806
  in newborn, 42-43
Claw-hand deformity
  in Charcot-Marie-Tooth disease, 590f, 591
  in Hurler syndrome, 26, 27f
  in newborn, 44, 45f
Claw-toe deformity, 841-843, 843f
Clear cell sarcoma, 654
Cleft lip and palate, 8f, 49, 49f, 868-870, 868t, 869f
Clinodactyly, 7f
Cloacal anomaly, 671, 672f
Cloacal exstrophy, 545, 545f, 667f
Clostridium tetani, 501
Closure time, 424, 425
Clotting factor deficiencies, 202
Club hand, radial, 826, 826f
Clubbing
  causes of, 618, 620t
  with cough, 606
  digital, 127, 128f, 129f
Clubfoot, 8f
  congenital, 836-838, 837f
  versus normal foot, 838f
"Clue cells," in bacterial vaginosis, 704, 705f
Coagulation cascade, 425, 426f
Coagulation disorders, epistaxis in, 910
Coagulopathy, 425-427, 426f
  acquired, 427
  heritable, 425-426, 426f, 427f
Coarctation of the aorta
  balloon angioplasty for, 155-156, 156f
  echocardiography in, 146, 148f
  radiographic appearance of, 137, 137f
  rib notching in, 138, 140f
Coats disease, 743, 743f
Codon, 20
Cognitive development, 73-76, 73f-75f, 76t
  delayed, 76, 76t
  in visual impairment, 91, 92
Cognitive impairment
  in Apert syndrome, 879
  in cerebral palsy, 84
  in Down syndrome, 10
  in fragile X syndrome, 16-17
Coil embolization, of collaterals, 158
Coin rubbing, 202, 203f
COL1A1/COL1A2 genes, 844
Cold abscess, in skeletal tuberculosis, 493f, 494
Cold sore, 453, 453f
Cold urticaria, 114, 115f
Colitis, ulcerative, 392, 394f-397f
Collapse-consolidation infiltrates, in tuberculosis, 492, 493f
Collaterals, closure of, 158

Collodion baby, 280, 320, 321f
Coloboma
  in CHARGE association, 27, 27f
  of eyelid, 728, 729f
  of iris, 736, 737f
  of retina, 741, 741f
Colonic atresia, 637-638, 638f
Colonic stricture, 643, 644f
Color vision, abnormalities of, 748
Comedonal acne, 313, 313f
Common variable immunodeficiency, 118
Compartment syndrome, fracture and, 794, 811-812
Complement system disorders, 124
Complex regional pain syndrome, 272
Computed tomography (CT)
  of abdominal mass, 649
  in AIDS, 503, 505f
  in choanal atresia, 903, 904f
  in cystic fibrosis, 614, 615f
  in Dandy-Walker malformation, 577, 578f
  in head trauma, 196
  in hydranencephaly, 577, 578f
  in hydrocephalus, 576, 577f
  in mastoiditis, 894, 894f
  in nasal dermoids, 905, 905f
  in orbital cellulitis, 919, 919f
  of parapharyngeal abscess, 927, 928f
  of retropharyngeal abscess, 926, 927f
  of simple renal cyst, 541, 541f
  in sinusitis, 914, 916f
  in Sturge-Weber syndrome, 571, 572f, 573
  in tuberous sclerosis, 570, 571f
Concussion, return to play after, 865
Conduct disorder, 90
Condylar fracture, 799t, 801f
Condylomata acuminata, 224, 226f, 701-702, 701f
Condylomata lata, 702, 703f
  in congenital syphilis, 500
Congenital anomalies, 6-9, 6t, 7f, 8f. *See also* Congenital malformation(s).
  anorectal, 670-674
  branchial, 662, 663f
  cardiac, in Apert syndrome, 879
  classification of, 6-7
  cloacal, 671, 672f
  of cornea, 734, 734f
  craniofacial
    affecting skull, 872-882, 873t, 874f-880f
    mandibular, isolated, 886-887, 887f
    midfacial, 882-886, 882f-885f
  in Down syndrome, 9-10, 9f
  of external ear, 46, 46f
  of female genitalia, 556-559, 557f-559f
  of hands and feet, 45-46, 46f
  history in, 7
  of male genitalia, 547-556, 548f-556f
  midline defects as, 46-47, 47f
  in newborn assessment, 44-47
  of optic nerve, 750, 750f
  pancreatic, 383, 384f
  physical examination in, 7, 9
  renal, 520-522, 521f-523f
  of urachus, 538, 539f
Congenital cervical spinal atrophy, 591, 591f
Congenital heart disease. *See* Heart disease, congenital.
Congenital infections. *See* Infection.
Congenital malformation(s), 6-7. *See also* Association(s); Multiple malformation syndrome.
  bronchopulmonary foregut, 627-630, 629f, 630f
  central nervous system, 575-581, 576f-581f
  cough in, 601-602, 601f
  in inborn errors of metabolism, 24-26, 25f, 26t
  vascular
    in biliary atresia, 399, 399f
    capillary and capillary/venous, 328-329, 329f
    in occult spinal dysraphism, 579, 580f

Conjunctiva, laceration of, 752
Conjunctivitis. *See also* Keratoconjunctivitis.
  in adenovirus infection, 446, 447f
  allergic, 112-113, 113f, 114f, 733
  bacterial, 732, 733f
  follicular, 732, 732f
  hemorrhagic, 733-734, 733f
  in Kawasaki syndrome, 268, 268f
  neonatal, 731-732, 732f
  papillary, 113, 114f, 732, 732f
  phlyctenular, 733, 733f
  in rubeola, 443, 444f
  vernal, 113, 113f, 114f
  viral, 732-733, 733f
Connective tissue disease
  genetic, 21-24, 22f, 23f
  mixed, 262, 263t
Constipation, 385, 387f
  abdominal pain in, 711t
  in newborn, 54
Contact burns, 178, 179f
Contact dermatitis
  allergic, 287-288, 290f, 291f
  "id" reaction in, 288, 292f
  irritant, 287
  management of, 288, 290
  periauricular, 894, 895f
  photocontact and phototoxic, 288, 292f
  vulvar, 694
Contact forces, head injuries caused by, 191, 192
Contusions. *See* Bruises.
Convergence insufficiency, exotropia and, 722
Cooley anemia, 408, 408f, 532
Coombs-positive hemolytic anemia, 411, 413f
COPD (chronic obstructive pulmonary disease), 111
Copper deficiency, 210, 381, 382f
Cornea
  abnormalities of, 734-735, 734f-735f
  abrasions of, 752-753, 753f
  blood staining of, 753, 753f
  dermoids of, 734, 734f
  developmental anomalies of, 734, 734f
  edema of, in glaucoma, 735, 735f
  ulcers of, 734, 735f
Corneal light reflex test, 723, 724f
Cornelia de Lange syndrome, 28-29, 29f
Coronal suture, 867, 868f
Coronal synostosis, 875, 875f
Coronary artery aneurysm, in Kawasaki syndrome, 270, 270f
Cortical calcification, in congenital toxoplasmosis, 497, 497f
Cortical tubers, in tuberous sclerosis, 570, 572f
Corticosteroids
  chronic, complications of, 108, 109f
  for contact dermatitis, 290
  for irritant diaper dermatitis, 296
  for juvenile dermatomyositis, 265
  for keloids, 315
  topical
    complications of, 345-346, 346f
    for lichen planus, 297
    for scabies, 310
    for seborrheic dermatitis, 285
Cortisol
  excess of, 361-362, 362f, 363f
  synthesis of, 365f
Coryza, 606
Costello syndrome, 30
Cotton-wool spot, 257, 257f, 745
Cough, 597, 599-606
  causes of, age and, 599-604, 600t
  diagnostic approach to, 606, 606t
  with digital clubbing, 606
  evaluation of, 605-606, 605t
  in infant, 599-602, 600f-602f
  in preschooler, 602-604, 603f-604f
  psychogenic (habit), 604
  in school age to adolescence, 604, 605f
  sputum examination and, 605, 606
Cover-uncover test, 13f, 723-724, 724f

Cow's milk
  bioactive substances in, 377t
  iron deficiency anemia from, 405
Coxa plana, 830, 830f
Coxsackie hand-foot-and-mouth disease, 446, 448, 448f
Coxsackievirus herpangina, 476t
Crab lice, 310-311, 312f
Crackles, 598
Cradle cap, 285, 287f
Cradle position
  classic, 58f, 59
  cross-, 58-59, 58f
Cranial abnormalities, in mental retardation, 85
Cranial bruit, 129t
Cranial sutures
  anatomy of, 867, 868f
  premature fusion of. *See* Craniosynostosis.
  widened, in increased intracranial pressure, 581, 582f
Craniofacial anatomy and embryology, 867-868, 868f
Craniofacial anomalies
  affecting skull, 872-882, 873t, 874f-880f
  mandibular, isolated, 886-887, 887f
  midfacial, 882-886, 882f-885f
Craniomandibular dysfunction, 778-779
Craniopharyngioma, 352, 353f, 440, 583, 584f
Craniosynostosis, 872-882
  complex, syndromic, 876-882, 877f-880f, 877t
  etiology of, 873
  incidence of, 873
  primary versus secondary, 872
  simple, nonsyndromic, 873-876, 874f-877f
  skull shape nomenclature in, 872-873, 873t
Crawling, 69, 69f
Creeping, 69, 69f
CREST syndrome, 259, 261f
Cretinism, 357-358, 357f
Cricoarytenoid joint examination, 242-243
Cri-du-chat syndrome, 6t
Crohn disease, 392, 394f-396f, 647, 648f, 655, 657f
Cross-cradle, in breastfeeding, 58-59, 58f
Croup, 606-607, 607f, 929-930, 929f, 930t
Crouzon syndrome, 879, 880f, 881, 893f
Cruising, 69-70, 69f
Crush injury, of distal phalanx, 808, 809f
Crying, as trigger for abusive behavior, 164
Cryptorchidism, 366, 537
  with hypospadias, 537, 538f
CT. *See* Computed tomography (CT).
Cubitus valgus, 786, 786f
Cubitus varus, 786, 786f
Cultural practices, and healing practice bruises, 202, 203f
Culture
  in tonsillopharyngitis, 923
  in tuberculosis, 496
  in vulvovaginitis, 680, 681t
Cupping, 202, 203f
Curetting, for molluscum contagiosum, 314
Cushing syndrome, 361-362, 362f, 363f
Cutaneous sensory innervation (dermatomes), 563, 564f-565f
Cutaneous urinary diversion, 541, 542f-544f
Cutis aplasia, 47, 47f
Cutis congenita, aplasia, 341, 342f
Cutis marmorata, 319-320, 320f
Cyanosis
  examination for, 127, 128f, 129f
  in respiratory distress, 50, 51f
Cyclosporine
  gingival hyperplasia from, 762
  hirsutism from, 531
Cyst(s)
  Baker, 245, 247, 247f, 835, 835f
  bone, fracture in, 209, 210f
  branchial cleft, 478t, 661, 661f
  bronchogenic, 601, 608, 608f, 633f

Cyst(s) (*Continued*)
  choledochal, 399, 399f, 648, 654, 656f
  dental lamina, 760, 760f
  eruption, 762, 762f
  gastrointestinal duplication, 651, 651f
  gingival, in newborn, 760, 760f
  median raphe, 552, 552f
  omental, 651, 652f
  orbital, 751, 751f
  ovarian, 369, 647, 648f, 651, 655, 710t
  paraurethral, 558, 559f
  posterior fossa, in Dandy-Walker
      malformation, 577, 578f
  preauricular, 658, 895, 897f
  renal, simple, 540-541, 541f. *See also*
      Polycystic kidney disease.
  scalp, 658, 658f
  splenic, 654, 657f
  thymic, 661, 661f
  thyroglossal duct, 478t, 660, 660f
  urachal, 538, 539f
  vallecular, 933, 935f
Cystic acne, 313, 313f
Cystic adenomatoid malformation, 626, 628-
    629, 628f, 629f
Cystic fibrosis, 392, 397f-398f, 398, 610,
    612-616
  versus asthma, 111
  complications of, 614, 614f
  cough in, 602
  diagnosis of, 614-616
  failure to thrive in, 236
  genetic factors in, 610, 612
  presentations of, 612-614, 613f-614f, 613t
  radiographic and CT findings in, 614, 615f
Cystic hygroma, 623, 625f
Cystic renal dysplasia, 524t, 525-526, 526f,
    539-540, 541f
Cystinosis, 527-529, 529f
  corneal, 734, 734f
  ocular findings in, 747
Cystinuria, 516, 517f
Cystitis, bacterial, 519-520, 520f, 520t
Cystourethrogram, 518, 519f, 536, 536f
Cytomegalovirus infection, 476t
  congenital, 498, 498f, 599, 600f
  retinochoroiditis in, 744-745, 745f

D
Dacryoadenitis, 730, 731f
Dacryocele, 731, 731f
Dacryocystitis, 731, 731f
Dactylitis
  blistering distal, 206, 298, 299f
  in sickle cell disease, 416, 416f
Damus-Stansel-Kaye procedure, 153, 153f
Dance, injury prevention in, 858t
Dandy-Walker malformation, 576-577, 578f
Deceleration forces, head injuries caused by,
    191-192
Deep tendon reflexes, 563, 566f
Deep venous thrombosis, 427-428, 427f
Deformation, 7
Deformational plagiocephaly, 870-872, 871f
Degloving injury, orofacial, 772, 772f
Deletion, chromosome, 3, 3f
Deletion 22q11.2, 6t
Demineralization from disuse, 209, 209f
Dennie sign, in allergic rhinitis, 99-100, 100f
Dental abscess, 769, 769f, 770f
Dental anatomy, 755, 756f
Dental caries, 235f, 236-237, 766-767, 767f
Dental development, 755-758, 757f-759f
Dental diastema, 761f
Dental enamel defects, 764, 764f, 765f
Dental examination, 755, 756f
Dental history, 755
Dental lamina cyst, 760, 760f
Dental trauma, 770-771, 774-775, 775f-776f
Dentinogenesis imperfecta, 764-765, 765f, 845
Denys-Drash syndrome, 364, 529, 530f

Depigmentation
  in piebaldism, 335-336, 336f
  in vitiligo, 334, 336f
Deprivation amblyopia, 724, 726f
Dermal sinus, congenital, 46-47, 47f
Dermatitis
  atopic, 280-284
    differential diagnosis of, 283
    herpes simplex infection with, 284, 452,
        453f
    IgE level in, 122-123
    keratosis pilaris in, 281, 283f
    lichenification in, 282f
    phases of, 281, 281f-282f
    pityriasis alba in, 283, 283f
    treatment of, 283-284
  contact
    allergic, 287-288, 290f, 291f
    "id" reaction in, 288, 292f
    irritant, 287
    management of, 288, 290
    periauricular, 894, 895f
    photocontact and phototoxic, 288, 292f
    vulvar, 694
  diaper
    candidal, 295, 296f, 466, 505f
    irritant, 294-295, 295f
    from neglect, 235f
    psoriatic, 277, 296, 297f
    seborrheic, 296
    staphylococcal, 295-296, 296f
    tinea, 296-297, 297f
  "fleabite," of newborn, 317-318, 319f
  in Job syndrome, 285-286, 288f
  juvenile plantar-palmar, 284-285, 285f
  from neglect, 233, 234f
  in pityriasis rosea, 286-287, 289f
  rhus, 287, 290f
  seborrheic, 285, 286f, 287f
Dermatomal distribution, in herpes zoster,
    453, 454f
Dermatomes, 563, 564f-565f
Dermatomyositis, juvenile, 262-265
  calcinosis in, 263, 263f, 264
  disease markers in, 264
  magnetic resonance imaging in, 264-265,
      265f
  muscle weakness in, 263
  pneumatosis intestinalis in, 265, 265f
  rash in, 263, 264f
Dermatophyte infection, 291-294. *See also*
    Tinea *entries*.
Dermographism, 114, 115f
Dermoids, 478t
  corneal, 734, 734f
  midline scalp or back, 658, 658f
  nasal, 904-905, 905f
  orbital, 751, 751f
Descemet membrane break, in glaucoma, 735,
    736f
Desensitization, for drug reactions, 98
Desmarres lid retractor, 752, 753f
Desquamating agents, for tinea versicolor, 294
Desquamation
  in congenital syphilis, 500, 500f
  in Kawasaki syndrome, 268, 269f
  in staphylococcal scalded skin syndrome,
      457, 457f
  in staphylococcal scarlet fever, 457-458,
      458f
  in streptococcal scarlet fever, 455, 456f
  in toxic shock syndrome, 458f, 459
Development. *See also* Growth.
  of antigravity muscular control, 66-67, 68f,
      69f
  assessment of. *See* Developmental
      assessment.
  of athletic skills, 849-850, 850t
  of attachment, 79
  in attention-deficit hyperactivity disorder,
      89-91, 90t
  in autism, 87-88
  in cerebral palsy, 81-84, 82f-84f, 82t

Development (*Continued*)
  cognitive, 73-76, 73f-75f, 76t
    delayed, 76, 76t
    in visual impairment, 91, 92
  of complex fine motor skills, 72, 72f
  of complex gross motor patterns, 70
  dental, 755-758, 757f-759f
  of early sensory processing, 73, 73f
  of early skills in speech perception and
      production, 76-77, 77f
  fine motor, 70-73, 70f-73f, 91
  gross motor, 65-70, 66f-69f, 66t, 69t
    delayed, 70, 70t
    in visual impairment, 91
  of head control, 66, 67f
  of head righting, 66-67, 68f
  of immune system, 115-116, 116f
  of intelligible and fluent language, 77-78,
      78t
  of involuntary grasp, 70, 70f
  language. *See* Language development.
  of locomotion, 67, 69-70, 69f, 69t
  of logical thinking, 75, 75f
  in mental retardation, 84-87, 86f
  of musculoskeletal system, 781-783, 782f,
      783f
  normal, principles of, 65
  of parachute response, 67, 69f
  of primitive reflexes, 65-66, 66f, 66t
  of protective equilibrium response, 66-67,
      66t, 68f
  pubertal, 349, 350f, 351, 351f-352f
  of receptive and expressive language
      responses, 77, 78t
  of sense of self, 80-81, 80f
  of sensorimotor intelligence, 73-74, 74f, 75f
  of sitting/standing posture control, 66, 68f
  social, 79-81, 79f, 80f, 92
  of symbolic capabilities, 74-75
  of trunk control, 66, 67f, 68f
  in visual impairment, 91-92, 91t
  of voluntary grasp, 71, 71f, 72f
Developmental assessment
  cognitive, 75-76, 76t
  fine motor, 72-73, 73f
  gross motor, 70
  hearing, 88, 88f
  language, 78-79
  screening tests in, 65
  social, 81
  surveillance in, 65
Developmental delay/disabilities
  evaluation of, 81-92
  global, 70t
  remediable disorders associated with, 76t
Developmental milestones
  fine motor, 70-73, 70f-73f
  gross motor, 65-70, 66f-69f, 66t, 69t
  receptive and expressive language, 78t
Dexamethasone suppression test, in Cushing
    syndrome, 361-362, 363f
Dextrocardia, 134, 134f
Diabetes insipidus
  central, 356
  nephrogenic, 356
Diabetes mellitus, 369-371
  joint mobility in, 370-371, 371f
  retinopathy in, 746
  short stature and, 370
  skin lesions in, 371, 371f
Diamond-Blackfan anemia, 410
Diaper dermatitis
  candidal, 295, 296f, 466, 505f
  irritant, 294-295, 295f
  from neglect, 235f
  psoriatic, 277, 296, 297f
  seborrheic, 296
  staphylococcal, 295-296, 296f
  tinea, 296-297, 297f
Diaphragmatic hernia, congenital, 625-626,
    628f
Diaphyseal fracture, 186-187, 186f-189f, 799f,
    799t

Diarrhea, 388-389
Diastematomyelia, in occult spinal dysraphism, 579, 580f
Diazoxide, hirsutism from, 531
DiGeorge syndrome, 6t, 118-119, 119f
hypocalcemia and, 359
physical findings in, 130, 130t
Digit. *See also* Finger; Toe.
clubbing of, 127, 128f, 129f
duplication of, 45, 46f
supernumerary, 45, 46f
Digital desquamation, in Kawasaki syndrome, 268, 269f
Digital pitting scars, in scleroderma, 261, 261f
Dimercaptosuccinic acid (DMSA) scan, 520, 520f
Diphallus, 551, 551f
Diplegia, spastic, 83-84, 84f
Diplopia, 581, 718
Discoid lupus erythematosus, 258
Diskitis, juvenile, 486-488, 489f
Dislocations, 812-814, 812f-814f. *See also specific sites.*
Disruption, 7
Disseminated intravascular coagulation, 424
disease triggers of, 418t
in Kasabach-Merritt syndrome, 424, 424f
in microangiopathic hemolytic anemia, 418, 418f
Districhiasis, 726, 728f
Diuresis renography, in ureteropelvic junction obstruction, 539, 540f
Diverticulum
esophageal, 478t
Meckel, 643-644, 644f, 645f
urachal, 538
Döhle bodies, 421-422, 422f
Doppler ultrasonography, in renal venous thrombosis, 518, 518f
Double aortic arch, 137-138, 138f
"Double bubble" sign, in duodenal atresia, 637, 637f
Double elevator palsy, 723
Double vision, 581, 718
Down syndrome, 9-11, 9f, 10f
brush spots in, 738
congenital anomalies in, 9-10, 9f
etiology of, 10-11, 10f
facial abnormalities in, 85, 87f
growth charts for, 85, 86f
leukemoid reaction in, 419, 421
maternal age and, 10, 10t
physical findings in, 129-130, 130t
Doxycycline, for Rocky Mountain spotted fever, 462
Drash syndrome, 529
"Drooping lily" sign, in adrenal neuroblastoma, 653, 654f
Drug allergy, 98, 99f
Drug eruptions
fixed, 304, 305f
morbilliform, 304, 305f
Duane syndrome, 720, 721f
Duchenne muscular dystrophy, 588-589, 588f-590f, 588t
Ductus arteriosus, patent
closure of, 158, 158f
heart size in, 136
Duhaime infant model, shaken baby syndrome and, 193
Duodenal atresia, 637, 637f
Duodenal hematoma, 199, 199f
Duodenal obstruction, from midgut volvulus, 637, 637f
Dwarfism, camptomelic, 364
Dye dermatitis, 287, 291f
Dyschromatopsia, 748
Dyserythropoietic anemia, congenital, 410, 412f
Dyshidrotic eczema, 284, 284f
Dyslexia, 89
Dysmenorrhea, 711t

Dysmorphic features
approach to evaluation of, 6-9, 6t, 7f, 8f
in mental retardation, 85
Dysostosis
acrofacial, 883-884, 884f
mandibulofacial, 882-883, 882f
Dyspepsia, functional, 383
Dysphagia, 390-391, 390f, 391f
Dysplasia, 7
Dystrophic epidermolysis bullosa, 315, 321-322, 322f
Dystrophic nail, 344, 344f
Dystrophin, 588
Dysuria, noninfectious, 690t

E
"E game," 714-715
Eagle-Barrett syndrome, 521, 521f, 537-538, 538f
Ear. *See also* Hearing *entries.*
anatomy of, 889, 890f
angioedema of, 894, 895f
cellulitis of, 894, 895f
examination of, 889-892, 891f, 892f
external
anatomy of, 889, 890f
atresia of, 896f
cleaning of, 889, 891f
congenital anomalies of, 46, 46f
deformity of, 894-896, 896f, 897f
discharge from, 433, 434f, 893, 893f
discoloration of, 894, 894f, 895f
disorders of, 892-893, 893f-897f
displacement of pinna of, 893-894, 894f, 895f
foreign body in, 893, 893f, 896, 897f
in newborn assessment, 35-36, 36f
internal, anatomy of, 889, 890f
lop, 896f
middle. *See also* Tympanic membrane.
anatomy of, 889, 890f
cholesteatoma of, 901, 902f
disorders of, 896-902, 898f-902f
inflammation of, 897-900. *See also* Otitis media.
protection of, 900-901
Ear creases, 433
Ear pits, 46, 46f, 433
Ear tags, 46, 46f, 896f
Earplugs (ear defenders), 900-901
Ebstein's anomaly, box-shaped heart in, 135, 136f
Ecchymoses, 423f, 777, 778f
Echocardiography, in congenital heart disease, 144-146, 145f, 148f
Ecthyma, 466, 467f
Ectodermal dysplasia, of scalp, 47, 47f
Ectopia cordis, 664
Ectopia lentis, 740, 740f
Ectopic pregnancy, 710t
Ectopic ureter, 558, 558f
Ectrodactyly, 8f
Ectropion, 684, 684f, 728, 729f
Eczema. *See also* Dermatitis, atopic.
dyshidrotic, 284, 284f
lip-licking, 285, 285f
nummular, 284, 284f
thumb-sucking, 285, 285f
Eczema herpeticum, 284, 452, 453f
Edema. *See also* Angioedema.
angioneurotic, 607
of aryepiglottic folds, 618, 619
cerebral
increased intracranial pressure in, 582, 582f
in shaken baby syndrome, 195, 197f
of cornea, in glaucoma, 735, 735f
of eyelid
in minimal change disease, 514, 514f
in mononucleosis, 450, 450f
in Henoch-Schönlein purpura, 266, 267f

Edema *(Continued)*
in Kawasaki syndrome, 268, 269f
in kwashiorkor, 375, 377f
in minimal change disease, 514, 514f, 515f
of optic disc, 582, 582f, 749, 749f
Egg allergy, 97, 98t
"Egg on a string" heart shadow, 135, 135f
"Egg on its side" heart, 135, 136f
Ehlers-Danlos syndrome, 21, 23f, 23t, 24, 204
Elbow
carrying angle of, 786, 786f
dislocation of, 814, 814f
examination of, 243, 244f, 786, 786f
fracture involving, 801f-803f, 806-807, 807f, 808f
fracture-dislocation of, 814, 814f
nursemaid's, 816-817, 816f, 817f
Electrocardiography
after radiofrequency catheter ablation, 143, 143f
of atrioventricular septal defect, 138, 141f
of complete heart block, 144, 144f
in congenital heart disease, 138-144, 140t, 141f-144f
of premature atrial contractions, 140, 142f
of premature ventricular contractions, 140, 142f
of prolonged QT syndrome, 143, 144f
of supraventricular tachycardia, 140, 142, 143f
of tricuspid atresia, 141f
of ventricular tachycardia, 143, 144f
of wandering atrial pacemaker, 140, 142f
Electroencephalography
in absence seizure, 593-594, 593f
in infantile spasm, 594, 594f
ELISA assay, in HIV infection, 503
Elliptocytosis, hereditary, hemolytic anemia in, 412-413, 414f
Ellis-van Creveld syndrome, 130, 130f, 130t
Embolization of collaterals, 158
Emesis. *See* Vomiting.
EMLA cream, in gynecologic examination of prepubertal patient, 680
Emmetropia, 716, 716f
Emotional abuse, 238
Emphysema
lobar, 610, 612f, 629, 629f, 630f
subcutaneous
in asthma, 107-108, 108f
in cystic fibrosis, 614, 614f
Empyema, intrathoracic, 631, 633f
Enamel defects, 764, 764f, 765f
Encephalocele, 8f
nasal, 904, 904f
in occult spinal dysraphism, 579, 580f
Encephalopathy, in glutaric aciduria, 213
End ureterostomy, 541, 542f
Endobronchial tuberculosis, 492, 493f
Endocarditis
bacterial
retinopathy in, 745-746, 745f, 746f
signs of, 132-133, 133f
Libman-Sacks, in systemic lupus erythematosus, 255-256
Endocrine disorders, 347-372
diabetes mellitus and, 369-371
failure to thrive in, 236
hypercalcemia and, 359
hypocalcemia and, 359-360
hypoglycemia and, 371-372
hypophosphatemia and, 360
obesity and, 372, 372t, 373f
syndromes associated with, 370t
Endocrine system
adrenal glands in, 361-364
gonads in, 364-369
hypothalamus and pituitary gland in, 351-356
parathyroid glands in, 359
thyroid gland in, 356-359

Endoscope, nasal, 902-903, 903f
Endurance training, 857
Enema, barium, in gastrointestinal obstruction, 634, 634f
Energy metabolism disorders, 30-31, 31t
Enmeshment, in idiopathic musculoskeletal pain syndromes, 273
Enteralgic gait, 790
Enterocolitis
milk protein, 98
necrotizing, 643, 643f
Enteropathy, gluten sensitive, 236, 389-390, 389f, 390f
Enteroviral syndromes, 448
Enthesitis, 253
Entropion, 726, 729f
Eosinophil(s), normal values for, 419t
Eosinophilia, 101, 101t, 419f
Eosinophilic esophagitis, 391, 391f
Eosinophilic fasciitis, 259
Eosinophilic gastroenteritis, 98
Eosinophilic granuloma. See Langerhans cell histiocytosis.
Ependymoma, 440, 583, 584f
Epiblepharon, 726, 728, 729f
Epicondylar fracture, 799t, 803f, 806-807
Epidemic keratoconjunctivitis, 732-733, 733f
Epidemic parotitis, 463-464, 463f
Epidermal necrolysis, toxic, 98, 300-301, 301f
Epidermal nevus, 332, 333f, 574, 574f
Epidermoid cysts, of orbit, 751, 751f
Epidermolysis bullosa, 320-322
dystrophic, 321-322, 322f
epidermolytic, 321, 321f
junctional, 321, 321f
Epidermolytic hyperkeratosis, 280, 281f
Epididymal cyst, 555, 555f
Epididymis, appendix, 552
torsion of, 553, 554f
Epididymitis, 464, 553-554, 555f
Epidural abscess, 916, 918f
Epidural hematoma, 583, 585, 585f
Epiglottitis, 927-929, 928f, 929f
Epilepsy
infantile spasm in, 594, 594f
seizure in, 593-594, 593f, 593t
Epinephrine
for anaphylaxis, 94, 96f
racemic, for croup, 929-930
EpiPen, 94, 96f
Epiphyseal maturation, 347, 781, 782f, 783f
Epiphysis
fractures of, 781, 799t, 800f
slipped capital femoral, 830-832, 831f
Epispadias, 545-546, 545f
Epistaxis, 424, 909-911, 909f-911f
Epitrochlear lymph nodes, 477, 481f
Epstein pearls, 760, 760f
Epstein-Barr virus, 441, 450
Epulis, congenital, 760, 760f
Equilibrium response, protective, 66-67, 66t, 68f
Equine gait, 791
Erb palsy, in newborn, 44, 45f
Ergometry, bicycle, 621
Eruption cyst/hematoma, 762, 762f
Erysipelas, 471, 471f
Erythema
in juvenile rheumatoid arthritis, 248f
in Kawasaki syndrome, 268, 269f
in serum sickness–like reaction, 304, 304f
in urticaria, 302-304, 303f
Erythema infectiosum, 448-449, 449f
Erythema marginatum, 131-132, 133f
Erythema migrans, in Lyme disease, 253, 254f, 461-462, 461f
Erythema multiforme, 98, 298-299, 299f, 301
Erythema nodosum, 302, 303f
Erythema toxicum neonatorum, 317-318, 319f
Erythroblastopenia, transient, 410, 410t

Erythroblastosis fetalis, tooth discoloration in, 766, 766f
Erythrocyte(s)
aplasia of, 410, 410t, 412f
casts of, in poststreptococcal glomerulonephritis, 512, 512f
count of, 510
function of, 403
mean corpuscular volume (MCV) of, 404t
morphologic evaluation of, 403, 404f
production of, 403, 404f
Erythroderma
in staphylococcal scalded skin syndrome, 457, 457f
in toxic shock syndrome, 458, 458f
Erythrophagocytosis, 422, 423f
Esodeviations, 718-721, 719f-721f
Esophageal atresia
pure, 625, 627f
with tracheoesophageal fistula, 624-625, 626f, 627f
Esophageal diverticulum, 478t
Esophageal dysmotility, in CREST syndrome, 259, 261f
Esophageal foreign body, 934, 936, 936f
Esophageal mucosal biopsy, 634
Esophageal pH probe, 634
Esophageal stricture, 390-391, 391f
Esophageal varices, 644
Esophagitis, eosinophilic, 391, 391f
Esophagram, barium, 634, 635f
in double aortic arch, 137-138, 138f
Esotropia
accommodative, 719, 720f
infantile, 719, 719f
nonaccommodative, 719, 720f
sixth cranial nerve palsy and, 719-720
Estrogen cream, for labial adhesions, 685
Ethmoid sinus, 911, 912f
Eutectic mixture of local anesthetics (EMLA) cream, in gynecologic examination of prepubertal patient, 680
Evidence collection, in sexual abuse cases, 225-228, 227t
Ewing sarcoma, 434, 439, 441f
Ex utero intrapartum treatment of (EXIT) procedure, 623, 625f
Exanthem subitum, 449-450, 449f
Exanthems
bacterial, 454-463, 456f-463f
meningococcal, 459-461, 459f-460f
morbilliform, 304, 305f
staphylococcal, 457-459, 457f-459f
viral, 298, 298f, 443-454, 444f-455f
Exercise testing, 621
Exodeviations, 721-722, 722f
Exon, 20
Exophthalmometer, 750, 751f
Exophthalmos, in Graves disease, 357, 357f
Exotropia, 722, 722f
Exstrophy
classic bladder, 541, 544f
cloacal, 545, 545f
epispadias and, 545-546, 545f
Extensor tendon injury, 808, 809f
Extensor tendon overpull, 787, 787f
Extracranial hemorrhage, in newborn, 42
Extrahepatic biliary atresia, 398-399, 399f
Extraocular motion testing, 563, 565f
Extraocular muscles, innervation of, 718, 718f
Extremity
lower
examination of, 787-791, 788f-790f, 792f
musculoskeletal disorders of, 828-843, 829f-843f
upper
examination of, 784-787, 784f-787f, 787t
musculoskeletal disorders of, 825-828, 825f-828f
Extremity pain, with ligamentous laxity, 817-818, 817f
Extrinsic allergic alveolitis, 111-112

Eye. See also Ocular entries; Vision; specific structures.
aniridia of, 432-433, 433f
anterior chamber of, 735-736, 735f, 736f
black, after forehead contusion, 202, 202f
conjunctiva of, 731-734, 732f-734f
embolism to, 745-746, 745f
eyelid and adnexae of, 725-730, 726f-730f
injuries to, 752-754, 752f-754f
lacrimal gland and nasolacrimal drainage system of, 730-731, 730f-731f
movements of, disorders of. See Strabismus.
phorias and tropias of, 718
raccoon, in neuroblastoma, 432, 433f
refractive errors of, 716-717, 716f, 717f
vergence movements of, 718
Eyelash abnormalities, 726, 728f, 729f
Eyelid
anatomy of, 725, 726f
ankyloblepharon of, 728
blepharitis of, 728
coloboma of, 728, 729f
ectropion of, 728, 729f
edema of
in minimal change disease, 514, 514f
in mononucleosis, 450, 450f
entropion of, 726, 729f
inflammation of, 728, 729f, 730f
laceration of, 752, 752f
ptosis of, 725-726, 727f
retraction of, 752, 753f

F
Fabry disease, 529, 529f
Face. See also Craniofacial entries; Orofacial entries.
anatomy and embryology of, 867-868, 868f
lesions of, 658-659, 659f
trauma to. See Orofacial trauma.
Facial abnormalities. See also Facies.
in mental retardation, 85, 87f
in 22q11 syndrome, 119, 119f
Facial cellulitis, 474, 769, 770f
Facial clefting, 8f, 49, 49f, 868-870, 868t, 869f
Facial infection, periorbital cellulitis from, 918, 918f
Facial muscles, central motor control of, 586, 586f
Facial nerve palsy, in newborn, 44, 44f
Facial skeleton, 867-868, 868f
Facial weakness, 586, 587f
Facies
in Cornelia de Lange syndrome, 28, 29f
in Hurler syndrome, 26, 27f
in Noonan syndrome, 29
in scleroderma, 261, 262f
in sickle cell disease, 416, 416f
Factor V Leiden mutation, thrombosis in, 428
Factor IX deficiency, 425-426
Factor VIII deficiency, 425-426
Failure to thrive, 233-238, 375, 377-378, 377t, 379f, 380-381
in AIDS, 503, 504f
anthropometric measurements in, 378, 379f, 379t, 380f, 380t
clinical observations of, 375, 376f-378f
etiology of, 377t
evaluation of, 237
laboratory tests in, 237, 377-378
organic causes of, 235-237, 238t
psychosocial, 74f, 233-235, 233f-235f
in renal disorders, 509
treatment of, 237, 378-381, 380f-383f
Familial Mediterranean fever, 272
Fanconi anemia, 428, 428f
Farmer's lung, 111
Fasciitis
eosinophilic, 259
necrotizing, 474-475, 474f
Fascioscapulohumeral muscular dystrophy, 588t

Fat malabsorption, 377, 380-381
Fat necrosis, in newborn, 43, 43f
Fecalith, 647, 647f
Feeding, vomiting and, 634
Feeding problems, as trigger for abusive behavior, 164
Femoral anteversion, 832, 832f
Femoral hernia, 670, 670f
Femoral lymph nodes, 477
Femur
    fracture of, 796f, 797f
    pseudotumor of, 427f
Ferritin, serum
    in chronic inflammatory states, 408-409
    in iron deficiency anemia, 406
Fertility, pelvic inflammatory disease and, 708
Fetal alcohol syndrome, 30, 30f, 85
Fetal blood, maternal blood versus, Apt-Downey test for, 642
Fetal hydronephrosis, 536, 536f
Fever
    familial Mediterranean, 272
    in Kawasaki syndrome, 268
    periodic
        in PFAPA syndrome, 272, 768-769
        syndromes associated with, 272
    rheumatic, 131-132, 133f, 241
    Rocky Mountain spotted, 462-463, 463f
    in roseola infantum, 449
    scarlet
        staphylococcal, 457-458, 458f
        streptococcal, 454, 455-457, 456f
    in systemic-onset juvenile rheumatoid arthritis, 249-250
    in tularemia, 481
FGFR (fibroblast growth factor receptor) gene mutations, craniofacial syndromes associated with, 877, 877t
Fibroadenoma, of breast, 665
Fibrocystic breast disease, 665
Fibromatosis coli, 662-663, 663f, 664f
Fibromatosis gingivae, 762
Fibromyalgia, 272
Fibular fracture, distal, Salter-Harris type I, 794, 794f
Fifth disease, 448-449, 449f
Fine motor development, 70-73, 70f-73f, 91
Fine needle aspiration, 661
Fine pincer grasp, 71, 71f, 72f
Finger
    Boutonnière (buttonhole) deformity of, 827, 827f
    clubbing of, in AIDS, 503, 506f
    fracture of, 807-809, 808f-809f
    mallet, 828, 828f
    swan-neck deformity of, 828, 828f
Fire ant sting, 97
FISH (fluorescence in situ hybridization), 5-6, 5f, 6t
Fish allergy, 97, 98t
Fistula
    perineal, 670, 671f
    rectourethral, 670-671, 671f
    tracheoesophageal
        cough in, 601, 601f
        with esophageal atresia, 624-625, 626f, 627f
        isolated, 625, 627f
    vulvovaginitis from, 695
Fitz-Hugh-Curtis syndrome, 709-710
Fixation reflex, 713, 715f
Flaring, in respiratory distress, 50
Flat warts, 313, 314f
Flatfoot
    in congenital vertical talus, 839-840, 840f
    physiologic, 841, 841f
"Fleabite" dermatitis, of newborn, 317-318, 319f
Flow-volume curves, 618, 620-621, 620f, 621f
Fluconazole, for tinea capitis, 342
Fluorescence in situ hybridization (FISH), 5-6, 5f, 6t

Folate/folic acid deficiency, megaloblastic anemia and, 409
Follicle stimulating hormone (FSH), 354-355, 355f
Follicular conjunctivitis, 732, 732f
Folliculitis, 465, 465f
    vulvar, 698
Fontan procedure, 150, 150f
Fontanelle
    anterior, 867, 868f
    bulging
        in central nervous system tumors, 431-432, 432f
        in meningococcal meningitis, 459, 459f
    posterior, 867, 868f
Food allergy
    IgE-mediated, 97-98, 97f, 98t
    non–IgE-mediated, 98
Foot
    athlete's, 292, 294f
    calcaneovalgus, 840-841, 841f
    cavus, 841-843, 842f
    club, 8f
        congenital, 836-838, 837f
        versus normal foot, 838f
    congenital anomalies of, 45-46, 46f
    disorders of, 836-843
    examination of, 247, 247f
    flat
        in congenital vertical talus, 839-840, 840f
        physiologic, 841, 841f
    fracture of, 809-810, 810f
    ganglion of, 841, 842f
    interphalangeal joints of, 247
    normal, radiography of, 838f
    rocker-bottom, 839, 840f
Foot progression angle, 791, 792f
Football hold, in breastfeeding, 57-58, 58f
Forceps delivery, fat necrosis and, 43, 43f
Forchheimer spots, in rubella, 443
Forearm, bowing deformity of, 798f
Foregut malformations, bronchopulmonary, 627-630, 629f, 630f
Forehead contusion, black eyes after, 202, 202f
Foreign body
    aspiration of, 111, 111f, 930-931, 931f, 932f
    bronchial, 633f
    esophageal, 934, 936, 936f
    in external auditory canal, 893, 893f, 896, 897f
    inhaled, 602, 603f
    nasal, 907, 907f
    in vagina, 230-231, 231f, 695
Formula-feeding
    bioactive substances in, 377t
    stools in, 53, 53f
Forward bend test, 785, 785f, 819, 820f
Fovea, 713, 714f
Fracture(s), 791-812
    accidental, 207-208
    anatomic classification of, 799, 799f-803f, 799t
    articular, 799t, 800f
    avulsion
        pelvic, 811, 811f
        of tibial spine, 815, 815f, 816
    bowing, 795, 795t, 798f
    boxer's, 809, 809f
    from child abuse, 180-188, 182f-190f. See also Child abuse, fractures in.
    of clavicle, 187, 189f, 796f, 805-806
        in newborn, 42-43
    comminuted, 795, 795t, 797f
    compartment syndrome and, 794, 811-812
    compression/distraction (three-point bending), 187, 188f
    conditions associated with or mimicking, 209-211, 210f-212f
    condylar, 799t, 801f
    dental, 774, 775, 774f, 775f
    diagnosis of, 791-795, 793f, 794f
    diagnostic imaging of, 188-190, 190f
    diaphyseal, 186-187, 186f-189f, 799f, 799t

Fracture(s) (Continued)
    differential diagnosis of, 207-211, 209f-212f
    of distal fibula, Salter-Harris type I, 794, 794f
    of distal radius, 798f
    elbow and, 801f-803f, 806-807, 807f, 808f
    epicondylar, 799t, 803f, 806-807
    epiphyseal, 781, 799t, 800f
    of femur, 796f, 797f
    of finger, 807-809, 808f-809f
    of foot, 809-810, 810f
    greenstick, 795, 795t, 798f
    of hand, 188, 190f, 807-809, 808f-809f
    head injury and, 184
    healing of, 181-182, 182f, 184, 185f
    of humerus, 208, 796f, 803f
    impacted, 795, 795t, 797f
    intercondylar, 799t, 800f
    lap belt, 810-811, 810f
    lateral condylar, 801f, 806
    LeFort, 777-778, 777f, 778f
    long bone, 184, 186-187, 186f-189f
    longitudinal, 794f, 795, 795t
    of mandible, 776-777, 776f
    of maxilla, 777-778, 777f, 778f
    metacarpal, 188, 190f, 809, 809f
    metaphyseal, 22f, 23f, 182-183, 182f, 183f, 799f, 799t
    metatarsal, 190f, 809-810, 810f
    midfacial, 777-778, 777f, 778f
    Monteggia, 814, 814f
    multiple, bone scan in, 184, 185f
    nasal, displaced, 908, 908f
    oblique, 186-187, 187f, 795, 795t, 796f
    orbital floor, 752, 752f
    pathologic, 811
        conditions associated with, 208-209, 209f, 210f
    patterns of, 794f-798f, 795-799, 795t
    pelvic avulsion, 811, 811f
    periosteal stripping as, 184, 186, 186f
    phalangeal, 190f, 807-809, 808f-809f
    physeal, 799-804, 799t, 801f
    plastic deformation, 798f
    of proximal phalanx, 188, 190f, 797f
    of radial neck, 807, 807f
    radiography of, 795
    rib, 183-184, 184f, 185f, 200, 201f
    Salter-Harris classification of, 799, 803-804, 803t, 804f-805f
    skull, 194, 194f, 195f, 894, 895f
    spiral, 186, 186f, 795, 795t, 796f
    subcapital, 799t, 803f
    supracondylar, 187, 189f, 799t, 802f, 806, 808f
    toddler's, 795, 806, 806f
    of tooth, 774-775, 774f, 775f
    torus, 187, 187f, 795, 795t, 798f
    transcondylar, 806
    transverse, 187, 187f, 795, 795t, 796f, 809, 810f
    treatment principles in, 804-805
    vertebral, 188, 190f, 810-811, 810f
Fracture-dislocation
    of elbow, 814, 814f
    of hip, 812, 812f
Fragile X syndrome, 15-17, 16f, 16t, 17f
Frameshift mutation, 20
Francisella tularensis, 481
Free erythrocyte protoporphyrin (FEP)
    in iron deficiency anemia, 406
    in lead poisoning, 407
Frenulum
    abnormalities of, 761, 761f
    persistent, 659
Friction alopecia, 339-340, 340f
Friction rubs, 598
Friedreich ataxia, 132t
Frog-leg positions, 217-218, 679f
Frontal sinus, 911, 913f
Frontal sinusitis, 916, 918f
Fundoplication, 635

Fungal infection
   of nail, 344, 344f
   of oral cavity, 770, 771f
   of scalp, 341-342, 343f
   of skin, 291-297
Furuncle, 468, 468f

G
Gait
   antalgic, 790
   disturbances of, 790-791
   equine, 791
   evaluation of, 790-791
   steppage, 791
   Trendelenburg, 791
Galactokinase deficiency, 739-740
Galactorrhea, 355
Galactosemia, 739-740, 739f
Galeazzi sign, in developmental hip
      dislocation, 828
Gallbladder dilation, in Kawasaki syndrome,
      270, 270f
Gallstones, 383, 384f, 648
Gamekeeper's thumb, 814, 815f
Ganglion
   of foot, 841, 842f
   of wrist, 826-827, 826f
Gangliosidosis, 747, 747f
Gangrene, streptococcal, 474-475, 474f
Gas exchange, 622, 622t
Gastric emptying scan, 617, 619f
Gastric ulceration, 643, 643f
Gastritis, 383, 383f, 384f
Gastrocnemius stretch, 862f
Gastroenteritis, eosinophilic, 98
Gastroesophageal reflux, 385, 388, 388t
   aspiration in, 618, 619f
   cough in, 602
   failure to thrive in, 237
   otolaryngologic manifestations of, 903, 936,
      937f
   signs and symptoms of, 597
   stridor in, 607
   surgery for, 635
   vomiting and, 634-635, 635f
Gastrointestinal. *See also* Intestinal *entries.*
Gastrointestinal bleeding, 641-645
   causes of, 391-392, 392t, 393f, 642t
   in infant, 642-643, 643f, 643t, 644f
   in older children, 645, 646f
   in toddlers, 643-645, 644f-646f
Gastrointestinal disorders, 382-398
   failure to thrive and, 235
   functional, 382-383
   in scleroderma, 262
Gastrointestinal duplication cyst, 651, 651f
Gastrointestinal obstruction, 398, 398f, 632,
      634-641. *See also* Vomiting.
Gastrointestinal trauma, 391, 392f
Gastroschisis, 666-667, 667f
Gene(s). *See also* Chromosome(s).
   imprinted, abnormalities of, 18-20, 18f, 19f
   nature of, 20
Genetic disorders, 1-32
   of connective tissue, 21-24, 22f, 23f
   dysmorphic, approach to evaluation of, 6-9,
      6t, 7f, 8f
   failure to thrive in, 236
   fluorescence in situ hybridization in, 5-6,
      5f, 6t
   metabolic, 24-26, 25f, 26t
   newborn screening for, 31-32
   single-gene, 20-21
Genetic syndromes, cardiac findings in, 132t
Genetic testing, in cystic fibrosis, 614-615,
      616
Genital examination, 535
Genital tract
   lower, sexually transmitted disease of,
      703-708
   obstruction of, 685-687, 686f, 687t

Genital trauma, 560-561, 561f, 687-689,
      688f-690f
   accidental, 230, 231f
   frictional, 694, 694f
   moderate, 688-689, 689f
   severe, 690, 690f
   from sexual abuse, 221, 222f, 688, 688f
   superficial perineal injuries in, 687-688,
      688f
Genital ulcers
   in Behçet's disease, 271, 272f
   herpetic, 703, 704f
   syphilitic, 702, 702f
Genital warts, 313-314, 701-702, 701f
Genitalia
   ambiguous
      causes of, 560f
      congenital adrenal hyperplasia and, 363
      evaluation of, 364-366, 366f, 367f, 559
      imperforate anus and, 559, 560f
      in Smith-Lemli-Opitz syndrome, 25, 25f
   female. *See also* Gynecologic *entries.*
      congenital anomalies of, 556-559,
         557f-559f
      development of, 675-676, 675f-678f, 678t
      in gestational age assessment, 36, 37f
      lesions of, 556-559, 557f-559f
      normal appearance, 675f-677f
      trauma to, 561
   male
      anomalies of, 547-556, 548f-556f
      development of, 349, 350f, 351f
      in gestational age assessment, 36
      trauma to, 560-561, 561f
Genitourinary disorders, 509, 535-563
Gentian violet, for thrush, 60
Genum valgum, 833, 834f
Genum varum, 359, 361f, 832-833, 833f
Geographic tongue, 760-761, 761f
GER. *See* Gastroesophageal reflux.
Germ cell tumor, 437
German measles. *See* Rubella.
Gestational age
   appropriate for, 37, 39f
   assessment of, 33-37, 35f-38f
      arm recoil in, 37
      breast tissue in, 35, 36f
      cartilaginous development in, 35-36,
         36f
      external ear in, 35-36, 36f
      female genitalia in, 36, 37f
      growth abnormalities in, 37-40, 39f
      hair in, 34, 36f
      heel-to-ear maneuver in, 37, 38f
      knee flexion in, 37, 38f
      male genitalia in, 36
      neuromuscular maturity in, 37, 37f, 38f
      physical maturity in, 33-36, 35f-37f
      posture in, 37, 37f
      scarf sign in, 37, 38f
      skin in, 33-34, 36f
      sole creases in, 34-35, 36f
      square-window test in, 37, 37f
   large for, 37, 39-40, 39f
   small for, 37, 39f
Gestations, multiple
   placental evaluation in, 41, 41f
   size discordance in, 39, 39f
Gianotti-Crosti syndrome, 453-454, 455f
Giant nevomelanocytic nevus, 329, 330f
Giant papillary conjunctivitis, 113, 114f
Gigantism, 39, 85, 354
Gingiva
   abscess of, 769, 769f, 770f
   fibromatosis of, 762
   pericoronitis of, 757, 769-770, 771f
Gingival crevice, 755
Gingival cyst, in newborn, 760, 760f
Gingival hyperplasia, 761-762
   from cyclosporine, 762
   idiopathic, 762
   in leukemia, 433, 435f
   from phenytoin, 762, 762f

Gingivitis
   acute necrotizing ulcerative, 770, 771f
   in puberty, 758, 758f
Gingivostomatitis, herpetic, 451, 452f,
      767-768, 767f
Glaucoma, 573, 573f, 735-736, 735f, 736f
Glenn procedure, 150, 150f
Glioblastoma, 583, 584f
Glioma
   brainstem, 440-441, 583, 584f
   intranasal, 433, 435f
   optic nerve, 567, 751, 752f
Globe
   anatomy of, 713, 714f
   displacement of, 750, 751f
   injury to, 753, 753f
Glomerulonephritis
   acute, 513
   chronic, 512, 512f, 513
   membranoproliferative, 513
   mesangial proliferative, 513
   poststreptococcal, 512, 512f, 513
   rapidly progressive, 513
Glomerulopathy, membranous, 513
Glomerulosclerosis, focal, 513
Glossitis
   benign migratory, 760-761, 761f
   in vitamin B_{12} deficiency, 410, 412f
Glossopexy, for Pierre-Robin sequence, 887
Glucocorticoids
   excess of, 361-362, 362f, 363f
   synthesis of, 365f
Glucose-6-phosphate dehydrogenase
      deficiency, hemolytic anemia in, 417,
      417f, 417t
Glucosuria, 510
Glue dermatitis, 287, 291f
Glutaric aciduria, 213, 214f
Gluten sensitive enteropathy, 236, 389-390,
      389f, 390f
Glycogen storage disease, kyphosis in, 821,
      823f
Goiter, 356, 357f, 358, 358f, 478t, 660,
      661f
Goldenhar syndrome, 728, 729f, 884-886,
      886f
Gonadal dysgenesis, 365, 367f
   mixed, 560f
Gonadotropin-dependent precocious puberty,
      366-367
Gonadotropins, 354-355, 355f, 369
Gonads, 364-369
Gonococcal infection, disseminated, 706,
      707f
Gonorrhea, 692t, 697t, 705-706, 706f, 707f
   culture for, 680
   skin lesions in, 706, 708f
Goodell sign, 711
Gottron's papules, in juvenile
      dermatomyositis, 263, 264f
Gower maneuver, 588, 589f
Gower sign, 791
Granuloma
   eosinophilic. *See* Langerhans cell
         histiocytosis.
   pyogenic, 327-328, 328f
   of tympanic membrane, 901, 902f
   umbilical, 668
Granuloma annulare, 316, 319f
Granulomatosis, Wegener, 265
Granulomatous disease, chronic, 123, 123f
Grasp
   involuntary, 70, 70f
   voluntary, 71, 71f, 72f
Grasp reflex, 49, 50f
Graves disease, 357, 357f, 478t
Graves speculum, 683, 683f
Great arteries, transposition of, arterial switch
      for, 151, 151f
Great vessels, in congenital heart disease,
      136-138, 137f-139f
Griseofulvin, for tinea, 292, 342
Groin, examination of, 535-536, 535f

Gross motor development, 65-70, 66f-69f, 66t, 69t
  delayed, 70, 70t
  in visual impairment, 91
Growth. *See also* Development.
  abnormal
    in juvenile rheumatoid arthritis, 252-253
    in newborn assessment, 37-40, 39f
    in psychosocial failure to thrive, 233, 233f
  excessive, in newborn, 39-40
  failure of. *See* Failure to thrive.
  normal, 347-351, 348f, 349t, 350f, 351f-352f
Growth arrest lines, in acute lymphoblastic leukemia, 438, 439f
Growth charts, 347, 348f
Growth curve
  in acquired hypothyroidism, 358, 358f
  in constitutional growth delay, 347, 350f, 379f
  in Crohn disease, 392, 394f
  in Down syndrome, 85, 86f
  in failure to thrive, 379f
  in Turner syndrome, 369, 370f
Growth deceleration. *See* Short stature.
Growth delay, constitutional, 347, 350f, 369
Growth hormone
  deficiency of, 236, 353-354, 353f, 354f
  excess of, 354
  regulation of, 353, 354f
Growth restriction, intrauterine, 37-39, 39f
Growth retardation, generalized, 38, 39f
Grunting
  differential diagnosis of, fractures in, 190
  in respiratory distress, 50, 51f
Gunstock deformity, 786, 786f
Guttate psoriasis, 277, 278f
Gymnastics, injury prevention in, 858t
Gynecologic anatomic terminology, 221t
Gynecologic examination
  of adolescent or pubertal patient, 220f, 681-685, 681t, 682t, 683f-684f
    equipment for, 683, 683f
    history in, 681, 682t, 683
    indications for, 681, 681t, 682t
    technique in, 683-685, 683f
  in evaluation for sexual abuse, 217-220, 217f-222f
  in evaluation for sexually transmitted disease, 700-701
  of prepubertal patient, 676, 678-681, 678f-679f
    labial adhesions and, 685, 686f
    laboratory studies in, 680, 681t
    patient positions for, 217-218, 218f, 219f
Gynecomastia, 15f, 665, 665f

H
Haab striae, in glaucoma, 735, 736f
Haemophilus influenzae, buccal cellulitis in, 473, 473f
Hair
  disorders of, 337-343
  fungal infection of, 341-342, 343f
  loss of. *See* Alopecia.
  structural defects of, 342-343, 344f
Hair collar sign, in aplasia cutis congenita, 341, 342f
Hair follicles, superficial infection of, 465, 465f
Hair pulling, 340, 341f
Hairy patch, in occult spinal dysraphism, 579, 579f
Halo nevus, 331, 331f
Hamartoma, in tuberous sclerosis, 570, 572f
Hamartomatous nevus, 332, 333f
Hamartomatous polyps, 645, 646f
Hamstring stretch, 861f

Hand
  claw
    in Charcot-Marie-Tooth disease, 590f, 591
    in Hurler syndrome, 26, 27f
    in newborn, 44, 45f
  congenital anomalies of, 45-46, 46f
  examination of, 244, 244f, 245f, 786-787, 787f
  flexibility of, in scleroderma, 261, 262f
  fracture of, 188, 190f, 807-809, 808f-809f
  radial club, 826, 826f
Hand-foot-and-mouth disease, coxsackie, 446, 448, 448f
Hand-Schüller-Christian disease, 432
Harlequin eye, in coronal synostosis, 875
Hashimoto thyroiditis, 478t, 660, 661f
Head and neck lesions, 655-656, 657t, 658-663
Head bobbing, 594-595
Head circumference. *See also* Macrocephaly; Microcephaly.
  intrauterine growth restriction and, 38
  in mental retardation, 85
Head control, 66, 67f
Head lice, 310-311, 312f
Head righting, 66-67, 68f
Head trauma
  from child abuse, 190-196, 192f-198f
    clinical picture of, 194-195, 194f-197f
    differential diagnosis of, 211-213, 214f
    morbidity and mortality associated with, 190-191
    neuroimaging of, 195-197, 198f
    pathophysiology and biomechanics of, 191-192
    pathophysiology of shaking and, 192-194, 192f, 193f
  fracture and, 184
  increased intracranial pressure in, 583, 585, 585f
Headache
  allergic sinus (vacuum), 920
  in increased intracranial pressure, 581
  in Rocky Mountain spotted fever, 462
Hearing assessment, 88, 88f
Hearing loss
  in Alport syndrome, 527, 527f
  in cerebral palsy, 84
  conditions associated with, 88-89, 89t
  in congenital cytomegalovirus infection, 498
  disabling effects of, 89t
Heart. *See also* Cardiac.
  abnormal positions of, 134, 134f, 135f
  abnormal shape and size of, 134-136, 135f-136f
Heart block, complete, electrocardiography of, 144, 144f
Heart disease
  congenital, 127-158
    chest radiography in, 133-138, 134f-140f
    echocardiography in, 144-146, 145f, 148f
    electrocardiography in, 138-144, 141f-144f
    heart murmur and, 129, 129f, 129t
    interventional cardiac catheterization in, 153-158, 154f-158f
    laboratory diagnostic aids in, 133-146
    physical diagnosis of, 127-133, 128f-133f, 129t, 130t, 132t
    surgical treatment of, 146, 149-153, 149f-153f
    syndromes associated with, 129-131, 130t, 132t
  failure to thrive in, 236
Heart murmur, 127, 129, 129f, 129t
Heel-to-ear maneuver, 37, 38f
Hegar sign, 711
Height. *See also* Stature.
  growth rate and, 349t
  percentiles for, 348f
  target, estimation of, 347
Heinz body hemolytic anemia, 414-415, 416f
Helicobacter pylori gastritis, 383, 384f

Helmet therapy
  in deformational plagiocephaly, 872
  in sagittal synostosis, 873
Hemangioendothelioma, Kaposiform, 327
Hemangioma, 478t
  congenital
    noninvoluting (NICH), 327, 327f
    rapidly involuting (RICH), 327, 328f
  deep, 324, 325f
  of head and neck, 658, 658f, 659, 659f
  infantile, 322, 324-327, 324f-327f
    natural history of, 324, 324f
    in PHACES syndrome, 325, 325f
    with visceral involvement, 325
  involuting, 324f, 325f
  of larynx or trachea, 607
  lumbosacral, in occult spinal dysraphism, 579, 580f
  mixed, 324-325, 325f
  orbital capillary, 750-751, 751f
  superficial (strawberry), 324, 324f
  ulcerated, 327, 327f
Hemangiomatosis, 325, 325f
Hematocolpos, imperforate hymen and, 686, 686f
Hematogenous cellulitis, 473, 473f, 917-918
Hematologic disease, 403-429
Hematoma
  duodenal, 199, 199f
  epidural, 583, 585, 585f
  eruption, 762, 762f
  oral mucosal, 778f
  perineal, 688, 689f
  septal, 908, 909f
  subdural. *See* Subdural hematoma.
  subgaleal
    in child abuse, 167, 170f
    in newborn, 42
  extracranial, in newborn, 42
  vaginal, 688, 689f
Hematuria, 509, 514-515, 516f
Hemifacial microsomia, 884-886, 886f, 893f
Hemi-Fontan procedure, 150, 150f
Hemihypertrophy, in cancer, 438, 440f
Hemiplegic cerebral palsy, 83, 83f
Hemoglobin
  disorders of, 414-417
  levels of, by age, 404t
Hemoglobin C disease, 417
Hemoglobin SC disease, 417
Hemolytic anemia, 410-418
  acanthocytic (echinocytic), 413, 414f
  Coombs-positive, 411, 413f
  in glucose-6-phosphate dehydrogenase deficiency, 417, 417f, 417t
  Heinz body, 414-415, 416f
  in hemoglobin C disease, 417
  in hemoglobin SC disease, 417
  in hemoglobinopathies, 414-417
  in hereditary elliptocytosis, 412-413, 414f
  in hereditary spherocytosis, 411-412, 413f, 414f
  in malaria, 418, 418f
  microangiopathic, 417-418, 418f, 418t
  morphologic abnormalities in, 412t
  in pyruvate kinase deficiency, 417
  red cell enzymatic defects and, 417, 417f
  in sickle cell disease, 415-417, 415f, 416f
  target cells in, 413-414, 415f
  unstable hemoglobin variants and, 414-415, 416f
Hemolytic uremic syndrome, 418, 645
Hemophagocytic lymphohistiocytosis, 429
Hemophilia, 202, 203f, 425-426, 426f, 427f
Hemorrhage. *See also* Bleeding.
  adrenal, 200, 200f
  in bacterial endocarditis, 132, 133f
  extracranial, in newborn, 42
  intracranial, spontaneous, 583, 585f
  retinal. *See* Retinal hemorrhage.
  subconjunctival, 733-734, 733f
  subungual, 345, 345f
  vitreous, 740-741, 741f
Hemorrhagic conjunctivitis, 733-734, 733f

Hemorrhagic varicella, 445, 447f
Hemorrhoids, 674
Hemosiderosis, pulmonary, 603-604, 604f
Hemostasis, acquired disorders of, 427
Hemotympanum, 894, 895f
Henna dermatitis, 287-288, 291f
Henoch-Schönlein purpura, 203-204, 265-266, 304-307, 513-514, 645
  arthritis in, 266, 267f
  edema in, 266, 267f
  gastrointestinal symptoms in, 266, 534, 646f
  renal disorders in, 266, 305
  skin lesions in, 266, 266f, 267f, 305, 306f, 513, 514f
Hepatic fibrosis, congenital, 401, 401f
Hepatitis, autoimmune, 400
Hepatoblastoma, 437, 654, 656f
Hepatocellular carcinoma, 437
Hepatosplenomegaly, 436f, 437
Herald patch, in pityriasis rosea, 287, 289f
Hereditary hemorrhagic telangiectasia, 910-911, 911f
Hereditary motor-sensory neuropathy type I, 590-591, 590f
Hermaphrodism, true, 560f
Hernia
  Bochdalek, 625
  congenital diaphragmatic, 625-626, 628f
  femoral, 670, 670f
  inguinal, 668-669, 669f
  intestinal obstruction from, 641
  involving abdominal wall, 667f
  Morgagni, 625, 626, 628f
  paraduodenal (paracolic), 641
  umbilical, 667-668, 668f
Herpangina, 448, 448f
Herpes labialis, 453, 453f
Herpes simplex virus (HSV), 451-453, 476t
  culture for, 680
  genital, 224, 692t, 697t, 703, 704f
  gingivostomatitis from, 451, 452f, 767-768, 767f
  keratitis in, 734-735, 735f
  neonatal, 498-499, 499f
  ocular, 452, 452f
  in patients with eczema, 452, 453f
  periocular lesions in, 728, 730, 730f
  primary, 451-452, 452f
  recurrent, 452-453, 453f
  retinochoroiditis in, 745
Herpes zoster, 453, 454f, 768, 768f
Herpetic whitlow, 452, 452f
Hertel exophthalmometer, 750, 751f
Heterochromia, 432, 433f
Heterochromia iridis, 737, 737f
Heterophil antibodies, in mononucleosis, 451
Heterozygous gene locus, 1
Hidradenitis suppurativa, 468-469, 469f
Hinman-Allen syndrome, 547, 547f
Hip
  dislocation of, 812-813, 813f
    in cerebral palsy, 843, 844f
    congenital, 33, 34f, 47, 48f
    developmental, 828-829, 829f
  examination of, 245, 246f, 247f, 787-788, 788f
  fracture-dislocation of, 812, 812f
Hip adductor stretch, 861f
Hip flexor stretch, 861f
Hirschberg corneal light reflex test, 723, 724f
Hirschsprung disease, 385, 387f, 638-639, 639f, 640f
Hirsutism, in mental retardation, 85
Histiocytosis. See Langerhans cell histiocytosis.
HIV/AIDS, 502-506
  clinical manifestations of, 503, 504f-506f
  diagnosis of, 503, 506
  failure to thrive in, 503, 504f
  genital infections in, 697t, 708
  immune abnormalities in, 503, 503t
  nephrotic syndrome in, 514
  treatment of, 506
  vertical transmission of, 502-503

Hives (urticaria), 302-304, 303f
Hodgkin disease, 478t
Holoprosencephaly, 352, 353f
Holt-Oram syndrome, 130, 130t, 131f
Homologues, 1
Homozygous gene locus, 1
Honeybee sting, 96-97, 97f
Hordeolum, 728, 729f
Horner syndrome
  anisocoria in, 749
  heterochromia iridis in, 737, 737f
Hornet sting, 97
Horseshoe kidney, 522, 523f
HOTV visual acuity tests, 714, 715f
HPV. See Human papillomavirus (HPV).
HSV. See Herpes simplex virus (HSV).
Huffman speculum, 683, 683f
Human herpesvirus 6, 449-450, 449f
Human immunodeficiency virus (HIV). See HIV/AIDS.
Human papillomavirus (HPV)
  characteristics of, 697t
  sexual abuse and, 224, 226f
  vaccine for, 685
  vaginal discharge in, 692t
  warts in, 313-314, 314f, 701-702, 701f
Humerus, fracture of, 208, 796f, 803f
Huntington disease, 17
Hurler syndrome, 26, 27f, 422, 423f
Hurler-Scheie syndrome, 26
Hutchinson sign, 345
Hutchinson teeth, in congenital syphilis, 501
Hydranencephaly, 577, 578f
Hydrocele, 556, 556f, 670, 670f
  in newborn, 48, 49f
Hydrocephalus, 575-576, 577f
  benign external, 212-213
Hydrometrocolpos, 559, 559f
Hydronephrosis
  congenital, 649-650
  fetal, 536, 536f
  in megaureter, 539, 540f
  postnatal, 536, 537f
  in ureteropelvic junction obstruction, 539, 540f
1α-Hydroxylase deficiency, 360, 361t
17-Hydroxylase deficiency, 369
21-Hydroxylase deficiency, 363
Hygroma
  cystic, 623, 625f
Hymen
  abnormalities of, from sexual abuse, 221, 222f
  development of, 675, 675f, 676f, 677f
  examination of, 218, 219f
  imperforate, 655, 657f, 685-687, 686f
  normal anatomic variations in, 228-229, 228f, 677f
Hymenal flaps, 228, 228f
Hymenoptera stings, 308, 308f
Hymenoptera venom, hypersensitivity reactions to, 94-97, 97f
Hyper IgE syndrome, 122-123, 122f, 123f, 285-286, 288f
Hyper IgM syndrome, 122
Hyperbilirubinemia
  conjugated
    neonatal, 398-399, 398t, 399f, 400f
    in older child, 399-401, 401f
  unconjugated
    neonatal, 398
    in older child, 399, 400t
Hypercalcemia, 359
Hypercalciuria, 515-516
Hyperdontia, 763, 763f
Hyperexplexia, 594
Hyperimmunoglobulin D periodic fever syndrome (HIDS), 272
Hyperinsulinemia, hypoglycemia and, 371-372
Hyperkeratosis, epidermolytic, 280, 281f
Hyperlipoproteinemia, familial type II, 132t
Hyperopia, 716-717, 716f, 717f

Hyperparathyroidism, 359, 532
Hyperpigmentation
  in acanthosis nigricans, 336, 337f
  differential diagnosis of, 204-205, 204f, 205f
  in epidermal nevus syndrome, 574, 574f
  in incontinentia pigmenti, 322, 323f
  in juvenile dermatomyositis, 263, 263f
  in neurofibromatosis 1, 566, 567f
  postinflammatory, 204, 204f, 332-333, 334f
  in scleroderma, 260f, 262
  in subungual hemorrhage, 345, 345f
Hyperprolactinemia, 355
Hypersensitivity disorders. See also Allergy.
  classification of, 93, 94t
  skin lesions in, 113-115, 114f, 115f
  type I, 93-98, 94f, 95f, 96f
  urticaria as, 303
Hypersensitivity pneumonitis, 111-112
Hypersensitivity reactions
  to drugs, 98, 99f
  to food, 97-98, 97f, 98t
  to hymenoptera venom, 94-97, 97f, 308, 308f
  to insect bites, 309
  to insect stings, versus cellulitis, 473
Hypersensitivity vasculitis, 265
Hypertelorism, 725
Hypertension
  epistaxis in, 911
  hirsutism and, 531
  portal, 644-645, 645f
  pulmonary, left-to-right shunt associated with, 138, 139f
  in renal artery stenosis, 530-531, 531f
  renovascular, 509
  in systemic lupus erythematosus, 257
Hyperthyroidism, 236, 357, 357f
Hypertrophic pyloric stenosis, 635, 635f, 636f
Hypervitaminosis A, 210-211
Hyphema, 316, 753, 753f
Hypocalcemia, 359-360, 360f, 361f, 361t
Hypocalcification of dental enamel, 764, 764f, 765f
Hypodontia, 763, 764f
Hypogammaglobulinemia
  congenital, 117, 117f
  transient, of infancy, 117, 118f
Hypoglycemia, 371-372
  in Beckwith-Wiedemann syndrome, 372, 372f
  fasting, 371f, 371t
  hyperinsulinemia and, 371-372
  ketotic, 372
  postprandial, 371t
Hypogonadism, 369
Hypoparathyroidism, 359
Hypophosphatasia, 360
Hypophosphatemia, 360, 361t
Hypophosphatemic rickets, 527, 528f
Hypopigmentation
  in albinism, 335
  in ash-leaf spots, 334, 336f
  in piebaldism, 335-336, 336f
  postinflammatory, 332-333, 334f
  in scleroderma, 260f, 262
  in vitiligo, 334, 336f
Hypopituitarism, 236
  central nervous system abnormalities and, 351-352, 353f
  growth hormone for, 353-354
  midline defects and, 353, 353f
Hypoplasia of dental enamel, 764, 764f
Hypoplastic left heart syndrome, 149, 149f
Hypospadias, 8f, 547, 548f
  cryptorchidism with, 537, 538f
  in Smith-Lemli-Opitz syndrome, 25, 25f
Hypothalamic hypogonadism, 369
Hypothalamic tumors, 583, 584f
Hypothalamus, 351-356
Hypothyroidism, 357-359
  acquired, 358-359, 358f
  congenital, 236, 357-358, 357f
Hypotonic cerebral palsy, 84

Hypotonic infant, 592, 592f, 592t
Hypoxic/ischemic injury
  in inflicted head injury, 194
  in shaken baby syndrome, 195, 198f
Hypsarrhythmia, 594, 594f

I

Ice hockey, injury prevention in, 858t
Ichthyosis
  collodion baby and, 280, 320, 321f
  epidermolytic hyperkeratosis form of, 280,
    281f
  lamellar, 280, 280f
  X-linked, 279, 280f
Ichthyosis vulgaris, 279, 279f
Icterus. *See* Jaundice.
Immersion burns, in child abuse, 175, 178,
  178f, 178t
Immotile cilia syndrome, 124-125, 125f
Immune globulin, intravenous, for Stevens-
  Johnson syndrome and toxic epidermal
  necrolysis, 301
Immune system, development of, 115-116, 116f
Immunodeficiency
  in AIDS, 503, 503t
  in ataxia-telangiectasia, 574
  categories of, frequencies of, 116f
  cellular, 118-119, 119f
  combined
    partial, 122-123, 122f, 123f
    severe, 119-122, 120t, 121f
  common variable, 118
  complement system, 124
  humoral, 117-118, 117f, 118f
  laboratory screening tests for, 117, 117t
  mucosal barrier–related, 124-125, 125f
  phagocytic, 123-124, 123f, 124f
  primary
    classification of, 120t
    presentation of, 116-117, 116f, 117f
  warning signals of, 117f
Immunoglobulin(s), serum, ontogeny of, 118f
Immunoglobulin A deficiency, selective, 118
Immunoglobulin E
  excess of, 122-123, 122f, 123f
  in type I hypersensitivity disorders, 93, 94f
Immunoglobulin G subclass deficiency, 118
Immunoglobulin M, excess of, 122
Immunotherapy, for hymenoptera sensitivity,
  95-96
Impact forces, head injuries caused by, 191, 192
Imperforate anus, 8f, 521, 522f, 670-671, 671f-
  673f, 673
  ambiguous genitalia and, 559, 560f
Imperforate hymen, 655, 657f, 685-687, 686f
Impetigo, 207, 298, 465-466, 465f, 466f
  breastfeeding and, 60, 60f
  bullous, 207, 465, 466f
  vulvar, 698
Imprinting, disorders of, 18-20, 18f, 19f
Inborn errors of metabolism. *See* Metabolic
  disorders.
Incontinentia pigmenti, 322, 323f, 574-575
Infant. *See also* Newborn.
  acute hematogenous osteomyelitis in, 483,
    483f
  cough in, 599-602, 600f-602f
  of diabetic mother, 39, 39f
  gastroesophageal reflux in, 385
  gastrointestinal bleeding in, 642-643, 643f,
    643t, 644f
  head injury vulnerability of, 191
  Henoch-Schönlein purpura in, 267f
  hydrocephalus in, 576, 577f
  hypotonic, 592, 592f, 592t
  jaundice in, 398-399, 398t, 399f, 400f
  post-term, skin in, 34, 36f
  premature
    breastfeeding of, 61-63, 61f, 62f
    retinopathy in, 743, 744f
    skin assessment in, 34, 36f

Infant *(Continued)*
  sudden death of, 161, 616
  visual acuity of, 73
  vomiting in, 634-639
Infantile acropustulosis, 301-302, 302f
Infantile esotropia, 719, 719f
Infantile hemangioma, 322, 324-327,
  324f-327f
  natural history of, 324, 324f
  in PHACES syndrome, 325, 325f
  with visceral involvement, 325
Infantile perianal pyramidal protrusion, 231,
  232f
Infantile scabies, 309, 311f
Infantile spasm, 594, 594f
Infection, 443-506. *See also specific sites and
  types.*
  bacterial
    of bone and joint, 482-491, 483f-490f
    exanthematous, 454-463, 456f-463f
    of oral cavity, 769-770, 769f-771f
    of skin and soft tissue, 298, 299f, 464-
      475, 465f-474f
  congenital, 496-506, 497f-506f, 599-601
  dermatophyte, 291-294. *See also* Tinea.
  exanthematous, 443-463
  fungal
    of nail, 344, 344f
    of oral cavity, 770, 771f
    of scalp, 341-342, 343f
    of skin, 291-297
  perinatal, 496-506, 497f-506f
  tuberculous. *See* Tuberculosis.
  viral
    exanthematous, 443-454, 444f-455f
    of oral cavity, 767-769, 767f-768f
    of skin, 298, 298f
  yeast, breastfeeding and, 59-60, 60f
Infestation
  lice, 310-311, 312f, 701
  scabies, 309-310, 310f-312f, 701
Infiltration, skin, 313-316
Inflammation
  chronic, microcytic anemia and, 408-409
  pigmentation disorders after, 204, 204f,
    332-333, 334f
Inflammatory abdominal mass, 655, 657f
Inflammatory bowel disease, 392, 394f-397f,
  711t
Inflammatory pseudocyst, 655
Inguinal disorders, 668-670, 669f-671f
Inguinal hernia, 668-669, 669f
Inguinal lymph nodes, 477, 477f, 479f
Inguinal lymphadenopathy, in syphilis, 702,
  702f
Injury. *See* Trauma.
Injury patterns, in child abuse, 167-200
Insect bites and stings, 307-309, 307f-309f
  hypersensitivity reactions to, 94-97, 97f, 473
  papular urticaria from, 204, 207, 207f, 308-
    309, 309f
  treatment principles for, 309
  urticaria pigmentosa and, 316
  vesiculation after, 205-206, 206f, 302, 302f
Insulin resistance, 372, 373f
Intelligence quotient (IQ), 76
Intercondylar fracture, 799t, 800f
Interdental papillae, 755
Interdental septae, 755
Interphalangeal joint
  dislocation of, 814, 814f
  of foot, 247
  proximal, 244, 245f
Intersex anomalies, 537, 538f, 559. *See also*
  Genitalia, ambiguous.
Interstitial pneumonitis, 602, 602f
Intervertebral disc, herniated, 822, 824-825,
  824f
Intestinal. *See also* Gastrointestinal *entries.*
Intestinal atresia, 637-638, 638f, 666, 667f
Intestinal diversion, 541, 543f
Intestinal malrotation, 388, 389f, 635, 635f,
  637, 637f

Intestinal obstruction, 398, 398f, 632,
  634-641
Intestinal pseudo-obstruction, 645, 645f
Intoeing, 791, 836, 836f
Intra-atrial baffle, for transposition of the
  great arteries, 150-151, 151f
Intracranial hemorrhage, spontaneous, 583,
  585f
Intracranial mass, 582-583, 583f
Intracranial pressure, increased, 581-586
  in brain abscess, 583, 584f
  causes of, 582-586, 582f-586f
  in central nervous system tumors, 431-432,
    432f, 583, 583f
  double vision in, 581
  papilledema in, 582, 582f
  signs and symptoms of, 581-582, 582f
Intracranial tumors, 440, 583, 583f
Intraocular pressure, increased, in glaucoma,
  736
Intraoral mass, 433, 434f
Intraoral rhabdomyosarcoma, 433, 434f
Intraperitoneal air, free, 643, 643f
Intraspinal lesions, in occult spinal
  dysraphism, 579, 580f
Intrathoracic injuries, 200, 201f, 213
Intrauterine growth restriction, 37-39, 39f
Intravaginal ridges, 228-229, 228f
Introital polyps, 557, 558f
Intron, 20
Intussusception, 383, 385, 386f, 639-641,
  640f, 641f
Inverse pityriasis, 287
Inversion, chromosome, 3, 3f
Iris
  abnormalities of, 736-738, 737f, 738f
  absence of, 736-737, 737f
  coloboma of, 736, 737f
  Lisch nodules of, 737
  pigmented hamartomas of, in
    neurofibromatosis 1, 566, 568f
Iritis, 737, 737f, 740, 740f, 753
Iron deficiency anemia, 405-406, 405f, 406f
  lead poisoning and, 407
Irritability
  differential diagnosis of, fractures in, 190
  in roseola infantum, 449
Irritable bowel syndrome, 383, 711t
Isomerism, atrial, 134, 135f
Isotretinoin, for acne, 313
Isthmic spondylolisthesis, 821, 823f
Itraconazole, for tinea capitis, 342
Ivermectin, for scabies, 310
Ixodes tick, 461

J

Jaccoud arthropathy, in systemic lupus
  erythematosus, 257
Jackson-Weiss syndrome, 881
Jadassohn nevus sebaceus, 332, 333f, 574,
  574f
Janeway lesions, in bacterial endocarditis,
  132, 133f
Jantene procedure, for transposition of the
  great arteries, 151, 151f
Jargon, 77
Jatene procedure, for transposition of the
  great arteries, 151, 151f
Jaundice
  in infant, 398-399, 398t, 399f, 400f
  in older child, 399-401, 400t, 401f
  physiologic, 398
Jaw, Burkitt lymphoma of, 433, 434f
Jaw-winking, 726, 728f
Jejunoileal atresia, 637-638, 638f
Jeune syndrome, 529, 529f
Job syndrome, 285-286, 288f
Joint(s)
  dislocation of, 812-814, 812f-814f
  hypermobility of, in Ehlers-Danlos
    syndrome, 23f, 24

Joint(s) (*Continued*)
  infection of, 488-491, 489t, 490f. *See also* Septic arthritis.
  pain in, 241. *See also* Arthritis.
  physical examination of, 241-247, 242f-247f, 242t, 243t, 784
Junctional epidermolysis bullosa, 321, 321f
Junctional nevus, 331, 331f
Juvenile rheumatoid arthritis (JRA). *See* Rheumatoid arthritis, juvenile.

K
Kallman syndrome, 369
Kaposi sarcoma, in AIDS, 503, 506f
Kaposi varicelliform eruption, 452, 453f
Kaposiform hemangioendothelioma, 327
Kartagener syndrome, 124-125, 125f
Karyotype, 1, 2f
Kasabach-Merritt syndrome, 327, 418, 424, 424f, 658
Kawasaki syndrome, 266-270
  coronary artery aneurysm in, 270, 270f
  diagnostic criteria for, 267t
  differential diagnosis of, 270, 271t
  gallbladder dilation in, 270, 270f
  laboratory studies in, 270
  ophthalmologic findings in, 268, 268f
  oral findings in, 268, 268f
  skin findings in, 268, 268f, 269f
  urethral meatus inflammation in, 269, 269f
Kayser-Fleischer rings, 400, 401f
Keloids, 315, 315f
Keratitis
  herpes simplex, 734-735, 735f
  interstitial, in congenital syphilis, 501
Keratoconjunctivitis
  atopic, 113, 113f
  epidemic, 732-733, 733f
  in herpes simplex infection, 452
Keratolytics
  for epidermolytic hyperkeratosis, 280
  for lamellar ichthyosis, 280
Keratopathy, band, in juvenile rheumatoid arthritis, 252, 252f
Keratosis pilaris, in atopic dermatitis, 281, 283f
Kerion, 341, 343f, 470
Kerner-Morrison syndrome, 430
Ketoconazole, for tinea capitis, 342
Ketones, 510
Ketotic hypoglycemia, 372
Kidney. *See also* Renal *entries*.
  horseshoe, 522, 523f
  polycystic. *See* Polycystic kidney disease.
Kleeblattschädel, 873, 873t, 881
Klinefelter syndrome, 13-15, 15f, 369
Klippel-Feil syndrome, 329, 522, 523f, 818, 819f
Klippel-Trénaunay syndrome, 573, 573f
Klumpke palsy, in newborn, 44, 45f
Knee
  examination of, 245, 247, 247f, 788-790, 789f-790f
  knock, physiologic, 833, 834f
  penetrating injury of, 793, 793f
  sprains of, 815f, 816
Knee-chest position, 218, 218f, 219f
Knock-knee, physiologic, 833, 834f
Koebner phenomenon
  in juvenile rheumatoid arthritis, 250
  in psoriasis, 277, 279f
KOH (potassium hydroxide) preparation
  in bacterial vaginosis, 704
  in candidal vulvovaginitis, 699
  in gynecologic examination, 685
  in tinea capitis, 341, 343f
  in tinea corporis, 292, 293f, 294f
  in tinea diaper dermatitis, 297
  in tinea pedis, 292
  in tinea versicolor, 294, 295f
  in *Trichomonas vaginalis*, 704

Koilonychia, in iron deficiency anemia, 406, 406f
Komoto syndrome, 725, 727f
Konno procedure, 151, 152f, 153
Konno-Rastan procedure, 153, 153f
Koplik spots, 443, 444f
Kwashiorkor, 375, 377f, 378f
Kyphoscoliosis, in Ehlers-Danlos syndrome, 24
Kyphosis, 785, 785f, 821, 822f, 823f

L
Labia
  fused, with enlarged clitoris, 8f
  hypertrophy of, 556, 557f
  separation maneuvers of, 218, 680
Labial adhesions, 229, 229f, 556-557, 557f, 685, 686f, 693
  thickening of, from sexual abuse, 221, 222f
Laceration
  in child abuse, 173, 175f, 176f, 179-180, 181f
  genital, 688, 688f
  orofacial, 772, 772f, 773f
Lachman test, 789-790, 790f
Lacrimal gland, 730-731, 730f-731f
Lactic acidosis, in mitochondrial diseases, 31
Lambdoid suture, 867, 868f
Lambdoid synostosis, 875-876, 877f
Lamellar ichthyosis, 280, 280f
Langerhans cell histiocytosis, 316, 318f
  otorrhea in, 433, 434f
  skin lesions in, 430-431, 431f
Language development
  delay or disturbance in, 78-79, 88-89, 88f, 89f
    physical examination in, 88-89, 88f
    prognosis in, 89
  early skills in, 76-77, 77f
  specific disabilities in, 88, 89
  in visual impairment, 91-92
Lanugo, 34, 36f
Lap belt fracture, 810-811, 810f
Laparoscopy, in Meckel diverticulum, 644, 645f
Large for gestational age (LGA), 37, 39-40, 39f
Laryngeal cleft, 601
Laryngeal examination, 931-932, 933f
Laryngeal hemangioma, 607
Laryngeal lesions, respiratory distress in, 623
Laryngeal papillomatosis, 607, 608f, 934, 935f
Laryngeal web, 601, 607, 608f
Laryngocele, 478t
Laryngomalacia, 607, 607f, 932-933, 934f, 935f
Laryngoscopy, 931-932, 933f
Laryngotracheobronchitis, 606-607, 607f, 929-930, 929f, 930t
Lasix renal scan, in ureteropelvic junction obstruction, 539, 540f
Lateral condylar fracture, 801f, 806
Lead poisoning, microcytic anemia from, 406-408, 407f
Learning problems, self image and, 81
Lecithin-cholesterol acyltransferase deficiency, target cells in, 414
LeFort fractures, 777-778, 777f, 778f
Leg
  bowed
    physiologic, 832-833, 833f
    in rickets, 359, 361f
  stork, in Charcot-Marie-Tooth disease, 590, 590f
Leg length
  inequality of, gait disturbances from, 790-791
  measurement of, 247, 248f, 787-788, 788f
Legg-Calvé-Perthes disease, 830, 830f
Length, intrauterine growth restriction and, 38

Lens of eye
  abnormalities of, 738-740, 738f-740f, 738t, 739t
  dislocation of, 740, 740f
  opacification of. *See* Cataract.
  subluxation of, 740
Lenticular myopia, in diabetes mellitus, 746
Leptomeningeal angiomatosis, in Sturge-Weber syndrome, 573
Letter charts, 715
Leukemia, 418, 420f, 478t
  acute lymphoblastic, 420f, 428-429, 438, 439f
  acute myelogenous, 420f
  acute myeloid, 429
  chronic myelogenous, 438
  gingival hyperplasia in, 433, 435f
  leukemic lines in, 211, 212f
  musculoskeletal system in, 438, 439f
  pancytopenia in, 428-429
Leukemoid reaction, 418, 419, 420f, 421
Leukocoria
  differential diagnosis of, 738, 738t. *See also* Cataract.
  in retinoblastoma, 432, 432f
Leukocyte(s)
  casts of, in glomerulonephritis, 512, 512f, 513
  counts of, 403, 419, 420t
  morphologic abnormalities of, 421, 421f
Leukocyte adhesion deficiency, 123-124, 124f
Leukocyte alkaline phosphatase level (LAP) score, 419
Leukocyte esterase test, 510
Leukocytoclastic vasculitis, 265
Leukoerythroblastosis, 419, 421f
Leukorrhea, physiologic, 676, 678f, 691, 692t
Levocardia, 134, 134f
Leydig cell hypoplasia, 365
Libman-Sacks endocarditis, in systemic lupus erythematosus, 255-256
Lice, 310-311, 312f, 701
Lichen planus, 297, 297f
Lichen sclerosus, 230, 230f, 695-696, 696f
Lichen striatus, 297-298, 298f
Lichenoid papules, in Gianotti-Crosti syndrome, 454, 455f
Lidocaine, topical, in gynecologic examination of prepubertal patient, 680
Ligamentous injuries
  dislocations as, 812-814, 812f-814f
  sprains as, 814-816, 815f, 815t
  subluxations as, 816-817, 816f, 817f
Ligamentous laxity, extremity pain with, 817-818, 817f
Limb-girdle muscular dystrophy, 588t
Linear scleroderma, 259, 260f
Linear sebaceous nevus of Jadassohn, 574, 574f
Lingual thyroid gland, 659
Lip
  cleft, 49, 49f, 868-870, 868t, 869f
  cracked, in Kawasaki syndrome, 268, 268f
  laceration of, 772, 773f
  traumatic ulceration of, 773, 773f
Lipid-laden macrophage test, 618, 619f
Lip-licking eczema, 285, 285f
Lipoma
  intraspinal, in occult spinal dysraphism, 579, 580f
  subcutaneous, in occult spinal dysraphism, 579, 579f
Lisch nodules, 566, 568f, 737
Lissencephaly, 6t
Lithotomy position, 218, 679f
Livedo reticularis, in systemic lupus erythematosus, 255
Liver
  cancer of, 437
  congenital fibrosis of, 401, 401f
  injury to, in child abuse, 199

Liver disease
   in cystic fibrosis, 398
   hyperbilirubinemia in, 399-401, 401f
   target cells in, 414
   tooth discoloration in, 765, 765f
   xanthomas in, 399, 400f
Lobar emphysema, 610, 612f, 629, 629f, 630f
Locomotion, development of, 67, 69-70, 69f, 69t
Logical thinking, development of, 75, 75f
Long bone fracture, 184, 186-187, 186f-189f
Loop ureterostomy, 541, 542f
Lop ear, 896f
Lower extremity
   examination of, 787-791, 788f-790f, 792f
   musculoskeletal disorders of, 828-843,
      829f-843f
Lumbar stretch, 861f
Lumbosacral hemangioma, in occult spinal
      dysraphism, 579, 580f
Lung. *See also* Pulmonary *entries;* Respiratory
      entries.
Lung bud anomalies, 627-630, 629f, 630f
Lung volume, measurement of, 618, 620-621,
      620f, 621f
Lupus anticoagulant (LAC), 427, 428
Lupus erythematosus
   discoid, 258
   neonatal, 258, 258f
   subacute cutaneous, 258
   systemic. *See* Systemic lupus erythematosus.
Lupus-like reaction, drug-induced, 258
Luteinizing hormone (LH), 354-355, 355f
Lyme arthritis, 253, 254f, 462
Lyme disease, 461-462, 461f
Lymph node(s)
   axillary and epitrochlear, 477, 481f
   cervical, 475, 476f, 477
   femoral, 477
   inguinal, 477, 477f, 479f
   superficial regional, 475, 477
Lymph node regions, 433-434, 435f
Lymphadenitis
   actinomycotic, 478t
   acute suppurative, 477, 479, 479f
   associated with animal or vector contact,
      480-482, 481f
   diagnosis of, 482
   versus lymphadenopathy, 475
   mycobacterial, 479-480, 480f
   in PFAPA syndrome, 272
   tuberculous, 479-480, 480f, 495
Lymphadenopathy, 433-434, 435f
   versus adenitis, 475
   cervical, 475, 476f, 477, 477f
      benign reactive, 661, 661f, 662f
      diagnostic approach to, 482
      differential diagnosis of, 478t, 661-662,
         662f
      infectious causes of, 475, 476t
      in mononucleosis, 450
   inguinal, in syphilis, 702, 702f
   reactive, 475
Lymphangioma, 478t, 623, 625f, 659, 659f
Lymphangitis, 470-471, 470f
Lymphoblast(s), 420f
Lymphoblastic leukemia, acute, 420f, 428-
   429, 438, 439f
Lymphocyte(s)
   atypical, 421, 421f
   normal values for, 419t
Lymphocytic interstitial pneumonitis, 602,
   602f
Lymphocytosis, 419f, 451
Lymphohistiocytosis, hemophagocytic, 429
Lymphoid interstitial pneumonitis, in AIDS,
   503, 505f, 506f
Lymphoma
   Burkitt, 433, 434f
   Hodgkin's, 478t
   non-Hodgkin's, 478t, 654, 662, 662f
      of abdomen, 437, 437f
      pleural effusion in, 436, 436f
   of tonsil, 924, 925f

Lymphopenia, in severe combined
      immunodeficiency, 121, 121f
Lymphoproliferative disorder, post-transplant,
   441
Lysosomal storage diseases, 25-26, 26t

M

Macrocephaly, 575-577, 575t, 576f-578f
Macrodont, 763, 764f
Macroglossia, 7f
Macro-orchidism, in fragile X syndrome, 17,
   17f
Macrophage activation syndrome, in
      systemic-onset juvenile rheumatoid
      arthritis, 251, 251f, 251t
Macula
   anatomy of, 713, 714f
   cherry red spot in, 746, 746f, 747, 747f
Magnetic resonance imaging (MRI)
   in head trauma, 196, 198f
   in juvenile dermatomyositis, 264-265,
      265f
   in neurofibromatosis 1, 567, 569f
   in tuberous sclerosis, 570, 572f
   of vascular ring, 627, 628f
Malabsorption
   carbohydrate, 388
   in celiac disease, 389-390, 389f, 390f
   fat, 377, 380-381
      growth failure and, 235-236
   protein, 377
Malar rash, in systemic lupus erythematosus,
   254-255, 254f, 255f
Malaria, hemolytic anemia in, 418, 418f
Malathion, for pediculosis, 311
Malformation. *See* Congenital
   malformation(s).
Malignancy. *See* Cancer; Leukemia; Tumor(s).
Mallet finger, 828, 828f
Malnutrition. *See* Failure to thrive.
Malrotation, 388, 389f, 635, 635f, 637, 637f
Malt-worker's lung, 111
Mandible
   fractures of, 776-777, 776f
   hypoplasia of
      in Nager syndrome, 884
      in Pierre-Robin sequence, 886
Mandibulofacial dysostosis, 882-883, 882f
Mantoux test, 491, 491f, 495, 495t
Marasmus, 375, 376f
Marcus Gunn jaw, 726, 728f
Marcus Gunn pupil, 748, 748f
Marfan syndrome, 21, 22f, 130, 130t, 131f
Marie-Foix maneuver, 83f
Marshall syndrome, 272, 768-769
Mass(es). *See also* Tumor(s).
   abdominal, 436-437, 436f-437f, 649-655.
      See also Abdominal mass.
   adrenal, 651
   cervical, 623, 625f
   chest wall, 434, 435f
   intracranial, 582-583, 583f
   intraoral, 433, 434f
   mediastinal, 623-625, 625t, 626f, 627f
   nasal, 433, 435f, 904, 904f
   neck
      lateral, 661-663, 661f-664f
      midline, 659-661, 660f-661f
   ovarian, 655
   paravertebral, 434, 435f
   pharyngeal, 623, 625f
   testicular, 438, 438f
   tympanic membrane, 901, 902f
MASS phenotype, 21
Mastitis
   breastfeeding and, 60, 60f
   in infant, 665
Mastocytoma, 315, 316f
Mastocytosis, cutaneous, 315-316, 316f,
   317f
Mastoiditis, 893-894, 894f

Maternal age
   Down syndrome and, 10, 10t
   Klinefelter syndrome and, 14-15
Maternal blood, swallowed, 642
Maxilla
   fractures of, 777-778, 777f, 778f
   hyperplasia of
      in sickle cell disease, 415-416, 416f
      in thalassemia major, 408, 408f
Maxillary sinus, 911, 912f
Maximum oxygen uptake (VO_{2max}), 857
May-Hegglin anomaly, 422, 422f
McCune-Albright syndrome
   café-au-lait spots in, 337, 338f, 566
   precocious puberty in, 367, 368f
Measles
   German. *See* Rubella.
   nine-day or red, 443, 444f
Meatal bridges, 549, 550f
Meatal stenosis, 549, 549f
Meckel diverticulum, 643-644, 644f, 645f
Meckel scan, 644, 644f
Meconium
   aspiration of, 52, 52f
   failure to pass, 52-53
   passage of, 52, 53f, 671, 672f
   staining from, 43, 43f
Meconium ileus, 392, 397f, 634, 634f, 638,
   639f
   in cystic fibrosis, 612-613, 613f
Meconium peritonitis, 634, 634f, 638, 639f
Median raphe cyst, 552, 552f
Mediastinal crunch, in asthma, 108
Mediastinal mass, 623-625, 625t, 626f, 627f
Mediastinal tumor, 434, 435f, 436, 436f
Medullary cystic disease, 526
Medullary sclerosis, 181, 182f
Medulloblastoma, 440
Megakaryocytes, 424, 425f
Megaureter, 539, 540f
Melanoma, 331-332, 331f, 431, 431f. *See also*
   Nevomelanocytic nevus.
   differential diagnosis of, 332, 332f
   nevus and, 331-332, 331f
Melanosis, transient neonatal pustular, 318,
   320f
Melanotic neuroectodermal tumor of infancy,
   760, 761f
Melanotic spots of Peutz-Jeghers syndrome,
   645, 646f
MELAS syndrome, 31, 32f
Membranoproliferative glomerulonephritis,
   513
Meningismus, 459, 459f
Meningitis
   aseptic, in Lyme disease, 462
   bacterial, 585, 585f
   meningococcal, 459, 459f
   in tuberculosis, 494
Meningocele, 844
Meningococcal meningitis, 459, 459f
Meningococcemia
   acute, 459-460, 460f
   chronic, 460-461
Meningoencephalitis, in mumps, 464
Meningomyelocele, 8f
Menkes' kinky hair syndrome, 210
Mental illness, child abuse and, 164t
Mental retardation, 84-87, 86f
   in cerebral palsy, 84
   cranial abnormalities in, 85
   facial abnormalities in, 85, 87f
   growth pattern in, 85, 86f
   physical examination in, 85, 87
   prognosis in, 87
   skin findings in, 85
Mentzer index, 406
MERRF syndrome, 31
Mesangial proliferative glomerulonephritis,
   513
Mesenteric tears, in child abuse, 199,
   200f
Mesoblastic nephroma, 650

Metabolic disorders
  genetic, 24-26, 25f, 26t
  kyphosis in, 821, 823f
  retinopathy in, 746-747, 747f
Metabolic syndrome, 372
Metacarpal fracture, 809, 809f
Metacarpophalangeal joint, 244, 245f
Metaphyseal flaring, in rickets, 359, 361f
Metaphyseal fracture, 22f, 23f, 182-183, 182f, 183f, 799f, 799t
Metaphyseal lucencies, in acute lymphoblastic leukemia, 438, 439f
Metatarsal fracture, 809-810, 810f
Metatarsophalangeal joint, 247
Metatarsus varus (adductus), 838-839, 839f, 840f
Methylene tetrahydrofolate reductase (MTHFR) gene mutation, 428
Metopic suture, 867, 868f
Metopic synostosis, 875, 876f
Metronidazole, for *Trichomonas vaginalis,* 704
Microangiopathic hemolytic anemia, 417-418, 418f, 418t
Microcephaly, 577-578, 579t
Microcornea, 734, 734f
Microdont, 763, 764f
Micrognathia, in juvenile rheumatoid arthritis, 242, 243f
Micropenis (microphallus), 550, 550f
Microphthalmia, 738-739
Microretrognathia, 7f
Midarm circumference, 379f
Midfacial anomalies, 882-886, 882f-885f
Midfacial fracture, 777-778, 777f, 778f
Midgut volvulus, 637, 637f
Midline defects, 46-47, 47f
  hypopituitarism and, 353, 353f
  and occult spinal dysraphism, 578-581, 579f-581f
  perineal, 231, 232f
Midline hand play, 71, 71f
Midline neck mass, 659-661, 660f-661f
Milia, 314-315, 315f, 322f
Miliaria crystallina, 301, 301f
Miliaria rubra, 301, 301f
Miliary tuberculosis, 493-494, 494f
Milk
  breast, bioactive substances in, 54. *See also* Breastfeeding.
  cow's
    bioactive substances in, 377t
    iron deficiency anemia from, 405
Milk allergy, 97, 98t
Milk protein enterocolitis, 98
"Milk" scan, 617, 619f, 635
Miller-Dieker phenotype, with lissencephaly, 6t
Mineralocorticoids, synthesis of, 365f
Minimal change disease, 513, 514, 514f, 515f
Minoxidil, hirsutism from, 531
Missense mutation, 20
Mist therapy, for croup, 929
Mitochondrial DNA mutations, 30-31, 31t
Mitosis, 1, 2f
Mitral stenosis, cardiac catheterization for, 154
Mixed connective tissue disease, 262, 263t
Molecular cytogenetic syndromes, 15-17
Molluscum contagiosum, 314, 314f
  in AIDS, 503, 505f
  eyelid lesions in, 730
  sexually transmitted, 702
Mongolian spots, 204, 204f, 317, 319f
Monilethrix, 342, 344f
Moniliasis, 770, 771f
Monocytes, normal values for, 419t
Monocytosis, 419f
Mononucleosis, 450-451, 476t
  atypical lymphocytes in, 421, 421f
  clinical features of, 450-451, 450f
  diagnosis of, 451
  differential diagnosis of, 451
Monorchism, congenital, 537

Monospot test, 451
Monteggia fracture, 814, 814f
Morbilliform drug eruptions, 304, 305f
Morgagni hernia, 625, 626, 628f
Moro reflex, 49-50, 51f, 65, 66f
Morphea, in scleroderma, 259, 260f
Mosaicism, 2-3, 3f, 333-334, 335f
Motor development
  fine, 70-73, 70f-73f, 91
  gross, 65-70, 66f-69f, 66t, 69t
    delayed, 70, 70t
    in visual impairment, 91
Motor skills, sports-related, 849-850, 850t
Motor-sensory neuropathy, hereditary, 590-591, 590f
Mouth. *See also* Oral *entries.*
  trench, 770, 771f
MRI. *See* Magnetic resonance imaging (MRI).
Mucocele, 762, 762f
Mucocutaneous lymph node syndrome, 267. *See also* Kawasaki syndrome.
Mucolipidoses, ocular findings in, 747
Mucopolysaccharidosis, 26
  cardiac findings in, 132t
  classification of, 26, 26t
  retinopathy in, 746-747
  type I, 26, 27f
Mucosal barrier disorders, 124-125, 125f
Mucosal ulceration, in systemic lupus erythematosus, 255, 256f
Mucous membrane changes, in rheumatic disease, 241, 242t
Mucous patches
  in congenital syphilis, 500
  in syphilis, 702, 703f
Muenke syndrome, 881
Mulberry molars, in congenital syphilis, 501
Mullerian duct, persistent, 366
Multiple endocrine neoplasia (MEN) syndrome
  type 1, hyperparathyroidism in, 359
  type 2A and 2B, pheochromocytoma in, 363-364
Multiple gestations
  placental evaluation in, 41, 41f
  size discordance in, 39, 39f
Multiple malformation syndrome, 7
  Cornelia de Lange syndrome as, 28-29, 29f
  fetal alcohol syndrome as, 30, 30f
  Noonan syndrome as, 29-30
Mumps, 463-464, 463f
Murmur, 127, 129, 129f, 129t
Muscle biopsy, in juvenile dermatomyositis, 265
Muscle enzymes, elevated, in juvenile dermatomyositis, 264
Muscle strength
  evaluation of, 241, 242f, 243t, 587-588
  grading of, 784, 784t
Muscle tone, in cerebral palsy, 82, 82f, 83f
Muscle weakness
  gait disturbances from, 791
  in juvenile dermatomyositis, 263
  in neuromuscular disease, 586
Muscular dystrophy(ies)
  Becker, 588, 588t
  cardiac findings in, 132t
  clinical features of, 588t
  Duchenne, 588-589, 588f-590f, 588t
Muscular hypertrophy, in myotonia congenita, 591, 591f
Muscular pseudohypertrophy, in Duchenne muscular dystrophy, 589, 590f
Muscular ventricular septal defect, 144, 146f
Musculoskeletal disorders
  in cancer, 438-440, 439f-441f
  categories of, 781
  generalized, 843-848, 843f-849f
  history in, 783-784
  of lower extremity, 828-843, 829f-843f
  of neck, 818, 818f, 819f
  physical examination in, 784-791. *See also* Musculoskeletal examination.

Musculoskeletal disorders *(Continued)*
  of spine, 818-825, 820f-824f
  sports-related. *See* Sports injuries.
  traumatic, 791-818. *See also* Fracture(s); Ligamentous injuries; Sports injuries.
  of upper extremity, 825-828, 825f-828f
Musculoskeletal examination, 784-791
  of ankle, 790
  of elbow, 786, 786f
  gait assessment in, 790-791, 792f
  of hip, 787-788, 788f
  of knee, 788-790, 789f-790f
  lower extremity, 787-791, 788f-790f, 792f
  regional, 784-790
  in rheumatic disease, 241-247, 242f-248f, 242t, 243t
  of shoulder, 786
  strength testing in, 241, 242f, 243t, 587-588, 784, 784t
  of thoracolumbar spine, 785-786, 785f, 786f
  of trunk and neck, 784-785
  upper extremity, 784-787, 784f-787f, 787t
  of wrist and hand, 786-787, 787f
Musculoskeletal pain syndromes, idiopathic, 272-273
Musculoskeletal system
  development of, 781-783, 782f, 783f
  examination of. *See* Musculoskeletal examination.
Mustard procedure, for transposition of the great arteries, 150-151, 151f
Mutations
  mitochondrial DNA, 30-31, 31t
  types of, 20-21
Mycobacterial lymphadenitis, 479-480, 480f
Mycobacterial tuberculosis, 662, 662f
Mycoplasma infection, genital, 708
Mycoplasma pneumoniae infection, 604, 605f
Myelogenous leukemia
  acute, 420f
  chronic, 438
Myeloid leukemia, acute, 429
Myelomeningocele, 844, 845f
Myocarditis, in congenital toxoplasmosis, 497
Myofascial pain, 272
Myoglobinuria, bruises and, 171, 175f
Myopia, 716, 716f, 717, 717f
  lenticular, in diabetes mellitus, 746
Myotonia congenita, 591-592, 591f, 592f
Myotonic dystrophy, 17, 588t

N
Nager syndrome, 883-884, 884f
Nail(s)
  disorders of, 343-345, 344f-345f
  dystrophic, 344, 344f
  fungal infection of, 344, 344f
  paronychia of, 343-344, 344f
  plummer, 357
  psoriatic, 345, 345f
  Scotch-plaid pitting of, 337, 345, 345f
  spooning of, in iron deficiency anemia, 406, 406f
  trauma to, 344-345, 344f, 345f
NARES (nonallergic rhinitis with eosinophilia syndrome), 101, 101t
NARP syndrome, 31
Nasal bleeding, 424, 909-911, 909f-911f
Nasal congestion, 903
Nasal crease, in allergic rhinitis, 100, 100f
Nasal deformities, in newborn, 43-44, 44f
Nasal dermoids, 904-905, 905f
Nasal disorders, 903-911
Nasal encephalocele, 904, 904f
Nasal endoscope, 902-903, 903f
Nasal examination, 902-903, 903f
Nasal foreign body, 907, 907f
Nasal fracture, displaced, 908, 908f
Nasal mass, 433, 435f, 904, 904f

Nasal obstruction
    acquired forms of, 905-908, 906f-908f
    in allergic rhinitis, 100, 100f
    congenital causes of, 903-905, 904f-905f
Nasal papilloma, 905, 905f
Nasal polyps, 613, 613f, 907-908, 908f
Nasal trauma, 908-909, 908f, 909f
    after delivery, 43-44, 44f
    from child abuse, 180, 181f
Nasogastric tube, in upper airway obstruction, 623, 624
Nasolacrimal drainage system, 730-731, 730f-731f
Nasolacrimal duct obstruction, 731, 731f
Nasolacrimal sac mucocele, 731, 731f
Nasopharyngeal angiofibroma, juvenile, epistaxis in, 911, 911f
Nasopharyngeal culture, in tonsillopharyngitis, 923
Nasopharyngitis, in gastroesophageal reflux, 903
Near response, 718
Neck
    disorders of, 936-937
    examination of, 245, 245f, 784-785
    masses of
        lateral, 661-663, 661f-664f
        midline, 659-661, 660f-661f
    musculoskeletal disorders of, 818, 818f, 819f
Neck exercises, in deformational plagiocephaly, 872
Necrobiosis lipoidica diabeticorum, 371, 371f
Necrotizing cellulitis, 474-475, 474f
Necrotizing enterocolitis, 643, 643f
Necrotizing fasciitis, 474-475, 474f
Needle aspiration, 661
Neglect, 232-237. *See also* Child abuse.
    failure to thrive from
        differential diagnosis of, 235-237, 238t
        evaluation and management of, 237
        physical findings in, 233-235, 233f-235f
    reporting of, 238-239
    risk factors for, 162-163, 162t-164t, 232-233
Neisseria meningitidis, 459
Neonate. *See* Newborn.
Nephritis, 512-514, 512f. *See also* Glomerulonephritis.
    in Henoch-Schönlein purpura, 305
    hereditary progressive, 527, 527f, 528f
    in systemic lupus erythematosus, 257, 257t
Nephrogenic diabetes insipidus, 356
Nephrolithiasis, 515-517, 515t, 517f
Nephroma, mesoblastic, 650
Nephronophthisis, juvenile, 526
Nephrostomy, 541, 544f
Nephrotic syndrome, 512-514, 512f, 514f, 515f
Neural tube, abnormal closure of, 578-581, 579f-581f. *See also* Midline defects.
Neuroblastoma
    abdominal, 436, 436f, 437
    adrenal, 651, 652f-654f, 653
    cervicothoracic, 432, 433f
    metastatic to orbit, 751, 751f
    paravertebral, 434, 435f
    pelvic, 650f
    pseudorosette formation in, 429f
    raccoon eyes in, 432, 433f
    skin lesions in, 430, 430f, 431f
Neurocranium, 867, 868f
Neurocutaneous abnormality, in mental retardation, 85
Neurocutaneous syndromes, 564, 566-585, 567f-574f
Neurocysticercosis, increased intracranial pressure in, 585-586, 586f
Neurofibroma, 315, 315f, 751
Neurofibromatosis, 430
    café-au-lait spots in, 336-337, 338f
    Lisch nodules in, 737
    with Noonan syndrome, 30
    renal artery stenosis in, 530, 531f, 567-568

Neurofibromatosis *(Continued)*
    type 1, 315, 315f, 564, 566-568, 566t, 567f-569f
    type 2, 568-569, 569t
Neurogenic bladder, 546, 547f
Neurohypophysis, 356, 356f
Neurologic dysfunction
    failure to thrive and, 235
    in occult spinal dysraphism, 579, 581
Neurologic examination, 563-564, 564f-566f
Neurologic soft signs, 90, 90t
Neuromuscular disease, 586-592, 588f-592f
Neuromuscular maturity, in gestational age assessment, 37, 37f, 38f
Neuropathic pain, 272
Neurovesical dysfunction, 546, 547f
Neutrophil(s)
    abnormalities of, 421-422, 421f-423f
    hereditary giant, 421
    in megaloblastic anemia, 409, 410f
    normal values for, 419t
Neutrophilia, 419f
Nevomelanocytic nevus
    acquired, 330-331, 331f
    congenital, 329-330, 330f
    giant, 329, 330f
Nevus
    blue, 332, 332f
    compound, 331, 331f
    halo, 331, 331f
    hamartomatous, 332, 333f
        epidermal, 332, 333f, 574, 574f
    junctional, 331, 331f
    melanoma and, 331-332, 331f
    nevomelanocytic
        acquired, 330-331, 331f
        congenital, 329-330, 330f
        giant, 329, 330f
    Spitz, 332, 332f
Nevus depigmentosus, 334, 336f
Nevus flammeus, 329, 329f
Nevus sebaceus of Jadassohn, 332, 333f, 574, 574f
Nevus simplex, 329, 329f
Nevus spilus, 330, 330f
Newborn. *See also* Infant.
    abdominal mass in, 649-651, 650f-652f
    breast abscess in, 469, 469f
    breastfeeding and, 54-63. *See also* Breastfeeding.
    congenital epulis in, 760, 760f
    conjunctivitis in, 731-732, 732f
    Coombs-positive hemolytic anemia in, 411
    gingival cyst in, 760, 760f
    goiter in, 358, 358f
    heart murmur in, 127
    herpes simplex infection in, 498-499, 499f
    hyperbilirubinemia in, 398-399, 398t, 399f, 400f
    lupus erythematosus in, 258, 258f
    neurologic examination of, 564
    scalp abscess in, 469-470, 470f
    skin disorders in, 317-322, 319f-323f
    tetanus in, 501-502, 502f
    thrombocytopenia in, 424
    transient pustular melanosis in, 318, 320f
    transient tachypnea in, 50, 52f
    vitamin K deficiency in, 427
    vomiting in, 634-639
Newborn assessment, 33-63
    amniotic bands in, 47, 48f
    arm recoil in, 37
    birth trauma and, 42-44, 42f-45f
    breast tissue in, 35, 36f
    cartilaginous development in, 35-36, 36f
    congenital anomalies and, 44-47. *See also* Congenital anomalies.
    congenital hip dislocation in, 33, 34f, 47, 48f
    external ear in, 35-36, 36f
    female genitalia in, 36, 37f
    general techniques for, 33, 34f, 34t
    gestational age in, 33-37, 35f-38f

Newborn assessment *(Continued)*
    growth abnormalities in, 37-40, 39f
    hair in, 34, 36f
    heel-to-ear maneuver in, 37, 38f
    historical database in, 33, 34f, 34t
    knee flexion in, 37, 38f
    lanugo in, 34, 36f
    male genitalia in, 36
    neuromuscular maturity in, 37, 37f, 38f
    oral clefts in, 49, 49f
    physical maturity in, 33-36, 35f-37f
    placenta in, 40-41, 40f, 41f
    posture in, 37, 37f
    primitive reflexes in, 49-50, 49f-51f
    respiratory distress and, 50, 51f, 52, 52f
    scarf sign in, 37, 38f
    scrotal swelling in, 48, 49f
    skin in, 33-34, 36f
        post-term, 34, 36f
        premature, 34, 36f
    sole creases in, 34-35, 36f
    square-window test in, 37, 37f
    stools in, 52-54, 53f
    umbilical hernia in, 47-48, 48f
Newborn screening, for genetic disorders, 31-32
NF1 gene, 566
NF2 gene, 569
NICH lesion (noninvoluting congenital hemangioma), 327, 327f
Nickel dermatitis, 287, 290f
Nikolsky sign, 457
Nipple discharge, 665
Nipple evaluation, pinch test in, 55, 55f
Nipple shield, 55-56, 56f
Nipple trauma, 57, 57f, 59, 59f
Nitrite test, 510
Nodules
    Bohn, 760, 760f
    Lisch, 566, 568f, 737
    pulmonary, 434, 436f
    subcutaneous
        in juvenile rheumatoid arthritis, 251
        in rheumatic fever, 132, 133f
    thyroid, 356, 660, 660f
Non-Hodgkin's lymphoma, 478t, 654, 662, 662f
    of abdomen, 437, 437f
    pleural effusion in, 436, 436f
Nonsense mutation, 20
Nonsteroidal anti-inflammatory drugs (NSAIDs), for erythema nodosum, 302
Noonan syndrome, 29-30
    differential diagnosis of, 30
    physical findings in, 130, 130t, 131f
Norwood procedure, 149, 149f
Nose. *See* Nasal *entries.*
Nuchal rigidity, in meningococcal meningitis, 459, 459f
Nucleic acid amplification tests (NAATs), 680
Null mutation, 21
Nummular eczema, 284, 284f
Nursemaid's elbow, 816-817, 816f, 817f
Nursing. *See* Breastfeeding.
Nursing bottle caries, 235f, 236-237, 767, 767f
Nursing bottle-sucking habits, 758
Nursing system, supplemental, 62-63, 62f
Nutrition
    normal, 375, 376t
    parenteral
        complications of, 381, 382f
        in gastrointestinal tract injury, 378-380, 380f
        indications for, 381
Nutritional deficiencies. *See also* Failure to thrive.
    physical signs of, 380t
    treatment of, 378-381, 380f-383f
Nutritional status assessment, 375-381, 376f-382f
    anthropometric, 378, 379f, 379t, 380f, 380t

Nutritional status assessment *(Continued)*
  in failure to thrive, 378, 379f, 379t, 380f, 380t
  grading in, 379t
Nystatin, for thrush, 59

O

Obesity, 372, 372t, 373f
  in mental retardation, 85
  in Prader-Willi syndrome, 18, 19f
Object permanence, 74, 74f
Object recognition cards, 714, 715f
Obliterative bronchiolitis, 610, 612f
Obstructive sleep apnea, 616, 879
Ocular abnormalities
  in Sturge-Weber syndrome, 573, 573f
  in systemic lupus erythematosus, 257, 257f
Ocular allergy, 112-113, 113f, 114f
Ocular herpes simplex infection, 452, 452f
Ocular trauma, 752-754, 752f-754f
Oculo-auriculo-vertebral spectrum, 884-886, 886f
Oculocutaneous albinism, 335
Oculomotor nerve (CN III) palsy, exotropia in, 722, 722f
Oligodendroglioma, 583, 583f
Oligohydramnios, 41, 41f
Omental cyst, 651, 652f
Omphalitis, 645
Omphalocele, 665-666, 666f, 667, 667f
Omphalomesenteric duct remnants, 641, 642f, 668, 668f
Oncology, 429-441. *See also* Cancer.
Onychomycosis, 344, 344f
Oophoritis, in mumps, 464
Ophthalmia neonatorum, 731-732, 732f
Ophthalmologic examination, 563, 565f, 716-717, 716f, 717f
  in juvenile rheumatoid arthritis, 252, 252f, 252t
Ophthalmologic findings, in Kawasaki syndrome, 268, 268f
Oppenheim technique for checking Babinski reflex, 563, 566f
Oppositional defiant disorder, 90
Opsoclonus-myoclonus syndrome, 430
Optic cup enlargement, 736, 736f
Optic nerve, 747-750
  atrophy of, 750, 750f
  developmental anomalies of, 750, 750f
  disorders of, color vision abnormalities in, 748
  functional assessment of, 748, 748f
  glioma of, 567, 751, 752f
  hypoplasia of, 750, 750f
  inflammation of, 749
  papilledema of, 582, 582f, 749, 749f
  pseudopapilledema of, 717, 717f, 749-750
Optic neuritis, 749
Oral abnormalities, in sexual abuse, 222-223
Oral allergy syndrome, 97
Oral cavity. *See also* Dental; Tooth (teeth).
  burns involving, 772, 773f
  disorders of, 755-779
    developmental, 760-765, 761f-765
    natal and neonatal, 758, 760, 760f-761f
  infections of
    bacterial, 769-770, 769f-771f
    fungal, 770, 771f
    viral, 767-769, 767f-768f
  in newborn, 755-756
Oral examination, 755, 756f
Oral findings, in Kawasaki syndrome, 268, 268f
Oral habits
  craniomandibular dysfunction and, 779
  harmful, 758, 759f
Oral history, 755
Oral injuries, in child abuse, 179-180, 181f
  differential diagnosis of, 213
Oral mucosa, laceration of, 772, 772f

Oral structures, normal, 755-758, 756f-759f
Oral ulcers
  in Behçet's disease, 271
  in coxsackie hand-foot-and-mouth disease, 446, 448f
  in herpes simplex infection, 451, 452f
  traumatic, 773, 773f
Orbit
  anatomy of, 917f
  cellulitis of, 919, 919f
  dermoid and epidermoid cysts of, 751, 751f
  disorders of, 750-751, 751f-752f
  neuroblastoma metastatic to, 751, 751f
  pseudotumors of, 751
  rhabdomyosarcoma of, 432, 433f, 751
  tumors of, 750-751, 751f
Orbital capillary hemangioma, 750-751, 751f
Orbital cellulitis, 919, 919f
Orbital floor fracture, 752, 752f
Orchitis, mumps, 464
Orofacial findings, in cancer, 433-434, 434f-435f
Orofacial trauma, 770-778
  assessment of, 770-771
  to dentition, 774-775, 775f-776f
  to soft tissue, 771-773, 772f-773f
  to supporting structures, 775-778, 776f-778f
Orofaciodigital syndrome, 896f
  frenula abnormalities in, 761, 761f
Oropharyngeal disorders, 920-925, 920f-925f
Oropharyngeal examination, 920
Oropharyngeal obstruction, 623, 624f, 625f
Oropharyngeal trauma, penetrating, 921-925, 925f
Orthopedic disorders. *See* Musculoskeletal disorders.
Orthopedic examination. *See* Musculoskeletal examination.
Orthophoria, 724
Ortolani maneuver, 33, 34f
Ortolani sign, in developmental hip dislocation, 828
Os vesalianum, 809, 810f
Osgood-Schlatter disease, 834-835, 835f
Osler nodes, in bacterial endocarditis, 132, 133f
Osler-Weber-Rendu disease, epistaxis in, 910-911, 911f
Osmotic fragility testing, in hereditary spherocytosis, 412, 414f
Ossification centers
  age at onset, 781, 782f, 783f
  secondary, 809, 810f
Osteoarthropathy
  hypertrophic, in cancer, 438, 440f
  in inflammatory bowel disease, 392, 397f
Osteodystrophy, Albright hereditary, 359, 360f
Osteogenesis imperfecta, 20-21, 24, 844-848
  classification of, 844-845
  diagnosis of, 848
  differential diagnosis of, 848
  fracture in, 208-209
  subdural hematoma and, 213
  treatment of, 848
  type I, 845, 846f
  type II, 845-846, 846f
  type III, 846-847, 847f
  type IV, 847
  type V, 847
  type VI, 847
  type VII, 847-848
Osteomyelitis, 482-488, 483f-489f
  acute
    from contiguous spread, 484
    diagnosis of, 484, 485f, 486f
    from hematogenous spread, 483-484, 483f, 484f
  chronic, 486, 488f
  subacute, 485-486, 487f
  vertebral, 486, 488, 489f
Osteopenia
  in cancer, 438, 439f
  in osteogenesis imperfecta, 845, 846f

Osteoporosis, idiopathic juvenile, versus osteogenesis imperfecta, 848
Osteosarcoma, 434, 439, 441f
Otitis externa, 893, 893f
Otitis media
  acute, 897-900, 899f-900f
    with bullous myringitis, 899, 899f
    classic findings in, 898-899, 899f
    with perforation, 899-900, 900f
  in Apert syndrome, 878
  chronic-recurrent, 900, 901f
  with effusion, 900, 900f
    hearing loss in, 89
  in facial clefting, 870
  pathogens in, 897-898, 899f
  serous, 900f
Otolaryngologic examination, 889, 890f
Otorrhea, 433, 434f, 893, 893f
Otoscopy
  ear, 889, 897, 898f
  nasal, 902
Out-toeing, 791
Ovarian cyst, 369, 647, 648f, 651, 655, 710t
Ovarian mass, 655
Ovarian torsion, 647, 648, 648f, 710t
Ovarian tumor, 647-648, 648f
Overuse injuries, 856
Oxycephaly, 873, 873t
Oxygen uptake, maximum, 857
Oxytocin, 356

P

Pacifier-sucking habits, 758, 759f
Pain, in juvenile diskitis, 486
Pain syndromes, idiopathic musculoskeletal, 272-273
Palate
  cleft, 49, 49f, 868-870, 868t, 869f, 920-921, 920f-922f
  high-arched, 921, 922f
  laceration of, 772, 773f, 925, 925f
  submucous cleft of, 921, 922f
Pallor, 430
  in anemia, 404, 405f
Palmar crease, 46
Pancreatic anomalies, 383, 384f
Pancreatic insufficiency, in cystic fibrosis, 392, 397f, 610
Pancreatic pseudocyst, 383, 384f, 648, 649f
Pancreatitis, 383, 384f, 648
  in cystic fibrosis, 614
  in mumps, 464
Pancytopenia, 428-429, 428f, 429f
Panhypopituitarism, 236
Panniculitis, popsicle, 473, 473f
Papanicolaou (Pap) smear
  in HPV infection, 702
  recommendations for, 681
  technique for, 684-685
Papillae, interdental, 755
Papillary conjunctivitis, 113, 114f, 732, 732f
Papilledema, 194f, 582, 582f, 749, 749f
Papilloma, nasal, 905, 905f
Papillomatosis, laryngeal, 607, 608f, 934, 935f
Papular acrodermatitis, 453-454, 455f
Papular urticaria, 204, 207, 207f, 308-309, 309f
Papules
  in cat-scratch disease, 481, 481f
  in incontinentia pigmenti, 322, 323f
Papulosquamous disorders, 277-298
Parachute response, 67, 69f
Paraduodenal (paracolic) hernia, 641
Parallel play, 79
Paralumbar prominence, in scoliosis, 818, 819, 820f
Paranasal sinuses
  developmental changes in, 911, 912f, 913f
  inflammation of. *See* Sinusitis.
Paraneoplastic syndromes, 429-430
Parapharyngeal abscess, 926-927, 928f
Paraphimosis, 551

Parathyroid glands, 359
Parathyroid hormone, 359
Paraurethral cyst, 558, 559f
Paravertebral mass, 434, 435f
Parental risk factors for child abuse and
    neglect, 162-163, 162t-164t, 232-233
Parenteral nutrition
    complications of, 381, 382f
    in gastrointestinal tract injury, 378-380, 380f
    indications for, 381
Parinaud syndrome, 583
Paronychia, 343-344, 344f, 468, 468f
Parotitis, 894
    bacterial, 464, 464f
    epidemic, 463-464, 463f
Paroxysmal movement disorders, 594-595
Paroxysmal nocturnal hemoglobinuria, 428
Parry-Romberg syndrome, 259
Pars planitis, 740, 740f
Partial thromboplastin time (PTT), 425, 426f
Parvovirus B19, 448
Pasteurella multocida adenitis, 480
Pastia lines, in streptococcal scarlet fever, 455,
    456f
Patella
    anterior, disorders of, 835-836
    examination of, 247
Patellar dislocation, 813, 813f
Patent ductus arteriosus
    closure of, 158, 158f
    heart size in, 136
Patent urachus, 538, 539f
Pavlik harness, for developmental hip
    dislocation, 829
Peak expiratory flow rate (PEFR), in asthma,
    102, 103f, 104
Peanut allergy, 97, 98t
Peau d'orange lesion, in erysipelas, 471, 471f
Pectus carinatum, 663, 664f
    in Marfan syndrome, 21, 22f
Pectus excavatum, 138, 663, 664f
Pedersen speculum, 683, 683f
Pediculosis, 310-311, 312f
Pedophile, 214
Pelger-Huët anomaly, 421, 421f
Pelvic appendiceal abscess, 694-695, 694f
Pelvic avulsion fracture, 811, 811f
Pelvic bones, osteomyelitis of, 483
Pelvic examination. See Gynecologic
    examination.
Pelvic inflammatory disease, 708-710, 709f,
    709t, 710t
Pelvic neuroblastoma, 650f
Pelvic tumors, 655
Penis
    buried, 548, 549f
    double, 551, 551f
    length of, age and, 550, 550f
    small, 550, 550f
    torsion of, 548, 549f
    trauma to, 560, 561f
    webbed, 548, 549f
Peptic ulcer disease, 383, 383f, 384f
Perforation, orofacial, 772
Periapical abscess, 769, 769f, 770f
Periauricular cellulitis, 894, 895f
Pericarditis
    in systemic lupus erythematosus, 255
    tuberculous, 495
Pericoronitis, 757, 769-770, 771f
Perifollicular abscess, 468, 468f
Perihepatitis, 709-710
Perimembranous ventricular septal defect,
    144, 145f
Perinatal infections. See Infection.
Perineal fistula, 670, 671f
Perineal midline fusion defects, 231, 232f
Perineum
    hematoma of, 688, 689f
    lesions of, in sexually transmitted disease,
        701-703, 701f-703f
    median raphe cyst of, 552, 552f
    moderate to severe trauma to, 689, 690f

Perineum (Continued)
    poor aeration in, maceration secondary to,
        693-694, 693f
    poor hygiene in, irritation secondary to,
        693, 693f
    superficial injuries of, 687-688, 688f
Periodic fever
    in PFAPA syndrome, 272, 768-769
    syndromes associated with, 272
Periorbital cellulitis
    diagnostic studies in, 919
    from facial infection, 918, 918f
    from hematogenous seeding, 917-918
    from sinusitis, 916-917, 918f
Periorbital erythema, in sinusitis, 914, 914f
Periosteal stripping injury, 184, 186, 186f
Peripheral blood smear, 403, 404f
Peripheral nerve damage, in newborn, 44, 44f
Peritonsillar abscess, 923-924, 924f
Periungual abscess, 468, 468f
Periungual fibroma, in tuberous sclerosis, 570,
    571f
Permethrin
    for pediculosis, 311
    for scabies, 310
Pertussis, pneumonia in, 600-601, 600f
Pes cavus, 841-843, 842f
Pes planus, 841, 841f
Petechiae, 430
    differential diagnosis of, 167, 168, 170f,
        172f, 202, 203f
    in meningococcemia, 459, 460f
    in newborn, 43, 43f, 423f
    in Rocky Mountain spotted fever, 462, 463f
Peutz-Jeghers syndrome, 337, 645, 646f
PFAPA (periodic fever, aphthous stomatitis,
    pharyngitis, and adenitis) syndrome, 272,
    768-769
Pfeiffer syndrome, 879, 880f, 881
PHACES syndrome, 325, 325f
Phagocytic disorders, 123-124, 123f, 124f
Phakomatoses, 564, 566-585, 567f-574f
Phalangeal fracture, 807-809, 808f-809f
Phalanx
    distal, crush injury of, 808, 809f
    proximal, fracture of, 797f
Phallus, agenesis of, 366, 367f
Pharyngeal mass, 623, 625f
Pharyngeal wall, posterior, penetration of,
    925, 925f, 926, 927f
Pharyngitis
    acute, 921-923, 923f
    streptococcal, 476t
Pharyngotonsillitis, in mononucleosis, 450,
    450f
Pharynx, examination of, 920
Phenytoin, gingival hyperplasia from, 762, 762f
Pheochromocytoma, 363-364
Phlyctenular conjunctivitis, 733, 733f
Phonemes, and intelligibility, 78t
Phorias, 718, 723-724, 724f
Photocontact and phototoxic dermatitis, 288,
    292f
Photophobia, in rubeola, 443, 444f
Phthiriasis, 730, 730f
Phthisis bulbi, 740, 740f
Phyllodes tumors, 665
Physeal injuries, 799-804, 799t, 801f
    Salter-Harris classification of, 799, 803-804,
        803t, 804f-805f
Physical abuse. See Child abuse.
Physical maturity, in gestational age
    assessment, 33-36, 35f-37f
Phytophotodermatitis, 204, 204f, 288
Piebaldism, 335-336, 336f
Pierre-Robin sequence, 623, 624f, 886-887,
    887f, 920f
Pigmentary disorders, 332-337, 334f-338f.
    See also Hyperpigmentation;
    Hypopigmentation.
Pigmentary mosaicism, 333-334, 335f
Pili torti, 342-343, 344f
Pilonidal sinus, 46, 47f

Pimecrolimus, for atopic dermatitis, 283-284
Pinch test, in nipple evaluation, 55, 55f
Pineal region tumors, 583, 583f
Pinna
    displacement of, 893-894, 894f, 895f
    erythema of, 894, 894f, 895f
Pinworms, vulvovaginitis from, 698-699, 699f
Pituitary gland, 351-356. See also
    Hypopituitarism.
    anterior, 352-355, 353f-355f
    ectopic, 356, 356f
    hormones of, 353-355, 353f-355f
    posterior, 356, 356f
Pityriasis, inverse, 287
Pityriasis alba, 283, 283f
Pityriasis rosea, 286-287, 289f
PKD. See Polycystic kidney disease (PKD).
Placenta
    circumvallate, 40, 40f
    dichorionic, diamniotic, 41, 41f
    infarction of, 40-41, 40f
    monochorionic, monoamniotic, 41, 41f
    premature separation of, 40, 40f
    velamentous cord insertion into, 40, 40f
Plagiocephaly, 870-872, 871f, 873, 873t, 875
Plague, bubonic, 481-482
Plain films. See Radiography.
Plantar warts, 313, 314f
Plantar-palmar dermatitis, juvenile, 284-285,
    285f
Plasmodium vivax malaria, 418f
Plastic deformation, 798f
Platelet(s)
    disorders of, 424-425, 424f-425f
    function testing of, 425
    giant, 424, 424f
    normal range of, 424
Play, social, 79-80, 80f
Pleural effusion
    malignant, 434, 436, 436f
    in non-Hodgkin's lymphoma, 436, 436f
    in systemic lupus erythematosus, 256, 256f
    in tuberculosis, 492
Plexiform neuroma, 566, 568f, 751
Plummer nails, 357
Pneumatic otoscopy, 889, 897, 898f
Pneumatocele, in hyper IgE syndrome, 122,
    123f
Pneumatosis intestinalis, 265, 265f, 643, 644f
Pneumocystis jiroveci pneumonia, 503, 505f,
    601
Pneumogram, 622
Pneumomediastinum
    in asthma, 107-108, 108f
    in cystic fibrosis, 614, 614f
Pneumonia
    congenital, 50, 52, 52f, 599-601, 600f
    Pneumocystis jiroveci, 503, 505f, 601
Pneumonitis
    hypersensitivity, 111-112
    interstitial, 602, 602f
    lymphocytic interstitial, 602, 602f
    lymphoid interstitial, in AIDS, 503, 505f,
        506f
Pneumoperitoneum, 643
Pneumothorax, 630-631, 632f
    in asthma, 107, 108f
    noisy, 108
Poison ivy, 287, 290f
Poland syndrome, 663-664, 664f
Polyarteritis nodosa, 265, 530-531, 531f
Polycystic kidney disease (PKD), 523-526
    autosomal dominant, 524-525, 525f
    autosomal recessive, 523-524, 524f, 525f
    in cystic renal dysplasia, 525-526, 526f
    syndromes associated with, 523, 524t
Polycystic ovarian syndrome, 369
Polydactyly, 8f, 45, 46f
Polymerase chain reaction
    in fragile X syndrome, 17
    in HIV infection, 503, 506
Polyostotic fibrous dysplasia, in McCune-
    Albright syndrome, 367, 368f

Polyps
  adenomatous, 645, 646f
  introital, 557, 558f
  juvenile, 645, 646f
  nasal, 613, 613f, 907-908, 908f
  of tympanic membrane, 901, 902f
Pompe disease, cardiac findings in, 132t
Popliteal cyst, 245, 247, 247f, 835, 835f
Popsicle panniculitis, 473, 473f
Porphyria, tooth discoloration in, 766, 766f
Portal hypertension, 644-645, 645f
Port-wine stain, 329, 329f
  in Klippel-Trénaunay syndrome, 573, 573f
  in Sturge-Weber syndrome, 570-571, 572f
Posterior drawer test, 789, 789f
Posterior fat pad sign, 802f, 807, 808f
Posterior fontanelle, 867, 868f
Posterior fossa cyst, in Dandy-Walker
    malformation, 577, 578f
Posterior urethral valves, 521-522, 522f, 536-
    537, 536f, 537f, 650, 650f
Posterior uveitis, 740
Posthitis, 551
Post-translational gene modification, 20
Post-transplant lymphoproliferative disorder,
    441
Postural kyphosis, 821
Potassium hydroxide preparation. *See* KOH
    (potassium hydroxide) preparation.
Pott puffy tumor, 916, 918f
Pott shunt, 149, 149f
Potter sequence, 526-527, 527f
Poverty, child abuse or neglect and, 161-162,
    162t, 233
PPD test, 491, 491f, 495, 495t
Prader-Willi syndrome, 18-19, 18f, 19f
Preauricular sinus and cyst, 658, 895, 897f
Preauricular skin tag, 46, 46f
Precocious puberty, 366-369, 368f
Prednisone, for recurrent aphthous ulcers, 769
Pregnancy, 710-712
  alcohol consumption and, 30, 30f
  breast changes in, 54-55, 54f
  ectopic, 710t
  rubella exposure during, 444-445
  signs and symptoms of, 710-712, 711t
  tests for, 711, 712t
Prehension, development of, 71, 71f, 72f
Prehn sign, 552, 554
Premature atrial contractions, 140, 142f
Premature infant
  breastfeeding of, 61-63, 61f, 62f
  retinopathy in, 743, 744f
  skin assessment in, 34, 36f
Premature pubarche, 368-369, 368f
Premature thelarche, 368, 368f
Premature ventricular contractions, 140, 142f
Preputial adhesions, 549-550, 550f
Priapism, 416, 416f, 438, 551, 551f
Prickly heat, 301, 301f
Primitive reflexes, 49-50, 49f-51f, 65-66, 66f,
    66t, 83
Processus vaginalis, abnormalities of, 668-
    669, 669f
Progeria, cardiac findings in, 132t
Prolactin, 355
Prolonged QT syndrome, 143, 144f
Proptosis
  in Graves disease, 357, 357f
  retro-orbital, 432, 433f
Protective equilibrium response, 66-67, 66t,
    68f
Protein
  malabsorption of, 377
  in urine, 510
Protein C deficiency, 427-428, 427f
Protein S deficiency, 428
Protein-energy malnutrition, 375, 376f-378f
Proteinuria, in nephrotic syndrome, 514
Prothrombin gene variant, 428
Prothrombin time (PT), 425, 426f
Proximal interphalangeal joint, 244, 245f
Proximal phalanx fracture, 797f

Proximal tibia, angular varus deformity of,
    834, 834f
Prune-belly syndrome, 521, 521f, 537-538, 538f
Pseudarthrosis, of clavicle, congenital, 210f,
    825-826, 825f
Pseudocyst
  inflammatory, 655
  pancreatic, 383, 384f, 648, 649f
Pseudohypoparathyroidism, 359, 360f
Pseudomonas septicemia, ecthyma
    gangrenosum in, 466, 467f
Pseudopapilledema, 717, 717f, 749-750
Pseudorosette, in neuroblastoma, 429f
Pseudostrabismus, 721, 721f
Pseudotumor
  of femur, 427f
  of orbit, 751
Pseudotumor cerebri, 585
Pseudovitamin D–deficient rickets, 360, 361t
Psoriasis, 277-279, 278f
  diaper dermatitis as, 277, 296, 297f
  guttate, 277, 278f
Psoriatic arthritis, 253, 253f
Psoriatic nails, 345, 345f
Psychosocial failure to thrive, 74f, 233-235,
    233f-235f
Psychosocial history, in idiopathic
    musculoskeletal pain syndromes, 273
Ptosis, 725-726, 727f
Pubarche, premature, 368-369, 368f
Pubertal gynecomastia, 665, 665f
Puberty
  delayed, 369
    constitutional growth delay and, 347
    in Turner syndrome, 369
  physiology of, 349, 350f, 351, 351f-352f
  precocious, 366-369, 368f
Pubic hair
  development of
    female, 350f, 351, 352f
    male, 350f, 351, 352f
    premature, 368-369, 368f
  shaving of, 694
Pulmonary artery, anomalous left, 138, 139f
Pulmonary artery sling, 138, 139f
Pulmonary atresia
  cardiac catheterization for, 153-154, 154f
  tetralogy of Fallot with, "egg on its side"
    heart in, 135, 136f
Pulmonary blastoma, 629, 630f
Pulmonary disorders, 102-112, 597-622. *See
    also* Respiratory *entries*.
  chronic obstructive, 111
  in cystic fibrosis, 614, 614f
  diagnostic techniques in, 618, 620-622
  failure to thrive in, 236
  history in, 597
  physical examination in, 597-598, 598f
  radiographic evaluation of, 598-599, 599f
  in systemic lupus erythematosus, 256-257,
    256f
Pulmonary fibrosis, in scleroderma, 261, 262f
Pulmonary function tests, 606, 618, 620-621,
    620f, 621f
  in asthma, 104-105, 105f
  in preparticipation sports examination, 854
Pulmonary hemosiderosis, 603-604, 604f
Pulmonary hypertension, left-to-right shunt
    associated with, 138, 139f
Pulmonary nodules, 434, 436f
Pulmonary sequestration, 601, 601f, 629-630,
    631f
Pulmonary stenosis
  balloon angioplasty for, 155, 155f, 156
  cardiac catheterization for, 153-154, 154f
  radiographic appearance of, 136, 137f
  tetralogy of Fallot with, "boot-shaped"
    heart in, 135, 135f
Pulmonary tuberculosis, 492-493, 493f
Pulmonary vascularity, in congenital heart
    disease, 138, 139f, 140
Pulmonary venous return, total anomalous,
    138, 140f

Pulse, examination of, 127
Pulsus paradoxus, in asthma, 106, 106t
Pupil(s)
  examination of, 748, 748f
  Marcus Gunn, 748, 748f
  unequal size of, 748-749
Pupillary membranes, persistent, 737, 737f
Purpura, 430, 430f
  Henoch-Schönlein. *See* Henoch-Schönlein
    purpura.
  idiopathic thrombocytopenic, 202, 203f
  in meningococcemia, 459-460, 460f
  thrombotic thrombocytopenic, 418, 423f
Pustulosis
  cephalic (neonatal acne), 318-319, 320f
  transient neonatal, 318, 320f
Pyelography, in adrenal neuroblastoma, 653,
    654f
Pyelostomy, cutaneous, 541, 542f
Pyloric stenosis, 385, 387f, 388f
  hypertrophic, 635, 635f, 636f
Pyoderma gangrenosum, in inflammatory
    bowel disease, 392, 397f
Pyogenic arthritis, 253
Pyogenic granuloma, 327-328, 328f
Pyruvate dehydrogenase deficiency, 31
Pyruvate kinase deficiency, 417

Q

QRS complex, prolonged, 142, 143f
QT interval, prolonged, 143, 144f
Quadriceps stretch, 861f
Quadriplegia, 83-84, 84f

R

Raccoon eyes, in neuroblastoma, 432, 433f
Rachitic rosary, in rickets, 360, 361f
Radial club hand, 826, 826f
Radial head, subluxation of, 816-817, 816f,
    817f
Radial neck, fracture of, 807, 807f
Radiofrequency catheter ablation, 143, 143f
Radiography
  of adrenal neuroblastoma, 653, 653f
  in allergic bronchopulmonary aspergillosis,
    609, 609f
  in asthma, 107-108, 108f
  of cardiac apex and situs discordance, 134,
    134f, 135f
  chest, 598-599, 599f
  in clubfoot, 837f, 838
  in congenital cystic adenomatoid
    malformation, 609-610, 609f
  in congenital heart disease, 133-138,
    134f-140f
  in congenital lobar emphysema, 629, 629f
  in congenital syphilis, 500-501, 500f
  in congenital toxoplasmosis, 497, 497f
  in congenital vertical talus, 840, 840f
  contrast
    in double aortic arch, 137-138, 138f
    of esophagus, 634, 635f
    in gastrointestinal obstruction, 634, 634f
    in swallowing study, 617, 617f
  in croup, 606-607, 607f, 929, 930f
  in cystic fibrosis, 614, 615f
  in epiglottitis, 929, 929f
  of epiphyseal maturation, 347
  of esophageal foreign body, 934, 936f
  of foot, 838f
  of foreign body aspiration, 931, 931f, 932f
  of foreign body inhalation, 602, 603f
  of fracture, 795
  in gastrointestinal obstruction, 634, 634f
  of great vessels, 136-138, 137f-139f
  in head trauma, 195-196
  of heart shape and size abnormalities, 134-
    136, 135f-136f
  of hip dislocation, 828, 829f
  in intussusception, 640-641, 641f

Radiography (Continued)
in knee trauma, 793, 793f
in lead poisoning, 406, 407f
in lobar emphysema, 610, 612f
in lymphocytic interstitial pneumonitis, 602, 602f
in malrotation, 637, 637f
in Mycoplasma pneumoniae infection, 604, 605f
in obliterative bronchiolitis, 610, 612f
in osteomyelitis, 484, 485-486, 485f, 487f
panoramic, 776, 776f
in pneumatosis intestinalis, 643, 644f
in pulmonary disorders, 598-599, 599f
in pulmonary hemosiderosis, 603, 604f
of pulmonary vascularity, 138, 139f, 140f
of retropharyngeal abscess, 926, 927f
in septic arthritis, 490, 490f
in sinusitis, 914, 915f
of skeletal abnormalities, 138, 140f
skull
in increased intracranial pressure, 581, 582f
in macrocephaly, 575, 576f
in thalassemia major, 408, 408f
in tuberculosis, 492, 493f
in tuberculous spondylitis, 495, 495f
Radius, distal, fracture of, 798f
Ranula, 659, 659f, 762-763, 763f
Rape, 215, 227t
Rapid slide tests, in mononucleosis, 451
Rash. See Skin lesions.
Rastelli procedure, 151, 152f
Raynaud's phenomenon
in CREST syndrome, 259, 261f
in systemic sclerosis, 261
Reading disorder, 89
Reagin tests, in syphilis, 702
Rectourethral fistula, 670-671, 671f
Rectovaginal examination, 685
Rectovaginal fistula, 695
Rectum. See also Anorectal entries.
bimanual examination of, 751
prolapse of, 392, 398, 398f, 613, 613f, 673, 673f
suction biopsy of, in Hirschsprung disease, 639, 640f
Red blood cells. See Erythrocyte(s).
Red diaper syndrome, 510
Red strawberry tongue, in streptococcal scarlet fever, 455, 456f
Refeeding syndrome, 380
Reflex(es)
asymmetrical tonic neck, 65-66, 66f, 83-84
bulbocavernosus, 535
corneal light, 723, 724f
deep tendon, 563, 566f
fixation, 713, 715f
Moro, 49-50, 51f, 65, 66f
primitive, 49-50, 49f-51f, 65-66, 66f, 66t, 83
white pupillary, 738, 738t
Reflex hand grasp, 70, 70f
Reflex sympathetic dystrophy, 272
Reflux
gastroesophageal. See Gastroesophageal reflux.
vesicoureteral, 518, 519f, 536f
with ureteropelvic junction obstruction, 539, 540f
Reflux rhinitis, 903
Refractive errors, 716-717, 716f, 717f
Regurgitation, versus vomiting, 632
Rehabilitation, after sports injuries, 864-865
Reilly bodies, 422, 423f
Renal angiomyolipoma, 521, 521f, 570
Renal anomalies, 520-522, 521f-523f
Renal artery stenosis
hypertension in, 530-531, 531f
in neurofibromatosis, 567-568
Renal calculi, 515-516
Renal colic, 515
Renal cyst, simple, 540-541, 541f. See also Polycystic kidney disease (PKD).

Renal disorders, 509-533
developmental, 520-522, 521f-523f
failure to thrive in, 236
glomerular, 512-514, 512f, 514f, 515f
hematuria in, 509, 514-515, 516f
in Henoch-Schönlein purpura, 266, 305
hereditary and metabolic, 522-530
history and physical examination in, 509
polycystic. See Polycystic kidney disease (PKD).
in systemic lupus erythematosus, 257, 257t
in tuberous sclerosis, 570
urinalysis in, 510-512, 511f, 512f, 512t
Renal dysplasia
cystic, 524t, 525-526, 526f, 539-540, 541f
multicystic, 526, 539-540, 541f, 650, 651f
Renal ectopy, crossed, 522, 523f
Renal failure, chronic
anemia in, 532, 533f
growth failure in, 509, 532-533
renal osteodystrophy in, 531-532, 532f
Renal scan
in multicystic renal dysplasia, 540, 541f
in ureteropelvic junction obstruction, 539, 540f
Renal tubular acidosis, 516, 518f
Renal venous thrombosis, 517-518, 518f, 650, 651f
Renography, diuresis, in ureteropelvic junction obstruction, 539, 540f
Renovascular hypertension, 509
hirsutism and, 531
in renal artery stenosis, 530-531, 531f
Respiratory alternans, 597
Respiratory disease. See Pulmonary disorders.
Respiratory distress
classic syndrome of, 50, 51f
clinical evaluation of, 623, 624f
extrathoracic, 632
grunting, flaring, and retractions in, 50, 51f
in newborn, 50, 51f, 52, 52f
in Pierre-Robin sequence, 886
severity, estimation of, 926, 926t
symptoms of, 102
thoracic causes of, 623-632, 626f-633f
from upper airway obstruction, 623, 624f, 625f
Respiratory infection
versus asthma, 110-111
upper, in early infancy, 903
Respiratory rate, normal, 107t
Restraint injury, in child abuse, 173, 177f
Reticulocyte, 403, 404f
Retina
cherry red spot on, 34, 34f, 35f, 746, 746f, 747, 747f
coloboma of, 741, 741f
detachment of, 743, 744f
developmental abnormalities of, 741-743, 741f-743f
disorders of, 741-747, 741f-747f
leukemic infiltration in, 746
myelinated nerve fibers of, 741, 741f
Retinal artery occlusion, central, 745-746, 746f
Retinal hemorrhage, 745, 745f, 754
differential diagnosis of, 212-213, 214f
in shaken baby syndrome, 192, 193-194, 193f
Retinal telangiectasis, 743, 743f
Retinal toxocariasis, 745, 745f
Retinitis, 744. See also Retinochoroiditis.
Retinitis pigmentosa, 743, 743f
Retinoblastoma, 432, 432f, 747, 747f
Retinochoroiditis, 744-745, 744f, 745f
Retinoic acid, for acne, 313
Retinoids, for epidermolytic hyperkeratosis, 280
Retinopathy
diabetic, 746
in metabolic disorders, 746-747, 747f
of prematurity, 743, 744f
in rubella syndrome, 744, 745f
sickle cell, 746, 746f

Retractions, in respiratory distress, 50, 51f
Retro-orbital proptosis, 432, 433f
Retropharyngeal abscess, 926, 927f
Retropharyngeal air dissection, 925, 925f
Return to play, after sports injuries, 864-865
Reversal sign, 195, 198f
Rhabdomyosarcoma, 434, 439-440, 478t, 654, 655f
of bladder, 546f
cardiac, in tuberous sclerosis, 570
intraoral, 433, 434f
of orbit, 432, 433f, 751
otorrhea in, 433
Rheumatic disease, 241-273
joint examination in, 241-247, 242f-247f, 242t, 243t
leg length in, 247, 248f
musculoskeletal examination in, 241-247, 242f-248f, 242t, 243t
musculoskeletal history in, 241, 242f
Rheumatic fever, 131-132, 133f, 241
Rheumatoid arthritis, juvenile, 248-254
arthritis in, 241, 250, 251, 251f
cardiac involvement in, 253
diagnostic criteria for, 248, 248t
differential diagnosis of, 253-254, 253f, 253t, 254f
extraarticular manifestations of, 252-253, 252t
growth abnormalities in, 252-253
iritis in, 737, 737f
joint examination in, 248f, 249, 249f, 250f
macrophage activation syndrome in, 251, 251f, 251t
micrognathia in, 242, 243f
ophthalmologic examination in, 252, 252f, 252t
pauciarticular onset, 248f, 249f, 249t, 251-252
polyarticular onset, 248f, 249t, 251
rash in, 250, 250f
systemic-onset, 248f, 249-251, 249t, 250f, 251f, 251t
uveitis in, 251-252, 252f
Rheumatoid factor, in juvenile rheumatoid arthritis, 251
Rhinitis
allergic, 98-102, 99f-101f, 101t
with postnasal discharge, 919-920
nonallergic, with eosinophilia, 101, 101t
reflux, 903
vasomotor, 101, 101t
Rhinitis medicamentosa, 101
Rhonchi, 598
Rhus dermatitis, 287, 290f
Rib fracture, 183-184, 184f, 185f, 200, 201f
Rib hump, in scoliosis, 818, 819, 820f
Rib notching, in coarctation of the aorta, 138, 140f
Ribonucleoprotein
in mixed connective tissue disease, 262
in systemic lupus erythematosus, 258
RICH lesion (rapidly involuting congenital hemangioma), 327, 328f
Rickets, 210, 211f, 380, 381f
hypophosphatemic, 360, 361t, 527, 528f
laboratory findings in, 361t
pseudovitamin D–deficient, 360, 361t
vitamin D–deficient, 359-360, 361f, 361t
Rickettsia rickettsii, 462
Rieger syndrome, 734
Right middle lobe syndrome, 603
Right ventricular hypertrophy, 138-139
Ringworm, 291-292, 293f, 294f, 341-342, 343f
Risus sardonicus, in neonatal tetanus, 501, 502f
Rocker-bottom foot, 839, 840f
Rocky Mountain spotted fever, 462-463, 463f
Rooting reflex, 49, 49f
Roseola infantum, 449-450, 449f
Ross procedure, 151, 152f
Roth spot, 745, 745f
Rubber dermatitis, 287, 291f

Rubella, 443-445, 444f, 445f, 476t
  congenital, 497-498, 498f
  pregnancy and, 444-445
Rubella syndrome, retinopathy in, 744, 745f
Rubeola, 443, 444f
Rubinstein-Taybi syndrome, 896f
Rumination syndrome, 385
Rusty pipe syndrome, in breastfeeding, 61, 61f

S

Saccades, 717-718
Sacrococcygeal teratoma, 437, 438f, 651, 652f
Sacroiliac joint
  examination of, 245, 246f
  septic arthritis of, 489-490
Saddle-nose deformity, 908, 909f
Saethre-Chotzen syndrome, 881-882
Safety gear, sports-related, 856, 857t
Sagittal suture, 867, 868f
Sagittal synostosis, 873-875, 874f
St. Vitus dance, 595
Saliva, aspiration of, 617, 617f, 618f
Salivagram, 617, 618f
Salivary calculus, 763, 763f
Salivary gland lesions, 659, 659f
Salmon patch, 328-329, 329f
Salpingitis, 709
Sandifer syndrome, 385, 936
Sarcoma. *See also* Rhabdomyosarcoma.
  bone, 434, 439, 441f
  clear cell, 654
  Ewing, 434, 439, 441f
  Kaposi, in AIDS, 503, 506f
  soft tissue, 439-440
Sarcoma botryoides, 437, 438f
Scabies, 309-310, 310f-312f, 701
Scalded skin syndrome, staphylococcal, 298, 301, 457, 457f
Scalds
  accidental, 205, 205f
  inflicted, 175, 178, 178f, 178t
Scalp
  abscess of, 469-470, 470f
  dermoid cyst of, 658, 658f
  ectodermal dysplasia of, 47, 47f
  fungal infection of, 341-342, 343f
  hemangioma of, 658, 658f
  seborrhea of, 285, 287f
Scaphocephaly, 873, 873t
Scaphoid abdomen, 625, 627f
Scapular winging, in Duchenne muscular dystrophy, 589, 589f
Scarf sign, 37, 38f
Scarlet fever
  staphylococcal, 457-458, 458f
  streptococcal, 454, 455-457, 456f
Scarring alopecia, 340
Scheie syndrome, 26
Scheuermann disease, 821, 822f
Schmidt syndrome, 362
Schober test, 245, 246f
Scimitar syndrome, 134, 134f
Scissoring, in cerebral palsy, 82, 82f
Sclerae, blue, in osteogenesis imperfecta, 845, 846f
Sclerocornea, 734
Sclerodactyly
  in diabetes mellitus, 370-371, 371f
  in scleroderma, 261, 261f
Scleroderma, 258-262
  cardiac involvement in, 262
  classification of, 259, 259t
  in CREST syndrome, 259, 261f
  diagnostic criteria for, 261, 261f, 262f
  en coup de sabre, 259, 260f
  gastrointestinal involvement in, 262
  linear, 259, 260f
  localized, 258, 259, 259f, 260f, 261
  morphea in, 259, 260f
  skin lesions in, 260f, 261-262, 261f

Sclerosis
  glomerular, 513
  medullary, 181, 182f
  systemic, 258, 259, 259t
  tuberous, 334, 336f, 521, 521f, 569-570, 569t, 570f-572f
Sclerosus, lichen, 230, 230f, 695-696, 696f
Scoliosis, 785, 785f, 818-821
  angular, in neurofibromatosis 1, 566, 568f
  causes of, 818-819, 819t
  diagnosis of, 819-820, 820f
  diskogenic, 824f
  paravertebral mass in, 434, 435f
Scotch-plaid pitting of nails, 337, 345, 345f
Screening tests
  in developmental assessment, 65
  for immunodeficiency, 117, 117t
Scrotum
  acute, 552
  lesions of, 551-552, 669-670, 670f
  median raphe cyst of, 552, 552f
  swelling of
    chronic, 554-556, 555f-556f
    in minimal change disease, 514, 515f
  trauma to, 560, 561f
  ulcers of, in Behçet's disease, 271, 272f
Scurvy, 210, 211f
Sebaceous gland hyperplasia, neonatal, 318-319, 320f
Seborrhea, in Langerhans cell histiocytosis, 430, 431f
Seborrheic dermatitis, 285, 286f, 287f
Second impact syndrome, 865
Secundum atrial septal defect, 144, 145f
Sedimentation rate, in acute osteomyelitis, 484
Seizure
  absence, 593-594, 593f
  complex partial, 593
  generalized, 593
  simple partial, 593
  in Sturge-Weber syndrome, 573
Selenium sulfide shampoo, for tinea capitis, 342
Self-awareness, definition of, 80-81, 80f
Seminal products, after sexual abuse, 222, 224f
Senning procedure, for transposition of the great arteries, 150-151, 151f
Sensorimotor intelligence, development of, 73-74, 74f, 75f
Sensory innervation, cutaneous, 563, 564f-565f
Sensory processing, early, 73, 73f
Sepsis, meningococcal, 459-461, 460f
Septal deviation or dislocation, 908, 909f
Septal hematoma, 908, 909f
Septal remnants, 228, 228f
Septic arthritis, 488-491, 489t, 490f
Septo-optic dysplasia, 352, 353f
Sequence, 7
Serum sickness, 98, 99f
Serum sickness–like reaction, 304, 304f
Sexual abuse, 213-232
  acute traumatic findings in, 221-222, 223f, 224f
  anal and perianal abnormalities in, 223, 223f
  differential diagnosis of, 228-232, 228f-232f
  documentation of, 218-219, 220f, 225-228, 227t
  epidemiology of, 213-214
  false accusations of, 215
  genital trauma in, 221, 222f, 688, 688f
  history-taking in, 215-216, 216f
  internal injuries in, 219
  modes of presentation in, 216-217, 217t
  oral abnormalities in, 222-223
  perineal abnormalities in, 221, 222f

Sexual abuse *(Continued)*
  physical examination in
    general anesthesia for, 219-220
    patient positions for, 217-218, 218f, 219f
    perianal, 220-221
    perineal, 217-220, 217f-222f
  physical findings in, 221-225, 222f-226f
  seminal products after, 222, 224f
  sexualized behavior and, 214-215
  sexually transmitted disease from, 223-225
  specimen collection in, 225-228, 227t
  substitute chief complaint in, 217, 217t
Sexual development, 349, 350f, 351, 351f-352f. *See also* Puberty.
Sexual differentiation, 364-366, 366f, 367f
Sexual health care guidelines, for females, 682t
Sexualized behavior, 214-215
Sexually transmitted disease, 223-225, 690t, 697-698, 697t, 699-710
  approach to, 699-701
  in prepubertal patients, 699-700
  sexual abuse and, 223-225
Shagreen patch, in tuberous sclerosis, 569-570, 571f
Shaken baby syndrome, 745, 745f
  clinical picture of, 194-195, 194f-197f
  pathophysiology of, 192-194, 192f, 193f
Shampoo
  antiseborrheic, 285
  selenium sulfide, for tinea capitis, 342
Sheridan-Gardiner visual acuity tests, 714, 715f
Shigella, vulvovaginitis from, 698
Shingles, 453, 454f, 768, 768f
Short stature
  causes of, 347, 349t
  diabetes mellitus and, 370
  evaluation of, 347, 349
  mental retardation and, 85
Shoulder
  dislocation of, 813-814, 813f
  examination of, 243, 243f, 786
  strengthening exercises for, 860f
  stretching exercises for, 862f
Shoulder separation, 816
Shuddering attacks, 594
Shunt procedures, for tetralogy of Fallot, 146, 149, 149f
Sialadenitis, 478t
Sialolithiasis, 763, 763f
Sickle cell disease, 415-417, 415f, 416f
  priapism in, 551
  retinopathy in, 746, 746f
Side-lying position, in breastfeeding, 58f, 59
Sideroblastic anemia, 409, 409f
"Silk glove" sign, 669
Single ventricle, palliative procedures for, 149-150, 150f
Single-gene disorders, 20-21
Sinus
  paranasal, 911, 912f, 913f
  pilonidal, 46, 47f
  preauricular, 658, 895, 897f
  urogenital, posteriorly displaced, 560f
Sinus headache, allergic, 920
Sinus tachycardia, 142
Sinus tract, in occult spinal dysraphism, 579, 579f
Sinus venosus defect, 144, 145f
Sinusitis, 911-916
  ancillary diagnostic methods in, 914-915, 915f, 916f
  versus atopic disorders, 919-920
  versus cellulitis, 473
  clinical presentation in, 912, 914, 914f
  complications of, 915-916, 918f
  conditions predisposing to, 912
  periorbital cellulitis from, 916-917, 918f
  treatment of, 914, 915
Sipple syndrome, 363-364
Sitting/standing posture control, 66, 68f
Situs ambiguous, 135f

Situs inversus, 134, 134f
Situs solitus, 134, 134f
Skeletal. *See also* Bone; Musculoskeletal *entries.*
Skeletal abnormalities
  in congenital heart disease, 138, 140f
  in neurofibromatosis 1, 566-567, 568f
Skeletal injury. *See* Fracture(s).
Skeletal tuberculosis, 494-495, 495f
Skin
  anatomy of, 275, 275f
  atrophy of, corticosteroid-induced, 345, 346f
  examination of, 275-277, 277t, 276f
  in gestational age assessment, 33-34, 36f
  hyperextensibility of, in Ehlers-Danlos syndrome, 21, 23f
  sensory innervation of, 563, 564f-565f
  topical therapy complications of, 345-346, 346f
Skin bridges, after circumcision, 549-550, 550f
Skin findings
  in Kawasaki syndrome, 268, 268f, 269f
  in kwashiorkor, 375, 378f
  in mental retardation, 85
Skin folds, redundant, in Beare-Stevenson syndrome, 881
Skin infection
  abscess of, 467-470, 468f-470f
  bacterial, 298, 299f, 464-475, 465f-474f
  fungal, 291-297
  viral, 298, 298f
Skin lesions. *See also* Exanthems; specific types, e.g., Café-au-lait spots.
  in acne, 312-313, 313f
  anatomic depth of, 275-277, 277t
  in bacterial endocarditis, 132, 133f
  in cancer, 430-431, 430f-432f
  in congenital infections, 498f, 499f
  in diabetes mellitus, 371, 371f
  erythematous, 302-307. *See also* Erythema.
  evaluation of, 275-277, 277t, 276f
  in gonorrhea, 706, 708f
  in Henoch-Schönlein purpura, 266, 266f, 267f, 305, 306f, 513, 514f
  in hypersensitivity disorders, 113-115, 114f, 115f
  in inflammatory bowel disease, 392, 397f
  from insect bites and stings. *See* Insect bites and stings.
  in juvenile dermatomyositis, 263, 264f
  in juvenile rheumatoid arthritis, 250, 250f
  in Kawasaki syndrome, 268, 268f, 269f
  in kwashiorkor, 375, 378f
  in Langerhans cell histiocytosis, 430-431, 431f
  in lice infestation, 310-311, 312f
  in Lyme arthritis, 253, 254f
  morbilliform, 304, 305f
  in neonate, 317-322, 319f-323f
  in neuroblastoma, 430, 430f, 431f
  nevus, 329-332. *See also* Nevus.
  papulosquamous, 277-298
  pigmentary, 332-337, 334f-338f
  rash patterns in, 275, 277f
  in rheumatic disease, 241, 242t
  in scabies infestation, 309-310, 310f-312f
  in scleroderma, 260f, 261-262, 261f
  in staphylococcal scalded skin syndrome, 457, 457f
  in syphilis, 702, 703f
  in systemic lupus erythematosus, 254-255, 254f, 255f
  in tuberous sclerosis, 521, 521f
  vascular, 322, 324-329
  vesiculopustular, 298-302
Skin striae, corticosteroid-induced, 345, 346f
Skin tag
  perianal, 231-232, 232f
  preauricular, 7f, 46, 46f
Skin testing, allergy, 93, 95f, 95t
Skin tumors and infiltrations, 313-316

Skull
  abnormal shape of, nomenclature for, 872-873, 873f
  anatomy and embryology of, 867-868, 868f
  craniofacial anomalies affecting, 872-882, 873t, 874f-880f
  fracture of, 194, 194f, 195f, 894, 895f
Slashing wounds, in child abuse, 173, 176f
Sleep apnea, obstructive, 616, 879
Sleep position, deformational plagiocephaly and, 870-871
Sleep studies, 622
Slipped capital femoral epiphysis, 830-832, 831f
Small for gestational age (SGA), 37, 39f
Small intestinal atresia, 637-638, 638f
Small intestinal tears, in child abuse, 199, 200f
Smiling, early, 78, 79f
Smith-Lemli-Opitz syndrome, 24-25, 25f
Smith-Magenis syndrome, 6t
Snellen letter chart, 715
Snuffles, in congenital syphilis, 500
Soccer, injury prevention in, 858t
Social development, 79-81, 79f, 80f, 92
Sodomy, 220f
Soft neurologic signs, 90, 90t
Soft palate laceration, 772, 773f
Soft tissue developmental abnormalities, oral, 760-763, 761f-763f
Soft tissue infection
  abscess of, 467-470, 468f-470f
  bacterial, 464-475, 465f-474f
Soft tissue injuries, orofacial, 771-773, 772f-773f
Soft tissue sarcoma, 439-440
Softball, injury prevention in, 858t
Soleus stretch, 862f
Solo syndrome, 39, 85
Southern blot, in fragile X syndrome, 17, 17f
SOX9 gene mutation, in ambiguous genitalia, 364
Spasm, infantile, 594, 594f
Spasmus nutans, 595
Spastic diplegia, 83-84, 84f
Spastic quadriplegia, 843, 843f
Spasticity, gait disturbances from, 791, 792f
Special Olympics, 859
Specific gravity (SG), 510, 512
Specimen collection, in sexual abuse, 225-228, 227t
Speculum, 683, 683f
Speech. *See* Language development.
Spermatic cord, torsion of, 552-553, 553f
Spermatocele, 555, 555f
Sphenoid sinus, 911, 913f
Spherocytes, in Coombs-positive hemolytic anemia, 411, 413f
Spherocytosis, hereditary, hemolytic anemia in, 411-412, 413f, 414f
Sphingolipidoses, retinopathy in, 747, 747f
Spider bites, 308, 308f
Spider nevi, 400, 401f
Spina bifida cystica, 844, 845f
Spinal cord, tethered, 581, 581f
Spinal dysraphism, occult, 578-581, 579f-581f
Spinal tumors, 440
Spine
  cervical
    congenital atrophy of, 591, 591f
    fusion of, 879
    examination of, 245, 245f, 246f
    musculoskeletal disorders of, 818-825, 820f-824f
    thoracolumbar, 785-786, 785f, 786f
Spinobulbar muscular atrophy, 17
Spirometry, 618, 620-621, 620f, 621f
Spitz nevus, 332, 332f
Spleen, injury to, in child abuse, 199
Splenectomy, target cells and, 414
Splenic cyst, 654, 657f
Splenomegaly, 654, 657f
Splinting, for fracture, 792

Spondylitis, tuberculous, 494-495, 495f
Spondyloarthropathy, versus juvenile rheumatoid arthritis, 253, 253f
Spondylolisthesis, 821-822, 823f, 824f
Sports, 849-865
  athletic skill development and, 849-850, 850t
  for children with chronic health conditions, 857, 859-861, 859t, 863t-864t, 864
  classification of, 855t
  conditioning and training for, 857, 859t, 860f-862f
  disease-specific benefits of, 859t
  increasing organization of, 849
  injury risk in, 855-856, 855t
  participation clearance for, 853f, 855
    in children with chronic health conditions, 860-861
  preparticipation examination for, 850-855
    cardiopulmonary portion of, 851, 854
    in children with chronic health conditions, 859-860
    documentation of, 851, 852f-853f
    formats/sites of, 851
    goals of, 851
    musculoskeletal screening for, 854, 854f
  risk reduction and injury prevention in, 856-857, 857t, 858t-859t
  safety gear and field safety modifications for, 856, 857t
  strength training for, 857, 859t, 860f
  stretching exercises for, 857, 861f-862f
Sports injuries
  prevention of, 856-857, 857t, 858t-859t
  rehabilitation and return to play after, 864-865
  risk of, 855-856, 855t
Sprains, 814-816
  of ankle, 815-816, 815f
  classification of, 815t
  evaluation and management of, 816
  of knee, 815f, 816
Sprengel deformity, 825, 825f
Spur cell anemia, 413, 414f
Sputum examination, 605, 606
Squamous cell carcinoma, 431, 432f
Square-window test, 37, 37f
SRY gene mutation, in ambiguous genitalia, 364
Stab wounds, in child abuse, 173, 176f
Staphylococcal exanthems, 457-459, 457f-459f
Staphylococcal infection
  in impetigo, 465, 466f
  lymphadenitis in, 477
  of skin and soft tissue infection, 464
Staphylococcal scalded skin syndrome, 457, 457f
Staphylococcal scarlet fever, 457-458, 458f
Startle disease, 594
Stature. *See also* Height.
  percentiles for, 348t
  short
    causes of, 347, 349t
    diabetes mellitus and, 370
    evaluation of, 347, 349
    in mental retardation, 85
Steeple sign, in croup, 606-607, 607f, 929, 930f
Steppage gait, 791
Sternal cleft, 664
Sternoclavicular joint examination, 243
Sternocleidomastoid muscle, fibrous dysplasia of, 662-663, 663f, 664f
Steroid biosynthesis pathway, 365f
Steroids. *See* Corticosteroids.
Stethoscope, differential, 598, 598f
Stevens-Johnson syndrome, 98, 300-301, 300f
Stiffness, gait disturbances from, 791
Stigmata signs, in scoliosis, 819-820, 820f
Still's disease, 248f, 249-251, 249t, 250f, 251f, 251t
Still's murmur, 129t
Stings. *See* Insect bites and stings.

Stools
  "currant jelly," in intussusception, 639, 641f
  examination of, in diarrhea, 388
  newborn, 52-54, 53f
"Stork bite," 328-329, 329f
Stork-leg appearance, in Charcot-Marie-Tooth
    disease, 590, 590f
Strabismic amblyopia, 725, 726f
Strabismus, 432, 717-725
  in cerebral palsy, 84
  false, 721, 721f
  head posture and, 718
  tests for, 723-724, 724f, 725f
Straddle injuries, 230, 231f, 688, 688f
Straight leg raising test, 786, 786f
Stranger anxiety, 79
Strangulation injury, in child abuse, 173, 177f
Strawberry hemangioma, 324, 324f
Strawberry tongue, in Kawasaki syndrome,
    268, 268f
Strength testing, in musculoskeletal
    examination, 241, 242f, 243t, 587-588,
    784, 784t
Strength training, for sports, 857, 859t, 860f
Streptococcal gangrene, 474-475, 474f
Streptococcal infection
  in erysipelas, 471, 471f
  glomerulonephritis after, 512, 512f, 513
  in impetigo, 465, 465f, 466
  lymphadenitis in, 477
  of skin and soft tissue infection, 464
  in tonsillopharyngitis, 922, 923, 923f
Streptococcal pharyngitis, 476t
Streptococcal scarlet fever, 454, 455-457, 456f
Streptococcal vulvovaginitis, 698, 698f
Stress, craniomandibular dysfunction and,
    779
Stretching exercises, for sports, 857, 861f-862f
Striae, steroid-induced, 345, 346f
Stridor, 102
  causes of, 606-608, 607f-608f, 607t
  hysterical (psychogenic), 608
String sign, in pyloric stenosis, 385, 388f
Sturge-Weber syndrome, 329, 570-571, 572f-
    573f, 573
Stye, 728, 729f
Subaortic stenosis, Damus-Stansel-Kaye
    procedure for, 153, 153f
Subcapital fracture, 799t, 803f
Subconjunctival hemorrhage, 733-734, 733f
Subcutaneous atrophy, corticosteroid-induced,
    345, 346f
Subcutaneous disorders, diagnosis of, 277
Subcutaneous emphysema, in asthma, 107-
    108, 108f
Subcutaneous nodules
  in juvenile rheumatoid arthritis, 251
  in rheumatic fever, 132, 133f
Subdural hematoma
  in child abuse, 195, 196f
  differential diagnosis of, 212-213, 214f
  magnetic resonance imaging of, 196, 198f
  in shaken baby syndrome, 192, 192f, 195,
    196f
Subependymal astrocytoma, in tuberous
    sclerosis, 570, 572f
Subgaleal hematoma
  in child abuse, 167, 170f
  in newborn, 42
Subglottic disorders, airway obstruction in,
    929-931, 929f-932f
Subglottic stenosis, 607, 932, 933f, 934f
Subluxation
  of lens, 740
  of radial head, 816-817, 816f, 817f
Subperiosteal new bone formation, in fracture
    healing, 181, 182f, 186f
Subtalar joint examination, 247, 247f
Subungual hemorrhage, 345, 345f
Sucking habits, harmful, 758, 759f
Sucking reflex, 49, 50f
Sudden infant death syndrome, 161, 616
Suffocation, in child abuse, 161

Sunsetting sign, in hydrocephalus, 576, 577f
Superficial venous distention, 437, 437f
Superior vena cava syndrome, 436, 436f
Supernumerary digit, 45, 46f
Supernumerary tooth, 763, 763f
Supracondylar fracture, 187, 189f, 799t, 802f,
    806, 808f
Supraglottic disorders, airway obstruction in,
    926-929, 927f-929f
Supraglottitis, 927-929, 928f, 929f
Supraventricular tachycardia
  electrocardiography of, 140, 142, 143f
  radiofrequency catheter ablation for, 143,
    143f
  versus sinus tachycardia, 142
  Wolff-Parkinson-White syndrome in, 142,
    143f
Surveillance, developmental, 65
Swallowing study, barium contrast, 617, 617f
Swan-neck deformity, of finger, 828, 828f
Sweat test, in cystic fibrosis, 615
Sweaty sock syndrome, 284-285, 285f
Swimming, injury prevention in, 858t
Swinging flashlight test, 748, 748f
Swiping, 71, 71f
Sydenham chorea, 595
Symbolic capabilities, development of, 74-75
Sympathetic dystrophy, reflex, 272
Sympathetic ophthalmia, 744
Syndactyly, 45-46, 46f, 827, 827f, 878f, 879
Syndrome of inappropriate ADH secretion
    (siADH), 356
Syndrome X, 372
Synostosis. See also Craniosynostosis.
  coronal, 875, 875f
  lambdoid, 875-876, 877f
  metopic, 875, 876f
  sagittal, 873-875, 874f
Syphilis
  characteristics of, 697t
  congenital, 499-501, 500f
  primary, 702, 702f
  retinochoroiditis in, 745
  secondary, 702, 703f
Systemic lupus erythematosus, 254-258
  alopecia in, 255, 256f
  antibodies found in, 258, 258f, 258t
  arthritis in, 241, 257
  cardiac involvement in, 255-256
  central nervous system involvement in, 257,
    257f
  classification criteria of, 254, 254t
  livedo reticularis in, 255
  mucosal ulceration in, 255, 256f
  ocular manifestations of, 257, 257f
  pulmonary involvement in, 256-257, 256f
  rash in, 254-255, 254f, 255f
  renal involvement in, 257, 257t
  vasculitis in, 255, 256f
Systemic sclerosis, 258, 259, 259t
Systolic ejection murmur, 129t

T
T cell(s), development of, 116, 116f
T cell disorders, 118-119, 119f
  with B cell disorders
    partial, 122-123, 122f, 123f
    severe, 119-122, 120t, 121f
Tachycardia
  sinus, 142
  supraventricular, 140, 142, 143, 143f
  ventricular, 143, 144f
Tachypnea, transient, of the newborn, 50, 52f
Tacrolimus, for atopic dermatitis, 283-284
Talipes equinovarus, 836-838, 837f
Tampon use, toxic shock syndrome and, 458
Tanner staging, 349, 351, 351f-352f
Tanning, patterned, 204-205, 205f
Tarsal navicular, accessory, 841, 842f
Tay-Sachs disease, 747, 747f
Teeth. See Dental; Tooth (teeth).

Telangiectasia
  in ataxia-telangiectasia, 573, 573f
  in CREST syndrome, 259, 261f
  hereditary hemorrhagic, 910-911, 911f
  in juvenile dermatomyositis, 264f
Telangiectasis, retinal, 743, 743f
Telecanthus, 725
Telegraphic speech, 77
Teller Acuity Cards, 714
Telogen effluvium, 337, 339f
Temporal bone defects, 892, 893f
Temporomandibular joint
  dysfunction of, 778-779
  examination of, 242, 243f
  in Treacher Collins syndrome, 883
Tennis, injury prevention in, 858t
Teratogens, multiple malformations associated
    with, 30, 30f
Teratoma, 437, 438f, 478t, 651, 652f
Terbinafine, for tinea capitis, 342
Terson syndrome, 754
Testicular appendages, 552
  torsion of, 553, 554f, 669-670, 670f
Testis
  mass of, 438, 438f
  trauma to, 560-561, 561f
  tumors of, 556, 556f
  undescended, 535, 554
Testosterone, synthesis of, 365f
Tetanus, neonatal, 501-502, 502f
Tetracycline, tooth discoloration from, 765-
    766, 766f
Tetralogy of Fallot
  complete repair for, 149, 149f
  echocardiography in, 146, 148f
  with pulmonary atresia, "egg on its side"
    heart in, 135, 136f
  with pulmonic stenosis, "boot-shaped"
    heart in, 135, 135f
  shunt procedures for, 146, 149, 149f
Thalassemia major, 408, 408f, 532
Thalassemia minor, 406
Thalassemia trait, 408
Thelarche, premature, 368, 368f
Thenar eminence percussion, in myotonia
    congenita, 592, 592f
Therapeutic exercises, after sports injuries,
    865
Thomas test, 788, 788f
Thoracic dystrophy, asphyxiating, 529, 529f
Thoracolumbar spine, 785-786, 785f, 786f
Throat culture, in tonsillopharyngitis, 923
Thrombocytopenia, 424-425, 424f-425f
Thrombocytopenia-absent radius (TAR)
    syndrome, 425, 425f
Thrombocytopenic purpura, idiopathic, 202,
    203f
Thrombosis
  arterial, 427
  venous
    deep, 427-428, 427f
    renal, 517-518, 518f, 650, 651f
Thrombotic disorders, 427-428, 427f
Thrombotic thrombocytopenic purpura, 418,
    423f
Thrush, 770, 771f
  in AIDS, 505f
  in newborn, 59-60, 60f
Thumb
  congenital trigger, 827, 827f
  gamekeeper's, 814, 815f
Thumb sucking, 758, 759f
Thumb-sucking eczema, 285, 285f
Thymic cyst, 661, 661f
Thyroglossal duct cyst, 478t, 660, 660f
Thyroid cancer, 356, 434, 478t
Thyroid gland, 356-359
  agenesis of, 358
  ectopic, 358, 358f
  examination of, 356, 357f
  lingual, 659
Thyroid goiter, 356, 357f, 358, 358f, 478t, 660,
    661f

Thyroid hormones
  deficiency of, 236, 357-359, 357f, 358f
  excess of, 357, 357f
  resistance to, 359
Thyroid nodule, 356, 660, 660f
Thyroiditis, Hashimoto, 478t, 660, 661f
Thyroid-stimulating hormone (TSH), 355, 355f
  resistance to, 359
Thyroxine (T₄), 356
Thyroxine-binding globulin (TBG), 356
Tibia, proximal, angular varus deformity of, 834, 834f
Tibial torsion, internal, 836, 836f
Tibial tubercle, traction apophysitis of, 834-835, 835f
Tics, 594
Tinea capitis, 341-342, 343f
  versus folliculitis, 465
  versus streptococcal impetigo, 466
Tinea corporis, 291-292, 293f, 294f
Tinea pedis, 292, 294f
Tinea versicolor, 292, 294, 295f, 332-333
Tinidazole, for *Trichomonas vaginalis,* 704
Toddler's diarrhea, 389
Toddler's fracture, 795, 806, 806f
Toe, claw, 841-843, 843f
Toe-to-heel sequence, 791
Toe-walking, 83, 84, 84f, 791
Toilet-training, 81
Tongue
  geographic, 760-761, 761f
  laceration of, 772, 773f
  strawberry, in Kawasaki syndrome, 268, 268f
  in streptococcal scarlet fever, 455, 456f
Tongue lip adhesion, for Pierre-Robin sequence, 887
Tongue tie, 659, 761, 761f
Tonsil(s)
  abscess or cellulitis involving, 923-924, 924f
  hypertrophy of, 905-907, 906f
  lymphoma of, 924, 925f
  size of, grading of, 922f
Tonsillitis
  acute, 921-923, 923f
  recurrent, 923
Tooth (teeth). *See also* Dental *entries.*
  anatomy of, 755, 756f
  avulsion of, 775, 775f
  caries of, 766-767, 767f
  concrescence of, 763
  congenital absence of, 763, 764f
  crowns of, injuries to, 774, 774f, 775f
  development of, 755-758, 757f-759f
  discoloration of, 765-766, 765f-766f
  displacement injuries to, 775, 775f
  double, 757, 757f
  examination of, 755, 756f
  fracture of, 774-775, 774f, 775f
  fusion of, 763
  gemination (twinning) of, 763-764, 764f
  inappropriate loosening of, 433
  injuries to, 770-771, 774-775, 775f-776f
  maldevelopment of, in congenital syphilis, 501
  mixed, 757, 757f
  morphologic disturbances of, 763-764, 764f
  natal, 758, 760, 760f
  permanent, 758, 758f, 759f
  primary, 756-757, 757f, 759f
  reimplantation of, 775, 775f
  size abnormalities of, 763, 764f
  structure of, 755, 756f
  supernumerary, 763, 763f
  supporting structures of, trauma to, 775-778, 776f-778f
Topical anesthesia
  dermatitis from, 287, 291f
  in gynecologic examination of prepubertal patient, 680
Topical skin therapy, complications of, 345-346, 346f
TORCH infection, 744-745, 744f, 745f

Torticollis
  congenital, 818, 818f
  in deformational plagiocephaly, 871
  in peritonsillar abscess, 924, 924f
Torulopsis infection, vulvovaginitis in, 699
Total anomalous pulmonary venous return, 138, 140f
Tourette syndrome, 594
Tourniquet injury
  accidental, 207, 207f
  in child abuse, 173, 177f
  differential diagnosis of, 47f
Townes-Brocks syndrome, 28
Toxic epidermal necrolysis, 98, 300-301, 301f
Toxic granulations, 421, 422f
Toxic shock syndrome, 458-459, 458f
Toxocariasis, retinal, 745, 745f
Toxoplasmosis, 476t
  congenital, 496-497, 497f
  retinochoroiditis in, 744, 744f
Trachea
  hemangioma of, 607
  vascular compression of, 934, 935f
Tracheitis, bacterial, 930
Tracheoesophageal fistula
  cough in, 601, 601f
  with esophageal atresia, 624-625, 626f, 627f
  isolated, 625, 627f
Tracheostomy, for Pierre-Robin sequence, 887
Tracheotomy, for croup, 930
Track and field, injury prevention in, 859t
Traction alopecia, 340, 340f
Transaminase level, in child abuse, 200
Transbronchial biopsy, 622
Transcondylar fracture, 806
Transcription, gene, 20
Transient neonatal pustular melanosis, 318, 320f
Transitional stools, 53, 53f
Translation, gene, 20
Translocation, chromosome, 3-4, 3f
Transplantation, lymphoproliferative disorder after, 441
Transposition of the great arteries
  arterial switch for, 151, 151f
  corrected, valentine-shaped heart in, 135, 136f
  echocardiography in, 146, 147f
  "egg on a string" heart shadow in, 135, 135f
  intra-atrial baffle for, 150-151, 151f
Trantas dots, 113, 114f
TRAPS (tumor necrosis factor receptor–associated periodic fever syndrome), 272
Trauma
  abdominal, 198-200, 199f, 200f
  birth, 42-44, 42f-45f. *See also* Birth trauma.
  bruising and. *See* Bruises.
  dental, 770-771, 774-775, 775f-776f
  gastrointestinal, 391, 392f
  genital. *See* Genital trauma.
  head. *See* Head trauma.
  intrathoracic, 200, 201f, 213
  laryngeal, 934f
  musculoskeletal, 791-818. *See also* Fracture(s); Ligamentous injuries; Sports injuries.
  nail, 344-345, 344f, 345f
  nasal. *See* Nasal trauma.
  nipple, 57, 57f, 59, 59f
  ocular, 752-754, 752f-754f
  orofacial, 770-778. *See also* Orofacial trauma.
  oropharyngeal, penetrating, 921-925, 925f
Treacher Collins syndrome, 882-883, 882f, 893f
Tree nut allergy, 97, 98t
Treitz ligament, in malrotation, 637, 637f
Trench mouth, 770, 771f
Trendelenburg gait, 791
Trendelenburg test, 788, 788f
Treponema pallidum, 499
Triceps skinfold, 380f
Trichiasis, 726

Trichomonas vaginalis, 680, 692t, 697t, 703-704, 705f
Trichorrhexis nodosa, 339, 340f
Tricuspid atresia
  electrocardiography in, 138, 141f
  palliative procedures for, 149-150, 150f
Trigger thumb, congenital, 827, 827f
Trigonocephaly, 873, 873t, 875, 876f
Triiodothyronine (T₃), 356
Trinucleotide repeat disorders, 16, 17
Triploidy, 4
Trismus
  in neonatal tetanus, 502f
  in peritonsillar abscess, 924, 924f
Trisomy 1, 11t, 12-13, 12f
Trisomy 13, 11-12
  cardiac defect in, 130t
  neutrophil abnormalities in, 421, 422f
  physical manifestations of, 11-12, 11f, 11t
Trisomy 16, 4
Trisomy 18, 130t
Trisomy 21. *See* Down syndrome.
Trochlear nerve (CN IV) palsy, cyclovertical eye deviation in, 723, 723f
Tropias, 13f, 718, 724, 725f
Truncus arteriosus
  Rastelli procedure for, 151, 152f
  right aortic arch in, 137, 137f
Trunk, physical examination of, 784-785
Trunk control, development of, 66, 67f, 68f
Trypsinogen test, in cystic fibrosis, 614
Tryptase, serum, in anaphylaxis, 93
TSC1/TSC2 genes, 569
Tuberculin skin test, 491, 491f, 495, 495t
Tuberculosis, 491-496
  adenitis in, 495
  in adolescent, 495
  case finding in, 496
  diagnosis of, 496
  endobronchial, 492, 493f
  extrapulmonary, 494-495, 495f
  latent, 492
  lymphadenitis in, 479-480, 480f
  lymphohematogenous spread of, 493-494
  meningitis in, 494
  miliary, 493-494, 494f
  mycobacterial, 662, 662f
  pathogenesis of, 491-492
  pericarditis in, 495
  pleural effusion in, 492
  primary pulmonary, 492-493, 493f
  skeletal, 494-495, 495f
  spondylitis in, 494-495, 495f
  transmission of, 491
  treatment of, 496
Tuberous sclerosis, 334, 336f, 521, 521f, 569-570, 569t, 570f-572f
Tularemia, 481
Tumor(s). *See also* Cancer; Mass(es).
  bone, 439, 441f
  central nervous system, 431-432, 432f, 440-441, 583, 583f
    hypopituitarism in, 352
    in neurofibromatosis, 567, 569
  germ cell, 437
  mediastinal, 434, 435f, 436, 436f
  orbital, 750-751, 751f
  ovarian, 647-648, 648f
  pelvic, 655
  phyllodes, 665
  Pott puffy, 916, 918f
  precocious puberty associated with, 367-368
  skin, 313-316
  testicular, 556, 556f
  Wilms, 437-438, 653-654, 654f
Tumor necrosis factor receptor, periodic fever associated with, 272
Tumor necrosis factor receptor–associated periodic fever syndrome (TRAPS), 272
Turf toe, 345, 345f
Turner syndrome, 4, 13, 14f, 130t, 131, 369, 369f, 370f, 370t, 896f

Turribrachycephaly, 879
Turricephaly, 873, 873t
  22q11 syndrome, 118-119, 119f
Twins
  placental evaluation in, 41, 41f
  size discordance in, 39, 39f
TWIST gene mutation, in Saethre-Chotzen
    syndrome, 881
Tympanic membrane
  angulation of, 889, 891f
  distortions of, 901-902, 902f
  granulomas or polyps of, 901, 902f
  mass lesions involving, 901, 902f
  normal, 896-898, 898f
  perforation of, 896, 897f, 899-900, 900f
Tympanometry, 889, 892f
Tympanostomy tubes, 900, 901f
Tzanck smears
  in herpes simplex infection, 451
  in viral exanthems, 298, 298f

U
Ulcer(s)
  aphthous, recurrent, 768-769, 768f
  corneal, 734, 735f
  in ecthyma, 466, 467f
  gastric, 643, 643f
  genital
    in Behçet's disease, 271, 272f
    herpetic, 703, 704f
    syphilitic, 702, 702f
  mucosal, in systemic lupus erythematosus,
      255, 256f
  oral
    in Behçet's disease, 271
    in coxsackie hand-foot-and-mouth
        disease, 446, 448f
    in herpes simplex infection, 451, 452f
    traumatic, 773, 773f
  peptic, 383, 383f, 384f
  in tularemia, 481
Ulcerated hemangioma, 327, 327f
Ulcerative colitis, 392, 394f-397f
Ulcerative gingivitis, acute necrotizing, 770,
    771f
Ultrasonography
  in multicystic renal dysplasia, 540, 541f
  in renal venous thrombosis, 518, 518f
Umbilical cord, delayed separation of, in
    leukocyte adhesion deficiency, 123
Umbilical granuloma, 668
Umbilical hernia, 47-48, 48f, 667-668,
    668f
Undernutrition. *See* Failure to thrive.
Upper extremity
  examination of, 784-787, 784f-787f, 787t
  musculoskeletal disorders of, 825-828,
      825f-828f
Urachus
  abscess of, 538, 539f
  anomalies of, 538, 539f
  patent, 538, 539f
Ureaplasma urealyticum infection
  genital, 708
  pneumonia in, 601
Ureter
  ectopic, 558, 558f
  enlargement of, 539, 540f
Ureterocele, prolapse of, 557-558, 558f
Ureteropelvic junction obstruction, 539, 540f,
    649-650, 650f
Ureterostomy, 541, 542f
Urethral meatus inflammation, in Kawasaki
    syndrome, 269, 269f
Urethral prolapse, 230, 230f, 557, 557f, 695,
    696f
Urethral syndrome, in *Chlamydia trachomatis*
    infection, 708
Urethral valves, posterior, 521-522, 522f,
    536-537, 536f, 537f, 650, 650f
Urethritis, in gonorrhea, 705

Urinalysis, 510-512, 511f, 512f, 512t
  casts in, 511f, 512, 512f
  crystals in, 511f, 512
  enhanced, 520, 520f, 520t
  gross inspection in, 510, 512t
  microscopic examination in, 511f, 512
  screening by dipstick in, 510, 512
Urinary collecting system, duplication of,
    522, 523f, 558, 558f
Urinary diversion, cutaneous, 541, 542f-544f
Urinary retention, 546, 546f
Urinary tract dilation, antenatal, 536, 536f,
    537f
Urinary tract infection, 519-520, 520f, 520t
Urogenital disorders, 509, 535-563
Urogenital sinus, posteriorly displaced, 560f
Urogenital tract, in cancer, 437-438, 438f
Urologic disorders, 535-563
Urticaria, 113-115, 114f, 115f, 302-304, 303f
  cold, 114, 115f
  papular, 308-309, 309f
Urticaria pigmentosa, 315-316, 317f
Uveitis
  anterior, 737, 737f, 740, 740f
  intermediate, 740, 740f
  in juvenile rheumatoid arthritis, 251-252,
      252f
  in Kawasaki syndrome, 268, 268f
  posterior, 740
Uvula, bifid, 921, 922f
Uvulitis, 923, 924f

V
Vaccine, for human papillomavirus infection,
    685
Vacuum headache, allergic, 920
Vagina
  congenital obstruction of, 558-559, 559f
  discharge from
    disorders causing, 692t
    specimen collection for, 680, 681t, 691
  foreign body in, 230-231, 231f, 695
  hematoma of, 688, 689f
  normal or nonpathogenic flora in, 693t
  pH level in, 684
Vagina introitus, examination of, 535-536
Vaginoscopy, 680
Vaginosis, bacterial, 692t, 704-705, 705f
Valentine-shaped heart, 135, 136f
Vallecular cyst, 933, 935f
Variceal bleeding, 645
Varicella, 445, 446f, 447f
  disseminated, 118, 119f, 445, 447f
  hemorrhagic, 445, 447f
  in immunocompromised host, 445, 447f
  superinfection with, 445, 447f
  vulvovaginitis from, 698
Varicocele, 554-555, 555f
Vascular abnormalities, epistaxis in, 910-911,
    911f
Vascular malformations
  in biliary atresia, 399, 399f
  capillary and capillary/venous, 328-329,
      329f
  in occult spinal dysraphism, 579, 580f
Vascular ring, 610, 611f, 623, 624f, 627, 628f
Vascular skin lesions, 322, 324-329
Vasculitides, systemic, 265-273, 265t
Vasculitis
  hypersensitivity, 265
  leukocytoclastic, 265
  purpuric lesions in, 203-204
  in systemic lupus erythematosus, 255, 256f
  urticarial, 304
Vasomotor rhinitis, 101, 101t
Vaso-occlusive crisis, in sickle cell disease, 416
Vasopressin, 356
VATER/VACTERL association, 28, 28f
Velocardiofacial syndrome, 6t, 118-119, 119f,
    130, 130t
Vena cava syndrome, superior, 436, 436f

Venous distention, superficial, 437, 437f
Venous hum, 129t
Venous stenosis, balloon angioplasty for, 156
Venous thrombosis
  deep, 427-428, 427f
  renal, 517-518, 518f, 650, 651f
Ventricle(s)
  hypertrophy of, 138-139
  single, palliative procedures for, 149-150,
      150f
Ventricular contractions, premature, 140, 142f
Ventricular septal defect
  closure of, 157, 157f
  echocardiography in, 144, 145f, 146f
  heart size in, 136
Ventricular tachycardia, 143, 144f
Ventriculoperitoneal shunt, inflammatory
    pseudocyst and, 655
Vergence movements, 718
Vernal conjunctivitis, 113, 113f, 114f
Verruca plana, 313, 314f
Verruca vulgaris, 313, 313f
Vertebral body dysplasia, in neurofibromatosis
    1, 566, 568f
Vertebral fracture, 188, 190f
Vertebral osteomyelitis, 486, 488, 489f
Vertical eye deviation, 719, 719f, 722-723,
    723f
Vertical talus, congenital, 839-840, 840f
Vesical dysfunction
  neurogenic, 546, 547f
  non-neurogenic, 547, 547f
Vesicostomy, cutaneous, 541, 543f
Vesicoureteral reflux, 518, 519f, 536f
  with ureteropelvic junction obstruction,
      539, 540f
Vesicovaginal fistula, 695
Vesiculation, after insect bites, 205-206, 206f
Vesiculopustular disorders, 298-302
Vincent infection, 770, 771f
Viral arthritis, 253-254
Viral conjunctivitis, 732-733, 733f
Viral infection
  exanthematous, 298, 298f, 443-454,
      444f-455f
  of oral cavity, 767-769, 767f-768f
  of skin, 298, 298f
Visceral situs and cardiac apex, discordance
    of, in congenital heart disease, 134, 134f,
    135f
Viscerocranium, 867-868, 868f
Vision
  color, abnormalities of, 748
  double, 581, 718
  impaired, development and, 91-92, 91t
  screening of, 715-716
Visual acuity
  best corrected, 715
  of infant, 73
  measurement of, 713-716, 715f
  normal values for, 715
Visual axes, misalignment of. *See* Strabismus.
Visual cortex, 713, 714f
Visual evoked potential or response (VEP or
    VER), 713-714, 715f
Visual field assessment, 713
Visual pathways, 713, 714f
Visual system, anatomy of, 713, 714f
Vitamin A
  deficiency of, 380-381
  excess of, 210-211
Vitamin B$_{12}$ deficiency, megaloblastic anemia
    and, 409-410, 412f
Vitamin C deficiency, 210, 211f
Vitamin D deficiency, 210, 211f, 380, 381f
Vitamin D–deficient rickets, 359-360, 361f,
    361t
Vitamin E deficiency, 381, 413
Vitamin K deficiency, 381, 427
Vitelline bands, 641, 642f
Vitiligo, 334, 336f
Vitreous, persistent hyperplastic primary, 741,
    742f

...age, 740-741, 741f
...function, wheezing in, 609
Vocal cord paralysis, 607-608, 933-934, 935f
Vocal fremitus, 598
Voiding, dysfunctional, 547, 547f
Volar plate injury, 808-809, 809f
Volvulus, 388, 389f
  midgut, 637, 637f
  in utero, 667f
Vomiting, 385, 388, 632, 634-641
  bilious
    with abdominal distention, 637-639,
      638f-640f
    differential diagnosis of, 632, 634, 634f
    without abdominal distention, 635, 635f,
      637, 637f
  in increased intracranial pressure, 581
  in neonates and infants, 634-639
  nonbilious, in neonates and infants, 634-
    635, 635f, 636f
  in older infants and children, 639-641
  versus regurgitation, 632
Von Willebrand disease, 202-203, 425, 426
Vulvar erythema, 229
Vulvar folliculitis, 698
Vulvar impetigo, 698
Vulvitis, allergic, 694
Vulvovaginal complaints in adolescents, 691
Vulvovaginitis, 229
  candidal, 699, 700f
  chemical irritant, 694, 694f
  conditions mimicking, 695-696
  from gastrointestinal pathogens, 698-699,
    699f
  infectious, 690t, 696-710, 697t
  laboratory testing of, 680, 681t, 691
  noninfectious, 690t, 691, 693-695
  prepubertal, 689-691, 690f, 690t
  from respiratory and/or skin pathogens,
    698, 698f
  sexually transmitted, 690t, 697-698, 697t,
    699-710. *See also* Sexually transmitted
    disease.
  streptococcal, 698, 698f

W
Waardenburg syndrome, 336
WAGR syndrome, aniridia in, 432, 433f
Walking, development of, 69-70, 69f
Wandering atrial pacemaker, 140, 142f
Warthin-Starry silver stain, 662, 662f
Warts, 313-314, 314f, 701-702, 701f
Wasp sting, 97
Waterhouse-Friderichsen syndrome, 459
Waterston shunt, 149, 149f
Watson syndrome, 30
Weakness
  gait disturbances from, 791
  in juvenile dermatomyositis, 263
  in neuromuscular disease, 586
Weapons, in child abuse, 164t, 169, 174f
Wegener granulomatosis, 265
Weight
  body mass index cutoff points for, 349t
  intrauterine growth restriction and, 38
  stature percentiles by, 348f
West syndrome, 594
Wheezing, 102, 597, 598
  chronic, causes of, 608-610, 609f, 609t,
    611f-612f
  differential diagnosis of, 108-111, 109f,
    109t, 110t, 111f
Whitaker test, in ureteropelvic junction
  obstruction, 539
White blood cells. *See* Leukocyte(s).
White pupillary reflex, 738, 738t
White strawberry tongue, in streptococcal
  scarlet fever, 455, 456f
Williams syndrome, 130t, 131
Wilms tumor, 437-438, 653-654, 654f
Wilson disease, 400, 401f
Wimberger sign, in congenital syphilis, 500f,
  501
Wiskott-Aldrich syndrome, 122, 122f
Wolf syndrome, 336
Wolff-Parkinson-White syndrome, 142, 143,
  143f
Wolf-Hirschhorn syndrome, 6t
Wolfram syndrome, 356

Wood's lamp examination
  of ash-leaf spots, 334, 336f
  of child abuse bruises, 171, 175f
  in tinea versicolor, 294
  in vitiligo, 334
Wormian bones, in osteogenesis imperfecta,
  845, 846f
Wound-related cellulitis, 471-473, 472f
Wrestling, injury prevention in, 859t
Wrist
  examination of, 244, 244f, 786-787, 787f
  ganglion of, 826-827, 826f
Wryneck, 818, 818f
WT1 gene mutation, in ambiguous genitalia,
  364

X
X chromosome, 1
  inactivation of, 16, 16f
Xanthogranuloma, juvenile, 316, 318f,
  737-738, 738f
Xanthomas, in liver disease, 399, 400f
X-linked ichthyosis, 279, 280f
X-linked mental retardation, 16
XXX females, 15
XXY males, 14
XY/XXY males, 14
XYY males, 15

Y
Y chromosome, 1
Yeast infection, breastfeeding and, 59-60,
  60f
Yellow jacket sting, 96, 97f
Yersinia pestis, 481-482

Z
Zidovudine, 506